Noyes' Knee Disorders

Surgery, Rehabilitation, Clinical Outcomes

Noyes'
Knee
Disorders
Surgery, Rehabilitation, Clinical Outcomes

Editor

Frank R. Noyes, MD

Chairman and CEO
Cincinnati Sportsmedicine and Orthopaedic Center
President and Medical Director
Cincinnati Sportsmedicine Research and Education Foundation
Clinical Professor (Volunteer)
Department of Orthopaedic Surgery
University of Cincinnati College of Medicine
Cincinnati, Ohio

Associate Editor

Sue D. Barber-Westin, BS

Director, Clinical and Applied Research
Cincinnati Sportsmedicine Research and Education Foundation
Cincinnati, Ohio

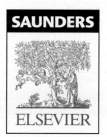

SAUNDERS

ELSEVIER

SAUNDERS
ELSEVIER

1600 John F. Kennedy Blvd.
Ste 1800
Philadelphia, PA 19103-2899

NOYES' KNEE DISORDERS: SURGERY, REHABILITATION,
CLINICAL OUTCOMES

ISBN: 978-1-4160-5474-0

Notice

Knowledge and best practice in this field are constantly changing. As new research and experience broaden our knowledge, changes in practice, treatment and drug therapy may become necessary or appropriate. Readers are advised to check the most current information provided (i) on procedures featured or (ii) by the manufacturer of each product to be administered, to verify the recommended dose or formula, the method and duration of administration, and contraindications. It is the responsibility of the practitioner, relying on their own experience and knowledge of the patient, to make diagnoses, to determine dosages and the best treatment for each individual patient, and to take all appropriate safety precautions. To the fullest extent of the law, neither the Publisher nor the Editors assumes any liability for any injury and/or damage to persons or property arising out of or related to any use of the material contained in this book.

The Publisher

Library of Congress Cataloging-in-Publication Data

Knee disorders : surgery, rehabilitation, clinical outcomes / editor,
Frank R. Noyes ; associate editor, Sue D. Barber-Westin. --1st ed.
   p.; cm.
  Includes bibliographical references.
  ISBN 978-1-4160-5474-0
1. Knee--Surgery. 2. Knee--Surgery--Patients--Rehabliitation. I.
Noyes, Frank R. II. Barber-Westin, Sue D.
  [DNLM: 1. Knee Injuries--surgery. 2. Joint Diseases--rehabilitation.
3. Joint Diseases--surgery. 4. Knee Injuries--rehabilitation. 5. Knee
Joint--surgery. WE 870 K6734 2009]
  RD561.K5745 2009
  617.5'82059--dc22   2009007993

Acquisitions Editor: Kimberly Murphy
Developmental Editor: Anne Snyder
Design Direction: Steven Stave

Working together to grow
libraries in developing countries

www.elsevier.com | www.bookaid.org | www.sabre.org

ELSEVIER   BOOK AID International   Sabre Foundation

Printed in China

Last digit is the print number: 9 8 7 6 5 4 3 2 1

DEDICATION

To JoAnne, my loving and precious wife,
and to all our families.

Contributors

Thomas P. Andriacchi, PhD
Professor, Stanford University, Stanford; Research Career Scientist, VA Palo Alto Research and Development, Bone and Joint Research Center, Palo Alto, California
Human Movement and Anterior Cruciate Ligament Function: Anterior Cruciate Ligament Deficiency and Gait Mechanics

John Babb, MD
Staff Orthopedic Surgeon, Mid-America Orthopedics, Wichita, Kansas
Medial and Anterior Knee Anatomy

Sue D. Barber-Westin, BS
Director, Clinical and Applied Research, Cincinnati Sportsmedicine Research and Education Foundation, Cincinnati, Ohio
Anterior Cruciate Ligament Primary and Revision Reconstruction: Diagnosis, Operative Techniques, and Clinical Outcomes; Scientific Basis of Rehabilitation after Anterior Cruciate Ligament Autogenous Reconstruction; Rehabilitation of Primary and Revision Anterior Cruciate Ligament Reconstructions; Risk Factors for Anterior Cruciate Ligament Injuries in the Female Athlete; Lower Limb Neuromuscular Control and Strength in Prepubescent and Adolescent Male and Female Athletes; Decreasing the Risk of Anterior Cruciate Ligament Injuries in Female Athletes; Function of the Posterior Cruciate Ligament and Posterolateral Ligament Structures; Posterior Cruciate Ligament: Diagnosis, Operative Techniques, and Clinical Outcomes; Posterolateral Ligament Injuries: Diagnosis, Operative Techniques, and Clinical Outcomes; Rehabilitation of Posterior Cruciate Ligament and Posterolateral Reconstructive Procedures; Medial and Posteromedial Ligament Injuries: Diagnosis, Operative Techniques, and Clinical Outcomes; Rehabilitation of Medial Ligament Injuries; Meniscus Tears: Diagnosis, Repair Techniques, and Clinical Outcomes; Meniscus Transplantation: Diagnosis, Operative Techniques, and Clinical Outcomes; Rehabilitation of Meniscus Repair and Transplantation Procedures; Primary, Double, and Triple Varus Knee Syndromes: Diagnosis, Osteotomy Techniques, and Clinical Outcomes; Rehabilitation after Tibial and Femoral Osteotomy; Correction of Hyperextension Gait Abnormalities: Preoperative and Postoperative Techniques; Operative Options for Extensor Mechanism Malalignment and Patellar Dislocation; Prevention and Treatment of Knee Arthrofibrosis; The Cincinnati Knee Rating System; The International Knee Documentations Committee Rating System; Rating of Athletic and Daily Functional Activities after Knee Injuries and Operative Procedures; Articular Cartilage Rating Systems

Asheesh Bedi, MD
Fellow, Shoulder Surgery and Sports Medicine, Hospital for Special Surgery, New York, New York
Biology of Anterior Cruciate Ligament Graft Healing

Geoffrey A. Bernas, MD
Clinical Assistant Professor of Orthopaedic Surgery, Department of Orthopaedic Surgery, University at Buffalo, Buffalo; University Sports Medicine, Orchard Park, New York
Management of Acute Knee Dislocation before Surgical Intervention

Lori Thein Brody, PT, PhD, SCS, ATC
Graduate Program Director, Orthopaedic and Sports Physical Therapy, Rocky Mountain University of Health Professions, Provo, Utah; Senior Clinical Specialist, UW Health, Madison, Wisconsin
Aquatic Therapy for the Arthritic Knee

William D. Bugbee, MD
Associate Professor, University of California, San Diego; Attending Orthopaedic Surgeon, and Director, Cartilage Transplant Program, Scripps Clinic, La Jolla, California
Valgus Malalignment: Diagnosis, Osteotomy Techniques, and Clinical Outcomes; Osteochondral Grafts: Diagnosis, Operative Techniques, and Clinical Outcomes

Terese L. Chmielewski, PhD, PT, SCS
Assistant Professor, Department of Physical Therapy, and Affiliate Assistant Professor, Department of Orthopaedics and Rehabilitation, University of Florida, Gainesville, Florida
Neuromuscular Retraining after Anterior Cruciate Ligament Reconstruction

A. Lee Dellon, MD, PhD
Professor of Plastic Surgery and Professor of Neurosurgery, Johns Hopkins University; Director, The Dellon Institutes for Peripheral Nerve Surgery, Baltimore, Maryland
Knee Pain of Neural Origin

Alvin Detterline, MD
Orthopaedic Surgeon, Sports Medicine, Towson Orthopaedic Associates, Baltimore, Maryland
Medial and Anterior Knee Anatomy

Eric W. Fester, MD
Assistant Professor of Surgery, Uniformed Services University of the Health Sciences, Bethesda, Maryland; Clinical Assistant Professor of Orthopaedic Surgery, Wright State University, Dayton, Ohio; Chief, Orthopaedic Sports Medicine, Wright-Patterson Medical Center, Wright-Patterson Air Force Base, Ohio
Lateral, Posterior, and Cruciate Knee Anatomy

Freddie Fu, MD
Chairman and David Silver Professor of Orthopedic Surgery, University of Pittsburgh School of Medicine; Chief of Orthopaedics, Department of Orthopaedic Surgery, University of Pittsburgh Medical Center, Pittsburgh, Pennsylvania
Scientific and Clinical Basis for Double-Bundle Anterior Cruciate Ligament Reconstruction in Primary and Revision Knees

Simon Görtz, MD
Research Fellow, Department of Orthopaedic Surgery, University of California, San Diego, La Jolla, California
Valgus Malalignment: Diagnosis, Osteotomy Techniques, and Clinical Outcomes; Osteochondral Grafts: Diagnosis, Operative Techniques, and Clinical Outcomes

Edward S. Grood, PhD
Director, Biomechanics Research, Cincinnati Sportsmedicine Research and Education Foundation; Professor Emeritus, Department of Biomedical Engineering, Colleges of Medicine and Engineering, University of Cincinnati, Cincinnati, Ohio
The Scientific Basis for Examination and Classification of Knee Ligament Injuries; Knee Ligament Function and Failure

Timothy P. Heckmann, PT, ATC
Co-Director of Rehabilitation, Cincinnati Sportsmedicine and Orthopaedic Center; Rehabilitation Consultant, Cincinnati Sportsmedicine Research and Education Foundation, Cincinnati, Ohio
Scientific Basis of Rehabilitation after Anterior Cruciate Ligament Autogenous Reconstruction; Rehabilitation of Primary and Revision Anterior Cruciate Ligament Reconstructions; Rehabilitation of Posterior Cruciate Ligament and Posterolateral Reconstructive Procedures; Rehabilitation of Medial Ligament Injuries; Rehabilitation of Meniscus Repair and Transplantation

Procedures; Rehabilitation after Tibial and Femoral Osteotomy; Correction of Hyperextension Gait Abnormalities: Preoperative and Postoperative Techniques

Susan Jordan, MD
Assistant Professor of Orthopaedic Surgery, University of Pittsburgh School of Medicine; University of Pittsburgh Medical Center, Pittsburgh, Pennsylvania
Scientific and Clinical Basis for Double-Bundle Anterior Cruciate Ligament Reconstruction in Primary and Revision Knees

Anastassios Karistinos, MD
Assistant Professor, Baylor College of Medicine; Physician/Surgeon, Veterans Administration Hospital, and Ben Taub General Hospital, Houston, Texas
Graft Options for Anterior Cruciate Ligament Revision Reconstruction

Jennifer Kreinbrink, BS
Research Technician Associate, Orthopaedic Surgery, University of Michigan Health System, Ann Arbor, Michigan
Gender Differences in Muscular Protection of the Knee

Scott Lephart, PhD, ATC
Associate Professor, University of Pittsburgh; Director, Neuromuscular Research Laboratory, Pittsburgh, Pennsylvania
Differences in Neuromuscular Characteristics between Male and Female Athletes

Thomas Lindenfeld, MD
Adjunct Professor, Department of Biomedical Engineering, and Volunteer Instructor Professor, Department of Orthopaedics, University of Cincinnati; Associate Director, Cincinnati Sportsmedicine and Orthopaedic Center, and Cincinnati Sportsmedicine Research and Education Foundation, Cincinnati, Ohio
Diagnosis and Treatment of Complex Regional Pain Syndrome

Frank R. Noyes, MD
Chairman and CEO, Cincinnati Sportsmedicine and Orthopaedic Center; President and Medical Director, Cincinnati Sportsmedicine Research and Education Foundation; Clinical Professor (Volunteer), Department of Orthopaedic Surgery, University of Cincinnati College of Medicine; Previous Adjunct Professor, Noyes Tissue Engineering and Biomechanics Laboratory, Department of Biomedical Engineering, University of Cincinnati College of Engineering, Cincinnati, Ohio
Medial and Anterior Knee Anatomy; Lateral, Posterior, and Cruciate Knee Anatomy; The Scientific Basis for Examination and Classification of Knee Ligament Injuries; Knee Ligament Function and Failure; Anterior Cruciate Ligament Primary and Revision Reconstruction: Diagnosis, Operative Techniques, and Clinical Outcomes; Scientific Basis of Rehabilitation after Anterior Cruciate

Ligament Autogenous Reconstruction; Rehabilitation of Primary and Revision Anterior Cruciate Ligament Reconstructions; Risk Factors for Anterior Cruciate Ligament Injuries in the Female Athlete; Lower Limb Neuromuscular Control and Strength in Prepubescent and Adolescent Male and Female Athletes; Decreasing the Risk of Anterior Cruciate Ligament Injuries in Female Athletes; Function of the Posterior Cruciate Ligament and Posterolateral Ligament Structures; Posterior Cruciate Ligament: Diagnosis, Operative Techniques, and Clinical Outcomes; Posterolateral Ligament Injuries: Diagnosis, Operative Techniques, and Clinical Outcomes; Rehabilitation of Posterior Cruciate Ligament and Posterolateral Reconstructive Procedures; Medial and Posteromedial Ligament Injuries: Diagnosis, Operative Techniques, and Clinical Outcomes; Rehabilitation of Medial Ligament Injuries; Meniscus Tears: Diagnosis, Repair Techniques, and Clinical Outcomes; Meniscus Transplantation: Diagnosis, Operative Techniques, and Clinical Outcomes; Rehabilitation of Meniscus Repair and Transplantation Procedures; Primary, Double, and Triple Varus Knee Syndromes: Diagnosis, Osteotomy Techniques, and Clinical Outcomes; Rehabilitation after Tibial and Femoral Osteotomy; Correction of Hyperextension Gait Abnormalities: Preoperative and Postoperative Techniques; Operative Options for Extensor Mechanism Malalignment and Patellar Dislocation; Prevention and Treatment of Knee Arthrofibrosis; Diagnosis and Treatment of Complex Regional Pain Syndrome; The Cincinnati Knee Rating System; The International Knee Documentations Committee Rating System; Rating of Athletic and Daily Functional Activities after Knee Injuries and Operative Procedures; Articular Cartilage Rating Systems

Lonnie E. Paulos, MD
Research Associate, Department of Health, Leisure and Exercise Science, University of West Florida; Medical Director, and Physician/Surgeon, Andrews-Paulos Research and Education Institute, Gulf Breeze Hospital, Andrews Institute Surgical Center, Pensacola Beach, Florida
Graft Options for Anterior Cruciate Ligament Revision Reconstruction

Lars Peterson, MD, PhD
Professor of Orthopaedics, University of Goteborg; Department of Orthopaedics, Sahlgrenska University Hospital, Gothenburg, Sweden
Autologous Chondrocyte Implantation

Michael M. Reinold, PT, DPT, ATC, CSCS
Rehabilitation Coordinator and Assistant Athletic Trainer, Boston Red Sox; Coordinator of Rehabilitation Research and Education, Division of Sports Medicine, Department of Orthopedic Surgery, Massachusetts General Hospital, Boston, Massachusetts
Rehabilitation after Articular Cartilage Procedures

Dustin L. Richter, BS
Medical Student, University of New Mexico School of Medicine, Albuquerque, New Mexico
Classification of Knee Dislocations

Scott A. Rodeo, MD
Professor and Co-Chief, Shoulder and Sports Medicine Service, Hospital for Special Surgery; Professor, Weill Cornell Medical College, New York, New York
Biology of Anterior Cruciate Ligament Graft Healing

David L. Saxton, MD
Clinical Faculty, University of Oklahoma Health Sciences Center, Oklahoma City, Oklahoma
Diagnosis and Treatment of Complex Regional Pain Syndrome

Sean F. Scanlan, MS
Stanford University, Stanford; Postdoctoral Fellow, VA Palo Alto Research and Development, Bone and Joint Research Center, Palo Alto, California
Human Movement and Anterior Cruciate Ligament Function: Anterior Cruciate Ligament Deficiency and Gait Mechanics

Robert C. Schenck, Jr., MD
Professor and Chair, Department of Orthopaedic Surgery, University of New Mexico School of Medicine; Head Team Physician, Department of Athletics, University of New Mexico, Albuquerque, New Mexico
Classification of Knee Dislocations

Timothy Sell, PhD, PT
Assistant Professor, University of Pittsburgh; Associate Director, Neuromuscular Research Laboratory, Pittsburgh, Pennsylvania
Differences in Neuromuscular Characteristics between Male and Female Athletes

Wei Shen, MD, PhD
Post-doctoral Associate, University of Pittsburgh, Pittsburgh, Pennsylvania
Scientific and Clinical Basis for Double-Bundle Anterior Cruciate Ligament Reconstruction in Primary and Revision Knees

Justin P. Strickland, MD
Physician's Clinic of Iowa, Cedar Rapids, Iowa
Lateral, Posterior, and Cruciate Knee Anatomy

Robert A. Teitge, MD
Professor, Wayne State University, Detroit; Chief, Orthopaedic Surgery, DMC Surgery Hospital, Madison Heights, Michigan
Patellofemoral Disorders: Correction of Rotational Malalignment of the Lower Extremity

Kelly L. Vander Have, MD
Assistant Professor, University of Michigan, Ann Arbor, Michigan
Anterior Cruciate Ligament Reconstruction in Skeletally Immature Patients

C. Thomas Vangsness, Jr., MD
Professor, Keck School of Medicine, University of Southern California, Los Angeles, California
Allografts: Graft Sterilization and Tissue Banking Safety Issues

Daniel C. Wascher, MD
Professor, Department of Orthopaedics, University of New Mexico, Albuquerque, New Mexico
Classification of Knee Dislocations

Kevin E. Wilk, DPT, PT
Adjunct Assistant Professor, Marquette University, Milwaukee, Wisconsin; Vice President, Education, and Associate Clinical Director, Physiotherapy Associates, Birmingham, Alabama; Rehabilitation Consultant, Tampa Bay Rays, Tampa, Florida
Neuromuscular Retraining after Anterior Cruciate Ligament Reconstruction; Rehabilitation after Articular Cartilage Procedures

Edward M. Wojtys, MD
Professor, Department of Orthopaedic Surgery, Chief, Sports Medicine Service, and Medical Director, MedSport, University of Michigan, Ann Arbor, Michigan
Anterior Cruciate Ligament Reconstruction in Skeletally Immature Patients; Gender Differences in Muscular Protection of the Knee; Management of Acute Knee Dislocation before Surgical Intervention

Preface

I am grateful to all of the contributors to this book on Knee Disorders, which is appropriately subtitled "Surgery, Rehabilitation, Clinical Outcomes." The chapters reflect the writings and teachings of the scientific and clinical disciplines required for the modern treatment of clinical afflictions of the knee joint. The goal of the writers of each chapter is to present rational evidence-based treatment programs based on published basic science and clinical outcomes to achieve the most optimal outcomes for our patients.

The "KEY" to understanding the different disorders of the knee joint encountered in clinical practice truly rests on a multiple disciplinarian approach and includes a comprehensive understanding of knee anatomy, biomechanics, kinematics, and biology of soft tissue healing. Restoration of knee function then requires a precise diagnosis of the functional abnormality of the involved knee structures, a surgical technique that is precise and successful, and a rehabilitation program directed by skilled professionals to restore function and avoid complications. Each chapter follows a concise outline of indications, contraindications, physical examination and diagnosis, step-by-step open and arthroscopic surgical procedures, clinical outcomes, and analysis of relevant published studies.

The first two chapters comprise an anatomic description of the structures of the knee joint. The photographs and illustrations represent the result of many cadaveric dissections to document knee anatomic structures. It was a pleasure to have four of our fellows (class of 2008-2009) involved in these dissections which resulted in two superb instructional anatomic videos that already have received awards and are included in the DVD. Numerous anatomic textbooks and publications were consulted during the course of these dissections to provide to the best of our ability accurate anatomic descriptions, realizing there is still ambiguity in the nomenclature used for certain knee structures. Special thanks to Joe Chovan who is a wonderful and highly talented professional medical illustrator. Joe attended anatomic dissections and worked hand-in-hand with us to produce the final anatomic illustrations. Joe and I held weekly to bi-monthly long working sessions for over two years that resulted in the anatomic and medical illustrations throughout this book that are unique, highly detailed, and believed to be anatomically accurate.

All surgeons appreciate that surgical procedures come and go, replaced by newer techniques that are more successful as techniques are discarded that may have proven inadequate by long-term clinical outcome studies. I am reminded that the basic knowledge of anatomy, biomechanics, kinematics, biology, statistics, and validated clinical outcome instruments always remain as our light-posts for patient treatment decisions. For this reason, there is ample space devoted in chapters to these scientific disciplines. Equally, the description of surgical techniques is presented in a step-by-step approach, with precise details by experienced surgeons on the critical points for each surgical technique to achieve a successful patient outcome. It is hoped that surgeons in training will appreciate the necessity for the basic science and anatomic approach that, combined with surgical and rehabilitation principles, is required to become a true "master of knee surgery and rehabilitation".

There is a special emphasis placed in each of the major book sections on rehabilitation principles and techniques including pre-operative assessment, postoperative protocols, and functional progression programs to restore lower limb function. We have published comprehensive rehabilitation protocols in this book that have been used and continually modified over many years which direct the postoperative treatment of our patients. My co-author on these sections, Tim Heckmann, is a superb physical therapist. We have worked together treating patients in a wonderful harmonious relationship for nearly 30 years. In addition, there are special programs for the female athlete to reduce the risk of an ACL injury. Sportsmetrics, a non-profit neuromuscular training and conditioning program developed at our Foundation, is one of the largest women's knee injury prevention programs in the United States and has been in existence for over 15 years. A number of scientists, therapists, athletic trainers, and physicians at our Foundation have been involved in the research efforts and publications of this program. All centers treating knee injuries in athletes are reminded of the importance of preventive neuromuscular and conditioning programs whose need has been well established by many published studies.

The entire staff at Cincinnati Sportsmedicine and Orthopaedic Center and the Foundation functions in a team effort, working together in various clinical, research, and rehabilitation programs. The concept of a team approach is given a lot of attention; and those who have visited our Center have seen the actual programs in place. This team effort is appreciated by all including patients, staff, surgeons, physical therapists, athletic trainers, administrative staff, and clinical research staff. Our administrative staff, directed by a superb clinical operations manager Linda Raterman, manages five major MD-PT-ATC orthopedic centers. As the President and CEO, I have been freed of many of the operational administrative duties because of this excellent staff, allowing time required for clinical and research responsibilities. I have been blessed to be associated with a highly dedicated group of orthopedic partners who, besides providing excellent patient care and lively discussions at our academic meetings, have donated a defined income "tithing" every year for funding research and clinical education programs at our Foundation.

Nearly all of the patients treated at the Knee Institute are entered into prospective clinical studies by a dedicated clinical research group directed by Sue Barber-Westin and Cassie Fleckenstein. The staff meticulously tracks patients over many years to obtain in published studies a 90 to 100% follow-up. I invite you to read the forward of Sue Barber-Westin who has performed such an admirable and dedicated job in bringing our clinical outcome studies to publication. It is only through her efforts that we have been successful in large prospective clinical outcome studies. In each chapter, the results of these outcome studies are rigorously compared with other authors' publications. The research and educational staff work with fellows and students from many different disciplines including physicians, therapists, trainers and biomedical students. There have been 125 Orthopedic and Sportsmedicine Fellows who have received training at our Center. The scientific contribution of fellowship research projects are acknowledged numerous times in the chapters. Our staff enjoys the mentoring process and from a personal note, this has been one of my greatest professional joys.

In regard to mentoring, one might ask where the specialty of orthopedics (or any medical specialty) would be today without the professional mentoring "system" that trains new surgeons and advances our specialty, providing for a continuum of patient treatment approaches and advances. The informal dedication of the teacher to the student, often providing wisdom and guidance over many years, is actually contrary to capitalistic principles as the hours of dedication are rarely if ever compensated. It is the gift from one generation to another and I mention this specifically as I hope that I have been able to repay in part the mentors who provided this instruction and added time and interest for my career. I graduated from the University of Utah with a philosophy degree which provided an understanding of the writings and wisdom of the great scientists and "thinkers" of our times, taught by superb educators in premedical courses and philosophy. I received an M.D. degree from George Washington University and am thankful to the dedicated teachers who laid a solid medical foundation for their students and taught the serious dedication and obligation that physicians have in treating patients. I was fortunate to be accepted for internship and residency at the University of Michigan and remember the opportunity to be associated with truly outstanding clinicians and surgeons. Under the mentorship of the chairman William S. Smith, M.D., I and my fellow residents knew one of the finest orthopedic surgeons and dedicated teachers one could be associated with who was a truly humble man that inspired decades of orthopedic residents. Many graduates of this program have continued as orthopedic educators and researchers, which is a great tribute to Bill Smith and his mentorship. My fellow residents remember one of his many favorite sayings provided to remind residents of the need for humility. After a particularly enthusiastic lecture or presentation by a prominent surgeon and glowing statements of admiration, Bill Smith would say with a wink and smile, "He puts his pants on one leg at a time just like you do".

After orthopedic residency, I accepted a four-year combined clinical and research biomechanics position at the Aerospace Medical Research Laboratories with the United States Air Force in Dayton, Ohio. The facilities and veterinary support for biomechanical knee studies were unheralded and it was here that some of the first high strain-rate experiments on mechanical properties of knee ligaments were performed using the unique laboratory testing equipment available. I am indebted to Victor Frankel and Albert Burstein, the true fathers of biomechanics in the United States, as they guided me in these formative years of my career. I was particularly fortunate to have a close association with Al Burstein who mentored me in the discipline of orthopedic biomechanics. This research effort also included professors and students at the Air Force Institute of Technology. I am grateful to all of them for instructing me in the early years of my research training. As biomechanics was just in its infancy, it was obvious that substantive research was only possible with a combined MD-PhD team approach.

One of the most fortunate blessings in my professional life is the relationship I have had with Edward S. Grood, Ph.D. I established a close working relationship with Ed nd we currently have the longest MD-PhD (or PhD-MD) team that I know of which is still active today as we conduct the next round of knee ligament function studies using sophisticated three-dimensional robotic methodologies. We worked together in establishing one of the first Biomechanical and Bioengineering programs in the country at the University of Cincinnati College of Engineering, and I greatly appreciated that it was named the Noyes Biomechanics and Tissue Engineering Laboratory. This initial effort expanded with leadership and dedicated faculty and resulted in a separate Bioengineering Department within the College of Engineering with a complete program for undergraduate and graduate students. Dr. Grood pioneered this effort with other faculty and developed the educational curriculum for the five-year undergraduate program. Many students of this program have completed important research advances that are referenced in this book. David Butler, Ph.D. joined this effort in its early years and contributed important and unique research works that are also credited throughout the chapters. This collaborative effort of many scientists and physicians resulted in three Kappa Delta awards, the Orthopedic Research and Education Clinical Research award, AOSSM Research Awards, and the support of numerous grants from NIH, NSF, and other organizations. Thomas Andriacchi, Ph.D. collaborated on important clinical studies that provided an understanding of joint kinematics and gait abnormalities. It has been an honor to have Tom associated with our efforts throughout the years.

My finest mentors were my parents, a dedicated and loving father, Marion B. Noyes, M.D. who was a true renaissance surgeon entirely comfortable doing thoracic, general surgery, and orthopedics and who, as Chief Surgeon, trained decades of surgical residents. Early in my life, I read through classic Sobotta anatomic textbooks and orthopedic textbooks which remain in my library with his writings and notations along side. Later in my training, I was fortunate to scrub with him on surgical cases. My loving mother, a nurse by training, was truly God's gift to our family for many generations as she provided unqualified love and sage and expert advice to our entire family with knowledge, wisdom, and the admiration of all of us living into her nineties. She expected excellence, performance, and adherence to a rigorous value system. These are also the attributes of the most wonderful gift of all, the opportunity to go through life with a loving and true soul mate, my wife JoAnne Noyes that I remain eternally grateful and devoted. Our family includes a fabulous daughter and son-in-law, two wonderful grandchildren, my devoted son who graduated in Physics and mentors me in nuclear and atomic matters outside my reach, and a third wonderful and dedicated son and daughter-in-law with three additional grand-children. Together, with JoAnne and all our brothers and sisters, we enjoy wonderful family events together. As I look back on my career, it is the closeness of family and friends that has provided the greatest enrichment.

In closing I wish to specially thank Kim Murphy, the Publishing Director of Elsevier and their staff who are true professionals and were a joy to work with in completing this textbook. Given all the decisions that must be made in bringing a textbook to publication, at the end of the process the Elsevier team made everything work in a harmonious manner always striving for the highest quality possible.

FRANK R. NOYES, MD

Preface

My interest in conducting clinical research stemmed from my experience of undergoing open knee surgery as a collegiate athlete 30 years ago. Although the operation was done in an expert manner, it was followed by inadequate rehabilitation and a poor outcome. Three years later, the experience was repeated except that the patient education process was markedly improved, as was the postoperative therapy program, which produced a successful result. The tremendous contrast between these experiences prompted a lifelong interest in helping patients who face the difficulty of dealing with knee problems. Having undergone arthroscopic surgery recently, I can personally attest to the incredible advances sports medicine has achieved in the past three decades. However, it is important to acknowledge that there is still much to learn and understand regarding the complex knee joint.

My initial experience with research involved collecting and analyzing data from a prospective randomized study on the effect of immediate knee motion after ACL allograft reconstruction with Dr. Noyes and our rehabilitation staff. The experience was remarkable for the time Dr. Noyes spent mentoring me on all aspects of clinical studies, including critical analysis of the literature, correct study design, basis statistics, and manuscript writing. The scientific methodology adopted by Drs. Noyes and Grood, along with our center's philosophy of the physician-rehabilitation team approach, provided an extraordinary opportunity to learn and work with those on the forefront of orthopaedics and sports medicine. My second major project, used as the thesis for my undergraduate work, involved the analysis of functional hop testing. Dr. Noyes and our statistical consultant, Jack McCloskey, were invaluable in their assistance and efforts to see the investigations through to completion. I remain grateful for these initial stimulating experiences, which provided the basis and motivation for my research career.

The clinical outcomes sections of the chapters of this textbook represent a compilation of knowledge from studies involving thousands of patients from both our center and other published cohorts. We have attempted to justify the recommendations for treatment based in part on the results of our clinical studies which used a rigorous rating system to determine outcome. The development and validation of the Cincinnati Knee Rating System was a major research focus for Dr. Noyes and I for several years. As a result, we have long advocated that "outcome" must be measured using many factors including the patient perception of the knee condition along with valid functional, subjective, and objective measures. Although this topic has come under recent debate, we continue to strongly believe

in this philosophy for many reasons. For instance, the purpose of an ACL reconstruction is to restore stability to the knee joint as measured by anterior tibial translation, the pivot-shift test, and knee function during strenuous activities. Some knee rating systems allow results of this operation to be rated as "excellent" or "good" even if the graft itself has failed (return of a positive pivot shift test). Patients in the short-term may appear to have a functional knee; however, over time a failed graft will cause problems and may require revision. A comprehensive evaluation that includes physical examination, knee arthrometer testing, function testing, and a subjective questionnaire is required to truly determine if an ACL reconstruction has been successful.

Even more compelling is the necessity to conduct long-term clinical studies with at least a 10-year follow-up evaluation. These studies must include all of the factors described (especially radiographs and in some cases, MRI) to determine the long-term sequela of various injuries and disorders. Simply collecting data from questionnaires does not, in our opinion, provide a scientific basis for treatment recommendations. At our Center, we will continue to conduct clinical research in this manner in our efforts to advance the state of knowledge of the knee joint and provide the best patient care possible.

Another area of particular research interest of mine over the years has been in the field of rehabilitation. In fact, the first clinical study I participated in was initiated while I worked on the physical therapy staff for two years. Having been a patient myself, I had a strong interest in studying the effects of different rehabilitation treatment programs on clinical outcomes. At our Center, we have always held the belief that postoperative rehabilitation is just as important as the operative procedure for a successful resolution of a problem. I have enjoyed working with Tim Heckmann in these studies for many years, as well as many other therapists, assistants, and athletic trainers who are all vital to the success of our rehabilitation research and clinical programs.

Many individuals have contributed to the success of our clinical research program over our nearly 30-year tenure and it is not possible to name them all. However, I want to especially recognize Jennifer Riccobene who, for 15 years, has doggedly tracked down and assisted hundreds of patients from all over the U.S. and beyond with their clinical research visits. Cassie Fleckenstein manages the studies in Cincinnati, keeping track of a multitude of tasks including fellowship involvement in research which has been a cornerstone of this program since the early 1980s. Our administrative department, especially Linda Raterman, has been particularly supportive of our research efforts and deserve recognition. Various institutions in Cincinnati have contributed financial support to our clinical studies over the years, including Jewish Hospital, the Deaconess Hospital Foundation, and Bethesda Hospital. We are grateful for the statistical expertise provided by Marty Levy of the University of Cincinnati and Jack McCloskey of the University of Dayton.

Finally, I'd like to thank my family - my husband Rick and my children, Teri and Alex for their support during this endeavor. I hope this textbook will be of value to many different types of health professionals for many years to come.

SUE BARBER-WESTIN

Foreword

It has been my observations over the years that Frank Noyes has three fundamental beliefs, or organizing principles, around which he has dedicated his professional life, and which explain the contents of this book. These are:

1. *Diagnosis and treatment of patient disorders should be strongly informed by knowledge gained from basic science studies.*
2. *The outcome of surgical treatment is critically dependent on rehabilitation therapy.*
3. *Advancement of medical care, both surgical and non-surgical, requires carefully conducted outcome studies that account for differences in outcome caused by the type and intensity of a patient's activities and avoid bias due to the loss of patients to follow-up.*

These core beliefs help explain the many research studies he and his colleagues conducted. The results of these studies and their clinical correlations, along with the broader base of knowledge developed by numerous investigators, form the foundation of Dr. Noyes' approach to the diagnosis and treatment of knee disorders.

This book details the approaches Dr. Noyes has developed to the diagnosis and treatment of knee disorders, along with the scientific foundations on which his approaches are based. The result is a valuable reference book for both physicians and physical therapists who care for patients with knee disorders. The inclusion of supporting basic science data also makes this book an excellent reference for any investigator or student who is interested in improving the care provided patients with knee disorders by further advancing knowledge of the normal and pathologic knee.

Although the title is "Noyes' Knee Disorders", and the content in large part reflects his clinical approaches and research, it also includes the clinical approaches and research results of other leading surgeons and physical therapists. There is, however, a common thread in that the clinical approaches presented include the scientific foundations on which they are based. Further, the reader will find that the chapters that present the research of Dr. Noyes and his colleagues also include results of other leading scientific investigators. The studies included were selected to fill in gaps and provide a broader perspective in areas where a consensus has not yet been developed.

The quality of the content of this book is complimented by the quality of its production. Each chapter has "Critical Points" sections that focus the reader's attention on the main walk-away messages. There has been extensive use of color to enhance readability, particularly in the presentation of data. Great care has been taken to make the anatomical drawings and medical illustrations accurate and to carefully label all illustrations and photographs. The care put into the production by the publisher reflects the high standard and care Dr. Noyes brings to those projects he undertakes, including the care delivered to his patients and his dedication to advancing care through carefully conducted basic science and clinical research studies. While one result of the publisher's and Dr. Noyes' efforts is the book's visual appeal, it was not the goal. Rather, the visual appeal is a by-product of their efforts to provide the reader a useful text in which the content is easily understood and accessible to the reader.

This book presents much of the research conducted by Dr. Noyes and his collaborators, including much of my own research. I would like to take this opportunity to express my appreciation and gratitude to Frank Noyes for the opportunity of collaboration, for the time and energy he has devoted to our collaboration, and to the significant financial support he and his partners have provided our research. I first met Frank in 1973 when he was stationed with the 6570th Aerospace Medical Research Laboratory, located at Wright Patterson Air Force base just outside Dayton, OH. I had recently received my PhD and was working at the University of Dayton Research Institute. It was there we met thanks to the efforts of a mutual friend and colleague George "Bud" Graves. It was also in Dayton we did our first collaborations that led to our paper on the age-related strength of the anterior cruciate ligament. In 1975 we moved to the University of Cincinnati, thanks to the encouragement of Edward Miller, M.D., then Head of the Division of Orthopaedics at the University of Cincinnati. This move was made possible by the generosity of Nicholas Giannestras, M.D. and many other orthopaedic surgeons in the community who provided support to initiate a Biomechanics Laboratory. It was in Cincinnati where we initiated our first study on whole knee biomechanics and designed and initiated our studies on primary and secondary ligamentous restraints. We were fortunate to have David Butler join our group in late 1976 and complete the study in progress on the ACL and PCL restraints, a study for which he later received the Kappa Delta Award.

In addition to working with excellent colleagues, I have been fortunate to work with many engineering students, orthopaedic residents, post-doctoral students, sports medicine fellows, and visiting professors. Without their combined intellectual contribution and hard work, I would not have been able to have completed many of the studies which are included in this text. They all have my sincerest appreciation for their support and contributions.

EDWARD S. GROOD, PHD
Director, Biomechanics Research
Cincinnati Sportsmedicine Research
and Education Foundation
Professor Emeritus, Department of Biomedical Engineering
Colleges of Medicine and Engineering
University of Cincinnati
Cincinnati, Ohio

Foreword

It is a true privilege to write this Foreword for *Noyes' Knee Disorders: Surgery, Rehabilitation, Clinical Outcomes* by Dr. Frank Noyes. The objective of this book was to produce an all-inclusive text on the knee joint that would include a multi-discipline approach to the evaluation and treatment of knee disorders. The textbook was designed to provide both basic and clinical sciences to enhance the readers' knowledge of the knee joint.

The knee joint continues to be one of the most researched, written about, and talked about subject in orthopaedics and/or sports medicine. Even with the extensive literature available, Dr. Noyes and Ms. Barber-Westin have done a masterful job pulling a tremendous amount of information together into over 1200 pages, with over 3,000 references and more than 1,000 figures in one comprehensive textbook. There are numerous chapters on the anatomy and biomechanics of various knee structures. There are specific and detailed sections on the evaluation and treatment of specific knee lesions, including the ACL, PCL, articular cartilage, patellofemoral joint, the menisci, and other structures. There are numerous chapters on the rehabilitation for each of the various knee disorders, and even a section on the gender disparity in ACL injuries. Furthermore, there is a thorough section on clinical outcomes – which is a much needed area for clinicians to understand and utilize.

I have had the true pleasure of knowing Dr. Noyes for over 20 years and he has always practiced medicine employing several principles. These include a scientific basis (evidence) to support his treatment approach, a team approach to treatment, meticulous surgery, and the attitude to always do what is best for the patient. He has applied these key principles into this outstanding textbook. Dr. Noyes has always been a proponent of a team approach to the evaluation and treatment of patients with knee disorders. This book illustrates this point beautifully with thorough chapters written by biomechanists, orthopaedic surgeons, and physical therapists. Furthermore, Dr. Noyes has always searched for the "best treatments" for the patient, seeking clinical evidence to support the treatment.

As they have done over a hundred times before in published manuscripts and chapters, Dr. Noyes and Ms. Barber-Westin have teamed up to provide us with an outstanding reference book. This outstanding text will surely remain on every knee clinician's desk for a very long time. It should be read and studied by physicians, physical therapists, athletic trainers, and anyone involved in treating patients with knee disorders. This book will surely be a favorite for all practitioners.

This is a great contribution to the literature.

Thank you Dr. Noyes for the guidance you have and continue to give us,

KEVIN E WILK, DPT, PT
Adjunct Assistant Professor
Marquette University
Milwaukee, Wisconsin
Vice President, Education, and
Associate Clinical Director
Physiotherapy Associates
Birmingham, Alabama

Contents

Knee Anatomy

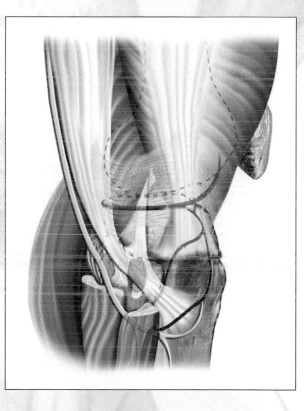

Chapter 1

Medial and Anterior Knee Anatomy

Alvin Detterline, MD ■ *John Babb*, MD ■ *Frank R. Noyes*, MD

MEDIAL ANATOMY OF THE KNEE

The medial anatomy of the knee consists of several layers of structures that work together to provide stability and function. Authors have used a variety of anatomic terms and descriptions that, unfortunately, have created ambiguity and confusion regarding this area of the knee. Two anatomic classifications or descriptions have been proposed to aid in the understanding of the relationships of the medial knee structures. These include a layered approach,[46] which describes the qualitative relationship of each medial structure, and a more quantitative description,[28] which details the exact attachment site and origin of each structure. In this chapter, both approaches are presented; however, emphasis is on the precise anatomic relationships that provide a more thorough understanding of the structures compared with the layered approach.

Medial Layers of the Knee

The three-layer description of the medial anatomy of the knee was proposed by Warren and Marshall.[46] In this approach, layer 1 consists of the deep fascia or crural fascia; layer 2 includes the superficial medial collateral ligament (SMCL), medial retinaculum, and the medial patellofemoral ligament (MPFL); and layer 3 is composed of the deep medial collateral ligament (DMCL) and capsule of the knee joint (Fig. 1–1). For this chapter, the term *medial collateral ligament* (MCL) has been selected instead of tibial collateral ligament because it represents the term most commonly used in the English literature. The medial structures identified as important in preventing lateral patellar subluxation are the MPFL and the medial patellomeniscal ligament, which inserts onto the inferior third of the patella to the anterior portion of the medial meniscus and runs adjacent to the medial fat

pad. The medial parapatellar retinaculum and so-called medial patellotibial ligament (thickening of the anterior capsule inserting from the inferior aspect of the patella to the anteromedial aspect of the tibia) are retinacular tissues that have been described; however, these structures are not believed important to providing patellar stability.

The layered approach is important because the ligaments and soft tissues on the medial side of the knee are not discrete, individual structures like the SMCL, but rather, fibrous condensations within tissue planes.[46] This qualitative description of anatomy assists in understanding the spatial relationships of these structures and how they function to support the knee.[48] It is equally important to understand the quantitative anatomy from precise measurements of the attachments and origins of each individual structure. The complex medial anatomy of the knee has been illustrated in the past with oversimplification of the soft tissue attachments to bone and other structures, which makes it difficult to compare the origins, insertions, and courses of the many separate structures among studies.[3,4,12,15,30,41,46] LaPrade and coworkers[28] recently published detailed quantitative measurements that provide a better understanding of the medial knee anatomy.

Layer 1: Deep Fascia

Layer 1 (see Fig. 1–1) consists of the deep fascia that extends proximally to invest the quadriceps, posteriorly to invest the two heads of the gastrocnemius and cover the popliteal fossa, and distally to involve the sartorius muscle and sartorial fascia. Anteriorly, layer 1 blends with the anterior part of layer 2, approximately 2 cm anterior to the SMCL.[46] Inferiorly, the deep fascia continues as the investing fascia of the sartorius and attaches to the periosteum of the tibia. Layers 1 and 2 are always

FIGURE 1–1. Medial layers of the knee. The gracilis and semitendinosus lie between layers 1 and 2.

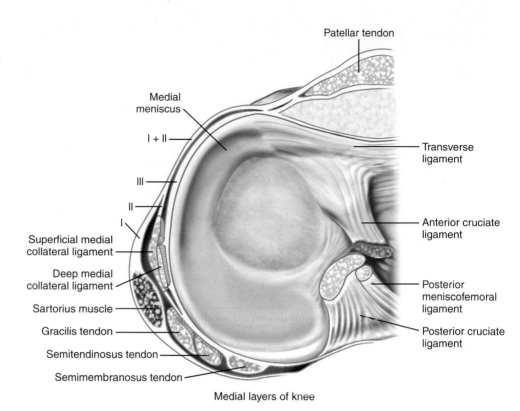

Medial layers of knee

distinct at the level of the SMCL unless extensive scarring has occurred.[46] The gracilis and semitendinosus tendons are discrete structures that lie between layers 1 and 2 and are easily separated from these two layers. However, according to Warren and Marshall,[46] these tendons will occasionally blend with the fibers in layer 1 anteriorly before they insert onto the tibia. As depicted in Figure 1–2, dissections and clinical experience of the authors of this chapter concur in that there is a blending of layer 1 with a confluence of the semitendinosus and gracilis tendons at their common insertion onto the tibia; however, they are easily found as discrete structures more posteriorly. Thus, it is the recommendation of the authors of this chapter that when attempting to harvest the semitendinosus and gracilis tendons for an anterior cruciate ligament reconstruction, these tendons initially be identified 2 to 3 cm posterior and medial to the anterior tibial spine. This will allow for easier visualization of the tendons, which can then be traced to their insertions on the anterior tibia to allow for maximal tendon length at the time of harvest.

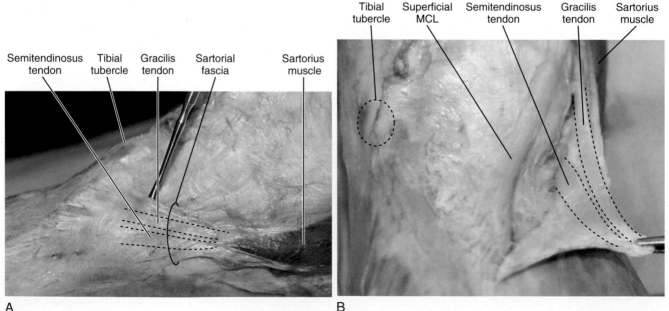

A   B

FIGURE 1–2. A, Sartorius fascia of layer 1 overlies the gracilis and semitendinosus tendons. **B,** Gracilis and semitendinosus tendons lie within the pes anserine fascia.

Layer 2: SMCL and Posterior Oblique Ligament

The SMCL is a well-defined structure that spans the medial joint line from the femur to tibia. According to LaPrade and coworkers,[28] the SMCL does not attach directly to the medial epicondyle of the femur, but is centered in a depression 4.8 mm posterior and 3.2 mm proximal to the medial epicondyle center. Other studies have described the MCL attaching directly to the medial epicondyle of the femur.* The confusion lies in the confluence of fibers that reside in the area of the medial epicondyle that make it difficult to identify the precise attachment site of the SMCL. As shown in Figure 1–3, the authors agree with LaPrade and coworkers[28] that the main fibers of the SMCL attach to an area just posterior and proximal to the medial epicondyle; but the origin of the SMCL is rather broad and, thus, there are also superficial fibrous strands attaching anterior on the medial epicondyle and posterior in a depression on the medial femoral condyle.

The posterior fibers of the SMCL overlying the medial joint line, both above and below the joint, change orientation from vertical to a more oblique pattern that forms a triangular structure with its apex posterior,[4,30] eventually blending with the fibers of the posterior oblique ligament (POL; Fig. 1–4). LaPrade and coworkers[28] described two anatomic attachment sites of the SMCL on the tibia. The first is located proximally at the medial joint line and consists mainly of soft tissue connections over the anterior arm of the semimembranosus. The second attachment site is further distal on the tibia, attaching directly to bone an average of 61.2 mm from the medial joint line. In the authors' experience, there is a consistent attachment of the proximal portion of the SMCL to the soft tissues surrounding the anterior arm of the semimembranosus, but a discrete attachment to bone is found only distally (see Fig. 1–4).

The gracilis and semitendinosus lie between layers 1 and 2 at the knee joint. The sartorius drapes across the anterior thigh and into the medial aspect of the knee invested in the sartorial fascia in layer 1. The insertion of the sartorius, as described by Warren and Marshall,[46] consists of a network of fascial fibers connecting to bone on the medial side of the tibia, but does not appear to have a distinct tendon of insertion such as the underlying gracilis and semitendinosus. However, LaPrade and coworkers[28] located the gracilis and semitendinosus tendons on the deep surface of the superficial fascial layer, with each of the three tendons attaching in a linear orientation at the lateral edge of the pes anserine bursa.

In the authors' experience, the sartorial fascia has a broad insertion onto the anteromedial border of the tibia and, with sharp dissection at its insertion, the underlying distinct tendons of the gracilis and semitendinosus are easily visualized (see Fig. 1–2). At the level of the joint, layers 1 and 2 are easily separated from each other over the SMCL. However, farther anteriorly, layer 1 blends with the anterior part of layer 2 along a vertical line 1 to 2 cm anterior to the SMCL.[46]

Also within layer 2 is the MPFL that courses from the medial femoral condyle to its attachment onto the medial border of the patella. This is a flat, fan-shaped structure that is larger at its patellar attachment than at its femoral origin, with a length averaging 58.3 mm (47.2–70.0 mm).[38] Controversy exists regarding where the MPFL attaches at the medial femoral condyle. LaPrade and coworkers[28] noted that the MPFL attaches

primarily to soft tissues between the attachments of the adductor magnus tendon and the SMCL, with an attachment to bone 10.6 mm proximal and 8.8 mm posterior to the medial epicondyle. Steensen and associates,[40] from a dissection of 11 knees, believed the MPFL attaches along the entire length of the anterior aspect of the medial epicondyle. Smirk and Morris[30] described a variable origination of the MPFL on the femur. In dissections of 25 cadavers, the MPFL attached solely to the posterior aspect of the medial epicondyle, approximately 1 cm distal to the adductor tubercle in 44% of specimens. The adductor tubercle was included in the origin in 4%, the adductor magnus tendon in 12%, the area posterior to the adductor magnus tendon in 20%, and a combination of these in 4%. In 16% of the specimens, the MPFL attached anterior to the medial epicondyle.

In the authors' experience, the MPFL attaches in a depression posterior to the medial epicondyle and blends with the insertion of the SMCL (Fig. 1–5). The anterior attachment of the MPFL consists of both attachments to the undersurface of the vastus medialis obliquus (VMO) and the proximal medial border of the patella. The work of Steensen and associates[40] demonstrated that the VMO does not overlap the MPFL, with the exception in 3 of 11 knees in which only 5% of the width of the MPFL was deep to the VMO. However, LaPrade and coworkers[28] reported that the distal border of the VMO attaches along the majority of the proximal edge of the MPFL before inserting onto the superomedial border of the patella. The midpoint of the MPFL attachment is located 41% of the length from the proximal tip of the patella along the total patellar length. The experience of the authors of this chapter is that the MPFL attaches to the proximal third of the patella, with the majority of the ligament connected to the distal portion of the VMO with fibrous bands (see Fig. 1–5).

The adductor magnus and medial gastrocnemius tendons also contribute to the medial anatomy of the knee; both attach on the medial femoral condyle. Similar to the SMCL attachment, the confluence of fibers over the medial femoral condyle makes it difficult to precisely identify the exact location of each attachment (Fig. 1–6). The adductor magnus tendon is a well-defined structure, attaching just superior and posterior to the medial epicondyle near the adductor tubercle. LaPrade and coworkers[28] reported the adductor magnus does not attach directly to the adductor tubercle, but rather to a depression located an average of 3.0 mm posterior and 2.7 mm proximal to the adductor tubercle. The adductor magnus also has fascial attachments to the capsular portion of the POL and medial head of the gastrocnemius.

The medial gastrocnemius tendon inserts in a confluence of fibers in an area between the adductor magnus insertion and the insertion of the SMCL (Fig. 1–7A). LaPrade and coworkers[28] described a gastrocnemius tubercle on the medial femoral condyle in this region; however, these authors stated that the tendon does not attach to the tubercle, but to a depression just proximal and posterior to the tubercle. In addition, fascial expansions from the lateral aspect of the medial gastrocnemius tendon form a confluence of fibers with the distal extent of the adductor magnus tendon in addition to the capsular arm of the POL (see Fig. 1–7A).

Layers 2 and 3 blend together in the posteromedial corner of the knee along with additional fibers that extend from the semimembranosus tendon and sheath that form the posteromedial capsule (see Fig. 1–7). LaPrade and coworkers[28] used the term

---

*See references 3, 4, 23, 30, 32, 33, 37, 39, 44, 46.

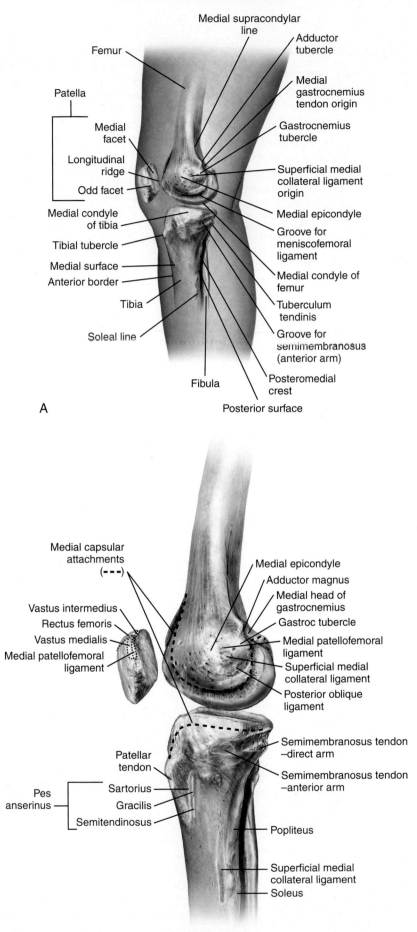

FIGURE 1–3. A, Osseous landmarks of the knee (medial view). **B**, Soft tissue attachments to bone (medial knee).

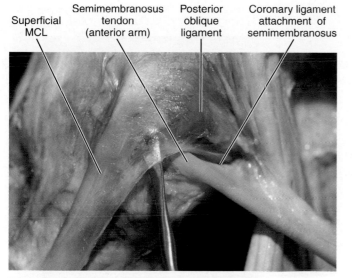

FIGURE 1-4. Oblique fibers of the superficial medial collateral ligament (SMCL) blend with the posterior oblique ligament (POL). Note the coronary ligament attachment from the anterior arm of the semimembranosus.

posterior oblique ligament (POL) for this same structure and described each of the three fascial attachments similar to Hughston and colleagues' original description.[21,22] The superficial arm of the POL runs parallel to both the more anterior SMCL and the more posterior distal expansion of the semimembranosus. Proximally, the superficial arm blends with the central arm; distally, it blends with the distal expansion of the semimembranosus as it attaches to the tibia.[28]

The central arm is the largest and thickest portion of the POL,[28] running posterior to both the superficial arm of the POL and the SMCL. It courses from the distal portion of the semimembranosus and is a fascial reinforcement of the meniscofemoral and meniscotibial portions of the posteromedial capsule. LaPrade and coworkers[28] noted that this structure has a thick attachment to the medial meniscus. As the central arm courses along the posteromedial aspect of the joint, it merges with the posterior fibers of the SMCL and can be differentiated from the SMCL by the different directions of the individual fibers. The distal attachment of the central arm is primarily to the posteromedial portion of the medial meniscus, the meniscotibial portion of the capsule, and the posteromedial tibia.[28]

The capsular portion of the POL is thinner than the other portions of this structure and fans out in the space between the central arm and the distal portions of the semimembranosus tendon. The capsular portion blends posteriorly with the posteromedial capsule of the knee and the medial aspect of the oblique popliteal ligament (OPL).[28] It attaches proximally to the fibrous bands of the medial gastrocnemius tendon and fascial expansions of the adductor magnus tendon, with no osseous attachment identified.

The superficial portion of the POL is rather thin and appears to represent a confluence of fibers from the SMCL and the semimembranosus more distally. The capsular portion appears to represent a confluence of fibers from the semimembranosus, adductor magnus, and medial gastrocnemius (see Fig. 1-7). The central arm appears more robust, having contributions from the semimembranosus and medial gastrocnemius.

Controversy remains on whether three separate distinct anatomic structures make up the POL. Other authors[36] have not found three distinct structures and note that with tibial rotation, different portions of the posteromedial capsule appear under tension but are not anatomically separate structures.

Semimembranosus

Controversy exists with respect to the exact number of attachments of the semimembranosus tendon at the knee joint.[5,6,8,22,24,25,27,34,46] However, it appears that three major attachments have been consistently identified. The common

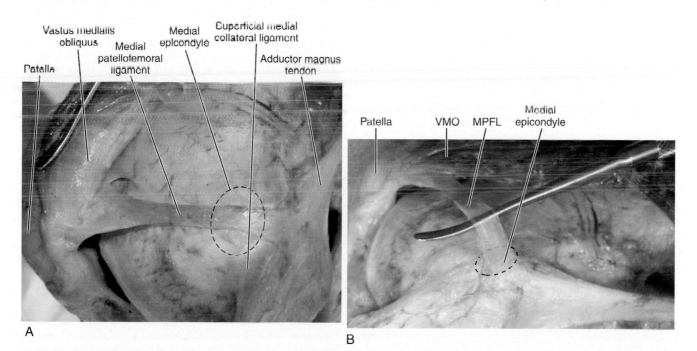

FIGURE 1-5. **A**, Medial patellofemoral ligament (MPFL) inserts into a depression behind the medial epicondyle and blends with fibers of the SMCL. **B**, Fibrous bands from the vastus medialis oblique (VMO) muscle connect to the MPFL before it inserts into the patella.

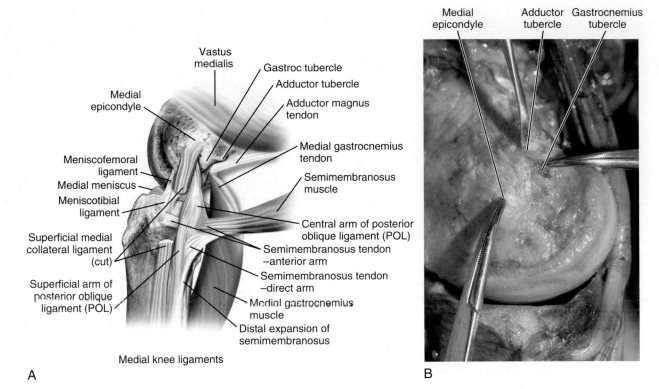

A Medial knee ligaments

B

FIGURE 1–6. A, Insertions onto the medial femoral condyle of the adductor magnus, medial head of the gastrocnemius, and the POL with its three divisions: capsular, central, and superficial arms. **B,** Osseous anatomy of the medial femoral condyle with the medial epicondyle, adductor tubercle, and gastrocnemius tubercle.

semimembranosus tendon bifurcates into a direct and anterior arm just distal to the joint line. LaPrade and coworkers[28,29] described the direct arm attaching to an osseous prominence called the *tuberculum tendinis*, approximately 11 mm distal to the joint line on the posteromedial aspect of the tibia. These authors also noted a minor attachment of the direct arm that extends to the medial coronary ligament along the posterior horn of the medial meniscus (see Fig. 1–4). A thinning of the capsule or capsular defect may be identified just distal to the femoral attachment of the medial head of the gastrocnemius and proximal to the direct arm of the semimembranosus. This is often the site of the formation of a Baker cyst.

Warren and Marshall[46] believed the semimembranosus tendon sheath and not the tendon itself extends distally over the popliteus muscle and inserts directly into the posteromedial aspect of the tibia, with some fibers coalescing with SMCL fibers inserting in the same region. These authors contend that these fibers do not have functional significance, because no change was found in the position or tension of the MCL when those fibers were transected. LaPrade and associates[29] separated the distal tibial expansion into a medial and a lateral division. Both divisions originating on the coronary ligament of the posterior horn of the medial meniscus are located on either side of the direct arm of the semimembranosus. The divisions then course distally to cover the posterior aspect of the popliteus muscle and insert onto the posteromedial aspect of the tibia, forming an inverted triangle. These authors noted that the medial division attaches just posterior to the SMCL, whose fibers coalesce with the superficial arm of the POL (as previously noted by Hughston and colleagues[22]) rather than the MCL.

In the authors' experience, as shown in Figure 1–8, the semimembranosus tendon sheath and not the tendon itself comprises

the distal tibial expansion, which includes a medial and a lateral division with a central raphae separating the two. The anterior arm of the semimembranosus courses deep to the SMCL and attaches directly to bone just distal to the medial joint capsule on the tibia (Fig. 1–9). There are fibrous connections between the SMCL and the anterior arm of the semimembranosus, but only the anterior arm of the semimembranosus has an osseous attachment in this region. Because both the direct and the anterior arms of the semimembranosus anchor directly to bone and attach distal to the tibial margin of the medial joint capsule, these are not considered part of either layer 2 or layer 3 as described by Warren and Marshall.[46]

The third major attachment of the semimembranosus is the OPL. Warren and Marshall[46] described the semimembranosus tendon sheath as forming fiber tracts that make up the OPL, although they admit some collagen fibers may come from the tendon itself. LaPrade and associates[29] described a lateral expansion off the common semimembranosus tendon, just proximal to its bifurcation into the direct and anterior arms, that coalesces to form a portion of the OPL, in addition to the capsular arm of the POL. As shown in Figure 1–10A–B, it is difficult to appreciate distinct structures making up the origin of the OPL because of the significant confluence of fibers in the region. However, there are fibers originating from both the semimembranosus tendon and its sheath that contribute to its origin.

The OPL is described as a broad fascial band that courses laterally and proximally across the posterior capsule. LaPrade and associates[29] noted two distinct lateral attachments of the OPL (proximal and distal). The proximal attachment is broad, extending to the fabella, the posterolateral capsule, and the plantaris (see Fig. 1–10). It does not attach directly to the lateral femoral

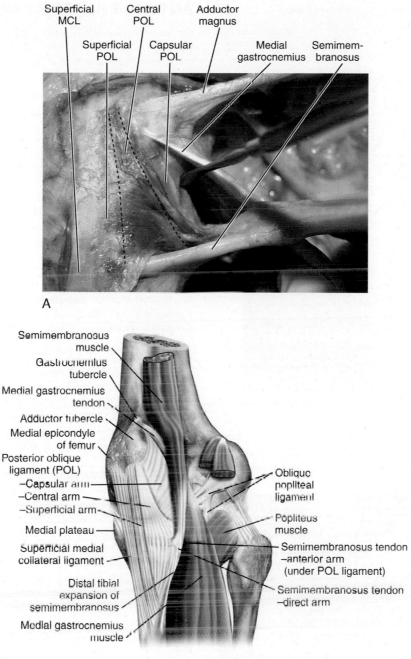

Superficial MCL   Central POL   Adductor magnus

Superficial POL   Capsular POL   Medial gastrocnemius   Semimembranosus

A

Semimembranosus muscle
Gastrocnemius tubercle
Medial gastrocnemius tendon
Adductor tubercle
Medial epicondyle of femur
Posterior oblique ligament (POL)
—Capsular arm
—Central arm
—Superficial arm
Medial plateau
Superficial medial collateral ligament
Distal tibial expansion of semimembranosus
Medial gastrocnemius muscle

Oblique popliteal ligament
Popliteus muscle
Semimembranosus tendon
—anterior arm (under POL ligament)
Semimembranosus tendon
—direct arm

B   Posterior oblique ligament (POL)

FIGURE 1–7. A, Insertions onto the medial femoral condyle of the adductor magnus, the medial head of the gastrocnemius, and the POL with its three divisions: capsular, central, and superficial arms. **B,** Anatomy of the POL with its three divisions.

condyle. The distal attachment is on the posterolateral aspect of the tibia, just distal to the posterior root of the lateral meniscus, but not directly attaching to the lateral meniscus as described by Kim and coworkers.[27] It is theorized that this may serve a functional role limiting hyperextension, but this has not been demonstrated in any biomechanical study to date.

LaPrade and associates[29] also described a proximal capsular arm of the semimembranosus as a thin aponeurosis that traverses medially to laterally along the superior border of the OPL. As it courses laterally, it blends with the posterolateral capsule and inserts on the distal lateral femur just proximal to the capsular insertion while at the same time extending fibers to the short head of the biceps femoris tendon (see Fig. 1–10B–C).

Layer 3: DMCL and Knee Capsule

The capsule of the knee joint is thin anteriorly and envelopes the fat pad. In this area, the capsule is easily separated from the overlying superficial retinaculum until it reaches the margin of the patella, where it is difficult to separate the capsule from the overlying superficial structures.[46] Under the SMCL lies a vertical thickening of the knee capsule known as the *distal medial collateral ligament* (DMCL). The DMCL crosses the joint from the distal femur to the medial meniscus and inserts into the proximal tibia at sites adjacent to the articular surfaces of the femur and tibia. These separate divisions of the DMCL are named the *meniscofemoral* and *meniscotibial* ligaments. Warren

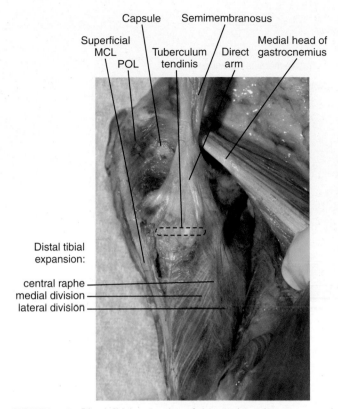

Capsule   Semimembranosus

Superficial
MCL   Medial head of
          Tuberculum   Direct   gastrocnemius
     POL   tendinis   arm

Distal tibial
expansion:

central raphe
medial division
lateral division

FIGURE 1–8. Distal tibial expansion of the semimembranosus tendon sheath with its medial and lateral divisions.

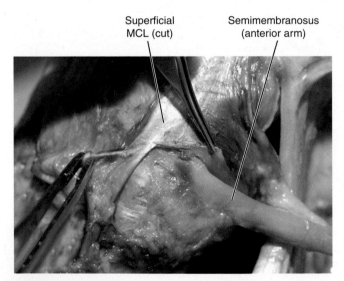

Superficial   Semimembranosus
MCL (cut)   (anterior arm)

FIGURE 1–9. SMCL is cut to show the anterior arm of the semimembranosus attachment to bone.

and Marshall[46] noted that the meniscofemoral portion of the DMCL had a discrete attachment onto the distal femur at its articular margin. Similarly, the meniscotibial portion of the DMCL, also known as the *coronary ligament*, is easily separated from the overlying SMCL in layer 2 before attaching to the tibia at its articular margin (Fig. 1–11).

The deepest structure on the medial side is the capsule of the knee, which envelopes the entire joint and extends proximally up to the suprapatellar pouch and distally to the attachment site of the meniscotibial ligament on the tibia–articular cartilage border.[46]

ANTERIOR ANATOMY OF THE KNEE

Several anatomic relationships and structures are important to recognize because they are critical to understanding the mechanics of the extensor mechanism and may be involved in several pathologic conditions.

Quadriceps Mechanism

The quadriceps consists of the rectus femoris, adjacent to the vastus medialis and lateralis on either side, and the vastus intermedius deep (Fig. 1–12). The rectus femoris is located centrally and superficially in the quadriceps mechanism and widens distally as it approaches the superior aspect of the patella. Reider and colleagues[35] found the width of the rectus femoris tendon to be 3 to 5 cm at the proximal pole of the patella. Some of the rectus tendon fibers insert into the superior aspect of the patella, but the majority continue over the anterior surface of the patella and are continuous with the patellar tendon distally. This is in contrast to the other components of the quadriceps mechanism that do not commonly contribute directly to the patellar tendon. The vastus medialis has fibers that run parallel to the rectus femoris fibers, called the *vastus medialis longus*, and others that run obliquely in relation to the rectus, termed the *vastus medialis obliquus* (VMO) according to Lieb and Perry.[31] Conlan and coworkers[7] described the VMO originating from the medial intermuscular septum and the adductor longus tendon proximal to the adductor tubercle. The angle of the obliquity of the VMO fibers varies considerably. Reider and colleagues[35] found a range of 55° to 70° in a cadaveric study. This variability in obliquity has been implicated in patellar maltracking.

The muscle of the vastus medialis extends distally and often becomes tendinous only millimeters from its patellar insertion. Reider and colleagues[35] noted that some fibers insert directly into the patella, whereas others course more distally and contribute to the medial retinaculum. Conlan and coworkers[7] contended that some fibers of the VMO extend more distally and actually contribute to the patellar tendon. As shown in Figure 1–12, the vast majority of the VMO fibers either attach directly onto the patella or extend more distally to make up the medial retinaculum. The most medial fibers of the medial retinaculum converge into the medial border of the patellar tendon, but do not provide a significant contribution to the patellar tendon fibers.

The vastus lateralis muscle is divided similarly to the vastus medialis with a longus and an obliquus portion. The insertions of the longus and obliquus tendons are quite variable, according to Hallisey and associates.[16] These authors contended that the amount of vastus lateralis tendon that travels over the anterior cortex of the patella and contributes to the patellar tendon distally is variable. In some cases, the lateralis tendon fibers remain lateral to the patella and interdigitate with the fibers of the iliopatellar tract without contributing to the patellar tendon (Fig. 1–13). The insertion of the obliquus fibers is also variable according to Hallisey and associates.[16] These authors found that in some specimens, the obliquus tendon fibers insert into the vastus lateralis longus fibers proximal to the patella; in others, they blend into the iliopatellar tract before inserting on the patella. As shown in Figure 1–13, it is the experience of the authors of this chapter that the most medial fibers of the lateralis obliquus tend to coalesce with the fibers of the longus, whereas

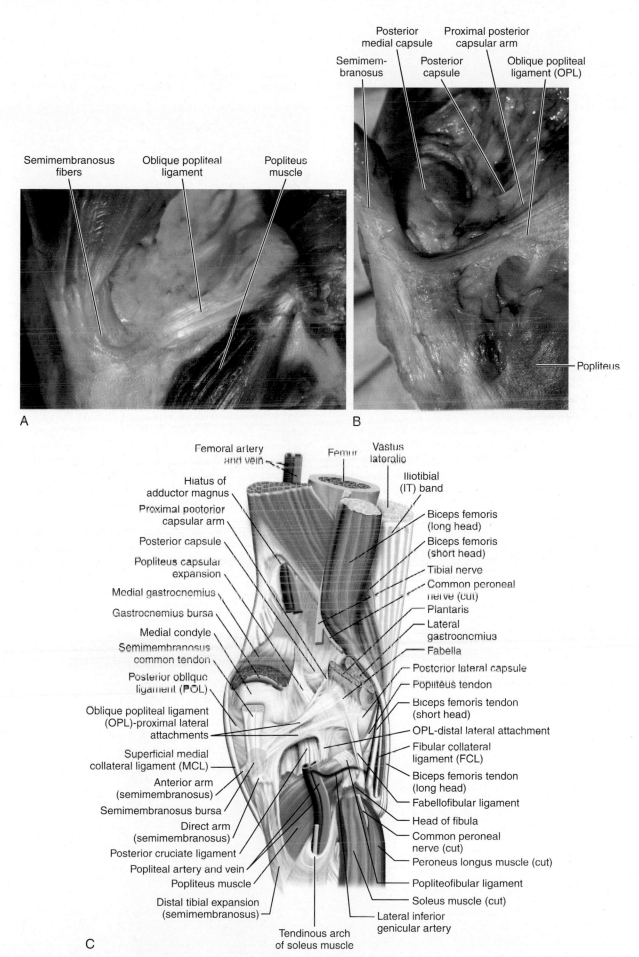

FIGURE 1-10. **A**, Semimembranosus fibers contribute to the oblique popliteal ligament (OPL). **B**, OPL fans across the posterior knee with its multiple fibrous divisions. **C**, Posterior knee showing the divisions of the OPL.

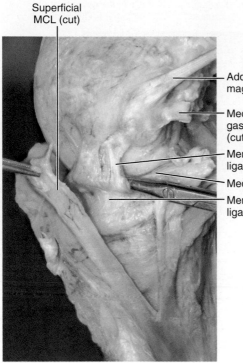

FIGURE 1–11. SMCL is cut to show the deep medial collateral ligament with its two divisions: meniscofemoral and meniscotibial.

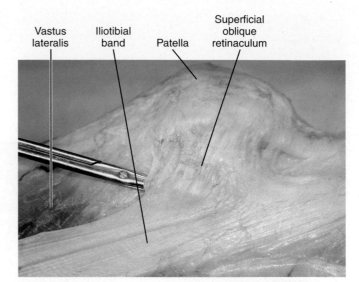

FIGURE 1–13. Longitudinal fibers of the vastus lateralis blend with fibers of the superficial oblique retinaculum.

the most lateral obliquus fibers coalesce with the iliopatellar tract. The vastus lateralis does not provide a significant contribution to the patellar tendon.

The fibers of the lateralis run more parallel to the rectus femoris fibers than to the vastus medialis (see Fig. 1–12). The average obliquity of the lateralis fibers is 31°, according to Reider and colleagues.[35] The lateralis fibers also become tendinous

more proximally than the medialis, an average of 2.8 cm proximal to the patella.[35] The angle of insertion of the obliquus fibers is rather variable, with an average of 48.5° in men and 38.5° in women.[30]

The vastus intermedius is deep to the rectus femoris, inserts directly into the proximal pole of the patella, and blends with the fibers of the medialis and lateralis that insert in similar fashion. Previous descriptions of the quadriceps tendon insertion depict a trilaminar arrangement of fibers, with the rectus femoris contributing the most superficial fibers, the medialis and lateralis contributing the middle layer, and finally, the intermedius contributing the deepest fibers. Reider and colleagues[35] described the inserting fibers as more of a coalescence rather

FIGURE 1–12. Extensor mechanism of knee shows the vastus lateralis, vastus medialis, and rectus femoris. Note the long tendon insertion of the vastus lateralis onto the proximal patella.

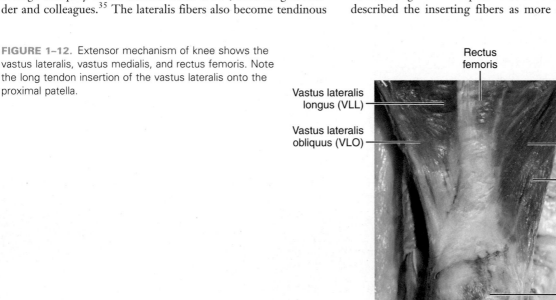

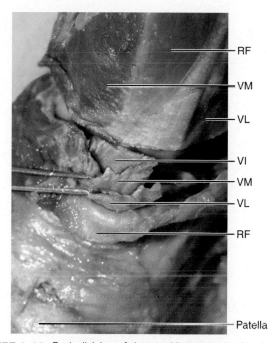

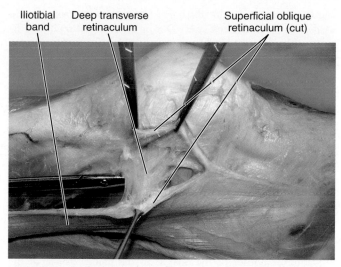

FIGURE 1–15. Deep transverse fibers of the iliopatellar tract.

FIGURE 1–14. Each division of the quadriceps mechanism is dissected proximal to the patella. RF, rectus femoris; VI, vastus intermedius; VL, vastus lateralis; VM, vastus medialis.

than distinct layers as previously described. It is the authors' experience that the quadriceps tendon is a coalescence of fibers at the proximal pole of the patella, but as one travels a few centimeters proximal, four distinct layers to the quadriceps tendon can be identified and separated from one another (Fig. 1–14). When harvesting a quadriceps tendon graft, it is important that all layers are identified.

Fascial Layers

Confusion arises when attempting to describe the various layers of the anterior knee structures because different nomenclature is used for both the medial and the lateral parapatellar tissues. This description will break down the layers both medially and laterally and then attempt to assimilate each as they form a confluence over the anterior aspect of the patella.

Lateral

The most superficial layer laterally, termed the *aponeurotic layer* by Terry and colleagues,[43] is composed of the superficial fascia of the vastus lateralis and biceps femoris. These fibers, termed *arciform fibers*, travel transversely across the anterior aspect of the patella to blend at the midline with the superficial fascia of the sartorius, which begins medially.

The next layer is termed the *superficial layer* by Terry and colleagues.[43] It is made up of the iliopatellar tract, which connects the iliotibial band to the patella.[13,45] The iliopatellar tract has been further subdivided into a superficial and a deep layer by Fulkerson and Gossling[13] who described two different fiber orientations. The most superficial is termed the *superficial oblique retinaculum* because its fiber orientation is oblique. This tract inserts along the lateral border of the patella (see Fig. 1–13). In addition, there are deep transverse fibers that also

connect the iliotibial band with the lateral aspect of the patella (Fig. 1–15). In this deeper, more transverse tract is the patellotibial ligament, which originates just proximal to Gerdy's tubercle on the tibia and inserts on the inferior portion of the lateral aspect of the patella.[13] Just deep to this ligament is the lateral meniscopatellar ligament, which runs between the anterior horn of the lateral meniscus and the inferior aspect of the patella. It is a thickening of the anterolateral capsule. The deepest layer on the lateral side is the capsular-osseous layer, which anchors the iliotibial band to the femur through the lateral intermuscular septum and travels anteriorly to the patella. Some authors[26,43,45] contended that it includes the lateral patellofemoral ligament, but the experience of the authors of this chapter is that a distinct ligament is not present.

As shown in Figure 1–16, the capsular-osseous layer of the iliotibial tract has a femoral attachment proximal to the lateral epicondyle. At the level of the lateral epicondyle is a bursa deep to the iliotibial tract. It is the authors' experience that there commonly is an identifiable nerve, which is called the *lateral*

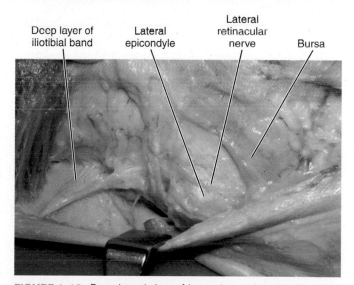

FIGURE 1–16. Deep lateral view of knee shows the capsular-osseous layer of the iliotibial band with bursa.

retinacular nerve, within this bursa that may play a role in pain associated with runner's knee. During an iliotibial tract lengthening procedure for recalcitrant runners' knee, it is the authors' belief that while the iliotibial bursa is excised, the lateral retinacular nerve should be identified and cut posterior to the lateral epicondyle to prevent recurrence of this painful condition.

Medial

The superficial fascia of the vastus medialis and sartorius form the most superficial layer medially. This aponeurotic layer travels laterally over the anterior aspect of the patella to merge with the same layer from the lateral side.

The next layer is considered to be the same as layer 2 as described by Warren and Marshall.[46] This is composed of the MPFL and the SMCL. In this layer is the medial retinaculum, which is defined as the VMO fibers running transversely from the anterior border of the SMCL to the medial aspect of the patella. The medial patellotibial ligament is also found in this middle layer (Fig. 1–17). According to Conlan and coworkers,[7] it originates on the inferior portion of the medial aspect of the patella and travels distally and posteriorly to insert on the anteromedial aspect of the tibia. The deepest structure found on the anteromedial aspect of the knee is the medial meniscopatellar ligament, which is a thickening of the capsule that runs between the anterior horn of the medial meniscus and the inferior portion of the medial border of the patella[7] (Fig. 1–18).

Prepatellar

The fascial layer covering the quadriceps is termed the *fascia lata*. Dye and coworkers[11] noted that the fascia lata extends distally as the most superficial layer overlying the patella after the skin and subcutaneous tissue. These authors described the fascia lata as an extremely thin layer that has little structural integrity, but visible transverse fiber orientation. This is in contrast to the intermediate layer overlying the patella, which has an oblique fiber orientation proximally and becomes more transverse distally over

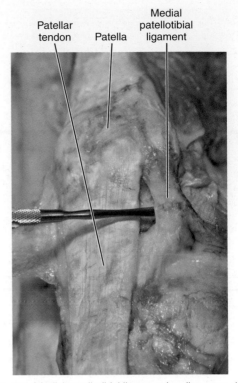

FIGURE 1–17. Medial patellotibial ligament is adjacent to the patellar tendon.

the patellar tendon. Dye and coworkers[11] described the intermediate layer consisting of tendinous fibers from the vastus medialis and lateralis, in addition to the superficial fibers of the rectus femoris that extend over the anterior aspect of the patella.

The deepest layer anterior to the patella is composed of the deeper fibers of the rectus femoris that extend distal to the proximal pole of the patella and are intimately associated with the anterior cortex of the patella as they continue to contribute to the fibers of the patellar tendon (Fig. 1–19).

FIGURE 1–18. Posterior anatomy of the patella with adjacent capsular thickenings and fat pads with the medial and lateral meniscopatellar ligaments.

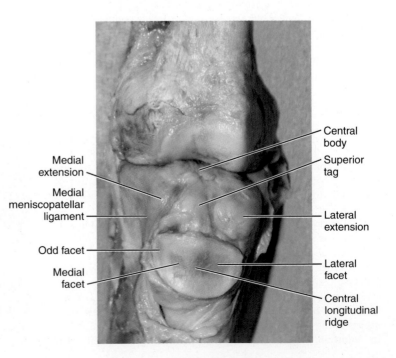

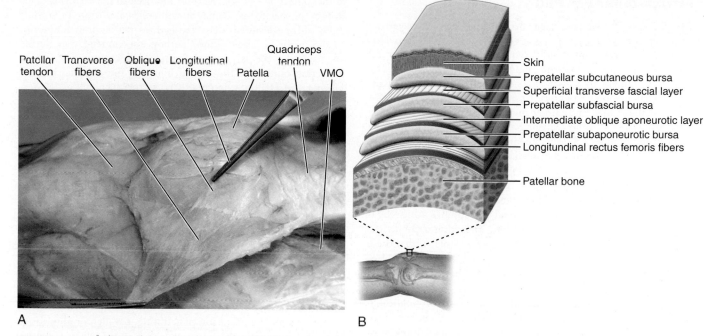

FIGURE 1–19. **A**, Fascia layers of the anterior knee. **B**, Layers of the anterior knee.

Dye and coworkers[11] noted that these layers form three separate bursae superficial to the patella. The most superficial is termed the *prepatellar subcutaneous bursa* (between the skin and the superficial fascia lata). The middle bursa is termed the *prepatellar subfascial bursa* (between the superficial fascia lata and the oblique intermediate layer). Finally, the deepest bursa is called the *prepatellar subaponeurotic bursa* (between the intermediate and the deep aponeurotic layers). It should be noted that no bursa exists between the deepest aponeurotic layer and the anterior cortex of the patella, as others have suggested.[23a]

Patella

The patella is a sesamoid bone deeply associated with the quadriceps tendon, as previously described (Fig. 1–20). The articular surface of the patella is often divided into facets based on longitudinal ridges. The major longitudinal ridge divides the medial and the lateral facets of the patella. A second longitudinal ridge near the medial border of the patella separates the medial facet from a thin strip of articular surface known as the *odd facet* (see Fig. 1–18). Wiberg[47] classified the morphology of patellae into three major types based upon the position of the longitudinal ridges. Type I patella have medial and lateral facets that are equal in size. Type II patella have a medial facet slightly smaller than the lateral facet. Type III patella have a very small and steeply angled medial facet, whereas the lateral facet is broad and concave. According to Dye and coworkers,[11] type II patella are the most common (present in 57% of knees) followed by type I (24%), and type III (19%).

Patellar Tendon

The patellar tendon courses between the inferior pole of the patella and the tibial tubercle (see Fig. 1–17). This tendon consists mostly of fibers from the rectus femoris, as previously mentioned.

The structure inserts on the proximal tibia, just distal to the most proximal portion of the tibial tubercle. It blends medially and laterally with the fascial expansions of the anterior surface of the tibia and the iliotibial band. Dye and coworkers[11] reported an average length of 46 mm, with a range of 35 to 55 mm.

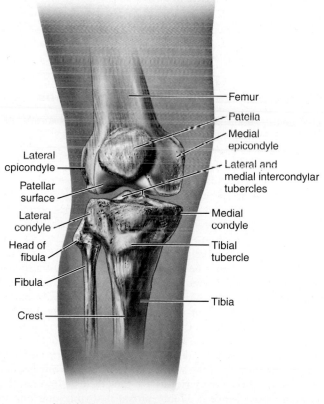

Anterior knee bony landmarks

FIGURE 1–20. Bony landmarks of the anterior knee.

Infrapatellar Fat Pad

The infrapatellar fat pad is an intracapsular, but extrasynovial structure; the deepest portion is covered by a synovial layer. This structure has been consistently identified to have a thick central body, with thinner medial and lateral extensions (see Fig. 1–18). It has attachments to the inferior pole of the patella proximally, the patellar tendon and anterior capsule anteriorly, the anterior horns of the medial and lateral menisci plus the proximal tibia inferiorly, and the intercondylar notch posteriorly via the ligamentum mucosum.[14] The ligamentum mucosum is an embryonic remnant separating the medial and lateral compartments of the knee. It has two alar folds that attach to the infrapatellar fat pad, allowing it to maintain its position in the joint.[17]

Gallagher and associates[14] identified two clefts in the infrapatellar fat pad: a horizontal cleft, found just inferior to the ligamentum mucosum, and a vertical cleft, located anterior to the superior tag of the central body. It has been postulated that these clefts may play a role in reducing the friction between the anterior capsule and the femoral condyles, but they also may be a location for loose bodies to hide.

Inflammation in the infrapatellar fat pad has been implicated as a source of anterior knee pain. Hoffa's disease is characterized by inflammation and hypertrophy, with subsequent trapping of the fat pad between the patellar tendon and the femoral condyles.[14] The treatment frequently consists of resection of the fat pad, but this has been associated with a decrease in patellar blood supply.[20] The fat pad may also become inflamed after arthroscopic surgery because of portal placement. This may lead to fibrous scarring, which can limit motion and serve as a source for residual pain.[10] Fibrous scars that occur after arthroscopy have a 50% resolution rate after one year.[42] It is recommended that portal placement be well medial and lateral to the patellar tendon borders so that damage to the central body and superior tag can be minimized in order to limit this potential complication.[14]

Superficial Neurovascular Structures

The medial inferior genicular artery traverses beneath the SCML after branching from the popliteal artery (Figs. 1–21 and 1–22). It can be visualized on the anterior border of the SMCL as it courses toward the patellar tendon and medial meniscus. This vascular structure may be encountered during any dissection on the medial aspect of the knee, most notably, during a posteromedial approach for meniscal repair. If identified in the approach, it must be retracted or cauterized to provide a clear approach to the medial meniscus.

Other important structures located on the medial side of the knee are the saphenous nerve with its sartorial and infrapatellar branches, the medial femoral cutaneous nerve, and the medial retinacular nerve (Fig. 1–23). These nerves may be easily injured with medial dissection of the knee. It has been reported that injury to the saphenous nerve occurs in 7% to 22% of patients during arthroscopic meniscal repair.[2] According to Dunaway and colleagues,[9] cadaver dissections in 42 knees revealed that the sartorial branch of the saphenous nerve consistently became extrafascial between the sartorius and the gracilis. However, this location varied between 37 mm proximal to the joint line to 30 mm distal to the joint line, with the nerve being extrafascial

at the joint only 43% of the time and deep to the sartorius fascia in 66% of specimens. Dunaway and colleagues[9] noted that only 2.8% of the specimens dissected had a sartorial branch anterior to the sartorius fascia. These authors recommend that during an inside-out medial meniscus repair, staying anterior during dissection minimizes the risk of injury to the sartorial branch. Horner and Dellon[18] described the sartorial branch as the terminal branch of the saphenous nerve that passes 3 cm posterior to the central point of the medial condyle of the femur and continues to the medial aspect of the foot alongside the saphenous vein.

The infrapatellar branch of the saphenous nerve may also be easily damaged with indiscriminate dissection on the medial aspect of the knee, leading to postoperative pain and paresthesia. Postoperative numbness, paresthesia, or hypersensitivity in the distribution of the infrapatellar branch of the saphenous nerve has been reported in the literature[38]: 21% in the Mayo Clinic series, 51.5% in the Iowa series, and 40% in the Alberta series.[19] The risk of damage is increased by the varying course of the nerve. The infrapatellar branch of the saphenous nerve may have four different courses at the level of the medial joint line, which are described by the nerve's relationship to the sartorius muscle. The nerve may be posterior, penetrating, parallel, or anterior to the sartorius, with the most common type being posterior (62.2%).[1] Arthornthurasook and Gaew-im[1] reported that the infrapatellar branch of the saphenous nerve is an average distance of 40.6 mm from the medial epicondyle when the nerve exits and travels posterior to the sartorius. Horner and Dellon[18] described the infrapatellar branch separating from the saphenous nerve in the proximal third of the thigh in 17.6% of specimens, in the middle third in 58.8%, and in the distal third of the thigh in 23.5%. This nerve innervates not only the patella but also the anterior-inferior capsule.[18]

Horner and Dellon[18] described the medial femoral cutaneous nerve traveling superficially to the sartorius muscle in 39.1% of knees. However, this nerve often travels in Hunter's canal and perforates the sartorius (30.4% of knees) or continues in Hunter's canal and exits deep to the sartorius (30.4% of knees). The termination of this nerve is the most superficial constant branch that eventually bisects the patella to form a prepatellar plexus before continuing to the lateral aspect of the knee and pairing with the infrapatellar branch of the saphenous nerve proximal to the knee joint.

The medial retinacular nerve has also been described as residing on the medial aspect of the knee near the vastus medialis. The vastus medialis is innervated by branches from the femoral nerve. The terminal branch of the nerve to the vastus medialis ends as the medial retinacular nerve. According to Horner and Dellon,[18] this nerve may traverse within the vastus medialis (90% of knees) or lie superficial to its fascia (10% of knees). The nerve enters the knee capsule beneath the medial retinaculum, 1 cm proximal to the adductor tubercle, and sends a branch to the MCL.[18] This nerve was not identified in dissections performed by the authors of this chapter.

Indiscriminate dissection on the medial side of the knee could easily damage any one of these described nerves, leading to the pathology already noted. Painful neuromas and complex regional pain syndrome can turn a successful operation into a complicated pain syndrome. Horner and Dellon[18] advised that the surgeon be aware of these pitfalls and recognize the possibility that symptomatology may result from damage to one or

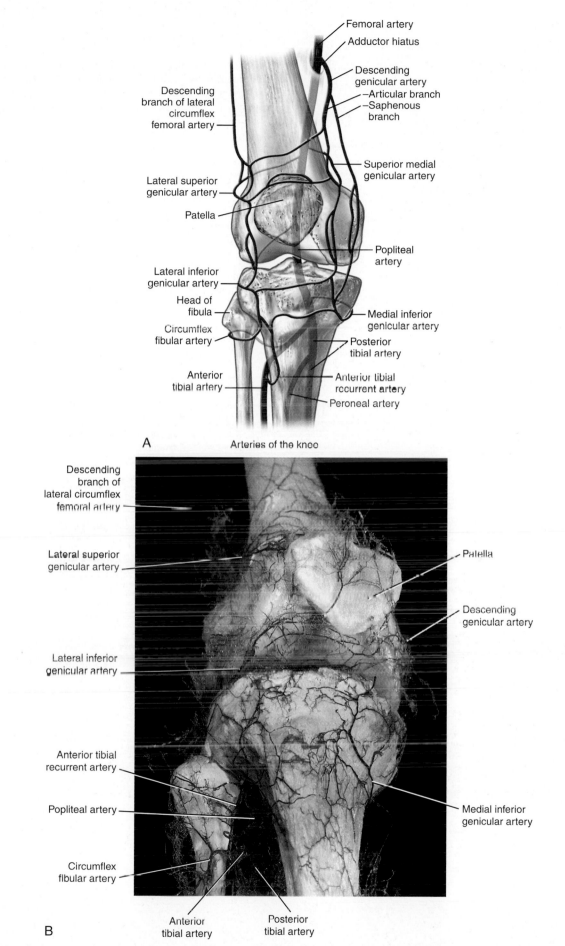

FIGURE 1–21. **A,** Arterial vasculature of the knee. **B,** Detailed vascularity shown after specialized injection technique. *(Unpublished from Kaderly RF, Butler DL, Noyes FR, Grood ES: The three-dimensional vascular anatomy of the human knee joint.)*

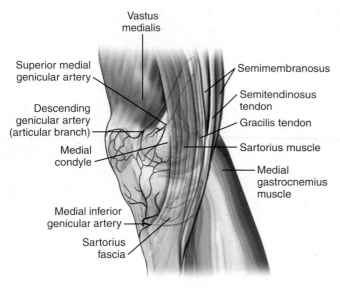

Medial knee arteries

FIGURE 1–22. Path of the medial inferior genicular artery.

more nerves that require diagnostic nerve blocks at multiple sites to identify the pathology. Unnecessary subsequent surgeries for postoperative pain may be prevented by identifying the true cause of pain, which may very well be the result of nerve damage. A neurectomy may be required when a nerve block provides only temporary relief of pain.[18]

CONCLUSIONS

The anterior and medial anatomy of the knee has frequently been oversimplified or poorly described in the literature. It is the authors' hope that this chapter has allowed the reader a greater appreciation for the anatomic relationships present and their potential implications in various knee conditions. A key to successful operative repair and reconstruction of the medial side of the knee is detailed knowledge of anatomy of its structures.

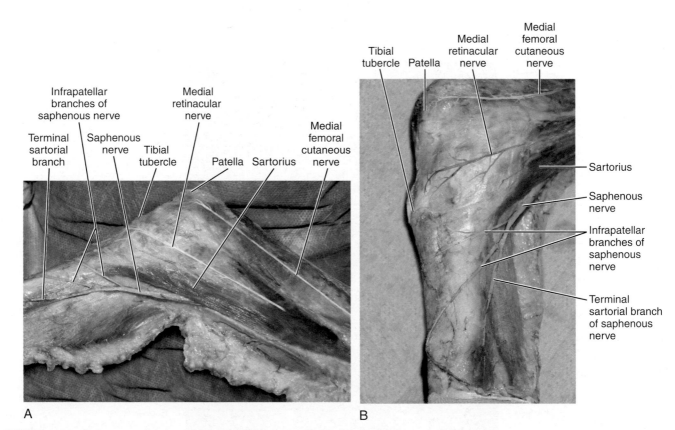

FIGURE 1–23. A, Anteromedial view of the superficial nerves. **B,** Medial view of the superficial nerves.

REFERENCES

1. Arthornthurasook, A.; Gaew-Im, K.: Study of the infrapatellar nerve. *Am J Sports Med* 16:57–59, 1988.
2. Austin, K. S.; Sherman, O. H.: Complications of arthroscopic meniscal repair. *Am J Sports Med* 21:864–869, 1993.
3. Brantigan, O. C.; Voshell, A. F.: The mechanics of the ligaments and menisci in the knee joint. *J Bone Joint Surg* 23A:44–61, 1941.
4. Brantigan, O. C.; Voshell, A. F.: The tibial collateral ligament: its function, its bursae, and its relation to the medial meniscus. *J Bone Joint Surg Am* 25:121–131, 1943.
5. Cave, A. E.; Porteous, C. J.: A note on the semimembranosus muscle. *Ann R Coll Surg Engl* 24:251–256, 1959.
6. Cave, A. E.; Porteous, C. J.: The attachments of m. semimembranosus. *J Anat* 9Z(Pt 4):638, 1958.
7. Conlan, T.; Garth, W. P.; Lemons, J. E.: Evaluation of the medial soft-tissue restraints of the extensor mechanism of the knee. *J Bone Joint Surg* 75:682–693, 1993.
8. Cross, M. J.: Proceedings: the functional significance of the distal attachment of the semimembranous muscle in man. *J Anat* 118(pt 2): 401, 1974.
9. Dunaway, D. J.; Steensen, R. N.; Wiand, W.; Dopirak, R. M.: The sartorial branch of the saphenous nerve: its anatomy at the joint line of the knee. *Arthroscopy* 21:547–551, 2005.
10. Duri, Z. A.; Aichroth, P. M.; Dowd, G.: The fat pad. Clinical observations. *Am J Knee Surg* 9:55–66, 1996.
11. Dye, S. F.; Campagna-Pinto, D.; Dye, C. C.; et al.: Soft-tissue anatomy anterior to the human patella. *J Bone Joint Surg Am* 85:1012–1017, 2003.
12. Fischer, R. A.; Arms, S. W.; Johnson, R. J.; Pope, M. H.: The functional relationship of the posterior oblique ligament to the medial collateral ligament of the human knee. *Am J Sports Med* 13:390–397, 1985.
13. Fulkerson, J. P.; Gossling, H. R.: Anatomy of the knee joint lateral retinaculum. *Clin Orthop Relat Res* 153:183–188, 1980.
14. Gallagher, J.; Tierney, P.; Murray, P.; O'Brien, M.: The infrapatellar fat pad: anatomy and clinical correlations. *Knee Surg Sports Traumatol Arthrosc* 13:268–272, 2005.
15. Haimes, J. L.; Wroble, R. R.; Grood, E. S.; Noyes, F. R.: Role of the medial structures in the intact and anterior cruciate ligament-deficient knee. Limits of motion in the human knee. *Am J Sports Med* 22:402–409, 1994.
16. Hallisey, M. J.; Doherty, N.; Bennett, W. F.; Fulkerson, J. P.: Anatomy of the junction of the vastus lateralis tendon and the patella. *J Bone Joint Surg Am* 69:545–549, 1987.
17. Hardaker, W. T.; Whipple, T. L.; Bassett, F. H., 3rd: Diagnosis and treatment of the plica syndrome of the knee. *J Bone Joint Surg Am* 62:221–225, 1980.
18. Horner, G.; Dellon, A. L.: Innervation of the human knee joint and implications for surgery. *Clin Orthop Relat Res* 301:221–226, 1994.
19. Huckell, J. R.: Is meniscectomy a benign procedure? A long-term follow-up study. *Can J Surg* 8:254–260, 1965.
20. Hughes, S. S.; Cammarata, A.; Steinmann, S. P.; Pellegrini, V. D., Jr.: Effect of standard total knee arthroplasty surgical dissection on human patellar blood flow in vivo: an investigation using laser Doppler flowmetry. *J South Orthop Assoc* 7:198–204, 1998.
21. Hughston, J. C.: The importance of the posterior oblique ligament in repairs of acute tears of the medial ligaments in knees with and without an associated rupture of the anterior cruciate ligament. Results of long-term follow-up. *J Bone Joint Surg Am* 76:1328–1344, 1994.
22. Hughston, J. C.; Andrews, J. R.; Cross, M. J.; Moschi, A.: Classification of knee ligament instabilities. Part I. The medial compartment and cruciate ligaments. *J Bone Joint Surg Am* 58:159–172, 1976.
23. Hughston, J. C.; Eilers, A. F.: The role of the posterior oblique ligament in repairs of acute medial (collateral) ligament tears of the knee. *J Bone Joint Surg Am* 55:923–940, 1973.
23a. International Anatomical Nomenclature Committee. Nomina anatomica. Authorized by the 12th International Congress of Anatomists in London, 1985. 6th ed. Edinburgh: Churchill Livingstone, 1989.
24. Kaplan, E. B.: Factors responsible for the stability of the knee joint. *Bull Hosp Joint Dis* 18:51–59, 1957.
25. Kaplan, E. B.: Some aspects of functional anatomy of the human knee joint: an integral part of the deep capsular layer (layer III). *Clin Orthop Relat Res* 23:18–29, 1962.
26. Kaplan, E. B.: The iliotibial tract. *J Bone Joint Surg* 40A:817–832, 1958.
27. Kim, Y. C.; Yoo, W. K.; Chung, I. H.; et al.: Tendinous insertion of semimembranosus muscle into the lateral meniscus. *Surg Radiol Anat* 19:365–369, 1997.
28. LaPrade, R. F.; Engebretsen, A. H.; Ly, T. V.; et al.: The anatomy of the medial part of the knee. *J Bone Joint Surg Am* 89:2000–2010, 2007.
29. LaPrade, R. F.; Morgan, P. M.; Wentorf, F. A.; et al.: The anatomy of the posterior aspect of the knee. An anatomic study. *J Bone Joint Surg Am* 89:758–764, 2007.
30. Last, R. J.: Some anatomical details of the knee joint. *J Bone Joint Surg Br* 30:683–688, 1948.
31. Lieb, F. J.; Perry, J.: Quadriceps function. An anatomical and mechanical study using amputated limbs. *J Bone Joint Surg* 50A:1535–1548, 1968.
32. Loredo, R.; Hodler, J.; Pedowitz, R.; et al.: Posteromedial corner of the knee: MR imaging with gross anatomic correlation. *Skeletal Radiol* 28:305–311, 1999.
33. Moore, K. L.; Dalley, A. F.: Clinically oriented anatomy. In: *Lower Limb.* New York: Williams & Wilkins, 1999; pp. 503–663.
34. Muller, W. (ed): *The Knee: Form, Function and Ligament Reconstruction.* New York: Springer-Verlag, 1983.
35. Reider, B.; Marshall, J. L.; Koslin, B.; et al.: The anterior aspect of the knee joint. An anatomical study. *J Bone Joint Surg* 63A:351–356, 1981.
36. Robinson, J. R.; Sanchez-Ballester, J.; Bull, A. M.; et al.: The posteromedial corner revisited. An anatomical description of the passive restraining structures of the medial aspect of the human knee. *J Bone Joint Surg Br* 86:674–681, 2004.
37. Sims, W. F.; Jacobson, K. E.: The posteromedial corner of the knee: medial-sided injury patterns revisited. *Am J Sports Med* 32:337–345, 2004.
38. Smirk, C.; Morris, H.: The anatomy and reconstruction of the medial patellofemoral ligament. *Knee* 10:221–227, 2003.
39. Standring, S. (ed): *Gray's Anatomy: The Anatomical Basis of Clinical Practice.* 39th ed. New York: Churchill Livingstone, 2005.
40. Steensen, R. N.; Dopirak, R. M.; McDonald, W. G., 3rd: The anatomy and isometry of the medial patellofemoral ligament: implications for reconstruction. *Am J Sports Med* 32:1509–1513, 2004.
41. Sullivan, D.; Levy, I. M.; Sheskier, S.; et al.: Medial restraints to anterior-posterior motion of the knee. *J Bone Joint Surg* 66A:930–936, 1984.
42. Tang, G.; Niitsu, M.; Ikeda, K.; et al.: Fibrous scar in the infrapatellar fat pad after arthroscopy: MR imaging. *Radiat Med* 18:1–5, 2000.
43. Terry, G. C.; Hughston, J. C.; Norwood, L. A.: The anatomy of the iliopatellar band and iliotibial tract. *Am J Sports Med* 14:39–45, 1986.
44. Thompson, J. C. (ed): *Netter's Concise Atlas of Orthopaedic Anatomy.* Teterboro, NJ: Icon Learning Systems, 2002.
45. Vieira, E. L.; Vieira, E. A.; da Silva, R. T.; et al.: An anatomic study of the iliotibial tract. *Arthroscopy* 23:269–274, 2007.
46. Warren, L. F.; Marshall, J. L.: The supporting structures and layers on the medial side of the knee: an anatomical analysis. *J Bone Joint Surg Am* 61:56–62, 1979.
47. Wiberg, G.: Roentgenographic and anatomic studies on the femoropatella joint. *Acta Orthop Scand* 12:319–410, 1941.
48. Yoshiya, S.; Kuroda, R.; Mizuno, K.; et al.: Medial collateral ligament reconstruction using autogenous hamstring tendons: technique and results in initial cases. *Am J Sports Med* 33:1380–1385, 2005.

Chapter 2

Lateral, Posterior, and Cruciate Knee Anatomy

Justin P. Strickland, MD ■ *Eric W. Fester*, MD ■ *Frank R. Noyes*, MD

INTRODUCTION

The posterior and lateral anatomy of the knee joint presents a challenge to even the most experienced knee surgeon. Knowledge of the bony topography will result in a greater number of anatomic ligament reconstructions (Fig. 2–1). A lack of familiarity leads to hesitancy when performing approaches in these areas of the knee. The inherent anatomic complexity of this region is further complicated by variations in terminology found in the orthopaedic literature. Work by LaPrade and coworkers[23,24,26] and others have attempted to clarify the nomenclature used to describe these structures, allowing for better communication among surgeons. These advances also facilitate more accurate biomechanical studies.

In posterolateral reconstructive procedures, the anatomic relationships of the fibular collateral ligament (FCL), popliteus muscle-tendon-ligament complex (PMTL), popliteofibular ligament (PFL), and the posterolateral capsule are particularly important. These structures function together to resist lateral joint opening, posterior subluxation of the lateral tibial plateau with tibial rotation, knee hyperextension, and varus recurvatum (see Chapter 20, Function of the Posterior Cruciate Ligament and Posterolateral Ligament Structures).[11,45,47]

The goals of this chapter are to (1) accurately describe all relevant structures and their relationships to one another, (2) provide confidence to the knee surgeon when encountering the posterolateral aspect of the knee, and (3) apply knowledge of these structures to provide a base for safe and efficient surgical approaches to the posterolateral aspect of the knee.

ILIOTIBIAL BAND

The iliotibial band (ITB) is a large fascial expansion that originates on the anterior superior iliac spine, covering the tensor fascia lata muscle proximally and extending along the lateral aspect of the thigh. Distally, the ITB has been divided into three separate layers: superficial, deep, and the capsulo-osseous layer.[50,64] A portion of the superficial layer, called the *iliopatellar band*, extends anteriorly to the lateral aspect of the patella (Fig. 2–2).[62] This band is important for proper patellofemoral tracking by resisting abnormal medial patella translation (medial glide).[23] The majority of the superficial layer continues distally to insert on Gerdy's tubercle. The deep layer connects the medial portion of the superficial layer to the lateral intermuscular septum of the distal femur. The most distal fibers of the deep layer continue to attach to the posterior aspect of the lateral femoral condyle (Fig. 2–3).[64] The capsulo-osseous layer extends more medial and distal to the deep layer to merge with fibers from the short head of the biceps to form the biceps–capsulo-osseous iliotibial tract confluens.[63] The capsulo-osseous layer continues distally, creating a sling posterior to the lateral femoral condyle to attach posterior and proximal to Gerdy's tubercle.

In knee extension, the ITB is anterior to the axis of rotation and helps maintain extension. When the knee is flexed to 90°, the ITB moves posterior to the axis of rotation. The anteroposterior (AP) position of the ITB with knee flexion contributes to the pivot shift phenomena with an anterior cruciate ligament (ACL) rupture.[16] The posterior portion of the ITB tibiofemoral attachment is recreated in the lateral extra-articular ACL reconstruction.[23,50]

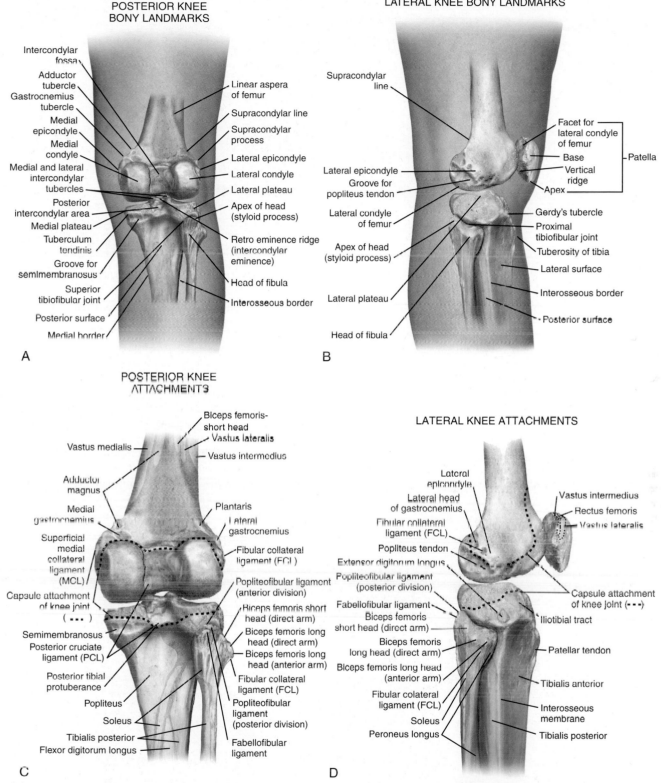

POSTERIOR KNEE
BONY LANDMARKS

Intercondylar fossa
Adductor tubercle
Gastrocnemius tubercle
Medial epicondyle
Medial condyle
Medial and lateral intercondylar tubercles
Posterior intercondylar area
Medial plateau
Tuberculum tendinis
Groove for semimembranosus
Superior tibiofibular joint
Posterior surface
Medial border

Linear aspera of femur
Supracondylar line
Supracondylar process
Lateral epicondyle
Lateral condyle
Lateral plateau
Apex of head (styloid process)
Retro eminence ridge (intercondylar eminence)
Head of fibula
Interosseous border

A

LATERAL KNEE BONY LANDMARKS

Supracondylar line
Lateral epicondyle
Groove for popliteus tendon
Lateral condyle of femur
Apex of head (styloid process)
Lateral plateau
Head of fibula

Facet for lateral condyle of femur
Base
Vertical ridge
Apex
Patella
Gerdy's tubercle
Proximal tibiofibular joint
Tuberosity of tibia
Lateral surface
Interosseous border
Posterior surface

B

POSTERIOR KNEE
ATTACHMENTS

Vastus medialis
Adductor magnus
Medial gastrocnemius
Superficial medial collateral ligament (MCL)
Capsule attachment of knee joint (•••)
Semimembranosus
Posterior cruciate ligament (PCL)
Posterior tibial protuberance
Popliteus
Soleus
Tibialis posterior
Flexor digitorum longus

Biceps femoris-short head
Vastus lateralis
Vastus intermedius
Plantaris
Lateral gastrocnemius
Fibular collateral ligament (FCL)
Popliteofibular ligament (anterior division)
Biceps femoris short head (direct arm)
Biceps femoris long head (direct arm)
Biceps femoris long head (anterior arm)
Fibular collateral ligament (FCL)
Popliteofibular ligament (posterior division)
Fabellofibular ligament

C

LATERAL KNEE ATTACHMENTS

Lateral epicondyle
Lateral head of gastrocnemius
Fibular collateral ligament (FCL)
Popliteus tendon
Extensor digitorum longus
Popliteofibular ligament (posterior division)
Fabellofibular ligament
Biceps femoris short head (direct arm)
Biceps femoris long head (direct arm)
Biceps femoris long head (anterior arm)
Fibular colateral ligament (FCL)
Soleus
Peroneus longus

Vastus intermedius
Rectus femoris
Vastus lateralis
Capsule attachment of knee joint (- - -)
Iliotibial tract
Patellar tendon
Tibialis anterior
Interosseous membrane
Tibialis posterior

D

FIGURE 2–1. A, Bony anatomy of the posterior knee joint. **B,** Bony anatomy of the lateral knee joint. **C,** Key anatomic attachments of the posterior aspect of the knee with the joint capsule outlined. **D,** Key anatomic attachments of the lateral aspect of the knee with the joint capsule outlined.

During flexion, the ITB moves posteriorly, exerting an external rotational and posteriorly directed force on the lateral tibia, contributing to the reduction in the pivot shift test. The ITB and lateral capsule are important structures that resist internal tibia rotation (see Chapter 3, The Scientific Basis for Examination and Classification of Knee Ligament Injuries). In extension, the ITB acts as a secondary restraint to varus stress.[3] In severe lateral knee ligament injuries, the ITB may become abnormally

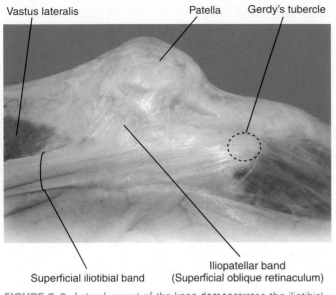

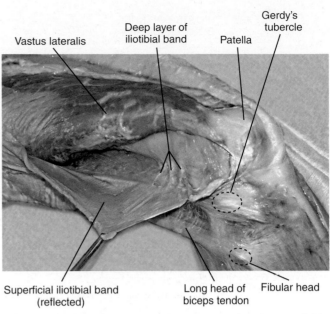

FIGURE 2–2. Lateral aspect of the knee demonstrates the iliotibial band (ITB) with its distal insertion on Gerdy's tubercle and the iliopatellar fibers.

FIGURE 2–3. Deep fibers of the ITB are exposed as the superficial ITB is split and retracted posteriorly.

lengthened, and at the time of surgery, distal advancement at Gerdy's tubercle is indicated. A bursa between the ITB and the lateral femoral epicondylar region may become inflamed and produce pain. The lateral retinacular nerve courses just posterior to the bursa and may also become symptomatic.

FCL

For this chapter, the term *fibular collateral ligament* has been selected instead of lateral collateral ligament because it represents the term most commonly used in anatomy textbooks[23,55] and several studies.[22,26,28,58,68,70] The FCL is a cord-like ligament that runs from the lateral femoral epicondyle to the fibular head (Fig. 2–4). When performing an anatomic FCL reconstruction, it is imperative that the surgeon understands the relationship of the FCL to its surrounding structures. On the femur, the FCL originates approximately 14 mm anterior[26] and slightly distal to the attachment of the lateral gastrocnemius tendon. This tendon is a key landmark during FCL

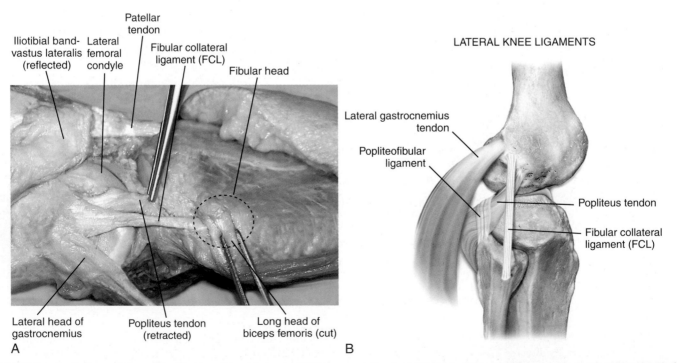

FIGURE 2–4. A, Gross picture of the fibular collateral ligament (FCL) demonstrates its relationship to the popliteus tendon and the lateral head of the gastrocnemius. **B,** The FCL and its relationship to the popliteus tendon and the lateral head of the gastrocnemius.

FIBULAR HEAD ATTACHMENTS

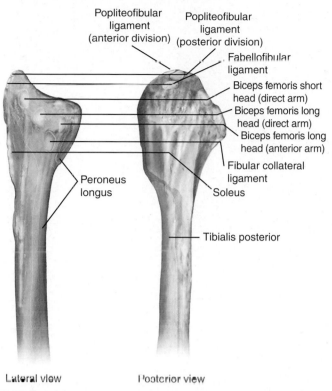

Popliteofibular ligament (anterior division)

Popliteofibular ligament (posterior division)

Fabellofibular ligament

Biceps femoris short head (direct arm)

Biceps femoris long head (direct arm)

Biceps femoris long head (anterior arm)

Fibular collateral ligament

Soleus

Peroneus longus

Tibialis posterior

Lateral view

Posterior view

FIGURE 2–5. Lateral view of the knee demonstrates the FCL insertion onto the proximal fibula distal to the fibular styloid.

reconstruction because it is frequently spared during a posterolateral corner knee injury.[64] In addition, the FCL attaches proximal and posterior to the popliteus femoral insertion. Distally, it attaches to the lateral aspect of the fibular head just medial to the anterior arm of the long head of the biceps tendon.

In 2003, LaPrade and associates[26] published a quantitative anatomic study that described the FCL and its relationship to osseous landmarks and other posterolateral structures of the knee. These authors reported that the FCL does not originate directly off of the lateral epicondyle, but attaches approximately 1.4 mm proximal and 3.1 mm posterior to the epicondyle, residing in a small bony depression. The average distance between the FCL and the popliteus attachments on the femur was 18.5 mm. The ligament travels distally to insert 8.2 mm posterior to the anterior margin of the fibular head and 28.4 mm distal to the tip of the fibular styloid process (Fig. 2–5).[26] The distal 25% of the FCL is surrounded by the FCL–biceps femoris bursa, which has been implicated as a possible source of lateral knee pain.[10] The bursa is covered by the anterior arm of the long head of the biceps.[24]

The FCL is the primary restraint to varus loads at all degrees of flexion.[11] In a cadaveric sectioning study, Grood and colleagues[11] reported that the limit for varus angulation was normal as long as the FCL was intact. In addition, for large changes in external rotation to occur, the popliteus tendon, PFL, posterolateral capsule, and the FCL must all be injured.[67] Thus, the FCL provides significant resistance to external rotation. The FCL is a secondary restraint to internal rotation at higher flexion angles (see Chapter 3, The Scientific Basis for Examination and Classification of Knee Ligament Injuries).

FABELLOFIBULAR LIGAMENT

The fabellofibular ligament begins at the lateral aspect of the fabella (or posterior aspect of the supracondylar process of the lateral femur if a fabella is absent) and inserts distally on the posterolateral edge of the fibular styloid (Fig. 2–6).[4] It attaches posterior and lateral to the insertion of the PFL. Proximally, the fabellofibular ligament is a continuation of the capsular arm of the short head of the biceps tendon.[63,64] The fabellofibular ligament is termed the *short lateral ligament* in the absence of a fabella.[21] Throughout this text, this structure is referred to as the *fabellofibular ligament*. The size of the fabellofibular ligament has been directly correlated to the presence of a bony fabella.[23,36,51] When a bony fabella is present, the ligament is more robust, with the opposite being true when the fabella is cartilaginous or absent.

The fabellofibular ligament has been identified in several studies in a variable percentage of patients.[4,26,51,59,65] Sudasna and Harnsiriwattanagit[60] reported that the fabellofibular ligament was present in 68% percent of individuals. Minowa and coworkers[36] identified a fabellofibular ligament in 51.4% of cadaver knees. Diamantopoulos and associates[4] found the fabellofibular ligament in 40% of knees dissected using microsurgical techniques. In contrast, LaPrade[23] believes that the fabellofibular ligament is present in all knees owing to the fact that, by definition, it is the distal extension of the capsular arm of the short head of the biceps. This was confirmed by a recent article[27] describing these authors' anatomic findings. Functionally, the fabellofibular ligament is taut in extension.[65] Thus, it can be inferred that it provides resistance to knee hyperextension. However, to date, no biomechanical studies have been published that describe the function of the fabellofibular ligament.

FABELLA

The fabella, or "little bean," is a bony or cartilaginous structure nestled in the posterolateral aspect of the knee. It is generally believed to reside in the tendon of the lateral head of the gastrocnemius, however, many structures merge at the fabella (Table 2–1). The fabella ranges in size from approximately 5 mm to over 20 mm in diameter, with the majority (70%) being oval in shape.[36,16] There are varying reports on the incidence of the fabella. Earlier radiographic studies appear to underestimate the true prevalence of the fabella compared with more recent cadaveric and histologic studies (Table 2–2). This structure is present bilaterally in approximately 80% of cases. The fabella has been implicated as a cause of posterior knee pain in multiple conditions including chondromalacia fabella, "fabella syndrome," fracture of the fabella, impingement after total knee arthroplasty, and peroneal nerve irritation.[8,10,29,32,33,49,66] Thus, the fabella and surrounding structures represent a rare but potential source of posterolateral knee pain.

PMTL COMPLEX

The PMTL is an intricate anatomic conglomerate made up of the popliteus muscle, the PFL, the femoral insertion of the popliteus tendon, the popliteomeniscal fascicles and soft tissue attachments to the lateral meniscus, and the proximal tibia. The crucial components for posterolateral stability include the

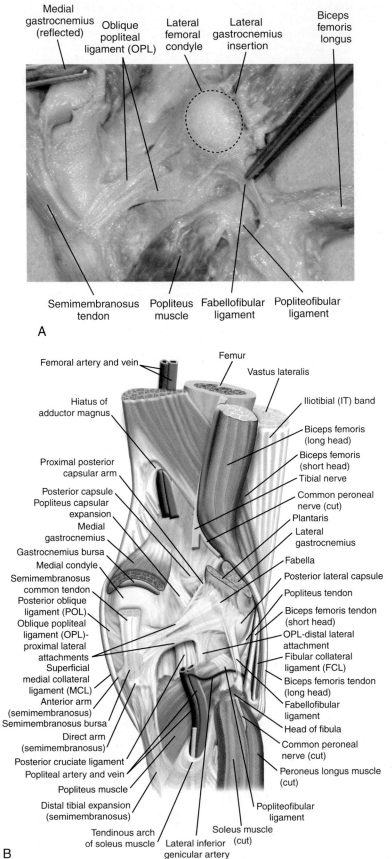

Medial gastrocnemius (reflected)
Oblique popliteal ligament (OPL)
Lateral femoral condyle
Lateral gastrocnemius insertion
Biceps femoris longus

Semimembranosus tendon
Popliteus muscle
Fabellofibular ligament
Popliteofibular ligament

A

Femoral artery and vein
Femur
Vastus lateralis

Hiatus of adductor magnus
Iliotibial (IT) band

Biceps femoris (long head)

Proximal posterior capsular arm
Biceps femoris (short head)
Tibial nerve

Posterior capsule
Popliteus capsular expansion
Common peroneal nerve (cut)

Medial gastrocnemius
Plantaris

Gastrocnemius bursa
Lateral gastrocnemius

Medial condyle
Fabella

Semimembranosus common tendon
Posterior lateral capsule

Posterior oblique ligament (POL)
Popliteus tendon

Oblique popliteal ligament (OPL)- proximal lateral attachments
Biceps femoris tendon (short head)

Superficial medial collateral ligament (MCL)
OPL-distal lateral attachment

Anterior arm (semimembranosus)
Fibular collateral ligament (FCL)

Semimembranosus bursa
Biceps femoris tendon (long head)

Direct arm (semimembranosus)
Fabellofibular ligament

Posterior cruciate ligament
Head of fibula

Popliteal artery and vein
Common peroneal nerve (cut)

Popliteus muscle
Peroneus longus muscle (cut)

Distal tibial expansion (semimembranosus)
Popliteofibular ligament

Tendinous arch of soleus muscle
Lateral inferior genicular artery
Soleus muscle (cut)

B

FIGURE 2–6. **A**, Posterior aspect of the knee with forceps holding the fabellofibular ligament. This ligament originates on the posterior aspect of the lateral femoral condyle and inserts on the fibular head. **B**, The posterior aspect of the knee.

TABLE 2–2   Published Incidence of Fabella

Reference	N	Methodology	Prevalence
Pancoast[46]	529	Radiographs	12.3%
Falk[7a]	1023	Radiographs	12.9%
Sutro[60]	700	Radiographs	11.5%
Pritchett[48a]	600	Radiographs	35% in patients with OA, 15% in patients without OA
Minowa et al.[36]	212	Cadavers/histology	85.8% (74% bony, 26% cartilaginous)
LaPrade et al.[23]	100	Cadavers/histology	100% (38% bony, 62% cartilaginous)

OA, osteoarthritis.

popliteus tendon and the PFL. These structures act in concert with the FCL and posterolateral capsule to prevent excessive external rotation and varus rotation of the knee.[11,45] Restoration of only a portion of these structures may result in residual instability.[42] This is discussed in detail in Chapter 22, Posterolateral Ligament Injuries: Diagnosis, Operative Techniques, and Clinical Outcomes, including the anatomic reconstruction of the FCL, popliteus tendon, and PFL.[38–41]

The popliteus muscle originates on the posterior tibia just proximal to the soleal line and proceeds lateral and proximal to insert on the lateral femoral condyle (see Fig. 2–6B). The popliteus tendon proceeds proximally through a hiatus in the coronary ligament of the lateral meniscus, then deep to the FCL to ultimately insert anterior and distal to the insertion of the FCL (see Fig. 2–4). As referenced earlier, LaPrade and associates[26] reported that the popliteus inserted an average of 18.5 mm from the FCL on the femur. Staubli and Birrer[56] further described the anatomy of the popliteus tendon at the level of the knee joint. Three attachments of the popliteus tendon to the lateral menisci (termed the *popliteomeniscal fascicles*) were noted that include the anteroinferior, posterosuperior, and posteroinferior fascicles (Fig. 2–7). These fascicles provide stability to the lateral meniscus and, when torn, lead to abnormal translation of the lateral meniscus.[25,54] This may lead to mechanical symptoms and lateral knee pain. In Chapter 28, Meniscus Tears: Diagnosis, Repair Techniques, and Clinical Outcomes, the repair techniques for the lateral meniscus and popliteomeniscal fascicles are described.

LaPrade and colleagues[27] described a thickening of the posterior joint capsule that extends from the medial aspect of the popliteus musculotendinous junction to the posteromedial aspect of the intercondylar notch of the femur, termed the *proximal popliteus capsular expansion* (see Fig. 2–6B). The study reported this structure to be present in all dissections, and the authors of this chapter have also found it to be a constant structure. This structure may provide an additional restraint to knee external tibial rotation and hyperextension.

The PFL originates at the musculotendinous junction of the popliteus and attaches to the medial aspect of the fibular head (Fig. 2–8), where it lies deep to the fabellofibular ligament. Of clinical significance, the inferior lateral geniculate artery

POPLITEOMENISCAL FASCICLES

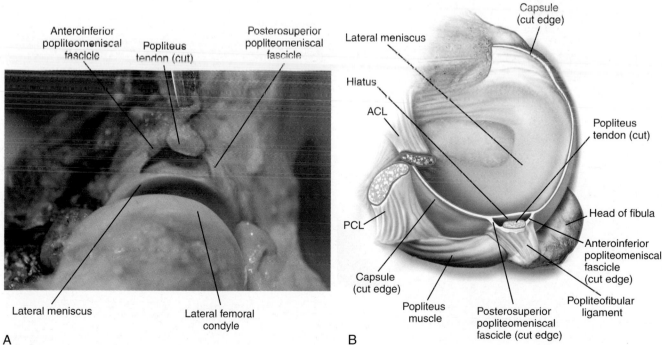

FIGURE 2–7. A, The popliteus tendon is cut at the level of the joint with its surrounding popliteomeniscal fascicles. The posterosuperior fascicle and anteroinferior fascicle secure the popliteus tendon to the lateral meniscus. The lateral femoral condyle is labeled for reference. **B,** The popliteus tendon and its surrounding popliteomeniscal fascicles.

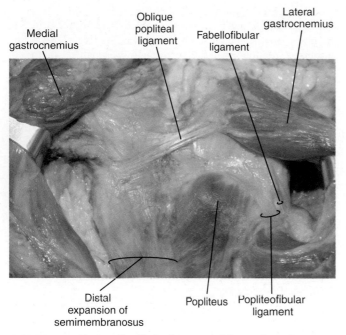

Medial gastrocnemius / Oblique popliteal ligament / Fabellofibular ligament / Lateral gastrocnemius

Distal expansion of semimembranosus / Popliteus / Popliteofibular ligament

FIGURE 2–8. The popliteofibular ligament originates from the popliteus muscle and attaches to the medial aspect of the fibula. The lateral head of the gastrocnemius is being retracted proximally.

courses between these two structures. The artery is frequently encountered during exposure of the posterolateral corner of the knee, especially during the approach for an inside-out lateral meniscus repair (Fig. 2–9). The artery is protected, if possible, and, if injured, requires cauterization to prevent postoperative hematoma formation. The PFL consists of two divisions, an anterior and a posterior division.[26] LaPrade and associates[26] found that the average width of the anterior division's attachment at the fibular styloid was 2.6 mm, and the posterior division's width at the fibular styloid attachment was 5.8 mm. Thus, the posterior division may contribute more significantly than the anterior division to stability of the posterolateral aspect of the knee.

BICEPS FEMORIS

The biceps femoris is a fusiform muscle comprising two heads: long and short. The long head originates from the ischial tuberosity and is innervated by the tibial division of the sciatic nerve. The short head originates from the lateral aspect of the linea aspera of the femur and is innervated by the peroneal division of the sciatic nerve.[50] Distally, the two heads of the biceps lie just posterior to the ITB (Fig. 2–10). Both heads of the biceps have complex attachments to the posterolateral aspect of the knee. These distinct attachments are described and shown in Tables 2–3 and 2–4. In the authors' experience (in cadaveric dissections and at surgery), many of the attachments blend together distally and are difficult to identify as separate structures. The peroneal nerve lies just distal and posterior to the biceps, curving around the fibular neck. The biceps flexes the knee and also externally rotates the leg when the knee is flexed.[51]

There are varying descriptions of the anatomy of the biceps and the number of attachments.[19,20,34,51,63] Terry and LaPrade[63] described five attachments of the long head of the biceps, including two tendinous and three fascial components (Fig. 2–11; see also Table 2–3). The two tendinous components (direct and anterior arms) and one of the fascial components (lateral aponeurotic expansion) make up the key portion of the long head anatomy. The other fascial components are the reflected arm and the anterior aponeurotic expansion.

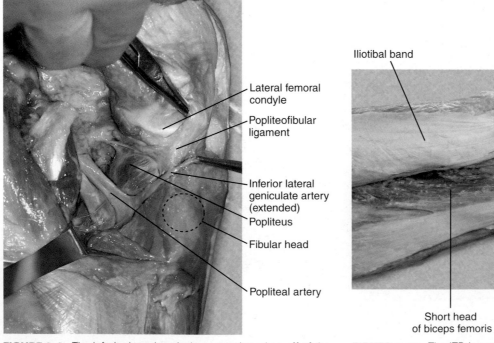

Lateral femoral condyle

Popliteofibular ligament

Inferior lateral geniculate artery (extended)

Popliteus

Fibular head

Popliteal artery

FIGURE 2–9. The inferior lateral geniculate artery branches off of the popliteal artery and runs superficial to the popliteofibular ligament. The fabellofibular ligament has been removed to better demonstrate the inferior lateral geniculate artery.

Iliotibial band / Patella / Fibular head

Short head of biceps femoris / Long head of biceps femoris / Peroneal nerve

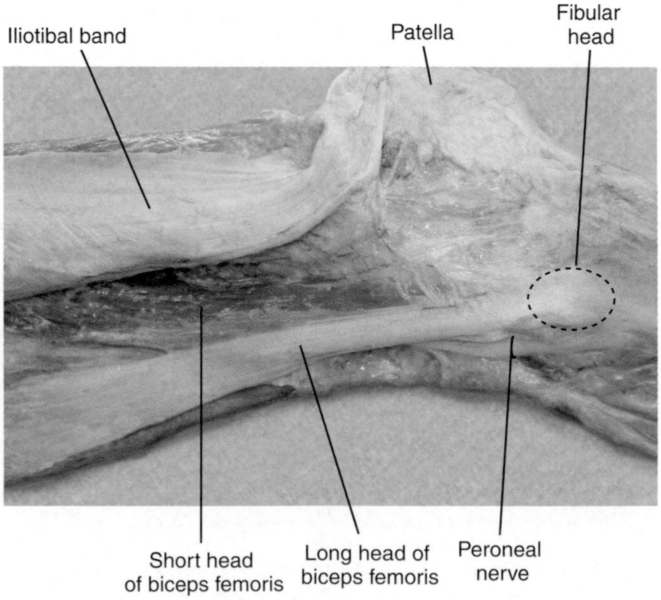

FIGURE 2–10. The ITB is retracted superiorly demonstrating the short head of the biceps attaching to the long head tendon and inserting onto the fibular head. The peroneal nerve is seen posterior to the biceps.

TABLE 2–3 Five Components of the Long Head of the Biceps Femoris

Component	Attachment
Reflected arm	Posterior edge of ITB
Direct arm	Posterolateral edge of the fibula
Anterior arm	Lateral fibular head, FCL, anterior aponeurotic expansion
Lateral aponeurotic expansion	FCL
Anterior aponeurotic expansion	Anterior compartment of the leg

FCL, fibular collateral ligament; ITB, iliotibial band.

TABLE 2–4 Six Components of the Short Head of the Biceps Femoris

Component	Attachment
Proximal muscular attachment	Anteromedial aspect of the long head
Capsular arm	Posterolateral knee capsule
Capsulo-osseus layer	Proximolateral tibia
Direct arm	Fibular head
Anterior arm	Proximolateral tibia
Lateral aponeurotic expansion	FCL

FCL, fibular collateral ligament.

complex attachment and some important anatomic points. A portion of the anterior arm inserts onto the lateral aspect of the fibular head, and the rest continues distally just lateral to the FCL. Just proximal and at this fibular insertion, portions of the anterior arm ascend anteriorly to form the lateral aponeurotic expansion that attaches to the posterior and lateral aspect of the FCL. Here, a small bursa separates the anterior arm from the distal fourth of the FCL. The anterior arm thus forms the lateral wall of this bursa.[63] This is an important surgical landmark because a small horizontal incision can be made here, 1 cm proximal to the fibular head, to enter this bursa and locate the insertion of the FCL into the fibular head (Fig. 2–12).[23] The anterior arm then continues distally over the FCL, forming the anterior aponeurosis, which covers the anterior compartment of the leg.

The short head of the biceps courses just deep (or medial) and anterior to the long head tendon, sending a majority of its proximal muscular fibers to the long head tendon itself.[63] It has six distal attachments (Fig. 2–13; see also Table 2–4). The most important attachments are that of the direct arm, the anterior arm, and the capsular arm.

The capsular arm originates just prior to the short head reaching the fibula. It then continues deep to the FCL to insert onto the posterolateral knee capsule and fabella. Here, the fibers of the capsular arm continue distally as the fabellofibular ligament.[63] Just distal to the capsular arm, a capsulo-osseous layer forms a fascial confluence with the ITB (the biceps–capsulo-osscous–iliotibial tract confluens). The direct arm of the short head inserts onto the fibular head just posterior and proximal to the direct arm of the long head tendon. The anterior arm then continues medial or deep to the FCL, partially blends with the anterior tibiofibular ligament, and inserts onto the tibia 1 cm posterior to Gerdy's tubercle. This site is also the attachment of

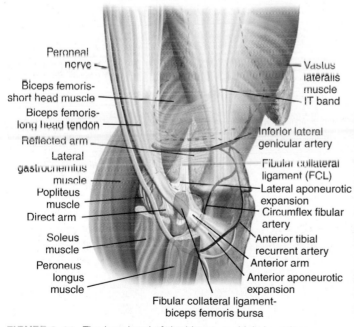

BICEPS FEMORIS LONG HEAD LIGAMENTO

Peroneal nerve
Biceps femoris-short head muscle
Biceps femoris-long head tendon
Reflected arm
Lateral gastrocnemius muscle
Popliteus muscle
Direct arm
Soleus muscle
Peroneus longus muscle
Vastus lateralis muscle
IT band
Inferior lateral genicular artery
Fibular collateral ligament (FCL)
Lateral aponeurotic expansion
Circumflex fibular artery
Anterior tibial recurrent artery
Anterior arm
Anterior aponeurotic expansion
Fibular collateral ligament-biceps femoris bursa

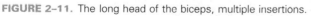

FIGURE 2–11. The long head of the biceps, multiple insertions.

The most proximal component is the reflected arm. It originates just proximal to the fibular head and ascends anteriorly to insert on the posterior edge of the ITB. The direct arm inserts onto the posterolateral edge of the fibula just distal to the tip of the styloid (see Fig. 2–5).[23] The anterior arm has a more

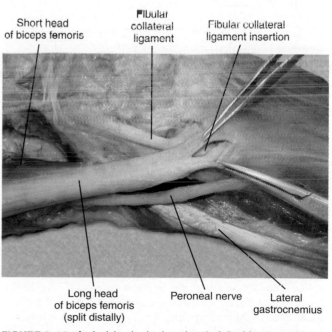

Short head of biceps femoris
Fibular collateral ligament
Fibular collateral ligament insertion
Long head of biceps femoris (split distally)
Peroneal nerve
Lateral gastrocnemius

FIGURE 2–12. An incision in the long head of the biceps tendon reveals the insertion of the FCL as it lies deep to the tendon. The peroneal nerve is in close proximity as it lies superficial to the lateral gastrocnemius.

BICEPS FEMORIS SHORT HEAD LIGAMENTS

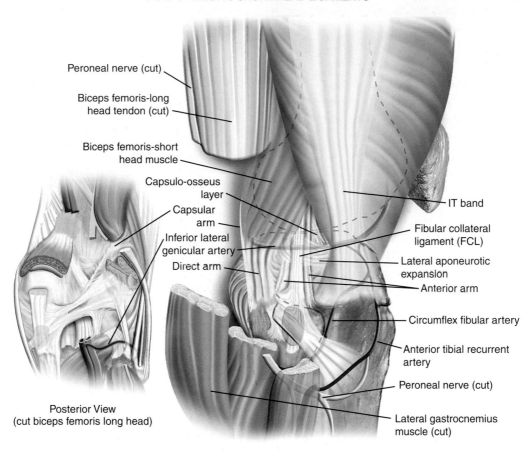

FIGURE 2–13. The insertion of the short head of the biceps tendon.

the mid-third lateral knee capsule.[63] It is important clinically because an avulsion fracture can be seen here in ACL injuries, known as a *Segond fracture*.[52,63] Finally, the lateral aponeurotic expansion of the short head inserts onto the medial aspect of the FCL (versus this expansion of the long head that inserts onto the posterior aspect of the FCL).[63]

THE FIBULAR HEAD

The fibular head is a key anatomic and structural component to the posterolateral knee. It is easily palpable in most patients and is thus an excellent anatomic reference point. In the literature, incomplete descriptions of the anatomy and insertion of structures of the proximal fibula exist. Six key structures attach to the fibular head: three tendons and three ligaments (Table 2–5; see also Fig. 2–5). The PFL attaches to the tip of the fibular styloid. Just distal and lateral, the fabellofibular ligament attaches on the slope of the styloid. The FCL, as mentioned previously, attaches proximally 28 mm distal to the styloid and 8 mm from the anterior cortex of the fibula, depending of course on specimen size variations.[26] A portion of the anterior arm of the long head of the biceps attaches to the lateral aspect of the fibular head. The direct arms of the long and short heads of the biceps attach to the posterior aspect of the fibular head, the long head being just lateral to that of the short head.

TABLE 2–5	Key Structures That Attach to the Fibular Head
Structure	**Location on Fibular Head**
LH biceps, direct arm	Posterolateral edge (lateral and distal to the styloid)
LH biceps, anterior arm	Posterolateral edge (slightly distal and lateral to the direct arm of the LH)
SH biceps, direct arm	Posterior edge (lateral to the styloid, medial to the direct arm of the LH)
Popliteofibular ligament	Medial aspect of the styloid
Fibular collateral ligament	Anterolateral edge (28 mm distal to the styloid, 8 mm posterior to the anterior edge of the fibula)
Fabellofibular ligament	Lateral to the tip of the styloid

LH, long head; SH, short head.

THE KNEE CAPSULE

The knee capsule envelopes the joint, extending from the articular margin of the femur to the tibia (see Fig. 2–1C and D). On the tibia, it inserts 4 to 14 mm below the articular surface. The most distal attachment at the tibia is located at the posteromedial and posterolateral aspect.[2] Some authors[50] have identified a thickening of the capsule laterally, naming this the *mid-third*

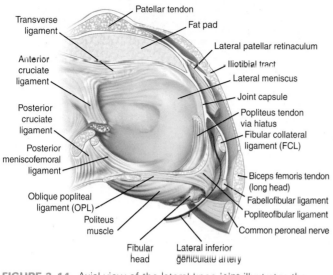

FIGURE 2–14. Axial view of the lateral knee joint illustrates the trilaminar relationship of the various posterolateral structures.

lateral capsular ligament. This ligament is divided into two components. The meniscofemoral component and meniscotibial component extend from the femur and tibia, respectively, to attach to the lateral meniscus.[50] The lateral retinacular nerve, a branch of the sciatic nerve, courses along the surface of the lateral capsule (Fig. 2–14).

ACL

The ACL (Figs. 2–15 and 2–16) is the primary restraint to anterior translation of the tibia at all degrees of flexion.[44] It also limits coupled internal rotation and anterior translation of the tibia, measured by the pivot shift and/or flexion-rotation drawer tests.[43,44] Various descriptions, nomenclature, and anatomic reference points of the ACL are present in the literature. Early descriptions date back to the 1800s.[69] Since then, numerous studies describing ACL anatomy have been published (Table 2–6). The average length of the ACL is 38 mm, and the average width is 11 mm. The ACL has a larger attachment site than its central dimensions. Although some authors describe a separate anteromedial and posterolateral bundle, the authors of this chapter do not believe an anatomic separation exists. Some authors such as Edwards and coworkers[5,6] (see Table 2–6) divide the ACL into two functional bundles. However, as discussed in Chapter 7, Anterior Cruciate Ligament Primary and Revision Reconstruction: Diagnosis, Operative Techniques, and Clinical Outcomes, this represents an oversimplification of fiber function. The ACL, like the posterior cruciate ligament (PCL), is a continuum of fibers of different lengths and attachment characteristics.

The ACL originates on the medial aspect of the lateral femoral condyle (Figs. 2–17 and 2–18). The origin has been described as an oval or a semicircle, approximately 18 mm long and 10 mm wide, lying just behind a bony ridge known as *resident's ridge*.[17] It is anterior to the posterior cartilage of the lateral femoral condyle (Fig. 2–19A). Multiple referencing systems have been used to describe the ACL femoral attachment including clock systems, quadrant or grid systems, and measurements based on the posterior articular cartilage (see Chapter 7, Anterior Cruciate Ligament Primary and Revision Reconstruction: Diagnosis, Operative Techniques, and Clinical Outcomes).

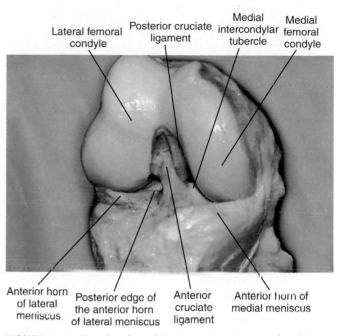

FIGURE 2–15. Anterior view of the knee demonstrates the oblique orientation of the anterior cruciate ligament (ACL) originating on the sidewall of the lateral femoral condyle.

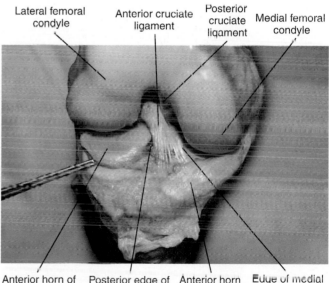

FIGURE 2–16. Anterosuperior view of the knee demonstrates the ACL tibial insertion.

The ACL inserts onto the tibia in the anterior intercondylar area (AIA) in a roughly oval to triangular pattern. The insertion fans out, especially anteriorly, at the tibial insertion and has been described as a "duck's foot" (see Fig. 2–19B).[48] The AP dimension of the insertion is approximately 18 mm, and the mediolateral dimension is 10 mm. The anterior border of the ACL is approximately 22 mm from the anterior cortex of the tibia and 15 mm from the anterior edge of the articular surface. Its center is approximately 15 to 18 mm anterior to the retroeminence

TABLE 2–6　ACL Anatomy Investigations

Reference	N	Methods of Evaluation	Tibial Insertion	Femoral Insertion	Bundle Separation Techniques	Anteromedial Bundle Characteristics	Posterolateral Bundle Characteristics	Anatomic References	Conclusions
Edwards et al.[6]	22	Photographic computer analysis		Attachment for both bundles is 14 mm long, 7 mm wide	Separated bluntly by different tensioning patterns during ROM	Extends to posteroproximal limit of the femoral notch, 10:00–11:30, 4.3 mm from posterior edge of notch	9:00–10:30, 8.9 mm from posterior edge of notch		For double-bundle reconstruction, place AMB at 11:00 and 5 mm in, PLB at 10:00 and 9 mm in
Siebold et al.[53a]	50	Photographic computer analysis	Average footprint of 114 mm² (range, 67–259), in AIA		Separated with a probe based on fiber orientation	Tibial footprint of 67 mm², 5 mm posterior to anterior border of native ACL	Tibial footprint of 52 mm², 6 mm posterior to anterior border of native ACL, 5 mm anterior to posterior horn of lateral meniscus	Medial border of AMB is on anteromedial rim of medial tibial condyle, lateral border of PLB is on anterolateral rim of lateral tibial condyle	Large variability, AMB and PLB insertions cannot be exactly anatomically reconstructed; use native landmarks of the patient
Luites et al.[30a]	35	Gross, 3-D electromagnetic tracking system	Medial part of AIA, 229 mm²	Medial surface of the lateral wall, 184 mm²	Separated bluntly by different tensioning patterns during ROM with anterior load applied at 90°	7.2 mm from posterior edge of femoral notch with 81 mm² surface area; on tibia inserted medially along cartilage edge of medial tibial condyle, 136 mm²	8.8 mm from posterior edge of notch, "about half of the notch height," 103 mm² surface area; on tibia bounded by anterior horn of lateral meniscus, 93 mm²		Use arthroscopic landmarks for anatomic reconstruction (notch height and depth on femoral side; anterior horn of lateral meniscus and cartilage edge of condyles on tibial side)
Heming et al.[15a]	12	Gross	18.5 mm long and 10.3 mm wide, center of insertion is 15 mm from tibial notch of PCL, medial border is 1.9 mm from medial plateau articular cartilage	18.4 mm long and 9.5 mm wide, posterior border 4 mm from cartilage border of notch, 10:14–11:23	Not done			PCL, articular cartilage border of medial tibial plateau	Transtibial drilling methods miss central footprints and produce vertical grafts, drill femoral tunnel through anteromedial portal or use two-incision technique

Study	n	Method	Dimensions / Center Location	Separation			Landmarks	Comments
Ferretti et al.[7b]	7,60, 15	Histologic in 7 fetuses, arthroscopic in 60 ACL reconstruction cases, gross and 3-D laser photography for 16 cadavers	17.2 mm long and 9.9 mm wide (~96.8 mm²)	Separated bluntly by different tensioning patterns during ROM	120 mm² footprint on femoral side	7-8 mm² footprint on femoral side	Lateral bifurcate bridge between femoral attachments of the AMB and PLB, ACL femoral insertion posterior to lateral intercondylar ridge	"Resident's ridge" should be called lateral intercondylar ridge, use anteromedial portal to view femoral insertion, AMB and PLB separated by bony bridge
Edwards et al.[5]	55	Photographic computer analysis	18 mm long and 9 mm wide, center was 15 mm anterior to over-the-back ridge and 5 mm lateral from medial tibial spine	Separated bluntly by different tensioning patterns during ROM	17 mm anterior to over-the-back ridge, 5 mm lateral to medial tibial spine	10 mm anterior to over-the-back ridge, 4 mm lateral to medial tibial spine	Over-the-back interspinous ridge just anterior to PCL attachment (a.k.a. the RER), lateral border of medial tibial spine	Use over-the-back ridge and medial tibial spine as landmarks for anatomic ACL tibial placement
Colombet et al.[1a]	7	Gross and radiographic	17.5 mm long and 12.7 mm wide	Separated bluntly by different tensioning patterns during ROM	Tibia: 17.5 mm anterior to RER Femur: proximal and anterior in femoral notch extending up to over-the-top position	Tibia: 8.4 mm posterior to center of AMB Femur: adjacent to AMB, "skirting" articular surface	AMB at 36% on Amis and Jakob's line, PLB at 52%; RER is curved just anterior to tibial attachment of PCL	Can use intraoperative fluoroscopy and postoperative radiographs to evaluate tunnel placement, do not rely on PCL for ACL tibial placement (will place graft too posterior)—use RER
Takahashi et al.[61a]	32	Photographic computer analysis and radiographic		Bluntly with forceps	Tibia: 29% of distance from anterior to posterior cartilage surface, 44% of distance medial to lateral, 67 mm² Femur 7.6 mm anterior to cartilage of lateral femoral condyle, 4.1 mm from roof of notch, 67 mm²	Tibia: 32% of distance from anterior to posterior cartilage surface, 52% of distance medial to lateral, 52 mm² Femur: 7 mm anterior to cartilage of lateral femoral condyle, 11.2 mm from roof of notch, 56 mm²	Tibial center of ACL is 32% from anterior margin of articular surface, 48% from anterior cortex	Can use lateral radiograph to evaluate tunnel placement

Continued

TABLE 2–6   ACL Anatomy Investigations—Cont'd

Reference	N	Methods of Evaluation	Tibial Insertion	Femoral Insertion	Bundle Separation Techniques	Anteromedial Bundle Characteristics	Posterolateral Bundle Characteristics	Anatomic References	Conclusions
Harner et al.[14]	5,10	Laser micrometer	Oval, 136 mm², 3.5 x larger than mid-substance of ligament	Circular, 113 mm², 3.5 x larger than mid-substance of ligament	Separated bluntly by different tensioning patterns during ROM	Tibia: anteromedial to PLB Femur: proximal (or deep) to PLB	Tibia: posterolateral to AMB Femur: distal (or shallow) to AMB		Separate bundles less distinct than PCL, functional division, large insertional footprints
Staubli and Rauschning[57]	10, 35	Gross and microcryosectional (10), MRI (35)	21.2 mm from anterior tibial margin (41%–44% of width)		Not done			Percentage of tibial width on MRI for ACL center	Place ACL graft in center of ACL footprint at 41%–44% of tibial width, parallel to inclination angle of notch
Girgis et al.[9]	44	Gross, calipers	Wide area adjacent to medial articular surface and attached to anterior horn of lateral meniscus, starts 15 mm in from anterior articular edge	Semicircle, 23 mm long, starts 4 mm in from posterior of notch and 1 mm in from roof of notch, weaker than tibial insertion	Not done			Tibial insertion just anterior and lateral to medial intercondylar tubercle, well-marked slip to anterior horn of lateral meniscus	Differential tensioning of areas of native ACL during ROM, average length and width of 38 mm and 11 mm

ACL, anterior cruciate ligament; AIA, anterior intercondylar area; AMB, anteromedial bundle; MRI, magnetic resonance imaging; PCL, posterior cruciate ligament; PLB, posterolateral bundle; RER, retroeminence ridge; ROM, range of motion; 3-D, three-dimensional.

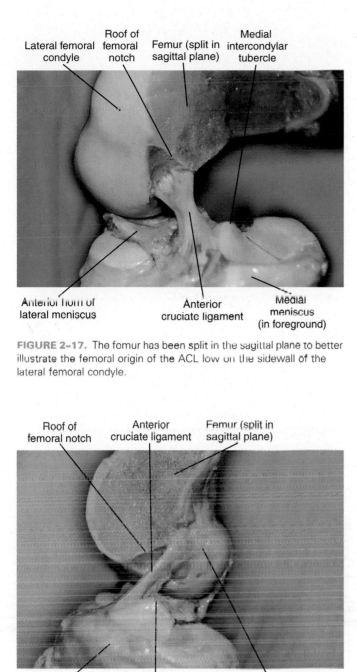

FIGURE 2-17. The femur has been split in the sagittal plane to better illustrate the femoral origin of the ACL low on the sidewall of the lateral femoral condyle.

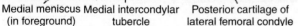

FIGURE 2-18. The femoral origin of the ACL pictured from a lateral perspective. The posterior fibers, and thus the posterolateral bundle origin, are not well visualized.

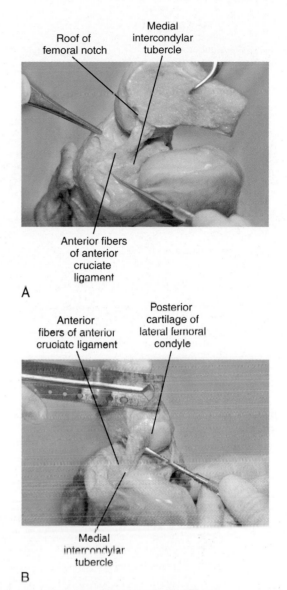

FIGURE 2-19. Lateral view of the ACL. **A**, Note the distance from the posterior cartilage of the lateral femoral condyle to the ACL. **B**, The same specimen is in 90° of flexion. The anterior extension of the tibial insertion of the ACL is well visualized.

ridge (RER) (Fig. 2-20). Edwards and coworkers[5] described the RER (a.k.a. the over-the-back interspinous ridge) as a transverse ridge on the apex of the posterior slope of the tibial plateau, just anterior to the PCL. Different terms are used for the bony topography of the proximal tibia (Fig. 2-21). The term retroeminence ridge is referred to as the *intercondylar eminence* in gross anatomy texts.[1,55] The medial and lateral tibial spines are referred to as the *medial* and *lateral intercondylar tubercles*.[1] The ACL insertion is just lateral to the tip of the medial intercondylar tubercle, and therefore, it inserts not on the tip of the medial intercondylar tubercle, but on the lateral slope. The anterior horn of the lateral

meniscus is a useful landmark during an arthroscopic ACL reconstruction. Over 50% of the ACL inserts anterior to the posterior edge of the anterior horn of the lateral meniscus (Fig. 2-22). Using radiography and magnetic resonance imaging (MRI), Staubli and Rauschning[57] showed that the center of the insertion is 44% of the width from anterior to posterior of the proximal tibia. For ACL reconstruction, we recommend placing the graft at the tibial and femoral attachment sites, as discussed in Chapter 7, Anterior Cruciate Ligament Primary and Revision Reconstruction: Diagnosis, Operative Techniques, and Clinical Outcomes.

PCL

The PCL is the primary restraint to posterior translation of the tibia at all degrees of flexion. Numerous studies describing PCL anatomy have been published (Table 2-7). Various descriptions, nomenclature, and anatomic reference points are present in the

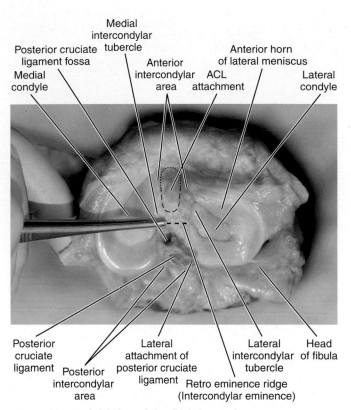

Medial intercondylar tubercle
Posterior cruciate ligament fossa
Medial condyle
Anterior intercondylar area
ACL attachment
Anterior horn of lateral meniscus
Lateral condyle

Posterior cruciate ligament
Posterior intercondylar area
Lateral attachment of posterior cruciate ligament
Retro eminence ridge (Intercondylar eminence)
Lateral intercondylar tubercle
Head of fibula

FIGURE 2–20. Axial view of the tibial plateau demonstrates the anterior insertion of the ACL. Notice the ACL's tibial insertion in relation to the medial tibial spine and the retroeminence ridge.

TIBIAL PLATEAU BONY LANDMARKS

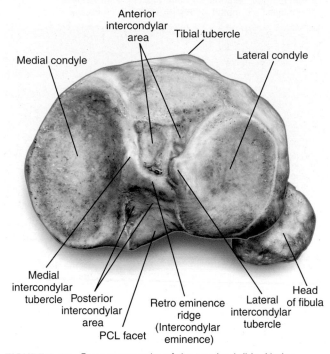

Medial condyle
Anterior intercondylar area
Tibial tubercle
Lateral condyle

Medial intercondylar tubercle
Posterior intercondylar area
PCL facet
Retro eminence ridge (Intercondylar eminence)
Lateral intercondylar tubercle
Head of fibula

FIGURE 2–21. Bony topography of the proximal tibia. Notice the relative posterior position of the intercondylar eminence and the trapezoidal shape of the posterior cruciate ligament (PCL) fossa.

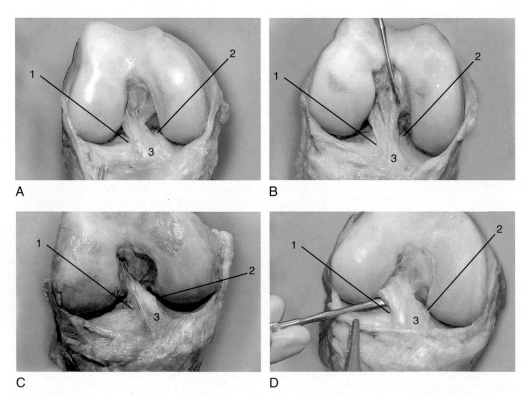

A

B

C

D

FIGURE 2–22. A–D, Anterosuperior views of a series of four knees show that greater than 50% of the ACL (3) inserts anterior to the posterior edge of the anterior horn of the lateral meniscus (1). Medial intercondylar tubercle (2). Note in **B** that arbitrary clefts can sometimes be seen in the ACL, not seen in **A, C,** and **D. D,** The transverse ligament connecting the anterior horns of the medial and lateral menisci is shown.

TABLE 2–7 PCL Anatomy Investigations

Reference	N	Methods of Evaluation	Tibial Insertion	Femoral Insertion	Bundle Separation Techniques	Anterolateral Bundle Characteristics	Posteromedial Bundle Characteristics	Anatomic References	Conclusions
Moorman et al.[37a]	14	Gross, histologic, radiographic	Posterior half of PCL facet. Mean AP dimension of 15.6 mm					Center of tibial insertion 7 mm anterior to posterior cortex of PCL facet	PCL facet is a consistent, radiographically recognizable landmark to identify PCL tibial insertion
Lopes et al.[30]	20	Gross, 3-D laser photography		Average area of footprint 209 mm². Shortest distance from articular edge to center of ALB is 7 mm, to PMB is 8 mm	Separated bluntly by different tensioning patterns during ROM. Distance between centers femoral attachments of bundles is 11 mm	Femoral footprint area 118 mm²	Femoral footprint area 90 mm²	Medial intercondylar ridge proximal to PCL attachment in 18 of 20 knees. Medial bifurcate ridge in 8 of 20 knees that separate PMB and ALB	Osseous landmarks may be used as a guide for anatomic femoral tunnel placement during PCL reconstructions
Edwards et al.[7]	39	Photographic computer analysis	ALB covered entire "posterior intercondylar fossa". PMB was distal and lateral to ALB. No anatomic separation of bundles	Maximal AP length was 22 mm. Center of ALB to articular edge is 7 mm, center of PMB to articular edge is 10 mm when parallel to femoral long axis	Separated bluntly by different tensioning patterns during ROM	Tibial insertion AP length 8 mm, width 9 mm. Center of femoral insertion 10:20 when parallel to femoral long axis	Tibial insertion AP length 6 mm, width 10 mm. Center of femoral insertion 8:30 when parallel to femoral long axis		Accurate knowledge of bundles of the PCL is essential to develop successful reconstruction techniques
Takahashi et al.[61]	32 femur 33 tibia	Photographic computer analysis	Distance from articular plane to center of PMB is 4.6 mm. Center of ALB is on or very close to articular plane	ALB is 9.6 mm from anterior articular surface and 4.8 mm from notch. PMB is 10.6 mm from anterior articular surface and 11.4 mm from notch	No mention of separation techniques	Femoral area of insertion is 58 mm². Tibial area of insertion is 46.7 mm²	Femoral area of insertion is 64.6 mm². Tibial area of insertion is 115.8 mm²		Better understanding of anatomy will lead to better outcomes in PCL reconstruction

Continued

TABLE 2-7   PCL Anatomy Investigations—Cont'd

Reference	N	Methods of Evaluation	Tibial Insertion	Femoral Insertion	Bundle Separation Techniques	Anterolateral Bundle Characteristics	Posteromedial Bundle Characteristics	Anatomic References	Conclusions
Sheps et al.[53]	10	Gross	Trapezoidal insertion with medial length 128 mm, lateral 160 mm, superior side 107 mm, and inferior side 169 mm		Two independent bundles could not be identified Grossly visualized different tensioning patterns with knee ROM	Inserts at superior and lateral aspect of PCL fossa	Inserts at inferior and medial aspect of fossa	Medial and lateral walls of PCL fossa ~5 mm deep Palpable ridge present at inferior extent of PCL fossa Four corners of tibial insertion were palpable with probe from back and front of knee	These reference points could potentially aid in placement of an anterolateral and posteromedial tibial tunnel for a two-tibial tunnel PCL reconstruction
Mejia et al.[35]	12	Gross with use of solder wire and photographic record	AP diameter averaged 14 mm and mediolateral averaged 14.4 mm	Extends past midline in the notch to 11:21 position Originates from 11:30 to 4:00 o'clock position Can be divided into anterior, middle, and posterior portions Bulk of PCL found in middle portion	Continuous fan-shaped appearance, not possible to discern discreet fiber bundle geometry			Described four different methods to describe PCL femoral attachment Most accurate representation achieved when lines perpendicular to cartilage surface and parallel to femoral shaft were used Location of center of clock face should be identified with knee at 90° of flexion	More than one reference system needed to accurately describe femoral origin of PCL
Makris et al.[31]	24	Microsurgical dissection with operative microscope	AP diameter averaged 31 mm, proximodistal diameter averaged 11 mm from anterior and central part and 6 mm from posterior part		No artificial separation of bundles Four partially separated fiber regions: anterior, central, posterolongitudinal, and posterooblique	Anterior and central fibers make up bulk of ligament Anterior fibers are most nonisometric and tensioned at 30° to 90° of flexion	Posterior fibers only make up 15% of PCL but were most isometric and remained in tension in extension and deep flexion	Average length of PCL 38 mm AP diameter at midsection is 5 mm, mediolateral is 14 mm	Four partially separated fiber regions identified but functionally distinct Findings during arthroscopic examination of the PCL may aid in decision making

Study	No.	Technique	Cross-sectional area		Bundle determination	Insertion finding 1	Insertion finding 2	Additional findings	Conclusions
Harner et al.[14]	5 measured mid-substance, 10 insertional	Laser micrometer, digitization of insertion	Average area was 153 mm² ALB and PMB separated as per their names	Average area was 128 mm² ALB and EMB separated with line running from proximal to distal	Separated based on tensioning patterns throughout ROM of knee	53% of tibial insertion, 52% of femoral insertion. Average tibial area insertion is 70 mm², femoral area insertion is 74 mm²	47% of tibial insertion, 48% of femoral insertion. Average tibial area insertion is 62 mm², femoral area insertion is 69 mm²		Can be functionally separated into two components with distinct insertions. Insertions are significantly larger than mid-substance
Morgan et al.[37b]	20 (in vivo during TKA)	Gross, calipers			No mention of how bundles were determined.	Originated 13 mm posterior to cartilage-wall interface and 13 mm inferior to cartilage-roof interface	Originated 8 mm posterior to cartilage-wall interface and 20 mm inferior to cartilage-roof interface	PCL insertions three times larger than mid-substance area. Tibial insertion is 117% of ACL tibial insertion. Femoral insertion is 121% of ACL femoral insertion	Reconstruction that reconstructs both major bands of PCL utilizes three tunnels: one tibial and two femoral defined by reference points in this study
Harner et al.[15]	8	Laser micrometer			No mention of bundles		PCL is widest in its mediolateral direction. Cross-sectional area increased from tibia to femur. Cross-sectional area 50% larger than ACL proximally, 20% larger distally		In situ geometry of ligament should be useful in modeling of human knee. Knowledge of PCL shape and size may aid in graft selection during reconstruction

ACL, anterior cruciate ligament; ALB, anterolateral bundle; AP, anteroposterior; PCL, posterior cruciate ligament; PMB, posteromedial bundle; ROM, range of motion; 3-D, three-dimensional; TKA, total knee arthroplasty.

literature. One of the first anatomic studies was conducted in 1975 by Girgis and associates.[9] Earlier studies focused on femoral and tibial attachment sites as well as cross-sectional area and length of the PCL. The PCL is a large ligament with fan-shaped insertion sites. The average length of the PCL is 38 mm, and the average width is 13 mm.[9] The insertion sites are three times the cross-sectional area than its mid-substance area.[14] The PCL's insertion sites are larger than the corresponding insertion sites of the ACL.[15]

With the advent of the two-bundle description of PCL anatomy, more recent studies have attempted to arbitrarily separate two functional bundles based on differing tensioning patterns throughout the range of motion of the knee.[7,14,30,61] However, some studies have been unable to identify discreet geometric bundles.[31,35,53] These descriptions have focused on separate anterolateral (AL) and posteromedial (PM) bundles in hopes to more accurately reconstruct the PCL; however, the authors of this chapter believe that the two-bundle representation of the PCL oversimplifies PCL fiber function. The PCL is a continuum of fibers of different lengths and attachment characteristics that are more accurately described in Chapter 20, Function of the Posterior Cruciate and Posterolateral Ligament Structures. Inconsistency in the size and description of the two bundles exists in the literature owing to the fact that these are not distinct anatomic structures. The bundle nomenclature is used to reference other publications that have used this terminology.

The PCL inserts on the tibia up to 1 cm distal to the posterior articular cartilage surface in the midportion of the tibia in the coronal plane (Figs. 2–23 and 2–24). Its insertion is rectangular or trapezoidal. One published study[37] described the PCL attaching to the "PCL facet" of the posterior proximal tibia. This insertion area has also been termed the *posterior intercondylar fossa* or the *PCL fossa*.[7] The AP dimension of the tibial insertion is approximately 15 mm (14–16 mm) in length. The mediolateral dimension is approximately 10 to 16 mm in width.

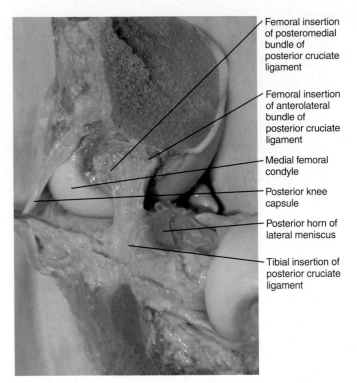

FIGURE 2–24. Posterior oblique view of the knee demonstrates how some fibers of the PCL coalesce with the posterior horn of the lateral meniscus.

The inferior base is wider, contributing to its trapezoidal shape. The center of the PCL tibial attachment lies 7 mm anterior to the posterior cortex of the PCL fossa. Sheps and colleagues[53] described palpable landmarks of the four corners of the PCL fossa as well as a ridge present at the inferior extent of the tibial insertion. Harner and coworkers[14] believe that the AL and PM bundles contribute equally to the tibial insertion area of the PCL. However, Takahashi and associates[61] found the majority of the tibial insertion to be made up of the PM bundle (115.8 mm² vs. 46.7 mm²). The medial meniscal root lies anterior and along the medial aspect of the PCL fossa and must be protected during PCL reconstruction.[18] The capsule attachment at the distal aspect of the PCL fossa (see Fig. 2–1C) is an important anatomic landmark because PCL graft reconstructions are placed at the most distal aspect of the fossa. Through dissections, the authors of this chapter have noted a coalescence of fibers with the posterior horn of the lateral meniscus that is distinct from the meniscofemoral ligaments (MFLs).

The femoral insertion of the PCL is highly variable. It attaches to the medial intercondylar wall in a half-moon– or bullet-shaped fashion (Figs. 2–25 to 2–27). Multiple reference points have been used to describe this insertion, including clock positions perpendicular to the cartilage surface, clock measurements parallel to the femoral shaft, clock measurements parallel to the intercondylar roof, and radial measurements from the intercondylar roof.[7,35] More than one measurement should be used to describe the PCL femoral insertion accurately.[35] Edwards and colleagues[7] used a grid measurement scale to describe the femoral attachment. The area of femoral insertion varies widely from approximately 125 mm² to over 200 mm².[14,30] The AL bundle attaches "higher" onto the wall with a portion of its fibers crossing the midline. Edwards and colleagues[7] found the

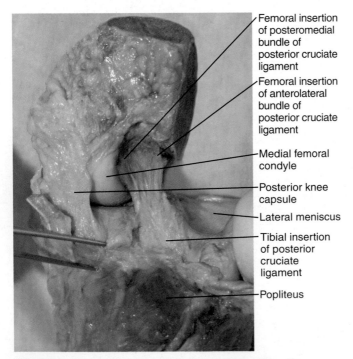

FIGURE 2–23. Posterior view of the knee demonstrates the trapezoidal insertion of the PCL attachment to the tibial plateau.

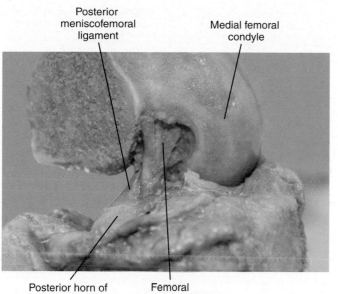

FIGURE 2–25. View of the medial femoral condyle demonstrates the smaller posteromedial bundle of the PCL compared with the larger anterolateral bundle.

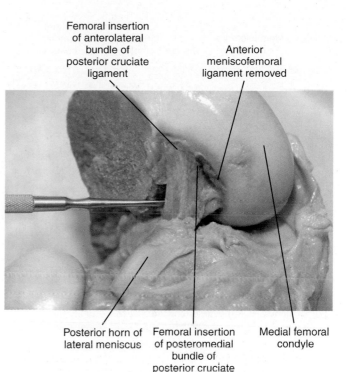

FIGURE 2–27. View of the medial femoral condyle with the anterior meniscofemoral ligament removed to demonstrate the femoral insertion of the PCL. Notice that the anterolateral bundle inserts closer to the articular cartilage than does the posteromedial bundle.

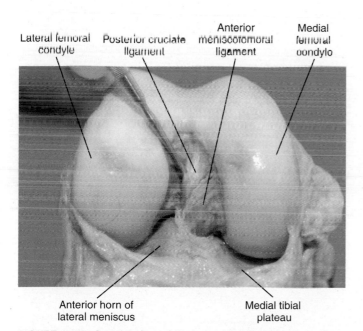

FIGURE 2–26. Anterior view of the knee demonstrates the large femoral insertion of the PCL.

AL bundle's femoral insertion centered at the 10:20 position when referenced parallel to the femoral shaft. The PM center corresponded to the 8:30 position. The AL bundle is generally closer to the articular cartilage of the medial femoral condyle, with its center 7 mm from the edge, and the center of the PM bundle is approximately 8 to 11 mm from the edge of the cartilage. Harner and coworkers[14] found equal distributions of the AL and PM bundles to the femoral insertion area. However, Lopes and coworkers[30] found the AL bundle contributes 118 mm^2 compared with the PM bundle's contribution of 90 mm^2. These investigators also described a medial bifurcate ridge (present in 8 of 20 cadavers) that separates the AL and PM bundles' femoral insertions. The variation between studies reflects the lack of a true anatomic separation of the PCL into bundles, which does not accurately describe PCL fiber function (see Chapter 20, Function of the Posterior Cruciate and Posterolateral Ligament Structures).

Besides the contribution of the PCL to knee stability, the MFLs contribute as secondary restraints to resist posterior tibial translation. Two MFLs may exist: the anterior meniscofemoral ligament of Humphrey (aMFL) and/or the posterior meniscofemoral ligament of Wrisberg (pMFL) (Figs. 2–28 to 2–32). The aMFL originates from the posterior horn of the lateral meniscus and travels anterior to the PCL, attaching close to the articular cartilage of the medial femoral condyle. The pMFL travels posterior to the PCL and attaches near the intercondylar roof. Gupte and associates[12] described three main anatomic clues to distinguish the MFLs from the PCL. These include the insertional anatomy of the femur, the increased obliquity of the fibers of the MFLs compared with the PCL fibers, and a cleavage plane between the MFLs and the PCL. Gupte and colleagues[13] found the aMFL to be present in 74% of cadaveric knees and the pMFL in 69% of knees. Ninety-three percent of specimens were found to have at least one MFL. In a separate report, Gupte and associates[12] described an arthroscopic "meniscal tug test" to distinguish the MFLs from the PCL, thus avoiding the misdiagnosis of partial versus complete PCL rupture.

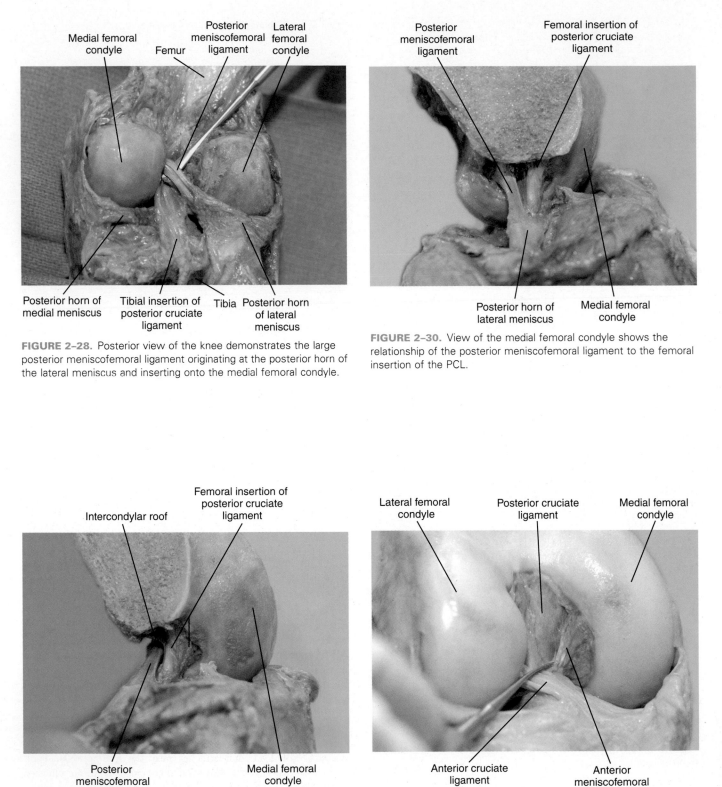

FIGURE 2–28. Posterior view of the knee demonstrates the large posterior meniscofemoral ligament originating at the posterior horn of the lateral meniscus and inserting onto the medial femoral condyle.

FIGURE 2–30. View of the medial femoral condyle shows the relationship of the posterior meniscofemoral ligament to the femoral insertion of the PCL.

FIGURE 2–29. View of the medial femoral condyle shows the relationship of the posterior meniscofemoral ligament to the femoral insertion of the PCL.

FIGURE 2–31. Gross view of the anterior aspect of the knee demonstrates the anterior meniscofemoral ligament inserting anterior to the PCL on the medial femoral condyle.

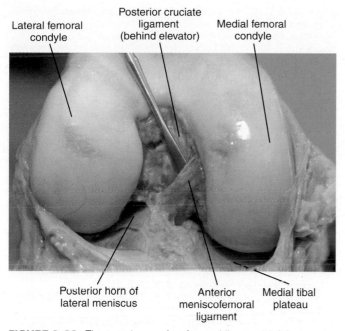

Lateral femoral condyle

Posterior cruciate ligament (behind elevator)

Medial femoral condyle

Posterior horn of lateral meniscus

Anterior meniscofemoral ligament

Medial tibial plateau

FIGURE 2–32. The anterior meniscofemoral ligament originates at the posterior horn of the lateral meniscus inserting onto the intercondylar wall of the medial femoral condyle.

CONCLUSION

The posterior and lateral aspects of the knee are difficult anatomic areas for the orthopaedic surgeon owing, in part, to the varied nomenclature in the literature. This chapter has attempted to clarify these terms based on the most recent references. Illustrations have been used as needed to point out the key structures. An axial view of the proximal tibia summarizes the nomenclature and anatomy (see Fig. 2–14).

REFERENCES

1. Clemente, C. D. (ed.): *Anatomy: A Regional Atlas of the Human Body.* Baltimore: Lippincott, Williams & Wilkins, 2007.
1a. Colombet, P.; Robinson, J.; Christel P.; et al.: Morphology of anterior cruciate ligament attachments for anatomic reconstruction: a cadaveric dissection and radiographic study. *Arthroscopy* 22:984–992, 2006.
2. DeCoster, T. A.; Crawford, M. K.; Kraut, M. A.: Safe extracapsular placement of proximal tibia transfixation pins. *J Orthop Trauma* 18(8 suppl):S43–S47, 2004.
3. DeLee, J. C.; Drez, D.; Noyes, F. R.; et al.: The role of high tibial osteotomy in the anterior cruciate-deficient knee with varus alignment. In DeLee, J. C.; Drez, D.; Miller, M. D. (eds.), *Orthopaedic Sports Medicine. Principles and Practice.* Philadelphia: W. B. Saunders, 2003; p. 1900.
4. Diamantopoulos, A.; Tokis, A.; Tzurbakis, M.; et al.: The posterolateral corner of the knee: evaluation under microsurgical dissection. *Arthroscopy* 21:826–833, 2005.
5. Edwards, A.; Bull, A. M.; Amis, A. A.: The attachments of the anteromedial and posterolateral fibre bundles of the anterior cruciate ligament: part 1: tibial attachment. *Knee Surg Sports Traumatol Arthrosc* 15:1414–1421, 2007.
6. Edwards, A.; Bull, A. M.; Amis, A. A.: The attachments of the anteromedial and posterolateral fibre bundles of the anterior cruciate ligament: part 2: femoral attachment. *Knee Surg Sports Traumatol Arthrosc* 16:29–36, 2008.
7. Edwards, A.; Bull, A. M.; Amis, A. A.: The attachments of the fiber bundles of the posterior cruciate ligament: an anatomic study. *Arthroscopy* 23:284–290, 2007.
7a. Falk, G. D.: Radiographic observations on the incidence of fabella. *Bull Hosp Joint Dis* 24:127–129, 1963.
7b. Ferretti, M.; Ekdahl, M.; Shen, W.; Fu, F. H.: Osseous landmarks of the femoral attachment of the anterior cruciate ligament: an anatomic study. *Arthroscopy* 23:1218–1225, 2007.
8. Frey, C.; Bjorkengen, A.; Sartoris, D.; Resnick, D.: Knee dysfunction secondary to dislocation of the fabella. *Clin Orthop Relat Res* 222:223–227, 1987.
9. Girgis, F. G.; Marshall, J. L.; Monajem, A. L.: The cruciate ligaments of the knee joint. Anatomical, functional and experimental analysis. *Clin Orthop* 106:216–231, 1975.
10. Goldenberg, R. R.; Wild, E. L.: Chondromalacia fabellae. *J Bone Joint Surg Am* 24:688–690, 1952.
11. Grood, E. S.; Stowers, S. F.; Noyes, F. R.: Limits of movement in the human knee. Effect of sectioning the posterior cruciate ligament and posterolateral structures. *J Bone Joint Surg Am* 70:88–97, 1988.
12. Gupte, C. M.; Bull, A. M.; Atkinson, H. D.; et al.: Arthroscopic appearances of the meniscofemoral ligaments: introducing the "meniscal tug test." *Knee Surg Sports Traumatol Arthrosc* 14:1259–1265, 2006.
13. Gupte, C. M.; Smith, A.; McDermott, I. D.; et al.: Meniscofemoral ligaments revisited. Anatomical study, age correlation and clinical implications. *J Bone Joint Surg Br* 84:846–851, 2002.
14. Harner, C. D.; Baek, G. H.; Vogrin, T. M.; et al.: Quantitative analysis of human cruciate ligament insertions. *Arthroscopy* 15:741–749, 1999.
15. Harner, C. D.; Livesay, G. A.; Kashiwaguchi, S.; et al.: Comparative study of the size and shape of human anterior and posterior cruciate ligaments. *J Orthop Res* 13:429–434, 1995.
15a. Heming, J. F.; Rand, J. Steiner, M. E.: Anatomical limitations of transtibial drilling in anterior cruciate ligament reconstruction. *Am J Sports Med* 35:1708–1715, 2007.
16. Hoppenfeld, S.: The knee. In Hoppenfeld, S.; deBoer, P. (eds.): *Surgical Exposures in Orthopedics: The Anatomic Approach.* Philadelphia: J. B. Lippincott, 1994; pp. 455–478.
17. Hutchinson, M. R.; Ash, S. A.: Resident's ridge: assessing the cortical thickness of the lateral wall and roof of the intercondylar notch. *Arthroscopy* 19:931–935, 2003.
18. Kantaras, A. T.; Johnson, D. L.: The medial meniscal root as a landmark for tibial tunnel position in posterior cruciate ligament reconstruction. *Arthroscopy* 18:99–101, 2002.
19. Kaplan, E. B.: Comparative anatomy of the extensor digitorum longus in relation to the knee joint. *Anat Rec* 131:129–149, 1958.

20. Kaplan, E. B.: Surgical approach to the lateral (peroneal) side of the knee joint. *Surg Gynecol Obstet* 104:346–356, 1957.

21. Kaplan, E. B.: The fabellofibular and short lateral ligaments of the knee joint. *J Bone Joint Surg Am* 43:169–179, 1961.

22. LaPrade, R. F.: Anatomic reconstruction of the posterolateral aspect of the knee. *J Knee Surg* 18:167–171, 2005.

23. LaPrade, R. F. (ed.): *Posterolateral Knee Injuries. Anatomy, Evaluation, and Treatment.* 238, New York: Thieme, 2006; p. 38.

24. LaPrade, R. F.; Hamilton, C. D.: The fibular collateral ligament–biceps femoris bursa. An anatomic study. *Am J Sports Med* 25:439–443, 1997.

25. LaPrade, R. F.; Konowalchuk, B. K.: Popliteomeniscal fascicle tears causing symptomatic lateral compartment knee pain: diagnosis by the figure-4 test and treatment by open repair. *Am J Sports Med* 33:1231–1236, 2005.

26. LaPrade, R. F.; Ly, T. V.; Wentorf, F. A.; Engebretsen, L.: The posterolateral attachments of the knee: a qualitative and quantitative morphologic analysis of the fibular collateral ligament, popliteus tendon, popliteofibular ligament, and lateral gastrocnemius tendon. *Am J Sports Med* 31:854–860, 2003.

27. LaPrade, R. F.; Morgan, P. M.; Wentorf, F. A.; et al.: The anatomy of the posterior aspect of the knee. An anatomic study. *J Bone Joint Surg Am* 89:758–764, 2007.

28. LaPrade, R. F.; Tso, A.; Wentorf, F. A.: Force measurements on the fibular collateral ligament, popliteofibular ligament, and popliteus tendon to applied loads. *Am J Sports Med* 32:1695–1701, 2004.

29. Larson, J. E.; Becker, D. A.: Fabellar impingement in total knee arthroplasty. A case report. *J Arthroplasty* 8:95–97, 1993.

30. Lopes, O. V., Jr.; Ferretti, M.; Shen, W.; et al.: Topography of the femoral attachment of the posterior cruciate ligament. *J Bone Joint Surg Am* 90:249–255, 2008.

30a. Luites, J. W.; Wymenga, A. B.; Blankevoort, L.; Kooloos, J. G.: Description of the attachment geometry of the anteromedial and posterolateral bundles of the ACL from arthroscopic perspective for anatomical tunnel placement. *Knee Surg Sports Traumatol Arthrosc* 15:1422–1431, 2007.

31. Makris, C. A.; Georgoulis, A. D.; Papageorgiou, C. D.; et al.: Posterior cruciate ligament architecture: evaluation under microsurgical dissection. *Arthroscopy* 16:627–632, 2000.

32. Mangieri, J. V.: Peroneal-nerve injury from an enlarged fabella. A case report. *J Bone Joint Surg Am* 55:395–397, 1973.

33. Marks, P. H.; Cameron, M.; Regan, W.: Fracture of the fabella: a case of posterolateral knee pain. *Orthopedics* 21:713–714, 1998.

34. Marshall, J. L.; Girgis, F. G.; Zelko, R. R.: The biceps femoris tendon and its functional significance. *J Bone Joint Surg Am* 54:1444–1450, 1972.

35. Mejia, E. A.; Noyes, F. R.; Grood, E. S.: Posterior cruciate ligament femoral insertion site characteristics: importance for reconstructive procedures. *Am J Sports Med* 30:643–651, 2002.

36. Minowa, T.; Murakami, G.; Kura, H.; et al.: Does the fabella contribute to the reinforcement of the posterolateral corner of the knee by inducing the development of associated ligaments? *J Orthop Sci* 9:59–65, 2004.

37. Moorman, C. T., 3rd; LaPrade, R. F.: Anatomy and biomechanics of the posterolateral corner of the knee. *J Knee Surg* 18:137–145, 2005.

37a. Moorman, C. T., 3rd; Murphy Zane, M. S.; Bansai, S., et al.: Tibial insertion of the posterior cruciate ligament: a sagittal plane analysis using gross, histologic, and radiographic methods. *Arthroscopy* 24:269–275, 2008.

37b. Morgan, C. D.; Kalman, V. R.; Grawl, D. M.: The anatomic origin of the posterior cruciate ligament: Where is it? Reference landmarks for PCL reconstruction. *Arthroscopy* 13:325–331, 1997.

38. Noyes, F. R.; Barber-Westin, S. D.: Posterolateral knee reconstruction with an anatomical bone–patellar tendon–bone reconstruction of the fibular collateral ligament. *Am J Sports Med* 35:259–273, 2007.

39. Noyes, F. R.; Barber-Westin, S. D.: Surgical reconstruction of severe chronic posterolateral complex injuries of the knee using allograft tissues. *Am J Sports Med* 23:2–12, 1995.

40. Noyes, F. R.; Barber-Westin, S. D.: Surgical restoration to treat chronic deficiency of the posterolateral complex and cruciate ligaments of the knee joint. *Am J Sports Med* 24:415–426, 1996.

41. Noyes, F. R.; Barber-Westin, S. D.: Treatment of complex injuries involving the posterior cruciate and posterolateral ligaments of the knee. *Am J Knee Surg* 9:200–214, 1996.

42. Noyes, F. R.; Barber-Westin, S. D.; Albright, J. C.: An analysis of the causes of failure in 57 consecutive posterolateral operative procedures. *Am J Sports Med* 34:1419–1430, 2006.

43. Noyes, F. R.; Grood, E. S.: Classification of ligament injuries: why an anterolateral laxity or anteromedial laxity is not a diagnostic entity. *Instr Course Lect* 36:185–200, 1987.

44. Noyes, F. R.; Grood, E. S.; Butler, D. L.; Malek, M.: Clinical laxity tests and functional stability of the knee: biomechanical concepts. *Clin Orthop* 146:84–89, 1980.

45. Noyes, F. R.; Stowers, S. F.; Grood, E. S.; et al.: Posterior subluxations of the medial and lateral tibiofemoral compartments. An in vitro ligament sectioning study in cadaveric knees. *Am J Sports Med* 21:407–414, 1993.

46. Pancoast, H. K.: Radiographic statistics of the sesamoid in the tendon of the gastrocnemius. *Univ Penn Med Bull* 22:213, 1909.

47. Pasque, C.; Noyes, F. R.; Gibbons, M.; et al.: The role of the popliteofibular ligament and the tendon of popliteus in providing stability in the human knee. *J Bone Joint Surg Br* 85:292–298, 2003.

48. Petersen, W.; Zantop, T.: Anatomy of the anterior cruciate ligament with regard to its two bundles. *Clin Orthop Relat Res* 454:35–47, 2007.

48a. Pritchett, J. W.: The incidence of fabellae in osteoarthritis of the knee. *J Bone Joint Surg Am* 66:1379–1380, 1984.

49. Robertson, A.; Jones, S. C.; Paes, R.; Chakrabarty, G.: The fabella: a forgotten source of knee pain? *Knee* 11:243–245, 2004.

50. Sanchez, A. R., 2nd; Sugalski, M. T.; LaPrade, R. F.: Anatomy and biomechanics of the lateral side of the knee. *Sports Med Arthrosc* 14:2–11, 2006.

51. Seebacher, J. R.; Inglis, A. E.; Marshall, J. L.; et al.: The structure of the posterolateral aspect of the knee. *J Bone Joint Surg Am* 64:536–541, 1982.

52. Segond, P.: Reserches cliniques et experimentales sure es epachernents sanquins de genou par entarse. *Prog Med* 7:297, 1879.

53. Sheps, D. M.; Otto, D.; Fernhout, M.: The anatomic characteristics of the tibial insertion of the posterior cruciate ligament. *Arthroscopy* 21:820–825, 2005.

53a. Siebold, R.; Ellert, T.; Metz, S.; Metz, J.: Tibial insertions of the anteromedial and posterolateral bundles of the anterior cruciate ligament: morphometry, arthroscopic landmarks, and orientation model for bone tunnel placement. *Arthroscopy* 24:154–161, 2008.

54. Simonian, P. T.; Sussmann, P. S.; van Trommel, M.; et al.: Popliteomeniscal fasciculi and lateral meniscal stability. *Am J Sports Med* 25:849–853, 1997.

55. Standring, S. (ed.): *Gray's Anatomy: The Anatomical Basis of Clinical Practice.* New York: Churchill Livingstone, 2005.

56. Staubli, H.-U.; Birrer, S.: The popliteus tendon and its fascicles at the popliteal hiatus: gross anatomy and functional arthroscopic evaluation with and without anterior cruciate ligament deficiency. *Arthroscopy* 6:209–220, 1990.

57. Staubli, H. U.; Rauschning, W.: Tibial attachment area of the anterior cruciate ligament in the extended knee position. Anatomy and cryosections in vitro complemented by magnetic resonance arthrography in vivo. *Knee Surg Sports Traumatol Arthrosc* 2:138–146, 1994.

58. Strauss, E. J.; Ishak, C.; Inzerillo, C.; et al.: Effect of tibial positioning on the diagnosis of posterolateral rotatory instability in the posterior cruciate ligament–deficient knee. *Br J Sports Med* 41:481–485; discussion 485, 2007.

59. Sudasna, S.; Harnsiriwattanagit, K.: The ligamentous structures of the posterolateral aspect of the knee. *Bull Hosp Jt Dis Orthop Inst* 50:35–40, 1990.

60. Sutro, C. J.; Sutro, W. H.: Two concepts. I: The third femoral condyle. *Bull Hosp Jt Dis Orthop Instr* 51:40–46, 1991.

61. Takahashi, M.; Matsubara, T.; Doi, M.; et al.: Anatomical study of the femoral and tibial insertions of the anterolateral and posteromedial bundles of human posterior cruciate ligament. *Knee Surg Sports Traumatol Arthrosc* 14:1055–1059, 2006.

61a. Takahashi, M.; Doi, M.; Abe, M.; et al.: Anatomical study of the femoral and tibial insertions of the anteromedial and posterolateral bundles of human anterior cruciate ligament. *Am J Sports Med* 34:787–792, 2006.

62. Terry, G. C.; Hughston, J. C.; Norwood, L. A.: The anatomy of the iliopatellar band and iliotibial tract. *Am J Sports Med* 14:39–45, 1986.

63. Terry, G. C.; LaPrade, R. F.: The biceps femoris muscle complex at the knee. Its anatomy and injury patterns associated with acute anterolateral-anteromedial rotatory instability. *Am J Sports Med* 24:2–8, 1996.
64. Terry, G. C.; LaPrade, R. F.: The posterolateral aspect of the knee. Anatomy and surgical approach. *Am J Sports Med* 24:732–739, 1996.
65. Watanabe, Y.; Moriya, H.; Takahashi, K.; et al.: Functional anatomy of the posterolateral structures of the knee. *Arthroscopy* 9:57–62, 1993.
66. Weiner, D.; Macnab, I.; Turner, M.: The fabella syndrome. *Clin Orthop Relat Res* 126:213–215, 1977.
67. Wroble, R. R.; Grood, E. S.; Cummings, J. S.; et al.: The role of the lateral extra-articular restraints in the anterior cruciate ligament–deficient knee. *Am J Sports Med* 21:257–262; discussion 263, 1993.
68. Yoon, K. H.; Bae, D. K.; Ha, J. H.; Park, S. W.: Anatomic reconstructive surgery for posterolateral instability of the knee. *Arthroscopy* 22:159–165, 2006.
69. Zantop, T.; Petersen, W.; Sekiya, J. K., et al.: Anterior cruciate ligament anatomy and function relating to anatomical reconstruction. *Knee Surg Sports Traumatol Arthrosc* 14:982–992, 2006.
70. Zhao, J.; He, Y.; Wang, J.: Anatomical reconstruction of knee posterolateral complex with the tendon of the long head of biceps femoris. *Am J Sports Med* 34:1615–1622, 2006.

Classification and Biomechanics

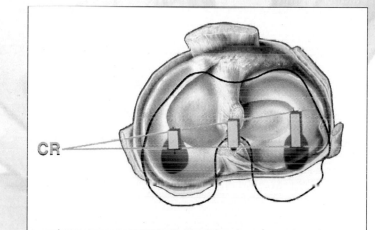

Chapter 5

The Scientific Basis for Examination and Classification of Knee Ligament Injuries

Frank R. Noyes, MD ■ *Edward S. Grood*, PhD

CLASSIFICATION SYSTEM FOR KNEE LIGAMENT INJURIES

Many different classification systems for knee ligament injuries have been proposed in the sports medicine literature.[20,21,31,32,42] A series of studies conducted by the authors enabled the development of an algorithm for the diagnosis and classification of these injuries based on kinematic and biomechanical data.[8,14–17,36–42,55,60] The purpose of this chapter is to summarize these studies and provide the clinician with the proper examination techniques that allow precise diagnosis of abnormal knee motions, subluxations, and ligament injuries.

The purposes of a classification system are to (1) make accurate distinctions between separate pathologic conditions in laboratory and clinical studies and (2) provide a common descriptive tool for investigators who wish to present cases and describe the outcome of treatment programs. A system that allows two or more discrete types of injuries to be grouped as a single entity does not allow the association of a unique natural history or surgical result with the anatomic defect on the actual pathologic condition being treated.

The classification scheme developed from the authors' investigations is based on seven concepts:

1. The final diagnosis of knee ligament injuries is based on the specific anatomic defect derived from the abnormal motion limits and joint subluxations.
2. Ligaments have distinct mechanical functions to provide limits to tibiofemoral motions and the types of motions that occur between opposing cartilage surfaces.

3. Although there are six degrees of freedom (DOF), the manual stress examinations are designed to test just one or two limits at a time.
4. Ultimately, the clinical examination must be analyzed by a six-DOF system to detect abnormalities.
5. Together, the ligaments and joint geometry provide two limits (opposite directions) for each DOF.
6. Rotatory subluxations are characterized by the separate compartment translations that occur to the medial and lateral tibial plateaus during the clinical test.
7. The damage to each ligament and capsular structure is diagnosed using tests in which the primary and secondary ligament restraints have been experimentally determined.[37]

In this chapter, the studies presented relate to the anterior cruciate ligament (ACL), posterior cruciate ligament (PCL), medial collateral ligament (MCL) and posteromedial structures, the iliotibial band (ITB), and the midlateral capsule. Studies related to the posterolateral structures (fibular collateral ligament [FCL], popliteus muscle-tendon-ligament, and posterolateral capsule) are presented in Chapters 20, Function of the Posterior Cruciate and Posterolateral Ligament Structures, and 22, Posterolateral Ligament Injuries: Diagnosis, Operative Techniques, and Clinical Outcomes.

Concept 1: The Final Diagnosis of Knee Ligament Injuries Is Based on the Specific Anatomic Defect Derived from the Abnormal Motion Limit and Joint Subluxation

The term *instability* has been used to describe an abnormal motion or motion limit that exists to the joint due to a ligament injury. This term has also been used to indicate symptomatic giving-way of the knee joint that occurs during activity. Giving-way may be caused by many factors including a ligament rupture, poor muscular control of the knee joint, altered neurologic function and control mechanisms, or mechanical problems such as a torn meniscus or loose body. In many cases, giving-way occurs because of multiple factors and the term *instability* does not precisely indicate the exact cause of the episode. Rather than a diagnosis of anterior instability, it is more appropriate to reduce the abnormality to a precise anatomic diagnosis such as ACL rupture. In addition, other ligament deficiencies, if present, should be identified.

The term *laxity* simply indicates looseness and may be applied to increases in joint motion or increases in ligament elongation. Therefore, the term *laxity* does not provide a diagnosis of a specific abnormality. The knee has a normal amount of laxity (play or motion) required for function. An abnormal amount of laxity may occur as a result of a ligament disruption. Laxity may also indicate a ligament injury in which the ligament has an increase in length or elongation during loading. The finding of abnormal laxity represents a clinical sign that does not provide a precise diagnosis. Instead, the specific anatomic defect of the ruptured ACL and associated injured ligaments or capsular structures should be recorded as the diagnosis. The goal of a comprehensive knee examination is to detect an increase in the amount of motion (translation or rotation) or an abnormal position (subluxation) to determine the specific anatomic defects that are present.

Concept 2: Ligaments Have Distinct Mechanical Functions to Provide Limits to Tibiofemoral Motions and the Types of Motions That Occur between Opposing Cartilage Surfaces

Ligaments have distinct mechanical functions to provide limits to the amount of tibiofemoral motion that determines the types of motions that occur between opposing cartilage surfaces. The limits of motion are the main focus because loss of this function and the consequent subluxation are the underlying deficits in ligament-injured knees. In addition, the change in limits of motion is the primary basis of diagnosis.

The ability of ligaments to limit tibiofemoral motion provides the geometric parameters within which the neuromuscular system is able to control the position of the knee during activity. Although focus is placed on the mechanical function of the ligaments and capsular structures, the reader should be cognizant of the potentially important role of ligaments in providing sensory feedback to the neuromuscular system.[24,53] Ligaments have three properties that affect their ability to limit joint motion: location of their attachment on the bones, just-taut length, and stiffness.

Tibiofemoral motions are limited along the line that connects the ligament's tibial and femoral attachments in the direction that loads the ligament. Ligaments are not able to limit motions perpendicular to their orientation or motions that cause them to become slack. Just-taut length is a determinant of joint laxity because it controls the amount of motion before the ligament begins to provide a resisting force. Because the two cruciate ligaments are required to limit anteroposterior (AP) translation, total AP translation is determined by the just-taut length of both ligaments.

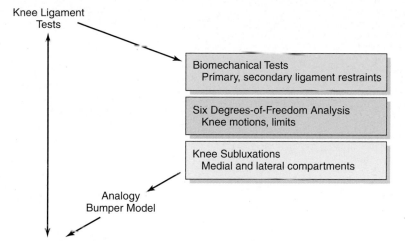

FIGURE 3–1. The results of clinical tests require specific biomechanical and kinematic principles for correct diagnosis of ligament defects. Ligament defects are defined by anatomic, functional, and severity categories. *(Reprinted from Noyes, F. R.; Grood, E. S: Classification of ligament injuries: why an anterolateral laxity or anteromedial laxity is not a diagnostic entity. In Griffin, P. [ed.]: AAOS Instructional Course Lectures, Vol. XXXVI. Chicago: American Academy of Orthopaedic Surgeons, pp. 185–200, 1987.)*

Ligament stiffness controls how much additional joint movement is required after the ligament has become taut to create a force large enough for the ligament to resist the applied load. Decreased ligament stiffness produces an increase in the motion limit because a greater motion is required before the ligament can develop a sufficient restraining force.

The kinematic and biomechanical concepts required to interpret clinical tests are shown in Figure 3–1. First, the appropriate clinical test must be selected to diagnose a specific ligament structural abnormality. Diagnostic information is obtained based on understanding the primary and secondary ligament restraint system. The results of the tests must be understood and communicated in terms of the six-DOF system that determines the abnormal motion limits. The medial and lateral tibiofemoral compartments are examined separately to determine the different types of subluxation. The final diagnosis of the ligament defect must be made in precise anatomic and functional terms and according to the severity of ligament failure (partial or complete).

Concept 3: Although There Are Six DOF, the Manual Stress Examinations Are Designed to Test Just One or Two Limits at a Time

Although there are six DOF, the knee ligament examination is specifically designed to test just one or two motion limits at a time. Combinations of these motions (coupled motions) are particularly important to the diagnosis of knee ligament injury because they occur during many of the manual stress examinations.

Translation of a rigid body (such as the tibia) is described by the motion of an arbitrarily selected point on the body. Typically, the AP translation is described by the motion of a point located midway between the medial and the lateral margins of the tibia. If only translation motions occur, the amount of motion does not depend upon which point is chosen, that is, whether the point is at the center of the knee or at the medial or lateral joint margin. This is because all points will move along parallel paths. However, when rotation and translation motions are combined, the amount of translation does depend upon which point is used. This can be seen by considering the four cases illustrated in Figure 3–2.

Figure 3–2B shows an anterior translation of 10 mm without associated tibial rotation. All points move anteriorly by the same amount. Figure 3–2C shows an internal rotation of 15° about an axis located midway between the spines of the intercondylar eminence. The point on the rotation axis is stationary while the lateral joint margin (edge) moves anteriorly and the medial margin posteriorly (see Fig. 3–2D). The amount of anterior and posterior motion of the points at the joint margin depends upon the amount of rotation and how far away the points are from the rotation axis (center of rotation). This illustrates that when translation is measured in the presence of a concurrent rotation, it is important to know at what point the translation was measured.

Concept 4: Ultimately, the Clinical Examination Must Be Analyzed by a Six-DOF System to Detect Abnormalities

The clinician who understands all of the possible motions in the knee joint that are normally limited by the knee ligaments will be able to perform manual stress tests and correctly determine the specific abnormality that is present. However, a diagnosis cannot be based solely on the abnormal motions detected. The diagnosis also requires knowledge of the biomechanical data regarding which ligaments limit each of the possible motions in the knee joint.

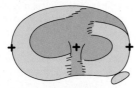

A. Reduced Position

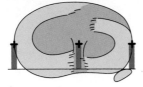

B. 10mm Anterior Translation

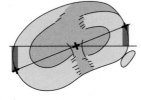

C. 15° Rotation About Joint Center

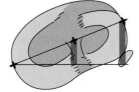

D. Combined Translation and Rotation

FIGURE 3–2. Combined anterior translation and tibial rotation. **A,** The tibial plateau is shown along with the contact area on the femur, indicated by the *shaded regions*. The tibia is in a reduced position. **B,** Anterior tibial translation of 10 mm. The amount of translation, shown by the *vertical bars*, is the same at the medial and lateral joint margins as it is at the center of the joint. **C,** 15° internal rotation about the joint center. Tibial contact is anterior on the lateral plateau and posterior on the medial plateau. The *bars* show the amount and direction of its translation at the medial-lateral joint lines. The amount of translation is approximately 10 mm in an average knee 80 mm wide. There is no translation at the center of the joint where the rotation axis is located. **D,** Combined tibial translation and rotation. A 10-mm anterior translation is combined with a 15° internal rotation at the medial aspect of the tibia. The center of the tibia translates anteriorly 10 mm, and the lateral joint margin translates 20 mm anteriorly. (**A–D,** *Redrawn from Grood, E. S.; Noyes, F. R.: Diagnosis of knee ligament injuries: biomechanical precepts. In Feagin, J. [ed.]:* The Crucial Ligaments. *New York: Churchill Livingstone, 1988, pp. 245–260.)*

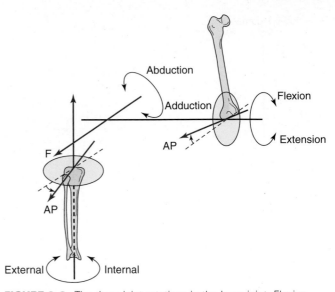

FIGURE 3–3. The three joint rotations in the knee joint. Flexion-extension occurs about the medially and laterally oriented axis in the femur. Internal and external tibial rotation occurs about an axis parallel to the shaft of the tibia. Abduction occurs about a third axis parallel to the femoral sagittal plane and also through the tibial transverse plane. *(Redrawn from Noyes, F. R.; Grood, E. S.: Classification of ligament injuries: why an anterolateral laxity or anteromedial laxity is not a diagnostic entity. In Griffin, P. [ed.]:* AAOS Instructional Course Lectures, Vol. XXXVI. *Chicago: American Academy of Orthopaedic Surgeons, 1987; pp. 185–200.)*

The field of science that describes the motions between objects is known as *kinematics*. A fundamental aspect of this field is the recognition that six possible motions may occur in three dimensions. Each of the six motions is discrete and separate from the other five motions. The six motions are referred to as *degrees of freedom* (DOF). The three rotational DOF in the knee joint are shown in Figure 3–3. Each rotation occurs about one axis: flexion-extension, internal-external, and abduction-adduction.

The flexion-extension axis is located in the femur and oriented in a pure medial-lateral direction perpendicular to the femoral sagittal plane. Rotation of the tibia about this axis does not have associated internal-external rotation or abduction-adduction motions.[17] Because these motions occur during flexion, the flexion-extension axis shown in Figure 3–3 does not correspond to the functional flexion axis. The functional flexion axis is skewed in the knee and changes its orientation as the knee is flexed. This skewed orientation accounts for the combined motions of flexion, abduction, and tibial rotation.

The internal-external tibial rotation axis is located in the tibia, parallel to the tibial shaft and perpendicular to the tibial transverse plane. Rotations about this axis are pure internal and external tibial rotation motions without any associated abduction-adduction or flexion-extension.

The abduction-adduction rotation axis is more difficult to visualize because it is not located in either bone and its orientation can change relative to both. This axis is always parallel to the femoral sagittal plane. When the knee is flexed, the orientation of the abduction axis changes relative to the femur as it rotates in the sagittal plane. The abduction axis is perpendicular to the tibial rotation axis and parallel to the tibial transverse plane.

There are three linear DOF in the knee joint referred to as *translations*. One simple approach to describing translations is to visualize relative sliding between the bones along each of the three rotational axes (Fig. 3–4). The sliding motion along the flexion-extension axis is the medial-lateral translation between the tibia and the femur. The sliding motion along the tibial rotation axis results in joint compression and distraction translation. Sliding motions along the abduction-adduction rotation axis produce AP translations. These are also commonly known as *drawer motions*.

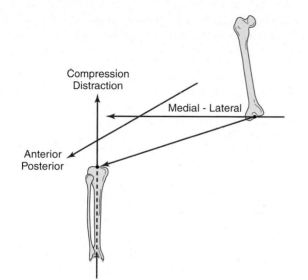

FIGURE 3–4. The three translations of the knee joint are motions of a point on the tibia parallel to each of the three axes. The point of the tibia used is located midway between the spines of the tibial plateau and is indicated by the *arrow* originating from the center point of the femur. Medial-lateral translation is motion of the point parallel to the flexion-extension axis. Anteroposterior (AP) translation is motion of the tibial point parallel to the abduction axis, and compression-distraction translation is motion of the point along the internal and external rotation axis. *(Redrawn from Noyes, F. R., Grood, E. S.: Classification of ligament injuries: why an anterolateral laxity or anteromedial laxity is not a diagnostic entity. In Griffin, P. [ed.]: AAOS Instructional Course Lectures, Vol. XXXVI. Chicago, American Academy of Orthopaedic Surgeons, 1987; pp. 185–200.)*

Therefore, six possible motions can occur in the knee, three rotations and three translations. Three axes are required to explain these six motions, one fixed in each bone, as shown in Figure 3–4. Each axis represents two DOF, one rotation occurring about the axis and the other a translation.

The purpose of the examination is to determine the specific increase in motion (amount and direction) of each clinically relevant DOF. In many cases, coupled motions occur in the knee joint, such as anterior translation combined with internal tibial rotation during Lachman testing, which is further increased on pivot shift testing. First, the examiner must understand the effect that ligament defects have upon each of these motions, because one or both may be increased. Second, both the amount of increased motion and the resulting subluxation of the tibial plateaus depend on the position of the knee joint, which is defined in terms of six DOF. Third, after a ligament is ruptured, an abnormal position usually is present in the axis of internal-external tibial rotation. This may be detected on examination and is helpful in diagnosing the ligament defect.

In order to understand the results of the clinical examination, a distinction must be made between abnormalities in joint motion and abnormalities in joint position (subluxation) that occur at the limit of the test. An abnormality in one or more motion limits can cause a subluxation of the knee joint. The subluxation depends on the direction and magnitude of the loads applied. Clinical tests are used to detect the motion limit and the final abnormal joint position. The examination usually detects a subluxation and not a complete knee dislocation, in which contact of the articulating surfaces of both tibiofemoral compartments is lost.

Concept 5: Together, the Ligaments and Joint Geometry Provide Two Limits (Opposite Directions) for Each DOF

Together, the ligaments and joint geometry provide two limits (opposite directions) for each DOF. All together, there are 12 possible limits of motion of the knee (Table 3–1). Injury to the structures that limit each motion increases joint laxity. The position of the joint at the final limits of motions (reflecting the ligament attachment sites) provides the information required for diagnosis. From a diagnostic standpoint, it would be ideal if each of the 12 limits of motion were controlled by a single ligamentous structure. Differential diagnosis could then be performed by evaluating each of the 12 limits separately. Clearly, this ideal situation does not exist. The ligaments, capsular structures, and joint geometry all work together and each contributes to limiting more than one motion. Thus, the problem of diagnosing knee injuries reduces to determining how to apply individual or combination motions to lengthen primarily a single ligament or capsular structure so that structure can be evaluated independently.

The ability to isolate each structure is the key to differential diagnosis of individual ligament injuries. The isolation of a structure is accomplished by placing the knee at the proper joint position (specifically, knee flexion angle and tibial rotation position) before the clinical stress test is performed. For example, the abduction (valgus) stress test is performed both in full extension and at 20° to 30° of flexion. In the flexed position, the posterior capsule becomes slack, which allows the examiner to primarily load the MCL and midmedial capsule. The evaluation of ACL function is performed at 20° of knee flexion[56] as opposed to the 90° position[29] commonly used many years ago because the 20° position more often results in increased anterior subluxation because secondary restraints are more slack and less able to block this motion. Diagnosis of an injury to a specific ligament is performed at a joint position at which other structures are the most lax and least able to block the abnormal subluxation from the ligament injury. The lax secondary restraints allow an increase in joint motion before they become taut and resist

TABLE 3–1	Twelve Limits of Knee Joint Motion
Motion Limit	**Structures Limiting the Motion**
Flexion	Ligaments, leg and thigh shape, joint compression
Extension	Ligaments and joint compression
Abduction	Ligaments and lateral joint compression
Adduction	Ligaments and medial joint compression
Internal rotation	Ligaments and menisci
External rotation	Ligaments and menisci
Medial translation	Bones (spines interlocking with femoral condyles) and ligaments (to prevent distraction)
Lateral translation	Bones (spines interlocking with femoral condyles) and ligaments (to prevent distraction)
Anterior translation*	Ligaments
Posterior translation*	Ligaments
Joint distraction	Ligaments
Joint compression	Bone, menisci, and cartilage

*Menisci, joint compressive effects after injury to primary restraint.

further joint motion. Thus, isolating a ligament so its integrity may be individually tested requires placing the knee in a position in which other supporting structures are slack.

Another example of the importance of selecting the joint position for clinical tests is the diagnosis of PCL injury. Figure 3–5 shows the amount of increased posterior tibial translation that occurs when the PCL is removed.[10,16,17] The increase in posterior translation is two to three times greater at 90° of flexion than at 20° of flexion. This phenomenon is easily understood using a bumper model analogy in which the amount of joint motion after a ligament is injured depends on the role and function of the remaining ligaments that must ultimately limit the joint motion (Fig. 3–6). Thus, the increase in joint motion that occurs when a ligament is injured reflects the amount of additional joint motion required before the remaining intact ligaments become stretched and are able to limit further motion.

Figure 3–7 illustrates the limits to internal tibial rotation in the knee joint.[16] At 30° flexion (see Fig. 3–7A), the limits to internal rotation are provided by posteromedial structures, lateral structures, and the ACL all working together. Sectioning either the ACL or the lateral structures produces a small increase in internal rotation. When both of these structures are cut together, a larger increase in internal rotation occurs. The further limit to internal rotation is the FCL, based upon its anatomy.

The ACL dominates at flexion angles less than 30°, whereas the lateral structures dominate at flexion angles greater than 30°. This can be explained by considering the changes that occur in ligament slackness with flexion and extension. As the knee is extended past 20°, the amount of AP translation decreases owing to reduction in the combined slackness of both cruciate ligaments. This brings these bumpers closer together. The posteromedial capsule (PMC) also tightens, moving its bumper anteriorly. This combination (see Fig. 3–7B) results in a decreased role of the anterolateral structures because the tibia can no longer rotate to the point where they become taut.

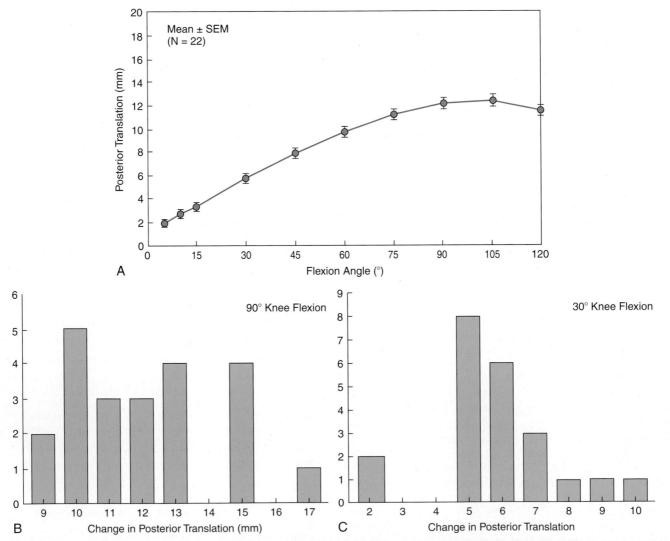

FIGURE 3–5. A, The increase in posterior translation is shown in 22 cadaveric knees under 100 N posterior force applied to the proximal tibia. The posterior force did not constrain the other degrees of freedom. The increase in posterior translation was 5.7 ± 0.4 mm at 30° flexion (**B**) and 12.1 ± 0.46 at 90° flexion (**C**). The data show that the majority of knees (15 of 22) that had the posterior cruciate ligament (PCL) sectioned alone had greater than 10 mm of increased posterior translation. This demonstrates the variability in knees in the physiologic tightness or slackness of the secondary restraints in resisting posterior tibial translation after PCL disruption. (*A–C, From J. T. Shearn and F. R. Noyes, unpublished data.*)

Effect of Knee Flexion on Posterior Bumpers

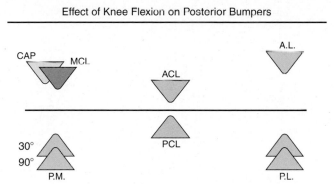

FIGURE 3–6. Effect of knee flexion on posterior bumpers. After loss of the PCL and as the knee is flexed, the posterior capsular structures become slack, allowing increased tibial displacement before they limit posterior translation. This is shown in the model by the more posterior position of the posteromedial and posterolateral bumpers at 90° compared with 30° of knee flexion. ACL, anterior cruciate ligament; AL, anterolateral restraints; CAP, capsule; MCL, medial collateral ligament; PL, posterolateral restraints; PM, posteromedial restraints. *(Redrawn from Grood, E. S.; Noyes, F. R.: Diagnosis of knee ligament injuries: biomechanical precepts. In Feagin, J. [ed.]: The Crucial Ligaments. New York: Churchill Livingstone, 1988; pp. 245–260.)*

With flexion beyond 30°, the lateral structures become progressively tighter and the posteromedial structures become progressively slack. This combination causes internal rotation to be limited first by the extra-articular restraints. This is consistent with laboratory results that showed that sectioning the ACL alone does not increase internal rotation when the knee is flexed between 40° and 80°.

Figure 3–8 illustrates the limits to external rotation. At 30° flexion, external rotation is limited only by the extra-articular restraints. On the lateral side, this includes all of the posterolateral structures, which act as a unit. Large increases in rotation do not occur until all structures are cut. At 90° flexion, the posterior capsule is slack and the PCL blocks significant increases in external rotation when the posterolateral structures are sectioned. In laboratory studies, external rotation increases an average of only 5.3° ± 2.6° when all of the posterolateral structures are sectioned and the PCL is intact. When the PCL is also sectioned, a large additional increase in external rotation occurs, ranging from 15° to 20°.

An example of the changes in motion limits in ACL ruptures is shown in Figure 3–9. In cadaver knees, cutting the ACL causes an abnormal increase in both anterior tibial translation and internal tibial rotation.[8] The increase in anterior tibial translation is the primary abnormality, because it increases 100% while there is a small increase in internal rotation (approximately 15%). Cutting the ACL alone produced a small but significant increase in internal rotation, greatest at 0° and 15° (Fig. 3–10). Subsequently, sectioning the ITB and lateral capsule produced statistically significant increases at 30° and greater.

Coupled motions (anterior tibial translation, internal tibial rotation) occur in cadaver knees after sectioning the ACL and lateral extra-articular structures. Coupled motions can be caused by factors intrinsic to the knee or by the manner in which the clinical test is performed. For instance, the amount of internal tibial rotation elicited depends on the amount of rotation the clinician applies during the examination. This is why it is difficult to obtain reproducible results with the Lachman and other

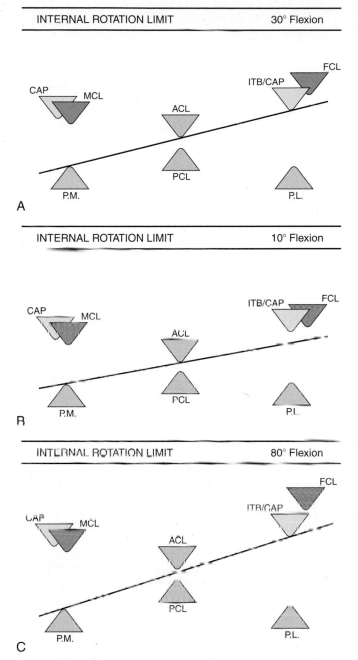

FIGURE 3–7. Limits to internal rotation. **A,** At 30° of flexion, internal rotation is limited by the ACL centrally and the lateral restraints. These structures limit anterior translation. In addition, the posterior translation of the medial plateau is limited by the posteromedial (PM) restraints. **B,** At 10° of flexion, the posterior bumpers move in closer toward the PCL owing to a reduction in the slackness present in the posterior capsule. In addition, the ACL bumper moves posteriorly as a result of tightening the ACL/PCL complex. Because of this, internal rotation of the tibia is now limited by the ACL centrally and the PM restraints alone. The tibia can no longer rotate far enough to engage the lateral restraints. **C,** At 80° flexion, the posterior bumpers move further posterior, reflecting the increased slackness in the posterior capsule. In addition, the distance between the ACL and the PCL bumpers has increased slightly to reflect the increased laxity of these structures. The medial and lateral structures are now moved posteriorly owing to tightening of the extra-articular restraints with knee flexion. Internal rotation is now limited by the lateral and PM restraints without direct involvement with the ACL. *(A–C, Redrawn from Grood, E. S.; Noyes, F. R.: Diagnosis of knee ligament injuries: biomechanical precepts. In Feagin, J. [ed.]: The Crucial Ligaments. New York: Churchill Livingstone, 1988; pp. 245–260.)*

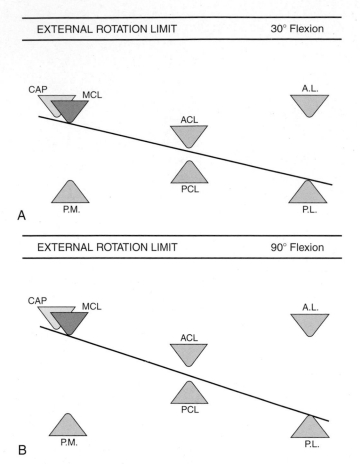

EXTERNAL ROTATION LIMIT — 30° Flexion

A

EXTERNAL ROTATION LIMIT — 90° Flexion

B

FIGURE 3–8. Limits to external rotation. **A,** At 30° flexion, the external rotation of the tibia is limited by the bumpers, which stop anterior translation of the medial plateau and posterior translation of the lateral plateau. Owing to the position of the structures, there is no direct involvement of either the ACL or the PCL in limiting external rotation. **B,** At 90° flexion, the posterior bumpers are moved posterior, reflecting the increased slack in the posterior capsule. Because of this, the PCL is nearly taut at the limit of external rotation. After removing the PL restraints, only a small increase in external rotation occurs at this flexion angle. *(A and B, Redrawn from Grood, E. S.; Noyes, F. R.: Diagnosis of knee ligament injuries: biomechanical precepts. In Feagin, J. [ed.]: The Crucial Ligaments. New York: Churchill Livingstone, 1988; pp. 245–260.)*

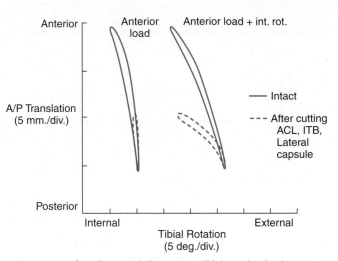

FIGURE 3–9. Anterior translation versus tibial rotation is shown during the Lachman-type anterior loading test at 15° of knee flexion. The amount of anterior tibial translation is shown *vertically* and the position of tibial rotation is shown *horizontally*. *(From Noyes, F. R.; Grood, E. S.: Classification of ligament injuries: why an anterolateral laxity or anteromedial laxity is not a diagnostic entity. In Griffin, P. [ed.]: AAOS Instructional Course Lectures, Vol. XXXVI. Chicago: American Academy of Orthopaedic Surgeons, 1987; pp. 185–200.)*

clinical tests. The KT-2000 provides an objective measurement of the amount of tibial translation measured at the center of the tibia. However, the millimeters produced by this device do not include the added millimeters of translation at the lateral tibiofemoral joint with added internal tibial rotation, such as that produced during the pivot shift test.

The amount of anterior tibial translation induced during anterior drawer testing is dependent upon the amount of internal or external tibial rotation applied at the beginning of the test (Fig. 3–11). The instrumented knee joint is shown for measuring rotations and translation motions during the clinical examination in Figure 3–12. This is because rotation tightens the extra-articular secondary restraints. The greatest amount of anterior or posterior tibial translation will be produced when the tibial is not forcibly rotated internally or externally, tightening extra-articular structures, during the clinical test. If the tibia is internally or externally rotated prior to the start of testing, the amount of tibial translation elicited will be smaller. Thus, the

clinician controls the amount of translation both by the initial rotational position of the tibia and by the amount of rotation imposed during the test. There is considerable variation in examination techniques of clinicians that makes all of the clinical tests highly subjective and qualitative, as is discussed.

The pivot shift[12] and flexion-rotation[44] drawer (Fig. 3–13) tests involve a complex set of tibial rotations and AP translations. At the beginning of the flexion-rotation drawer test, the lower extremity is simply supported against gravity (Fig. 3–14, position A). After ligament sectioning, both anterior tibial translation and internal rotation increase as the femur drops back and externally rotates into a subluxated position.[42] This position is accentuated as the tibia is lifted anteriorly (see Fig. 3–14, position B). At approximately 30° of flexion, the tibia is pushed posteriorly, reducing the tibia into a normal relationship with the femur (see Fig. 3–14, position C). This is the limit of posterior tibial translation resisted primarily by the PCL. From position C to position A, the knee is extended to produce the subluxated position again.

The rotational component of the test can be purposely accentuated by the examiner inducing a rolling motion of the femur. One advantage of the flexion-rotation drawer test is that it is not necessary to produce joint compression or add a lateral abduction force required in the pivot shift test. The rolling motion avoids the sometimes painful "thud/clunk" phenomenon induced in the pivot shift test. A finger may also be placed along the anterior aspect of the lateral and medial plateau and the tibiofemoral step-off palpated to provide a qualitative estimate of the millimeters of anterior tibial subluxation. The examiner can easily visualize the translation and rotation motions. Translation is observed by watching the forward motion of the tibial plateaus. Rotation is observed by watching the patella rotate externally with the femur in the subluxated position and internally in the reduced position.

The pivot shift and flexion-rotation drawer tests are graded only in qualitative terms because it is not possible to determine accurately the actual amount of internal tibial rotation or

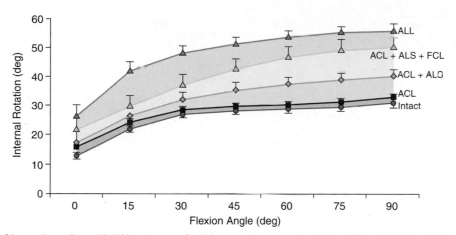

FIGURE 3–10. Limits of internal rotation with 5 Nm moment for intact specimens and with the ACL, ACL/ALS, ACL/ALS/FCL, and ALL structures (ACL/ALS/FCL/PLS) cut. Increases in internal rotation with the ACL cut are all statistically significant, but these increases are of such small magnitude that they are clinically unimportant. With ACL/ALS sectioning, increases in internal rotation are statistically significant at 30° of flexion and above. Statistically significant increases are found at 15° of flexion and above in the ACL/ALS/FCL cut state, and at all flexion angles of the ALL cut state. The effect of the PLS on restraining internal rotation in the extended knee can be seen by comparing the ACL/ALS/FCL curve and the ALL cut curve. The difference between these curves reflects sectioning the PLS. The largest differences are found at 15° and 30° of flexion. ALS, the iliotibial band and midlateral capsule; FCL, fibular collateral ligament; PLS, popliteus tendon and posterolateral capsule. *(Modified from Wroble, R. R.; Grood, E. S.; Cummings, J. S.; et al.: The role of the lateral extra-articular restraints in the anterior cruciate ligament–deficient knee. Am J Sports Med 21:257–262; discussion 263, 1993.)*

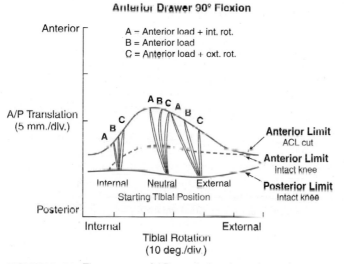

FIGURE 3–11. The amount of AP translation depends on the rotational position of the tibia at the beginning of the anterior drawer test. *(From Noyes, F. R.; Grood, E. S.: Classification of ligament injuries: why an anterolateral laxity or anteromedial laxity is not a diagnostic entity. In Griffin, P. [ed.]: AAOS Instructional Course Lectures, Vol. XXXVI. Chicago: American Academy of Orthopaedic Surgeons, 1987; pp. 185–200.)*

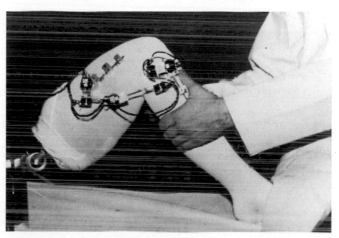

FIGURE 3–12. The six degrees-of-freedom electrogoniometer provides the clinician with immediate feedback on the motions induced during the manual drawer tests. *(From Noyes, F. R.; Grood, E. S.: Classification of ligament injuries: why an anterolateral laxity or anteromedial laxity is not a diagnostic entity. In Griffin, P. [ed.]: AAOS Instructional Course Lectures, Vol. XXXVI. Chicago, American Academy of Orthopaedic Surgeons, 1987; pp. 185–200.)*

anterior translation elicited. A fully positive pivot shift test (grade III) indicates a gross subluxation of the lateral tibiofemoral articulation along with an increased anterior displacement of the medial tibial plateau (Table 3–2). The amount of anterior subluxation elicited is indicative of rupture to the ACL and laxity to the secondary extra-articular restraints. The lateral tibial plateau demonstrates the greater subluxation in a positive pivot shift test, indicating that the lateral restraints (ITB, lateral capsule) are not functionally tight. This does not mean that these restraints are injured because a physiologic slackness of the ITB tibiofemoral attachments is normal at the knee flexion

position used in this test. These attachments are tightest at knee flexion angles of 45° and higher. Therefore, the majority of knees with an isolated ACL tear will have a positive pivot shift phenomenon.

In knees with a grade III pivot shift test, the amount of anterior tibial subluxation is so great that the posterior margin of the lateral tibial plateau impinges against the lateral femoral condyle and blocks further knee flexion during the test. The examiner must add both a maximal anterior force and an internal tibial rotation force to determine whether the maximum subluxation position can be reached. In revision ACL reconstructions, a combined intra-articular graft and extra-articular ITB surgical approach is often considered, as is discussed.[34]

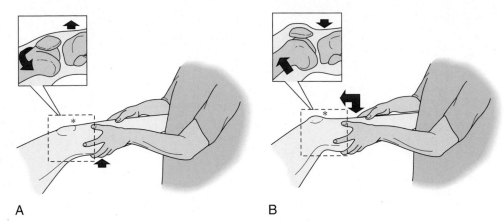

A   B

FIGURE 3–13. **A,** Flexion-rotation drawer test, subluxated position. With the leg held in neutral rotation, the weight of the thigh causes the femur to drop back posteriorly and rotate externally, producing anterior subluxation of the lateral tibial plateau. **B,** Flexion-rotation drawer test, reduced position. Gentle flexion and a downward push on the leg reduces the subluxation. This test allows the coupled motion of anterior translation–internal rotation to produce anterior subluxation of the lateral tibial condyle. (**A** and **B,** *Redrawn from Noyes, F. R.; Bassett, R. W.; Grood, E. S.; et al.: Arthroscopy in acute traumatic hemarthrosis of the knee. J Bone Joint Surg Am 62:687–695, 1980.*)

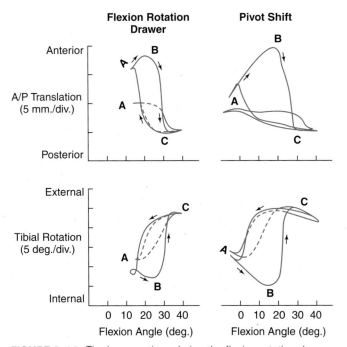

FIGURE 3–14. The knee motions during the flexion-rotation drawer and pivot shift tests are shown for tibial translation and rotation during knee flexion. The clinical test is shown for the normal knee (*open circle*) and after ligament sectioning (*dotted circle*). The ligaments sectioned were the ACL, iliotibial band (ITB), and lateral capsule. Position A equals the starting position of the test, B is the maximum subluxated position, and C indicates the reduced position. The pivot shift test involves the examiner applying a larger anterior translation load that increases the motion limits during the test. (*Redrawn from Noyes, F. R.; Grood, E. S.; Suntay, W. J.: Three-dimensional motion analysis of clinical stress tests for anterior knee subluxations. Acta Orthop Scand 60:308–318, 1989.*)

In a small percentage of knees with ACL ruptures, the classic "thud" or "clunk" will not be elicited during the pivot shift test. An experienced examiner will detect an increased slipping sensation in the knee (grade I), which indicates that the extra-articular secondary restraints are physiologically "tight," limiting the amount of anterior tibial subluxation or that a partial ACL tear exists.

Concept 6: Rotatory Subluxations Are Characterized by the Separate Compartment Translations That Occur to the Medial and Lateral Tibial Plateaus during the Clinical Test

A simple concept may assist in explaining the abnormal motions that occur after ACL rupture: rotatory subluxations can be classified according to the amount of anterior and posterior translation of each tibiofemoral compartment. Figure 3–15A shows a Lachman test performed on a knee in which the combined motions of anterior tibial translation and internal tibial rotation occur about a medially located rotation axis. In this example, only planar motion occurs; the ACL rupture doubles the amount of anterior tibial translation and slightly increases internal tibial rotation. The rotation axis shifts medially. The ratio of tibial translation to degrees of internal tibial rotation determines how far medially the axis of rotation shifts.

The abnormalities in tibial rotation and translation are easily expressed in terms of the different amounts of anterior translation that occur to the medial and lateral compartments (see Fig. 3–15B) in biomechanical tests. During the clinical tests, the clinician may qualitatively palpate and observe the anterior or posterior translation of each tibial plateau. The AP translation of each plateau is characterized instead of defining the individual components of translation, rotation, and rotation axis location that all lead to the anterior subluxation. The combined effect of the rotation and translation determines the translation of the medial and lateral tibiofemoral compartments.

The type of rotatory subluxations that occur depends on both the ligament injury and the knee flexion position. The subluxations of the medial and lateral compartment are usually recorded at two knee flexion positions, such as 20° and 90°. To be described later is the dial test for posterolateral injuries, in which the examiner determines whether increases in external tibial rotation reflect anteromedial or posterolateral tibial subluxations. It should be noted that rotatory subluxations are historically based on increases in tibial internal or external rotation and in only a few studies have the actual medial and lateral tibial subluxations in an AP direction been determined.[16,45] There are complex rotatory subluxations involving increases in translation, but in opposite directions of both the medial and the lateral compartments with combined medial and lateral ligament injuries.

TABLE 3–2   Classification of Pivot Shift Test Grades

Test Grade	Structures Involved			Positive Tests	Comments
	Anterior Cruciate Ligament	Iliotibial Band, Lateral Capsule	Modial Ligaments, Capsule		
Normal	Intact	Intact	Intact		
Grade I	Intact to slight increase in laxity	Intact	Intact	Lachman, flexion-rotation drawer, pivot shift "slip" but not "jerk"	Either physiologic laxity or partial ACL laxity allow subtle subluxation-reduction phenomena. Secondary ligament restraints limit the amount of joint subluxation. Subluxation is detected as a "slip," indicating increased lateral compartment translation.
Grade II	Ruptured	Intact to slight increase in laxity	Intact	All tests	Hallmark is an obvious "jump," "thud," or "jerk" with the gross subluxation-reduction during the test. There is either a normal physiologic laxity (lateral capsule, iliotibial band) or injured secondary restraints.
Grade III	Ruptured	Significant increase in laxity	May have increase in laxity	All tests	Hallmark is a gross subluxation with impingement of the posterior aspect of the lateral tibial plateau against the femoral condyle. The examiner must decrease internal rotational torque on the leg to allow lateral tibiofemoral reduction and further knee flexion.

Concept 7: The Damage to Each Ligament and Capsular Structure Is Diagnosed Using Tests in Which the Primary and Secondary Ligament Restraints Have Been Experimentally Determined

Tears to the ACL and injury to the extra-articular ligamentous and capsular structures may be diagnosed using the Lachman, pivot shift, and flexion-rotation drawer tests. These tests provide the basic signs that allow the clinician to determine which structures are injured based on abnormal motion limits and resultant joint subluxations. The tests are performed in knee flexion positions in which the secondary restraints are unable to resist abnormal motions so that maximum displacement (subluxation) of the joint is produced. Table 3–3 provides a general summary of the primary and secondary restraints for the major tests used in the clinical examination. Later in this chapter, the specific restraining function of the ligaments is discussed in detail.

The qualitative grading of the pivot shift phenomenon is illustrated in Figure 3–16 to explain how ligament structures resist combined tibiofemoral motions. The cruciate ligaments are represented by a set of central bumpers that limit the amount of AP translation. There are also medial and lateral sets of bumpers that resist medial and lateral tibiofemoral compartment translations. For the medial and lateral bumpers, different ligament structures commonly work together as systems to provide the resistance. The bumpers represent not the anatomic position of the ligament structures, but rather a visual schematic to show the final restraints to tibial motion, summarizing the effect of the ligaments, menisci, and capsular structures. The tension-retraining effect of the ligaments is replaced by an opposite mechanism, a compressive bumper.

In diagnosing abnormal knee motion limits, the Lachman test involves primarily tibial translation without significant tibial rotation, testing the central bumper represented by the ACL.

A bumper model representation of a partial ACL tear or an ACL-deficient knee with tight medial and lateral extra-articular restraints that limit the amount of anterior tibial translation is shown in Figure 3–16A. The amount of central and lateral tibial translation is only slightly increased. The bumper model illustrates how the anterior restraints limit motion during the flexion-rotation drawer test, which allows the maximal anterior excursion of the medial and lateral tibiofemoral compartments. In this knee, the pivot shift test is qualitatively listed as a grade I.

The most common type of anterior subluxation that occurs after an ACL rupture is shown in Figure 3–16B. The center of rotation shifts medially outside the knee joint, with a resultant increase in translation to both the medial and the lateral compartments, with the anterior subluxation of the lateral compartment being the greatest. The anatomic structures include the ACL and the lateral extra-articular restraints. In this knee, the pivot shift test is qualitatively listed as a grade II.

A knee with gross anterior subluxation is represented in Figure 3–16C. There is increased translation and subluxation to both the medial and the lateral compartments and the rotation axis shifts even further medially outside the knee joint. The pivot shift test is listed as a grade III, indicative of gross subluxation with impingement of the posterior aspect of the tibia against the femoral condyle. Partial damage to the medial ligamentous structures may be present.

LIGAMENTOUS RESTRAINTS TO AP TRANSLATION

In a series of biomechanical cadaveric experiments,[8] the ranked order of the importance of each knee ligament and capsular structure in resisting the clinical anterior and posterior drawer tests was determined, providing the primary and secondary restraints to specific knee motions. The ranked order was based on the force provided by each ligament in resisting AP translation.

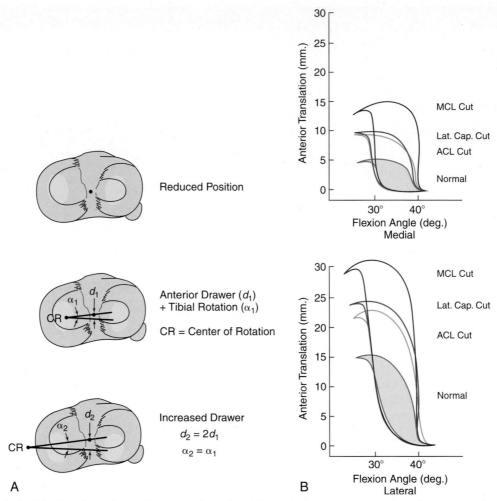

FIGURE 3–15. A, A simplification of the abnormal knee motions after ACL sectioning. An understanding of rotatory subluxations requires specifying changes in (1) position of the vertical axis of rotation and (2) displacement of the medial and lateral tibiofemoral compartments. The normal or subluxated position of the joint is determined by the degrees of rotation and the amount of translation. In the figure, an anterior pull is applied to the knee, which has an intact ACL. There is a normal anterior translation (d_1) and internal tibial rotation (a_1) about the center of rotation (CR). After ACL sectioning, there is a 100% increase in tibial translation (d_2) along with only a slight (15%) increase in internal tibial rotation (a_2). This shifts the axis of rotation medially and produces the subluxation of the lateral compartment and medial compartment, as demonstrated. Loss of the medial extra-articular restraints would result in a further medial shift in the axis of rotation. This would increase the anterior subluxation of the medial tibial plateau and lateral tibial plateau. **B,** The amount of anterior tibial translation is shown for the medial and lateral tibiofemoral compartments during the flexion-rotation drawer test in a cadaveric knee preparation using the instrumented spatial linkage and digitization of the tibia and femoral joint geometry. (**A,** *Redrawn from Noyes, F. R.; Grood, E. S.: Classification of ligament injuries: why an anterolateral laxity or anteromedial laxity is not a diagnostic entity. In Griffin, P. [ed.]: AAOS Instructional Course Lectures, Vol. XXXVI. Chicago: American Academy of Orthopaedic Surgeons, 1987; pp. 185–200;* **B,** *redrawn from Noyes, F. R.; Grood, E. S.; Suntay, W. J.: Three-dimensional motion analysis of clinical stress tests for anterior knee subluxations. Acta Orthop Scand 60:308–318, 1989.)*

Prior to these experiments, investigators performed studies in which selective sectioning of ligaments was conducted and the increases in anterior or posterior tibial displacement were measured.[5,6,11,13,19,28,29,47,50] For example, the displacement test was done by applying a force on an intact knee, cutting a ligament, repeating the test, and measuring the increase in displacement. One problem with this experimental design is that the increase in displacement is dependent on the order in which the ligaments are sectioned. If this order is altered, the measured increase in displacement will change. Therefore, it is not possible to define the function of a single ligament in a precise manner. In addition, the amount of residual joint displacement after ligament sectioning is dependent on the just-taut length of the remaining ligaments, which varies between physiologic "tight" and "loose" knee joints.

To solve these problems, a testing method was developed that allowed the restraining force of each individual ligament to be determined. A precise displacement was applied and the resultant restraining force measured. The reduction in restraining force that occurred after sectioning a ligament defined its contribution. Because the joint displacement was controlled, the contributions of the other ligaments and capsular structures of the knee to the resultant tibial displacement were not affected. Controlling and reproducing the joint displacement from test to test eliminated the effect of the cutting order of the structures. This is because the joint displacement controls the amount of ligament stretch and, thereby, its force. Reproducing the displacement reproduces the force in each ligament. This indicates that even after a single ligament is cut, the remaining structures are unaffected. The reader should distinguish the

TABLE 3–3   Ligamentous Restraints of the Knee Joint

	Primary Restraint				Secondary Restraint		
Clinical Test	Medial	Central	Lateral	Degrees	Medial	Central	Lateral
Anterior drawer	—	ACL	—	20/90	MCL	—	ALS
Anterior drawer + internal rotation	—	ACL	ALS	20/90	—	—	ALS + FCL
Anterior drawer + external rotation	MCL	ACL	—	20/90	PMC, MM	—	—
Flexion-rotation drawer, pivot shift	—	ACL	—	15	—	—	ALS + FCL
Posterior drawer	—	PCL	—	20/90	MCL	—	FCL + PMTL
Posterior drawer + external rotation	—	PCL	FCL + PMTL	30	—	—	LM
Posterior drawer + external rotation	PMC	PCL	FCL + PMTL	90	—	—	LM
Posterior drawer + internal rotation	—	—	—	20	—	—	ALS
Posterior drawer + internal rotation	PMC	PCL	—	90	—	—	ALS
Valgus	MCL + PMC	—	Bone	5	—	PCL + ACL	—
Valgus	MCL	—	Bone	20	PMC	PCL + ACL	—
Varus	Bone	—	FCL + PLC + PMTL	5	—	ACL + PCL	—
Varus	Bone	—	FCL + PMTL	20	—	ACL + PCL	PLC
External rotation	MCL	—	FCL + PMTL	30	PMC, MM	PCL	PLC
External rotation	MCL	PCL	PMTL + FCL	90	MM	—	PLC
Internal rotation	PMC	ACL	ALS	20	—	PCL	FCL
Internal rotation	PMC	ACL	ALS	90	—	PCL	FCL

ACL, anterior cruciate ligament; ALS, iliotibial band + anterior + midlateral capsule; FCL, fibular collateral ligament; MCL, superficial medial collateral ligament plus middle third deep capsule; LM, lateral meniscus; MM, medial meniscus; PCL, posterior cruciate ligament; PLC, posterolateral capsule (includes fabellofibular ligament); PMC, posteromedial capsule (includes posterior oblique ligament); PMTL, popliteus muscle tendon-ligament.

difference between these two testing methods in ligament sectioning studies, because the data provide different conclusions on ligament function.

Fourteen cadaver knees were tested from donors aged 18 to 65 years (mean, 42 yr). The knee specimens were mounted in an Instron Model 1321 biaxial servocontrolled electrohydraulic testing system (Fig. 3–17). A pair of grips was used for the femur and tibia that allowed for their precise position to be adjusted. First, the femur was secured with its shaft aligned along the axis of the load cell. The tibia was placed horizontally, with its weight supported by the lower grip. The output of the load cell was adjusted to zero to compensate for the weight of the upper grip and femur. The tibia was placed in a rotated position halfway between its limits of internal and external rotation. The output of the load cell was monitored while the tibia was secured in order to avoid pre-loading the ligaments. Single-plane anterior and posterior drawer tests were conducted by causing the actuator to move up and down without rotation. This is a constrained test in which coupled tibial rotation is purposely blocked. Specific details regarding the tests and data acquisition and statistical analyses are described in detail elsewhere.[8]

An AP drawer test is shown in Figure 3–18. Two curves are present, one for each direction of motion, as a result of the viscoelastic behavior of the knee ligaments. The peak restraining force of this specimen is approximately 500 N (112 lb) at 5 mm of drawer. The general shape of the force-displacement curve for the intact knee is nonlinear. The stiffness of the knee, or slope of the curve, is smallest near the neutral position and increases as the joint is displaced. The average restraining force in the intact knee is approximately 440 N (95 lb) at 90° of flexion and approximately 333 N

(75 lb) at 30° flexion. This is comparable with forces expected during moderate to strenuous activity and is well above the manual force applied during clinical drawer testing.[27,28]

The effect of sectioning the ACL is shown by the decrease in slope of the anterior curve and increase in displacement in Figure 3–18. Note that the anterior curve does not drop to zero owing to the presence of secondary ligament restraints. The ACL is the primary restraint to anterior translation (Fig. 3–19). Its contribution at displacements from 1 to 5 mm is shown in Figure 3–20. The percentages given above the bars are for 90° of knee flexion. Nearly identical results are shown at 30° of flexion, which represents the position of the knee during the Lachman test. No significant differences were found between 1 and 5 mm of drawer regardless of the trend toward increasing percentages at larger joint displacements.

The secondary restraints to anterior translation when the ACL is sectioned are shown in Table 3–4. The range in values for each structure demonstrates the large variation in results between specimens. No statistical difference was found among the percentages calculated. The contributions of the PCL, the anterior and posterior capsules, and the popliteal tendon were not included because they provided minimum restraining force.

It is important to characterize the effect of the ACL and secondary restraints on the coupled motions of anterior translation and internal-external tibial rotations. Figure 3–21 shows the effect of the lateral secondary restraints on both anterior translation and internal tibial rotation.

The PCL provides 94.3% ± 2.2% of the total restraining force at 90° of knee flexion, with similar findings at 30° of flexion (Fig. 3–22). No other structure contributes greater than 3% of

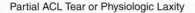

Partial ACL Tear or Physiologic Laxity

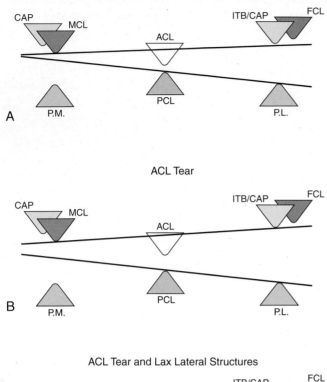

A

ACL Tear

B

ACL Tear and Lax Lateral Structures

C

FIGURE 3–16. A, Grade I pivot shift. There is anterior translation of the lateral compartment that is resisted by the ACL. There will be a slight increase in anterior translation with a partial ACL tear. Many knees with physiologic ACL laxity have a normal grade I pivot shift. Rarely, a knee will have excessively tight lateral structures that also limit anterior translation and, even with an ACL tear, there is only a grade I pivot shift phenomena. The *lower line* represents the posterior limit of tibial displacement. The *upper line* represents the anterior limit of tibial excursion resisted by the appropriate ligament bumpers. The millimeters of increased translation to the lateral-central-medial compartments is shown, reflecting the coupled motions of anterior translation and internal rotation. **B,** Grade II pivot shift. This is the usual finding after ACL disruption. The lateral extra-articular structures are physiologically lax between 0° and 45° of knee flexion, allowing for increased anterior translation of the lateral tibiofemoral compartment. The lesion may also involve injury to the lateral structures (ITB, lateral capsule). **C,** Grade III pivot shift. There is associated laxity of the lateral extra-articular restraints. There may also be associated laxity of the medial ligament structures. This allows for a gross subluxation of both the medial and the lateral tibial plateaus easily palpable during the pivot shift test, as well as the flexion-rotation drawer and Lachman tests. **(A–C,** *Redrawn from Noyes, F. R.; Good, E. S.: Classification of ligament injuries: why an anterolateral laxity or anteromedial laxity is not a diagnostic entity. In Griffin, P. [ed.]: AAOS Instructional Course Lectures, Vol. XXXVI. Chicago: American Academy of Orthopaedic Surgeons, 1987; pp. 185–200.)*

Critical Points LIGAMENTOUS RESTRAINTS TO ANTEROPOSTERIOR TRANSLATION

- This investigation was the first to introduce the concepts of primary and secondary ligament restraints to joint motion.
- A testing method was developed that allowed the restraining force of each individual ligament to be determined.
- A precise displacement was applied and the resultant restraining force measured.
- The reduction in restraining force that occurred after sectioning a ligament defined its contribution.
- The ACL is the primary restraint to anterior translation, providing 86% of the total restraining force.
- Secondary restraints to anterior tibial translation include the iliotibial tract and band, midmedial capsule, midlateral capsule, MCL, and FCL. No statistical difference exists among these structures in their contribution.
- The PCL provides 94% of the total restraining force of posterior tibial translation at 90° of knee flexion, with similar findings at 30° of flexion.
- The posterolateral capsule, popliteus tendon, and MCL provide the greatest secondary restraint to posterior tibial translation. The posterior medial capsule, FCL, and midmedial capsule provide only modest secondary restraining contribution.

ACL, anterior cruciate ligament; FCL, fibular collateral ligament; MCL, medial collateral ligament; PCL, posterior cruciate ligament.

the total restraint. The secondary restraints to posterior drawer after the PCL is sectioned (including the lateral meniscofemoral ligament when present) are shown in Table 3–5. The posterolateral capsule and popliteus tendon (combined contribution, 58.2%) and the MCL (15.7%) provided the greatest restraint. The posterior medial capsule, FCL, and midmedial capsule contributed only modest restraints. The combined restraint provided by the posterolateral capsule and popliteus tendon was significantly different from those provided by the other structures.

This investigation was the first to introduce the concepts of primary and secondary ligament restraints to joint motion. The cruciate ligaments are the primary restraints to AP drawer and provide approximately 90% of the total restraining force at 5 mm of joint displacement. The remaining structures provide only a small contribution. This study also made a distinction between clinical forces, which are small loads applied to the knee during a clinical examination, and functional forces, which are large in vivo loads experienced during moderate or strenuous activities (Fig. 3–23). The increase in joint displacement after the loss of either the ACL or the PCL depends on the forces applied to the knee. Whereas the light forces applied during a clinical test may produce only a slight increase in joint displacement, these increases are expected to be much larger under moderate or strenuous functional forces. Therefore, all clinical ligament examination tests do not predict the magnitude of joint displacement that may occur during functional activities.

LIGAMENTOUS AND CAPSULAR RESTRAINTS RESISTING MEDIAL AND LATERAL JOINT OPENING

The authors previously determined the ligaments and capsular structures that resist medial and lateral joint opening in cadaver knees. The ligaments were ranked in order of importance based on the percent of the total restraining force that each provides.

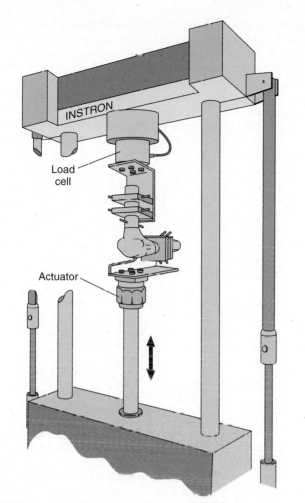

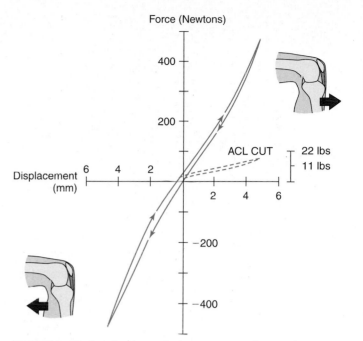

FIGURE 3–18. A typical force-displacement curve for anterior-posterior drawer in an intact joint (*solid line*) and after cutting the ACL (*broken line*). The *arrows* indicate the direction of motion. (*Redrawn from Butler, D. L., Noyes, F. R.; Grood, E. S.: Ligamentous restraints to anterior-posterior drawer in the human knee. A biomechanical study.* J Bone Joint Surg Am *62:259–270, 1980.)*

FIGURE 3–17. Cadaver knee mounted in 90° of flexion. The femur and tibia are potted in aluminum tubes. The femur is secured to the load cell above and the tibia is anchored to the moving actuator below. Single-plane anterior and posterior drawer is produced by vertical motion of the actuator. (*Redrawn from Butler, D. L.; Noyes, F. R.; Grood, E. S.: Ligamentous restraints to anterior-posterior drawer in the human knee. A biomechanical study.* J Bone Joint Surg Am *62:259–270, 1980.)*

The results are independent of the order in which ligaments are sectioned, allowing all ligaments to be studied in each cadaver knee. Most prior studies of knee ligament function were based on knee motion limits after cutting selected ligaments[6,19,28,58] or on the injury patterns associated with observed clinical pathologies.[5,9,20,21,25,33,46,47,54]

An Instron model-1321 biaxial testing system was used in which the femur was secured to the load cell with two grips that allowed its position to be adjusted.[15] The tibia was attached to the actuator through a plantar hinge mechanism that prevented axial rotation and flexion of the tibia during testing. Each knee was placed to the full-extended (hyperextended) position by applying a 5-Nm extension moment. The tests were performed with the knee flexed 5° and 25° from this position. Single-plane varus and valgus displacements were produced by causing the actuator to move up and down, but not rotate. The tests were done in a fixed manner that first produced medial and then lateral joint opening. A constant rate was used so that peak opening occurred in 1 second. A series of 25 conditioning tests that produced 6 mm of medial and 6 mm of lateral joint opening were done at the two knee flexion angles. Typically, the peak force changed less than 0.25% per cycle during

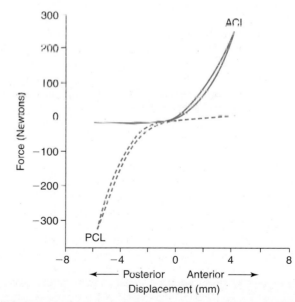

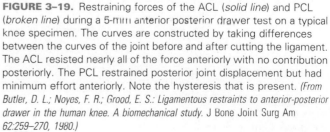

FIGURE 3–19. Restraining forces of the ACL (*solid line*) and PCL (*broken line*) during a 5-mm anterior posterior drawer test on a typical knee specimen. The curves are constructed by taking differences between the curves of the joint before and after cutting the ligament. The ACL resisted nearly all of the force anteriorly with no contribution posteriorly. The PCL restrained posterior joint displacement but had minimum effort anteriorly. Note the hysteresis that is present. (*From Butler, D. L.; Noyes, F. R.; Grood, E. S.: Ligamentous restraints to anterior-posterior drawer in the human knee. A biomechanical study.* J Bone Joint Surg Am *62:259–270, 1980.)*

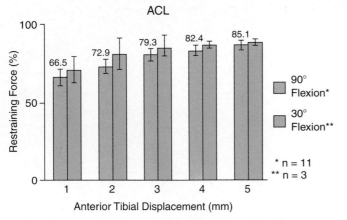

FIGURE 3–20. Anterior drawer in neutral tibial rotation. The restraining force of the ACL is shown for increasing tibial displacements at 90° and 30° of knee flexion. The mean value is shown, ± 1 standard error of the mean (SEM). Percentage values are given for 90° of flexion. No statistical difference was found between 90° and 30° or between 1 and 5 mm of displacement using the Welch modification of the Student t test (P > .05). (Redrawn from Butler, D. L.; Noyes, F. R.; Grood, E. S.: Ligamentous restraints to anterior-posterior drawer in the human knee. A biomechanical study. J Bone Joint Surg Am 62:259–270, 1980.)

the last 5 conditioning tests. Then, baseline tests were done at both knee flexion angles. A ligament was cut and the test repeated. The restraint due to the cut ligament was calculated to be the decrease that occurred in the joint restraining moment compared with the moment determined in the test prior to the ligament sectioning. This process was repeated after cutting other structures until the restraining moments due to all of the ligamentous and capsular structures had been measured. The medial and lateral tests were performed in 16 knees obtained from 11 cadavers 18 to 55 years old (mean, 36.8 yr).

In six other cadaver lower limbs, the three-dimensional motion of the knee joint was measured during the clinical examination for medial and lateral joint opening. The motions were determined first in the intact knee and then after a collateral ligament was sectioned to measure the increase in joint opening. The opposite collateral ligament was then sectioned and the increase in joint opening documented. The goals were to determine the actual motions produced in uninjured knees during a clinical examination and to evaluate the change in joint opening that occurred with cutting each collateral ligament. The knee motions were measured using the instrumented kinetic chain[55] (Fig. 3–24), which was positioned across the knee on the lateral side. The leg was positioned over the side of a table. The joint line was palpated with one hand while a force was applied at the ankle with the other hand. The force applied was not measured in order to conduct the examination in the normal

manner. In order to make these measurements, it was necessary to know the position of the ends of the instrumented chain with respect to the femur and tibia. These positions were established by performing a three-dimensional analysis using biplane radiographs.[7] Tests for reproducibility demonstrated that translational and rotational motions could be measured within ±0.5 mm and ±0.5°, respectively.

The ligaments and capsular structures studied were the ACL, PCL, superficial parallel fibers of the MCL, the FCL, the popliteus musculotendinous unit including the popliteofibular ligament (POP), the medial and lateral halves of the capsule (subdivided into anterior, middle, and posterior thirds), and the femorotibial portion of the ITB. The middle third of the medial capsule was considered to be the deep fibers of the MCL described by others.[54,59] The posterior third included the complex of capsular structures previously detailed[22,59] and the remaining portion of the medial portion of the capsule extending to the midpopliteal region (including the oblique popliteal ligament). The lateral half of the capsule was divided into the anterior third (from the lateral margin of the patellar tendon to Gerdy's tubercle), the middle third (from Gerdy's tubercle to just anterior to the FCL), and the posterior third (the popliteus muscle-tendon-ligament unit and the rest of the capsule extending back to the midpopliteal region).

Results

The results of a typical test on an intact knee and then after sectioning the MCL are shown in Figure 3–25. The curve marked "Intact" represents behavior after conditioning but before ligaments were sectioned. The restraining moment was greater during loading (*upper curve*) than during unloading (*lower curve*) owing to the viscoelastic properties of the ligaments.

During clinical testing in which varus and valgus forces of 45 N are applied at the ankle, a moment of approximately 18 Nm is produced at the knee. These moments produced a medial and lateral joint opening in the knee shown in Figure 3–26. When the MCL was cut (*"MCL CUT" curve*) and a valgus moment applied, the medial opening increased approximately 3 mm. The secondary restraints blocked further joint opening, because they were sufficient to resist the small forces typically induced during a clinical examination. The restraining moment produced by the MCL alone is shown in Figure 3–26.

Medial Restraints

The ligaments and capsular structures resisting 5 mm of medial joint opening are shown for 5° of flexion in Figure 3–27 and for 25° of flexion in Figure 3–28. The MCL was the primary restraint

TABLE 3–4	Comparison of Secondary Structures at Increased Anterior Displacement*				
	Iliotibial Tract and Band	**Midmedial Capsule**	**Midlateral Capsule**	**Medial Collateral Ligament**	**Fibular Collateral Ligament**
Mean ± SEM (%)	24.8 ± 4.7	22.3 ± 6.9	20.8 ± 5.4	16.3 ± 2.9	12.4 ± 3.3
Minimum (%)	9.8	3.4	1.6	8.1	7.0
Maximum (%)	44.4	43.6	36.9	29.4	25.2

*N = 6, anterior drawer of 12.2–16.3 mm at 90° of knee flexion.
†By Duncan's multiple range test, no statistical difference was found among the percentages for any of the structures shown (P > .05).
SEM, standard error of the mean.

at both knee flexion angles, providing 57.4% ± 3.5% of the total restraining moment at 5° and 78.2% ± 3.7% at 25° of flexion. The increase in contribution with flexion was due primarily to a decrease in the contribution of the posteromedial portion of the capsule, which became increasingly slack as flexion occurred. The anterior and middle parts of the medial half of the capsule provided weak secondary restraint limiting medial joint opening, equivalent to 7.7% ± 1.7% of the total restraint at 5° and to 4.0% ± 0.9% of the total at 25° with 5 mm of opening. The posterior portion of the medial half of the capsule provided 17.5% ± 2.0% of the total restraint at 5° and 5 mm of medial opening. At 25° of flexion, the restraint due to this part of the capsule dropped to 3.6% ± 0.8%. The effect of increasing medial joint opening on the contribution of the MCL is shown in Figure 3–29. At 5° of knee flexion, the contribution of the MCL decreased from 70.0% at 2 mm to 53.2% at 6 mm of opening.

Cruciate Ligaments

The medial restraint provided by the ACL and PCL in combination was 14.8% ± 2.1% of the total at 5° of flexion and 13.4% ± 2.7% at 25°. In nine specimens, the contribution of one cruciate was separated from that of the other (Table 3–6). At 25° flexion,

the PCL accounted for approximately 75% of the combined restraint exerted by the cruciates to medial opening, and the ACL accounted for 25%. This result did not depend on the order of cruciate sectioning. However, at 5° of flexion, the order of cruciate ligament sectioning affected the results. When the PCL was cut first, it accounted for approximately 70% of their combined restraint. When the PCL was cut after the ACL, its contribution was only 20% of their combined restraint. These findings indicate that the cruciates do not function independently of each other when the knee is near full extension.

Lateral Restraints

The average contributions of the lateral ligaments, lateral half of the capsule, and cruciate ligaments to the restraining moment at 5 mm of lateral joint opening are shown in Figure 3–30 at 5° of flexion and in Figure 3–31 at 25° of flexion. The FCL was the primary restraint limiting lateral opening of the joint at both knee flexion angles, providing 54.8% ± 3.8% of the total restraint at 5° of flexion and 69.2% ± 5.4% at 25°. The increased contribution of the FCL with knee flexion was due to a marked decrease in the restraint provided by the posterolateral capsule. There was a large variability in the data for the

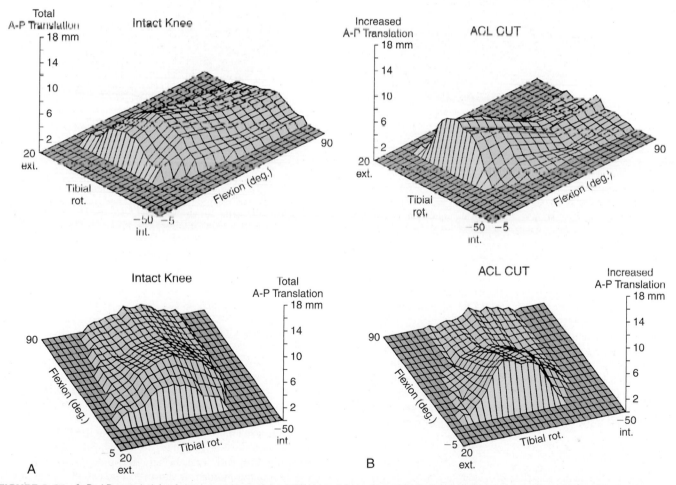

FIGURE 3–21. A–D, AP translation of the human knee joint (100 N load) from 0° to 90° flexion and under the maximal limits of internal and external tibial rotation (5 Nm torque) before and after selective cutting of ligaments. **A,** Intact knee shows maximum translation at low flexion positions and neutral rotation, two views of the same plot for one knee. **B,** Increased translation due to ACL sectioning occurs in low flexion positions, indicating that other soft tissue restraints are functioning at higher knee flexion positions.

Continued

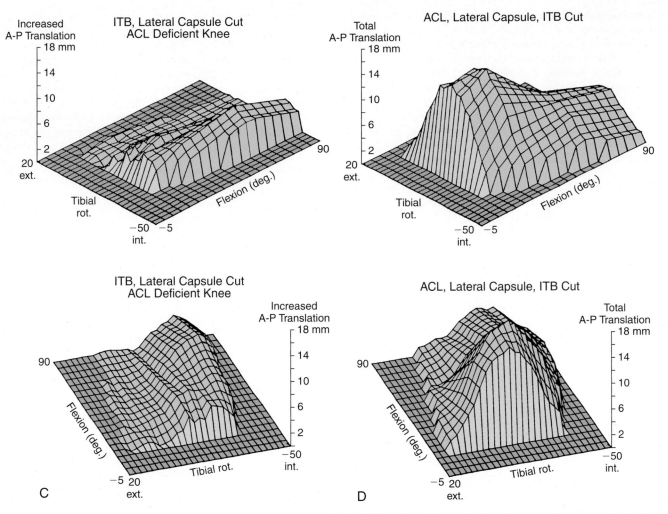

FIGURE 3–21—cont'd. **C,** Further increased translation after sectioning the ITB and lateral capsule. Note that the effect of sectioning these restraints occurs throughout knee flexion, but it is greatest at the higher flexion positions. This knee shows the effect of tight lateral extra-articular restraints because the initial increased translation after ACL sectioning was modest, and the translation markedly increased after the lateral structures were sectioned. **D,** The final total AP translation is shown for the ACL, lateral capsule, and ITB-sectioned knee, demonstrating major increases in translation throughout knee flexion. Increases in internal rotation of a lesser amount are also shown.

FCL, with its contribution ranging from 34.6% to 8.37% at 5° and from 40.5% to 94.7% at 25°. Still, the FCL provided a restraining moment greater than the combined moments of the entire lateral half of the capsule, the ITB, the popliteus tendon, and the cruciate ligaments.

The entire lateral half of the capsule provided 17.2% of the varus restraint at 5° of flexion (see Fig. 3–30) and 8.8% of this restraint at 25° (see Fig. 3–31). The anterior and middle thirds of the lateral half of the capsule contributed only a small secondary restraint, 4.1% ± 1.5% at 5° and 3.7% ± 1.5% at 25°. The posterolateral capsule became slack with flexion, and provided only 5.1% ± 1.3% of the total restraint at 25° of flexion.

Cruciate Ligaments

The cruciate ligaments together provided 22.2% ± 2.6% of the total restraining moment at 5° of flexion and 12.3% ± 4.2% at 25°. There was no effect on the order of cruciate sectioning. However, there was large variation in these data between specimens. The combined restraint of the cruciates ranged from 10.7% to 36.7% at 5° of flexion and from 1.9% to 45.7%

at 25° flexion. The ACL provided the greater portion of the combined restraining effects (Table 3–7) at both knee flexion angles.

Iliotibial Tract, Popliteus Tendon, and Biceps Tendon

The restraints limiting lateral opening caused by the ligament-like actions of the popliteus muscle tendon and ligament and of the femorotibial portion of the ITB were minimum at both knee flexion angles. Therefore, these structures were combined with the caution that the resulting data do not reflect larger in vivo restraining action of either structure owing to added in vivo muscle forces.

The effect of lateral opening on tension in the ITB and in the biceps tendon was investigated by applying a 225-N (50-lb) force to the ITB with a deadweight-and-pulley system. A curve of the restraining moment is shown in Figure 3–32 for an intact knee before and after the tension was applied. The tension produced an increase in the lateral restraining moment. The effect of the tension alone (Fig. 3–33) demonstrated that the applied force produced a nearly constant restraining moment, independent of the amount of lateral joint opening.

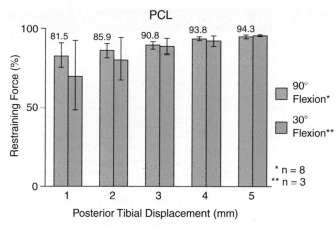

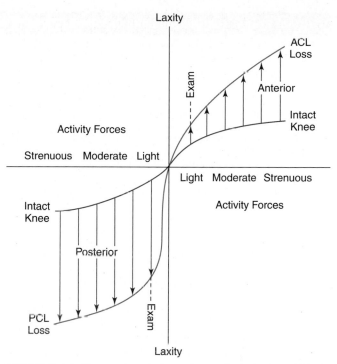

FIGURE 3–22. For posterior drawer in neutral tibial rotation, the percentage of total restraining force is shown for the PCL for increasing posterior tibial displacement at 90° and 30° of knee flexion. Mean values are shown, ⊥ 1 SEM. Percentage values are given for 90° of flexion. No statistically significant difference was observed between 90° and 30° of flexion or between 1 and 5 mm of displacement ($P > .05$). *(Redrawn from Butler, D. L.; Noyes, F. R.; Grood, E. S.: Ligamentous restraints to anterior-posterior drawer in the human knee. A biomechanical study. J Bone Joint Surg Am 62:259–270, 1980.)*

Location of Rotation Axes

The locations of the axes for varus valgus tests on the femur at 5° of flexion are shown in Figure 3–34. The tibia, which moves during the test, is drawn in the neutral position, corresponding to the beginning of the varus-valgus loading test. The rotation axes are located above the joint contact area on the lateral femoral condyle for valgus displacement and above the medial contact area for varus displacement. The lower points represent the rotation axes for the first half of the varus and valgus test (0–2.5 mm of joint opening). The upper points represent the axes for the last half of each test (2.5–5 mm of opening). For the total varus and valgus motion, the axes are located near the midpoints of the lines connecting the lower and upper points.[15]

The reader should note that the positions of the axes above the joint line indicate that a tibiofemoral sliding motion occurs during the loading test. The tibia slides laterally during a valgus test in the same direction as the applied force. The opposite sliding motion occurs during a varus test as the tibia moves medially. The proximal movement of the instant center reflects an increase in the amount of medial-lateral shear movement for each degree of varus-valgus rotation during the test. The increase in the amount of shear movement per degree of rotation occurs when the rotational stiffness of the joint increases more rapidly than its shear stiffness.[15]

FIGURE 3–23. Changes in anterior and posterior laxity in one knee specimen before and after loss of the cruciate ligaments. The laxities are shown for increasing activity force. Note the small increase in anterior laxity for a clinical anterior drawer test (Exam) performed with a forward pull. A large increase in laxity occurs for posterior drawer when the PCL is cut. *(From Butler, D. L.; Noyes, F. R.; Grood, E. S.: Ligamentous restraints to anterior-posterior drawer in the human knee. A biomechanical study. J Bone Joint Surg Am 62:259–270, 1980.)*

Joint Motions during Clinical Examination

The increases in joint opening after the collateral ligaments were sectioned are shown in Table 3–8. The increases in motion after cutting the FCL during varus testing were 0.84 ± 0.5 mm at 5° of flexion and 2.56 ± 0.8 mm at 25° of flexion. The greater amount of joint opening with flexion was explained by the loss of the restraint provided by the posterior portion of the capsule and the increase in the contribution of the FCL. However, the increases in motion at both knee flexion angles were small owing to the influence of the secondary restraints under the low forces applied during the clinical examination.

The increases in medial joint opening after the MCL was sectioned during valgus testing were larger. This was due to the larger contribution to varus-valgus restraint provided by the MCL in comparison with that provided by the FCL. The largest increase

TABLE 3–5 Comparison of Secondary Structures at Increased Posterior Displacement*					
	Posterolateral Capsule and Popliteus Tendon[†]	Medial Collateral Ligament	Posterior Medial Capsule	Fibular Collateral Ligament	Mid-Medial Capsule
Mean ± SEM (%)	58.2 ± 10.1	15.7 ± 5.2	6.9 ± 3.2	6.3 ± 4.7	6.2 ± 2.4
Minimum (%)	36.7	5.6	0	0	0
Maximum (%)	82.1	29.7	14.5	20.4	11.5

*$N = 4$; posterior drawer of 19.0–25.0 mm at 90° of knee flexion.
[†]By Duncan's multiple range test, only the posterolateral capsule and popliteus tendon were statistically different from all other structures ($P < .05$). Sectioned from femur, includes popliteofibular ligament.
SEM, standard error of the mean.

Critical Points LIGAMENTOUS AND CAPSULAR RESTRAINTS RESISTING MEDIAL AND LATERAL JOINT OPENING

The ligaments and capsular structures studied were the ACL, PCL, superficial parallel fibers of the MCL, the FCL, the popliteus musculotendinous unit (including the POP), the medial and lateral halves of the capsule (subdivided into anterior, middle, and posterior thirds), and the femorotibial portion of the ITB.

The middle third of the medial capsule was considered to be the deep fibers of the MCL.

The posterior third included the complex of capsular structures and the remaining portion of the medial portion of the capsule extending to the midpopliteal region (including the oblique popliteal ligament).

The lateral half of the capsule was divided into the anterior third (from the lateral margin of the patellar tendon to Gerdy's tubercle), the middle third (from Gerdy's tubercle to just anterior to the FCL), and the posterior third (the popliteus muscle-tendon-ligament unit and the rest of the capsule extending back to the midpopliteal region).

The MCL is the primary restraint to medial joint opening, providing 57% of the total restraining moment at 5° of flexion and 78% at 25° of flexion. The increase in contribution with flexion is due to a decrease in the contribution of the posteromedial portion of the capsule, which becomes increasingly slack as flexion occurs.

The medial restraint provided by the ACL and PCL in combination is 15% of the total at 5° of flexion and 13% at 25° of flexion.

The FCL is the primary restraint to lateral joint opening, providing 55% of the total restraint at 5° of flexion and 70% at 25° of flexion. The increased contribution of the FCL with knee flexion is due to a marked decrease in the restraint provided by the posterolateral capsule.

The cruciate ligaments together provide 22% of the total lateral restraining moment at 5° of flexion and 12% at 25° of flexion.

The restraints limiting lateral opening caused by the popliteus muscle tendon and ligament and of the femorotibial portion of the ITB are minimal at both knee flexion angles.

Only small joint openings may be demonstrated on clinical examination, even when the medial or lateral primary restraint is ruptured. A 5- to 8-mm increase measured clinically after an acute injury indicates significant collateral ligament injury, including the secondary restraints.

Rather than use grades to classify the injury, it is more accurate to define the degrees of injury as first, second, or third and then estimate the millimeters of increased joint opening at 5° and 25° of flexion.

The amount of medial or lateral joint opening detected upon clinical examination is only qualitative. The clinician should place a finger at the joint line to estimate the millimeters of joint opening and compare the finding with the opposite knee. If axial rotation of the tibia occurs owing to inadvertent rotation of the leg during the examination, the examiner may overestimate the amount of joint opening.

In cases of ACL rupture, the cradled position (holding the lower leg above the table) to induce varus or valgus tests should be avoided. The knee should be examined with the thigh supported by the examination table in a reduced position in which the weight of the leg prevents the anterior tibial subluxation.

ACL, anterior cruciate ligament; FCL, fibular collateral ligament; ITB, iliotibial band; MCL, medial collateral ligament; PCL, posterior cruciate ligament; POP, popliteofibular ligament.

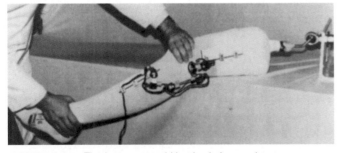

FIGURE 3–24. The instrumented kinetic chain, used to measure three-dimensional joint motion, is shown mounted across the knee on a cadaver lower limb. Each end of the chain is attached to a mounting platform made from pins 3.18 mm (1/8 inch) in diameter. The platforms are attached securely to each bone by three pins that pass through the skin, underlying muscle, and bone. The femur is attached to an angle plate by means of a rod cemented in the medullary canal and a mobile ball-and-socket joint that simulates the hip. The angle plate is secured to a table with C-clamps.

measured in medial joint opening was 5.5 mm in one knee at 30° of flexion; however, the average increase was less than 5 mm. Therefore, only small joint openings may be demonstrated on clinical examination even when the medial or lateral primary restraint is ruptured. A 5- to 8-mm increase measured clinically after an acute injury indicates significant collateral ligament injury, including the secondary restraints. The concept of a "grade I laxity" (defined as an up to 5-mm increase in medial or lateral joint opening) as not representing a significant injury is not supported by these data. This raises the need to carefully evaluate any increase in joint opening, because this represents significant damage to the

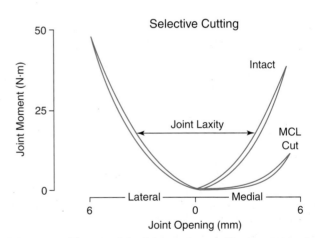

FIGURE 3–25. The restraining joint moment, in Newton-meters, is shown for a typical intact knee and for the same knee after selective cutting of the MCL. The test starts at the neutral position (0) with the knee intact. Six millimeters of medial opening is produced at a constant rate during 1 second. The knee then is returned to neutral and the same amount of lateral opening is produced. When the test is repeated after cutting the MCL the restraining moment to medial opening is markedly reduced, but there is no change during lateral opening. *(From Grood, E. S.; Noyes, F. R.; Butler, D. L.; Suntay, W. J.: Ligamentous and capsular restraints preventing straight medial and lateral laxity in intact human cadaver knees. J Bone Joint Surg Am 63:1257–1269, 1981.)*

restraining function of a primary collateral ligament. The treatment aspects of acute injuries to the medial and lateral knee ligaments are discussed in Chapters 22, Posterolateral Ligament Injuries: Diagnosis, Operative Techniques, and Clinical Outcomes,

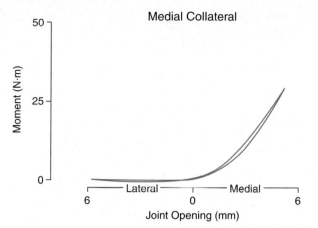

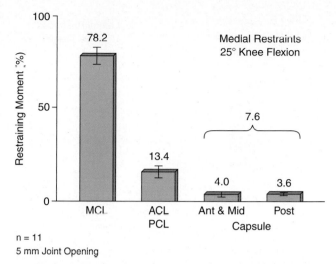

FIGURE 3–26. The curve for the restraining moment of the MCL alone versus joint opening. This curve was obtained by subtracting the curve after the L was cut from the curve for the intact knee shown in Figure 3–25. *(From Grood, E. S.; Noyes, F. R.; Butler, D. L.; Suntay, W. J.: Ligamentous and capsular restraints preventing straight medial and lateral laxity in intact human cadaver knees. J Bone Joint Surg Am 63:1257–1269, 1981.)*

n = 11
5 mm Joint Opening

FIGURE 3–28. The percent restraining contributions of the medial structures at 5 mm of opening and 5° of flexion. *(Redrawn from Grood, E. S.; Noyes, F. R.; Butler, D. L.; Suntay, W. J.: Ligamentous and capsular restraints preventing straight medial and lateral laxity in intact human cadaver knees. J Bone Joint Surg Am 63:1257–1269, 1981.)*

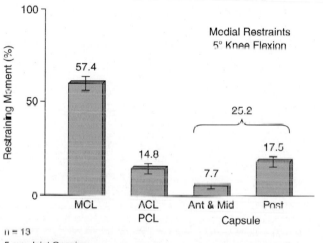

n = 13
5 mm Joint Opening

FIGURE 3–27. The average percent contributions to the medial restraints by the ligaments and capsule at 5 mm of medial joint opening and 5° of flexion. The *error bars* represent ± 1 SEM. *(Redrawn from Grood, E. S.; Noyes, F. R.; Butler, D. L.; Suntay, W. J.: Ligamentous and capsular restraints preventing straight medial and lateral laxity in intact human cadaver knees. J Bone Joint Surg Am 63:1257–1269, 1981.)*

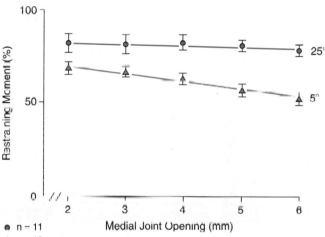

● n = 11
▲ n = 13

FIGURE 3–29. The percent contribution of the MCL to the restraints limiting medial joint opening in the range of 2–6 mm. The decrease with joint opening at 5° is statistically significant ($P < .005$; $r = 0.419$; $N = 65$). *(From Grood, E. S.; Noyes, F. R.; Butler, D. L.; Suntay, W. J.: Ligamentous and capsular restraints preventing straight medial and lateral laxity in intact human cadaver knees. J Bone Joint Surg Am 63:1267–1269, 1981.)*

and 24, Medial and Posteromedial Ligament Injuries: Diagnosis, Operative Techniques, and Clinical Outcomes. Table 3–9 shows the traditional classification system of the American Medical Association for medial and lateral ligament injury. A second-degree injury has only a few millimeters of joint opening, which is barely discernible. An increase up to 5 mm would represent a third-degree injury. Rather than use grades to classify the injury, it is more accurate to define the degrees of injury as first, second, or third and then estimate the millimeters of increased joint opening at 5° and 25° of flexion. Sequential increases of even 3 mm (rather than 5 mm) have important implications of injury to additional ligament structures that, in turn, effect treatment options.

A large amount of out-of-plane tibial rotation occurred during the clinical examination. The amount of axial rotation was typically greater than the total amount of medial-lateral joint

TABLE 3–6 Percentage of Restraining Moment Due to the Cruciate Ligaments for Medial Joint Opening*

Ligament	5° Knee Flexion PCL Cut before ACL (N = 3)	5° Knee Flexion PCL Cut after ACL (N = 6)	25° Knee Flexion (N = 9)
ACL	5.0 ± 2.6	12.0 ± 2.9	2.4 ± 0.6
PCL	10.2 ± 1.6	2.5 ± 0.8	7.8 ± 2.5
Both	15.2 ± 3.1	14.5 ± 3.0	12.2 ± 2.6

*Mean total medial restraining moment ± 1 SEM.
ACL, anterior cruciate ligament; PCL, posterior cruciate ligament.

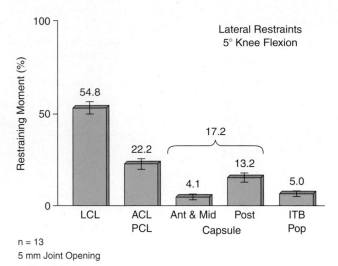

n = 13
5 mm Joint Opening

FIGURE 3–30. The average percent contribution to the lateral restraints by the ligaments and capsule at 5 mm of lateral joint opening and 5° of knee flexion. The error bars indicate ± 1 SEM. There was no tension on the ITB proximal to the lateral femoral condyle in these preparations. *(Redrawn from Grood, E. S.; Noyes, F. R.; Butler, D. L.; Suntay, W. J.: Ligamentous and capsular restraints preventing straight medial and lateral laxity in intact human cadaver knees. J Bone Joint Surg Am 63:1257–1269, 1981.)*

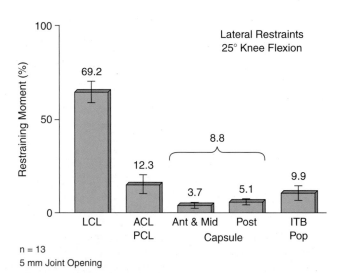

n = 13
5 mm Joint Opening

FIGURE 3–31. The percent contribution of the lateral structures at 5 mm of lateral joint opening and 25° of knee flexion. *(Redrawn from Grood, E. S.; Noyes, F. R.; Butler, D. L.; Suntay, W. J.: Ligamentous and capsular restraints preventing straight medial and lateral laxity in intact human cadaver knees. J Bone Joint Surg Am 63:1257–1269, 1981.)*

TABLE 3–7 Percentage of Restraining Moment Due to the Cruciate Ligaments for Lateral Joint Opening*		
Ligament	5° Knee Flexion	25° Knee Flexion
ACL	19.7 ± 2.7	10.3 ± 4.1
PCL	2.7 ± 0.7	4.1 ± 1.1
Both	22.4 ± 3.0	14.4 ± 4.7

*$N = 11$. Mean of total lateral restraint ± 1 SEM.
ACL, anterior cruciate ligament; PCL, posterior cruciate ligament.

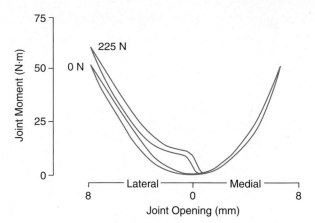

FIGURE 3–32. The effect of applying a 225-N force to the iliotibial tract. The force increases the lateral restraint (joint moment) and decreases lateral joint opening. *(From Grood, E. S.; Noyes, F. R.; Butler, D. L.; Suntay, W. J.: Ligamentous and capsular restraints preventing straight medial and lateral laxity in intact human cadaver knees. J Bone Joint Surg Am 63:1257–1269, 1981.)*

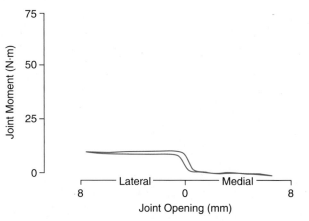

FIGURE 3–33. Difference curve shows the isolated lateral restraining effect of the force applied to the iliotibial tract. Note that the restraining action is independent of the amount of joint opening. *(From Grood, E. S.; Noyes, F. R.; Butler, D. L.; Suntay, W. J.: Ligamentous and capsular restraints preventing straight medial and lateral laxity in intact human cadaver knees. J Bone Joint Surg Am 63:1257–1269, 1981.)*

opening. In one knee, the joint opening (varus-valgus combined) near full extension was 2.5 mm and was accompanied by 4.5° of axial tibial rotation. At 30° flexion, the joint opening was 6.5 mm and was accompanied by 8.2° of axial tibial rotation.

The cruciate ligaments act as secondary restraints during medial and lateral opening. If one of the collateral ligaments and associate capsule is ruptured, then the cruciate ligaments become primary restraints. Because the cruciates are located in the center of the knee, close to the center of rotation, the moment arms are about one third of those of the collateral ligaments. Therefore, to produce restraining moments equal to the collateral ligaments, the cruciates have to provide a force three times larger than that of the collaterals.

The ITB functions as a single unit; when removed from its proximal pelvic attachments, the femorotibial portion becomes slack and incapable of restraining lesser amounts of lateral opening. The major function of the proximal muscle fibers appears to be the transmission of the tension maintaining a tautness of the ITB.[15] There appears to be two main sources of tension in the tract[23]:

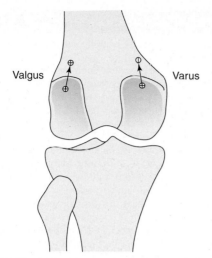

FIGURE 3–34. The instant centers for one-plane varus and valgus displacements of the knee at 5° of flexion. The instant centers are above the joint line, indicating a sliding motion at the tibiofemoral contact region. During valgus displacement, the instant center is on the lateral side; during varus displacement, it is on the medial side. The *arrows* indicate that the instant centers move proximally as the medial and lateral joint openings increase. (*From Grood, E. S.; Noyes, F. R.; Butler, D. L.; Suntay, W. J.: Ligamentous and capsular restraints preventing straight medial and lateral laxity in intact human cadaver knees. J Bone Joint Surg Am 63:1257–1269, 1981.*)

TABLE 3–8 Increase in Joint Opening after Sectioning of the Collateral Ligaments*

	Mean ± Standard Deviation (mm)	Range (mm)
Lateral		
5° flexion	0.84 ± 0.46	0.3–1.3
25° flexion	2.56 ± 0.80	1.7–3.7
Medial		
5° flexion	1.74 ± 0.69	0.4–2.3
25° flexion	3.90 ± 1.13	2.0–5.5

*$N = 5$. All numbers are in millimeters of joint opening; 1 mm is equivalent to approximately 1° of tibial angulation.

TABLE 3–9 Classification System of the American Medical Association

Sprain	Symptom	Signs	Tear Fibers
First degree	Mild	None	Minor
Second degree	Moderate	Slight abnormal motion	Partial
Third degree	Severe	Abnormal motion (3–15 mm)	Complete

Increase in medial-lateral joint opening (added by other investigators): Grade 1 (0–5 mm), Grade 2 (6–10 mm), Grade 3 (11–15 mm).

the passive ligament-like tension between the iliac and the femoral insertions of this structure and the active muscle forces transmitted by the tract. The passive ligament-like tension should increase during lateral joint opening. The ilium-to-tibia distance is so long, however, that lateral joint opening of a few millimeters would not be expected to produce much additional tension in the tract.[15]

Conclusions

The amount of medial or lateral joint opening detected upon clinical examination is only qualitative. The clinician should place a finger at the joint line to estimate the millimeters of joint opening and compare the finding with the opposite knee. If axial rotation of the tibia occurs because of inadvertent rotation of the leg during the examination, the examiner may overestimate the amount of joint opening. Associated internal or external tibial rotation may be falsely interpreted as additional medial or lateral joint opening. The amount of medial or lateral joint opening should always be measured during arthroscopy with the gap test to verify the preoperative diagnosis.

Recognition of axial rotation is especially important when assessing medial ligament injuries. Two types of tests have been described: one in which only an abduction moment is used for medial joint opening and a second type in which external rotation is produced by abducting and externally rotating the leg with the femur held stationary. The first test of medial joint opening more accurately assesses medial ligament damage and allows a diagnosis of ligament and capsular injury because it reproduces the known restraining function of structures proven under in vitro conditions. The second test, which allows a coupled medial joint opening with abduction and anterior tibial translation, may be used when there is an associated ACL rupture. The true millimeters of medial joint opening may be difficult to estimate when a coupled external rotation and anterior translation occurs.

In cases of ACL rupture, the cradled position (holding the lower leg above the table) to induce varus or valgus tests should be avoided. With the leg elevated, an anterior tibial displacement occurs.[35] The joint is partially subluxated and a medial to lateral rocking motion can be obtained that may be misinterpreted as increased medial or lateral joint opening. To prevent this, the knee should be examined with the thigh supported by the examination table in a reduced position in which the weight of the leg prevents the anterior tibial subluxation.

FUNCTION OF MEDIAL AND POSTEROMEDIAL LIGAMENTS IN ACL-DEFICIENT KNEES

The motion limits in normal knees and ACL-deficient cadaveric limbs were studied to define the role of the medial ligamentous structures in limiting anterior translation, abduction (degrees of medial joint opening), and external and internal tibial rotation.[18] The results provide a scientific basis for clinical tests for the diagnosis of combined ACL-MCL ruptures. A six-DOF instrumented spatial linkage at the knee joint was used to measure the motion limits under defined loading conditions using the techniques previously published.[55] The forces and moments in the experiment were: 100 N for anterior and posterior motion limits, 15 Nm for abduction-adduction limits, and 5 Nm for internal-external tibial rotation limits. After the motion limits were determined in the intact cadaveric knee, the ACL, MCL, and PMC were sectioned in different patterns to determine function when cut alone or after one of the other ligament structures. The ligaments cut were the ACL, superficial long fibers of the MCL (including deep medial one third meniscofemoral but not meniscotibial), and the entire PMC, including the posterior oblique portion.

The increases in motion limits are shown in Table 3–10. The changes in the anterior translation limits after the ligament

Critical Points FUNCTION OF MEDIAL AND POSTEROMEDIAL LIGAMENTS IN ACL-DEFICIENT KNEES

The motion limits in normal and ACL-deficient cadaveric limbs were studied to define the role of the medial ligamentous structures in limiting anterior translation, abduction (degrees or medial joint opening), and external and internal tibial rotation.

ACL sectioning alone allows only small increases in internal tibial rotation and no increases in external tibial rotation. When all medial structures (ACL intact) are sectioned, the abduction limit increases to only about 7°, or 7 to 8 mm of medial joint opening. This suggests that partial to complete ACL tears are required for further increases to occur in medial joint opening.

The MCL (and deep medial capsule) limits anterior tibial translation as a secondary restraint after the ACL is ruptured. A combined ACL-MCL injury has equal anterior translation at 30° and 90°, indicating the Lachman and 90° anterior drawer tests will show similar increases in anterior tibial translation, instead of only the major increase at 30° knee flexion.

In the ACL- and MCL-deficient knee, the Lachman test will show an absence of the normal coupled internal tibial rotation in contrast to the coupled rotation in the normal knee and the ACL-deficient knee.

The MCL is the primary restraint for external tibial rotation; however, the increase is small (4.6°–8.7° from 30°–90° of flexion). The increase in external rotation doubles when the PMC is also sectioned. Further increases in external rotation to approximately 15° occur when the ACL is also sectioned. The results validate the importance of performing the dial tibial rotation test to determine anterior subluxation of the medial tibial plateau with medial ligament injuries.

The combined MCL-PMC injury results in increases in external tibial rotation (9° at 30° of flexion), increases in internal tibial rotation (12° at 30° of flexion), and increases in abduction testing at 0° and 30° of flexion (6° and 9°, respectively).

The PMC is an important structure for stabilizing the extended knee under valgus loading (32% of the resistance).

The posterior drawer test for PCL rupture is performed in neutral tibial rotation to determine the maximum posterior tibial translation. When the posterior drawer is repeated in maximal internal rotation (in knees with a PCL rupture), the amount of posterior tibial translation will markedly decrease if the PMC is intact.

ACL, anterior cruciate ligament; MCL, medial collateral ligament; PMC, posterior medial capsule; PCL, posterior cruciate ligament.

---

sectioning procedures are shown in Figure 3–35. The typical pattern of a major increase in anterior translation at low flexion angles as compared with high flexion angles was statistically significant ($P < .001$). Note that subsequent sectioning of the MCL resulted in major increases in anterior translation at high flexion angles, with the amount of anterior translation equal at low flexion angles. This means that major increases in anterior translation at 90° knee flexion indicate that the secondary restraints are also insufficient. When the ACL was intact, there was no increase in anterior translation even when all of the medial ligament structures were sectioned.

TABLE 3–10 Increases in Motion Limits Relative to the Intact Knee That Occurred When the Indicated Structures Were Sectioned*

Limit	0° Flexion	15° Flexion	30° Flexion	60° Flexion	90° Flexion
Anterior (mm)					
ACL	5.8 ± 0.9[†]	9.4 ± 1.0[‡]	8.4 ± 1.9[†]	4.7 ± 2.1[§]	3.5 ± 1.6[§]
ACL & MCL	6.1 ± 2.0[†]	10.0 ± 2.4[†]	11.0 ± 2.9[†]	10.6 ± 3.5[†]	10.1 ± 4.2[§]
MCL & PMC	-0.5 ± 1.1	-0.3 ± 1.1	-0.5 ± 0.9	-0.1 ± 0.7	0.4 ± 1.1
ACL & MCL & PMC	8.7 ± 3.2[‡]	12.8 ± 4.3[‡]	14.4 ± 4.9[‡]	14.6 ± 5.7[‡]	12.5 ± 5.6[†]
External rotation (°)					
ACL	1.2 ± 1.4	0.7 ± 0.8	0.7 ± 0.6	0.7 ± 0.4	0.5 ± 0.5
MCL	2.5 ± 1.1[§]	3.3 ± 1.5[§]	4.6 ± 1.3[†]	8.0 ± 2.2[†]	8.7 ± 3.2[§]
PMC	1.6 ± 0.9	1.2 ± 1.2	0.9 ± 1.7	0.8 ± 2.5	0.8 ± 2.4
ACL & MCL	2.3 ± 0.4[‡]	3.2 ± 1.1[†]	4.6 ± 1.6[†]	7.3 ± 2.3[†]	7.5 ± 2.0[†]
MCL & PMC	6.8 ± 2.5[§]	7.2 ± 1.9[†]	9.0 ± 2.0[†]	13.6 ± 3.0[†]	15.0 ± 3.6[†]
ACL & MCL & PMC	10.9 ± 5.8[†]	12.7 ± 6.2[†]	14.7 ± 6.5[†]	16.7 ± 5.9[‡]	15.3 ± 5.1[‡]
Internal rotation (°)					
ACL	2.9 ± 1.0[†]	2.2 ± 0.9[§]	0.8 ± 0.9	0.5 ± 0.8	2.0 ± 2.6
MCL	0.5 ± 0.5	1.4 ± 0.7	2.1 ± 1.2	1.8 ± 0.3[‡]	1.5 ± 0.4[†]
PMC	3.4 ± 2.4	4.0 ± 2.3	2.7 ± 1.7	1.3 ± 0.7	1.4 ± 1.4
ACL & MCL	3.6 ± 1.5[§]	3.5 ± 1.4[§]	2.3 ± 1.3	2.4 ± 0.8[†]	2.1 ± 1.4
MCL & PMC	6.3 ± 5.8	11.6 ± 3.4[†]	9.3 ± 2.2[†]	3.9 ± 2.4	2.9 ± 1.5
ACL & MCL & PMC	12.7 ± 6.5[†]	13.2 ± 3.3[‖]	10.4 ± 2.1[‖]	4.5 ± 1.1[‖]	3.3 ± 1.2[‡]
Abduction (°)					
ACL	0.4 ± 0.2[§]	0.8 ± 0.5	0.6 ± 0.6	0.1 ± 0.3	0.0 ± 0.3
MCL	1.5 ± 0.9	3.3 ± 0.8[†]	4.1 ± 0.8[‡]	4.5 ± 0.8[‡]	3.8 ± 1.0[†]
PMC	0.4 ± 0.3	0.2 ± 0.6	0.4 ± 0.3	0.0 ± 0.9	0.4 ± 0.5
ACL & MCL	2.5 ± 1.1[§]	5.4 ± 2.6[§]	7.1 ± 3.6[§]	8.1 ± 4.0[§]	7.1 ± 2.8[§]
MCL & PMC	4.6 ± 1.9[§]	6.0 ± 1.4[†]	6.6 ± 0.9[‖]	5.8 ± 1.2[‡]	4.8 ± 1.1[†]
ACL & MCL & PMC	9.1 ± 4.6[†]	12.7 ± 4.8[‡]	14.4 ± 5.0[‡]	14.2 ± 4.5[‡]	12.1 ± 4.0[‡]

*Means, standard deviations.
[†]$P < .01$.
[‡]$P < .001$.
[§]$P < .05$.
[‖]$P < .0001$.
ACL, anterior cruciate ligament (6 donors); MCL, superficial medial collateral ligament (6 donors); PMC, posteromedial capsule, including the posterior oblique ligament (6 donors); ACL & MCL (6 donors); MCL & PMC (6 donors); ACL & MCL & PMC (9 donors).

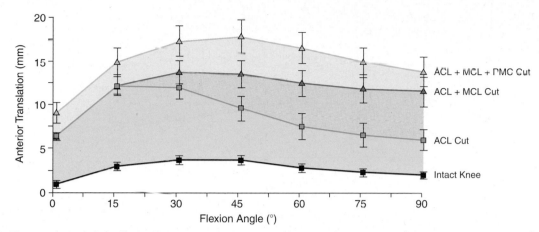

FIGURE 3–35. The anterior translation limits (*bottom curve*) when a 100-N anterior force was applied to control intact knees (11 donors). Sectioning the ACL (ACL Cut) increased the anterior limits more at 15° and 30° of flexion than at 90° of flexion (6 donors). When the superficial MCL was subsequently cut (ACL + MCL Cut), the anterior limit further increased in the flexed knee (6 donors). Subsequent cutting of the posteromedial capsule (PMC; *top curve*) produced an additional 2.4–4 mm increase over that for the ACL and MCL injury (9 donors). *Error bars* show the SEM. *(Modified from Haimes, J. L.; Wroble, R. H.; Grood, E. S.; Noyes, F. R · Role of the medial structures in the intact and anterior cruciate ligament–deficient knee. Limits of motion in the human knee. Am J Sports Med 22:402–409, 1994.)*

The changes in coupled internal and external tibial rotation during the anterior translation and abduction loading tests are shown in Table 3–11. The anterior loading produced a coupled internal tibial rotation, as expected. The coupled internal tibial rotation decreased after the ACL was sectioned, but still remained. However, sectioning the MCL produced a loss of the coupled internal rotation. This indicates the importance of the MCL in maintaining a rotation point for the coupled internal rotation to occur that is lost with MCL insufficiency, as already discussed. In pivot shift tests with a combined ACL-MCL injury, the magnitude of anterior tibial subluxation results in a grade III pivot shift (tibial impingement). In the abduction (valgus) test for medial joint opening, as long as there is an intact ACL, a coupled internal tibial rotation occurs. However, with an ACL and MCL injury, this internal tibial rotation with abduction is lost and there is an associated increase in external tibial rotation. These subtle changes in internal tibial rotation with combined ACL-MCL injuries are important, because the obligatory coupled rotation of anterior translation–internal tibial rotation is lost, which can be detected on clinical examination.

The increase in the external tibial rotation limit with ligament sectioning is shown in Figure 3–36. Sectioning of the MCL produced major increases in external tibial rotation that increased with each subsequent ligament sectioning. The MCL acted as the primary restraint to external tibial rotation at all flexion angles. Cutting just the PMC (ACL, MCL intact) did not result in any increase in external tibial rotation (see Table 3–10).

The increase in the internal tibial rotation limit is shown in Figure 3–37. Note that the internal tibial rotation limit increases in the intact knee with knee flexion. ACL sectioning produced small increases in internal rotation (<3°) at 0° and 15° knee flexion (see Table 3–10). Sectioning the PMC alone had no effect on internal tibial rotation; however, PMC sectioning after MCL and ACL sectioning produced a major increase in the internal limit from 0° to 45° knee flexion.

The changes in the abduction rotation limits in the intact knee and with ligament sectioning are shown in Figure 3–38. The MCL was the primary restraint; however, the data show only small increases in abduction (medial joint opening) with complete MCL sectioning, with further increases in the motion limits after the PMC was sectioned. The ACL cut allowed for even further increases in abduction, indicating that it is a secondary restraint after the medial ligaments (MCL, PMC) are cut.

The conclusions of this cadaveric study on the function of the ACL and medial ligament structures applied to the clinical diagnosis and function of ligament injuries are

1. ACL sectioning alone allows only small increases in internal tibial rotation and no increases in external tibial rotation. When all medial structures (ACL intact) were sectioned, the abduction limit increased to only about 7°, or 7 to 8 mm of medial joint opening. This suggests that partial to complete ACL tears are required for further increases to occur in medial joint opening (see Table 3–10).
2. The MCL (and deep medial capsule) limits anterior tibial translation as a secondary restraint after the ACL is ruptured. A combined ACL-MCL injury has equal anterior translation at 30° and 90°, indicating the Lachman and 90° anterior drawer tests will show similar increases in anterior tibial translation, instead of only the major increase at 30° knee flexion.

TABLE 3–11   Mean Degrees of Coupled Rotation during Anterior Translation and Abduction Tests for Intact Knees and after Ligament Sectioning*

	Anterior test flexion angle		Abduction test flexion angle		
	30°	**90°**	**0°**	**15°**	**30°**
Intact	−8.6	−10.6	−2.0	4.1	−6.9
ACL	−5.4	−5.0	−3.2	−7.0	−9.1
MCL	−11.7	−14.7	1.4	6.4	5.9
ACL & MCL	0.6	0.0	−0.5	−2.5	−4.2

*Negative numbers represent internal rotation and positive numbers represent external rotation. These numbers are the change in tibial rotation from the position of the tibia in the intact knee during passive flexion to the position of the tibia after application of anterior forces or abduction moments. Intact (11 donors); ACL cut (6 donors); MCL cut (6 donors); ACL & MCL cut (6 donors). ACL, anterior cruciate ligament; MCL, medial collateral ligament.

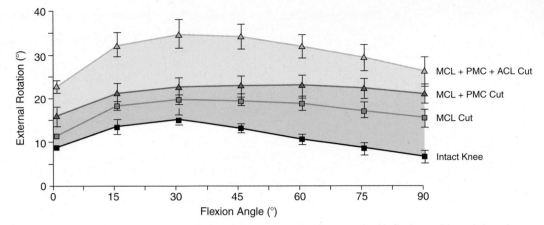

FIGURE 3–36. The external rotation limits in the intact knee (*bottom curve*) first increased with flexion to 30° and then decreased with further flexion (11 donors). Cutting just the superficial MCL (MCL Cut) increased the external rotation limits more in flexion than in extension (16 donors). Further cutting of the PMC (MCL + PMC Cut) produced a further increase in the external limit at all flexion angles, but the increase was again greater in flexion than in extension. Cutting the superficial MCL, the PMC, and the ACL allowed for a large increase in the external limit, particularly from 15° to 45° flexion (*top curve*). (*Modified from Haimes, J. L.; Wroble, R. R.; Grood, E. S.; Noyes, F. R.: Role of the medial structures in the intact and anterior cruciate ligament–deficient knee. Limits of motion in the human knee. Am J Sports Med 22:402–409, 1994.*)

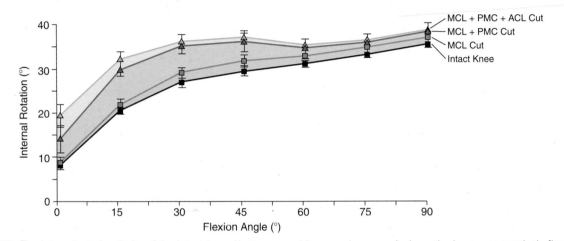

FIGURE 3–37. The internal rotation limits of the intact knee (*bottom curve*) increased progressively as the knee was passively flexed (11 donors). Cutting the superficial MCL (MCL Cut) produced only a small increase in the internal rotation limits (6 donors). Cutting the MCL and PMC (MCL + PMC Cut) caused large increases in the internal rotation limits from 0° to 45° of flexion (6 donors). Cutting the MCL, the PMC, and the ACL (*top curve*) caused similarly large increases in the internal limits from 0° to 45° of flexion relative to the intact knee (6 donors). However, these increases were not significantly different from those seen with the MCL and PMC cut. (*Modified from Haimes, J. L.; Wroble, R. R.; Grood, E. S.; Noyes, F. R.: Role of the medial structures in the intact and anterior cruciate ligament–deficient knee. Limits of motion in the human knee. Am J Sports Med 22:402–409, 1994.*)

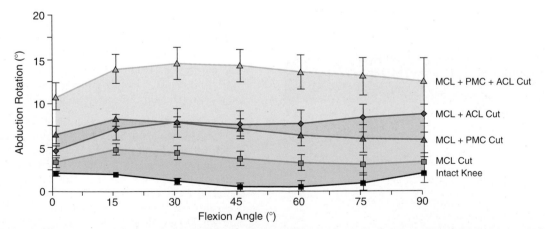

FIGURE 3–38. The abduction rotation limits (valgus opening) of the intact knee (*bottom curve*) (11 donors). Cutting only the MCL (MCL Cut) produced a small increase (approximately 2°–4°) in the abduction limit from 15° to 75° of flexion. Cutting the ACL (MCL + ACL Cut) increased the abduction limit (6 donors). Cutting the PMC in addition to the MCL (MCL + PMC Cut) with the ACL intact allowed for a further small but consistent increase (2°–3°) over the superficial MCL alone (6 donors). When compared with the intact knee, this injury combination increased the abduction limit approximately 6° to 7° at both 15° and 30° of flexion. Subsequently cutting the ACL (*top curve*) caused a large increase in the abduction limits at all flexion angles (9 donors). (*Modified from Haimes, J. L.; Wroble, R. R.; Grood, E. S.; Noyes, F. R.: Role of the medial structures in the intact and anterior cruciate ligament–deficient knee. Limits of motion in the human knee. Am J Sports Med 22:402–409, 1994.*)

3. In the ACL- and MCL-deficient knee, the Lachman test will show an absence of the normal coupled internal tibial rotation in contrast to the coupled rotation in the normal knee and the ACL-deficient knee.
4. The MCL is the primary restraint for external tibial rotation; however, the increase is small (4.6°–8.7° from 30°–90° of flexion). The increase in external rotation doubles when the PMC is also sectioned. Further increases in external rotation to approximately 15° occur when the ACL is also sectioned. The results validate the importance of performing the dial tibial rotation test (see Chapters 20, Function of the Posterior Cruciate Ligament and Posterolateral Ligament Structures, and 22, Posterolateral Ligament Injuries: Diagnosis, Operative Techniques, and Clinical Outcomes) to determine anterior subluxation of the medial tibial plateau with medial ligament injuries.
5. The combined MCL-PMC injury results in increases in external tibial rotation (9° at 30° of flexion), increases in internal tibial rotation (12° at 30° of flexion), and increases in abduction testing at 0° and 30° of flexion (6° and 9°, respectively). The increase in internal tibial rotation was previously recognized by Mueller[30] and is an interesting finding not commonly reported.

The results of the authors' studies are in agreement with recently published data in cadaveric knees. Robinson and coworkers[51] studied the superficial medial collateral ligament (SMCL) and deep medial collateral ligament (DMCL) and the PMC and measured the changes in motion limits under AP drawer, valgus, and internal external rotation loads by sequential MCL cutting in 18 cadaveric knees. These authors reported that the PMC limited valgus, internal rotation, and posterior drawer in extension, resisting 42% of a 150-N drawer force when the tibia was in internal rotation (Figs. 3–39 to 3–42). The SMCL resisted valgus at all angles and was dominant from 30° to 90° of flexion, plus internal rotation in flexion. The DMCL resisted tibial anterior translation of the flexed and externally rotated knee and was a secondary restraint to valgus.

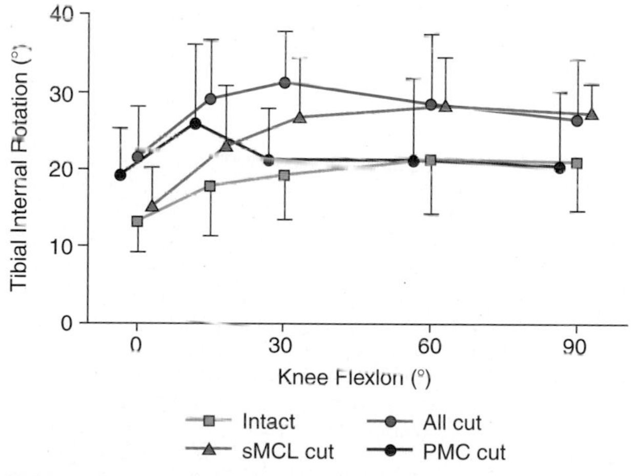

FIGURE 3–39. Tibial internal rotation motion limits with the knee intact ($n = 18$) and cutting the superficial medial collateral ligament (sMCL) alone ($n = 4$), posteromedial capsule (PMC) alone ($n = 4$), and sMCL, deep medial collateral ligament (dMCL), and PMC together ($n = 14$). These data show the reciprocal action of the sMCL and PMC restraining internal rotation at different angles of tibiofemoral flexion. *(From Robinson, J. R.; Bull, A. M.; Thomas, R. R.; Amis, A. A.: The role of the medial collateral ligament and posteromedial capsule in controlling knee laxity.* Am J Sports Med *34:1815–1823, 2006.)*

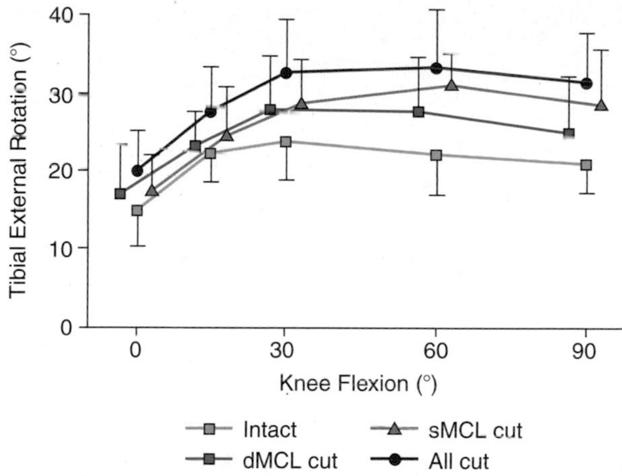

FIGURE 3–40. Tibial external rotation motion limits with the knee intact ($n = 18$) as well as changes caused by cutting either the superficial medial collateral ligament (sMCL) alone ($n = 4$) or the deep medial collateral ligament (dMCL) alone ($n = 6$) or after cutting both the whole MCL and the posteromedial capsule (PMC; $n = 14$). *(From Robinson, J. R.; Bull, A. M.; Thomas, R. R.; Amis, A. A.: The role of the medial collateral ligament and posteromedial capsule in controlling knee laxity.* Am J Sports Med *34:1815–1823, 2006.)*

These authors reaffirmed that the PMC is an important structure for stabilizing the extended knee under valgus loading (32% of the resistance). With knee flexion, the PMC slackens and the MCL becomes the dominant restraint. In the extended knee, with posterior drawer and internal rotation, the PMC tightens based on its attachments at the femur (just posterior to the adductor tubercle) and the posteromedial aspect of the tibia resisting 42% of the posterior load.

In the bumper model of ligament behavior previously discussed, applying an internal tibial rotation tightens the PMC and the SMCL, thereby increasing their resistance to posterior tibial displacement. The internal tibial rotation also tightens the ITB and the midlateral capsule. In essence, the tibia is placed in a highly constrained position with AP translation blocked by lateral and medial extra-articular structures.

The posterior drawer test for PCL rupture is performed in neutral tibial rotation to determine the maximum posterior tibial translation. When the posterior drawer test is repeated in maximal internal rotation (in knees with a PCL rupture), the amount of posterior tibial translation will markedly decrease if the PMC is intact. This can be used as a test to reaffirm that the medial secondary restraints are disrupted. However, more accurate medial joint opening tests at 5° and 25° of flexion provide the same and frequently more meaningful data.

In regard to the anatomic description in these biomechanical experiments, Robinson and associates[52] dissected the MCL and capsular structures in 20 cadaver knees and reported on the anatomy of the SMCL, DMCL, and PMC. In the PMC, there were oblique fibers, referred to as *capsular condensations*, that attached at the posterior margin of the SMCL femoral attachment at the femoral epicondyle, proceeding in a distal direction to blend in with the capsule and semimembranosus tendon sheath expansions. These capsular fibers tightened with internal tibial rotation, and the entire PMC tightened with knee extension. The authors reported that the three distinct bands corresponding to the posterior oblique ligament (POL) described by Hughston and Eilers[22] could not be identified, preferring instead to use the nomenclature of the PMC.

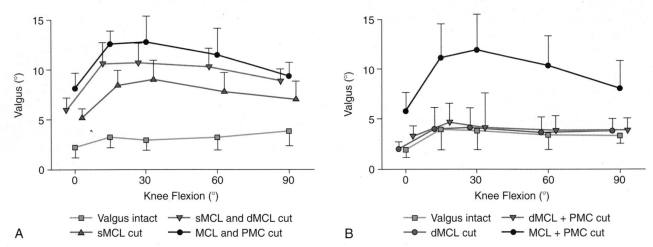

FIGURE 3–41. A, Valgus rotation produced by a 5-Nm moment of the intact knee and after sequential division of the posteromedial structures, superficial collateral ligament (sMCL), then deep medial collateral ligament (dMCL), then posteromedial capsule (PMC; $n = 4$). **B,** Valgus rotation with the knee intact and after sequential division of the posteromedial structures, dMCL, then PMC, then sMCL ($n = 6$). **(A** and **B,** From Robinson, J. R.; Bull, A. M.; Thomas, R. R.; Amis, A. A.: The role of the medial collateral ligament and posteromedial capsule in controlling knee laxity. Am J Sports Med 34:1815–1823, 2006.)

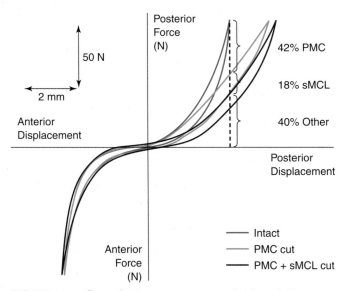

FIGURE 3–42. Force-displacement test: mean load vs. displacement curves for intact, posteromedial capsule (PMC)–deficient, and PMC + superficial medial collateral ligament (sMCL)–deficient knees tested at 0° of flexion with fixed tibial internal rotation. Load share calculated for 100-N posterior displacement force; $n = 4$. (From Robinson, J. R.; Bull, A. M.; Thomas, R. R.; Amis, A. A.: The role of the medial collateral ligament and posteromedial capsule in controlling knee laxity. Am J Sports Med 34:1815–1823, 2006.)

EFFECT OF SECTIONING THE MCL AND THE PMC ON POSTERIOR TIBIAL TRANSLATION

Ritchie and colleagues[49] studied in 14 cadaver knees the contribution of various structures in the PCL-deficient knee in resisting posterior tibial translation.[49] Single-plane posterior drawer tests were performed with the knee in neutral tibial rotation and in 20° of internal tibial rotation. The authors reported that with

Critical Points VARIABILITY BETWEEN CLINICIANS DURING CLINICAL KNEE LIGAMENT TESTING

An investigation was conducted with 11 experienced knee surgeons to determine differences in clinical examination testing techniques, accuracy in estimating knee displacements, and skill in diagnosing specific ligament injuries in knees with multiple abnormal motion limits.

Wide variability existed between examiners in the starting position of knee flexion and tibial rotation for AP displacement during the Lachman test and for the amount of tibial translation and rotation induced.

The starting position for the pivot shift test varied among examiners. As the knee was flexed, varying amounts of anterior tibial translation and internal tibial rotation were produced. Many examiners induced coupled motions of anterior tibial translation and internal tibial rotation to produce anterior tibial subluxation without constraining or enhancing either motion.

Most of the examiners' estimates were within 3 mm of the actual measured values in the laboratory during the medial joint space abduction test. Each examiner performed the tests at a different flexion angle and reached a different final tibiofemoral position in both the intact knee and the ACL/MCL-sectioned knee.

Large variations were found between examiners in the amount of internal and external tibial rotation induced during testing the ACL/MCL-sectioned knee. Each examiner performed the test at a different knee flexion angle and reached a different final rotation position.

Seven of the 11 examiners incorrectly diagnosed an injury to the posterolateral structures after the ACL and MCL were sectioned.

The pivot shift test must be considered qualitative in nature and imprecise in determining the results of ACL reconstructive procedures.

Examination test techniques must be standardized regarding the test conditions so that examiners conduct knee examinations in a similar manner.

The diagnosis of rotatory subluxations is highly subjective and requires a careful assessment of the AP position of the medial and lateral tibial plateaus relative to the femur.

ACL, anterior cruciate ligament; AP, anteroposterior; MCL, medial collateral ligament.

the knee in internal tibial rotation, posterior displacement was significantly less compared with that in neutral rotation when the SMCL was sectioned. The results showed that the SMCL was responsible for a decrease in posterior tibial translation in the PCL-deficient knee and not the PMC, including the POL.

ROLE OF THE POL

Petersen and coworkers,[48] in a cadaveric study using a robotic testing system, examined the restraint of the SMCL, the DMCL, the POL, and the PMC in resisting posterior tibial translation after PCL sectioning. The study reported that the POL has a much larger role than the SMCL and DMCL in resisting posterior tibial translation and internal tibial rotation. It should be noted that these two structures were first sectioned; no studies were done when the POL was sectioned first. This indicates there could be a sectioning artifact introduced in the study. Even so, there are posteromedial oblique capsular fibers from the lateral femoral condyle to the tibia, just posterior to the SMCL, that resist internal tibial rotation and posterior tibial translation (after PCL sectioning). The study concluded that there are discrete oblique fibers that form the middle arm of the POL described by Hughston and Eilers.[22] Of interest in this cadaveric study was the finding that a valgus loading of the knee joint close to knee extension (with PCL-deficiency) produced an increased posterior tibial translation of the medial compartment with absence of the POL and PMC.

Robinson and associates[52] conducted a cadaveric study of the medial and posteromedial structures and could not identify a distinct separate POL structure, but did identify an oblique portion of the PMC where fibers could be tensioned under internal tibial rotation loading. Robinson and coworkers[51] and Haimes and associates[18] studied the contribution of the PMC, which included the POL. Robinson and coworkers[51] reported that the PMC resisted 28% of the posterior tibial load when the tibia rotated freely in the extended knee, which rose to 42% when the tibia was subjected to internal rotation. These authors concluded that the PMC resisted posterior tibial translation close to full extension, and less so with knee flexion, which relaxes the PMC. With knee flexion, the SMCL resisted posterior tibial translation.

In knees with chronic PCL instability and associated medial and posteromedial ligament and capsular injury, the integrity of all the structures should be restored. Specific tests for increased internal tibial rotation using the dial test are performed.

VARIABILITY BETWEEN CLINICIANS DURING CLINICAL KNEE LIGAMENT TESTING

There is a well-appreciated difficulty in quantifying the amount of tibial displacements and rotations in the clinical knee examination, and the potential exists for considerable variability to occur among examiners. For this reason, any attempt to provide objective measurements, such as knee arthrometer or stress radiographs (even with these test limitations), is believed to be more accurate than comparing manual examination results among various clinicians.

An investigation was conducted with 11 experienced knee surgeons to determine differences in clinical examination testing

techniques, accuracy in estimating knee displacements, and skill in diagnosing specific ligament injuries in knees with multiple abnormal motion limits.[36,40] Knee joint positions and abnormal motions were measured in right-left cadaveric knees by a three-dimensional instrumented spatial linkage. A comparison was made of the clinicians' estimate of the knee motion limits and subluxations with the actual measured values. The three-dimensional limits of knee motion were measured in the laboratory under defined loading conditions before and after the clinicians' examination.

AP Displacement

Wide variability existed among examiners in the starting position of knee flexion and tibial rotation for AP displacement during the Lachman test (Fig. 3–43) and for the amount of tibial translation and rotation induced. Whereas some of the clinicians displaced the knee to the maximal displacement limits obtained in the laboratory, others failed to do so by a wide margin. The conclusion was reached that there was a wide variation in the loads applied among the examiners during the tests.

Pivot Shift Testing

The starting position for the pivot shift test varied among examiners, but was typically close to 5° extension (Fig. 3–44). As the knee was flexed, varying amounts of anterior tibial translation and internal tibial rotation were produced. During flexion, the maximal amount of internal tibial rotation was achieved first, followed by the maximal amount of anterior tibial translation. Although the amount of anterior translation of the lateral tibial plateau was similar among examiners, large differences existed among the clinicians (range, 6–16.9 mm) in the amount of maximum anterior translation of the medial tibial plateau. Examiners who produced the greatest amount of internal tibial rotation during the pivot shift test also significantly limited the amount of anterior translation of the medial tibial plateau ($R = -0.79$; $P < .01$).

The maximal amount of anterior tibial translation and the limits to anterior and posterior translation produced by each examiner are shown in Fig. 3–45. The normal and abnormal limits of tibial translation are shown before and after combined ACL and MCL ligament sectioning. The maximal amount of anterior translation (central point) ranged from 10 to 18 mm among examiners, and the maximal amount of anterior subluxation of the lateral tibial plateau ranged from 14 to 19.8 mm.

The mean value for maximal internal tibial rotation induced during the pivot shift test was $15.8 \pm 3.6°$ (range, 11°–24°). Maximal internal rotation occurred at an average knee flexion angle of $15.6° \pm 5.2°$ (range, 5°–23°). The limits to internal and external tibial rotation are shown in Figure 3–46. Two examiners exceeded the normal intact internal tibial rotation limit obtained under 5 Nm of torque. Only a slight increase occurred in the degrees of internal tibial rotation after the ACL and MCL were cut. Increases in external tibial rotation limits were also measured after ACL/MCL sectioning, which occurred during the tibial reduction phase of the pivot shift maneuver.

The tibial reduction phenomenon involved a posterior tibial translation and external tibial rotation. Three examiners (C, F, and I) produced the reduction phase with posterior tibial translation, uncoupling this motion from external tibial rotation.

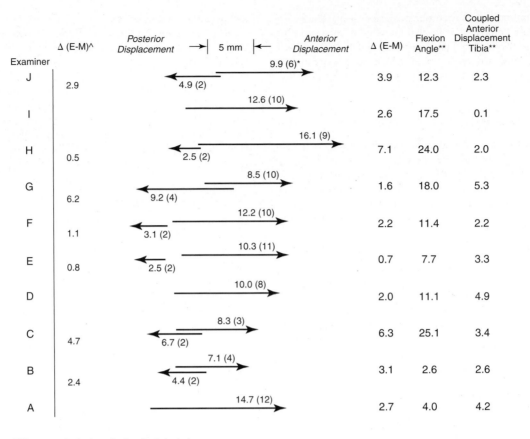

^ISL measured value (examiner's estimated value)
•Δ (E-M) = difference between estimate and measured
** Measured during anterior displacement test

FIGURE 3–43. The *bars* show the instrumented spatial linkage measured values for anterior and posterior displacement for each examiner. The *numbers above* and *below* each *bar* give the measured displacement; the examiner estimated values are given in *parentheses*. Starting position flexion angles and the coupled external rotation for the anterior displacement test are given for each examiner. *(From Noyes, F. R.; Cummings, J. F.; Grood, E. S.; et al.: The diagnosis of knee motion limits, subluxations, and ligament injury. Am J Sports Med 19:163–171, 1991.)*

Four examiners (A, B, C, and F) continued to flex the knee after reduction to about 80° of flexion. Five examiners accentuated the reduction event by producing the maneuver with 20° or less change in knee flexion, which resulted in the steepest decline in the translation and rotation curves.

A few examiners demonstrated variability during the pivot shift test in regard to enhancement of internal tibial rotation (Figs. 3–47 to 3–48). The millimeters of anterior translation of the medial, central, and lateral points varied depending on how the test was performed.

Medial-Lateral Joint Space Opening

During abduction and adduction rotation testing, the examiners were instructed to begin the tests with the femoral condyle in contact with the tibial plateau. Data from the medial joint space abduction test demonstrated that most of the examiners' estimates were within 3 mm of the actual measured values in the laboratory (Fig. 3–49). The starting flexion angle averaged 11.6° (range, 3.1°–21.3°). Each examiner performed the tests at a different flexion angle and reached a different final tibiofemoral position in both the intact knee and the ACL/MCL-sectioned knee (Fig. 3–50).

Internal-External Tibial Rotation

Large variations were found among examiners in the amount of internal and external tibial rotation induced during testing the ACL/MCL-sectioned knee. Although most of the examiners estimated the total amount of internal tibial rotation to within 5° of that measured in the laboratory, only one examiner provided such an estimate for the total amount of external tibial rotation. The knee flexion angle at the start of the test ranged from 1.9° to 35.3°. Each examiner performed the test at a different knee flexion angle and reached a different final rotation position.

Medial-Lateral Compartment Translations during External Tibial Rotation

After sectioning the ACL and MCL, the amount of external tibial rotation increased from 17.8° (intact knee) to 22.1°. Most of the examiners produced an increase in anterior translation of the medial tibial plateau during the external rotation test. The displacement of the medial and lateral tibial plateaus in both the intact and the ACL/MCL-sectioned states are shown in Figure 3–51. The average center of tibial rotation in both states was in the lateral tibiofemoral compartment. The lateral shift in the axis of tibial rotation is demonstrated in Figure 3–51B, along with the increase in anterior displacement (range, 3.0–8.5 mm) of the medial tibial plateau. Seven of the 11 examiners incorrectly diagnosed an injury to the posterolateral structures, even though the lateral tibial plateau did not displace further posteriorly.

Study Limitations and Conclusions

Limitations existed in these studies, including the use of cadaver limbs, which do not represent actual clinical conditions. Although whole lower limbs were used, with the hip replaced with a ball-and-socket joint, the muscles and capsular structures of the hip were removed, which may have affected femoral rotations. The forces or torques applied to the limb by each examiner were not directly measured, but inferred by comparing the joint displacements obtained in the clinical tests with those documented in the laboratory under defined loading conditions. The pivot shift test technique used by many examiners more closely replicated that which would be used while patients are under anesthesia and not during a clinical examination. The

gentler techniques, such as those induced during the flexion-rotation drawer test, avoid pain and apprehension while still inducing a subluxation-reduction phenomenon.

The investigation demonstrated that many examiners induced coupled motions during the pivot shift test of anterior tibial translation and internal tibial rotation to produce anterior tibial subluxation without constraining or enhancing either motion. These examiners produced a greater anterior subluxation of the medial and lateral tibial plateaus than those who induced greater amounts of internal tibial rotation, which significantly decreased anterior subluxation of the medial tibial plateau ($P < .01$; Fig. 3–52). The recommendation can, therefore, be made to avoid intentional enhancement of internal tibial rotation when performing this test to allow the tibia to subluxate in the least constrained manner.

The variability demonstrated among examiners in the maximal amount of anterior tibial subluxation produced during the pivot shift test may affect the final grade assigned. It is certainly possibly that one examiner would rate a knee as a grade II, and another examiner who applied a smaller force

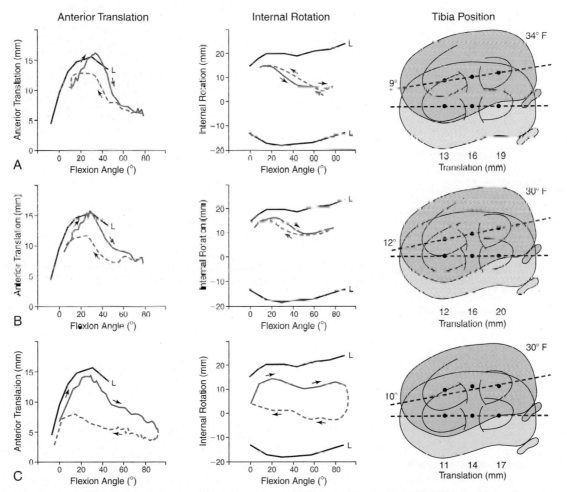

FIGURE 3–44. The tibial translations and rotations are shown for six examiners during the pivot shift test. The limit curve (L) for 100 N of anterior translation and 5 Nm of the tibial rotation is superimposed on the clinical test results. The test follows the *arrow* sequence of knee flexion to reach a maximum anterior subluxation, the reduction event, followed by knee extension to return to the starting position of the test. The tibial plateau drawings show the position of maximum anterior subluxation (based on tibial center reference point). The millimeters of anterior translation for the medial, central, and lateral tibial reference points are shown (subluxated position from neutral position). *(Redrawn from Noyes, F. R.; Grood, E. S.; Cummings, J. F.; Wroble, R. R.: An analysis of the pivot shift phenomenon. The knee motions and subluxations induced by different examiners. Am J Sports Med 19:148–155, 1991.)*

Continued

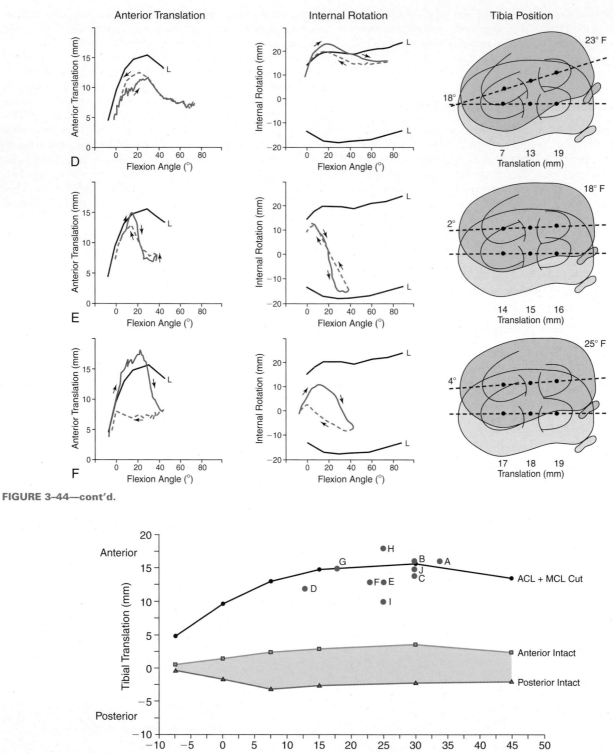

FIGURE 3–44—cont'd.

FIGURE 3–45. The anterior and posterior limits (central point) of tibial translation with a 100-N force are shown before and after ligament cutting. The *circles* represent the point at which the maximum amount of anterior translation occurred for each examiner. *(From Noyes, F. R.; Grood, E. S.; Cummings, J. F.; Wroble, R. R.: An analysis of the pivot shift phenomenon. The knee motions and subluxations induced by different examiners.* Am J Sports Med *19:148–155, 1991.)*

would rate the same knee as a grade I. Thus, the pivot shift test must be considered qualitative in nature and imprecise in determining the results of ACL reconstructive procedures. These results determined the need for a clinical testing device that could measure the anterior and posterior subluxations of the medial and lateral tibial plateaus under controlled loading conditions.

The tests for mediolateral joint space opening demonstrated wide variation among examiners in the starting position of the tibiofemoral compartment during abduction-adduction rotation

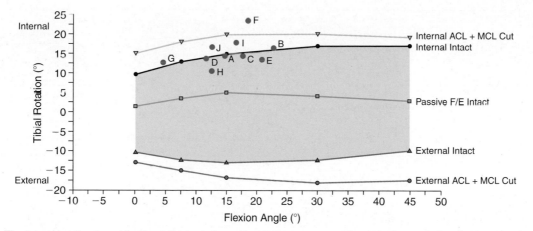

FIGURE 3–46. The internal and external limits of tibial rotation with a 5-Nm torque are shown before and after ligament cutting. The maximal amount of internal rotation is graphed for each examiner. *(From Noyes, F. R.; Grood, E. S.; Cummings, J. F.; Wroble, R. R.: An analysis of the pivot shift phenomenon. The knee motions and subluxations induced by different examiners. Am J Sports Med 19:148–155, 1991.)*

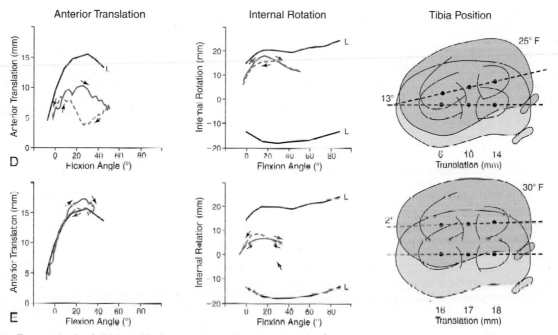

FIGURE 3–47. Two methods of tibial positioning are shown, first, by enhancing internal rotation during the pivot shift test and, second, by not enhancing internal tibial rotation. The enhanced internal tibial rotation limited anterior translation of the tibia. *(Redrawn from Noyes, F. R.; Grood, E. S.; Cummings, J. F.; Wroble, R. R.: An analysis of the pivot shift phenomenon. The knee motions and subluxations induced by different examiners. Am J Sports Med 19:148–155, 1991.)*

testing. The medial or lateral tibiofemoral compartment must be in the closed position initially in order for the examiner to be able to accurately estimate the amount of joint space opening.

Even though variation existed among examiners in the estimated displacements, 9 of the 11 clinicians correctly diagnosed the ACL/MCL injury. However, numerous errors were made in the diagnosis of other ligament injuries, most notably, to the posterolateral structures. An increase in external tibial rotation was interpreted by many examiners to be a result of a posterior subluxation of the lateral tibial plateau and, therefore, injury to the posterolateral structures. The abnormality was actually an anterior subluxation of the medial tibial plateau, created by sectioning the ACL and MCL. To avoid this misdiagnosis, the examiner should palpate the medial and lateral tibial plateaus

and their position relative to the femoral condyle in the maximum position of external and internal tibial rotation.[43,45] Because this provides only a qualitative estimate, the need exists for instrumented or radiographic methods to diagnose more accurately the complex rotatory subluxations of the knee joint.

Based on these investigations, the following conclusions and recommendations were reached: (1) examination test techniques must be standardized regarding the test conditions so that examiners conduct knee examinations in a similar manner, (2) wide variations among clinicians regarding how knee tests are performed may not allow the comparison of knee motion limits, (3) instrumented teaching models should be developed to increase reproducibility among examiners, (4) reliable quantification of clinical testing in the form of knee arthrometry or

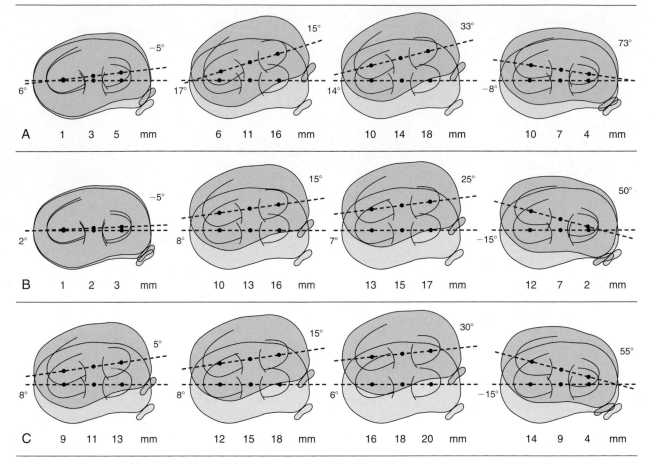

FIGURE 3–48. A, The pivot shift test is performed first enhancing internal rotation. The test is then repeated in **B** with the examiner not purposely enhancing internal rotation and in **C** with the tibia attempted to be held in a more externally rotated position. Actually, the tibia is not externally rotated in **B** and **C** until the end of the test. The millimeters of anterior translation of the medial, central, and lateral points vary depending on how the test is performed. *(**A–C,** From Noyes, F. R.; Grood, E. S.; Cummings, J. F.; Wroble, R. R.: An analysis of the pivot shift phenomenon. The knee motions and subluxations induced by different examiners. Am J Sports Med 19:148–155, 1991.)*

stress radiography should be required for reporting clinical results, and (5) the diagnosis of rotatory subluxations is highly subjective and requires a careful assessment of the AP position of the medial and lateral tibial plateaus relative to the femur.

DEFINITION OF TERMS FOR KNEE MOTIONS, POSITIONS, AND LIGAMENT INJURIES

Considerable discrepancy exists in the orthopaedic literature in the implied meanings of many terms commonly used to describe knee motions, positions, and ligament injuries. As a result, confusion may develop when clinicians communicate or compare the results of studies. In addition, the use of precise terminology is essential in the development of a valid ligament classification system, as described earlier in this chapter. In recognition of this problem, surgeons and scientists from two institutions conducted a study and made recommendations regarding the definitions of medical and engineering terms commonly used to describe the motion and position of the knee observed during clinical testing.[43]

A systematic format was adopted to (1) categorize the terminology used in major articles on knee ligament injuries, (2) compare terms used in the selected articles to determine whether unique definitions had evolved over time through common usage,

(3) review and compare definitions of these terms from a variety of primary, secondary, and tertiary sources, and (4) provide a recommendation for use of these terms in the orthopaedic literature. Dictionaries were considered primary sources[2,57]; textbooks,[26] secondary sources; and published articles, tertiary sources. Terms that had controversial or multiple definitions in the orthopaedic literature were classified according to the least ambiguous meaning based on simplicity and clarity.

The definitions of terms used to describe positions of the knee (position, dislocation, and subluxation) are shown in Table 3–12, and the terms used to describe motion of the knee (motion, displacement, translation, rotation, range of motion, limits of motion, coupled displacement and motion, constrained and unconstrained motion, force, moment, laxity, and instability) are shown in Table 3–13. The terms used to describe injury to the knee (sprain, rupture, and deficiency) are shown in Table 3–14.

It is important to note that motion and displacement of the knee are described by the combination of (1) the change in orientation of the tibia and (2) the motion or displacement of some reference or base point on the tibia. The change in orientation is quantified by the rotation of the tibia about the three independent axes (flexion-extension rotation, internal-external rotation, and abduction-adduction rotation) and the motion or displacement of the reference point on the tibia. The flexion-extension axis is located in the femur, and its orientation relative to the

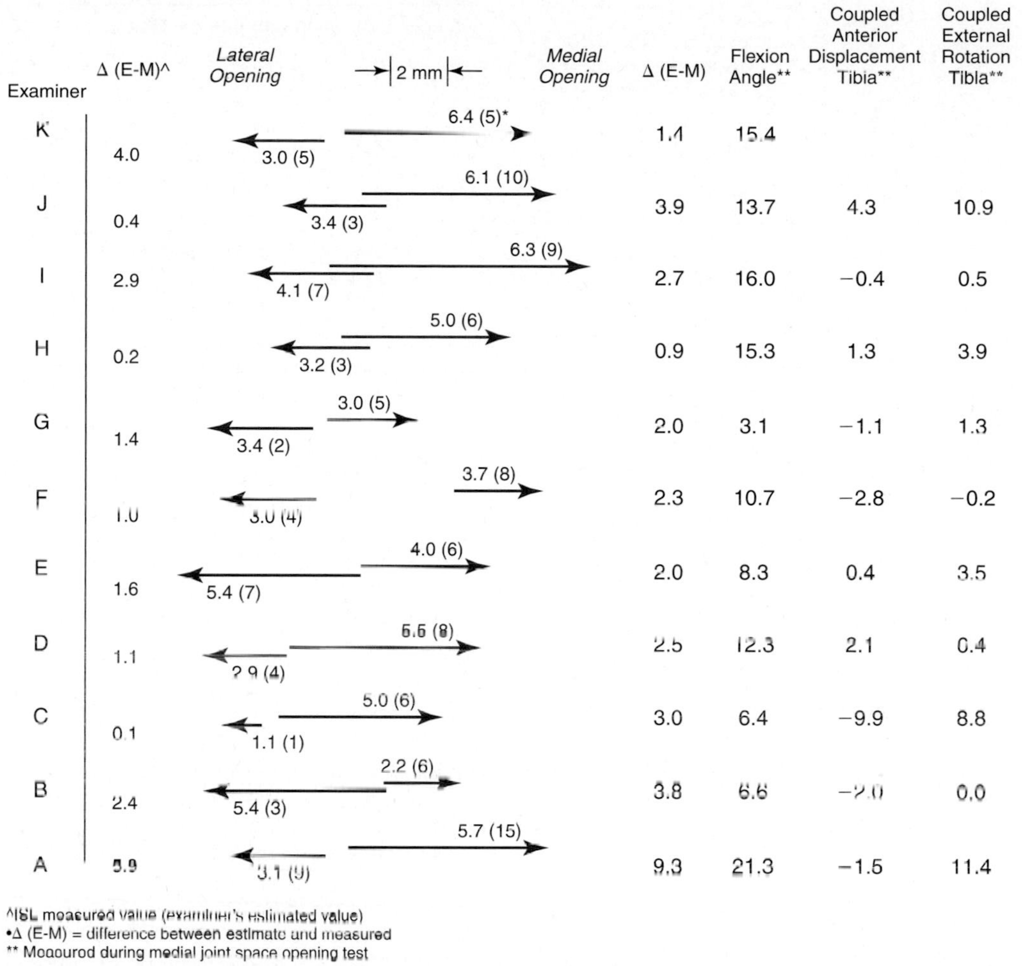

Examiner	Δ (E-M)^	Lateral Opening	→|2 mm|←	Medial Opening	Δ (E-M)	Flexion Angle**	Coupled Anterior Displacement Tibia**	Coupled External Rotation Tibia**
K	4.0	3.0 (5)		6.4 (5)*	1.4	15.4		
J	0.4	3.4 (3)		6.1 (10)	3.9	13.7	4.3	10.9
I	2.9	4.1 (7)		6.3 (9)	2.7	16.0	−0.4	0.5
H	0.2	3.2 (3)		5.0 (6)	0.9	15.3	1.3	3.9
G	1.4	3.4 (2)		3.0 (5)	2.0	3.1	−1.1	1.3
F	1.0	3.0 (4)		3.7 (8)	2.3	10.7	−2.8	−0.2
E	1.6	5.4 (7)		4.0 (6)	2.0	8.3	0.4	3.5
D	1.1	2.9 (4)		6.6 (8)	2.5	12.3	2.1	0.4
C	0.1	1.1 (1)		5.0 (6)	3.0	6.4	−9.9	8.8
B	2.4	5.4 (3)		2.2 (6)	3.8	6.6	−2.0	0.0
A	5.9	3.1 (9)		5.7 (15)	9.3	21.3	−1.5	11.4

^ISL measured value (examiner's estimated value)
•Δ (E-M) = difference between estimate and measured
** Measured during medial joint space opening test

FIGURE 3–49. The *bars* show the instrumented spatial linkage measured values for the medial and lateral joint space opening in the abduction-adduction rotation test for each examiner. The *numbers above* and *below* each bar give the measured displacement, the estimated value for each examiner are given in *parentheses*. Starting position flexion angles, coupled anterior tibial displacement, and the coupled external rotation for the abduction rotation test are given for each examiner. *(From Noyes, F. R.; Cummings, J. F.; Grood, E. S.; et al.: The diagnosis of knee motion limits, subluxations, and ligament injury. Am J Sports Med 19:163–171, 1991.)*

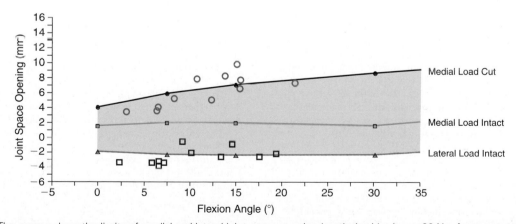

FIGURE 3–50. The *curves* show the limits of medial and lateral joint space opening (*vertical axis*) when a 20-Nm force was applied to the knee for both the intact and the sectioned states. The *circles* represent individual examiner final positions for the medial test on the ACL/MCL-sectioned knee. The *squares* represent individual examiner final positions for the lateral test on the ACL/MCL-sectioned knee. *(Modified from Noyes, F. R.; Cummings, J. F.; Grood, E. S.; et al.: The diagnosis of knee motion limits, subluxations, and ligament injury. Am J Sports Med 19:163–171, 1991.)*

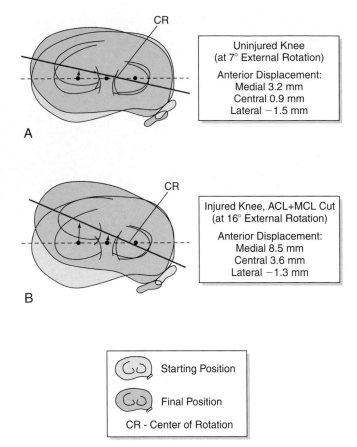

FIGURE 3–51. External rotation test in the uninjured knee (**A**) and after sectioning the ACL and MCL (**B**). The increase in external tibial rotation is shown (7°–16°). The figures show the increase in anterior displacement of the medial tibial plateau and the lateral shift in the axis of tibial rotation. (**A** and **B**, From Noyes, F. R.; Cummings, J. F.; Grood, E. S.; et al.: The diagnosis of knee motion limits, subluxations, and ligament injury. Am J Sports Med 19:163–171, 1991.)

Uninjured Knee
(at 7° External Rotation)

Anterior Displacement:
Medial 3.2 mm
Central 0.9 mm
Lateral −1.5 mm

Injured Knee, ACL+MCL Cut
(at 16° External Rotation)

Anterior Displacement:
Medial 8.5 mm
Central 3.6 mm
Lateral −1.3 mm

Starting Position

Final Position

CR - Center of Rotation

Anterior Translation with Internal Rotation

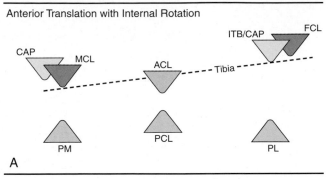

Anterior Translation with Enhanced Internal Rotation

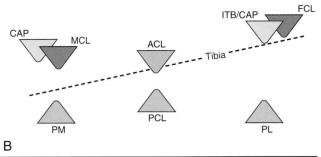

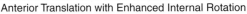

FIGURE 3–52. The bumper model of the knee joint is shown for the pivot shift test at approximately 20° of knee flexion. The central ACL bumper is not shaded, indicating ACL disruption. The tibial position line extends past this point, being limited by the medial and lateral bumpers. **A,** An anterior translation is combined with internal tibial rotation to reach a maximum anterior subluxation of the medial and lateral tibiofemoral compartments, resisted by the medial and lateral ligament restraints. **B,** Enhanced internal tibial rotation reduces the anterior translation of the central tibial region medial tibiofemoral compartment. CAP, medial capsular structures; ITB/CAP, iliotibial band + lateral capsular structures; MCL, medial collateral ligament; PL, posterolateral structures and fibular collateral ligament; PM, posteromedial capsular structures. (**A** and **B,** Modified from Noyes, F. R.; Grood, E. S.; Cummings, J. F.; Wroble, R. R.: An analysis of the pivot shift phenomenon. The knee motions and subluxations induced by different examiners. Am J Sports Med 19:148–155, 1991.)

Critical Points DEFINITION OF TERMS FOR KNEE MOTIONS, POSITIONS, AND LIGAMENT INJURIES

Considerable discrepancy exists in the orthopaedic literature in the implied meanings of many terms commonly used to describe knee motions, positions, and ligament injuries.

Motion and *displacement* of the knee are described by the combination of (1) the change in orientation of the tibia and (2) the motion or displacement of some reference or base point on the tibia.

The term *translation* in its purest form refers to the motion of a rigid body and not of a point. The use of this term to refer to a point has evolved from general usage. The location of the reference point for translation may be chosen arbitrarily. However, the amount of translation depends on which point is selected; any associated rotation could cause the reference points to move differently.

When applied to a ligament, the term *laxity* is used to indicate slackness or lack of tension. Laxity may be normal or abnormal; abnormal laxity may be congenital or result from an injury. The adjective *abnormal* should be used to indicate when laxity is pathologic.

Because the word *laxity* has many different meanings (in English), more precise terms should be used when possible to describe abnormalities in motion or position of the knee joint.

The term *instability* is commonly used to indicate a condition (physical sign) that is characterized by abnormal displacement of the tibia and to describe an anatomic structure, such as ACL instability. It is preferable to describe the specific defect of the ligament or structures and to provide separately the abnormal displacements of the tibia.

Considerable confusion exists regarding the definition of terms used to describe rotatory instability of the knee, such as anterolateral, posterolateral, anteromedial, and posteromedial. Whereas some authors use these terms to describe abnormal motions, others use them to describe an abnormal position of the knee joint.

The goal of the examination of the knee joint is to determine the motions, limits of motion, and initial and final positions of the joint that result from specified loading conditions. The outcome of the test should include the motions of the knee that occur, the abnormal motion limits, and the final tibiofemoral position.

ACL, anterior cruciate ligament.

TABLE 3–12   Definitions of Terms Used to Describe Positions of the Knee

Term	Etymology	Primary Source Definition	Secondary, Tertiary Source Definitions	Comments
Position	From Latin *ponere*, to put, to place*	1. Of the human body: bodily posture or the arrangement of parts of the body (body segment) as used for a particular examination or surgical procedure. 2. Of a point: the location of a point with respect to a reference system. 3. Of a rigid body: the position of a point or particle in the body and the orientation of the body.	The location of a point on the tibia, such as the medial tibial spine, can be described by three translational coordinates: anteroposterior, mediolateral, and proximodistal. These coordinates indicate where the point is located with respect to a reference coordinate system on the femur. The *orientation of a body* refers to how it is rotated relative to other body segments. The orientation of the tibia relative to the femur is described by the angles of flexion-extension, abduction-adduction (or varus-valgus rotation), and internal-external rotation.	The position of the tibia is crucial to correctly diagnosing knee ligament injuries. The starting position of the tibia during clinical tests determines the tension in each of the ligamentous and capsular structures. The final position of the tibia when maximum subluxation has been reached determines which ligaments are injured.
Dislocation	From Latin *de*, away from; *locare*, to place*	An abnormal position of the osseous structures forming a joint, such that there is no longer contact between the normally opposed, articulating surfaces. Synonym: luxation	The term *dislocation* has been used to indicate a complete noncontact position of either the medial and the lateral tibiofemoral compartments or the patellofemoral joint. This term can also be used to describe a noncontact position of only the medial or lateral tibiofemoral compartment.	Dislocations of the knee joint are typically classified according to the final tibial position: anterior, posterior, medial, lateral, or rotatory.
Subluxation	From Latin *sub*, under, beneath; *luxare*, to put out of joint^A	A partial dislocation in which there is an abnormal position of the osseous structures forming the joint, however, a portion of the opposing articulating surfaces are still in contact.	*Subluxation* has been used to indicate an incomplete or partial dislocation. This term has been used synonymously with abnormal motion. However, *subluxation* represents a position of the joint and not its motion. It is therefore incorrect to use this term to indicate abnormal motion.	Identifying and quantifying subluxation is difficult because the term does not have units. The clinician must describe a subluxation according to the position of the tibia relative to the femur. Rotatory subluxations are described by the rotation of the tibia and the position of any point on the tibia. Or, the anteroposterior position of a point may be specified on the medial and lateral tibial plateaus.

*From Traupman, J. C. (ed.): *New College Latin and English Dictionary.* New York: AMSCO School, 1966.

femur does not change. The internal-external rotation axis is located in the tibia, and its orientation relative to the tibia does not change. The abduction-adduction axis is perpendicular to both the flexion and the tibial rotational axes, and its orientation can change relative to both bones. The term *translation* in its purest form refers to the motion of a rigid body and not of a point. Therefore, the use of the term *translation* to refer to a point has evolved from general usage.

The location of the reference point for translation may be chosen arbitrarily. However, the amount of translation depends on which point is selected; any associated rotation could cause the reference points to move differently. The reference point frequently used to describe translation of the knee is located midway between the medial and the lateral margins of the joint. Some investigators use a point on the tibial condyle that is midway between the spines of the intercondylar eminence.

The range and limits of knee flexion-extension are commonly defined in the literature by three numbers that denote maximum hyperextension, the zero or neutral point, and maximum flexion.

For example, 5–0–145 describes a knee that goes from 5° hyperextension to 145° flexion. A knee that lacks 15° from full (0°) extension would be described as 0–15–145.

Most clinical examination tests are performed in a constrained manner, in which the motion of the knee joint is restricted. For instance, in the abduction and adduction tests, the coupled external or internal tibial rotations are blocked by the examiner in order to determine the medial and lateral joint openings that are caused only by the abduction-adduction motion. An advantage of a constrained test is that the specific motions are known and may be reproduced in the laboratory, allowing the primary and secondary ligamentous restraints to be experimentally determined. During the Lachman test, the examiner may constrain the amount of coupled internal rotation of the tibia. In the pivot shift test, the motions are unconstrained to allow maximal subluxation of the lateral tibiofemoral compartment. The specific ligaments and the importance of each in limiting the final position will depend on how these tests are performed. We described earlier in this chapter the diagnostic information obtained during

unit in a manner that allows in vitro data to be extrapolated to in vivo loading conditions. This does represent a problem because there are so many different in vivo loading conditions at the time of ACL failure that it is simply not possible to reproduce these conditions in the laboratory. There is less of a problem in studying the effect of one factor or variable on the mechanical properties of a ligament-bone unit because the same loading conditions are used throughout the experiment.

Effect of Strain Rate on Mechanical Properties

The strain rate describes the rate of deformation used in mechanical studies (length change/initial length per unit of time). The authors conducted a series of fast and slow strain-rate tests on ACL bone-ligament-bone specimens in rhesus monkeys.[56] A slow rate of deformation was chosen to represent the strain rates used in many prior in vitro experiments. A fast rate of deformation was chosen to represent the physiologic in vivo loading conditions to which ligaments may be subjected. The ligament units were tested as right-left pairs at the two strain rates to exclude animal variability. The femur and tibia were at an angle that corresponded to 45° of knee flexion to allow as nearly uniform loading of the ligament as possible. In this experiment, a distraction of the joint was produced. An alternative loading sequence would be to induce anterior translation. Both of these loading profiles have been used experimentally.

Dividing the extension rate by the initial length of the ligament produced approximate strain rates of $0.662 \ \text{sec}^{-1}$ at the fast rate and of $0.00662 \ \text{sec}^{-1}$ at the slow rate, a 100-fold difference. At the fast rate, the ligament underwent the initial 15% to 20% elongation in approximately 0.25 second.

An example of a load-versus-time record from a typical test at the fast strain rate is shown in Figure 4–17. The curves demonstrate an initial concave toe region, followed by a fairly linear region up to the first significant failure. At this point, the load

is termed the *linear load* because it denotes the approximate point at which the ligament preparation enters into the major failure region. Minor failures occur first, with a drop in load. Decreases in load after the linear load indicate successive failures until complete failure, at which time the load falls to zero. The maximum load occurs in the major failure region. The time axis is proportional to the relative displacement of the grips and represents elongation of the ligament after the compliance of the testing device and the grips are computed. Because the extension rate is known, specimen elongation at the linear load, maximum load, and zero load (complete failure) is determined. The area under the load-deformation curve indicates the energy absorbed by the specimen up to complete failure. The slope of the curve in the linear region provides the approximate stiffness of the preparation. It was not possible in this experiment to calculate the cross-sectional area of the ACL with any degree of reproducible accuracy. Force values are reported as load rather than as stress (force per unit area). Alternative experiments, discussed later, employ other testing configurations in which ligament strain is measured by sensitive optic techniques.

The anterior cruciate bone-ligament-bone specimens showed a complex and varied mode of failure. These included avulsion of minor to major bone fragments from insertion sites, failure at the bone-ligament interface without bone avulsion, and ligament failure that occurred initially by tensile pull-apart failure of fiber bundles and then by shear failure between the disrupted fibers. The predominant mode of failure of each specimen was classified as one of the following: (1) ligamentous failure, (2) tibial avulsion failure, (3) combined ligament failure–tibial avulsion fracture, (4) femoral avulsion fracture, or (5) combined ligament failure–femoral avulsion fracture.

A statistically significant difference was found in the predominant mode of failure of the specimens tested at the fast strain rate compared with those tested at the slow rate ($P < .05$; Fig. 4–18). At the fast rate, two thirds of the specimens demonstrated a ligamentous failure and 28% failed by tibial avulsion fracture. At the slow rate, 57% of the specimens failed by tibial avulsion fracture and 29% failed by ligamentous failure.

The results of the strain-rate properties according to the modes of failure are shown in Table 4–1. Under slow strain-rate

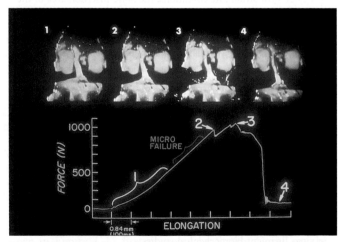

FIGURE 4–17. Oscillograph record of force vs. time for a tension test to failure of a rhesus femur-ACL-tibia preparation. A constant distraction rate was used so that the time axis was proportional to specimen elongation. The photographs, obtained from high-speed movies taken during the test, show the preparation at four stages of the test. *(From Butler, D. L.; Good, E. S.; Noyes, F. R.; Zernicke, R. F.: Biomechanics of ligaments and tendons. In Hutton, R. [ed.]: Exercise and Sports Science Review, Vol. 6. Philadelphia: Franklin Institute Press, 1978; pp. 125–182.)*

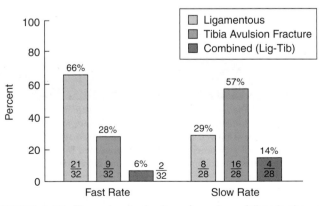

FIGURE 4–18. The major mechanism of specimen failure is shown for the 32 knees tested at the fast strain rate and the 28 knees tested at the slow strain rate. The difference in specimen failure at the two strain rates is statistically significant ($P < .05$). *(From Noyes, F. R.; DeLucas, J. L.; Torvik, P. J.: Biomechanics of anterior cruciate ligament failure: an analysis of strain-rate sensitivity and mechanisms of failure in primates. J Bone Joint Surg Am 56:236–253, 1974.)*

TABLE 4–1 **Strain-Rate Results by Failure Mode**

Strain Rate	N	Failure Mode	Maximum Load (kgf)	Strain to Maximum Load (%)	Energy (cm-kgf)	Strain to Failure (%)
Fast	21	Ligamentous	92.8 ± 17.5*	51.4 ± 7.5	39.8 ± 8.9	61.0 ± 8.9
	9	Tibial avulsion fracture	100.0 ± 19.3*	51.6 ± 7.0*	38.4 ± 13.2	55.0 ± 12.4
Slow	8	Ligamentous	93.0 ± 10.6*	47.8 ± 6.0*	39.9 ± 9.7†	59.0 ± 9.3†
	16	Tibial avulsion fracture	84.1 ± 20.1*	45.6 ± 7.4*	30.9 ± 9.3†	50.9 ± 8.0†

*Mean value significantly different from that of the same failure mode at the other strain rate.
†Mean value significantly different from that of the other failure mode at the same strain rate.
From Noyes, F. R.; DeLucas, J. L.; Torvik, P. J.: Biomechanics of anterior cruciate ligament failure: an analysis of strain-rate sensitivity and mechanisms of failure in primates. *J Bone Joint Surg Am* 56:236–253, 1974.

conditions, the bone-insertion area of the tibia was the weakest component, demonstrated by the reduced maximum load and energy absorbed to failure. At the fast strain rate, representing the more physiologic loading condition, the ligament and bone components failed at a similar maximum load and energy. The overall difference in strength properties was due in part to increased strength of the bone component at the fast rate. At the slow rate, failure by tibial avulsion fracture was interpreted as premature failure, indicating a decrease in the specimen's potential strength. The size of the animals was not a factor contributing to the predominant mode of failure. The different types of failure were distributed throughout each strain-rate group regardless of the weight of the animal. In addition, juvenile animals were not used, which could have biased the results toward a higher frequency of tibial avulsion fractures.

Analysis of Failure-Mode Mechanisms

Macroscopic Analysis

High-speed films of specimen loadings demonstrated that the mechanism of failure usually involved both the bony and the ligamentous components in a progressive manner until complete failure occurred. Sequential failure of ligament fibers commonly occurred first, prior to major tibial avulsion fractures. In other specimens, minor avulsion fractures were associated with major ligamentous failure (Fig. 4–19).

Microscopic Analysis

Microscopic analyses were conducted after the loading tests to define the mechanisms of specimen failure. Resorption changes at the bone-ligament interface, indicative of premature failure, were not visualized in any of the femoral or tibial insertion sites. Polarized light microscopy demonstrated that the ACL inserted at femoral and tibial sites through four well-defined zones of fibrocartilage (see Fig. 4–19).[17] The zonal arrangement at the insertion site represents a change in composition of the surrounding medium as the ligament collagen fibers (zone 1) pass through fibrocartilage (zone 2), across a blue line to mineralized fibrocartilage (zone 3), and into the bone (zone 4).

The specimens in this investigation demonstrated three histologic modes of failure, which were consistent with the macroscopic observations. First, ligamentous failure occurred by an initial tensile failure of collage fibers, followed by a pulling-apart shear failure of the disrupted fibers (Fig. 4–20). Rupture of collagen fiber bundles was also observed throughout the ligament.

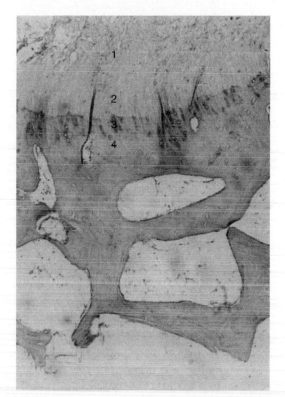

FIGURE 4–19. Photomicrograph after tibial avulsion mode of failure shows that cleavage occurred through cancellous bone below the more dense cortical bone at the site of ligament insertion. The zonal arrangement at the bone-ligament interface is shown. Ligament, zone 1; fibrocartilage, zone 2; mineralized fibrocartilage, zone 3; and bone, zone 4 (hematoxylin and eosin, x90). *(From Noyes, F. R.; DeLucas, J. L.; Torvik, P. J.: Biomechanics of anterior cruciate ligament failure: an analysis of strain-rate sensitivity and mechanisms of failure in primates. J Bone Joint Surg Am 56:236–253, 1974.)*

The ligament fiber microgeometry under the loading conditions in the experiment determined which fibers were subjected to the greatest deformation leading to the serial rupture of fibers and accounted for rupture of fibers in areas adjacent to intact fibers. Although branching between individual collagen fiber bundles was observed, the pulling-apart type of failure suggests that little in the way of cohesive properties exists between the major fiber bundles. A more explicit definition of the mechanism of failure of collagen tissues also involves the ultrastructural changes of fibrils and microfibrils under failure conditions.[56]

Second, avulsion fracture at the attachment site occurred most commonly through the cancellous bone immediately

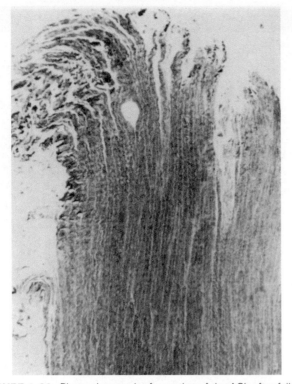

FIGURE 4–20. Photomicrograph of a portion of the ACL after failure. The mechanism of failure appeared to be a tensile, pulling-apart type of failure. The collagen fibers are shown to have ruptured at different portions of the ligament, giving an uneven cleavage line corresponding to the common "mop-end" gross appearance (trichrome, x45). *(From Noyes, F. R.; DeLucas, J. L.; Torvik, P. J.: Biomechanics of anterior cruciate ligament failure: an analysis of strain-rate sensitivity and mechanisms of failure in primates.* J Bone Joint Surg Am *56:236–253, 1974.)*

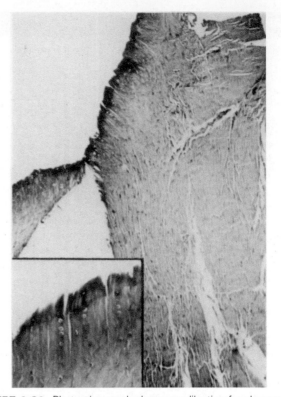

FIGURE 4–21. Photomicrograph shows predilection for cleavage at the ligament-bone interface to occur through the mineralized fibrocartilage zone, in this case just distal to the *blue line. Inset,* Columnar arrangement of chondrocytes (periodic acid–Schiff, x80). *(From Noyes, F. R.; DeLucas, J. L.; Torvik, P. J.: Biomechanics of anterior cruciate ligament failure: an analysis of strain-rate sensitivity and mechanisms of failure in primates.* J Bone Joint Surg Am *56:236–253, 1974.)*

beneath the dense cortical bone (Fig. 4–21). The minute gritty material sometimes just barely palpable on the end of the ligament after failure represented fragments of bone beneath the cartilaginous zone of ligament insertion.[56]

Third, cleavage at the ligament-bone interface showed a predilection for the fracture cleavage line to occur through the zone of mineralized fibrocartilage (zone 3) at or just distal to the blue line. Failure at this interface was the least common mode of failure. It was identified microscopically in 6 of 22 specimens; however, it represented only a minor part of the failure process, the major failure having occurred by either a ligamentous or a bone avulsion mode. Failure through the fibrocartilaginous zone was, therefore, never the major mode of specimen failure, but not infrequently accompanied the other two modes of failure.[56]

In summary, it was possible to classify the major mechanism of failure histologically, although minor modes of failure involved to different degrees all portions of the bone-ligament-bone unit. Thus, it was not unusual to find microscopic evidence of minor to moderate ligament disruption associated with major bone avulsion failures or vice versa.[56]

This study showed for the first time that an ACL-ligament-bone preparation failed at a higher load and at greater elongation, and absorbed significantly more energy, at a fast rate of deformation than at a slow rate. These findings show the time-dependent behavior of bone-ligament-bone preparations and questioned the results of prior ligament failure studies that often showed premature bone

failure at less than expected failure loads. At the slow deformation rate, the bone insertion area of the tibia was the weakest component. At the fast deformation rate, the ligament and tibial osseous component were balanced as to strength properties with an increased frequency of ligamentous failure.[56] The specimen under the fast-deformation rate withstood greater loads without premature osseous failure, allowing the ligament to participate in the failure process.[67] Even with expected viscoelastic effects in the ligament as a result of the higher strain rate, the strength of the bone increased faster than did an expected increase in strength of the ligament.[56]

Many cadaveric and experimental animal studies have reported the difficulty of producing ligamentous injuries and have traditionally stated that the bone is the weakest component of the bone-ligament-bone system.[34,52,73,78,79,84,85,93] Other than the difficulty in reproducing in the laboratory the complex loading and displacement conditions that occur in traumatic injuries, the deformation rate of the experimental tests and the effect of disuse-induced bone changes due to animal caging or aged cadavers are believed to be the major explanations for premature bone avulsion of the ligament-bone unit.[56]

In agreement with these results, Welsh and associates[89] demonstrated that the failure mode of a calcaneal–Achilles tendon unit changed from bone avulsion at low deformation rates to failure at the tendon-grip apparatus under high deformation rates. The ultimate load of the specimens in that investigation may not have been obtained because of the difficulty of clamping the tendons; however, the bone insertion site did not fail at the high strain rate despite the specimen reaching a higher load.

In cases of tibial avulsion fracture, the ligament failure component could not be appreciated on gross examination after the test. In view of the demonstrated elongation on the ligament in the region of failure, it is reasonable to expect damage to collagen fibers and blood vessels within the ligament, even though continuity remains. It is well appreciated that the visual determination of continuity of a ligament at surgery provides an inadequate determination of the extent of ligament damage that has actually occurred and its functional capacity. Such factors, among others, may contribute to the occasional unsatisfactory result in cases of partial ligament disruption with continuity and in cases of ligament reinsertion after bone avulsion.[56]

The fibrocartilaginous zone at the ligament insertion site is believed to be advantageous in producing a gradual change in mechanical properties, decreasing the stress-concentration effect of the ligament's insertion into the stiffer bone structure.[17] This zone protects against fatigue and shear failure at the bone-ligament junction, providing a composite structure with the addition of cartilage and mineralized fibrocartilage to the collagen network. The fibrocartilaginous ground substance may provide greater cohesion between fiber bundles and provide a mechanism for diffusion of load over the entire insertion site, avoiding the deleterious effects of stress concentration. Based on the microscopic analysis of specimen failure and the infrequent occurrence of failure through the fibrocartilaginous zone, the zonal insertion arrangement appears to be mechanically advantageous.[56]

EFFECTS OF IMMOBILIZATION AND DISUSE ON LIGAMENT BIOMECHANICAL PROPERTIES

It is well appreciated that immobility may lead to deleterious changes in bone, joint, and soft tissue.* The authors conducted a study to determine the effect of altered activity levels on the mechanical properties of ligaments in primates.[60] Whereas exercise is accepted as beneficial in preventing muscle atrophy and maintaining joint motion, its effect in preventing deterioration or strengthening a bone-ligament-bone unit had not been established. The study simulated certain clinical states of immobility and determined: (1) the effect of immobilization on the mechanical properties of a bone-ligament-bone unit, (2) the effect of an exercise program in preventing changes in these properties, and (3) the extent to which the changes remained after a 20-week reconditioning period. The reader is referred to the publication for the detailed explanation of the study.[60]

The rhesus animals were placed into four groups: (1) group I, control group, 30 knees; (2) group II, 9 animals immobilized for 8 weeks in total body plaster casts that included both lower limbs; (3) group III, 11 animals in which one lower limb was immobilized for 8 weeks and the other lower limb was exercised daily; and (4) group IV, 11 animals immobilized as in group II, reconditioned in room-sized gang cages for 5 months that were wide and deep and provided ample room for jumping and other activities.

*See references 4, 16, 22, 24, 26, 36, 41–43, 45, 46, 76.

Critical Points EFFECTS OF IMMOBILIZATION AND DISUSE ON LIGAMENT BIOMECHANICAL PROPERTIES

The authors conducted a study in primates to determine the effect of altered activity levels on the mechanical properties of ligaments.

The results showed that 8 wk of immobilization produced a marked decrease of nearly one half of the maximum failure load and significant weakening of a functional ligament unit.

The decrease in strength properties was associated with resorption of haversian bone and weakening of the cortex beneath the ligament's insertion site at both the tibia and the femur.

An exercise program had little effect in preventing the decline in the strength properties of the ligament unit during immobilization and only partial recovery in strength properties occurred after 20 wk of resumed activity.

After immobility, an extended period of time may be required before the functional capacity of a ligament unit returns to normal.

Disuse-induced changes after fracture or ligament reconstruction may extend well into the time period after which normal activity has been resumed by the patient.

The animals in exercise group (group III) performed an active pushing movement against resistance with one free lower extremity in response to a food-reward system. The pushing movement was from 90° of hip and knee flexion to 20° of hip and knee flexion. The foot and ankle were secured by a boot to an exercise apparatus, and with each successful stroke, the animals received a pellet of food. The animals performed the exercise diligently, and on occasion, food had to be restricted. The force required to perform the exercise was minimal initially and then gradually increased over the first 2 weeks so that the animals performed the task at least 600 times daily. The resistance, length of push, and number of repetitions were recorded daily. The animals usually depressed the apparatus 600 to 900 times daily against a resistance of 1.6 to 2.4 kg (about one third body weight).

The average daily work performed by each primate was $11,000 \pm 4000$ kg force cm (range, 6600–20,200). The average total work performed by each animal during the 8 weeks of immobilization was $6.19 \times 10^5 \pm 2.4 \times 10^5$ kg force-cm (range, $3.69 \times 10^5 – 1.11 \times 10^6$ kg force-cm). There was no significant correlation between the total amount of work each animal performed and the strength of the ligament preparation.

The results showed that 8 weeks of immobilization produced a marked decrease of nearly one half of the maximum failure load ($P < .001$; Table 4–2). No significant differences were found in ultimate failure load between the immobilized or the exercise group or between the right and the left ligament units from the exercised group. The failure load for the reconditioned animals indicates partial but incomplete recovery at 20 weeks (Fig. 4–22).

The data demonstrate that immobilization leads to significant weakening of a functional ligament unit. The exercise program had little effect in preventing the decline in the strength properties of the ligament unit during immobilization, and only partial recovery in strength properties occurred after 20 weeks of resumed activity. The decrease in strength properties was associated with resorption of haversian bone and weakening of the cortex beneath the ligament's insertion site at both the tibia and the femur.

The mechanism of failure of a ligament-bone unit after disuse-induced changes depends on the anatomic characteristics

TABLE 4–2   Effect of Immobilization, Exercise, and Reconditioning on Biomechanical Properties of Primate Femur–Anterior Cruciate Ligament–Tibia Complex Preparations*

Parameter	Control (*N* = 30)	Immobilized (*N* = 18)	Exercise Right (*N* = 11)	Exercise Left (*N* = 11)	Reconditioned (*N* = 22)	Statistical Analyses
Linear load (kgf)	78.04 ± 19.35	46.79 ± 15.88	47.66 ± 12.56	55.97 ± 15.87	64.37 ± 23.16	C-I $P < .001$; C-R $P < .05$ C-ER $P < .001$; I-R $P < .01$ C-EL $P < .01$; R-ER $P < .05$
Maximum load (kgf)	87.33 ± 19.40	53.14 ± 12.79	61.71 ± 8.60	61.38 ± 13.04	68.68 ± 18.35	C-I $P < .001$; C-R $P < .01$ C-ER $P < .001$; C-EL $P < .001$ I-R $P < .01$
Strain to linear load (%)	39.24 ± 8.52	33.00 ± 9.86	32.04 ± 10.48	36.28 ± 10.66	36.21 ± 9.91	C-I $P < .05$; C-ER $P < .05$
Strain to maximum load (%)	46.66 ± 8.63	43.88 ± 9.08	40.86 ± 8.23	41.64 ± 5.66	38.53 ± 7.80	C-R $P < .01$
Strain to failure (%)	60.47 ± 9.07	66.28 ± 16.72	58.80 ± 8.45	53.89 ± 7.36	58.03 ± 13.26	C-EL $P < .05$; ER-EL $P < .05$ I-EL $P < .05$
Energy to failure (cm-kgf)	34.02 ± 10.72	23.16 ± 5.27	23.88 ± 6.31	24.37 ± 5.61	26.53 ± 7.19	C-I $P < .001$; C-R $P < .01$ C-ER $P < .01$; C-EL $P < .01$

*Mean values and standard deviations for the mechanical test parameters in the control and experimental groups. Statistical comparisons of the mean values between groups are listed for those parameters significantly different from zero on t-test analysis at $P < .05$ (two-tailed test). Group comparisons not listed are not statistically significant.

C, control; I, immobilized; ER, exercise right; EL, exercise left (nonexercised limb in exercise group); R, reconditioned.

From Noyes, F. R.; Torvik, P. J.; Hyde, W. B.; DeLucas, J. L.: Biomechanics of ligament failure. II. An analysis of immobilization, exercise, and reconditioning effects in primates. *J Bone Joint Surg Am* 56:1406–1418, 1974.

at the ligament-bone insertion site. Most knee ligaments insert into bone through the well-defined zones of fibrocartilage previously described.[17,46,56,68] These zones appear to be protective, because subsynovial and subperiosteal (femoral site) resorption of bone was observed at the peripheral margins of the ligament insertion site but not at the ligament-bone junction. Ultimate failure of the ligament unit occurred either through the underlying cortical bone at the insertion site or through the body of the

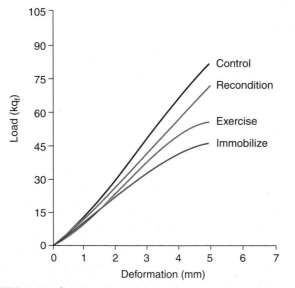

FIGURE 4–22. Calculated load-deformation curves show ligament behavior under loading for all specimens in each of the animal groups. A significant decrease in stiffness (slope of the load-deformation curve) of the ligament preparation is seen in specimens from the exercised and immobilized group. Partial recovery occurred at 20 weeks. *(From Noyes, F. R.; Torvik, P. J.; Hyde, W. B.; DeLucas, J. L.: Biomechanics of ligament failure. II. An analysis of immobilization, exercise, and reconditioning effects in primates. J Bone Joint Surg Am 56:1406–1418, 1974.)*

ligament (or at both of these locations), but not through the ligament-bone junction. This protective effect of the fibrocartilage probably also applies to tendons that have a similar type of attachment.[17,68,74] The zone also imposes a barrier to a vascular supply of the ligament from the bone beneath the insertion site.[68] The tibial attachment of the long fibers of the MCL is into the periosteum and Sharpy fibers without a fibrocartilaginous interface. Immobility has a pronounced effect on producing subperiosteal bone reabsorption that decreases the tibial MCL attachment site strength, resulting in premature failure prior to involving the ligament in the failure process.[41,43,46] Because of the premature attachment failure, the use of a MCL bone-ligament unit is not ideal and disuse-induced cage confinement of experimental animals induces this as a variable affecting the results. The authors agree with Laros and coworkers[46] that the reported increase in ligament strength above control values resulting from increased activity in animals may represent the prevention or reduction of the disuse effect of caging.

The effect of immobility on the ligament itself is of importance to its mechanical function. The change in the relationship between force and ligament elongation (stiffness) after immobilization correlated with the inactivity of the primates. The exercised ligament units were somewhat less affected than the fully immobilized specimens. Both groups were significantly different compared with the control group. The stiffness of the ligament unit in the reconditioned specimens had nearly returned to normal at 20 weeks, although the recovery in strength was incomplete. Other studies have shown a similar correlation between the general level of activity during confinement and the strength of a ligament unit.[1,46,78,80,85,93]

The clinical relevance of this study relates to the suggestion that after immobility, an extended period of time may be required before the functional capacity of a ligament unit returns to normal. Disuse-induced changes after fracture or ligament reconstruction may extend well into the time period after which normal activity has been resumed by the patient.

STRENGTH OF THE ACL: AGE-RELATED AND SPECIES-RELATED CHANGES

Important changes occur in the functional properties of bone-ligament units with age and, as well, differences from one animal species to another. The authors[57] conducted a study in which the mechanical properties of ACL specimens from humans and rhesus monkeys were determined in tension to failure under high strain-rate conditions. The age of the cadaver specimens ranged from 16 to 86 years. One of the purposes of the study was to determine whether discrepancies in strength and mechanisms of ligament failure between human and animal specimens were due to size differences, to variables in the human specimens such as age or disuse atrophy, or to certain experimental testing variables. In addition, human data are required to define the strength properties required for ACL graft replacements.

Comparison of Size Parameters

The mass of the rhesus animals was small in comparison to that of the human donors (Table 4–3). The ligament lengths and areas of the animals were approximately one half and one fourth those in the human donors, respectively.

Comparison of Structural Parameters

A typical force/elongation curve for one young and one older adult human specimen is shown in Figure 4–23. The mean values for the stiffness and strength parameters of the human and rhesus ligament specimens are shown in Table 4–4. A significant difference was found between the older and the younger human specimens. The preparations from the younger humans failed at a maximum force that was an average of 2.4 times that of the specimens from the older humans. The ligaments from the animals failed at force values higher than those of the older human specimens, despite an approximate fivefold difference in the respective cross-sectional areas of the ligaments.

Comparison of Material Properties

The data shown in Table 4–5 represent measurements of the mechanical properties of the ligament collagen as a material. They are normalizations of the structural parameters, adjusted for variations in the cross-sectional areas and lengths of the specimens. There were large differences in all parameters shown between ligaments from younger and older humans. The mean value for the elastic modulus of the ligaments from young adult humans was 1.7 times that of the ligaments from the older humans, but was significantly lower than the mean value for the ligaments from the animals.

The maximum stress and the strain energy to failure in the specimens from younger humans were 2.8 and 3.3 times the

Critical Points STRENGTH OF THE ACL: AGE-RELATED AND SPECIES-RELATED CHANGES

The authors conducted a study in which the mechanical properties of ACL specimens from humans and rhesus monkeys were determined in tension to failure under high strain-rate conditions.

The purposes of the study were to determine whether discrepancies in strength and mechanisms of ligament failure between human and animal specimens were due to size differences, to variables in the human specimens such as age or disuse atrophy, or to certain experimental testing variables.

The ligament lengths and areas of the animals were approximately one half and one fourth those in the human donors, respectively.

Significant differences were found between the older and the younger human specimens in stiffness, strength, and mechanical properties. Preparations from the younger humans failed at a maximum force that was an average of 2.4 times that of the specimens from the older humans.

Ligaments from the rhesus animals failed at normalized force values (to body mass) over three times higher than those of the younger human specimens.

The specimens from older humans showed a decrease in cortical thickness and trabecular bone at the insertion of the ligaments. Failure occurred by fracture through the cortical and underlying trabecular bone, owing to both age-related and probably disuse-induced changes.

respective values for the older human group. The maximum stress and the strain energy to failure in the ligaments from the animals were 1.8 and 1.9 times the respective values for the specimens from younger humans.

Age-related Changes

Statistically significant decreases were found with age in the elastic modulus, maximum stress, and strain energy for the specimens that failed by a ligamentous mode, in which prior antemortem effects were excluded, but not for the specimens from older humans that failed by premature bone–avulsion fracture, in which significant antemortem effects were suspected.

The regression equation (y) and correlation coefficient (r) for the specimens that failed by a ligamentous mode are shown in Figure 4–24. Maximum stress showed the highest correlation with age ($R = 0.863$; $P < .005$). A low correlation was found with strain energy to failure (0.75) and elastic modulus (0.712), but all correlations were statistically significant.

Histologic Findings

The change in mechanism of specimen failure with age from a ligamentous mode to bone–avulsion fracture correlated with histologic findings. The specimens from older humans showed a

TABLE 4–3	Anterior Cruciate Ligament Strength: Comparison of Size				
	Specimens (*N*)	Donor Mass (kg)	Length (mm)	Area (mm²)	Volume (ml)
Older human 48–86 yr	20	72.1 ± 24.6	27.5 ± 2.8	57.5 ± 16.2	1.60 ± 0.53
Younger human 16–26 yr	6	52.6 ± 0.52	26.9 ± 1.5	44.4 ± 9.7	1.21 ± 0.31
Rhesus monkey	25	7.0 ± 0.6	12.3	12.7 ± 1.71	0.156

From Noyes, F. R.; Grood, E. S.: The strength of the anterior cruciate ligament in humans and rhesus monkeys. Age-related and species-related changes. *J Bone Joint Surg Am* 58:1074–1082, 1976.

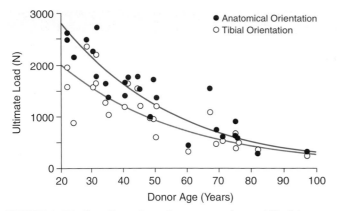

FIGURE 4–25. The effect of specimen age on femur-ACL-tibia complex (FATC) ultimate load. Data on ultimate load as a function of specimen age and orientation using a least squares curve fit demonstrated that the strength of the FATC decreases in an exponential manner. *(From Woo, S. L.-Y.; Hollis, J. M.; Adams, D. J.; et al.: Tensile properties of the human femur–anterior cruciate ligament–tibia complex. The effects of specimen age and orientation. Am J Sports Med 19:217–225, 1991.)*

TABLE 4–6 Effects of Specimen Age and Orientation on the Structural Properties of the Femur–Anterior Cruciate Ligament–Tibia Complex*

Age Group (yr)	Specimen Orientation	Stiffness[†] (N/mm)	Ultimate load[†] (N)	Energy Absorbed[†] (Nm)
Younger	Anatomic	242 ± 28	2160 ± 157	11.6 ± 1.7
(22–35)	Tibial	218 ± 27	1602 ± 167	8.3 ± 2.0
Middle	Anatomic	220 ± 24	1503 ± 83	6.1 ± 0.5
(40–60)	Tibial	192 ± 17	1160 ± 104	4.3 ± 0.5
Older	Anatomic	180 ± 25	658 ± 129	1.8 ± 0.5
(60–97)	Tibial	124 ± 16	495 ± 85	1.4 ± 0.3

*Mean ± SEM.
[†]Younger specimens have significantly higher values than older specimens ($P < .001$).
From Woo, S. L.-Y.; Hollis, J. M.; Adams, D. J.; et al.: Tensile properties of the human femur-anterior cruciate ligament-tibia complex. The effects of specimen age and orientation. *Am J Sports Med* 19:217–225, 1991.

and the results reflect a maturation process rather than aging, which were probably related to changes in insoluble collagen, increased intermolecular and intramolecular cross-linking, and increases in the collagen-to-glycosaminoglycan and collagen-to-water ratios.[73] The physiochemical and mechanical changes that occur in collagen after completion of maturation, which can be ascribed to an aging process in the absence of adverse environmental or disease factors, have not been defined.

EFFECT OF INTRA-ARTICULAR CORTICOSTEROIDS ON LIGAMENT PROPERTIES

The effect of an intra-articular, slightly soluble corticosteroid (methylprednisolone acetate) was investigated on the mechanical properties of a ligament unit.[58,59] ACL preparations from wild rhesus animals were used to determine the effect of corticosteroid dosage and time duration after administration.

Critical Points EFFECT OF INTRA-ARTICULAR CORTICOSTEROIDS ON LIGAMENT PROPERTIES

The effect of slightly soluble corticosteroid (methylprednisolone acetate) was investigated on the mechanical properties of a rhesus ACL ligament unit.

A direct steroid injection into the ligament resulted in statistically significant decreases in maximum load and energy to failure in both the large-dosage and the small-dosage groups.

The clinical implications are that a single direct injection of a slightly soluble steroid preparation has a marked effect on decreasing ligament functional properties, which remained up to 1 yr.

Intra-articular injections resulted in alterations in ligament behavior that were dependent on the dosage of the drug and the time that has elapsed after injection.

In the high-dosage group, the maximum failure load of the ligament unit decreased by 11% after 6 wk and 20% after 15 wk. In the low-dosage group, the maximum failure load of the ligament unit decreased by 9%.

In the high-dosage group, a significant decline in the stiffness of the ligament unit had occurred at 15 wk. No such decline was detected in the low-dosage group.

The clinical implications suggest that intra-articular, slightly soluble corticosteroids in high and frequent doses have the potential to alter ligament strength and function. The risk associated with such alterations may be minimal if infrequent, low-dose injections are administered.

Direct Steroid Injection into Ligament

In the first study, animals were divided into a control group, a sham control group (saline injection), a 20-mg large-dosage group, and a 4-mg small-dosage group (methylprednisolone acetate).[12,58] The large-dosage group was studied at 6 and 15 weeks after injection, and the small-dosage group was studied at 15 and 52 weeks. The FATC specimens were tested in tension to failure using a procedure previously described.[56]

Statistically significant decreases occurred in maximum load in the large-dosage (21% and 39% declines at 6 and 15 wk, respectively) and the small-dosage groups (27% at 15 wk, which remained comparable at 52 wk). In the large-dosage group, minimal decreases in energy to failure were found at 6 weeks, but significant declines (43%) were present at 15 weeks. In the small-dosage group, decreases occurred in energy to failure of 27% at both time intervals.

Intra-articular Steroid Injection

In the second investigation, two animal groups were studied.[59] The first group (high corticosteroid dosage) comprised 10 animals that received a total of three intra-articular injections of methylprednisolone acetate (6.0 mg/kg) into one knee. The injections were spaced 1 week apart. A sham procedure was performed on the opposite knee that consisted of an intra-articular saline injection in equal volume to that of the drug. These animals were sacrificed 6 weeks after the first injection. The second group (low corticosteroid dosage) comprised 12 animals that received two injections of a dosage one tenth that used in the other animal group (methylprednisolone acetate 0.6 mg/kg). The two injections were given 2 weeks apart, with a sham saline injection administered into the opposite knee. The animals were sacrificed 15 weeks after the first injection.

A load-versus-time record from a typical right and left specimen pair in an animal from the high corticosteroid dosage group

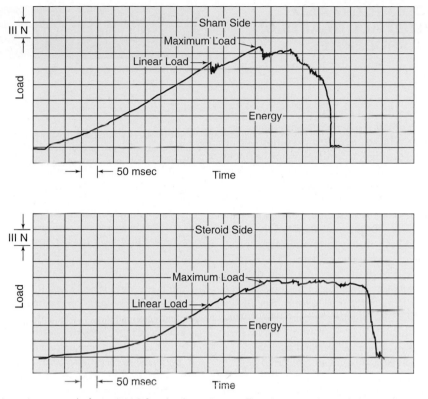

FIGURE 4-26. Typical load vs.-time records for a right-left pair of specimens. The sham specimen demonstrates normal behavior under loading. The steroid side demonstrates a decrease in stiffness (initial slope of the curve), failure at lower loads, and an increase in ligament elongation at complete failure. *(From Noyes, F. R.; Grood, E. S.; Nussbaum, N. S.; Cooper, S. M.: Effect of intra-articular corticosteroids on ligament properties: a biomechanical and histological study in rhesus knees. Clin Orthop 123:197–209, 1977.)*

is shown in Figure 4–26. The strain parameters are approximated owing to inherent errors in measuring ligament length and in using the tibia femur separation distance as a measure of ligament elongation during testing.

The histologic analysis of the failed ligament units showed no detectable corticosteroid effect in that the fibrocartilage zones at the ligament insertion sites were intact. There were no bone resorptive changes at the ligament attachment sites. On scanning electron microscopy, no alterations were found in the surface appearance of collagen fibers and fibrils in the ligaments that received the corticosteroid.[59]

The alterations in ligament behavior were dependent on the dosage of the drug and the time that has elapsed after injection. In the higher-dosage group, the maximum failure load of the ligament unit decreased by 11% after 6 weeks and 20% after 15 weeks. The stiffness of the ligament preparation showed a minimal decrease 6 weeks after injection; however, at 15 weeks, a significant decline had occurred. In the lower-dosage group, the maximum failure load of the ligament unit decreased by 9% and the energy absorbed prior to failure decreased by 8%. The decreases were found when the right-left specimen pairs were compared and were statistically significant. No significant change occurred in the stiffness of the ligament unit. These small changes suggest only slight alterations in the projected functional capacity of the ligament unit.

The specific ultrastructural mechanisms responsible for the alterations in ligament mechanical properties after administration of corticosteroid are unknown. There are known inhibitory effects of corticosteroids on the synthesis of glycosaminoglycans, proteins,

and collagen. Whether decreased collagen synthesis occurs owing to the drugs' effect on specific collagen precursors and enzymes or from a general inhibitory effect on overall protein synthesis is unknown. Corticosteroid preparations are known to alter fibroblast proliferation and metabolism. The cellular and subcellular effects are highly complex and beyond the scope of this chapter. The end result of these drugs is generally antianabolic and responsible for the adverse effect on wound and soft tissue healing.

The clinical implications of this study are suggestive that intra-articular, slightly soluble corticosteroids in high and frequent doses have the potential to alter ligament strength and function. The risk associated with such alterations may be minimal if infrequent, low-dose injections are administered. Alternatively, a single direct injection of a slightly soluble steroid preparation has a marked effect on decreasing ligament functional properties, which remained up to 1 year.

Wiggins and colleagues[90] and Walsh and coworkers[88] reported extensive studies on the effect of a steroid injection in human equivalent doses on the healing of a rabbit MCL model. Their data show statistically significant reductions in maximum failure loads and alteration in histologic properties compared with appropriate controls. The authors concluded that a single steroid injection at the site of a healing ligament would decrease or retard healing properties; however, they suggested that the effect was probably reversible. The authors reviewed a number of mechanisms for the deleterious effects. It should be noted that the studies were performed on a rabbit model that exhibits a known hypersensitivity to steroids that is more pronounced than that expected in other animals and humans.

EFFECT OF VASCULARIZED AND NONVASCULARIZED ACL GRAFTS ON BIOMECHANICAL PROPERTIES

After ACL graft reconstruction, there is marked cellular invasion that removes necrotic collagenous tissues with replacement collagenous fibers that are a ligament in a parallel fashion, but do not resemble the native microgeometry of the ACL. The question that has been posed is whether maintaining a vascular supply (and any concomitant neural innervation) of an ACL graft would limit the so-called necrotic phase of ligament remodeling and retain more normal ligament functional properties. An investigation was conducted to measure the mechanical properties of patellar tendon autografts used to replace the ACL in the cynomolgus monkey at four time periods up to 1 year.[11] The ACL was replaced with the medial half of the patellar tendon as a vascularized graft in one knee and as a nonvascularized (or free) graft in the contralateral knee. The 5-mm-wide medial patellar tendon free grafts were prepared through a standard medial parapatellar exposure. The vascularized grafts were prepared in a similar manner, except the medial retinacular vascular supply and a portion of the fat pad were preserved. The tibial attachment sites were prepared by producing a thin bony trough in the anteromedial aspect of the tibia to the site of the ACL attachment, and the ACL grafts with the vascularized pedicle were transposed into a bony trough. An identical tibial and femoral placement was used for the free grafts. Standard graft fixation methods were used. The knees were immobilized for 4 weeks at 30° of flexion followed by unrestricted activity in large cages.

Critical Points EFFECT OF VASCULARIZED AND NONVASCULARIZED ACL GRAFTS ON BIOMECHANICAL PROPERTIES

An investigation was conducted to determine whether maintaining a vascular supply (and any concomitant neural innervation) of an ACL graft would limit the so-called necrotic phase of ligament remodeling and retain more normal ligament functional properties.

The ACL was replaced with the medial half of the patellar tendon as a vascularized graft in one knee and as a nonvascularized (or free) graft in the contralateral knee in cynomolgus monkeys.

Both the vascularized and the nonvascularized grafts underwent significant reductions in structural mechanical and material properties as early as 7 wk after surgery.

Retention of a portion of the blood supply to the ligament is not sufficient to avoid a major reduction in ligament mechanical properties that occur in vivo after implantation.

Both the vascularized and the nonvascularized grafts underwent significant reductions in structural mechanical and material properties as early as 7 weeks after surgery. Stiffness values were as low as 24% to 28% of control ACL and medial patellar tendon values. Maximum force at 7 weeks was 16% of control ACL values, increasing to 39% of control maximum force by 1 year (Fig. 4–27A). Modulus and maximum stress showed even greater reductions and were only 34% and 26%, respectively, of control ACL values at 1 year (see Fig. 4–27B). The rate of return was slow up to 1 year for all variables studied. The changes in maximum force over time were generally consistent

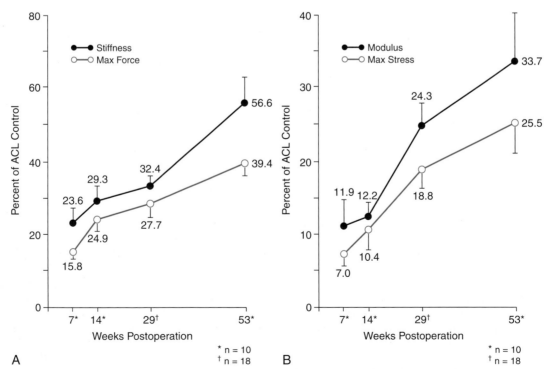

FIGURE 4–27. A, Normalized graft stiffness and maximum force (1 standard error of the mean [SEM]) are plotted against weeks postoperation. Note the more rapid increase in the stiffness values over time. By 1 year, stiffness and maximum force were 57% and 39% of control, respectively. **B,** Normalized graft modulus and maximum stress are plotted against weeks postoperation. No significant differences are present between the parameters at any time period. Modulus and maximum stress are lower than corresponding stiffness and maximum force in **A,** suggesting that the collagen material is both very compliant and weak. *(From Butler, D. L.; Grood, E. S.; Noyes, F. R.; et al.: Mechanical properties of primate vascularized vs. nonvascularized patellar tendon grafts; changes over time. J Orthop Res 7:68–79, 1989. Reprinted with permission of Wiley-Liss, Inc., a subsidiary of John Wiley & Sons, Inc.)*

with other studies that used free grafts, showing on a mechanical basis that an extended period of time is required for ACL graft remodeling and partial return of strength. The study concluded that retention of a portion of the blood supply to the ligament is not sufficient to avoid a major reduction in ligament mechanical properties that occur in vivo after implantation.

EFFECT OF CELLULAR NECROSIS AND STRESS-SHIELDING ON ACL HEALING AND RETENTION OF NATIVE ACL FIBER MICROARCHITECTURE

Jackson and associates[37-39] performed a series of landmark studies in a goat model in which the ACL was frozen in situ, producing cellular necrosis while retaining the normal fiber microarchitecture. Mechanical loading tests of the ACL bone-ligament-bone preparation at 6 months showed no difference in the maximum failure load, stiffness, or AP translation compared with those in untreated controls. The authors theorized that the large decreases in ACL mechanical properties and strength in experimental animals after ACL reconstruction could not be explained by cell death and devascularization.

To provide additional experimental information, a study was conducted in the authors' laboratory in which the previously described devitalized freeze model in the goat ACL was used and two conditions were added.[10] In one group of knees, the ACL tibial attachment was elevated by osteotomy and then replaced in its normal anatomic position. In a second group of knees, the ACL tibial attachment was osteotomized and replaced on the tibia 5 mm posterior to its normal attachment to study the effects of an altered loading state (stress-shielding) on ligament remodeling properties. The results of the ACL mechanical failure tests are summarized in Table 4–7. The stiffness, maximum force, and stress and modulus were greater in the anatomic placement group than in the posterior ACL placement group; however, they were still less than historical controls. Increased failures were noted at the tibial attachment site in the posterior ACL placement group.

TABLE 4–7   Mean Geometric, Structural, and Material Properties

	Anatomic Placement	Posterior Placement	SEM	Historical Controls
Length (mm)	20.4	21.5	0.7	18.2 ± 0.3
Area (mm^2)	31.2	23.0	3.3	17.7 ± 1.2
Stiffness (N/mm)	473.9*	315.8*	11.4	548.0 ± 31.0
Maximum force (N)	1625.0†	895.0†	246.8	2603.0 ± 213.0
Maximum stress (MPa)	59.4	35.9	22.9	155.0 ± 13.0
Modulus (MPa)	338.4	297.5	45.9	578.0 ± 51.0

*Significant difference ($P < .0005$) between anatomic and posterior placements.
†Significant difference ($P < .05$) between anatomic and posterior placements.
From Bush-Joseph, C. A.; Cummings, J. F.; Buseck, M.; et al.: Effect of tibial attachment location on the healing of the anterior cruciate ligament freeze model. *J Orthop Res* 14:534–541, 1996.

Critical Points EFFECT OF CELLULAR NECROSIS AND STRESS-SHIELDING ON ACL HEALING AND RETENTION OF NATIVE ACL FIBER MICROARCHITECTURE

Based on a series of studies,[37-39] Jackson et al concluded that large decreases in ACL mechanical properties and strength in experimental animals after ACL reconstruction could not be explained by cell death and devascularization.

Other experimental studies strongly suggest that the use of ACL ligament grafts, which have no similarity to the native ACL fiber organization and in vivo microstrains, results in replacement of the ACL graft with a scarlike disorganized collagen framework with marked loss of mechanical strength and stiffness.

Clinically, ACL grafts are limited in their ability to truly restore native ACL fiber microgeometry and, therefore, never function in a manner similar to that of a normal ligament. The grafts function to provide a gross checkrein to abnormal knee displacements.

The results of all of the studies* are summarized in Figure 4–28, which compares historical maximum failure loads in experimental animals with the frozen devitalized specimens in Jackson and associates' study[38] and the anatomic- and posterior-placed ACL preparations.[10] Although the anatomic-placed ACL (after tibial osteotomy) had a reduction in strength compared with the native frozen ACL, the strength was still greater than ACL graft reconstructions. The presumed loss of the normal stress and fiber loading in the posterior-placed ACL, in addition to tibial healing effects, produced marked reductions in all mechanical properties.

The results of these experimental studies strongly suggest that retaining the complex native microgeometry of the ACL provides a necessary stimulus for ligament remodeling. In addition, the use of ACL ligament grafts, which have no similarity to the native ACL fiber organization and in vivo microstrains, results in replacement of the ACL graft with a scarlike disorganized collagen framework with marked loss of mechanical strength and stiffness. Insofar as the results apply to clinical ACL reconstructions, the suggestion is that ACL grafts are limited in their ability to truly restore native ACL fiber microgeometry and, therefore, never function in a manner similar to that of a normal ligament. The authors hypothesize that ACL grafts function to provide a gross checkrein to abnormal knee displacements in contrast to the so-called fine-tuning of joint motions by a ligament fiber guiding microarchitecture mechanism. It is probable that even two-bundle graft constructs behave in a similar manner, replacing the collagen fiber mass of the ligament at tibial and femoral attachments. However, with remodeling, even two-bundle constructs have altered mechanical properties and function that do not approximate native ligament function.

ALLOGRAFTS AND AUTOGRAFTS: BIOMECHANICAL PROPERTIES AFTER IMPLANTATION AND EFFECT OF IRRADIATION

Multiple studies have been published on the biomechanical properties of autografts and allografts in experimental animal models.[3,10,20,37-40,70,71,77,83] The majority demonstrate that allografts have inferior results compared with those of autografts (and

---

*See references 11, 13–15, 33, 39, 48, 49, 55, 71, 77, 82, 92.

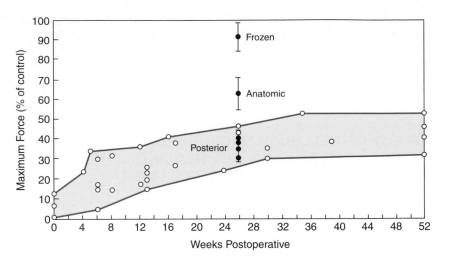

FIGURE 4–28. Maximum load to failure versus postoperative time. The range (*shaded region*) of means for allograft reconstructions (*open circles*) are from previously published studies. The mean (±SEM) for ligaments frozen and their tibial insertion moved 5 mm posterior (Posterior) lie within this range. Ligaments frozen and replaced in the anatomic position (Anatomic) have greater maximum loads but still less than for in situ freezing alone as reported by Jackson et al (Frozen). *(From Bush-Joseph, C. A.; Cummings, J. F.; Buseck, M.; et al.: Effect of tibial attachment location on the healing of the anterior cruciate ligament freeze model. J Orthop Res 14:534–541, 1996. Reprinted with permission of Wiley-Liss, Inc., a subsidiary of John Wiley & Sons, Inc.)*

contralateral controls) in regard to mechanical strength properties. In 1989, Thorson and colleagues[77] studied the 4-month postoperative mechanical properties of adult canines that received either bone-tendon-bone allografts or autografts. The allograft group showed a mean load to failure of only 17% of the contralateral control ligament, compared with 41% in the autograft group. Shino and coworkers,[70,71] in two studies using the canine model, reported that allografts had a mean maximum tensile load of approximately 30% that of contralateral controls 1 year postimplantation. Jackson and associates[39] reported in 1993 in a goat model that the strength of fresh frozen patellar tendon allografts was only 27% of controls at 6 months postimplantation. In contrast, the strength of patellar tendon autografts was 62% of control ACLs. The authors concluded that allograft remodeling is much slower than autograft

and suggested that patients who receive allografts should probably be protected against maximum activities for a longer period of time than those who receive autografts.

In another study in which freeze-dried bone-ACL-bone allografts were implanted, Jackson and associates[37] reported that the maximum load of the allografts was only 25% of the contralateral ACL controls at 1 year postimplantation. Figure 4–29[10] summarizes a number of allograft ACL reconstruction studies and demonstrates that all had mechanical properties in low ranges from 4 to 52 weeks postoperative. The healing effects of autografts and allografts are covered in greater detail in Chapter 5, Biology of ACL Graft Healing.

Critical Points ALLOGRAFTS AND AUTOGRAFTS: BIOMECHANICAL PROPERTIES AFTER IMPLANTATION AND EFFECT OF IRRADIATION

The majority of experimental studies demonstrate that allografts have inferior results compared with autografts (and contralateral controls) in regard to mechanical strength properties.

The effects of gamma irradiation on the mechanical and material properties of allografts have been studied in the goat model and human cadavers for many years.

- Effects of 2 and 3 Mrads of gamma irradiation on goat ACL bone–patellar tendon–bone in vitro properties: maximum stress, maximum strain, and strain energy were significantly reduced after 3 Mrads; however, there were no signification reductions after 2 Mrads of irradiation.
- Effects of 0 vs. 4 MRads of gamma irradiation on human cadavers: irradiation produced a small, but significant, decrease in graft length (0.6 mm). Irradiated grafts showed significant reductions in stiffness and maximum force.
- Effects of 4, 6, and 8 Mrads on goat ACL bone–patellar tendon–bone units: data showed the overall dose-dependent effects of irradiation on ligament mechanical properties; doses less than 2 Mrad had minimal effects.
- In vivo effect of 4 Mrad of gamma irradiation on bone–patellar tendon–bone units in goats at time 0 and 6 mo postimplantation: irradiation significantly altered structural but not material properties.

At present, there is no experimental data to show that the low-dose irradiation as used to secondarily sterilize allografts has a deleterious effect on graft mechanical properties.

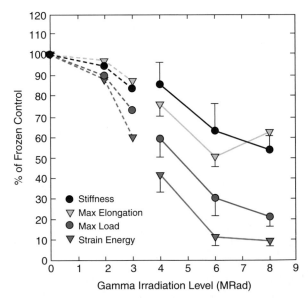

FIGURE 4–29. Average dose-dependent response curves for all four mechanical properties (*solid lines*), expressed as percentages of values for contralateral frozen controls. Normalized data for 2 and 3 Mrad (*broken lines*) from earlier studies are also shown. Those studies used different testing conditions. Note the nearly linear declines in all curves between 2 and 6 Mrad. *(From Salehpour, A.; Butler, D. L.; Proch, F. S.; et al.: Dose-dependent response of gamma irradiation on mechanical properties and related biochemical composition of goat bone–patellar tendon–bone allografts. J Orthop Res 13:898–906, 1995. Reprinted with permission of Wiley-Liss, Inc., a subsidiary of John Wiley & Sons, Inc.)*

The authors' laboratory has studied the effects of gamma irradiation on the mechanical and material properties of allografts in the goat model and in human cadavers. In the first study, Gibbons and colleagues[25] reported on the effects of 2 and 3 Mrads of gamma irradiation on goat ACL bone–patellar tendon–bone in vitro properties. The study reported that the maximum stress, maximum strain, and strain energy were significantly reduced after 3 Mrads; however, there were no signification reductions after 2 Mrads of irradiation (Table 4–8).

In a second study, the effects of a higher level of irradiation (4 Mrad) were studied on human cadaver donor (aged 18–59 yr) frozen patellar tendon-bone allografts and were compared with a frozen control graft (0 Mrad).[64] Irradiation produced a small, but significant, decrease in graft length (0.6 mm; $P < .01$; Table 4–9). The irradiated grafts showed significant reductions in stiffness ($P < .025$) and maximum force ($P < .001$).

In a third study, Salehpour and associates[66] studied the effects of 4, 6, and 8 Mrad (40,000, 60,000, or 80,000 Gys) of gamma irradiation on the in vitro properties of a bone–patellar tendon–bone allograft unit retrieved from mature female goats. On average, stiffness decreased by 18%, 40%, and 42% at 4, 6, and 8 Mrad, respectively ($P < .05$ for all comparisons). The data as a whole showed the overall dose-dependent effects of irradiation on ligament mechanical properties. Doses less than 2 Mrad have minimal effects. Recently, Schwartz and coworkers[69] examined the in vivo effect of 4 Mrad of gamma irradiation on bone–patellar tendon–bone units in adult goats at time 0 and 6 months postimplantation. The irradiation significantly altered structural but not material properties. Stiffness was reduced by 30% and maximum force by 21%, resulting in these parameters averaging 12% to 20% of normal ACL values (Table 4–10).

The authors concluded that 4 Mrad of gamma irradiation affect ACL allograft subfailure viscoelastic and structural properties but not material or biochemical properties over time. The ACL allografts of the 0 Mrad failed at 497 N (see Table 4–9),

TABLE 4–8   Dose-dependent Effects of Gamma Irradiation on Composite Unit Structural Mechanical Properties*

Composite Unit	N	Stiffness (N/mm)[†]	Max Force (N)[†]	Max Elongation (mm)[†]	Strain Energy (Nm)[†]
Frozen control	24	189.9 + 33.6	1406.1 ± 363.8	10.2 ± 1.5	8.2 ± 3.2
2 Mrad	12	179.3 ± 23.9	1261.8 ± 252.1	9.9 ± 1.8	7.2 ± 3.0
3 Mrad	12	158.2 ± 14.3[‡]	1206.2 ± 101.2[§‖]	8.9 ± 1.3[¶]	4.9 ± 1.1[‡§]

*Data are presented as means ± standard deviation (SD).
[†]$P < .05$ compared with control (based on one-sided Dunnett multiple comparison of irradiated to control).
[‡]$P < .005$ compared with control (based on contrasts for individual variables).
[§]$P < .05$ compared with control (based on ANOVA for all variables).
[‖]$P < .0005$ compared with control (based on contrasts for individual variables).
[¶]$P < .05$ compared with control (based on contrasts for individual variables).
From Gibbons, M. J.; Butler, D. L.; Grood, E. S.; et al.: Effects of gamma irradiation on the initial mechanical and material properties of goat bone-patellar tendon-bone allografts. *J Orthop Res* 9:209–218, 1991.

TABLE 4–9   Effects of 4 MRads of Irradiation on Human Patellar Tendon-Bone Allograft Length and Mechanical Properties

	Allograft Length before Irradiation (mm)	Allograft Length after Irradiation (mm)	Static Creep* (mm)	Peak Cyclic Creep[†] (mm)	Stiffness (kN/m)	Maximum Load (N)
Control	58.0 ± 6	—	0.4 ± 0.3	0.4 + 0.2	311 ± 51	2519 ± 131
Irradiated	57.6 + 6	57.0 ± 6	0.5 ± 0.3	0.5 ± 0.3	275 ± 52	1884 ± 330
Number of pairs	18	18	20	20	20	16
Significant (P)	—	0.01[‡]	—	—	0.025	0.001

*Measured at 90 N force after 10 min.
[†]Measured at 200 N force after 3600 cycles at 1 cycle/sec.
[‡]Preirradiation to postirradiation.
From Rasmussen, T. J.; Feder, S. M.; Butler, D. L.; Noyes, F. R.: The effects of 4 Mrad of gamma irradiation on the initial mechanical properties of bone-patellar tendon-bone grafts. *Arthroscopy* 10:188–197, 1994.

TABLE 4–10   Structural Properties of Anterior Cruciate Ligament Allografts 6 Months Postimplantation in Caprine Model

	Linear Stiffness (KN/m)	Maximum Force (N)	Elongation to Failure (mm)	Energy to Maximum Force (Nm)
0 Mrad, mean (SD) (n = 12)	123.2 (45.4)*	496.6 (144.6)*	8.2 (2.7)	1.6 (0.8)
4 Mrad, mean (SD) (n = 12)	86.3 (32.5)*	392.0 (165.2)*	7.6 (1.3)	0.9 (0.3)
0 Mrad as a percentage of normal ACL[†]	16.8 (732)	19.8 (2506)	172.1 (4.8)	29.8 (5.3)
4 Mrad as a percentage of normal ACL[†]	11.8	15.6	158.9	17.9

*$P < .05$ between 0 Mrad and 4 Mrad groups.
[†]Mean values for normal ACL based on prior published literature.
ACL, anterior cruciate ligament.
From Schwartz, H. E.; Matava, M. J.; Proch, F. S.; et al.: The effect of gamma irradiation on anterior cruciate ligament allograft biomechanical and biochemical properties in the caprine model at time zero and at 6 months after surgery. *Am J Sports Med* 34:1747–1755, 2006.

which in comparison with the first study of Gibbons and associates[25] showed a control graft of 1400 N maximum force. This suggests that the effects of the remodeling process, resulting in a weakened graft with altered mechanical properties as previously described, produced even more profound deleterious effects than the irradiation treatment. At present, there are no experimental data to show that the low-dose irradiation as used to secondarily sterilize allografts has a deleterious effect on graft mechanical properties. One clinical study[63] reported inferior outcomes in knees that received irradiated Achilles tendon allografts compared with knees that received frozen Achilles tendon allografts, and the authors recommended that other secondary sterilization methods be pursued. These concepts are further discussed in Chapter 7, ACL Primary and Revision Reconstruction: Diagnosis, Operative Techniques, and Clinical Outcomes. The authors prefer to obtain allografts for patients from tissue banks that use secondary chemical sterilization for bacterial contamination.

REFERENCES

1. Adams, A.: Effect of exercise upon ligament strength. *Res Q* 37:163–167, 1966.
2. Alm, A.; Ekstrom, H.; Stromberg, B.: Tensile strength of the anterior cruciate ligament in the dog. *Acta Chir Scand Suppl* 445:15–23, 1974.
3. Arnoczky, S. P.; Warren, R. F.; Ashlock, M. A.: Replacement of the anterior cruciate ligament using a patellar tendon allograft. An experimental study. *J Bone Joint Surg Am* 68:376–385, 1986.
4. Barfred, T.: Experimental rupture of the Achilles tendon. Comparison of experimental ruptures in rats of different ages and living under different conditions. *Acta Orthop Scand* 42:406–428, 1971.
5. Beynnon, B. D.; Fleming, B. C.; Johnson, R. J.; et al.: Anterior cruciate ligament strain behavior during rehabilitation exercises in vivo. *Am J Sports Med* 23:24–34, 1995.
6. Beynnon, B. D.; Johnson, R. J.; Fleming, B. C.; et al.: The measurement of elongation of anterior cruciate-ligament grafts in vivo. *J Bone Joint Surg Am* 76:520–531, 1994.
7. Beynnon, B. D.; Johnson, R. J.; Fleming, B. C.; et al.: The strain behavior of the anterior cruciate ligament during squatting and active flexion-extension. A comparison of an open and a closed kinetic chain exercise. *Am J Sports Med* 25:823–829, 1997.
8. Bradley, J.; FitzPatrick, D.; Daniel, D.; et al.: Orientation of the cruciate ligament in the sagittal plane. A method of predicting its length-change with flexion. *J Bone Joint Surg Br* 70:94–99, 1988.
9. Burmester, L. (ed.): Lehrbuch der Kinematik. Leipzig, Germany: A. Felix Verlag, 1888.
10. Bush-Joseph, C. A.; Cummings, J. F.; Buseck, M.; et al.: Effect of tibial attachment location on the healing of the anterior cruciate ligament freeze model. *J Orthop Res* 14:534–541, 1996.
11. Butler, D. L.; Grood, E. S.; Noyes, F. R.; et al.: Mechanical properties of primate vascularized vs. nonvascularized patellar tendon grafts; changes over time. *J Orthop Res* 7:68–79, 1989.
12. Butler, D. L.; Grood, E. S.; Noyes, F. R.; Zernicke, R. F.: Biomechanics of ligaments and tendons. In Hutton, R. (ed.): *Exercise and Sports Science Review*, Vol. 6. Philadelphia: Franklin Institute Press, 1978; pp. 125–182.
13. Butler, D. L.; Hulse, D. A.; Kay, M. D.; et al.: Biomechanics of cranial cruciate ligament reconstruction in the dog. II. Mechanical properties. *Vet Surg* 12:113–118, 1983.
14. Clancy, W. G.; Narechania, R. G.; Rosenberg, T. D.; et al.: Anterior and posterior cruciate ligament reconstruction in rhesus monkeys. A histological, microangiographic, and biomechanical analysis. *J Bone Joint Surg Am* 63:1270–1284, 1981.
15. Collins, H. R.; Hughston, J. C.; Dehaven, K. E.; et al.: The meniscus as a cruciate ligament substitute. *J Sports Med* 2:11–21, 1974.
16. Cooper, R. R.: Alterations during immobilization and regeneration of skeletal muscle in cats. *J Bone Joint Surg Am* 54:919–953, 1972.
17. Cooper, R. R.; Misol, S.: Tendon and ligament insertion. A light and electron microscopic study. *J Bone Joint Surg Am* 52:1–20, 1970.
18. Crisp, J. D. C.: Properties of tendon and skin. In Fung, Y. C.; Perrone, N.; Anliker, M. (eds.): *Foundations and Objectives*. Englewood Cliffs, NJ: Prentice-Hall, 1972; pp. 141–177.
19. Crowninshield, R.; Pope, M. H.; Johnson, R. J.: An analytical model of the knee. *J Biomech* 9:397–405, 1976.
20. Curtis, R. J.; Delee, J. C.; Drez, D. J., Jr.: Reconstruction of the anterior cruciate ligament with freeze-dried fascia lata allografts in dogs. A preliminary report. *Am J Sports Med* 13:408–414, 1985.
21. Elliott, D. H.: Structure and function of mammalian tendon. *Biol Rev Camb Philos Soc* 40:392–421, 1965.
22. Enneking, W. F.; Horowitz, M.: The intra-articular effects of immobilization on the human knee. *J Bone Joint Surg Am* 54:973–985, 1972.
23. Fick, R. (ed.): Anatomie und mechanik der gelenke. Part I: anatomie der gelenke; Part II: allgemeine gelenk- und muskelmechanik; Part III: apezielle gelenk- und muskelmechanik. Jena, Germany: Gustav Fischer, 1911.
24. Geiser, M.; Trueta, J.: Muscle action, bone rarefaction and bone formation: an experimental study. *J Bone Joint Surg Br* 40:282–311, 1958.
25. Gibbons, M. J.; Butler, D. L.; Grood, E. S.; et al.: Effects of gamma irradiation on the initial mechanical and material properties of goat bone–patellar tendon–bone allografts. *J Orthop Res* 9:209–218, 1991.
26. Ginsberg, J. M.; Eyring, E. J.; Curtiss, P. H., Jr.: Continuous compression of rabbit articular cartilage producing loss of hydroxyproline before loss of hexosamine. *J Bone Joint Surg Am* 51:467–474, 1969.
27. Grant, M. E.; Prockop, D. J.: The biosynthesis of collagen. 1. *N Engl J Med* 286:194–199, 1972.
28. Grood, E. S.; Hefzy, M. S.; Lindenfeld, T. N.: Factors affecting the region of most isometric femoral attachments. Part I: the posterior cruciate ligament. *Am J Sports Med* 17:197–207, 1989.
29. Harner, C. D.; Livesay, G. A.; Kashiwaguchi, S.; et al.: Comparative study of the size and shape of human anterior and posterior cruciate ligaments. *J Orthop Res* 13:429–434, 1995.
30. Harner, C. D.; Zerogeanes, J. W.; Livesay, G. A.; et al.: The human posterior cruciate ligament complex: an interdisciplinary study. Ligament morphology and biomechanical evaluation. *Am J Sports Med* 23:736–745, 1995.
31. Hefzy, M. S.; Grood, E. S.: Sensitivity of insertion locations on length patterns of anterior cruciate ligament fibers. *J Biomech Eng* 108:73–82, 1986.
32. Hefzy, M. S.; Grood, E. S.; Noyes, F. R.: Factors affecting the region of most isometric femoral attachments. Part II: the anterior cruciate ligament. *Am J Sports Med* 17:208–216, 1989.
33. Holden, J. P.; Grood, E. S.; Butler, D. L.; et al.: Biomechanics of fascia lata ligament replacements: early postoperative changes in the goat. *J Orthop Res* 6:639–647, 1988.
34. Horwitz, M. T.: Injuries of the ligaments of the knee joint. An experimental study. *Arch Surg* 38:946–954, 1939.
35. Hruza, Z.; Chvapil, M.; Dlouha, M.: The influence of age, sex and genetic factors on the mechanical and physico-chemical structural stability of collagen fibres in mice. *Gerontologia* 13:20–29, 1967.
36. Issekutz, B., Jr.; Blizzard, J. J.; Birkhead, N. C.; Rodahl, K.: Effect of prolonged bed rest on urinary calcium output. *J Appl Physiol* 21:1013–1020, 1966.
37. Jackson, D. W.; Grood, E. S.; Arnoczky, S. P.; et al.: Freeze-dried anterior cruciate ligament allografts. Preliminary studies in a goat model. *Am J Sports Med* 15:295–303, 1987.
38. Jackson, D. W.; Grood, E. S.; Cohn, B. R.; et al.: The effects of in situ freezing on the anterior cruciate ligament. An experimental study in goats. *J Bone Joint Surg Am* 73:201–213, 1991.
39. Jackson, D. W.; Grood, E. S.; Goldstein, J. D.; et al.: A comparison of patellar tendon autograft and allograft used for anterior cruciate ligament reconstruction in the goat model. *Am J Sports Med* 21:176–185, 1993.
40. Jackson, D. W.; Grood, E. S.; Wilcox, P.; et al.: The effects of processing techniques on the mechanical properties of bone–anterior cruciate ligament–bone allografts. An experimental study in goats. *Am J Sports Med* 16:101–105, 1988.
41. Jenkins, D. P.; Cochran, T. H.: Osteoporosis: the dramatic effect of disuse of an extremity. *Clin Orthop Relat Res* 64:128–134, 1969.
42. Kazarian, L. E.; Von Gierke, H. E.: Bone loss as a result of immobilization and chelation. Preliminary results in *Macaca mulatta*. *Clin Orthop Relat Res* 65:67–75, 1969.

43. Keim, H. A.: An analysis of periosteal attachment in human long bones of normal adults and adult paraplegics: an electron microscopic study. *Clin Orthop Relat Res* 54:207–214, 1967.

44. Kennedy, J. C.; Hawkins, R. J.; Willis, R. B.; Danylchuck, K. D.: Tension studies of human knee ligaments. Yield point, ultimate failure, and disruption of the cruciate and tibial collateral ligaments. *J Bone Joint Surg Am* 58:350–355, 1976.

45. Kharmosh, O.; Saville, P. D.: The effect of motor denervation on muscle and bone in the rabbit's hind limb. *Acta Orthop Scand* 36:361–370, 1965.

46. Laros, G. S.; Tipton, C. M.; Cooper, R. R.: Influence of physical activity on ligament insertions in the knees of dogs. *J Bone Joint Surg Am* 53:275–286, 1971.

47. Markolf, K. L.; Hame, S.; Hunter, D. M.; et al.: Effects of femoral tunnel placement on knee laxity and forces in an anterior cruciate ligament graft. *J Orthop Res* 20:1016–1024, 2002.

48. McFarland, E. G.; Morrey, B. F.; An, K. N.; Wood, M. B.: The relationship of vascularity and water content to tensile strength in a patellar tendon replacement of the anterior cruciate in dogs. *Am J Sports Med* 14:436–448, 1986.

49. McPherson, G. K.; Mendenhall, H. V.; Gibbons, D. F.; et al.: Experimental mechanical and histologic evaluation of the Kennedy ligament augmentation device. *Clin Orthop Relat Res* 196:186–195, 1985.

50. Menschik, A.: The basic kinematic principle of the collateral ligaments demonstrated on the knee joint. In Chapchal, G. (ed.): *Injuries of the Ligaments and Their Repair: Hand, Knee, Foot.* Stuttgart: Thieme, 1977; pp. 9–16.

51. Menschik, A.: [Mechanics of the knee-joint. 1 (author's trans.)]. *Z Orthop Ihre Grenzgeb* 112:481–495, 1974.

52. Miltner, L. J.; Hu, C. H.; Fang, H. C.: Experimental joint sprain. Pathologic study. *Arch Surg* 35:234–240, 1937.

53. Minns, R. J.; Soden, P. D.; Jackson, D. S.: The role of the fibrous components and ground substance in the mechanical properties of biological tissues: a preliminary investigation. *J Biomech* 6:153–165, 1973.

54. Mueller, W. (ed.): The Knee—Form, Function and Ligament Reconstruction. New York: Springer Verlag, 1983.

55. Ng, G. Y.; Oakes, B. W.; Deacon, O. W.; et al.: Biomechanics of patellar tendon autograft for reconstruction of the anterior cruciate ligament in the goat: three-year study. *J Orthop Res* 13:602–608, 1995.

56. Noyes, F. R.; DeLucas, J. L.; Torvik, P. J.: Biomechanics of anterior cruciate ligament failure: an analysis of strain-rate sensitivity and mechanisms of failure in primates. *J Bone Joint Surg Am* 56:236–253, 1974.

57. Noyes, F. R.; Grood, E. S.: The strength of the anterior cruciate ligament in humans and rhesus monkeys. Age-related and species-related changes. *J Bone Joint Surg Am* 58:1074–1082, 1976.

58. Noyes, F. R.; Grood, E. S.; Nussbaum, N. S.; Cooper, S. M.: Biomechanical and ultrastructural changes in ligaments and tendons after local corticosteroid injections. Proceedings of the Orthopaedic Research Society, 1975 Annual Meeting. *J Bone Joint Surg Am* 57:876, 1975.

59. Noyes, F. R.; Grood, E. S.; Nussbaum, N. S.; Cooper, S. M.: Effect of intra-articular corticosteroids on ligament properties: a biomechanical and histological study in rhesus knees. *Clin Orthop* 123:197–209, 1977.

60. Noyes, F. R.; Torvik, P. J.; Hyde, W. B.; DeLucas, J. L.: Biomechanics of ligament failure. II. An analysis of immobilization, exercise, and reconditioning effects in primates. *J Bone Joint Surg Am* 56:1406–1418, 1974.

61. O'Connor, J. T. S.; FitzPatrick, D.: Geometry of the knee. In Daniel, D.; Akeson, W.; O'Connor, J. (eds.): *Knee Ligaments: Structure, Function, Injury, and Repair.* New York: Raven, 1990; pp. 163–199.

62. Partington, F. R.; Wood, G. C.: The role of non-collagen components in the mechanical behaviour of tendon fibres. *Biochim Biophys Acta* 69:485–495, 1963.

63. Rappe, M.; Horodyski, M.; Meister, K.; Indelicato, P. A.: Nonirradiated versus irradiated Achilles allograft: in vivo failure comparison. *Am J Sports Med* 35:1653–1658, 2007.

64. Rasmussen, T. J.; Feder, S. M.; Butler, D. L.; Noyes, F. R.: The effects of 4 Mrad of gamma irradiation on the initial mechanical properties of bone-patellar tendon-bone grafts. *Arthroscopy* 10:188–197, 1994.

65. Rigby, B. J.; Hirai, N.; Spikes, J. D.; Eyring, H.: The mechanical properties of rat tail tendon. *J Gen Physiol* 43:265–283, 1959.

66. Salehpour, A.; Butler, D. L.; Proch, F. S.; et al.: Dose-dependent response of gamma irradiation on mechanical properties and related biochemical composition of goat bone–patellar tendon–bone allografts. *J Orthop Res* 13:898–906, 1995.

67. Sammarco, G. J.; Burstein, A. H.; Davis, W. L.; Frankel, V. H.: The biomechanics of torsional fractures: the effect of loading on ultimate properties. *J Biomech* 4:113–117, 1971.

68. Scapinelli, R.: Studies on the vasculature of the human knee joint. *Acta Anat (Basel)* 70:305–331, 1968.

69. Schwartz, H. E.; Matava, M. J.; Proch, F. S.; et al.: The effect of gamma irradiation on anterior cruciate ligament allograft biomechanical and biochemical properties in the caprine model at time zero and at 6 months after surgery. *Am J Sports Med* 34:1747–1755, 2006.

70. Shino, K.; Horibe, S.: Experimental ligament reconstruction by allogeneic tendon graft in a canine model. *Acta Orthop Belg* 57(suppl 2):44–53, 1991.

71. Shino, K.; Kawasaki, T.; Hirose, H.; et al.: Replacement of the anterior cruciate ligament by an allogeneic tendon graft. An experimental study in the dog. *J Bone Joint Surg Br* 66:672–681, 1984.

72. Sidles, J. A.; Larson, R. V.; Garbini, J. L.; et al.: Ligament length relationship in the moving knee. *J Orthop Res* 6:593–610, 1988.

73. Smith, J. W.: The elastic properties of the anterior cruciate ligament of the rabbit. *J Anat* 88:369–380, 1954.

74. Stilwell, D. L., Jr.; Gray, D. J.: The microscopic structure of periosteum in areas of tendinous contact. *Anat Rec* 120:663–677, 1954.

75. Strasser, H. (ed.): Lehrbuch der Muskel- und Gelenkmechanik. Berlin: Springer, 1913.

76. Thompson, R. C., Jr.; Bassett, C. A.: Histological observations on experimentally induced degeneration of articular cartilage. *J Bone Joint Surg Am* 52:435–443, 1970.

77. Thorson, E.; Rodrigo, J. J.; Vasseur, P.; et al.: Replacement of the anterior cruciate ligament. A comparison of autografts and allografts in dogs. *Acta Orthop Scand* 60:555–560, 1989.

78. Tipton, C. M.; James, S. L.; Mergner, W.; Tcheng, T. K.: Influence of exercise on strength of medial collateral knee ligaments of dogs. *Am J Physiol* 218:894–902, 1970.

79. Tipton, C. M.; Schild, R. J.; Flatt, A. E.: Measurement of ligamentous strength in rat knees. *J Bone Joint Surg Am* 49:63–72, 1967.

80. Tipton, C. M.; Schild, R. J.; Tomanek, R. J.: Influence of physical activity on the strength of knee ligaments in rats. *Am J Physiol* 212:783–787, 1967.

81. Trent, P. S.; Walker, P. S.; Wolf, B.: Ligament length patterns, strength, and rotational axes of the knee joint. *Clin Orthop Relat Res* 117:263–270, 1976.

82. van Rens, T. J.; van den Berg, A. F.; Huiskes, R.; Kuypers, W.: Substitution of the anterior cruciate ligament: a long-term histologic and biomechanical study with autogenous pedicled grafts of the iliotibial band in dogs. *Arthroscopy* 2:139–154, 1986.

83. Vasseur, P. B.; Rodrigo, J. J.; Stevenson, S.; et al.: Replacement of the anterior cruciate ligament with a bone-ligament-bone anterior cruciate ligament allograft in dogs. *Clin Orthop Relat Res* 219:268–277, 1987.

84. Viidik, A.: Biomechanics and functional adaptation of tendons and joint ligaments. In Evans, F. G. (ed.): *Studies on the Anatomy and Function of Bone and Joints.* Berlin: Springer Verlag, 1966; pp. 17–39.

85. Viidik, A.: Elasticity and tensile strength of the anterior cruciate ligament in rabbits as influenced by training. *Acta Physiol Scand* 74:372–380, 1968.

86. Viidik, A.: Functional properties of collagenous tissues. *Int Rev Connect Tissue Res* 6:127–215, 1973.

87. Vogel, H. G.: Correlation between tensile strength and collagen content in rat skin. Effect of age and cortisol treatment. *Connect Tissue Res* 2:177–182, 1974.

88. Walsh, W. R.; Wiggins, M. E.; Fadale, P. D.; Ehrlich, M. G.: Effects of a delayed steroid injection on ligament healing using a rabbit medial collateral ligament model. *Biomaterials* 16:905–910, 1995.

89. Welsh, R. P.; Macnab, I.; Riley, V.: Biomechanical studies of rabbit tendon. *Clin Orthop Relat Res* 81:171–177, 1971.

90. Wiggins, M. E.; Fadale, P. D.; Ehrlich, M. G.; Walsh, W. R.: Effects of local injection of corticosteroids on the healing of ligaments. A follow-up report. *J Bone Joint Surg Am* 77:1682–1691, 1995.

91. Woo, S. L.-Y.; Hollis, J. M.; Adams, D. J.; et al.: Tensile properties of the human femur–anterior cruciate ligament–tibia complex. The effects of specimen age and orientation. *Am J Sports Med* 19:217–225, 1991.

92. Yoshiya, S.; Andrish, J. T.; Manley, M. T.; Bauer, T. W.: Graft tension in anterior cruciate ligament reconstruction. An in vivo study in dogs. *Am J Sports Med* 15:464–470, 1987.

93. Zuckerman, J.; Stull, G. A.: Effects of exercise on knee ligament separation force in rats. *J Appl Physiol* 26:716–719, 1969.

Anterior Cruciate Ligament

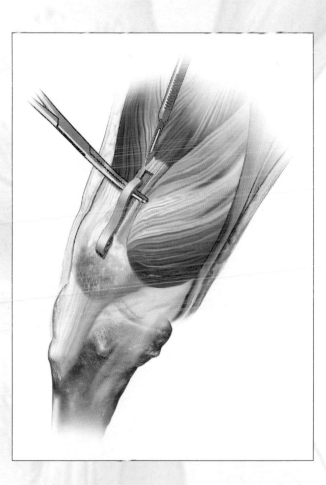

Chapter 5

Biology of Anterior Cruciate Ligament Graft Healing

Asheesh Bedi, MD ▪ *Scott A. Rodeo*, MD

INTRODUCTION

Anterior cruciate ligament (ACL) tears are common among athletes and may become functionally disabling knee injuries. Reconstruction of a torn ACL in order to restore function and limit injury to the menisci has become a common orthopaedic procedure. Despite advances in surgical techniques and the ability to implant an anatomic, isometric graft, ACL reconstruction is not a universally successful procedure. Rates of recurrent laxity 1 year postoperatively have been reported to be as high as 17%.[78]

Failure of graft integration and tendon-to-bone healing may be an important cause of recurrent laxity. The healing of tendon to bone is the basic requirement for the long-term survival of the graft.[12,24] Whether an autograft or an allograft tendon is used, biomechanical testing has shown that the initial strength of the graft material is superior to that of the intact ACL.[12,24] Therefore, the weakest link after reconstruction is not the graft itself, but rather the fixation points until graft osteointegration occurs. The intra-articular portion of the graft must also undergo remodeling and a process of "ligamentization" to form a structure that resembles a native ligament.[3,5,28,36,38]

Current techniques of ACL reconstruction require tendon-to-bone healing in a surgically created bone tunnel. There are no native sites in humans at which a tendon passes through a bone tunnel and, therefore, no analogous situation to the healing that is required after reconstruction. When a bone-tendon-bone graft is used for ACL reconstruction, graft fixation initially depends on bone-to-bone healing. However, tendon-to-bone healing still remains critical regardless of whether a soft tissue graft or a bone-tendon-bone graft is selected. The length of the tendinous portion of the bone-tendon-bone graft is greater than the intra-articular length of the native ACL, resulting in substantial tendon in the bone tunnel. Aperture fixation to minimize graft micromotion and tunnel widening requires tendon-to-bone healing with any graft.[38]

Because all grafts depend on tendon-to-bone healing, this chapter focuses on graft osteointegration and the process by which structural and functional continuity between the graft and the bone is achieved. The biologic and biomechanical environment in the bone tunnel results in formation of an attachment site that differs from the native ligament-bone insertion. The biology of this healing remains incompletely understood and is subject to a number of biomechanical and biologic influences. The current understanding of the biology of graft reconstruction is reviewed and potential strategies to enhance early graft integration are discussed.

NATIVE TENDON-BONE INSERTION

The ACL is an intra-articular, extrasynovial structure that acts to control anterior translation and rotational movements of the femur on a fixed tibia. It is composed of multiple fascicular collagen bundles enveloped in a sheath that contains vascular and neural elements.[4] The ACL inserts to bone via a direct type of insertion, similar to the transition seen from tendon to bone. Microscopic examination of the sites of bony attachment show interdigitation of the collagen fibers with bone through four distinct transition zones: tendon, unmineralized fibrocartilage, mineralized fibrocartilage, and bone (Fig. 5–1).[4,17,57,70] This graduated change in stiffness allows for transmission of complex mechanical loads from soft tissue to bone while minimizing peak stresses at any single point along the ligament. Cartilage-specific collagens including types II, IX, X, and XI are found in the fibrocartilage insertion site. Collagen X plays a key role in maintaining the interface between the mineralized and the unmineralized zones.[4,17,57,70]

TENDON-BONE INSERTION AFTER ACL RECONSTRUCTION

The overall structure, composition, and organization of a native ACL insertion site are not reproduced after ACL reconstruction and reflect an inability to recapitulate the events that occur during embryonic development with current surgical techniques. Rather than regenerating the four organized zones of direct insertion, the graft heals with an interposed zone of vascular, highly cellular granulation tissue between the graft and the tunnel wall (Fig. 5–2).[20,21,65] After 3 to 4 weeks, this interface tissue undergoes a maturation process until its matrix consists of oriented, Sharpey-like collagen fibers that bridge the bone to the graft (Fig. 5–3). The number and size of these collagen fibers positively correlate with the pull-out strength of the graft (Fig. 5–4). Graft attachment strength further improves as bone grows into the interface tissue and outer portion of the graft.[20,21,65]

The maturation process of a tendon graft in a bone tunnel was defined by Kanazawa and coworkers in a rabbit ACL model.[34] In the initial postoperative period, the graft-tunnel interface is filled with vascular granulation tissue containing type III collagen. Vascular endothelial growth factor (VEGF) and

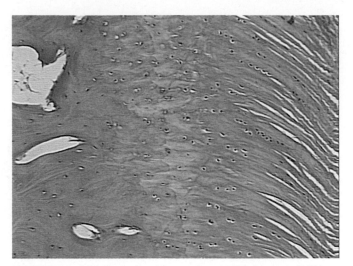

FIGURE 5–1. Histology of native anterior cruciate ligament (ACL) insertion to bone. Examination shows interdigitation of the collagen fibers with bone through four distinct transition zones: tendon, fibrocartilage, mineralized fibrocartilage, and bone.

fibroblast growth factor (FGF) are expressed, stimulating an influx of macrophages and enlarged fibroblasts. Chondroid cells accumulate along the walls of the bone tunnel and deposit type II collagen. The granulation tissue layer is degraded and becomes indistinct. The chondroid cells are gradually replaced with lamellar bone in a process similar to endochondral ossification.[34] The Sharpey-like fibers are composed of type III collagen and extend into the surrounding bone to resist shear stresses. The time interval for this process has been variably reported in the literature, ranging from 8 to 30 weeks.[34]

CHALLENGES OF TENDON-BONE HEALING AFTER ACL RECONSTRUCTION

The biology of healing between a grafted tendon and a bone tunnel remains incompletely understood. The biologic and biomechanical environments result in the formation of an inferior attachment site that is different from the organized, direct-type ACL insertion. Current work suggests a number of fundamental challenges that are responsible for the suboptimal healing response between tendon and bone instead of regeneration of the insertion site.[23] These factors include

1. The presence of inflammatory cells at the graft-tunnel interface that precipitates scar formation.
2. Slow and limited bony ingrowth into the graft from the tunnel walls, resulting in a biomechanically weaker attachment.
3. Insufficient number of undifferentiated stem cells at the healing tendon-bone interface.
4. Graft-tunnel micromotion that precludes the formation of a firm attachment at the tunnel aperture.
5. Lack of a coordinated gene-signaling cascade that directs healing toward regeneration rather than scar tissue formation in the postnatal organism.

Strategies to promote tendon-to-bone healing in ACL reconstruction focus on overcoming these challenges through modification of the biologic and biomechanical environment.

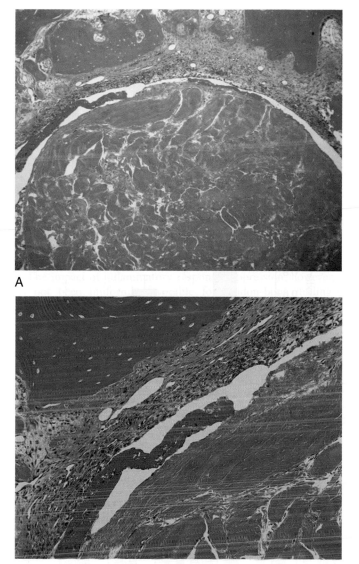

A

B

FIGURE 5–2. Insertion site histology 1–2 weeks after ACL reconstruction. Vascular, highly cellular granulation tissue is interposed as a layer between the graft and the tunnel wall.

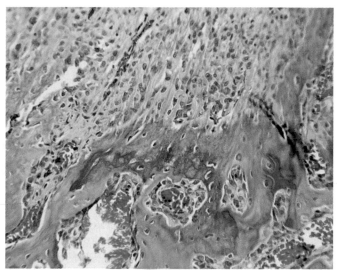

FIGURE 5–3. Insertion site histology 3–4 weeks after ACL reconstruction. The interposed tissue has matured with oriented, Sharpey-like collagen fibers bridging the tendon to bone.

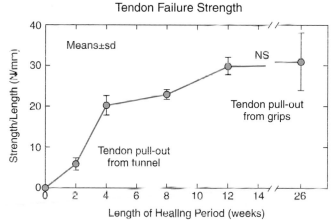

FIGURE 5–4. Pull-out strength of graft correlates with the number and size of bridging, Sharpey-like collagen fibers. (*From Rodeo, S. A.; Arnoczky, S. P.; Torzilli, P. A.; et al.: Tendon-healing in a bone tunnel. A biomechanical and histological study in the dog. J Bone Joint Surg Am 75:1795–1803, 1993.*)

MODULATION OF TENDON-BONE HEALING

Technical Factors

Adjustments can be made in the surgical technique of reconstruction to optimize tendon-to-bone healing. The fundamental principle is to maximize the surface area of the tendon-bone interface. Animal studies have shown that increasing the length of the bone tunnel positively correlates with the quality and strength of the reconstruction.[80] Minimizing graft tunnel mismatch by achieving as tight a fit as possible also improves healing.[22] In addition, maximizing circumferential contact area of the graft and tunnel (i.e., avoiding use of an interference screw) may improve healing.[73]

Critical Points MODULATION OF TENDON-BONE HEALING

- Maximizing the surface area of the tendon-bone interface by minimizing graft tunnel mismatch and using long bone tunnels can help to improve the chances of secure graft-bone healing.
- ACL graft-tunnel micromotion, often seen with suspensory fixation techniques, can preclude the formation of a secure attachment to the tunnel wall and is associated with osteoclast-mediated bone resorption and tunnel widening.
- The rapid inflammatory response after ACL reconstruction is highly complex and may trigger a cascade of events that favors fibrosis and scar formation over tissue regeneration, resulting in an inferior tendon-bone attachment site.
- Ingrowth of bone from the surrounding tunnel wall into the interface zone and graft is ultimately responsible for the improved biomechanical properties of the attachment site after healing is complete.
- Use of undifferentiated stem cells and/or cytokines at the tendon-bone interface may have a future role in promoting tissue regeneration and the restoration of native insertion site morphology after ACL reconstruction.

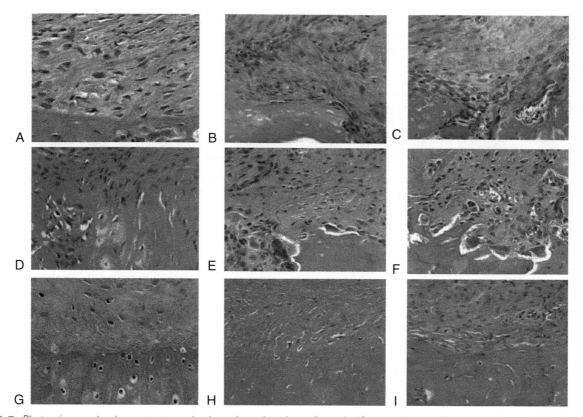

FIGURE 5–7. Photomicrographs demonstrate tendon-bone insertion site at 2 weeks (**A**, control group; **B**, celecoxib group; **C**, indomethacin group), 4 weeks (**D**, control group; **E**, celecoxib group; **F**, indomethacin group), and 8 weeks (**G**, control group; **H**, celecoxib group; **I**, indomethacin group) after surgery (hematoxylin and eosin, ×320). *(**A–I**, From Cohen, D. B.; Kawamura, S.; Ehteshami, J. R.; Rodeo, S. A.: Indomethacin and celecoxib impair rotator cuff tendon-to-bone healing. Am J Sports Med 34:362–369, 2006.)*

tendon. Biomechanical testing demonstrated higher tendon pull-out strength in the treated limbs relative to controls at 2 weeks. Ma and colleagues[41] delivered rhBMP-2 in an injectable calcium phosphate matrix to the bone tunnel in a rabbit ACL reconstruction model. Histologic analysis revealed a dose-dependent increase in bone formation at the tendon-bone interface and significantly narrower tunnel diameters (15%–45%) relative to the control group. Increased construct stiffness was also seen in the treatment group at 8 weeks postoperatively.[41] Martinek and associates[44] transected semitendinosus grafts in vitro with adenovirus-BMP-2 (Ad-BMP-2) and compared them with untreated controls in a rabbit ACL reconstruction model. These investigators demonstrated the formation of a fibrocartilaginous interface at the tendon-bone junction in the experimental group that was absent in the controls. Both stiffness and load-to-failure parameters were superior in the treatment group at 8 weeks. BMP-7 has also been shown to improve bone formation at the tendon-bone interface and load to failure at both 3 and 6 weeks postoperatively in an ovine reconstruction model.[1,45]

Further support for the role of BMPs in bone ingrowth around tendon graft comes from studies of BMP inhibition. Ma and colleagues[41] delivered noggin, a potent inhibitor of all BMP activity, to the healing tendon-bone interface using an injectable calcium phosphate matrix in a rabbit ACL reconstruction model. Noggin significantly inhibited new bone formation at the tendon-bone interface. Furthermore, a significant increase in the width of the fibrous tissue interface between tendon and bone was found in the noggin-treated animals (Fig. 5–8).

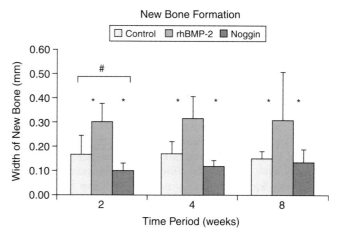

FIGURE 5–8. The width of new bone formation (mm ± SD) at the tunnel-graft interface after ACL reconstruction in a rabbit model. *Significant difference compared with rhBMP-2 group ($P < .05$). #Significant difference compared with the control group ($P < .05$). For each dosage of rhBMP-2 and noggin test, four rabbit limbs were used for histomorphometric analysis. *(Modified from Ma, C.; Kawamura, S.; Deng, X.; et al.: BMP-signaling plays a role in tendon-to-bone healing: A study of rhBMP-2 and noggin. Am J Sports Med 35:597–604, 2007.)*

The favorable effect of osteoinductive agents on tendon-bone healing in a tunnel is further supported by studies that have used tendons wrapped in periosteum. Transplantation of a long digital extensor tendon wrapped in periosteum into a tunnel in the proximal tibia was compared with controls in a rabbit model.[10,61] Improved biomechanical strength and bone and fibrocartilage formation at the tendon-bone interface were shown in the treated animals at 8 and 12 weeks. Ohtera and colleagues[61] completed further studies comparing fresh and frozen periosteum and demonstrated better histologic and biomechanical outcomes using fresh periosteal wraps. These findings support the hypothesis that the viable osteoinductive factors in the periosteum may contribute to the improved outcomes.

Osteoconductive agents have also been met with favorable outcomes in animal models. Calcium phosphate (CaP)–hybridized grafts used in a rabbit ACL reconstruction model demonstrated improved fibrocartilage and bone formation relative to animals treated with unhybridized grafts at 3 weeks postoperatively.[56] Furthermore, studies by Tien and coworkers[76] using injectable CaP cement in the femoral tunnel of a rabbit ACL reconstruction model showed improved bone formation and biomechanical strengths relative to controls at 1 and 2 weeks postoperatively.

Modulation of osteoclast activity in the bone tunnel is another technique of promoting bone formation at the tendon-bone interface. Furthermore, inhibition of osteoclast-mediated bone resorption offers a potential means by which to limit the bone tunnel expansion commonly seen after ACL reconstruction. One study demonstrated that increased knee laxity correlated with radiographic tunnel widening after ACL reconstruction using hamstring tendon.[25] The role of osteoclastic bone resorption on tendon-bone healing has been evaluated in a rabbit ACL reconstruction model.[15] Osteoprotegerin (OPG), a potent inhibitor of osteoclast activity, or receptor activator of nuclear factor κB ligand (RANKL), a potent stimulant of osteoclast formation, were delivered to the bone tunnels around a tendon graft using a CaP carrier matrix. A significantly greater amount of bone surrounding the tendon at the interface was seen in the OPG-treated limbs relative to controls and RANKL-treated limbs at all time points (Fig. 5–9).[15] Furthermore, biomechanical testing at 8 weeks demonstrated significantly increased stiffness of the femur-graft-tibia complex in the OPG-treated limbs compared with the RANKL-treated limbs.

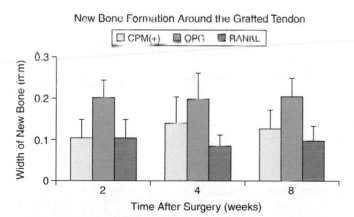

New Bone Formation Around the Grafted Tendon

□ CPM(+)   ▨ OPG   ■ RANKL

FIGURE 5–9. Fifteen New Zealand white rabbits underwent unilateral ACL reconstruction using an autologous semitendinosis tendon graft. Animals treated with osteoprotegerin (OPG) 100 μg had a significant ($P = .007$) increase in newly formed bone around the graft compared with the control group (0.16 ± 0.01 mm^2; 0.06 ± 0.02 mm^2). RANKL, receptor activator of nuclear factor κB ligand. (*Modified from Rodeo, S. A.; Kawamura, S.; Ma, C. B.; et al.: The effect of osteoclastic activity on tendon-to-bone healing: an experimental study in rabbits.* J Bone Joint Surg Am 89:2250–2259, 2007.)

Stem Cells

Undifferentiated, pluripotent mesenchymal cells, also termed *stem* cells, may be critical to stimulate tissue regeneration rather than scar formation at the tendon-bone interface. These cells retain the capacity to differentiate into various specialized cell types based on biologic signals in the local environment. Animal studies have tested the effects of local stem cell delivery on tendon-bone healing. Rabbit bone marrow stromal cells placed in a fibrin glue carrier were delivered to the tendon-bone interface of hallucis longus tendon in a calcaneal tunnel.[62] Histologic analysis revealed improved healing with fibrocartilaginous attachment between tendon and bone in the experimental group. Lim and associates[40] performed bilateral ACL reconstructions in a rabbit model and evaluated the role of mesenchymal stem cells (MSC) on the tendon-bone interface. The grafts coated with MSC demonstrated cartilage at the tendon-bone interface, whereas only fibrous tissue was observed at the interface in the contralateral control limbs. The interface stained positively for type II collagen in the MSC-treated grafts, and was similar in organization to a native, direct ligament insertion. Furthermore, biomechanical testing at 8 weeks demonstrated higher loads to failure and stiffness relative to controls.[40]

Further work is required to determine the mechanism by which pluripotent stem cells enhance tendon-bone healing. It is unknown whether these cells differentiate into fibrochondrocytes or if they produce cytokines that improve insertion site organization and tissue regeneration.

Modulation of Vascularity

Whereas vascularity is critical for the efficient delivery of oxygen and nutrients to support tissue healing, the precise role of local vascularity at the tendon-bone interface remains to be defined. Krivic and colleagues[37] demonstrated improved vascularity at the healing Achilles tendon–bone interface after treatment with gastric pentadecapeptide BPC 157 in a rat model. This improved vascularity correlated with favorable histologic and biomechanical properties of the tendon-bone interface. In contrast, however, a recent study examined the effect of VEGF on graft healing in an ovine ACL reconstruction model.[82] Although vascularity and cellularity were increased in the VEGF-soaked grafts relative to controls, the stiffness of the femur-graft-tibia complex was significantly inferior to controls at 3 months. Although only a single concentration of VEGF was utilized, the results present the possibility that excessive vascularity may adversely affect healing and the biomechanical properties of the tendon-bone interface.[82]

Modulation of MMPs

The MMPs are a family of zinc-dependent endoproteinases that play a critical role in tissue degradation, healing, and normal remodeling. They function both in an extracellular environment and through transmembrane and intracytoplasmic domains.[14] Inflammatory cytokines such as interleukin-1 (IL-1) and tumor necrosis factor (TNF) initiate the transcription and activation of MMPs from their zymogen form. Their catabolic, destructive activity is balanced, however, by TIMPs. TIMPs provide a check-and-balance mechanism to control the activity of these degradative enzymes and thereby maintain homeostasis of extracellular matrix formation and degradation that occurs with tissue remodeling.[18]

Synovial fluid tracking between the graft and the tunnel walls after ACL reconstruction is known to contain large amounts of collagenase and stromelysin. It has been theorized that these MMPs may have adverse effects on the tendon-bone interface, perhaps by limiting the formation of Sharpey-like collagen fibers. Demirag and coworkers[14] used α_2-macroglobulin, an endogenous inhibitor of MMPs, to study this hypothesis in a rabbit ACL reconstruction model. Each rabbit underwent bilateral ACL reconstruction with hamstring autograft. α_2-Macroglobulin was injected into one knee postoperatively and compared with the contralateral control limb. The interface tissue in treated specimens was more mature with significantly greater Sharpey-like fibers. Biomechanical studies demonstrated greater load to failure compared with controls at 2 and 5 weeks[14] (Fig. 5–10). Further studies are necessary to characterize the precise mechanism of action of MMPs at the tendon-bone interface. Nonetheless, this work provides preliminary evidence that modulation of MMP activity can improve graft-bone healing in a bone tunnel.

Modulation of Nitric Oxide

Nitric oxide is a free radical agent synthesized by nitric oxide synthase from L-arginine. It acts as a regulatory molecule both in cells and in the extracellular matrix. Studies have shown that it is induced during tendon healing in vitro, with a dose-dependent effect on fibroblast collagen production.[54,55] ACL ligament fibroblasts are uniquely able to produce more nitric oxide compared with other local fibroblasts, including those derived from the medial collateral ligament (MCL).[46] The influence of nitric oxide levels on tendon-bone healing after ACL reconstruction remains to be defined.

Effect of Hyperbaric Oxygen

Yeh and associates[81] recently studied the influence of hyperbaric oxygen (HBO) therapy on the graft-bone tunnel interface in a rabbit model. The HBO group was exposed to 100% oxygen at 2.5 atm pressure for 2 hours daily, 5 consecutive days a week.

The control group was exposed to normal air. The HBO group demonstrated increased neovascularization and an increased number of Sharpey fibers relative to controls. Furthermore, the HBO group achieved higher maximal pull-out strengths at 12 and 18 weeks relative to control specimens.[81] Although the mechanism of action is unclear, these preliminary results suggest that HBO therapy may improve tendon-bone healing after ACL reconstruction.

Modulation of Other Biologic Mediators

Future techniques to enhance tendon-bone healing after ACL reconstruction will be directed by an improved understanding of the biology of this healing process. Use of cytokines to provide important signals for tissue formation and differentiation, gene therapy techniques to provide sustained cytokine delivery, stem cells, or transcription factors to modulate endogenous gene expression represent some of these possibilities. *Scleraxis*, a transcription factor expressed in mesenchymal tendon progenitor cells, and *sox-9*, a transcription factor critical for chondrogenesis, are two such proteins that may play key roles in native tendon insertion site formation.

BONE-TO-BONE HEALING IN ACL AUTOGRAFT RECONSTRUCTION

Healing of a bone plug to the osseous tunnel walls after autograft ACL reconstruction is unique and unlike anywhere else in the body. The biomechanical and biologic environments in the graft tunnels present significant challenges to union.

The sequence of bone-tendon-bone autograft incorporation has been defined in animal models. Tomita and colleagues[77] compared healing of a soft tissue graft to a bone–patellar tendon–bone autograft in a canine model. The bone plug undergoes osteonecrosis and is gradually replaced by a process of creeping substitution (Fig. 5–11). Newly formed bone surrounding the plug is seen at 3 weeks. These investigators found pull-out strength of the bone–patellar tendon–bone graft to be superior to the soft tissue graft at 3 weeks, but not significantly different at 6 weeks. At 6 weeks, a change in the point of failure was noted from the graft-tunnel interface to the tendon-bone plug interface. Papageorgiou and coworkers[64] directly compared tendon-bone with bone-bone healing in a goat model. Bone–patellar tendon autografts were harvested; the soft tissue graft was placed in the tibial tunnel while the bone plug was secured in the femoral tunnel. Biomechanical testing at 3 weeks demonstrated universal failure of the tendon-bone interface with

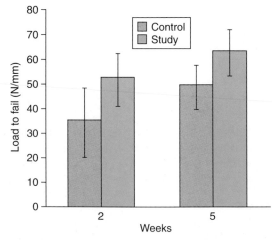

FIGURE 5–10. The ultimate load to failure was significantly greater in the α_2-macroglobulin–treated specimens than in the untreated control specimens at both 2 and 5 weeks ($P = .007$ and $P = .006$, respectively). *(Modified from Demirag, B.; Sarisozen, B.; Durak, K.; et al: The effect of alpha-2 macroglobulin on the healing of ruptured anterior cruciate ligament in rabbits. Connect Tissue Res 45:23–27, 2004.)*

Critical Points BONE-TO-BONE HEALING AFTER ACL AUTOGRAFT RECONSTRUCTION

- The process of bone plug incorporation after ACL reconstruction is complex and is characterized by osteonecrosis followed by creeping substitution and new host bone formation.
- Synovial fluid flow into the bone tunnels may interfere with healing at the tendon-bone interface.
- Regardless of whether a soft tissue or bone-tendon-bone graft is utilized, the critical healing at the intra-articular aperture that must occur to minimize graft micromotion usually requires tendon-bone healing.

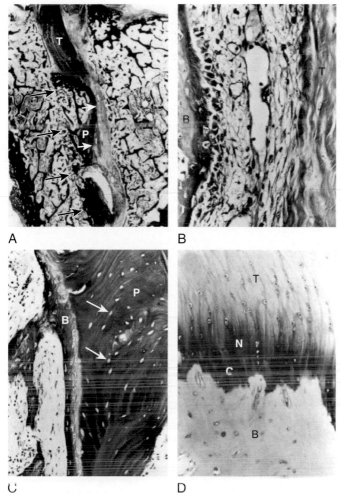

FIGURE 5–11. (**A**) The anterior portion of the bone plug–bony wall gap was filled with granulation tissue (*white arrows*), while the posterior aspect of the bone plug appeared to be in contact with the bony wall (*black arrows*) (T, patellar tendon; P, bone plug of the BPTB) (H&E, original magnification × 2). (**B**) In the granulation tissue around the intraosseous tendon portion, few collagen fibers are seen (B, bone wall; T, patellar tendon) (H&E, original magnification × 100). (**C**) In the bone plug of the BPTB graft, a number of empty lacunae (*white arrows*) that indicated bone necrosis were found, except for the superficial portion of the plug (B, bone wall; P, bone plug of the BPTB) (H&E, original magnification × 50). (**D**) At the tendon bone junction of the graft, both the noncalcified and calcified fibrocartilage layers appeared to be normal (T, patellar tendon; N, noncalcified fibrocartilage layer; C, calcified fibrocartilage layer; B, bone) (toluidine-blue, original magnification × 50). (*From Tomita, F.; Yasuda, K.; Mikami, S.; et al.: Comparisons of intraosseous graft healing between the doubled flexor tendon graft and the bone-patellar tendon-bone graft in anterior cruciate ligament reconstruction. Arthroscopy 17:461–476, 2001.*)

pull-out from the tibial tunnel. At 6 weeks, however, approximately 20% of cases demonstrated midsubstance failures. The remaining cases continued to be tibial tunnel graft pull-out. Histologic evaluation at 3 weeks confirmed creeping substitution with a necrotic bone plug surrounded by granulation tissue. Evaluation at 6 weeks revealed complete plug incorporation with bridging cancellous bone.[64]

Synovial fluid flows from the joint into the tunnels and can interfere with healing at the tendon-bone interface. The high quantities of MMPs and other proteolytic enzymes in synovial fluid can slow bone-tendon-bone and bone-bone healing. Berg and associates[9] evaluated the role of synovial fluid by drilling

femoral and tibial tunnels and leaving them empty in a rabbit ACL model. These authors found healing to occur most rapidly at points farthest away from the joint, whereas the slowest and most incomplete regions of healing were at the tunnel apertures. These findings are suggestive of a possible inhibitory effect of synovial fluid on healing in the tunnel.

It is critical to remember that whether a soft tissue or a bone-tendon-bone graft is used, the critical aperture fixation will usually require tendon-bone healing. The tendon length of a bone–patellar tendon–bone graft exceeds the native ACL length, such that a substantial portion of the tunnel, including the aperture zone, will contain tendon. Tendon-bone healing at the aperture, regardless of graft choice, is essential to minimize graft micromotion and subsequent risk of tunnel widening.

INTRA-ARTICULAR GRAFT HEALING IN ACL AUTOGRAFT RECONSTRUCTION

Ligamentization refers to the complex process of biologic incorporation and remodeling that occurs to the tendon after ACL reconstruction. Animal studies have attempted to define the phases of intra-articular graft healing that occur postoperatively. The graft goes through an initial phase of avascular necrosis. At 2 weeks, the graft demonstrates patches of necrosis, although the collagen architecture and scaffold remain intact.[2,3,36,63] By 4 weeks, the graft is almost entirely avascular and acellular. This phase, however, is followed by cellular repopulation from the host synovial cells. Biopsy at 3 months reveals extensive vascular proliferation and cellular repopulation. By 9 months, the graft histologically resembles the native ligament.[2,3,36,63]

Intra-articular healing has also been studied in other animal models. Oaks and colleagues[60] demonstrated remodeling to occur from the periphery toward the graft center. This was associated with a change from large-diameter to small-diameter collagen fibrils. This pattern of remodeling supports the hypothesis that healing is dependent on gradual revascularization and cellular repopulation from the host synovium. Arnoczky and coworkers[3] evaluated patellar tendon graft revascularization in a canine model. Initially the grafts were avascular, but by 6 weeks, they were completely ensheathed in a vascular synovial envelope. The soft tissues of the infrapatellar fat pad, the tibial remnant of the ACL, and the posterior synovial tissues contributed to this synovial vasculature. Intrinsic revascularization of the patellar tendon graft progressed from the proximal and distal portions of the graft centrally.[3] The tibial attachment of the patellar tendon graft did not contribute any vessels to the revascularization process. The contribution of the soft tissues of the knee to the revascularization process of the graft emphasized the importance of their preservation in maintaining the graft's viability.

Although animal models have provided insight into the process of ligamentization, the process has not been fully characterized in humans. Jackson and associates[28] concluded that an incorporated graft never replicates the native ACL and rather functions like a checkrein of organized scar tissue. Delay and

Critical Points INTRA-ARTICULAR GRAFT HEALING IN ACL AUTOGRAFT RECONSTRUCTION

- Intra-articular graft healing occurs by a process of remodeling that is dependent on revascularization and cellular repopulation from the host synovium.
- The incorporated graft does not achieve the organization or vascularity of the native ACL.

colleagues[13] described a case report of a bone–patellar tendon–bone autograft with avascular, acellular regions in the deep, distal graft 18 months after reconstruction. Rougraff and Shelbourne[69] performed patellar tendon graft biopsies on nine subjects 3 to 8 weeks after autogenous ACL reconstruction. Graft vascularity was present at 3 weeks and increased over the 8-week interval.

PRIMARY ACL HEALING AND REPAIR

Primary repair of the ACL after traumatic rupture was historically considered to be a viable surgical option. Outcome studies, however, have reported unacceptable rates of failure after primary surgical repair.[16] In their classic study, Feagin and Curl[16] reported a 94% rate of instability in patients at 5-year follow-up after primary suture and drill hole ACL repair. Marshall and coworkers[43] reported a 20% to 40% failure rate despite repair using a sophisticated, multiple-depth suture technique. Zysk and Refior[85] also reported modest outcomes in a study on middle-aged patients who underwent primary ACL repair and recommended that open primary repair be abandoned in favor of autogenous tissue reconstruction or augmentation. These results were recently corroborated by a Norwegian study that assessed long-term outcomes in a large series of patients who underwent primary ACL repair.[75] An open procedure using the original Palmer technique with nonabsorbable Bunnell sutures was performed in all cases. At 15 to 23 years postoperatively, 57% had greater than 3 mm of anterior translation on KT-1000 testing. The estimated rate of total failure was 27%. These results are in sharp contradistinction to the MCL, in which failure to primarily heal is the exception rather than the rule.

The poor rate of primary healing observed after ACL rupture is believed to be multifactorial in nature. One of the most salient factors is the intra-articular environment and synovial fluid that surrounds the ACL.[47–53,74] Studies by Murray and associates[47–53,74] elegantly demonstrated the differences in intra-articular (i.e., ACL) versus extra-articular (i.e., MCL) healing in a canine, central ACL wound model. An empty wound persists at the defect of an intra-articular ligament wound, whereas these wounds are rapidly filled with a fibrin-platelet scaffold in an extra-articular injury. This scaffold is critical to allow subsequent cellular repopulation, revascularization, and ligament remodeling into mature scar tissue. The lack of a scaffold in the intra-articular ligament wounds was associated with decreased inflammatory cytokines needed for the healing response, including fibrinogen, PDGF, TGF-β, and FGF.[47–53,74] Studies by Murray and associates[47–53,74] demonstrated that replacement of the central intra-articular ligament void with a collagen-platelet–rich plasma scaffold resulted in increased filling of the wound with repair tissue that

Critical Points PRIMARY ACL HEALING AND REPAIR

- Clinical outcomes studies have shown unacceptable rates of failure after primary ACL repair.
- The poor healing rate is believed to be multifactorial in nature, including an unfavorable, intra-articular biologic environment and altered cellular metabolism and function after injury.
- Augmentation with a collagen-platelet–rich plasma scaffold may offer future promise to improve healing after primary ligament repair.

had similar profiles of protein expression to matched, extra-articular ligament wounds. Biomechanical studies of suture ACL repair augmented with a collagen-platelet–rich scaffold in a porcine model have shown significant improvement in load to failure and linear stiffness at 4 weeks compared with unaugmented, control repairs.[47–53,74]

Other factors implicated in the poor ACL healing response include alterations in cellular metabolism after injury, cellular loss within the tissues after injury, and intrinsic deficiencies in ACL fibroblasts compared with fibroblasts in extra-articular ligaments. Murray and associates[47–53,74] defined the histologic changes that occur after ACL rupture. The human ACL undergoes four histologic phases: inflammation, epiligamentous regeneration, proliferation, and remodeling (Fig. 5–12). Although similar to the response to injury in other dense connective tissues, major exceptions include (1) formation of an alpha-smooth

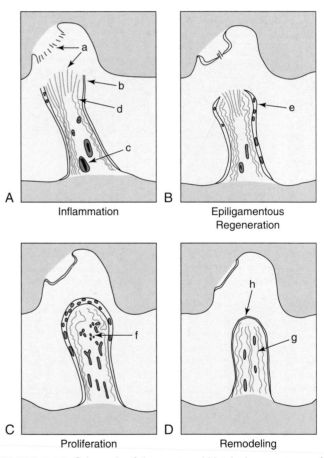

FIGURE 5–12. Schematic of the gross and histologic appearance of the four phases of the healing response in the human ACL. **A,** The inflammatory phase, showing mop-ends of the remnants (a), disruption of the epiligament and synovial covering of the ligament (b), intimal hyperplasia of the vessels (c), and loss of the regular crimp structure near the site of injury (d). **B,** The epiligamentous regeneration phase, involving a gradual recovering of the ligament remnant by vascularized, epiligamentous tissue and synovial tissue (e). **C,** The proliferative phase, with revascularization of the remnant with groups of capillaries (f). **D,** The remodeling and maturation phase, characterized by a decrease in cell number density and blood vessel density (g) and by retraction of the ligament remnant (h). (**A–D,** Modified from Murray, M. M.; Martin, S. D.; Martin, T. L.; Spector, M.: Histological changes in the human anterior cruciate ligament after rupture. J Bone Joint Surg Am 82:1387–1397, 2000.)

muscle actin-expressing synovial cell layer on the surface of the ruptured ends, (2) the lack of any tissue bridging the rupture site, and (3) the presence of an epiligamentous reparative phase that lasts 8 to 12 weeks.[47–53,74] The biology involved in intra-articular ligament healing will need to be further defined to overcome the obstacles to long-term success with primary ACL repair.

ALLOGRAFT HEALING IN ACL RECONSTRUCTION

An increasing desire to avoid the morbidity of graft harvest and to reduce operative times has led to a dramatic increase in the use of allografts as an alternative graft source in primary ACL reconstruction.[7] Allografts are also frequently used in revision procedures or multiligament reconstruction procedures. Good clinical outcomes have been reported with allograft reconstructions at 2 to 5 years follow-up, and multiple studies have found no significant subjective or objective difference in knee function after allograft versus autograft ACL reconstructions.[8] However, other studies have reported less favorable results after allograft reconstruction, particularly in the setting of chronic or revision knee surgery.[58,59]

Despite compatible clinical outcomes, animal studies have shown that allografts have a slower rate of incorporation, prolonged inflammatory response, and greater initial decrease in biomechanical properties compared with autografts.[2–6,29–33,84] The phases of healing, although delayed, resemble those of the autograft. The tendon-bone interface develops a fibrovascular granulation tissue interface that eventually undergoes bone ingrowth and develops Sharpey-like anchoring fibers.[2–6,32,33,84] The intra-articular graft undergoes ligamentization with a phase of avascular necrosis followed by cellular repopulation and vascular proliferation from host synovium. Donor DNA was entirely replaced by host DNA within 4 weeks in a goat reconstruction model. Revascularization starts at 3 weeks and progresses gradually over the next several weeks. Jackson and colleagues compared healing of patellar tendon autografts with fresh allografts in a goat ACL reconstruction model.[31–33] Although graft structural properties were similar at time zero, the allografts healed at a much slower rate. At 6 months, the autografts demonstrated a superior load to failure, larger increase in graft cross-sectional area, and better restraint to anteroposterior displacement. The allografts demonstrated a significantly greater decrease in their preimplantation structural properties.

Human studies have supported these findings of slower allograft incorporation. At 2 years postoperatively, biopsy studies have shown that the central portion of allografts can continue to be acellular.[27] Cellular repopulation of the entire graft was often seen only after 3 or more years after allograft reconstruction.[42]

Because of the relative hypocellularity of tendon allografts and current sterilization techniques, the host immune response is relatively limited. Major histocompatibility complex (MHC) antigens that incite a potent immune response are largely depleted. Matrix antigens, however, persist and can elicit an immune response that may contribute to the delayed incorporation and the pronounced alteration in structural properties after surgery.[68,79] The specific influences of such an immune response on the biology of ACL graft healing remains to be defined.

Critical Points ALLOGRAFT HEALING IN ACL RECONSTRUCTION

- Allografts demonstrate a slower rate of host incorporation, prolonged inflammatory response, and greater decrease in initial biomechanical properties than those of autografts in ACL reconstruction.
- Greater variability in clinical outcomes compared with autograft ACL reconstruction
- Higher failure rate when used for revision ACL reconstruction

---

CONCLUSION

This chapter presents the basic principles of the biology of ACL reconstruction and reviews potential techniques to improve graft healing. A sound understanding of the complex mechanism of tendon-to-bone healing offers new and exciting ways to manipulate the chemical and molecular mediators of the inflammatory response and to ultimately improve the quality of surgical and postoperative interventions.

REFERENCES

1. Anderson, K.; Seneviratne, A. M.; Izawa, K.; et al.: Augmentation of tendon healing in an intra-articular bone tunnel with use of a bone growth factor. *Am J Sports Med* 29:689–698, 2001.
2. Arnoczky, S. P.: Biology of ACL reconstructions: what happens to the graft? *Instr Course Lect* 45:229–233, 1996.
3. Arnoczky, S. P.; Tarvin, G. B.; Marshall, J. L.: Anterior cruciate ligament replacement using patellar tendon. An evaluation of graft revascularization in the dog. *J Bone Joint Surg Am* 64:217–224, 1982.
4. Arnoczky, S. P.: Anatomy of the ACL. *Clin Orthop* 172:19–25, 1983.
5. Arnoczky, S. P.; Warren, R. F.; Ashlock, M. A.: Replacement of the anterior cruciate ligament using a patellar tendon allograft. An experimental study. *J Bone Joint Surg Am* 68:376–385, 1986.
6. Arnoczky, S. P.; Rubin, R. M.; Marshall, J. L.: Microvasculature of the cruciate ligaments and its response to injury. An experimental study in dogs. *J Bone Joint Surg Am* 61:1221–1229, 1979.
7. Bach, B. R., Jr.; Aadalen, K. J.; Dennis, M. G.; et al.: Primary anterior cruciate ligament reconstruction using fresh frozen, nonirradiated patellar tendon allograft: minimum 2-year follow-up. *Am J Sports Med* 33:284–292, 2005.
8. Barrett, G.; Stokes, D.; White, M.: Anterior cruciate ligament reconstruction in patients older than 40 years: allograft versus autograft patellar tendon. *Am J Sports Med* 33:1505–1512, 2005.
9. Berg, E. E.; Pollard, M. E.; Kang, Q.: Interarticular bone tunnel healing. *Arthroscopy* 17:189–195, 2001.
10. Chen, C. H.; Chen, W. J.; Shih, C. H.; et al.: Enveloping the tendon graft with periosteum to enhance tendon-bone healing in a bone tunnel: A biomechanical and histologic study in rabbits. *Arthroscopy.* 19:290–296, 2003.
11. Cohen, D. B.; Kawamura, S.; Ehteshami, J. R.; Rodeo, S. A.: Indomethacin and celecoxib impair rotator cuff tendon-to-bone healing. *Am J Sports Med* 34:362–369, 2006.
12. Cooper, D. E.; Deng, X. H.; Burstein, A. L.; Warren, R. F.: The strength of the central third patellar tendon graft. A biomechanical study. *Am J Sports Med* 21:818–823; discussion 823–824, 1993.
13. Delay, B. S.; McGrath, B. E.; Mindell, E. R.: Observations on a retrieved patellar tendon autograft used to reconstruct the anterior cruciate ligament. *J Bone Joint Surg Am* 84:1433–1438, 2002.

14. Demirag, B.; Sarisozen, B.; Durak, K.; et al.: The effect of alpha-2 macroglobulin on the healing of ruptured anterior cruciate ligament in rabbits. *Connect Tissue Res* 45:23–27, 2004.

15. Dynybil, C.; Kawamura, S.; Kim, H. J.; et al.: [The effect of osteoprotegerin on tendon-bone healing after reconstruction of the anterior cruciate ligament: a histomorphological and radiographical study in the rabbit]. *Z Orthop Ihre Grenzgeb* 144:179–186, 2006.

16. Feagin, J. A., Jr.; Curl, W. W.: Isolated tear of the anterior cruciate ligament: 5-year follow-up study. *Clin Orthop Relat Res* 325:4–9, 1996.

17. Fujioka, H.; Thakur, R.; Wang, G. J.; et al.: Comparison of surgically attached and non-attached repair of the rat Achilles tendon-bone interface. Cellular organization and type X collagen expression. *Connect Tissue Res* 37:205–218, 1998.

18. Gomez, D. E.; Alonso, D. F.; Yoshiji, H.; Thorgeirsson, U. P.: Tissue inhibitors of metalloproteinases: structures, regulation and biological functions. *Eur J Cell Biol* 74:111–122, 1997.

19. Goodman, R. B.; Pugin, J.; Lee, J. S.; Matthay, M. A.: Cytokine-mediated inflammation in acute lung injury. *Cytokine Growth Factor Rev* 14:523–535, 2003.

20. Goradia, V. K.; Rochat, M. C.; Grana, W. A.; et al.: Tendon-to-bone healing of a semitendinosus tendon autograft used for ACL reconstruction in a sheep model. *Am J Knee Surg* 13:143–151, 2000.

21. Grana, W. A.; Egle, D. M.; Mahnken, R.; Goodhart, C. W.: An analysis of autograft fixation after anterior cruciate ligament reconstruction in a rabbit model. *Am J Sports Med* 22:344–351, 1994.

22. Greis, P. E.; Burks, R. T.; Bachus, K.; Luker, M. G.: The influence of tendon length and fit on the strength of a tendon-bone tunnel complex. A biomechanical and histologic study in the dog. *Am J Sports Med* 29:493–497, 2001.

23. Gulotta, L. V.; Rodeo, S. A.: Biology of autograft and allograft healing in anterior cruciate ligament reconstruction. *Clin Sports Med* 26:509–524, 2007.

24. Hamner, D. L.; Brown, C. H., Jr.; Steiner, M. E.; et al.: Hamstring tendon grafts for reconstruction of the anterior cruciate ligament: biomechanical evaluation of the use of multiple strands and tensioning techniques. *J Bone Joint Surg Am* 81:549–557, 1999.

25. Hantes, M. E.; Mastrokalos, D. S.; Yu, J.; Paessler, H. H.: The effect of early motion on tibial tunnel widening after anterior cruciate ligament replacement using hamstring tendon grafts. *Arthroscopy* 20:572–580, 2004.

26. Hays, P.; Kawamura, S.; Deng, X.; et al.: The role of macrophages in early healing of a tendon graft in a bone tunnel: an experimental study in a rat anterior cruciate ligament reconstruction model. *J Bone Joint Surg Am* 90:565–579, 2008.

27. Hortsman, J. K.; Ahmadu-Suka, F.; Norrdin, R. W.: Anterior cruciate ligament fascia lata allograft reconstruction: progressive histological changes towards maturity. *Arthroscopy* 9: 509–518, 1993.

28. Jackson, D. W.; Grood, E. S.; Goldstein, J. D.; et al.: A comparison of patellar tendon autograft and allograft used for anterior cruciate ligament reconstruction in the goat model. *Am J Sports Med* 21:176–185, 1993.

29. Jackson, D. W.; Simon, T. M.: Donor cell survival and repopulation after intra-articular transplantation of tendon and ligament allografts. *Microsc Res Tech* 58:25–33, 2002.

30. Jackson, D. W.; Grood, E. S.; Arnoczky, S. P.; et al.: Freeze-dried anterior cruciate ligament allografts. Preliminary studies in a goat model. *Am J Sports Med* 5:295–303, 1987.

31. Jackson, D. W.; Grood, E. S.; Cohn, B. T.; et al.: The effects of in situ freezing on the anterior cruciate ligament. An experimental study in goats. *J Bone Joint Surg Am* 73:201–213, 1991.

32. Jackson, D. W.; Simon, T. M.; Kurzweil, P. R.; Rosen, M. A.: Survival of cells after intra-articular transplantation of fresh allografts of the patellar and anterior cruciate ligaments. DNA-probe analysis in a goat model. *J Bone Joint Surg Am* 74:112–118, 1992.

33. Jackson, D. W.; Corsetti, J.; Simon, T. M.: Biologic incorporation of allograft anterior cruciate ligament replacements. *Clin Orthop Relat Res* 324:126–133, 1996.

34. Kanazawa, T.; Soejima, T.; Murakami, H.; et al.: An immunohistological study of the integration at the bone-tendon interface after reconstruction of the anterior cruciate ligament in rabbits. *J Bone Joint Surg Br* 88:682–687, 2006.

35. Kawamura, S.; Ying, L.; Kim, H. J.; et al.: Macrophages accumulate in the early phase of tendon-bone healing. *J Orthop Res* 23:1425–1432, 2005.

36. Kleiner, J. B.; Amiel, D.; Roux, R. D.; Akeson, W. H.: Origin of replacement cells for the anterior cruciate ligament autograft. *J Orthop Res* 4:466–474, 1986.

37. Krivic, A.; Anic, T.; Seiwerth, S.; et al.: Achilles detachment in rat and stable gastric pentadecapeptide BPC 157: promoted tendon-to-bone healing and opposed corticosteroid aggravation. *J Orthop Res* 24:982–989, 2006.

38. Kurosaka, M.; Yoshiya, S.; Andrish, J. T.: A biomechanical comparison of different surgical techniques of graft fixation in anterior cruciate ligament reconstruction. *Am J Sports Med* 15:225–229, 1987.

39. Leask, A.; Holmes, A.; Abraham, D. J.: Connective tissue growth factor: a new and important player in the pathogenesis of fibrosis. *Curr Rheumatol Rep* 4:136–142, 2002.

40. Lim, J. K.; Hui, J.; Li, L.; et al.: Enhancement of tendon graft osteointegration using mesenchymal stem cells in a rabbit model of anterior cruciate ligament reconstruction. *Arthroscopy* 20:899–910, 2004.

41. Ma, C.; Kawamura, S.; Deng, X.; et al.: BMP-signaling plays a role in tendon-to-bone healing: a study of rhBMP-2 and noggin. *Am J Sports Med* 35:597–604, 2007.

42. Malinin, T. I.; Levitt, R. L.; Bashore, C.; et al.: A study of retrieved allografts used to replace anterior cruciate ligaments. *Arthroscopy* 18:163–170, 2002.

43. Marshall, J. L.; Warren, R. F.; Wickiewicz, T. L.: Primary surgical treatment of anterior cruciate ligament lesions. *Am J Sports Med* 10:103–107, 1982.

44. Martinek, V.; Latterman, C.; Usas, A.; et al.: Enhancement of tendon-bone integration of anterior cruciate ligament grafts with bone morphogenetic protein-2 gene transfer. A histological and biomechanical study. *J Bone Joint Surg Am* 84:1123–1131, 2002.

45. Mihelic, R.; Pecina, M.; Jelic, M.; et al.: Bone morphogenetic protein-7 (osteogenic protein-1) promotes tendon graft integration in anterior cruciate ligament reconstruction in sheep. *Am J Sports Med* 32:1619–1625, 2004.

46. Murakami, H.; Shinomiya, N.; Kikuchi, T.; et al.: Up-regulated expression of inducible nitric oxide synthase plays a key role in early apoptosis after anterior cruciate ligament injury. *J Orthop Res* 24:1521–1534, 2006.

47. Murray, M. M.; Spindler, K. P.; Ballard, P.; et al.: Enhanced histologic repair in a central wound in the anterior cruciate ligament with a collagen-platelet-rich plasma scaffold. *J Orthop Res* 25:1007–1017, 2007.

48. Murray, M. M.; Spindler, K. P.; Abreu, E.; et al.: Collagen-platelet rich plasma hydrogel enhances primary repair of the porcine anterior cruciate ligament. *J Orthop Res* 25:81–91, 2007.

49. Murray, M. M.; Spindler, K. P.; Devin, C.; et al.: Use of a collagen-platelet rich plasma scaffold to stimulate healing of a central defect in the canine ACL. *J Orthop Res* 24:820–830, 2006.

50. Murray, M. M.; Bennett, R.; Zhang, X.; Spector, M.: Cell outgrowth from the human ACL in vitro: regional variation and response to TGF-beta1. *J Orthop Res* 20:875–880, 2002.

51. Murray, M. M.; Martin, S. D.; Martin, T. L.; Spector, M.: Histological changes in the human anterior cruciate ligament after rupture. *J Bone Joint Surg Am* 82:1387–1397, 2000.

52. Murray, M. M.; Martin, S. D.; Spector, M.: Migration of cells from human anterior cruciate ligament explants into collagen-glycosaminoglycan scaffolds. *J Orthop Res* 18:557–564, 2000.

53. Murray, M. M.; Spector, M.: Fibroblast distribution in the anteromedial bundle of the human anterior cruciate ligament: the presence of alpha-smooth muscle actin-positive cells. *J Orthop Res* 17:18–27, 1999.

54. Murrell, G. A.; Szabo, C.; Hannafin, J. A.; et al.: Modulation of tendon healing by nitric oxide. *Inflamm Res* 46:19–27, 1997.

55. Murrell, G. A.; Doland, M. M.; Jang, D.; et al.: Nitric oxide: an important articular free radical. *J Bone Joint Surg Am* 78:265–274, 1996.

56. Mutsuzaki, H.; Sakane, M.; Nakajima, H.; et al.: Calcium-phosphate-hybridized tendon directly promotes regeneration of tendon-bone insertion. *J Biomed Mater Res A* 70:319–327, 2004.

57. Niyibizi, C.; Sagarrigo Visconti, C.; Gibson, G.; Kavalkovich, K.: Identification and immunolocalization of type X collagen at the

ligament-bone interface. *Biochem Biophys Res Commun* 222:584–589, 1996.

58. Noyes, F. R.; Barber-Westin, S. D.; Roberts, C.: Use of allografts after failed treatment of rupture of the anterior cruciate ligament. *J Bone Joint Surg Am* 76:1019–1031, 1994.

59. Noyes, F. R.; Barber, S. D.: The effect of a ligament augmentation device on allograft reconstructions for chronic ruptures of the anterior cruciate ligament. *J Bone Joint Surg Am* 74:960–973, 1992.

60. Oaks, B. W.; Knight, M.; McLean, I. D.; et al.: Goat ACL autograft collagen remodeling: quantitative collagen fibril analysis over one year. In *Transactions of the Combined Meeting of the Orthopaedic Research Societies of USA, Japan, and Canada*, p. 60. October 21–23, 1991, Calgary, Alberta, Canada.

61. Ohtera, K.; Yamada, Y.; Aoki, M.; et al.: Effects of periosteum wrapped around tendon in a bone tunnel: a biomechanical and histological study in rabbits. *Crit Rev Biomed Eng* 28:115–118, 2000.

62. Ouyang, H. W.; Goh, J. C.; Lee, E. H.: Use of bone marrow stromal cells for tendon graft-to-bone healing: histological and immunohistochemical studies in a rabbit model. *Am J Sports Med* 32:321–327, 2004.

63. Panni, A. S.; Milano, G.; Lucania, L.; Fabbriciani, C.: Graft healing after anterior cruciate ligament reconstruction in rabbits. *Clin Orthop Relat Res* 343:203–212, 1997.

64. Papageorgiou, C. D.; Ma, C. B.; Abramowitch, S. D.; et al.: A multidisciplinary study of the healing of an intra-articular anterior cruciate ligament graft in a goat model. *Am J Sports Med* 29:620–626, 2001.

65. Rodeo, S. A.; Arnoczky, S. P.; Torzilli, P. A.; et al.: Tendon-healing in a bone tunnel. A biomechanical and histological study in the dog. *J Bone Joint Surg Am* 75:1795–1803, 1993.

66. Rodeo, S. A.; Kawamura, S.; Kim, H. J.; et al.: Tendon healing in a bone tunnel differs at the tunnel entrance versus the tunnel exit: an effect of graft-tunnel motion? *Am J Sports Med* 34:1790–1800, 2006.

67. Rodeo, S. A.; Suzuki, K.; Deng, X. H.; et al.: Use of recombinant human bone morphogenetic protein-2 to enhance tendon healing in a bone tunnel. *Am J Sports Med* 27:476–488, 1999.

68. Rodrigo, J.; Jackson, D.; Simon, T.; Muto, K.: The immune response to freeze-dried bone-tendon-bone ACL allografts in humans. *Am J Knee Surg* 6:47–53, 1993.

69. Rougraff, B. T.; Shelbourne, K. D.: Early histologic appearance of human patellar tendon autografts used for anterior cruciate ligament reconstruction. *Knee Surg Sports Traumatol Arthrosc* 7:9–14, 1999.

70. Sagarriga, H.; Visconti, C.; Kavalkovich, K.; et al.: Biochemical analysis of collagens at the ligament-bone interface reveals presence of cartilage specific collagens. *Arch Biochem Biophys* 328:135–142, 1996.

71. Sakai, H.; Fukui, N.; Kawakami, A.; Kurosawa, H.: Biological fixation of the graft within bone after anterior cruciate ligament reconstruction in rabbits: effects of the duration of postoperative immobilization. *J Orthop Sci* 5:43–51, 2000.

72. Singer, A. J.; Clark, R. A.: Cutaneous wound healing. *N Engl J Med* 341:738–746, 1999.

73. Singhatat, W.; Lawhorn, K. W.; Howell, S. M.; Hull, M. L.: How four weeks of implantation affect the strength and stiffness of a tendon graft in a bone tunnel: a study of two fixation devices in an extra-articular model in ovine. *Am J Sports Med* 30:506–513, 2002.

74. Spindler, K. P.; Murray, M. M.; Devin, C.; et al.: The central ACL defect as a model for failure of intra-articular healing. *J Orthop Res* 24:401–406, 2006.

75. Strand, T.; Molster, A.; Hordvik, M.; Krukhaug, Y.: Long-term follow-up after primary repair of the anterior cruciate ligament: clinical and radiological evaluation 15–23 years postoperatively. *Arch Orthop Trauma Surg* 125:217–221, 2005.

76. Tien, Y. C.; Chih, T. T.; Lin, J. H.; et al.: Augmentation of tendon-bone healing by the use of calcium-phosphate cement. *J Bone Joint Surg Br* 86:1072–1076, 2004.

77. Tomita, F.; Yasuda, K.; Mikami, S.; et al.: Comparisons of intraosseous graft healing between the doubled flexor tendon graft and the bone-patellar tendon-bone graft in anterior cruciate ligament reconstruction. *Arthroscopy* 17:461–476, 2001.

78. Tyler, T. F.; McHugh, M. P.; Gleim, G. W.; Nicholas, S. J.: Association of KT-1000 measurements with clinical tests of knee stability 1 year following anterior cruciate ligament reconstruction. *J Orthop Sports Phys Ther* 29:540–542, 1999.

79. Xiao, Y.; Parry, D. A.; Li, H.; et al.: Expression of extracellular matrix macromolecules around demineralized freeze-dried bone allografts. *J Periodontol* 67:1233–1244, 1996.

80. Yamazaki, S.; Yasuda, K.; Tomita, F.; et al.: The effect of intraosseous graft length on tendon-bone healing in anterior cruciate ligament reconstruction using flexor tendon. *Knee Surg Sports Traumatol Arthrosc* 14:1086–1093, 2006.

81. Yeh, W. L.; Lin, S. S.; Yuan, L. J.; et al.: Effects of hyperbaric oxygen treatment on tendon graft and tendon-bone integration in bone tunnel: biochemical and histological analysis in rabbits. *J Orthop Res* 25:636–645, 2007.

82. Yoshikawa, T.; Tohyama, H.; Katsura, T.; et al.: Effects of local administration of vascular endothelial growth factor on mechanical characteristics of the semitendinosus tendon graft after anterior cruciate ligament reconstruction in sheep. *Am J Sports Med* 34:1918–1925, 2006.

83. Yu, J. K.; Paessler, H. H.: Relationship between tunnel widening and different rehabilitation procedures after anterior cruciate ligament reconstruction with quadrupled hamstring tendons. *Chin Med J (Engl)* 118:320–326, 2005.

84. Zhang, C. L.; Fan, H. B.; Xu, H.; et al.: Histological comparison of fate of ligamentous insertion after reconstruction of anterior cruciate ligament: autograft vs allograft. *Chin J Traumatol* 9:72–76, 2006.

85. Zysk, S. P.; Refior, H. J.: Operative or conservative treatment of the acutely torn anterior cruciate ligament in middle-aged patients. A follow-up study of 133 patients between the ages of 40 and 59 years. *Arch Orthop Trauma Surg* 120:59–64, 2000.

Chapter 6

Human Movement and Anterior Cruciate Ligament Function: Anterior Cruciate Ligament Deficiency and Gait Mechanics

Thomas P. Andriacchi, PhD ▪ *Sean F. Scanlan*, MS

INTRODUCTION

The anterior cruciate ligament (ACL) plays an important role in stability of the knee primarily through its passive constraint to anterior tibial translation and tibial rotation. In addition, the ACL influences the dynamic function of the knee. For example, ambulatory changes have been associated with functional adaptations after loss of ACL function. The nature of these functional adaptations may be considered a potential functional marker for the ability to return to vigorous activities[3,28,29] as well as for secondary degenerative cartilage changes after ACL injury.[7]

Critical Points INTRODUCTION

The purpose of this chapter is

- To develop some fundamental gait analysis principles.
- To illustrate the application of gait analysis to the issues related to the evaluation and treatment of anterior cruciate ligament (ACL) injury.
- To describe the cause and implications of a change in muscle-generated moments after ACL injury.
- To describe kinematic changes at the knee during walking and the association of kinematics changes with emergence of premature osteoarthritis (OA) after ACL injury.
- To describe the influence of the adduction moment on the progression of knee OA and its implication for ACL-deficient patients with concomitant varus knee alignment and lateral ligament laxity.

Differences in the manner in which patients adapt their gait characteristics to the loss of the ACL provide a possible explanation for the variable outcome after this injury. It is likely that some patients can dynamically adapt to the loss of an ACL, whereas others will not adapt. The large variation in treatment selection and outcome[8,9] suggests a need for better methods of assessing the clinical and functional status of the patient after ACL rupture. Diagnostic methods for identifying a torn ACL have improved substantially; however, prognostic methods for assessing the probability of successful treatment are not yet available. Even quantitative laxity measurements obtained from devices such as the KT-1000 have not been predictive of clinical outcome.[36] Thus, variability in dynamic adaptations achieved through alteration in the patterns of muscle firing[1,23,34] during a particular activity provides a possible explanation for the differences in outcome of patients after ACL injury.

The variable natural history in the progression of degenerative joint disease suggests that some patients make appropriate functional adaptations for the loss of the ACL. The nature of these functional adaptations can differ substantially among patients who present with the same clinical status. Thus, the ability to identify and understand the nature and cause of changes in ambulatory function, or specifically gait characteristics, is an important consideration in the evaluation and treatment of ACL injury.

The purpose of this chapter is to discuss fundamental gait analysis principles and illustrate the application of gait analysis to the issues related to the evaluation and treatment of ACL injury. Specific examples are provided on the interaction between the passive function of the ACL and the change in muscle-generated moments, kinematics, and the relationship between kinematic changes and the emergence of premature osteoarthritis (OA). In addition, the influence of specific characteristics of gait in ACL-deficient patients with concomitant varus lower limb malalignment and lateral and posterolateral ligament deficiency are described.

JOINT KINETICS DURING GAIT AND THE ACL-DEFICIENT KNEE

An analysis of the kinetics (forces and moments) that act at the knee during walking provides useful insight into the functional changes associated with the ACL-deficient knee. In particular, the moments that act at the knee suggest the cause and potential effect of gait changes after ACL injury. For example, a reduction in the intersegmental moment tending to flex the knee (balanced by net quadriceps contraction) during walking was among the first changes in walking mechanics reported in the ACL-deficient knee.[10] The reduction of the net internal quadriceps moment is consistent with quadriceps muscle atrophy, which is frequently reported after ACL injury[40] and helps to explain why it is difficult to restore quadriceps strength in these knees. Thus, it is useful to examine the physical meaning and relevance of the intersegmental moment at the knee during walking. This section provides a summary of the methods used to determine the joint moments, an example of how to interpret the magnitude and pattern of the flexion-extension moment at the knee in context of the function of the knee flexors and extensors

during ambulation, and an example of how an analysis of the flexion-extension moment during walking can provide insight into the functional role of the ACL.

Definition of Intersegmental Moment

A *moment* is a vector quantity that can be considered a rotational force (lever arm x force) in the sense that it tends to produce a rotation about a specific point. Whereas moments can be calculated at any point, it is useful to use the joints between adjacent limb segments to define the moments that act on the body during walking. For example, the moment acting at the knee would be the intersegmental moment between the thigh and the shank. The external moment tending to flex or extend the joint is illustrated in Figure 6–1. The intersegmental moments are typically calculated from measurement of the foot-ground reaction forces (using a force platform) and the motion of markers placed on the limbs using an optoelectronic system for motion capture. The weight and inertial forces are often approximated by modeling the leg as a collection of rigid segments representing the thigh, shank, and foot. The reader should be aware of the assumptions used in performing these calculations.[5] Finally, the units of a moment are force and length. Therefore, it is useful when comparing different-sized subjects to express the intersegmental moments in nondimensional units by dividing the moment by the subject's height (ht) and body weight (bw). Thus, moments measured during gait are often expressed in units of percentage of the product of the body weight and height (% bw x ht), so that moments can be compared among subjects of different heights and weights.

Interpretation of Intersegmental Moment

The moment can be visualized in the context of the direction of the ground reaction vector relative to the position of the knee joint center (see Fig. 6-1). If the vector passes anterior to the

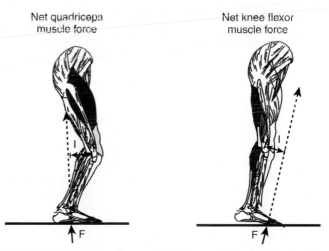

Net quadriceps muscle force   Net knee flexor muscle force

FIGURE 6–1. The intersegmental flexion-extension moment can be visualized by considering a ground reaction force vector that passes posterior to the knee will produce an external flexion moment that is balanced by a net internal quadriceps moment. When the vector passes anterior to the knee, an external extension moment is produced that must be balanced by a net internal flexor muscle moment.

knee, the moment will tend to extend the knee, whereas if the vector passes posterior to the knee, the moment will tend to flex the knee. As noted previously, the direction of the moment can be used to infer the net muscular moment. Thus, an external moment tending to flex the knee will be balanced by a net quadriceps moment. Previous studies have demonstrated that the external moments measured can be interpreted in terms of the loads on muscles, passive soft tissue, and joint surfaces.[32] In addition, the joint moments have been shown to be sensitive indicators of differences between normal and abnormal function.[3,10,31]

It is useful to examine the assumptions used as the basis for the interpretation of the joint moments during function. Mechanical equilibrium dictates that external forces and moments must be balanced by internal forces and moments. Internal forces generated by muscle, passive soft tissue, and joint contact force create these internal moments. If muscles act only synergistically when balancing the external moments, one could directly infer the internal muscle force in synergistic muscle groups. For example, the total force in the quadriceps needed to balance an external moment tending to flex the knee joint could be determined.[32] However, if antagonistic muscle activity is present, the external moment reflects the net balance between agonist and antagonist muscles. The force in the synergistic muscle group would be greater under these conditions. The external moment can, however, be used to obtain a conservative estimate or lower bound on the synergist muscle force. Throughout this chapter, external moments are described from the measurements taken in the laboratory and inferences are made in terms of the net muscular moment (see Fig. 6–1).

The Flexion-Extension Moment and the ACL-Deficient Knees

The normal temporal pattern of the flexion-extension moment during stance phase of walking can be interpreted in terms of the net quadriceps moment or net knee flexor muscle moment (hamstrings and/or gastrocnemius) during stance phase (Fig. 6–2). Typically, at heel strike, there is an external moment that tends to extend the knee joint, demanding a net knee flexor force. As the knee moves into midstance, the external moment reverses its direction, demanding a net quadriceps force. As the knee passes midstance, the moment again reverses its direction, demanding net flexor muscle force. Finally, in the pre-swing phase, the moment tends to flex the knee, demanding a net quadriceps muscle force. As previously noted, a reduction of the net quadriceps moment relative to normal is frequently seen in ACL-deficient subjects during level walking (see Fig. 6–2). Specifically, ACL-deficient subjects walk in a manner that has been interpreted as a tendency to avoid or reduce the demand on the quadriceps muscle.[10] Whereas the reduction in net quadriceps moment can be interpreted as either a reduction in the quadriceps or an increase in the knee flexor muscle moment, the fact that quadriceps atrophy is a common finding after ACL injury[20] supports the conclusion of a reduction in quadriceps contraction during walking.

The mechanics of the knee extensor mechanism suggests a possible cause for the inhibition of quadriceps contraction during walking. As illustrated in Figure 6–3, the anterior angulation of the patellar ligament insertion angle (PLIA) causes an anterior force to be applied to the tibia when the quadriceps

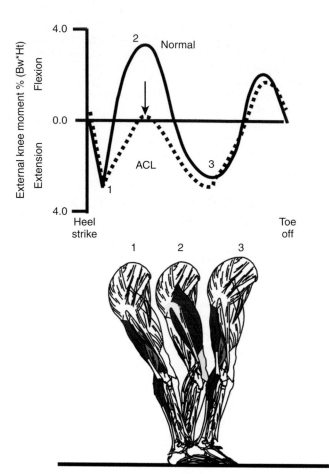

FIGURE 6–2. The pattern of the external flexion-extension moment during normal walking for anterior cruciate ligament (ACL)–deficient (*dashed line*) and normal (*solid line*) knees. Typically, patients with ACL-deficient knees have a reduced moment, tending to flex the knee (net quadriceps moment) during midstance. The figure of the leg indicates the position of the knee joint and the net muscular activation (*shaded area*) required to balance the external moment shown in the graph.

contracts. In the absence of the ACL, the tibia moves forward when the quadriceps contracts until the force is balanced by other secondary restraints to anterior tibial displacement, such as the medial collateral ligament, meniscus, or a hamstrings contraction. Thus, more anterior tibial translation could occur in ACL-deficient knees than in uninjured knees when the quadriceps contracts. The amount of anterior force is greatest at full extension because the PLIA has the largest anterior angle at full extension and this angle reduces as the knee flexes.[17,25] Thus, walking would produce a substantial component of anterior force owing to quadriceps contraction because the knee remains near full extension throughout stance phase, with maximum flexion angles less than 30°. A reduction in quadriceps contraction could eliminate large anterior tibial translations near full extension and prevent sensations of joint instability by the patient.

Interestingly, the magnitude of the net quadriceps moment can increase by more than a factor of 5 during jogging as compared with level walking (Fig. 6–4), yet the percentage change in the net quadriceps moment between ACL-deficient and normal

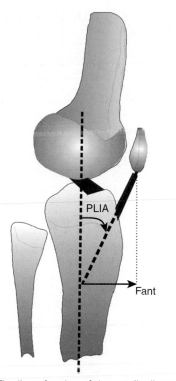

FIGURE 6–3. The line of action of the patellar ligament running from the posterior pole of the patella to the tibial tuberosity. The patellar ligament insertion angle (PLIA) is measured as the angle between the midshaft of the tibia and the line of action of the patellar ligament. With the knee in an extended position (as shown in the illustration), contraction of the quadriceps would transmit a relatively large anterior force (Γ_{ant}) to the proximal tibia.

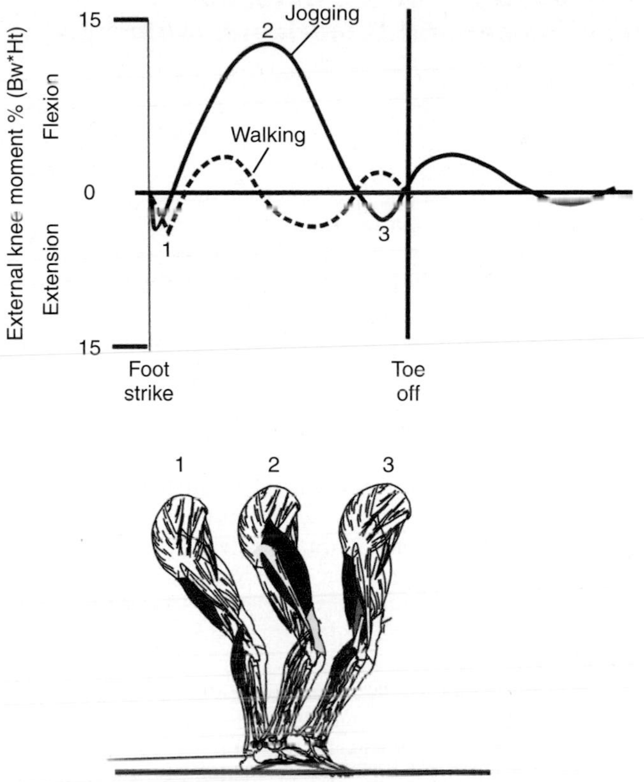

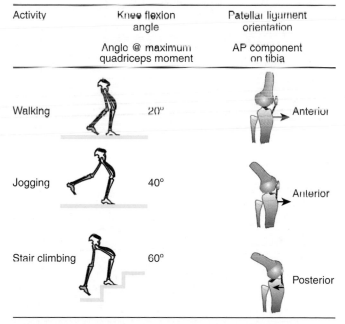

FIGURE 6–4. A comparison of the flexion-extension moments occurring during normal walking (*dashed line*) and jogging (*solid line*). The magnitude of the moment tending to flex the knee (net quadriceps moment) can be five times greater during jogging than during normal walking.

Activity	Knee flexion angle	Patellar ligament orientation
	Angle @ maximum quadriceps moment	AP component on tibia
Walking	20°	Anterior
Jogging	40°	Anterior
Stair climbing	60°	Posterior

FIGURE 6–5. The relationship between the knee flexion angle at which the maximum net quadriceps moment occurs during activities of daily living and the orientation of the patellar ligament relative to the tibia. As the knee moves from a relatively extended position (walking) to a more flexed position (stair climbing), the anteroposterior (AP) component of the patellar ligament shifts from an anterior orientation to a posterior orientation relative to the tibia.

subjects is substantially less during jogging than during walking.[10] The fact that the maximum net quadriceps moment during jogging occurs when the knee is at approximately 40° of flexion, as compared with 20° during level walking, might provide an explanation for the fact that patients with an ACL-deficient knee do not show a similar reduction in the net quadriceps moment during jogging compared with walking. Similarly, while ascending stairs, the maximum net quadriceps moment occurs at approximately 60° of flexion and thus the amount of reduction in the net quadriceps moment is small compared with that during level walking. The adaptations during activities of daily living appear to be dependent upon the angle of knee flexion when the greatest net quadriceps moment occurs. These observations suggest an interaction between the direction of pull of the patella ligament and the functional role of the ACL (Fig. 6–5). When the knee is near full extension, the patellar ligament places an anterior pull on the tibia. As the knee flexes beyond approximately 45°, the orientation of the patellar ligament reverses direction during the quadriceps contraction and places a posterior pull on the tibia. At deeper flexion angles, the contraction of the quadriceps acts to compensate for an absent ACL.

Thus, during level walking when the maximum net quadriceps moment occurs between 0° and approximately 20°, there is a greater tendency for the quadriceps contraction to produce an anterior pull on the tibia. The adaptation to avoid quadriceps contraction eliminates this anterior force component when the knee is near full extension (see Fig. 6–3).

The Anatomy of the Extensor Mechanism and Quadriceps Inhibition

The variation in the amount of reduction in the net quadriceps moment during walking can be explained by anatomic differences in the anatomy of the extensor mechanism as defined by the PLIA (see Fig. 6–3). As noted previously, the PLIA is of particular importance to the knee extensor mechanism because it determines the decomposition of quadriceps force into anterior and superior directions (see Fig. 6–3) while transferring the quadriceps contraction to the tibia. Previous studies confirmed this relationship by showing that the patellar ligament pulls the tibia anteriorly when the knee is near full extension and also that anatomic variations exist between individuals in both PLIA and the moment arm of the patellar ligament.[17] Thus, knees with larger PLIAs generate larger anterior forces on the tibia with the same level of quadriceps contraction.

More importantly, it has been shown that the PLIA negatively correlates to the peak knee flexion moment (balanced by net quadriceps moment) during walking in ACL-deficient knees,[35] whereas no correlation exists in uninjured contralateral knees of ACL-deficient patients (Fig. 6–6). The negative correlation between PLIA and the peak external knee flexion moment indicates that ACL-deficient knees with higher PLIAs significantly reduce usage of the quadriceps during walking. These results suggest that the subject-specific anatomy of the knee extensor mechanism provides a possible explanation for the variability[15] previously observed in adaptation of a quadriceps reduction strategy after ACL injury. This mechanism may explain the reduction in the external knee flexion moment, which is balanced by net quadriceps force, among ACL-deficient knees. This mechanism is further supported by the clinical observation of quadriceps atrophy in ACL-deficient subjects,[20] because reduced use of the quadriceps during walking should lead to muscle atrophy. However, the variability between individuals' adaptations to ACL injury suggests that other factors, such as PLIA, may influence which subjects adopt a strategy of quadriceps reduction.[13,28]

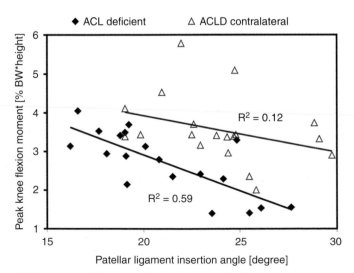

FIGURE 6–6. ACL-deficient knees show a significant negative correlation between peak external knee flexion moment (net quadriceps moment) and PLIA during normal walking. However, uninjured contralateral knees do not show a significant correlation.

KNEE KINEMATICS DURING WALKING AND ACL INJURY

The anatomy of the ACL suggests its potential role in determining the motion (kinematics) of the knee during ambulation. Clearly, passive function of the ACL for guiding motion and stabilizing the knee has been well documented. However, the analysis of the functional role of the ACL during dynamic in vivo ambulatory activities is more complex than for passive movements. The force generated by the ACL during passive stretch is relatively small compared with the magnitude of the muscle forces and extrinsic forces (load bearing) that occur during ambulation. Further, the ability to capture the movement of the knee under conditions that reflect natural movement remains a challenge. The kinematic role of the ACL during functional activities has been described for several weight-bearing activities.[4,16,22,37] The knee kinematics presented in this chapter focus primarily on walking. The mechanics of walking can provide valuable insights into the functional role of the ACL during locomotion.[6] Functional adaptation to the loss of the ACL can be detected during walking, because it has been suggested that patients can adapt patterns of locomotion that compensate for the loss of the ACL. In addition, walking is the most frequent ambulatory activity of daily living, and specific characteristics of this activity have been associated with cartilage thinning.[7,26] ACL rupture has been identified as a significant risk factor for premature knee OA. This chapter focuses on the internal-external rotation (IE) and anteroposterior (AP) translation that occur at the knee during walking. These secondary movements (IE, AP) of the knee are directly related to the function of the ACL and have been shown to change in patients with ACL-deficient knees during walking for the reasons described previously.

Critical Points KNEE KINEMATICS DURING WALKING AND ACL INJURY

- The motion (kinematics) of the knee is complex, and normal motion requires critical secondary movements of anteroposterior (AP) and internal-external (IE) rotation.
- The characteristics of the AP translation and IE rotation during walking provide a useful basis for understanding the pathomechanics of kinematic changes associated with the loss of the ACL.
- The swing phase of repetitive activities such as walking can provide useful insight into the functional role of the ACL because the passive force capacity of the ACL can have a substantial influence on the knee motion during non–weight-bearing whereas extrinsic forces and muscle forces dominate knee motion during the stance phase.
- The tibia translates forward and externally rotates as it extends during the terminal portion of swing phase in preparation for heel-strike positioning the tibia at an anterior position and in external rotation at heel strike.
- The normal external rotation and anterior translation of the tibia that occur as the knee extends during terminal swing is reduced in the absence of the ACL, and the tibia maintains this offset relative to normal throughout the stance phase of the walking cycle.
- The kinematic changes at the knee after ACL injury have been implicated as a factor in the cause of premature OA by shifting joint contact to regions in the cartilage that cannot adapt to the changes in the repetitive loads that occur during walking.

Methods for Defining and Measuring Knee Kinematics during Walking

The kinematics of human movement during walking is normally described in terms of relative motion between adjacent limb segments (Fig. 6–7). In practice, human gait is most often described in terms of the sagittal plane motion (flexion-extension). This practice has come as a consequence of the much larger motions in this plane, making these motions relatively easy to measure and perhaps most relevant to function. However, the motion at the knee is more complex than other major joints of the lower extremity, involving all six degrees of freedom (three rotations and three translations). The complexity of the kinematic analysis substantially increases when going from a sagittal plane analysis to a complete three-dimensional analysis. The appropriate interpretation of in vivo kinematic measurements requires a precise and physically meaningful definition of anatomic references. For the kinematics described in this chapter, the anatomic femoral coordinate system was located at the midpoint of the transepicondylar line of the distal femur, and the anatomic tibial coordinate system was set at the midpoint of a line connecting the medial and the lateral points of the tibial plateau. The AP translation was determined by calculating the displacement between the origins of the tibial coordinate system relative to a femoral coordinate system projected onto the AP axis of the tibia (see Fig. 6–7). IE rotations were measured by projecting the mediolateral femoral axis onto a plane created by the AP and mediolateral axes fixed in the tibia. Additional details of defining the system used in this chapter can be found in Andriacchi and Dyrby,[4] Andriacchi and coworkers,[5] and Dyrby and Andriacchi.[14]

AP Translation and IE Rotation of the Knee during Normal Walking

The flexion-extension motion of the knee is the primary motion of the joint because this movement is required for most ambulatory activities. However, AP translation and IE rotation are important secondary movements of the knee because these movements can influence the moment-generating capacity of the muscles[2] as well as the movement of the position of the tibial-femoral contact, all important for normal function. The AP translation and IE rotation of knee have been described for normal walking based on the coordinate system described previously.[4,14]

The characteristics of AP translation and IE rotation (see Fig. 6–7) provide a useful basis for understanding the pathomechanics of kinematic changes associated with the loss of the

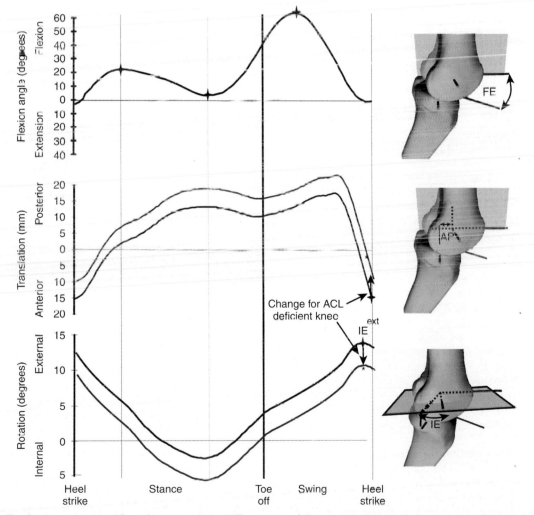

FIGURE 6–7. The flexion-extension, AP, and internal-external (IE) motions of the knee that occur during normal walking (expressed as the position of the tibia relative to the femur) for normal (*black line*) and ACL-deficient (*red line*) knees. The kinematic changes in the ACL-deficient knee are characterized by a posterior translation offset and an internal rotation offset.

ACL. During normal walking, the tibia is in an anterior position at heel strike that is the result of anterior tibial translation during the terminal portion of swing phase (see Fig. 6–7). During the major portion of stance phase, the tibia translates to a posterior direction. Finally, during the later portion of swing phase, the tibia moves in an anterior direction relative to the femur, reaching a maximum anterior position at or just before heel strike. In addition, at heel strike, the tibia is externally rotated and internally rotates through the major portion of stance phase. The tibia begins to externally rotate during swing phase as the knee extends prior to heel strike and reaches a maximum external rotation at or just before heel strike. The motion of the tibia during the terminal portion of swing phase reflects the natural screw-home motion[18] of the knee in which the tibia externally rotates as the knee extends. This natural screw-home movement occurs during the non–weight-bearing portion of the gait cycle in which the passive structure and joint surface drive the movement of the knee. As previously noted, during the weight-bearing stance phase of the walking cycle, the kinematics are driven by the extrinsic forces that act at the knee rather than the internal passive structures such as the ligaments. Thus, the swing phase of repetitive activities such as walking can provide useful insight into the functional role of the ACL because the passive force capacity can have a substantial influence on the knee motion during non–weight-bearing activities.

Kinematic Changes after ACL Injury

Kinematic changes at the knee during ambulation have been reported for patients with ACL-deficient knees.[4,16] In particular, the normal external rotation and anterior translation of the tibia that occur as the knee extends during terminal swing are reduced in the absence of the ACL. The tibia maintains this offset relative to normal throughout the stance phase of the walking cycle. These observations indicate that the ACL plays a critical role in the positioning of the knee at the end of swing phase[4] in preparation for heel strike during walking (see Fig. 6–7), suggesting a loss of the normal screw-home movement.[18] The loss of the screw-home movement at the end of swing phase produces an offset toward internal rotation in the average position of the tibia relative to the healthy knee that is maintained through stance phase. The reduced anterior displacement of the ACL-deficient knee at heel strike also appears to be related to modified kinematics during terminal swing phase. Thus, the transition between swing phase and stance is an important consideration in evaluating the ACL-deficient knee.[11,24]

ACL injury is associated with premature OA of the knee.[19–21,27] The kinematic changes at the knee after ACL injury have been implicated as a factor in the cause of premature OA in this population.[7] A shift in the rotational alignment near heel strike can shift the load-bearing contact to regions in the cartilage that have not adapted to the high loads occurring at heel strike. Typically, the thickest regions of the femoral and tibial load-bearing articular cartilage are aligned when the knee is at full extension.

The change in the rotational characteristics at the knee could cause specific regions of the cartilage to be loaded that were not loaded prior to the ACL injury. It has been suggested that the altered contact mechanics in the newly loaded regions could produce local degenerative changes to the articular cartilage.[12,40] As previously reported, cartilage in highly loaded areas is mechanically adapted relative to underused areas where

signs of fibrillation can be observed in healthy knees in relatively young subjects.[12,38] Thus, a spatial shift in the contact region could place loads on a region of cartilage that may not adapt to the rapidly increased load initiating degenerative changes.[39]

THE ADDUCTION MOMENT AT THE KNEE AND ACL INJURY

The external adduction moment during walking is a result of the line of action of the ground reaction force passing medial to the center of the knee (Fig. 6–8). The offset or lever arm of this force causes a moment that tends to adduct the knee during walking (Fig. 6–9). The adduction moment will influence the relative distribution of load (see Fig. 6–8) between the medial and the lateral compartments of the knee,[32] causing a higher force on the medial compartment relative to the lateral compartment. The adduction moment has become an ambulatory biomechanical marker for risk of progression of medial compartment OA at the knee.[7,26] In general, patients with a higher adduction moment have worse treatment outcome after high tibial osteotomy,[31] more severe disease,[33] and a higher rate of progression of OA.[26]

The Adduction Moment and OA at the Knee

The adduction moment during walking can be an important consideration in patients with ACL-deficient knees because OA in this group occurs most frequently in the medial compartment. It has been shown that patients with a varus angulation at the knee and ACL injury introduce additional problems that should be considered when making treatment decisions.[30] Varus angulation in conjunction with clinical indication of medial compartment OA, cartilage damage, or loss of medial meniscus

---

Critical Points THE ADDUCTION MOMENT AT THE KNEE AND ACL INJURY

- The external adduction moment during walking causes higher force on the medial compartment relative to the lateral compartment of the knee.
- The adduction moment has become an ambulatory biomechanical marker for risk of progression of medial compartment OA at the knee.
- The adduction moment is an important consideration in patients with ACL-deficient knees because OA in this group occurs most frequently in the medial compartment.
- In ACL-deficient patients with lateral joint laxity, a high adduction moment during walking makes the knee vulnerable to lateral joint opening in the absence of stabilizing muscle forces and can cause the entire force across the knee to be transmitted to the medial compartment.
- Varus angulation in conjunction with clinical indication of medial compartment OA, cartilage damage, or loss of medial meniscus function and a high adduction moment during walking is a potential indication for a high tibial osteotomy in patients with ACL-deficient knees.

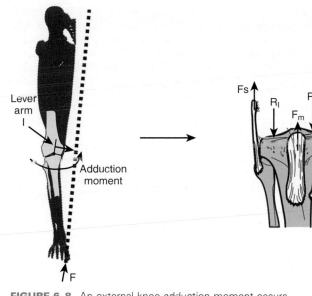

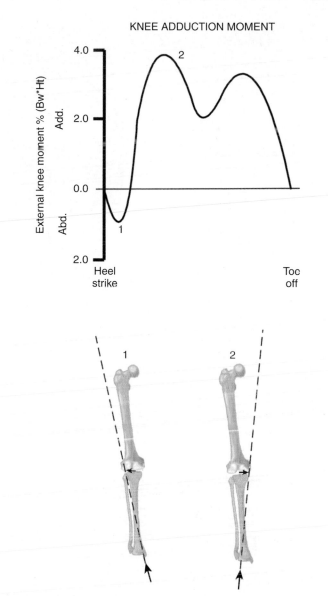

KNEE ADDUCTION MOMENT

FIGURE 6–8. An external knee adduction moment occurs during walking when the ground reaction force vector passes medial to the knee joint center in the frontal plane. The adduction moment will influence the relative distribution of load between the medial and the lateral compartments of the knee, with a high adduction moment resulting in a greater compressive load passing through the medial compartment relative to the lateral compartment.

function is a potential indication for high tibial osteotomy. Gait analysis can provide useful insight into those patients who are at greater risk for medial compartment OA.

The adduction moment during walking makes the knee vulnerable to lateral joint opening in the absence of stabilizing muscle forces. As illustrated in Figure 6–10, muscle contraction can dynamically stabilize the knee to resist a varus thrust and can compensate for lateral joint laxity. Thus, there is a potential interaction between the reduced quadriceps contraction, a high adduction moment, and lateral laxity[30] because a high adduction moment can produce a tendency to open the joint laterally in the absence of the stabilizing forces of muscle contraction (see Fig. 6–9). Based on the mechanics of walking, lateral laxity presents an additional risk in the presence of a varus malaligned knee, a high adduction moment, and reduced quadriceps activity because this combination of conditions can cause the entire force across the knee to be transmitted to the medial compartment. This combination of conditions places the medial compartment of the joint at greater risk for breakdown and should be considered in the overall clinical evaluation of patients with ACL injury.

FIGURE 6–9. The pattern of the external adduction-abduction moment during normal walking. Typically, an abduction moment occurs just after heel strike, and then an adduction moment is maintained throughout the rest of stance phase. The figure of the legs indicates the line of action of the ground reaction force vector relative to the frontal plane position of the knee joint. An external abduction moment is produced when the ground reaction force vector passes lateral to the knee joint center, and an adduction moment is produced when the vector passes medial to the knee joint center.

SUMMARY

The ambulatory characteristics of patients after ACL injury provide unique insight into the functional role of the ACL and provide information that can be helpful in treatment evaluation and planning. The nature and cause of the reduction of quadriceps muscle strength after ACL injury can be explained in part by the reduction of the moment sustained by the quadriceps during walking. The anatomy of the PLIA and the fact that quadriceps contraction creates the greatest anterior pull on the tibia when

the knee is near full extension (as during walking) provide a functional explanation for quadriceps reduction during level walking. Because the knee is more flexed during activities such as stair climbing or jogging, the PLIA has less anterior pull and there is a reduced need to adapt a pattern of movement to reduce quadriceps contraction unless there is secondary quadriceps weakness and the adaptation is to a weak quadriceps.

The kinematic changes at the knee during walking after ACL injury suggest that the ACL provides an important role in positioning the knee during the swing phase of walking. In

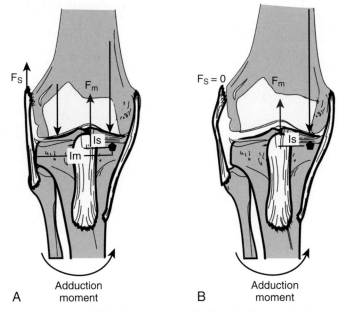

FIGURE 6–10. **A,** Muscle contraction (Fm) acting through the lever arm (lm), and competent lateral soft tissue structures (Fs) acting through the lever arm (ls), are capable of dynamically stabilizing the knee joint in the presence of a large moment, tending to adduct the knee (such as occurs during walking in the varus malaligned knee). **B,** However, the combination of weak extensor muscles and lateral joint laxity (Fs = 0) in the ACL-deficient knee can be potentially insufficient to resist a large adduction moment, resulting in opening of the lateral compartment and a concentration of the load across the medial compartment of the knee.

Critical Points SUMMARY

- Gait characteristics of patients after ACL injury provide unique insight into the functional role of the ACL and provide information that can be helpful in treatment evaluation and planning.
- The reduction of quadriceps muscle strength after ACL injury can be explained in part by the reduction of the moment sustained by the quadriceps during walking.
- The anatomy of the patellar insertion angle provides a functional explanation for quadriceps reduction during level walking.
- Kinematic changes have been implicated in the premature OA frequently reported in patients after ACL injury.
- Gait mechanics can provide insight into the treatment of the varus-aligned knee with ACL injury.

particular, patients with ACL injury demonstrate a rotational offset in the position of the tibia that is maintained during the stance phase of walking. This rotational offset has been implicated in the premature OA frequently reported in patients after

ACL injury. The rotational offset can cause a shift in the position of the articular cartilage contact between the femur and the tibia, and it has been suggested that the cartilage cannot adapt to this change in the local mechanical environment, causing the initiation of a degenerative process leading to OA.

Gait mechanics can also provide insight into the treatment of the varus malaligned knee with ACL injury. A high adduction moment during walking in patients with ACL deficiency and varus malaligned knees has been suggested as a consideration for high tibial osteotomy when symptoms of cartilage degradation are present.

Finally, this chapter has discussed how an analysis of ambulatory mechanics can provide insight into the pathomechanics of knee OA after ACL injury that cannot be obtained from other methods. Restoration of function and prevention of long-term comorbidities, such as OA and meniscus degeneration, are among the primary goals of treatment. Thus, quantitative analysis of function should be considered in the evaluation of new treatment modalities.

REFERENCES

1. Andriacchi, T. P.: Dynamics of pathological motion: applied to the anterior cruciate–deficient knee. *J Biomech* 23:99–105, 1990.
2. Andriacchi, T. P.: Functional analysis of pre and post-knee surgery. Total knee arthoplasty and ACL reconstruction. *J Biomech Eng* 115:575–581, 1993.
3. Andriacchi, T. P.; Birac, D.: Functional testing in the anterior cruciate ligament–deficient knee. *Clin Orthop Relat Res* 288:40–47, 1993.
4. Andriacchi, T. P.; Dyrby, C. O.: Interactions between kinematics and loading during walking for the normal and ACL-deficient knee. *J Biomech* 38:293–298, 2005.
5. Andriacchi, T. P.; Johnson, T. S.; Hurwitz, D. E.; Natarajan, R. N.: Musculoskeletal dynamics, locomotion, and clinical applications. In Mow, V. C.; Huiskes, R. (eds.): *Basic Orthopaedic Biomechanics and Mechano-Biology.* Philadelphia: Lippincott Williams & Wilkins, 2004; pp. 91–122.
6. Andriacchi, T.; Muendermann, A.: The role of ambulatory mechanics in the initiation and progression of knee osteoarthritis. *Curr Opin Rheumatol* 18:514–518, 2006.
7. Andriacchi, T. P.; Mundermann, A.; Smith, R. L.; et al.: A framework for the in vivo pathomechanics of osteoarthritis at the knee. *Ann Biomed Eng* 32:447–457, 2004.
8. Barber, S. D.; Noyes, F. R.; Mangine, R. E.; et al.: Quantitative assessment of functional limitations in normal and anterior cruciate ligament–deficient knees. *Clin Orthop Relat Res* 255:204–214, 1990.
9. Barrett. G. R.; Treacy, S. H.: The effect of intraoperative sometric measurement on the outcome of anterior cruciate ligament reconstruction. *Arthroscopy* 12:645–651, 1996.
10. Berchuck, M.; Andriacchi, T. P.; Bach, B. R.; Reider, B. R.: Gait adaptations by patients who have a deficient ACL. *J Bone Joint Surg Am* 72:871–877, 1990.
11. Beynnon, B. D.; Fleming, B. C.; Labovitch, R.; Parsons, B.: Chronic anterior cruciate ligament deficiency is associated with increased anterior translation of the tibia during the transition from non-weightbearing to weightbearing. *J Orthop Res* 20:332–337, 2002.
12. Bullough, P. G.: The pathology of osteoarthritis. In Moskowitz, R.; Howell, D.; Goldberg, V. (eds.): *Osteoarthritis Diagnosis and Medical/Surgical Management.* Philadelphia: W. B. Saunders, 1992; pp. 36–69.
13. Chmielewski, T. L.; Rudolph, K. S.; Fitzegeral, G. K.; et al.: Biomechanical evidence supporting a differential response to acute ACL injury. Clin Biomech 16:586–591, 2001.
14. Dyrby, C. O.; Andriacchi, T. P.: Secondary motions of the knee during weight bearing and non–weight bearing activities. *J Orthop Res* 22:794–800, 2004.
15. Ferber, R.; Osternig, L. R.; Woollacott, M. H.; et al.: Gait mechanics in chronic ACL deficiency and subsequent repair. *Clin Biomech* 17:274–285, 2002.
16. Georgoulis, A. D.; Papadonikolakis, A.; Papageorgiou C. D.; et al.: Three-dimensional tibiofemoral kinematics of the anterior cruciate

ligament–deficient and reconstructed knee during walking. *Am J Sports Med* 31:75–79, 2003.

17. Gross, M. T.; Tyson, A. D.; Burns, C. B.: Effect of knee angle and ligament insufficiency on anterior tibial translation during quadriceps muscle contraction: a preliminary report. *J Orthop Sports Phys Ther* 17:133–143, 1993.

18. Hallen, L. G.; Lindahl, O.: The "screw-home" movement in the knee-joint. *Acta Orthop Scand* 37:97–106, 1966.

19. Jacobsen, K.: Osteoarthrosis following insufficiency of the cruciate ligaments in man. A clinical study. *Acta Orthop Scand* 48:520–526, 1977.

20. Kannus, P.: Ratio of hamstring to quadriceps femoris muscles' strength in the anterior cruciate ligament insufficient knee. Relationship to long-term recovery. *Phys Ther* 68:961–965, 1988.

21. Kannus, P.; Jarvinen, M.: Posttraumatic anterior cruciate ligament insufficiency as a cause of osteoarthritis in a knee joint. *Clin Rheumatol* 8:251–260, 1989.

22. Li, G.; Defrate, L. E.; Rubash, H. E.; Gill, T. J.: In vivo kinematics of the ACL during weight-bearing knee flexion. *J Orthop Res* 23:340–344, 2005.

23. Limbird, T. J.; Shiavi, R.; Frazer, M.; Borra, H.: EMG profiles of knee-joint musculature during walking: changes induced by anterior cruciate ligament deficiency. *J Orthop Res* 6:630–638, 1988.

24. Ma, C. B.; Janaushek, M. A.; Vogrin, T. M.; et al.: Significance of changes in the reference position for measurements of tibial translation and diagnosis of cruciate ligament deficiency. *J Orthop Res* 18:176–182, 2000.

25. Matthews, L. S.; Sonstegard, D. A.; Henke, J. A.: Load bearing characteristics of the patello-femoral joint. *Acta Orthop Scand* 48:511–516, 1977.

26. Miyazaki, T.; Wada, M.; Kawahara, H.; et al.: Dynamic load at baseline can predict radiographic disease progression in medial compartment knee osteoarthritis. *Ann Rheum Dis* 61:617–622, 2002.

27. Nebelung, W.; Wuschech, H.: Thirty five years of follow-up of anterior cruciate ligament–deficient knees in high-level athletes. *Arthroscopy* 21:696–702, 2005.

28. Noyes, F. R.; Matthews, D. S.; Mooar, P. A.; Grood, E. J.: The symptomatic anterior cruciate–deficient knee. Part II: the results of rehabilitation, activity modification, and counseling on functional disability. *J Bone Joint Surg Am* 65:163–174, 1983.

29. Noyes, F. R.; Mooar, P. A.; Matthews, D. S.; Butler, D. L.: The symptomatic anterior cruciate–deficient knee. Part I: the long-term functional disability in athletically active individuals. *J Bone Joint Surg Am* 65:154–162, 1983.

30. Noyes, F. R.; Schipplein, O. D.; Andriacchi, T. P.; et al.: The anterior cruciate ligament–deficient knee with varus alignment. An analysis of gait adaptations and dynamic joint loadings. *Am J Sports Med* 20:707–716, 1992.

31. Prodromos, C. C.; Andriacchi, T. P.; Galante, J. O.: A relationship between gait and clinical changes following high tibial osteotomy. *J Bone Joint Surg Am* 67:1188–1194, 1985.

32. Schipplein, O. D.; Andriacchi, T. P.: Interaction between active and passive knee stabilizers during level walking. *J Orthop Res* 9:113–119, 1991.

33. Sharma, L.; Hurwitz, D. E.; Thonar, E. J.; et al.: Knee adduction moment, serum hyaluronic acid level, and disease severity in medial tibiofemoral osteoarthritis. *Arthritis Rheum* 41:1233–1240, 1998.

34. Shiavi, R.; Zhang, L. Q.; Limbird, T.; Edmondstone, M. A.: Pattern analysis of electromyographic linear envelopes exhibited by subjects with uninjured and injured knees during free and fast speed walking. *J Orthop Res* 10:226–236, 1992.

35. Shin, C. S.; Chaudhari, A. M.; Dyrby, C. O.; et al.: The patella ligament insertion angle influences quadriceps usage during walking of anterior cruciate ligament deficient patients. *J Orthop Res* 25:1643–1650, 2007.

36. Snyder-Mackler, L.; Fitzgerald, G. K.; Bartolozzi, A. R., 3rd; Ciccotti, M. G.: The relationship between passive joint laxity and functional outcome after anterior cruciate ligament injury. *Am J Sports Med* 25:191–195, 1997.

37. Tashman, S.; Kolowich, P.; Collon, D.; et al.: Dynamic function of the ACL-reconstructed knee during running. *Clin Orthop Relat Res* 454:66–73, 2007.

38. Wong, M. M.; Siegrist, M.; Cao, X.: Cyclic compression of articular cartilage explants is associated with progressive consolidation and altered expression pattern of extracellular matrix proteins. *Matrix Biol* 18:391–399, 1999.

39. Wu, J. Z.; Herzog, W.; Epstein, M.: Joint contact mechanics in early stages of osteoarthritis. *Med Eng Phys* 22:1–12, 2000.

40. Yao, J. Q.; Seedhom, B. B.: Mechanical conditioning of articular cartilage to prevalent stresses. *Br J Rheumatol* 32:956–965, 1993.

Chapter *7*

Anterior Cruciate Ligament Primary and Revision Reconstruction: Diagnosis, Operative Techniques, and Clinical Outcomes

Frank R. Noyes, MD ■ *Sue D. Barber-Westin*, BS

INDICATIONS

Anterior Cruciate Ligament Primary Reconstruction in Acute and Chronic Ruptures

Patients presenting with acute complete ruptures of the anterior cruciate ligament (ACL; >5 mm of increased anterior tibial translation and positive pivot shift test) are treated with rehabilitation until pain and swelling subside and joint motion and muscle function are restored. This delay markedly reduces the incidence of postoperative complications of knee motion limitations and muscle weakness. All patients with acute ruptures are profiled with regard to their desired future activity level to determine whether ACL reconstruction is warranted.[139] Those who wish to return to high-risk activities, including strenuous athletics or occupations involving pivoting, cutting, twisting, and turning, are considered for reconstruction. In patients with acute ACL ruptures and a concomitant displaced bucket-handle meniscus tear, surgery within 2 weeks is required to reduce the meniscus to a normal location and repair the tear. The ACL reconstruction may be performed at the same setting; however, knees with excessive swelling and pain undergo meniscus repair first. After an appropriate period of rehabilitation, ACL reconstruction is performed.

Patients involved in low-risk activities or who are willing to avoid strenuous athletic and occupational activities that place the knee at increased risk for giving-way episodes may not require ACL reconstruction. The patient is placed into a conservative treatment program that includes rehabilitation to regain muscle strength and neuromuscular function and counseling on the risk of future giving-way reinjuries and potential damage to the joint. Even with surgical reconstruction, patients are informed that an ACL rupture is a serious injury and it is unlikely that they will ever have a truly normal knee joint. The injury may also involve a bone bruise and chondral damage, with sequelae for future joint symptoms. The goal of conservative management is to prevent recurrent giving-way reinjuries, which are deleterious to the joint because they frequently result in

---

Critical Points INDICATIONS

- Complete anterior cruciate ligament (ACL) rupture: >5 mm of increased anterior tibial translation, positive pivot shift test.
- Profile patient for desired future activity level.
- High-risk activities (pivoting, cutting, twisting, turning): reconstruct.
- Acute ACL rupture and concomitant displaced bucket-handle meniscus tear: surgery within 2 wk to repair meniscus, usually concurrent ACL reconstruction.
- Low-risk activities, willing to avoid strenuous activities that place the knee at increased risk for giving-way episodes: conservative treatment.
- Partial ACL tears: <50% fibers torn, conservative treatment; >50% torn in athlete, consider graft augmentation.
- Revision ACL
  ○ Address all pathologies before surgery: lower limb malalignment, muscle atrophy, limitation knee motion, gait abnormalities, misplaced tunnels.
  ○ Goals, outcome of surgery depend on preexisting joint damage, associated procedures required.

---

meniscus tears and subsequent meniscectomy. It is important to categorize the knee joint as to the injury that has occurred. Repairable meniscus tears almost always indicate a concurrent ACL reconstruction. Otherwise, the success of the meniscus repair may be compromised.[40,108,157] DeHaven and coworkers[40] documented higher failure rates of meniscus repairs in knees with ACL deficiency than in knees with normal ACL function (46% and 5%, respectively) in a 10-year follow-up study. A grade III pivot shift and grossly positive Lachman test (increased ≥ 10 mm anterior tibial translation) indicate involvement of the secondary ligamentous restraints and, in the authors' experience, an increased risk of giving-way reinjuries with recreational activities. Patients with physiologic laxity of other ligaments or partial tears (second-degree) of medial or lateral ligaments frequently have a grossly positive pivot shift test, as discussed in Chapter 3, The Scientific Basis for Examination and Classification of Knee Ligament Injuries.

The rationale for the indications for ACL reconstruction is based on a study of 103 patients with chronic ACL ruptures.[141] These knees had no other ligament injuries and had not undergone reconstruction. The patients were evaluated a mean of 5.5 years after the initial knee injury; a subgroup of 39 patients presented an average of 11 years postinjury. This study was not a natural history study, because all patients sought treatment owing to symptoms. After the initial injury, 82% of the patients returned to sports activities, which gave an initial false impression of the seriousness of the ACL disruption. After 5 years, only 35% were continuing athletics, often with recurrent symptoms of pain or swelling. A significant reinjury occurred in 36 patients within 6 months and in 53 patients within the 1st year after the initial injury. Moderate to severe symptoms of pain, swelling, and/or giving-way were reported in 32 patients during walking, in 45 patients during activities of daily living, and in 73 patients during turning or twisting athletic activities. Giving-way occurred in 22 patients during walking, in 34 patients during recreational sports, and in 66 patients during strenuous sports. Knees that had undergone meniscectomy had a two- to fourfold increase in pain and swelling symptoms. Radiographic findings lagged behind clinical findings, because 44% of patients in the subgroup 11 years from injury had moderate to severe arthritic changes. The "ring" sign was noted, which represents an osteophyte (Fig. 7–1) that forms around the circumference of the lateral tibial plateau. This is associated with an absence of a pivot shift phenomena, but abnormal anterior tibial translation, because the lateral femoral condyle rotation is restrained by the osteophyte and increased concavity of the lateral tibial plateau.

In a follow-up study, 84 of the initial 103 patients underwent a repeat evaluation 3 years after initiating a conservative and activity modification treatment program.[139] The frequently quoted "rule of thirds" represents the outcome of this study regarding the effects of an ACL injury on subsequent functional activities. Approximately one third of the patients showed improvement in symptoms and functional limitations with daily or recreational activities, one third did not improve, and one third became worse with continuing symptoms and limitations. Thirty percent of the patients were noncompliant with the activity modification recommendations and stated they would continue athletics despite symptoms and the increased risk for future arthritis (labeled "knee abusers"). These patients had the poorest overall prognosis with conservative management. This general rule of thirds is not specific to individual patients with

Patients with a body mass index of 30 or greater are usually not surgical candidates. A history of prior infection with subsequent joint arthritis often contraindicates ACL revision. There may be associated medical conditions contraindicating surgery. The use of nicotine products is strongly discouraged and absolutely contraindicated if osteotomy alignment procedures are required.

CLINICAL BIOMECHANICS

Effect of ACL and Lateral Structures on Anterior Tibial Translation and Internal Tibial Rotation Limits

The function of the ACL is discussed in Chapter 3, The Scientific Basis for Examination and Classification of Knee Ligament Injuries. Additional information regarding the restoration of ACL function related to surgical techniques and graft placement issues are discussed in this section. The ACL is the primary restraint to anterior tibial translation, providing 87% of the total restraining force at 30° of knee flexion and 85% at 90° of flexion.[29] The iliotibial band (ITB), midmedial capsule, midlateral capsule, medial collateral ligament (MCL), and fibular collateral ligament (FCL) provide a combined secondary restraint to anterior tibial translation. The posteromedial (PM) and PL capsule structures provide added resistance with knee extension. The secondary restraints may become deficient after an ACL injury or repeat giving-way episode, resulting in increased symptoms.

The ACL resists the coupled motions of anterior tibial translation and internal tibial rotation along with the lateral structures. In the authors' laboratory, Wroble and colleagues[196] measured in ACL-deficient knees the simulated effect of lateral soft tissue injuries on internal tibial rotation and anterior tibial translation. The experimental design consisted of a six-degrees-of-freedom instrumented spatial linkage and loading of the knee joint under defined loads of 100 N anteroposterior (AP), 15 Nm varus-valgus, and 5 Nm internal-external tibial rotation torque. The limits of knee motions were determined in the intact knee and then after sectioning the ACL, ITB, lateral capsule, popliteus tendon and popliteofibular ligament, and PL capsule.

The effect of sectioning the ACL first, followed by the ITB and lateral capsule, is shown in Figure 7–2. Two distinct responses were measured. In the first set of knees (see Fig. 7–2A), there were only moderate increases in anterior tibial translation after ACL sectioning and negligible further increases after sectioning the ITB and lateral capsule. However, in the second set of knees (see Fig. 7–2B), much larger increases were noted in anterior tibial translation after sectioning the ACL and even greater increases were found after sectioning the ITB and lateral capsule. These findings are compatible with clinical tests after

---

Critical Points CLINICAL BIOMECHANICS

- ACL primary restraint anterior tibial translation.
- ITB, midmedial capsule, midlateral capsule, MCL, FCL combined secondary restraint.
- ACL resists coupled motions of anterior tibial translation and internal tibial rotation along with the lateral structures.
- Secondary restraints may become lax after reinjuries, may be physiologically loose or tight.
- Loss of ACL and lateral structures increases anterior tibial translation and internal tibial rotation.
- Increase in coupled motions shifts center of rotation to medial compartment.
- Concurrent injury to medial structures causes center of rotation to shift outside medial compartment, gross anterior subluxation of both compartments.
- Some authors provide evidence of two-bundle division of ACL, others argue that ACL fiber function is too complex to be artificially divided into two bundles.
- Characterization of ACL into two bundles represents gross oversimplification not supported by laboratory studies.
- With substantial anterior tibial loading or coupled motions, majority of ACL fibers are in a load-sharing configuration with different percentages as to fiber tensile loads.
- ACL is not isometric, all ACL fibers anterior to transitional zone lengthen with knee flexion, posterior fibers lengthen with knee extension.
- Function ACL fibers determined primarily by anterior-to-posterior direction (knee at extension), and secondarily by proximal-to-distal femoral attachment and anterior-to-posterior tibial attachment.
- Placement of graft too far in an anterior or a posterior femoral position has a large effect on deleterious lengthening and graft failure.

- Several studies report transtibial drilling techniques select a posterior tibial position, resulting in a vertical ACL graft orientation.
- Variation in ACL anatomy requires surgeon to outline the size and shape of the ACL attachment in each patient, if possible.
- Landmarks for ACL tibial attachment: medial tibial spine, posterior interspinous ridge (RER), attachment of lateral meniscus. PCL is poor landmark.
- Place guide pin eccentric and 2–3 mm anterior and medial to ACL center, avoiding posterior tibial attachment location.
- Limited anterior notchplasty often required with central ACL graft placement.
- Landmarks for ACL femoral attachment: posterior articular cartilage, Blumenstaat's line, resident's ridge, lateral femoral wall.
- Central anatomic ACL placement: femoral guide pin 2–3 mm above the midpoint of the proximal-to-distal length of the ACL attachment, 8 mm from the posterior articular cartilage edge. Define anatomic attachment with knee 20°–30° flexion.
- Majority in vitro robotic studies compare double-bundle graft with a less than ideal vertically placed single graft in a high femoral and posterior tibial location. This graft placement is not recommended.
- Studies of single ACL grafts in the more ideal central tibial and femoral anatomic attachment show restoration of rotational knee stability.
- There appears to be no distinct advantage of the more complex double-bundle technique over a well-placed central anatomic single-graft technique.
- Assessment of ACL graft function takes into account restoration of normal coupled motion limits of anterior tibial translation and internal tibial rotation. No current reliable measuring system is available to measure pivot shift test.

ACL, anterior cruciate ligament; FCL, fibular collateral ligament; ITB, iliotibial band; MCL, medial collateral ligament; PCL, posterior cruciate ligament; RER, retroeminence ridge.

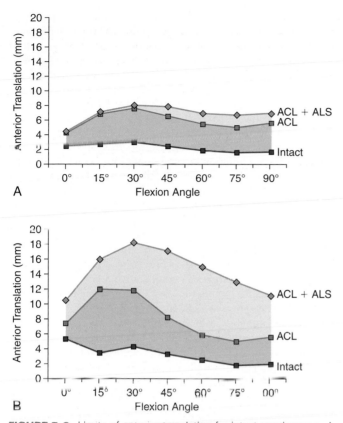

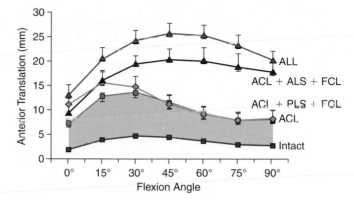

FIGURE 7–3. Limits of anterior translation for intact specimens and with serial sectioning of the ACL and lateral structures (100 N). Increases in anterior translation with sectioning the ACL are statistically significant at all flexion angles. For the ACL/PLS/FCL cut state, the only statistically significant increase was at 0° of flexion. For the ACL/ALS/FCL cut state, increases were statistically significant at 15° of flexion and above. Increases for the ALL cut state were statistically significant at all flexion angles. Anterior translation at 30° and 90° of flexion is approximately equal when the secondary lateral restraints are removed. ALS, iliotibial band, lateral capsule; FCL, fibular collateral ligament; PLS, posterolateral structures (popliteus tendon and popliteofibular ligament, posterolateral capsule). *(From Wroble, R. R.; Grood, E. S.; Cummings, J. S.; et al.: The role of the lateral extra-articular restraints in the anterior cruciate ligament–deficient knee. Am J Sports Med 21:257–262; discussion 263, 1993.)*

FIGURE 7–2. Limits of anterior translation for intact specimens and with the anterior cruciate ligament (ACL) and ACL/ALS cut (100 N). ALS, iliotibial band, lateral capsule. **A,** In these specimens, anterior translation in the intact state was low and, with sectioning of the ACL, moderate increases were found throughout the range of motion. Further sectioning of the ALS produced < 3 mm of increase in anterior translation, predominantly in the flexed knee. **B,** In this group of specimens, anterior translation in the intact state was higher than in the group of specimens shown in **A** at low flexion angles. After cutting the ACL, anterior translation was markedly increased in the 15°–30° of flexion range. After further sectioning of the ALS, large anterior translation increases were found at all flexion angles. **(A and B,** From Wroble, R. R.; Grood, E. S.; Cummings, J. S.; et al.: The role of the lateral extra-articular restraints in the anterior cruciate ligament–deficient knee. Am J Sports Med 21:257–262; discussion 263, 1993.)

ACL injury in which, in some knees, there may be only a moderate increase in anterior tibial translation, whereas in others, a much larger increase is present. This concept is discussed in Chapter 3, The Scientific Basis for Examination and Classification of Knee Ligament Injuries, using the analogy of the bumper model to simulate the effect of the secondary restraints on motion limits once the ACL is removed. Clinically, an ACL graft would be expected to be subjected to greater in vivo forces in the second set of knees without the unloading provided by relatively "tight" secondary restraints. The increase in the magnitude of anterior translation in these physiologically loose knees after loss of the anterolateral structures results in a grade III pivot shift phenomenon. These knees require a high-strength, securely fixated ACL graft to resist these major displacements, and autografts are highly recommended in these grossly unstable knees, as is discussed later.

The effect of sectioning the lateral and posterolateral structures (PLS) is shown in Figure 7–3.[196] Sectioning of the FCL or PLS (popliteus tendon, popliteofibular ligament, PL capsule) produced statistically significant, but small, increases in anterior tibial translation at low flexion angles. The combined ACL-ALS (anterolateral structures; ITB, anterior and middle portions of the lateral capsule)–FCL-sectioned knee had large increases in anterior tibial translation, with the greatest changes occurring at higher flexion angles.

The effect of sectioning the ACL and lateral structures on the limits of internal tibial rotation are shown in Figure 7–4. Sectioning of the ACL produced only a small increase in the final internal rotation limit. Sectioning of the ALS and the FCL produced a sequentially larger increase in internal tibial rotation. In select revision knees that have large increases in internal tibial rotation, the data support the role of a lateral extra-articular procedure to partially unload the ACL graft.

The conclusions from this study support the ACL as the primary restraint to anterior tibial translation. The data show the ultimate limit for internal tibial rotation is resisted by the lateral extra-articular structures that are tightened by the internal tibial rotation. The ACL limits internal rotation in the midrange of the envelope of tibial rotation, but not at the final limit of internal rotation. This is an important concept because clinical and biomechanical studies frequently attempt to measure increases in internal tibial rotation after ACL surgery in an attempt to quantify ACL graft function. Accordingly, this approach would not be expected to be successful. When the ITB and lateral capsule are physiologically slack, the FCL and ACL assume increased importance in limiting internal rotation. In summary, ACL function is ideally described by the restraining effect of limiting the coupled motions of internal tibial rotation and anterior tibial translation. A positive pivot shift test represents the effect of both of these increased motions, accounting for the anterior subluxation of the lateral and medial tibiofemoral compartment.

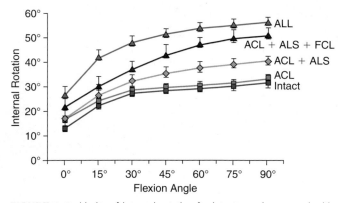

FIGURE 7–4. Limits of internal rotation for intact specimens and with the ACL, ACL/ALS, ACL/ALS/FCL, and ALL structures (ACL/ALS/FCL/PLS) cut (5 Nm). Increases in internal rotation with the ACL cut (statistically significant) are so small that they are clinically unimportant. With ACL/ALS sectioning, increases in internal rotation are statistically significant at 30° of flexion and above. Statistically significant increases are found at 15° of flexion and above in the ACL/ALS/FCL cut state and at all flexion angles for the ALL cut state. The effect of the PLS on restraining internal rotation in the extended knee can be seen by comparing the ACL/ALS/FCL curve and the ALL cut curve. The differences between these curves reflects sectioning the PLS. The largest differences are found at 15° and 30° of flexion. *(From Wroble, R. R.; Grood, E. S.; Cummings, J. S.; et al.: The role of the lateral extra-articular restraints in the anterior cruciate ligament–deficient knee. Am J Sports Med 21:257–262; discussion 263, 1993.)*

The motions that occur during the pivot shift maneuver are shown in Figure 7–5. At the beginning of the tests, the lower extremity is simply supported against gravity. After ACL disruption, both anterior tibial translation and internal tibial rotation increase as the femur drops back and externally rotates with subluxation of the lateral tibiofemoral compartment. This position is accentuated as the tibia is lifted anteriorly. At approximately 30° knee flexion, the tibia is pushed posteriorly, reducing the tibia into a normal position with the femur. From position C to position A (see Fig. 7–5B), the knee is extended to again produce the subluxated position. In addition to major increases in anterior tibial translation, there is also an increase in internal tibial rotation (midrange limit increase).

The effect of the ACL in providing rotational stability to the motions of anterior translation and internal tibial rotation is shown in Figure 7–6. After ACL sectioning, there is an increase in medial and lateral compartment translation as the center of rotation shifts from inside the knee joint to outside the medial compartment. The medial ligamentous structures influence the new center of rotation. With injury to the medial ligament structures, the center of rotation shifts so far medially that a rotational motion is essentially lost, resulting in a gross anterior subluxation of both compartments. The data show the important surgical concept of restoring injured medial and lateral ligament structures to restore anterior knee stability in conjunction with the ACL.

Division of the ACL into Anteromedial and Posterolateral Bundles

Controversy exists in published studies on the division of the ACL into two distinct fiber bundles. Some authors provide evidence of both an anatomic and a functional division, whereas others doubt that this division exists and argue that ACL fiber

function is too complex to be artificially divided into two bundles. In some studies,[4,32] the anteromedial (AM) bundle is identified functionally at its femoral location as the proximal half of the attachment (knee in extension) that tightens with knee flexion. The PL bundle is identified as the distal half of the ACL femoral attachment that tightens with knee extension. The PL bundle is described to relax with knee flexion, as the ACL femoral attachment changes from a vertical to a horizontal structure. The problem is that this classic description of a reciprocal tightening and relaxation of the AM and PL bundles occurs under no anterior loading conditions. With substantial anterior tibial loading, and in particular with a coupled motion of anterior translation and internal tibial rotation, the majority of the ACL fibers are brought into a load-sharing configuration to a differing percentage, as is presented later.

. The authors believe the characterization of the ACL into two fiber bundles represents a gross oversimplification not supported by biomechanical length-tension laboratory studies.[70,169] Zavras and coworkers[205] published a comparative study on previously published isometric points for the ACL and concluded that the ACL isometric zone was high and proximal in the ACL attachment, close to the posterior end of Blumensaat's line. This data, along with other studies, focused on placing grafts in the proximal aspect of the ACL attachment, in a so-called isometric position. The problem with applying published isometric data to the clinical situation is that the data are valid only for knee flexion-extension and do not indicate the most effective ACL graft position for controlling knee rotational loading as occurs during the pivot shift test. To date, data regarding the most effective graft positions to resist the coupled motions of anterior translation and internal rotation are not available. However, there are data on what graft placement positions are ineffective and should be avoided.

The length-tension behavior of ACL fibers is primarily controlled by the femoral attachment in reference to the center of femoral rotation, the coupled motions applied, the resting length of ACL fibers, and tibial attachment locations. In Chapter 3, The Scientific Basis for Examination and Classification of Knee Ligament Injuries, the concept of an isometric transition zone or contour plot is presented. The zone represents a central transition zone in which fibers undergo 2 mm of length change during knee flexion and extension. This zone is not an isometric zone, because the length change is not zero. All ACL fibers anterior to the zone lengthen with knee flexion, whereas the posterior fibers lengthen with knee extension. Under loading conditions, fibers in both the AM and the PL divisions contribute to resist tibial displacements. ACL fibers in the PL division attach in part posterior to the transitional zone and lengthen with knee extension. Note that the function of the ACL fibers is determined by the anterior-to-posterior direction (knee at extension) as well as the proximal-to-distal femoral attachment. Placement of a graft in an anterior or a posterior position has a large effect in producing deleterious lengthening and graft failure. The obvious example is a graft placed anterior to "residents' ridge," which is anterior to the femoral ACL attachment. The proximal-to-distal division used in two-bundle descriptions as the control of fiber length in knee flexion and extension oversimplifies the functional behavior of the ACL fibers, which are even more dependent on the AP femoral attachment.

The division of the ACL into two bundles was historically based on the tibial attachment site and not on a corresponding femoral attachment site. Recent studies project the tibial

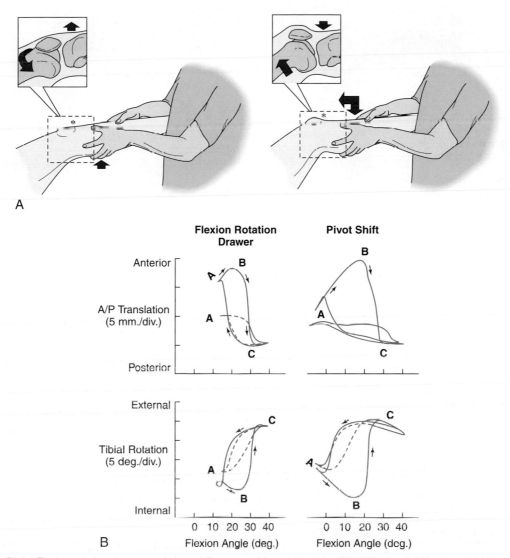

FIGURE 7–5. A, (Right) Flexion-rotation drawer and pivot shift tests, subluxated position. With the leg held in neutral rotation, the weight of the thigh causes the femur to drop back posteriorly and rotate externally, producing anterior subluxation of the lateral tibial plateau. (Left) Reduced position. Gentle flexion and a downward push on the leg reduces the subluxation. This test allows the coupled motion of anterior translation internal rotation to produce anterior subluxation of the lateral tibial condyle. **B,** The knee motions during the tests are shown for tibial translation and rotation during knee flexion. The clinical test is shown for the normal knee (*open circle*) and after ligament sectioning (*dotted circle*). The ligaments sectioned were the ACL, iliotibial band, and lateral capsule. Position A equals the starting position of the test, B is the maximum subluxated position, and C indicates the reduced position. The pivot shift test involves the examiner applying larger rotational loads, which increase the motion limits during the test. (**A,** From Noyes, F. R.; Bassett, R. W.; Grood, E. S.; et al.: Arthroscopy in acute traumatic hemarthrosis of the knee. J Bone Joint Surg Am 62:687–695, 1980; **B,** from Noyes, F. R.; Grood, E. S.; Suntay, W. J.: Three-dimensional motion analysis of clinical stress tests for anterior knee subluxations. Acta Orthop Scand 60:308–318, 1989.)

bundles onto two corresponding femoral sites. In these studies, to be described, the authors usually divide the ACL femoral attachment site at a midpoint into a corresponding AM and PL bundle. In the authors' opinion, there is not at present convincing anatomic data to support a division of the ACL into two separate bundles, although one study[50] reported a bony ridge between the two femoral attachment bundles. Because of the lack of a clear anatomic division of the ACL into two bundles, there is discrepancy among authors on anatomic descriptions of the ACL "bundles" and recommendations for the surgical technique on tibial and femoral tunnels for two bundle graft reconstructions.

Colombet and associates[32] measured the ACL femoral and tibial attachments of the AM and PL bundles in seven unpaired

cadaveric knees. The reference position of the retroeminence ridge (RER), representing the posterior interspinous ridge anterior to the posterior cruciate ligament (PCL) attachment, provided an important landmark for measuring from this point to the posterior ACL attachment. The tibial measurement points are shown in Figure 7–7 and the mean values are displayed in Table 7–1. Note the ACL extends posteriorly on the tibia to a distance 10.3 ± 1.9 mm from the RER line (coordinate bg). There is a discrepancy in the published text where this measurement is reported to be 7.1 mm. The mean length of the ACL (coordinate ag) was 17.6 ± 2.1 mm. The distance between the center of the AM and the center of the PL bundle (coordinate ef) was 8.4 ± 0.6 mm. The authors reported that the AM bundle was an average of 17.8 ± 1.7 mm anterior to the RER.

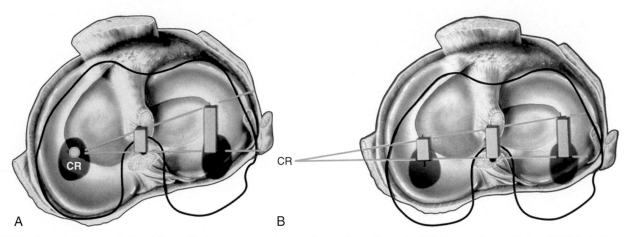

FIGURE 7–6. Intact knee and after ACL sectioning: response to coupled motions of anterior tibial translation and internal tibial rotation. **A**, Intact knee. The center of rotation may vary between the medial aspect of the PCL and the meniscus border, based on the loads applied and physiologic laxity of the ligaments. **B**, ACL sectioned; note shift in center of tibial rotation medially. The effect of the increase in tibial translation and internal tibial rotation produces an increase in medial and lateral tibiofemoral compartment translation (anterior subluxation). The millimeters of anterior translation of the tibiofemoral compartment represents the most ideal method to define knee rotational stability (see Chapter 3, The Scientific Basis for Examination and Classification of Knee Ligament Injury). The center of rotation under a pivot shift type of test shifts to the intact medial ligament structures. If these are deficient, the center of rotation shifts outside the knee joint.

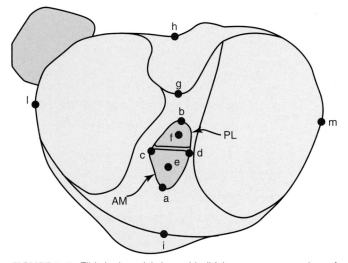

FIGURE 7–7. Tibia in the axial view with tibial measurement points of ACL attachment (a–m). a, Anterior extent; b, posterior extent; c, medial extent; d, lateral extent; e, projection of the center of the anteromedial (AM) bundle onto the ACL attachment area; f, projection of the center of the posterolateral (PL) bundle onto the ACL attachment area; g, retroeminence ridge; h, posterior border of the tibial plateau; i, anterior border of the tibial plateau; l, lateral border of the tibial plateau; m, medial border of the tibial plateau. *(From Colombet, P.; Robinson, J.; Christel, P.; et al.: Morphology of anterior cruciate ligament attachments for anatomic reconstruction: a cadaveric dissection and radiographic study. Arthroscopy 22:984–992, 2006.)*

The center of the ACL attachment was 19 mm anterior to the RER line. The center of the PL and AM bundles was determined to lie at 52% and 36% of the tibial width (line described by Amis and Jakob[5] that passes through the posterior corner of the tibial plateau and parallel to the medial tibial surface). The appearance of the ACL tibial attachments of the AM and PL bundles are shown in Figure 7–8 and represents a medial-to-lateral division, different from other authors who depict an anterior-to-posterior division.

The corresponding femoral attachments of the ACL from this study are shown in Figures 7–9 and 7–10 and the mean values are provided in Table 7–2. The overall length of the ACL was 18.3 ± 2.3 mm, with the center of the AM and PL bundles a mean of 8.2 mm apart and approximately 5 mm from the proximal and distal end of the ACL attachment. The authors recommended that the center of the PL bundle be located 8 mm lower and "shallower" in the notch than the center of the AM bundle. The femoral attachment was 2.5 mm from the articular cartilage. Using the grid system of Bernard and colleagues[19] (shown in Fig. 7–10), the center of the AM bundle was 26.4% ± 2.6%, and the center of the PL bundle was 32.3% ± 3.9% the length of Blumensaat's line.

In the most extensive study to date, Edwards and coworkers[45] defined the ACL tibial attachment in 55 cadaveric specimens. In Figure 7–11, the tibial bony landmarks are depicted. The "over-the-back" ridge (RER) again corresponds to the interspinous ridge just anterior and proximal to the PCL attachment. In Figure 7–12, the authors present their recommendations for best-fit central and two tunnel positions. The center of the ACL attachment was 15 ± 2 mm (range, 11–18 mm) from the RER at 36% of the AP depth of the tibia. The center of the PL bundle anterior from the RER was 10 ± 1 mm (range, 8–13 mm) and the AM bundle was 17 ± 2 mm (range, 13–19 mm), corresponding to 29% and 46% of the tibial depth, respectively. The authors noted, in disagreement with other publications, that they were not able to define two separate anatomic bundles. Instead, they defined two functional bundles by observing the tightening and slackening behavior of the ACL fibers during flexion and extension.

Stabuli and Rauschning[174a] reported the center of the ACL tibial attachment at 43% of the AP depth, which extended from 25% to 62% of the tibial width. These important landmarks provide a reference to measure lateral radiographs before and after ACL graft placement to avoid a posterior and vertical graft placement (Fig. 7–13). Siebold and associates[171] performed a cadaveric study in 50 knees and documented the ACL tibial insertion using a digital image analysis system and divided the ACL into AM and PL bundles. The average AP length of the ACL tibial attachment was 14 mm (range, 9–18 mm). The average male ACL tibial

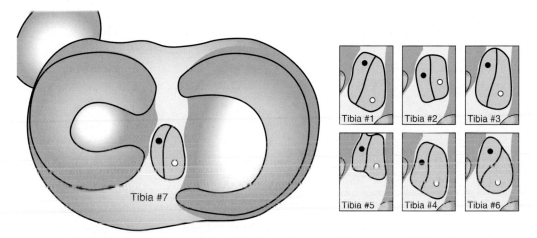

FIGURE 7–8. Appearances of the tibial ACL attachments. The projection of the central fibers of the AM bundle onto the attachment area is shown by a *white dot* (point e), and similarly, the projection of the central fibers of the PL bundle is shown by a *black dot* (point f). *(From Colombet, P.; Robinson, J.; Christel, P.; et al.: Morphology of anterior cruciate ligament attachments for anatomic reconstruction: a cadaveric dissection and radiographic study. Arthroscopy 22:984–992, 2006.)*

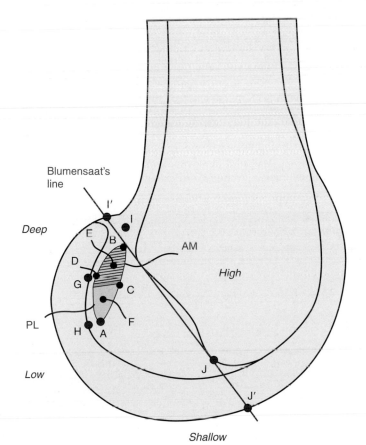

FIGURE 7–9. Femur in the sagittal view with femoral measurement points of the ACL attachment area (A–J). Both anatomic and corresponding surgical navigation terminology have been used for clarity. A, Distal border ("low" in the notch); B, proximal border ("high" in the notch); C, anterior border ("shallow" in the notch); D, posterior border ("deep" in the notch); E, projection of the center of the AM bundle onto the ACL attachment area; F, projection of the center of the PL bundle onto the ACL attachment area; G, posterior margin of the articular cartilage ("deep" in the notch); H, distal margin of the articular cartilage ("low" in the notch); I, "over-the-top" position ("high" in the notch); J, most anterior point of the roof of the notch. *(From Colombet, P.; Robinson, J.; Christel, P.; et al.: Morphology of anterior cruciate ligament attachments for anatomic reconstruction: a cadaveric dissection and radiographic study. Arthroscopy 22:984–992, 2006.)*

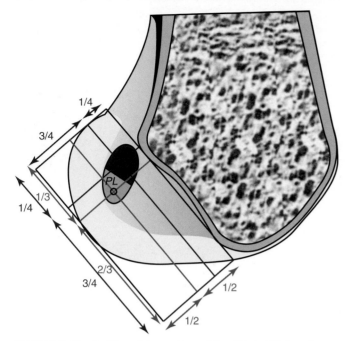

FIGURE 7–10. Position of the centers of the AM and PL bundles on the grid described by Bernard et al.[19] *(From Colombet, P.; Robinson, J.; Christel, P.; et al.: Morphology of anterior cruciate ligament attachments for anatomic reconstruction: a cadaveric dissection and radiographic study. Arthroscopy 22:984–992, 2006.)*

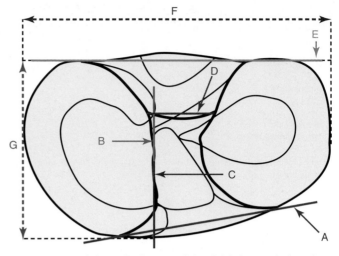

FIGURE 7–11. Schematic diagram of the tibial plateau depicts the landmarks used in this study. A, Anterior tibial surface; B, apex of medial tibial spine; C, lateral border of medial tibial spine; D, "over-the-back" ridge; E, posterior tibial axis; F, width; G, depth. *(From Edwards, A.; Bull, A. M.; Amis, A. A.: The attachments of the anteromedial and posterolateral fibre bundles of the anterior cruciate ligament: part 1: tibial attachment. Knee Surg Sports Traumatol Arthrosc 15:1414–1421, 2007; with kind permission of Springer Science+Business Media.)*

insertion area was 130 mm² versus the average female knee of 106 mm². The average AP length of the ACL footprint in females was 14 mm (range, 9–18 mm), and in males, 15 mm (range, 12–18 mm). The average width of the ACL in all knees was 10 mm. The study concluded that two tibial bone tunnels cannot be placed at the anatomic centers of the AM and PL bundles because the space is too narrow and the tunnels would overlap. This highlights the difficulty of the ACL double-bundle technique in re-creating the native ACL fiber attachment.

Zantop and colleagues[204] performed a cadaveric study in 20 knees that outlined the AM and PL bundle locations at the tibial and femoral sites. The authors arrived at different conclusions from those of Siebold and associates.[171] The tibia ACL division into the AM bundle was oriented from medial to lateral and occupied the anterior one half of the ACL footprint and was aligned with the anterior horn of the lateral meniscus. The center of the PL bundle was located 11 mm posterior and 4 mm medial to the anterior insertion of the lateral meniscus. The center of the AM bundle was located at 30% and the PL bundle was located at 40% on the lateral transtibial line.

Edwards and coworkers[46] described the anatomic locations of the ACL femoral attachments of the AM and PL bundles in a companion study in 22 cadaveric knees using a measurement grid system shown in Figure 7–14. The authors reported a wide variation in the size and shape of the ACL attachment and bundle arrangement that was selected (Fig. 7–15). Note that the AM and PL bundle divisions differ from the prior study. The femoral attachment was oriented at 37° to the long axis of the femur. The authors reported that the AM bundle extended to the posterior proximal limit of the femoral notch between the 10:30 and the 11:30 positions. The PL bundle was located between the 9:00 and the 10:30 positions. The authors reported that a 6-mm graft tunnel had the best fit if the AM bundle was located at 11 o'clock, 6 mm from the posterior outlet, and the PL bundle was located at 10 o'clock, 9 mm from the posterior outlet. The authors noted that other studies had different recommendations for the placement of two femoral tunnels in the double-bundle technique.

TABLE 7–2	Femoral Measurements Taken Directly from Cadaveric Specimens (mm)								
	AB	**CD**	**BE**	**AF**	**EF**	**BI**	**AH**	**DG**	**IJ**
Specimen 1	17.3	9.2	5.0	4.2	8.2	2.8	2.5	3.7	28.5
Specimen 2	14.2	7.2	4.5	3.5	5.7	3.2	2.2	2.7	23.0
Specimen 3	18.7	9.3	4.0	4.8	8.7	1.2	2.3	2.8	28.7
Specimen 4	20.2	12.8	5.3	6.7	9.5	0.2	3.0	2.5	31.2
Specimen 5	21.3	11.5	6.2	4.8	8.8	1.7	1.7	0.8	29.7
Specimen 6	18.8	14.5	7.8	5.2	8.5	3.0	6.2	3.7	27.3
Specimen 7	17.7	7.8	4.2	4.7	8.0	0.3	2.0	1.3	22.2
Mean	18.3	10.3	5.3	4.8	8.2	1.8	2.8	2.5	27.2
Standard deviation	2.3	2.7	1.3	1.0	1.2	1.3	1.5	1.1	3.4
Intraobserver error	1.1	1.1	0.4	0.7	0.8	0.9	0.9	0.7	2.5

From Colombet, P.; Robinson, J.; Christel, P.; et al.: Morphology of anterior cruciate ligament attachments for anatomic reconstruction: a cadaveric dissection and radiographic study. *Arthroscopy* 22:984–992, 2006.

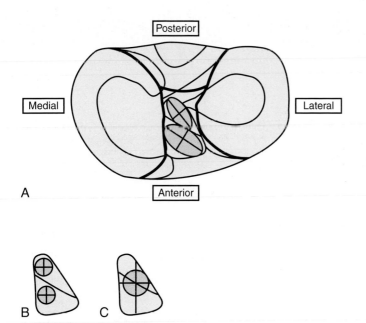

FIGURE 7–12. Schematic diagram of a left knee depicts the best-fit ellipses marking the centers of the AM and PL bundles (**A**); the positions of 6-mm tunnels placed in the posteromedial limits of the AM and PL bundles (**B**); and the center of the ACL attachment (**C**). *(From Edwards, A.; Bull, A. M.; Amis, A. A.: The attachments of the anteromedial and posterolateral fibre bundles of the anterior cruciate ligament: part 1: tibial attachment. Knee Surg Sports Traumatol Arthrosc 15:1414–1421, 2007; with kind permission of Springer Science+Business Media.)*

Rue and associates[159] in a cadaveric study used a transtibial-drilled femoral tunnel, placed at the 10:30 position, and determined the location of a single-graft femoral tunnel in relation to the AM and PL bundles. The authors placed the guide pin for the tibial tunnel approximately 7 mm anterior to the PCL, which would represent a posterior one third tibial attachment. The authors reported the transtibial drilling of the femoral tunnel resulted in the footprint of the AM occupying an average of 32% (range, 3%–49%) of the area of the tunnel, and the footprint of the PL bundle occupying an average of 26% (range, 7%–41%). In addition, the remainder of the area of the 10-mm tunnel did not overlap the ACL footprint. The wide ranges reported in this study for the location of the femoral tunnel in terms of the native ACL femoral attachment highlight the problems of using the tibial tunnel to drill the femoral tunnel.

Heming and colleagues[71] reported the ACL tibial and femoral footprints in 12 cadaveric knees (Fig. 7–16). Note in Figure 7–16C, the orientation of the clock face places the 9 to 3 o'clock horizontal line at the base of the femoral condyles and not within the center of the notch, which is typically used by other authors. A guide pin placed between the ACL anatomic femoral and tibial attachment centers (as in a transtibial drilling technique) was only possible if the tibial tunnel started in a medial position close to the joint line that would be too short to be functional for ACL grafts. The study concluded that transtibial drilling techniques resulted in a more vertical graft orientation.

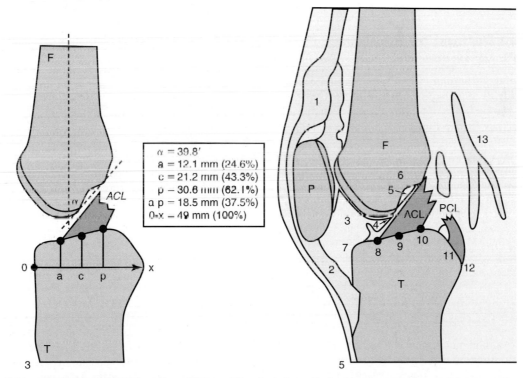

FIGURE 7–13. Schematic drawing of tibial insertion of ACL and its orientation with the knee in extension. In this cryosectional knee specimen (right knee, midsagittal plane, medial view at 0° of flexion, i.e., in the extended knee position, specimen 5), the inclination of a tangent constructed to the intercondylar roof formed an angle of 42° with respect to the midsagittal femoral shaft axis. The anterior limit of the ACL was located at 11 mm (23.4%), the central part at 20 mm (42.6%), and the posterior limit at 29 mm (61.7%) when determined from the anterior tibial margin and calculated over the total sagittal diameter of the tibia, which measured 47 mm (100%). F, femur; P, patella; T, tibia; 1, quadriceps tendon; 2, patellar tendon; 3, Hoffa's fat pad (corpus adiposum intrapatellare); 4, infrapatellar plica; 5, synovial fold of PCL; 6, roof of intercondylar fossa; 7, anterior tibial margin; 8, anterior limit of ACL; 9, central part of ACL; 10, posterior limit of ACL; 11, tibial attachment site of PCL at posterior intercondylar area; 12, posterior tibial margin at posterior intercondylar area; 13, popliteal artery. *(From Staubli, H. U.; Rauschning, W.: Tibial attachment area of the anterior cruciate ligament in the extended knee position. Anatomy and cryosections in vitro complemented by magnetic resonance arthrography in vivo. Knee Surg Sports Traumatol Arthrosc 2:138–146, 1994; with kind permission of Springer Science+Business Media.)*

FIGURE 7–14. A, Measurement lines drawn parallel to the femoral shaft at the o'clock positions. **B,** Measurement lines drawn parallel to the femoral notch roof from the o'clock positions. **C,** The posterior condyle circle reference system. **D,** Measurement grid for describing the position of the centres of the two functional ACL bundle attachments, with numbered zones. *(A–D, From Edwards, A.; Bull, A. M.; Amis, A. A.: The attachments of the anteromedial and posterolateral fibre bundles of the anterior cruciate ligament: part 2: femoral attachment.* Knee Surg Sports Traumatol Arthrosc *online, 2007.)*

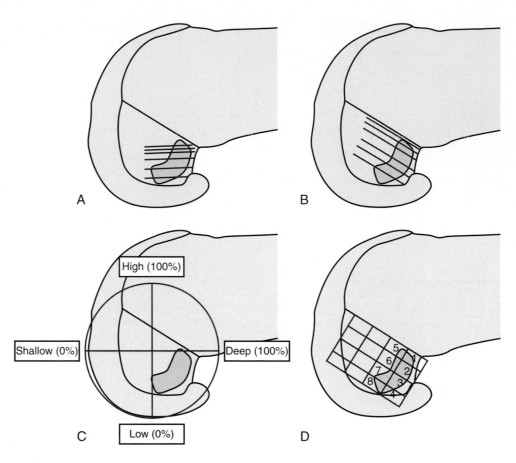

ACL Function Defined by the Role of AM and PL Divisions

Sakane and coworkers,[160] in one of the first cadaveric robotic studies, reported the PL bundle provided the primary restraint to anterior tibial translation at low flexion angles. Increasing forces were reported in the AM bundle with knee flexion; these remained lower than the calculated in situ forces of the PL bundle.

The role of the ACL bundles in restraining rotational motions was examined by Zantop and associates[203] in a robotic study. A 134-N anterior tibial load and a combined 10-Nm valgus and 4-Nm internal tibial torque were applied to cadaveric knees. Sectioning the PL bundle at 30° of flexion resulted in an approximately 7-mm increase in anterior tibial translation, whereas sectioning the AM bundle produced at 60° an approximately 9-mm increase in anterior translation. Similar data were reported at low flexion angles for the combined rotational loads. These data imply a near-absence of function of the remaining "intact" bundle. In contrast, Markolf and colleagues,[97] in a cadaveric study, reported that cutting the PL bundle resulted in an increase of only 1.1 mm at 10° flexion and 0.5 mm at 30° flexion. These authors questioned the need to reconstruct the PL bundle for restoration of normal ACL laxity.

Gabriel and coworkers,[55] in a robotic cadaveric experiment, removed all of the soft tissues to produce a femur-ACL-tibia specimen. For anterior tibial loading (Fig. 7–17), the AM bundle was reported to be nearly equal to the PL bundle at 15° of flexion, with increasing AM forces with knee flexion. Under the rotation loads of valgus and internal tibial rotation, the forces in the AM bundle exceeded those of the PL bundle (Fig. 7–18).

Li and associates[90] used MRI and fluroscopic images of subjects performing a lunge to create three-dimensional models in which the AM and PL ACL attachments were outlined. The study reported that the AM and PL bundles reached their maximum elongation between full extension and 30° of flexion and did not demonstrate a reciprocal behavior with knee flexion-extension.

Giron and colleagues,[61] in a cadaveric experiment, determined that a "deep" (proximal) femoral tunnel position could be achieved with either one of three techniques (double incision, transtibial, or anteromedial portal). However, Arnold and coworkers[9] showed in cadaveric experiments that the ACL is entirely attached to the lateral femoral wall and that this attachment position was not able to be accessed through a transtibial tunnel (40% AP tibial measurement). The transtibial tunnel method resulted in the guide pin and drill hole placed at the junction of the proximal ACL attachment and femoral roof (Fig. 7–19).

Mae and associates,[96] in a cadaveric knee study, used a robotic simulator to study the effect of single- versus two-femoral tunnel ACL graft reconstruction. A single tibial tunnel was placed in the center of the ACL tibial attachment. The locations of the single and two tunnels were described at the 1:00 and 2:30 positions. The data for AP laxity and AP in situ graft forces at 44 N graft pretension showed little difference between the single- and the double-bundle grafts, both of which produced a mild to moderate overconstraint that limited anterior tibial translation. The study reported on the load-sharing between the normal ACL bundles (Fig. 7–20), which demonstrated that the PL bundle functioned more at low flexion angles, equal to the AM bundle at 10° of flexion, with a further increase in AM bundle function with increasing knee flexion. A study of load-sharing between the two bundles of a simulated pivot shift type of loading was not performed.

Yagi and colleagues[199] compared single- and double-bundle ACL hamstring reconstructions. A double-looped single-bundle

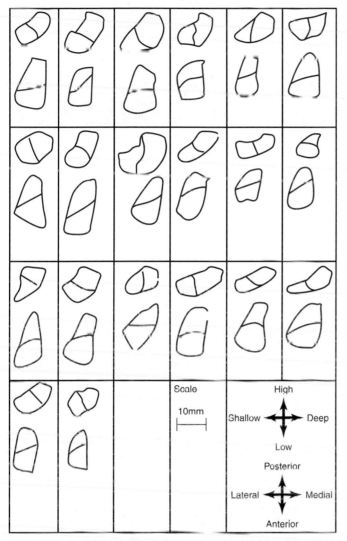

FIGURE 7-15. ACL attachment outlines on the femur and the corresponding outlines on the tibia; femur above tibia in each case; all shown for the right knee. *(From Edwards, A.; Bull, A. M.; Amis, A. A. The attachments of the anteromedial and posterolateral fibre bundles of the anterior cruciate ligament. part 2: femoral attachment. Knee Surg Sports Traumatol Arthrosc online, 2007.)*

hamstring graft was placed at approximately the 11 o'clock position and tensioned to 44 N, whereas each bundle of the double-bundle graft was tensioned to 44 N. The double-bundle graft had a total of 88 N of tension versus 44 N for the single-graft reconstruction. In response to a 134-N anterior load at 30° of flexion, the data showed an unexplained residual anterior tibial translation (intact, 6.4 mm ± 2.4 mm: single-bundle, 10.2 ± 2.5 mm), which would not be anticipated from a single graft in terms of resisting translation. The finding of a lax single graft most likely explains the reported decreased ability of the single graft to resist the combined rotation-translation motions.

Petersen and coworkers[146] concluded that the location of the ACL double-bundle grafts in clinical studies varied markedly at both the femoral and the tibial sites. In a cadaveric study, Petersen and coworkers[146] found that a two-tunnel tibial technique provided an advantage in resisting combined rotatory loads, simulating the pivot shift (anterior tibial translation, 7.5 mm vs. 9.5 mm, 30° flexion, 5 Nm internal rotation, 10 Nm valgus torque). Of note, the single tibial tunnel and graft was placed 7

to 8 mm anterior to the PCL; the authors stated that this was a position recommended by some surgeons.[74,107] As previously discussed, the posterior tibial tunnel position results in a more vertical ACL graft, with portions of the graft possibly even posterior to the native ACL tibial attachment. The addition of a second graft placed in a more anterior tibial position within the ACL footprint would be expected to provide better resistance to the loading conditions. Although the data do not provide evidence for a double-bundle ACL procedure, it does provide evidence to avoid placement of a single ACL graft in the posterior one third of the ACL tibial attachment.

Yamamoto and associates[200] conducted a cadaveric robotic study that compared a single ACL graft placed in the 10:00 position on the lateral wall with an anatomic double-bundle reconstruction. This is one of the few published studies in which a single-graft lateral wall placement was used, avoiding a more proximal graft placement. Similar loading conditions were used as in the other robotic studies (anterior tibial load 134 N, combined rotatory load 10 Nm valgus and 5 Nm internal tibial torque). There was no statistical difference in the anterior tibial translation or in situ force at 30° knee flexion between the intact ACL, the single bundle, or the anatomic double-bundle reconstructions. Under the combined rotatory loading conditions, there were no differences in anterior tibial translation, internal tibial rotation, and ACL in situ graft forces, which is in direct contrast to other robotic experiments.

Markolf and colleagues[98] measured in cadaver knees a simulated pivot shift in the intact knee and then after single-bundle and double-bundle ACL reconstruction. The single-bundle reconstruction (placed at the anatomic AM bundle site) restored mean tibial rotations and lateral plateau displacements to levels similar to those of the intact knee, whereas the double-bundle reconstructions reduced coupled rotations and displacements to levels less than those in the intact knee. The authors concluded that the overconstraint induced by the double-bundle reconstructions has unknown clinical consequences and that the need for the added complexity of this procedure is questionable.

Cuomo and coworkers[38] reported on the effects of tensioning single- and double-bundle ACL reconstructions in cadaveric knees instrumented with a six-degrees-of-freedom system under defined loading conditions (anterior translation, 90 N; 5 Nm internal rotation torque). Different flexion positions were used for tensioning each of the grafts in the double-bundle construct. The single graft was tensioned at 20° knee flexion. All grafts had sufficient tension applied to restore the intact knee laxity (translation). Tensioning each of the grafts individually (AM bundle at 90°, PL bundle at 20°, varying which was tensioned first) resulted in overconstraining AP translation. In contrast, tensioning both the AM and the PL grafts simultaneously at 20° provided the best match for the intact knee AP translation throughout knee flexion. The data show the difficulty in tensioning two ACL grafts at the time of surgery in terms of matching the intact ACL load-sharing between fibers. With anterior loading, both the AM and the PL fibers participate in load-sharing, but at different percentages, as already discussed. For single-bundle ACL grafts placed within the center of the femoral and tibial attachments, higher overall graft tension occurred under anterior loading compared with the two graft bundles tensioned at 20° flexion. Importantly, the data show that tensioning of the AM and PL grafts under low tensions (20 N) provided the best results. The single graft required 38 ± 27 N to restore the native knee laxity.

FIGURE 7–16. A, Right knee ACL tibial insertion. Measurements are the mean for the anterior-posterior length, medial-lateral width 10 mm from the posterior margin, distance from the PCL notch, and distance to the medial plateau articular cartilage. **B**, Right knee ACL femoral insertion. Measurements are the mean for the length, width 10 mm from the proximal margin, distance to the articular cartilage, and angle to the long axis of the femur in the sagittal plane. **C**, Right knee ACL femoral insertion in the coronal plane with the knee flexed 90°. The ACL insertion spanned the clock face from 10:14 to 11:23. The vertical 12 o'clock axis was perpendicular to the 3- to 9-o'clock axis drawn between the posterior femoral condyles. The vertical axis extended superiorly from a point midway between the walls of the notch to the apex of the notch. (**A–C**, *From Heming, J. F.; Rand, J.; Steiner, M. E.: Anatomical limitations of transtibial drilling in anterior cruciate ligament reconstruction.* Am J Sports Med *35:1708–1715, 2007.)*

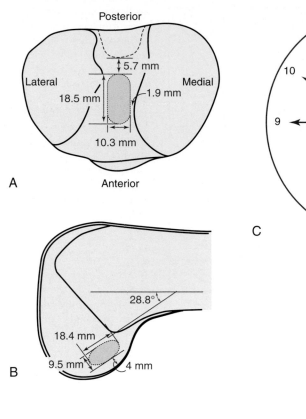

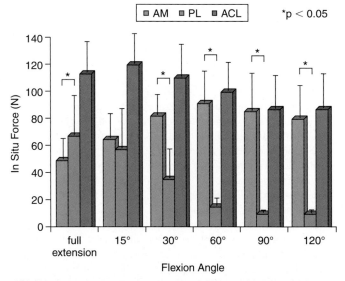

FIGURE 7–17. In situ force in the intact ACL and its AM and PL bundles in response to 134 N anterior tibial load. *(From Gabriel, M. T.; Wong, E. K.; Woo, S. L.; et al.: Distribution of in situ forces in the anterior cruciate ligament in response to rotatory loads.* J Orthop Res *22:85–89, 2004; reprinted with permission of Wiley-Liss, Inc., a subsidiary of John Wiley & Sons, Inc.)*

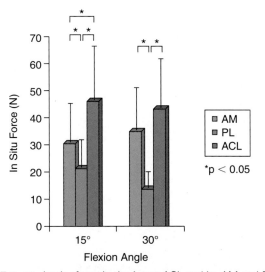

FIGURE 7–18. In situ force in the intact ACL and its AM and PL bundles in response to combined rotatory load (10 Nm valgus and 5 Nm internal tibial torque). *(From Gabriel, M. T.; Wong, E. K.; Woo, S. L.; et al.: Distribution of in situ forces in the anterior cruciate ligament in response to rotatory loads.* J Orthop Res *22:85–89, 2004; reprinted with permission of Wiley-Liss, Inc., a subsidiary of John Wiley & Sons, Inc.)*

Scopp and associates,[164] in cadaveric experiments, reported that a more oblique femoral tunnel placement (60° from vertical) was more effective in resisting internal rotational torques (difference 4.4°, 6.5 Nm) than a "standard" tunnel placement (30° from vertical). The femoral tunnel was drilled using a transtibial technique and, most likely, a posterior tibial tunnel placement. Anterior tibial translation values were not restored to normal (increased 2.5 and 2.2 mm, standard and oblique femoral tunnels).

Simmons and colleagues[172] in cadaver experiments showed the deleterious effects of a more vertical tibial tunnel (70°, 80°) with impingement against the PCL and higher graft tension. A more oblique tibial tunnel and femoral tunnel in the 60° coronal plane did not impinge against the PCL. The study recommended a posterior tibial tunnel placement and more proximal ACL femoral attachment with use of a transtibial drilling technique, again showing the predominance of studies in the literature in which a more vertical graft orientation results.

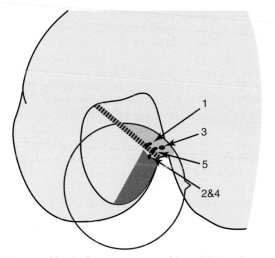

FIGURE 7–19. Notch view, summary guiding pinholes; knees no. 1–5, schematic drawing. *(From Arnold, M. P.; Kooloos, J.; van Kampen, A.: Single-incision technique misses the anatomical femoral anterior cruciate ligament insertion: a cadaver study. Knee Surg Sports Traumatol Arthrosc 9:194–199, 2001; with kind permission of Springer Science+Business Media.)*

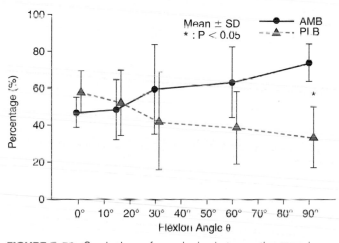

FIGURE 7–20. Graph shows force sharing between the normal ACL bundles under 100 N of anterior load. *(From Mae, T.; Shino, K.; Miyama, T.; et al.: Single- versus two-femoral socket anterior cruciate ligament reconstruction technique: biomechanical analysis using a robotic simulator. Arthroscopy 17:708–716, 2001.)*

Arnold and coworkers[10] showed in cadavers that the passive ACL tension flexion-extension tension curve was not reproduced by femoral tunnels placed at the 10 and 11 o'clock position, but was reproduced by grafts in the 9 o'clock–positioned tunnels. A posterior tibial tunnel was used in this experiment.

In summary, a majority of in vitro robotic studies compare a double-bundle graft construct to a hybrid proximal femoral and posterior tibial orientation of a more vertical single-bundle graft construct and not a centrally placed femoral and tibial graft construct. Therefore, the published data apply specifically to this type of single-graft construct and show as expected that a vertical single graft is not positioned to resist rotational loading. It may be concluded that there are sufficient experimental data to recommend that this hybrid graft orientation be avoided in clinical practice.

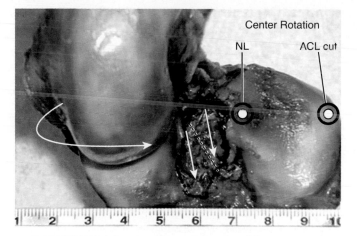

FIGURE 7–21. The ACL attachment on the tibia is outlined, along with an approximated center of tibial rotation. After ACL sectioning, the center of tibial rotation shifts medially, restrained in part by the medial ligament structures. The ACL tibial fibers are divided into AM and PL bundles. It should be noted that the AM bundle is anatomically positioned to limit the coupled motions of internal tibial rotation and anterior translation under loading conditions; this effect has been frequently underestimated in biomechanical studies.

There are incomplete in vitro data on the comparison of a anatomic single-graft construct (within central tibial and femoral tunnels) with a double-bundle construct.[94] There are also incomplete experimental data on the function of individual regions of ACL fibers in resisting coupled motions as occurs in the pivot shift phenomena, which is an important area for future study (Fig. 7–21). Other biomechanical studies reviewed show that a single ACL graft placed within the anatomic femoral and tibial attachments (avoiding a high femoral and posterior tibial position) restores rotatory stability and question the need for a double-bundle procedure.[98]

One theoretical advantage of a double-graft construct tensioned appropriately is that there is initially less graft tension in each of the graft strands compared with the overall tension in a single graft. Stated differently, a single graft will always exhibit much higher graft tension to resist anterior loading than two graft arms in which load-sharing occurs. There is also the theoretical advantage of tensioning the two graft strands at different knee flexion positions to exhibit a different percentage of sharing of the overall tension than a single graft. From an experimental standpoint, either a single-graft or a double-graft construct can be tensioned to restore normal motion limits; however, this may occur at the expense of high graft tensions, particularly in a single-graft construct. Thus, the advantage of a double-graft construct (either ACL or PCL) is to restore normal knee motion limits under the lowest graft tensile loads, which is advantageous during the graft healing and remodeling. A graft under lower loads has the theoretical advantage of less risk in stretching out with return of the abnormal motion limits. In addition, an ACL or a PCL graft under higher tension under cyclical loading conditions is at high risk of graft stretching and failure.[167] Again, it should be noted that either one or two ACL grafts do not restore native ACL fiber length-tension properties.

Clinical Measurement of ACL Graft Function during and after ACL Surgery

The assessment of ACL graft function must take into account the restoration of the normal coupled motion limits of anterior tibial translation and internal tibial rotation. During KT-2000 testing, only anterior tibial translation is assessed. If the knee joint has a 3-mm or lower increase in anterior tibial translation over the opposite knee, it can be assumed that there is not a positive pivot shift because this amount of constraint to anterior tibial translation also limits internal rotation. Conversely, if greater than 5 mm of increased anterior tibial translation exists, there is usually an abnormal increase in internal tibial rotation that results in a positive pivot shift test and patient complaints of giving-way. The problem is in knees that demonstrate 3 to 5 mm of increased anterior tibial translation, which may represent 20% to 30% of patients in clinical investigations,[2,7,143,165,166] especially when allografts are used.[131] This mild to moderate increase in anterior tibial translation results in a mildly positive Lachman test with a hard endpoint. However, along with an increase in internal tibial rotation, these knees may demonstrate a positive pivot shift and giving-way symptoms. Because the pivot shift test is highly subjective and variable between examiners (see Chapter 3, The Scientific Basis for Examination and Classification of Knee Ligament Injuries), an author may report a successful result based on the KT-2000 (anterior tibial translation) or a pivot shift test, whereas another examiner may grade the knee as a failure based on the method by which the pivot shift test is performed. There is a pressing need for clinical examination tools that incorporate tibial translations and rotations and the resultant subluxations in millimeters of the medial and lateral tibiofemoral compartments under defined loading conditions.

Bull and associates[25] were among the first authors to report intraoperative measurement of tibial translations and rotations using a three-dimensional motion analysis system. Robinson and colleagues[156] performed an ACL double-bundle reconstruction using computerized navigation techniques in 22 patients. Both the AM and the PL bundles contributed to resisting anterior tibial translation during the pivot shift tests. However, the PL bundle was more important than the AM bundle in controlling abnormal tibial rotation. It is probable that the AM bundle was placed in a more vertical proximal position adjacent to the intercondylar roof. Computerized navigation techniques allow for a highly accurate measurement of knee translations and rotations that may lead to the most objective means to measure knee kinematics during surgery. However, the exact location of ACL grafts and the loads applied by the examiner are variables still to be determined.

In a frequently quoted study, Tashman and coworkers[179] devised a unique methodology of dynamic in vivo measurements of patients after ACL reconstruction on a treadmill while running downhill, employing a biplanar radiographic system to measure tibiofemoral displacements. The reconstructed knees showed an increase in mean values of external tibial rotation (3.8° ± 2.3°) and adduction (2.8° ± 1.6°). The effect of these small differences from a clinical standpoint is unknown and future studies are required that involve more dynamic rotational movements in comparison with straight-ahead running to measure the rotational kinematics of the knee joint. The specific ACL graft femoral and tibial tunnel placement was not identified in this study.

Ristanis and associates[155] assessed 11 patients after a bone–patellar tendon–bone (B-PT-B) reconstruction using kinematic data from a six-camera optoelectronic system obtained during a jump landing and pivoting maneuver. The ACL reconstruction did not restore tibial rotation to normal values of the opposite uninvolved extremity or controls. The femoral tunnel was placed through an AM approach with the knee joint flexed to 120° to achieve a 10 to 11 o'clock lateral wall position. The tibial tunnel was placed into the center of the ACL footprint. The authors noted the limitation of the study in the movement of skin markers accurately representing true tibiofemoral joint rotations.

Monaco and colleagues[106] in patients undergoing ACL reconstruction evaluated the effect of a single-bundle reconstruction with an extra-articular procedure to a double-bundle ACL reconstruction. Computerized navigation instrumentation was used in the operating room before and after the ACL procedures. The addition of the PL bundle after the AM bundle did not have an effect in reducing AP translation or the limit of internal tibial rotation, and there were no significant differences between the single- and the double-bundle reconstructions. The extra-articular reconstruction significantly reduced the internal tibial rotation limit, as would be expected. The tibial placement of the graft was performed with the guide pin 7 mm anterior to the PCL insertion into the posterior ACL attachment. The authors did not determine the effect of either graft configuration on the coupled motions of the pivot shift test but only on the limit of internal tibial rotation alone.

The authors' conclusions of single-graft versus double-bundle graft ACL studies are summarized in Table 7–3. The hypothesis presented is that an ideally placed single-graft construct (avoiding a vertical graft orientation) provides control of the abnormal pivot shift motions, avoiding the necessity and added complexity of a double-bundle graft reconstruction.

Recommended Tibial and Femoral ACL Graft Locations

Given the variation in ACL anatomic shapes between specimens, it is important during surgery to outline the individual size and shape of the ACL attachment for each knee. This can be done in a primary ACL reconstruction, but usually not in revisions. The cadaveric studies provide important anatomic reference landmarks. Because of the variation in ACL attachment shapes, it would be expected that there would exist variation between surgeons on the locations chosen for both single- and double-bundle ACL graft locations. Newer computer navigation techniques have been studied to aid in the placement of ACL grafts; however, it is unknown at present what anatomic points to select for graft tunnels that would correlate with clinical stability results.

The important landmarks for the ACL tibial attachments are the medial tibial spine, posterior interspinous ridge (RER) of the proximal PCL fossa, and the attachment of the lateral meniscus. The PCL is a poor soft tissue landmark for the posterior extent of the native ACL attachment. It should be noted that some authors[75] have advocated a guide pin and tibial tunnel placement 6 to 8 mm from the PCL, which would place the tibial tunnel in the posterior portion of the ACL. In some knees, the tibial tunnel would be posterior to the native ACL attachment and just a few millimeters from the RER or interspinous ridge. This posterior tibial tunnel produces a near-vertical ACL graft that would not be expected to resist rotational loads in obliterating the pivot shift phenomena, as already discussed.

TABLE 7–3 Authors' Conclusions of Single- versus Double-Bundle Anterior Cruciate Ligament Reconstructions

1. The ACL is not an isometric structure and the length-tension behavior of its fibers cannot be represented by a functional division into two fiber bundles. Native ACL function cannot be replicated by either single- or double-bundle grafts. Oversimplification of the ACL anatomy into two bundles is firmly established in the orthopaedic literature. However, some studies suggest that there is no true anatomic division. In the future, a better understanding of which ACL femoral and tibial attachment regions represent the most ideal graft placement sites (and their appropriate tensioning) and the surgeon's ability to reproduce these conditions at surgery will result in a distinct advance for ACL surgery.

2. A common recommendation for placement of a single ACL graft into the proximal femoral attachment and posterior one third tibial attachment (7–8 mm from the PCL fossa) does not provide adequate control of the coupled motions of the pivot shift and is not recommended.

3. Endoscopic transtibial techniques commonly result in ACL grafts placed into a proximal femoral position through a tibial tunnel that is too posterior. Grafts in this location provide control of anterior tibial translation, but not internal rotation as in the pivot shift phenomena, and are not recommended.

4. A single ACL graft appears to be most ideally placed in the central femoral and tibial attachments, using for the femoral tunnel an AM portal with the knee in hyperflexion or a two-incision technique. Transtibial endoscopic drilling techniques are not recommended.

5. The double-bundle ACL technique has the theoretical advantage of locating grafts and collagen fibers throughout the entire ACL anatomic attachment sites in contrast to single grafts. Robotic laboratory and clinical studies supporting ACL double-bundle grafts appear to reference the results to a specific hybrid single-bundle (proximal femoral, posterior tibia location), which would not be expected to resist rotational loading.

6. It has not been experimentally proved from robotic or clinical studies that there is any difference (resisting the abnormal motions of the pivot shift phenomena) between a well-placed anatomic single ACL graft compared and a well-placed anatomic double-bundle graft.

7. The concepts of ACL double-bundle grafts have prompted a worthwhile reevaluation of ACL anatomy and study of the ideal location for both single- and double-bundle grafts. The added operative complexity of a double-bundle graft is not required in comparison with a well-placed single centrally located anatomic graft. In addition, revision procedures for failed double-bundle ACL reconstructions may represent an added and unnecessary complexity.

8. ACL double-bundle techniques often use soft tissue allografts to achieve the desired graft cross-sectional area. Allografts pose the added problem of a higher failure rate owing to delayed graft incorporation and healing compared with autografts. Prospective, randomized level 1 clinical studies comparing anatomic single- and double-bundle autografts are required to provide clinical data without the added variables related to allografts.

9. ACL double-bundle techniques may be most applicable to specific clinical cases, such as revision ACL knees or high-grade partial ACL tears in which an augmentation graft may be added to the remaining ACL fibers.

10. Further clinical studies and objective clinical testing methods to measure rotational knee stability are required. Measurements of the coupled motions in the pivot shift test are required. The limits of anterior tibial translation of the lateral and medial tibiofemoral compartments with these coupled motions provide the best description of the anterior joint subluxations that occur and represent patient complaints of knee instability.

The ACL tibial attachment location recommended by the authors for a single graft is directly adjacent to the lateral meniscus anterior horn attachment as shown in Figure 7–22. The ACL attachment can be easily mapped at surgery based on the anatomic references provided. In some knees, the anterior extent of the ACL attachment may be obscured by soft tissues, and in these cases, the RER or posterior interspinous ridge of the PCL fossa is an important landmark. The center of the ACL will be 16 to 20 mm anterior to the RER or posterior interspinous ridge. The guide pin is most ideally placed eccentric and 2 to 3 mm anterior and medial to the true ACL center, because the ACL graft displaces to the posterior and lateral aspect of the tibial tunnel.[31] The eccentric tunnel places the majority of the graft within the central tibial attachment and avoids the posterior attachment location. It is important that an impingement of the graft with the anterior intercondylar notch does not occur because the circular graft may occupy a portion of the native flattened ACL tibial attachment. A limited anterior notchplasty is often required. In many ACL revision knees, the bony ridge posterior to the ACL attachment ("no-man's land"; Fig. 7–23) has been disrupted by a prior graft tunnel that extends 1 to

2 mm from the RER and requires a bone graft prior to the revision procedure. It is important that during the ACL tibial tunnel preparation (primary or revision surgery), the tibial drill not inadvertently penetrate into or beyond the posterior one third ACL attachment and adjacent posterior interspinous ridge to avoid a vertical graft orientation.

Important landmarks for the femoral attachment are the posterior articular cartilage, Blumensaat's line, and identification of the ACL attachment on the lateral femoral wall of the notch (in the regions outlined on the grid systems). Again, the emphasis is made that no ACL fibers extend to the intercondylar roof; all of the fibers are on the lateral wall.

For single grafts, the authors recommend a central anatomic ACL placement with the femoral guide pin 2 to 3 mm above the midpoint of the proximal-to-distal length of the ACL attachment and 8 mm from the posterior articular cartilage edge (see Fig. 7–23). A key is to define the ACL attachment at 20° to 30° of flexion with the arthroscope in the AM portal. After the joint is marked, the knee can be placed in 120° of flexion if an endoscopic technique is selected. A 9- to 10-mm-diameter tunnel occupies the central ACL attachment, leaving only the most

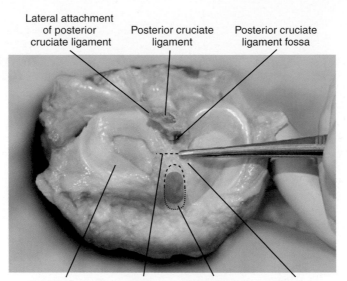

Lateral attachment of posterior cruciate ligament

Posterior cruciate ligament

Posterior cruciate ligament fossa

Anterior horn of lateral meniscus

Retro eminence ridge

Anterior fibers of anterior cruciate ligament

Medial intercondylar tubercle

A

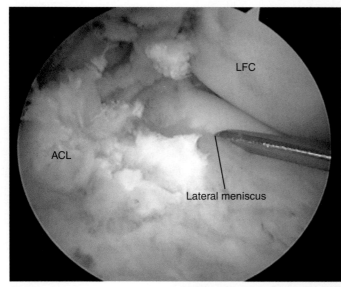

LFC

ACL

Lateral meniscus

B

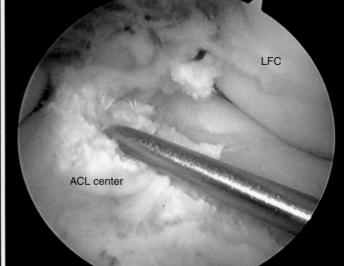

LFC

ACL center

C

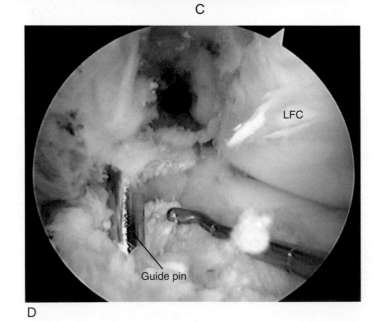

LFC

Guide pin

D

FIGURE 7–22. A, ACL tibial attachment is outlined along with the shaded region, indicating a central placement of an ACL graft and tibial tunnel. **B,** Arthroscopic ACL attachment anterior to the posterior edge of the lateral meniscus. **C,** Center of ACL attachment is marked and is anterior to the lateral meniscus posterior edge. **D,** Placement of central guide pin for single tunnel ACL reconstruction. FC, femoral condyle.

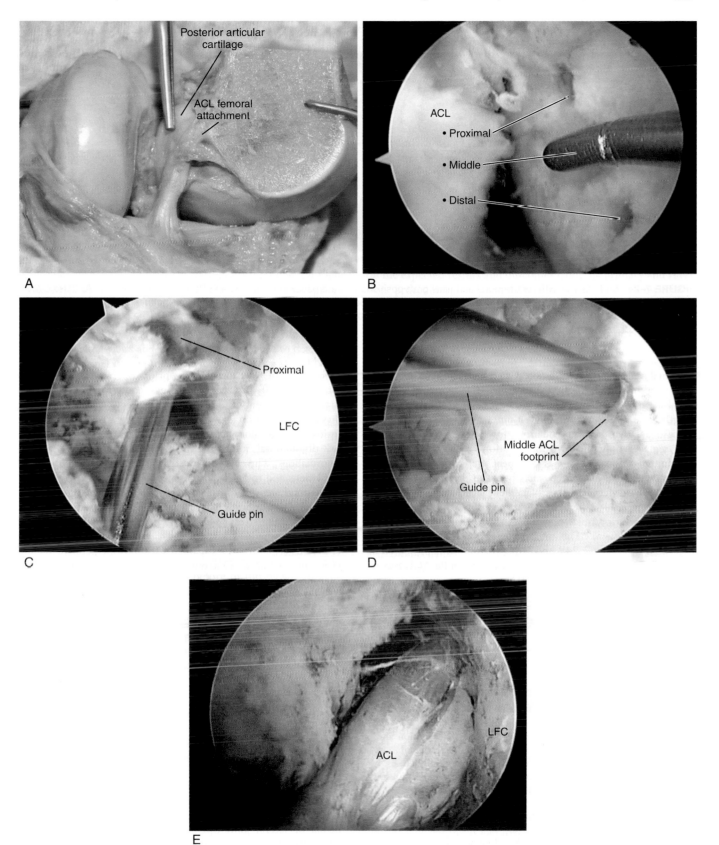

FIGURE 7–23. **A,** ACL femoral attachment shows the entire attachment on lateral wall of notch. **B,** Three points identified in proximal, middle, and distal portions of ACL attachment. **C,** Transtibial guide pin placement reaches only the proximal one third of ACL attachment with a portion of the femoral tunnel extending onto the notch roof when a central ACL tibial tunnel is used. **D,** ACL central point is reached with knee hyperflexion and AM portal or with a two-incision rear-entry technique. **E,** Final graft appearance on the lateral wall.

repeated at 4 hours and continued for 24 hours. A urinary indwelling catheter is not used unless there are specific indications. The patient's urinary output and total fluids are carefully monitored during the procedure and in the recovery room. The knee skin area is initialized by both the patient and the surgeon before entering the operating room, with a nurse observing the procedure. The identification process is repeated with all operative personnel with a "time out" before surgery to verify the knee undergoing surgery, procedure, allergies, antibiotic infusion, and special precautions that apply. All personnel provide verbal agreement.

A single femoral nerve block is administered preoperatively or in the recovery room, which markedly decreases the need for analgesic medication. The patient is instructed to use crutches with decreased weight-bearing for 24 hours owing to decreased quadriceps function. Bupivacaine (Marcaine) or lidocaine installation is not recommended because high local doses may alter chondrocyte function and viability.[68,84,184] A fluid inflow–pressure-regulated pump is recommended over gravity infusion because hemostasis can be controlled and tourniquet use avoided in most cases. An electrocautery device is always available to control bleeding points.

With the patient in a supine position on the operative table and all extremities well padded, a tourniquet is placed on the middle to proximal thigh (Fig. 7–25A). A leg holder is used for the initial arthroscopic examination to provide for maximum opening of the medial and lateral tibiofemoral compartments during the gap tests and to provide necessary distraction for a meniscus repair or partial resection. A leg holder provides better visualization of the posterior meniscus regions over a lateral post. A low-profile leg holder is used, which is pressed into the operative bed mattress to decrease posterior thigh pressure; this is removed after the initial diagnostic arthroscopic procedure. The knee portion of the bed is flexed 60° to 90° and the bed midportion is retroflexed 15° to allow flexion of the hips to relieve undue tension on the femoral neurovascular structures. The uninvolved extremity is placed in a well-cushioned padded holder. An alternative approach described in the literature is to place the uninvolved extremity in an abducted and flexed position with a thigh and leg holder.

After the arthroscopic procedures and removal of the leg holder, two positions may be used for the lower limb. The first is to adjust the operative bed to allow 90° of knee flexion. The knee can be flexed to 120° or more during the procedure, if necessary, by having the operative assistant flex the hip joint and knee joint. The second option is to position the operative bed flat and use an Alverado foot and leg holder or sandbag taped to the table to allow the knee joint to be flexed to the desired position (see Fig. 7–25B). The senior author prefers the second position when any associated medial, lateral, or PCL procedures are performed. The second position allows the surgical assistants to easily view and assist the associated ligament reconstructive procedures. With concurrent medial or lateral reconstructions, the surgical procedure is performed at 20° to 30° of flexion with a roll placed beneath the thigh. The knee joint can also be brought to full extension to determine that posterior capsular reconstructions do not constrain full knee extension.

Graft Harvest: B-PT-B Autograft

A tourniquet is inflated to 275 mm of pressure. This is usually the only time the tourniquet is inflated in the reconstructive procedure. A 3- to 4-cm vertical medial incision is made just adjacent to the medial border of the patella tendon, avoiding the tibial tubercle (Fig. 7–26). The incision is located just medial to the inferior pole of the patella. A proximal skin incision over the patella is not required because the patella is easily displaced distally during removal of the patella bone plug.

A cosmetic approach is used in which the plane beneath the subcutaneous tissues is dissected to allow for a limited skin incision. The skin incision is displaced proximally and distally as required for the graft harvest. Four vein retractors are placed into

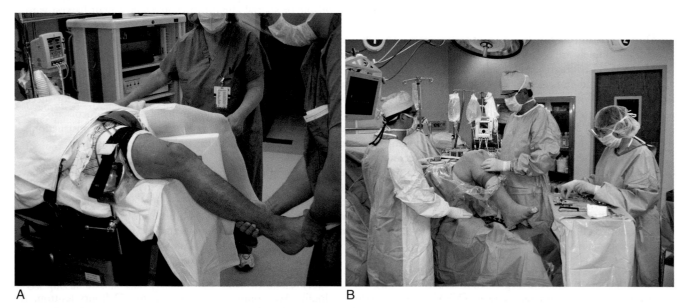

A   B

FIGURE 7–25. Initial operating room setup and patient positioning. **A,** Use of a thigh holder to achieve medial/lateral joint opening, particularly for meniscus repairs, that is removed for the ACL procedure. **B,** Patient in the supine position with a leg holder used to allow selected knee flexion positions, particularly hyperflexed position with AM portal pin placement for femoral tunnels.

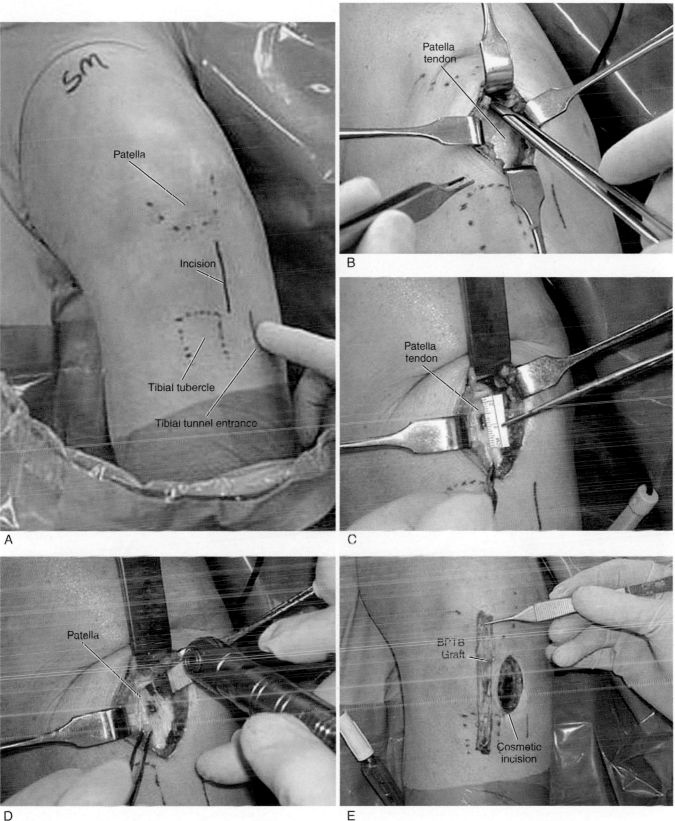

FIGURE 7–26. The technique the author recommends for harvest of a bone–patellar tendon–bone (B-PT-B) autograft. **A,** A 3- to 4-cm skin incision, just medial to the patellar tendon, is made to avoid the bony prominence of the patella and tibial tubercle. The index finger points to the planned tibial tunnel, which can be reached through this cosmetic incision. **B,** Mobilization of subcutaneous tissues to allow the cosmetically placed incision to be moved in a proximal-distal and medial fashion. Infrapatellar nerves when present are protected. **C,** A ruler measures the length of the patellar tendon and a 10-mm wide patellar tendon graft is marked by two or three ink dots. **D,** The patella is displaced distally and the patellar bone block removed. Note that the saw has a tape marking a 9-mm depth to prevent from cutting too deep into the patella. The saw is angled 10°–15° to produce a trapezoidal bone block. The saw carefully cuts the medial and lateral borders, making sure the bone beneath the tendon insertion has been cut to prevent a fracture of the graft. A similar technique is used for the tibial tubercle. **E,** Appearance of the graft after harvest.

Continued

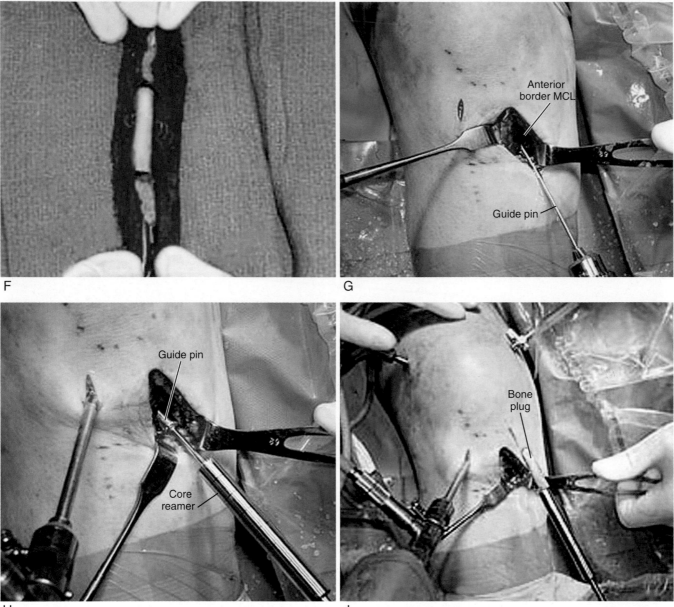

FIGURE 7–26—cont'd. **F,** Preparation of the graft. Two nonabsorbable No. 2 sutures are placed in a distal drill hole in each bone plug. The bone tendon junction is marked. The graft is wrapped in a blood-soaked sponge with the goal of maintaining viability of some tendon cells. **G,** The skin incision is displaced distally to reach the desired position for the coronal tibial tunnel, as described in the text. **H,** The core reamer is placed in the tibial tunnel for the graft harvest. **I,** The bone plug removed by the core reamer.

the proximal, distal, medial, and lateral aspects of the skin incision to allow for a rectangular skin opening for the graft harvest. A branch of the infrapatellar nerve may cross the middle of the patellar tendon and is preserved. The patient is advised preoperatively that there will be an area of decreased skin sensation just lateral to the patellar tendon because superficial nerve branches may be incised as a part of the procedure. An alternative technique is to use a proximal and distal skin incision, avoiding a vertical skin incision, which has less chance of a sensory skin loss but a greater chance of skin hypertrophic scar formation.

The retinaculum in the middle of the patellar tendon is incised and the dissection limited only to the midportion of the patellar tendon. The parapatellar tissues and blood supply to the tendon are not disturbed. The tendon should not be dissected to its edges because this damages the blood supply, particularly to the major vein and artery on the medial side of the tendon. In some knees, a branch of the infrapatellar nerve will cross the middle of the patella tendon and should be preserved. In these knees, the nerve provides a large area of cutaneous sensation over the lateral aspect of the knee. It should be noted that up to approximately one half of patients will later have an approximately 2-cm area of numbness just lateral to the patellar tendon from incision of small cutaneous nerve branches that are not visible during the procedure. Patients are warned of this potential loss of sensation preoperatively. The patellar retinaculum is carefully incised and reflected medially and laterally only for the width of the graft to be removed. The retinaculum is protected to allow for closure over the bone-grafted patellar defect. A similar procedure is used at the tibial tuberosity.

It is useful to have a precut 10-mm and 22-mm paper ruler held on a hemostat to place over the tendon and bone harvest sites to allow fine marks to be placed on the tissues to define graft dimensions.

The patellar tendon is incised in the midportion to the appropriate size, 9 to 10 mm. The patella is displaced distally into the wound using a forked retractor placed at the superior patellar margin. A powered handheld saw with a thin-width blade is marked with a SteriStrip 9 to 10 mm from the tip to prevent too deep a cut, which would weaken the patella. A trapezoidal bone block graft from the patella is removed by angling the fine saw 15° at each side of the cut. The bone cut is meticulous and proximally "cross-hatched," as a deep cut is avoided. The bone cut extends to the inferior pole, and care is taken to protect the insertion site of the patellar tendon. A 4-mm osteotome gently removes the patella bone block without wedging the sidewalls, which could induce a lateral fracture. A similar procedure is followed in the harvest of the tibial bone block.

The tourniquet is deflated, and a cotton sponge is placed in the wound. The graft is later wrapped in the blood-soaked sponge, which provides protection of the graft, maintains a moist blood environment, and may allow cells to survive in the graft-remodeling process. It would be incorrect to have the graft openly exposed on the back table, which would allow drying, cell death, and possible air contamination. A second surgeon prepares the graft to decrease operative time.

The bone blocks are prepared so they will pass easily through the tunnels. The diameter of the tunnels will be configured 1 mm larger than the diameter of the bone block. The bone-tendon junction of each graft is marked for later identification. The graft preparation involves one 2-mm drill hole placed one third of the way from the end of each bone block for sutures. The end sutures allow the graft to be passed into the tunnel. A suture placed into the midportion of the graft would tilt the bone block, making passage into the tunnels difficult. The tibial portion of the graft is identified and will be later passed in a retrograde manner through the tibial tunnel into the femoral tunnel. The bone block tip is fashioned into a bullet tip configuration for tibial tunnel passage. Two No. 2 nonabsorbable Fiber-wire (Arthrex, Naples, FL) sutures are passed into the distal one third tibial bone block. The graft is wrapped in a blood-soaked sponge.

At the conclusion of the ACL reconstruction, closure of the patellar tendon graft harvest site is performed. The patella tendon is loosely approximated with 2-0 absorbable sutures. A coring reamer used for the femoral tunnel provides a large dowel of cancellous bone to completely fill the patella and tibia defects. The bone-grafted sites are smoothed to remove any pressure points. It is important to place two horizontal mattress sutures at the inferior pole of the patella and at the superior tendon attachment at the tibia to create a buttress or pocket to maintain the position of the bone graft at each site. Otherwise, the bone graft may displace and be a source of pain because it is located in the tendon rather than the bony defect. The patella retinaculum is carefully closed to provide a soft tissue covering over the patella defect. The retinaculum over the tibial tuberosity is not as well defined; however, the soft tissues are closed using 2-0 absorbable horizontal mattress sutures.

The meticulous technique described for the B-PT-B graft procedure is an important part of the operative procedure.

The skin incision is medial to any bone prominences and does not extend over the patella. The dissection is limited entirely to that portion of the graft to be removed, protecting nerves and avoiding damage to the parapatellar vascular supply. The surgeon is seated, with the patient's foot in the surgeon's lap to directly visualize the wound and carefully control the saw blade. A headlight is always used to see the fine neural structures.

The use of the coring reamer (tibia or femoral tunnels) provides ample bone graft to completely fill the tibia and patella bone defects. The use of shavings or small amounts of bone obtained in the procedure is insufficient to completely fill these defects. If the tibial tuberosity defect is left partially unfilled, there will be ridges on either side of the defect that will prevent the patient from kneeling. If the defects are closed as described, kneeling with little to no discomfort is to be expected, equal to the opposite knee. In the authors' opinion, this point has not been sufficiently stressed in the literature. A completely filled graft harvest site at the patella and tibial tubercle is required. Saving bone chips during the ACL tunnel preparation usually results in insufficient bone for both harvest sites. The added time to use the coring reamer bone-graft harvesting instruments provides the benefit of a quality bone graft for both the patellar and the tibial sites. Commercially sold bone allografts are available; however, the authors prefer to use the patient's bone. The length of the bone block is 22 to 24 mm to facilitate passage.

Graft Harvest: QT-PB Autograft

A 5- to 6-cm longitudinal incision is made from the superior pole of the patella, extending to the midline proximally. The prepatellar retinaculum is reflected and protected for later closure over the grafted patellar defect. The quadriceps tendon and its junction with the vastus medialis obliquus and vastus lateralis obliquus (VLO) are identified. The proximal portion of the quadriceps tendon is identified and the graft harvest is carried 15 mm distal to the rectus femoris muscle-tendon attachment in order not to weaken this site. A 10-mm-wide tendon graft, through all three layers, is removed to a length of 60 to 70 cm (Fig. 7–27). The tendon attachment to the anterior superior pole of the patella is carefully identified and the synovial attachment protected. A power saw with the cutting blade marked with paper tape to a depth of 10 mm is used to cut the anterior cortex to produce a patellar bone graft 22 to 24 mm long by 9 to 10 mm wide. The bone graft is sized to 9 to 10 mm in diameter. The quadriceps tendon defect is closed with interrupted 0-Ethibond suture (Ethicon, Somerville, NJ). Two sutures of 0-nonabsorbable material are placed just proximal to the patellar bone defect to create a pocket for the bone graft obtained from the coring reamer. The core bone graft completely obliterates the patellar defect, and a meticulous closure of anterior tissues over the graft is performed, as already described.

Graft Harvest: STG Autograft

The STG graft harvest procedure is shown in Figure 7–28. A 3- to 4-cm oblique incision is made over the palpated pes tendons. The incision is cosmetic and the plane beneath the subcutaneous tissues carefully dissected. The surgeon is seated, the bed is flexed 60°, and a headlight is routinely used. The sartorius fascia is incised directly proximal to the semitendinosus and gracilis palpated tendons over the distal superficial medial collateral

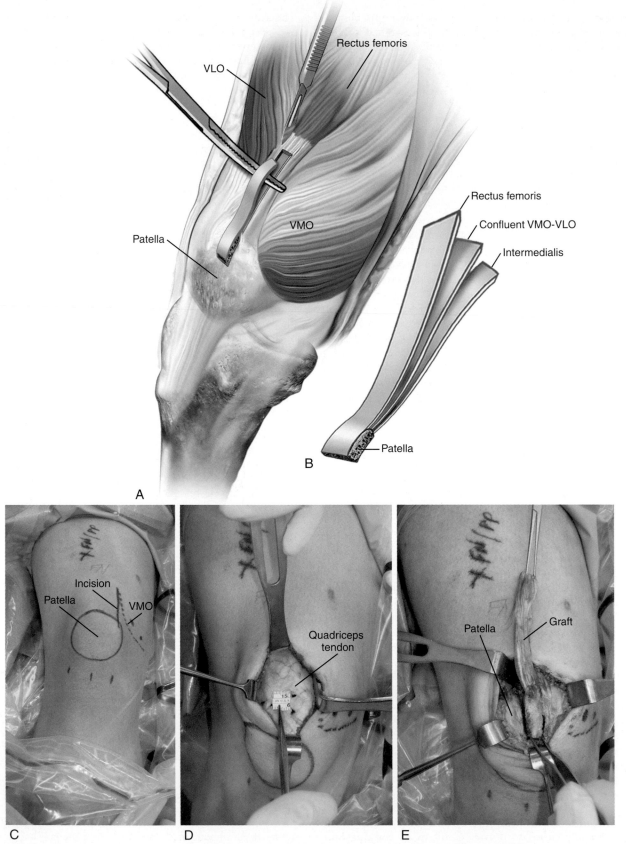

FIGURE 7–27. A, The quadriceps tendon and vastus medialis oblique and vastus lateralis oblique muscles are identified proximally. A 9- to 10-mm wide tendon graft, through all three layers, which has a length of 80–90 cm, is removed. The graft harvest does not extend to the muscle tendon junction. A patellar bone graft is fashioned to be approximately 22–24 mm long by 9–10 mm wide by 9–10 mm in diameter. **B,** Usually, all three layers are sutured together at the end of the graft (2-0 nonabsorbable suture) with a running suture on both sides of the graft. **C,** Surgical case, initial skin incision. **D,** Measurement of graft width. **E,** Final harvest.

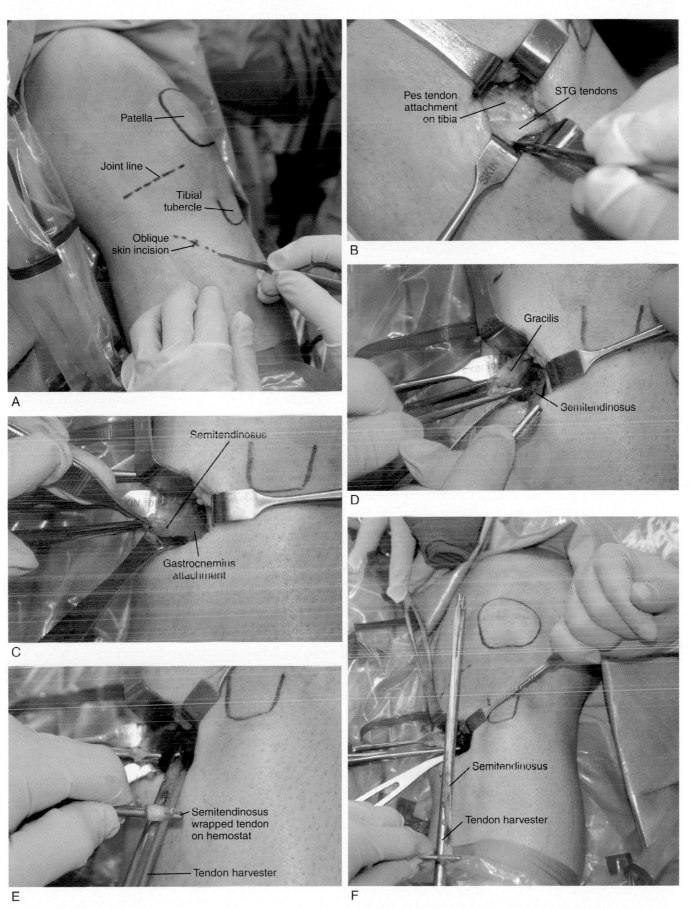

FIGURE 7–28. A, A 2-cm longitudinal or oblique incision at the AM tibia region. **B,** An L-shaped incision at the pes tendon tibial attachment is performed and the tendon flap is reflected to identify the semitendinosus-gracilis (STG) tendon. **C,** Dissection of soft tissue to identify the STG and remove the gastrocnemius secondary attachment. **D,** "Push-pull" test to confirm that the STG tendons are free of attachments. **E,** Harvest of the STG using a closed-end harvester to prevent premature transection of the STG. **F,** Appearance of the long semitendinosus tendon obtained at harvest.

Continued

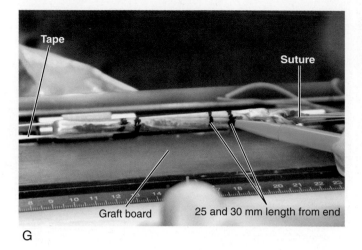

FIGURE 7–28—cont'd. G, Graft preparation with graft board. Nonabsorbable 3-mm tape at the proximal end and three 2-0 fiberwire fixation at the distal end. Running suture is used on each side of the STG graft.

ligament (SMCL) attachment. This provides a window and opening to protect the SMCL. The overlying fascia is incised proximally in the same oblique plane of the STG tendons.

It is worthwhile in the initial dissection to identify the STG tendons to protect them and not inadvertently section the tendons. This is best performed by extending the fascia, incise just above the gracilis tendon over its tibial insertion, and then at a 90° angle, lay back the insertion site distally. This allows the STG tendons to be viewed throughout their distal course to their tibial attachment. In most knees, the STG tendons are confluent and blend to make one tendinosus structure. Each tendon is identified and incised through the confluent distal tendon region. Each tendon is grasped at a 90° angle at its distal end and rolled two to three times around a straight hemostat, which allows tension to be placed on the tendon without producing damage.

The proximal extent of each tendon is palpated and superficial tissues removed, protecting the overlying sartorius fascia. The dissection plane is never carried close to the inferior sartorius or superior gracilis muscles to avoid injury to the saphenous nerve. The headlight provides excellent illumination in the proximal portion of the incision to protect any neurovascular structures. The proximal fascia about each tendon is bluntly dissected and the semitendinosus tendon attachment to the medial gastrocnemius fascia is incised. With tension on each tendon and a repetitive pulling motion, each tendon will freely displace 10 cm. It is important to determine that each tendon is completely free of tissues to allow the tendon harvester to pass freely. The closed-end graft harvester is passed along the trajectory of each tendon and each tendon is transected at 20 to 22 cm. There is a commercially available tendon harvester with a blunt tip that protects against inadvertent tendon transection and has a tendon cutter in its distal tip activated by the mechanism at the handle. The STG tendons are prepared (see Fig. 7–28). Each tendon is looped about a 3-mm tape and the tendon end sutured to itself with a No. 2 nonabsorbable suture. A third suture is added between both sutured tendon ends. A running 0-nonabsorbable suture is used to produce a tubed structure running from proximal to distal and then back to the

proximal starting point. A metal graft-tensioning board (25–30 N tension) is used rather than a graft preparation board with plastic holders because the latter is difficult to sterilize to avoid a graft contamination problem. The graft is marked 25 mm from each end, wrapped in a blood-soaked sponge, and placed in a secure place on the back table.

ITB Extra-articular Tenodesis

Two clinical studies (Noyes and Barber[112] and Ferretti and co-workers[49]) have shown statistically significant improvements in knee stability in knees with ACL revision or with gross instability and loss of secondary restraints that had an extra-articular tenodesis procedure for additional restraint of tibial internal rotation. The procedure is described here and the rationale for its use at the time of ACL reconstruction is discussed later in this chapter.

A lateral incision 8 to 10 cm in length is made at the midlateral aspect of the knee extending from Gerdy's tubercle to the tibia proximally. The skin incision is undermined by subcutaneous dissection to increase the skin mobility and shorten the incision for cosmetic purposes. A strip of ITB is incised proximal to distal from the posterior one third of the band, which is 12 mm wide and 18 to 20 cm long with the tibial attachment intact (Fig. 7–29).

The most isometric point on the proximal and posterior aspect of the lateral femoral condyle is located (see Fig. 7–29D) and tested by using a guide pin placed at the proximal and posterior aspect of the lateral femoral condyle. The point for the femoral attachment of the ITB is usually at the anatomic ITB deep fiber insertion to the femur. This region is usually just distal to the lateral intramuscular septum and posterior and proximal to the lateral epicondyle and anterior to the gastrocnemius tubercle lateral attachment. The error is to place the ITB graft too anterior, which blocks knee flexion. The posterior placement allows the ITB graft to undergo increasing tension with knee extension. This area is curetted to remove soft tissues to allow for the ITB strip to be in contact with the overlying bone.

It is important in tensioning the ITB graft not to overconstrain the joint and block normal internal tibial rotation. After the ACL procedure is completed, the extra-articular tensioning

---

Critical Points OPERATIVE TECHNIQUES: ILIOTIBIAL BAND EXTRA-ARTICULAR TENODESIS

- Lateral incision 8–10 cm in length at the midlateral aspect of the knee extending from Gerdy's tubercle proximally.
- Strip of iliotibial band (ITB) incised, 12 mm wide, 18–20 cm long, tibial attachment kept intact.
- Identify femoral attachment ITB—deep fiber insertion to femur, confirm isometric femoral point for screw placement.
- Knee 30° flexion, neutral tibial rotation.
- Loop ITB strip around soft tissue washer and screw and back to Gerdy's tubercle. Fixate graft at femoral site.
- Suture ITB strip to itself under only mild tension, including posterior ITB fibers.
- Take knee through internal-external tibial rotation to ensure no constraint to normal rotation.
- Close ITB absorbable sutures.
- Examine medial patellar medial glide for normal mobility, do not close or overtension lateral iliopatellar tissues.

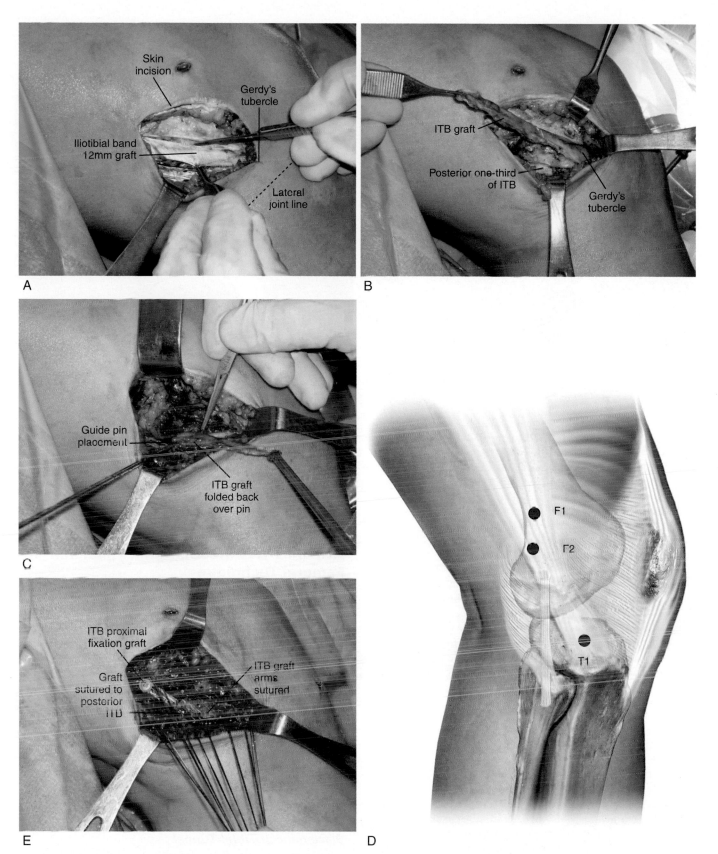

FIGURE 7–29. A, Cosmetic lateral incision is made just proximal to Gerdy's tubercle. A 10-mm strip along the posterior one half of the iliotibial band (ITB) is harvested. The proximal skin flap is undermined to obtain a 20-mm-long graft. **B,** The ITB graft (10 mm wide) is dissected distally to Gerdy's tubercle, where the tibial attachment is left intact. **C,** The ITB graft is looped around a guide pin placed just distal to the lateral intermuscular and proximal to the FCL attachment. The knee is flexed from 0 to 135°, neutral tibial rotation. **D,** The "isometric points" graft attachment sites for an extra-articular reconstruction measured by Kurosawa et al.[87a] The points T1–F1 provided the least change in length with knee flexion (maximum % of strain, 11.6 ± 3.0%). The points T1–F2 offer a second choice, except that there is an increase in the percentage of strain with knee flexion compared with that at T1–F1. **E,** The graft is looped around a soft tissue screw and washer and both graft ends are sutured to each other and to the remaining posterior ITB. This forms a strong femoral-tibial structure that both incorporates the graft and reproduces the normal posterior ITB femoral tibial attachments. The knee is in neutral tibial rotation and graft overtensioning is avoided.

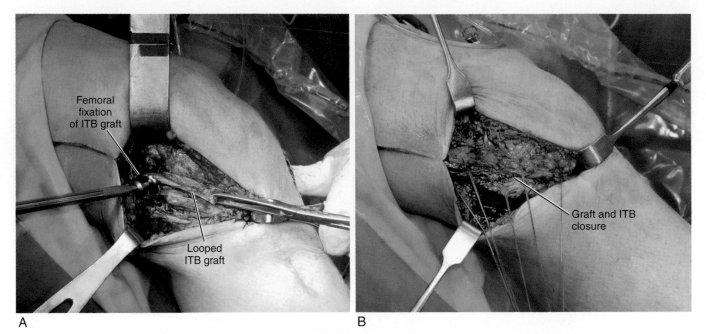

A   B

FIGURE 7–30. A, Extra-articular ITB graft is shown looped around a soft tissue screw and anchor in a second patient. **B,** Final closure of the overall remaining ITB to the looped ITB graft.

and fixation is performed. The knee is placed at 30° of flexion and neutral rotation. The ITB strip is fixated around a soft tissue washer (Fig. 7–30) and cancellous screw and brought back upon itself to Gerdy's tubercle. The screw is angulated anteriorly away from the ACL tunnel. The ITB strip is then sutured to itself with only mild tension applied to the ITB graft. The sutures are placed through the posterior one third of the remaining intact ITB just posterior to where the graft was harvested. This produces a strong restraint to abnormal internal tibial translation and anterior tibial translation. The knee is taken through a normal internal-external tibial rotation to ensure that there is no abnormal constraint to internal tibial rotation. The knee is flexed to 135°; usually, increasing knee flexion will provide for increased tension in the graft. There is no true isometric point for the femoral attachment of the graft for flexion-extension and tibial rotation motions. It is probable that even with precautions taken to not overconstrain knee motion, regaining full knee flexion may be more difficult when the extra-articular procedure is added.

The ITB is closed with absorbable sutures throughout the site where the graft was harvested. The patellar medial glide is examined at 30° knee flexion to ensure that closing the ITB does not limit the normal patellar mobility. The patella should have at least 10 mm of medial glide with a medially directed manual translation. If there is an abnormal restraint to medial patella mobility, a small lateral release is performed. The anterior fibers of the ITB, which make up the lateral retinaculum adjacent to the patella, are incised the required length to relieve the undue tension on these soft tissues due to closing the ITB defect, avoiding a release of the vastus lateralis tendon.

In the 1980s when extra-articular procedures were used frequently (instead of intra-articular ACL reconstruction), it was common for ITB reconstructive procedures to be routed underneath the FCL and then sutured to itself at Gerdy's tubercle (Cooker-Arnold procedure). This represents a nonanatomic placement of the ITB graft that does not restore the posterior

femoral-tibial ITB attachments that resist internal tibial rotation. In addition, there is concern that a soft tissue structure wrapped around the FCL could induce stretching of the FCL and allow for an increase in lateral joint opening. It is therefore recommended to secure the ITB graft to the femoral attachment discussed and to avoid looping the graft around the FCL.

ACL B-PT-B Graft Anatomic Tibial and Femoral Technique

A single-graft procedure is described in which the graft is located into the central anatomic tibial and femoral attachment locations, as already discussed. The graft placement for primary and revision knees specifically avoids the proximal ACL femoral attachment site and the posterior ACL tibial attachment site to avoid a vertical graft and allow the graft to resist rotational coupled motions in addition to anterior tibial translation (Fig. 7–31). This section describes using a single B-PT-B autograft or allograft procedure. The authors' clinical studies support the concept of a single-graft technique for primary and revision procedures. One exception in revision knees is when a double-bundle procedure may be used in a knee in which a prior vertical ACL graft placement was performed that limits anterior tibial translation and a second coronal graft is added to provide control of tibial rotation.

Placement of Tibial Tunnel

As previously described, the ideal central ACL tibial attachment location is directly adjacent and anterior to the posterior edge of the lateral meniscus anterior horn attachment (see Fig. 7–24). The ACL attachment can be easily mapped at surgery based on the anatomic reference maps provided, with the ACL center location based on the anterior-to-posterior and medial-to-lateral attachments. The anterior extent of the ACL attachment may be

Placement of Tibial Tunnel

- Define center ACL, usually 16–20 mm anterior to RER or interspinous ridge.
- Mark ACL center, usually adjacent and always anterior to posterior edge of lateral meniscus anterior horn attachment.
- Place guide pin eccentric and 2–3 mm anterior and medial to true ACL center.
- Determine graft length of patellar tendon on MRI.
- Two-incision technique allows graft length to be adjusted by proximal advancement of femoral tunnel.
- Place tibial tunnel in coronal manner, 55°–60° angle, tunnel length 35–40 mm.
- Begin tunnel adjacent to superficial MCL, 25–30 mm medial to tibial tubercle, 10 mm distal to proximal patellar tendon insertion.
- Use core reamer to obtain good-quality bone to fill graft bone defects.
- Drill tunnel, chamfer edges.
- Complete notchplasty as required, "worm's-eye" view scope in tibial tunnel, extend knee.

Placement of Femoral Tunnel

- Use either two-incision technique or anteromedial portal with knee hyperflexed 120°.
- Two-incision technique: Drill tunnel with retrograde or antegrade procedure.

- Identify ACL attachment with knee in 20°–30° flexion, scope anteromedial portal.
- Place guidewire central to ACL attachment. Always preserve 4 to 5 mm of posterior back wall of the tunnel so that the graft is not placed too far posteriorly. A guide pin placed 8 mm from the posterior articular cartilage at the central ACL attachment will have a 4 mm posterior back wall for a 8-mm graft.
- Drill tunnel, chamfer edges.

Graft Tunnel Passage, Conditioning, and Fixation

- Pass graft gently in retrograde, arthroscopically assisted.
- Bring graft proximally until bone is flush with tibia.
- Femoral position of graft at or just proximal to inside femoral tunnel.
- Fix femoral bone graft plug with interference screw.
- Condition graft, 44 N tension, flex knee 0°–135° 40 cycles.
- Verify position arthroscopically, no impingement.
- Place knee in 20° flexion, reduce tension to 10–15 N.
- Place interference screw tibia. Use additional sutures tied over suture post if required.
- Perform Lachman test, ensure no overconstraint.
- For STG graft, femoral fixation: Post with sutures and absorbable interference screw only if necessary; tibial fixation: Interference screw plus suture post.

ACL, anterior cruciate ligament; MRI, magnetic resonance imaging; RER, retroeminence ridge; STG, semitendinosus-gracilis tendons.

obscured by soft tissues, and the RER or posterior interspinous ridge of the PCL fossa is an important landmark. The center of the ACL will be 16 to 20 mm anterior to the RER or interspinous ridge. The guide pin is placed eccentric and 2 to 3 mm anterior and medial to the true ACL center as the ACL graft displaces to the posterior and medial aspects of the tibial tunnel.[31] This eccentric tunnel places the majority of the graft within the ideal central tibial attachment.

It is important to determine the graft length of the autograft or allograft to ensure that a mismatch does not occur in terms of tunnel and intra-articular length and graft length. The most common problem is with a patella alta and a B-PT-B length greater than 100 to 110 mm based on the patient's body habitus. The length of the patellar tendon is determined on preoperative lateral radiographs. The normal patellar length based on the Linclau technique[92] (patellar cartilage length to anterior vertical tibial prominence; see Chapter 41, Prevention and Treatment of Knee Arthrofibrosis) is a 1:1 ratio with the patellar tendon in the 35- to 45-mm range. The intra-articular ACL length is measured on the lateral MRI, and this length is matched with an autograft or allograft. It is possible to accommodate a shorter length patellar tendon by adjusting the proximity of the tibial tunnel. A patella alta with a tendon length greater than 50 mm is usable with the bone portion of the graft adjusted in the tibia and femoral tunnels. A two-incision technique allows adjustment of graft length by proximal advancement in the femoral tunnel and is ideal when there is graft mismatch due to an excessively long patellar tendon. In rare instances, with a long B-PT-B graft, the tibial bone plug is rotated 180° onto the tendon, sutured to the bone plug, and the tibial tunnel resized. The bone plug sutures are tied to a tibial post. With a graft length mismatch, the authors do not recommend removal of the bone plug to shorten overall graft length or multiple twisting of the graft.

The ideal tibial tunnel is placed in a coronal manner, at a 55° to 60° angle, allowing a tunnel length of 35 to 40 mm. The tunnel is begun just anterior and adjacent to the superficial MCL, and is usually 25 to 30 mm medial to the tibial tubercle and 10 mm distal to the most proximal point of the patellar tendon tibial tubercle insertion.

A core reamer is used to remove a tibial bone plug when a B-PT-B or QT-PB autograft is used to obtain a core of bone to fill the graft bone defects. As already described, the core reamer provides a more suitable graft material than drill reamings, and the bone defects are filled in an anatomic manner that results in the patient being able to kneel on the tibial bone harvest site.

The tunnel is drilled to the desired graft diameter and the joint tunnel edges chamfered to prevent graft abrasion.

Placement of Femoral Tunnel

As previously described, either a two-incision technique or an AM portal femoral tunnel placement with knee hyperflexion technique is used in primary and revision knees. Baer and associates[13] recently reported in a cadaver study that at least 110° of knee flexion is required for femoral tunnel drilling through the AM portal to avoid potential injury to the peroneal nerve, the lateral condylar articular surface, the FCL, and the popliteus tendon. The use of the AM portal to place the femoral tunnel has the problems in some knees of difficulty with visualization at 100° to 120° of flexion, the potential for the drill to damage the medial femoral condyle, and a shorter femoral socket which may be a problem with a B-PT-B autograft. As with any of the ACL techniques, operator experience is necessary to achieve a successful result.

In revision knees when the femoral tunnel is close to a prior tunnel, the two-incision procedure allows the guide pin to be more accurately placed and the tunnel divergence angle to be controlled more accurately than the endoscopic procedure.

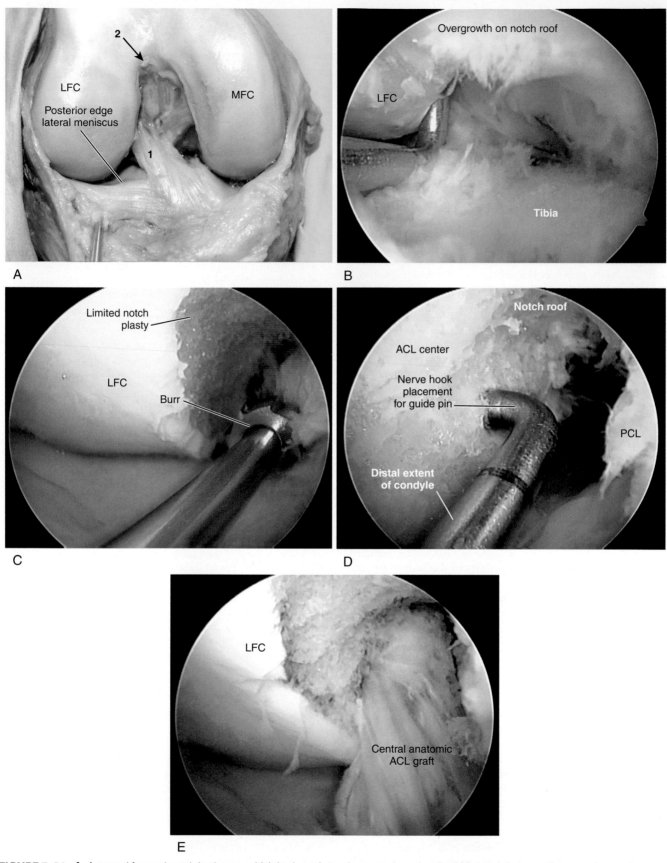

FIGURE 7–31. A, A normal femoral notch is shown, which is viewed at arthroscopy by using the AM portal. 1 shows the normal space between the lateral femoral condyle and the PCL, which is occupied by the ACL. 2 shows the normal anterior notch that should not impinge on the graft. **B,** Revision ACL with failed ACL graft shows overgrowth of the lateral notch and notch roof, requiring a limited notchplasty. **C,** The lateral notch wall is visualized entirely posteriorly to the articular cartilage of the femoral condyle. **D,** The ACL femoral attachment is mapped out and a central small hole is made for placement of the guide pin. The resident's ridge has been removed. The anterior notch region has not been disturbed. **E,** Final placement of a single-bundle graft within a central anatomic tibial and femoral placement that occupies over 75% of the attachment site.

Importantly, the two-incision procedure carries a smaller risk of placing a less than ideal femoral tunnel, because there have been cases in which endoscopic revision is performed and the tunnel breaks into the old tunnel, producing a more complex problem.

In the two-incision technique, there are two approaches based on the necessity to add additional suture after fixation at the femoral site. The two choices are to drill the tunnel in a retrograde or antegrade procedure. In the retrograde-drilling procedure (Fig. 7–32), a lateral incision of 2 to 3 cm in length is made at the posterior one third of the ITB. The posterior one third of the ITB is incised for 4 to 6 cm to allow exposure. The interval posterior to the vastus lateralis is entered and the muscle protected. An S retractor is placed beneath the VLO to gently lift the muscle anteriorly, avoiding entering the proximal joint capsule. The proximal edge of the lateral femoral condyle is bluntly palpated with an instrument (over-the-top location), and the goal is to locate the tunnel entrance just anterior and not distal to this point. A 15-mm periosteal incision is made and an elevator used to remove soft tissues from the site for the tunnel proximal entrance.

In most chronic ACL-deficient knees and revision knees, there is an overgrowth of cartilage and spur formation in the femoral notch, requiring a notchplasty to prevent ACL graft impingement. The notchplasty rules taught by the senior author since the mid 1980s and used in all the clinical studies reported later in this chapter are described in Table 7–5. In primary ACL knees, an anterior notchplasty of a few millimeters is almost always required owing to the central placement of the tibial tunnel and ACL graft within the central tibial attachment. A lateral notchplasty is performed when required when there is insufficient width (9–10 mm) between the PCL and the lateral femoral notch wall to accommodate the ACL graft.

The ACL femoral attachment is mapped based on the bony landmarks already described. The location of the guide pin for an ACL central femoral tunnel is shown in Figures 7–23, 7–24, 7–31, and 7–33. The guidewire is placed within the central ACL attachment, which is midway between the lateral notch roof and the distal articular cartilage edge (2:00 to 2:30 position), 8 mm from the posterior articular cartilage edge. Clock locations are actually an inaccurate description of the tunnel location.[45,47] With the central femoral tunnel, the posterior back wall is 3 to 4 mm thick and the graft occupies approximately two thirds to three fourths of the ACL footprint. Always preserve 4 to 5 mm of the posterior back wall of the tunnel so that the graft is not placed too far posteriorly. Grafts placed too far posteriorly will have increased tension with knee extension and may potentially block full extension. A guide pin placed 8 mm from the posterior articular cartilage at the central ACL attachment will have a 4 mm posterior back wall for a 8-mm graft. A guide pin placed 10 mm from the posterior articular cartilage at the central ACL attachment would have a 5 mm posterior back wall for a 10-mm graft. One key to define the ACL attachment is to place the knee in 20° to 30° of flexion viewed through the AM portal and map out the oval attachment and center point, measuring the distance to the posterior articular cartilage. Once the ideal center point is selected, the knee is flexed to the position desired. It is easier to mark out the ACL femoral attachment when it is viewed in a vertical plane rather than the horizontal attachment plane with knee flexion. The tunnel is drilled to the appropriate diameter for a snug graft fit in the tunnel. The edges of the tunnel are chamfered to prevent graft abrasion. The technique with a rear-entry guide drill is shown in Figure 7–33.

Graft Tunnel Passage, Conditioning, and Fixation

The graft is passed in a retrograde manner either with a Beath pin in the endoscopic technique (placed through the AM portal) or in the two-incision technique with a 20-gauge looped wire passed from the femur to the tibial tunnel. The graft is gently lifted up through the tibia and guided into the femoral tunnels with a nerve hook. The graft is marked at the bone-tendon junction to adjust its length in each tunnel. The graft is brought proximally until the bone is flush with the tibia. In most knees, the femoral portion of the graft is at or just proximal to the inside femoral tunnel. The femoral bone-graft plug is fixed with an interference screw of a metallic or absorbable type. Graft conditioning is performed by placing approximately 44 N tension on the distal graft sutures and flexing the knee from 0° to 135° for 30 to 40 flexion-extension cycles. The arthroscope is placed to verify that the graft position is ideal and there is no impingement against the lateral femoral condyle or notch with full hyperextension. Appropriate notchplasty is performed when necessary. The knee is placed at 20° flexion, and the tension on the graft is reduced to approximately 10 to 15 N in order to avoid overconstraining tibial AP translation. A finger is placed on the anterior tibia to maintain the posterior gravity position of the tibia. An alternative procedure is to fixate the graft with a larger graft tension at 0°; however, the senior author believes there is more control of graft tension at the partially flexed position. An interference screw (usually absorbable) is placed. In all revision knees and in primary ACL cases in which the interference screw fixation is not ideal or the screw resistance on placement is not acceptable, the sutures are tied over a suture post. The arthroscope is placed into the joint and final graft inspection performed. A Lachman test is performed, and there should be total AP translation motion of 3 mm, indicating that the graft has not been overtightened. If the graft has a "bowstring," tight appearance with little to no anterior tibial translation on testing, the distal tensioning and fixation procedure is repeated with less tension placed on the graft.

Li and associates[90] reported the ACL three-dimensional morphologic changes in humans during weight-bearing flexion using a fluoroscopic and MRI-based system. The ACL tibial insertion twisted internally relative to the femoral insertion. The ACL internal twist amounted to approximately 10° at full extension to 44° at 90° flexion. The data were based on insertion site measurements and not actual ACL fiber microgeometry. Even though some authors[5] have recommended an ACL graft orientation to reproduce an internal twist of the ACL fibers, this effect in terms of clinical outcome is unknown. The B-PT-B orientation is usually placed in the sagittal plane on the femur and tibia with the cancellous surface lateral in the femoral tunnel to lessen abrasion of the tendon against the femoral condyle.

Techniques Using Other Grafts

With all other grafts, the same procedure is used with the following exception. In the two-incision technique with an STG graft, a femoral post is always used with the sutures tied first at the femoral site about the post (35-mm, 4.0-mm cancellous self-cutting screw with washer). An absorbable interference screw is added if the graft tunnel interface is not tight. At the tibia, the interference screw is first placed, followed by the suture post fixation. Using the combined interference screw and suture post provides sufficient graft strength fixation for rehabilitation to proceed equal to the B-PT-B graft. An alternative technique for a four-strand STG graft

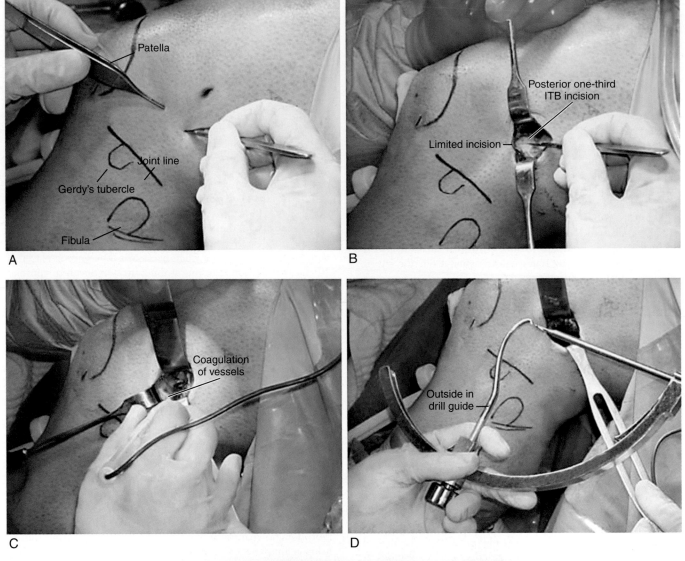

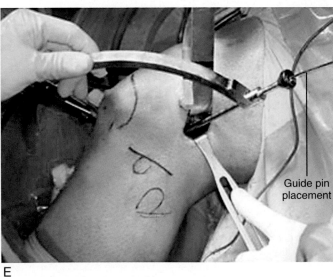

FIGURE 7–32. The ACL procedure for a two-incision technique. **A,** The anatomic landmarks. The joint line, tibial tubercle, and fibula are marked. **B,** The 2-cm incision that is made in the posterior one third of the ITB, as described in the text. **C,** Electrocoagulation of vessels. **D,** Commercially available drill guide. **E,** Placement of the guide pin.

TABLE 7–5   Notchplasty Techniques and Rules

1. The arthroscope is placed in the AM portal with instruments passed through a central portal (patellar tendon graft site or central patellar tendon portal). A mistake is to view the lateral wall of the notch through an anterolateral (AL) portal, which provides suboptimal visualization. In the presence of a prominent lateral resident's ridge, it is often difficult if not impossible to view or identify with accuracy the ACL femoral attachment through the AL portal. Place the knee at 20°–30° flexion to view the ACL attachment, not a high flexion angle where the ACL is in a horizontal plane.
2. Measure the clearance of the lateral notch wall to the PCL to ensure there is 9–10 mm clearance for the graft. Remove the shallow notch to obtain this clearance, starting distally and progressing proximally up to the top of the notch entrance. This ensures an adequate lateral graft notch clearance throughout knee flexion, preventing graft abrasion from a stenotic lateral notch wall. Usually only 2–3 mm of the lateral notch is removed, and aggressive resection of the lateral wall beyond this should be avoided.
3. To ensure that the height of the notch is sufficient and will not impinge, place the notchplasty burr at the central ACL tibial attachment and gently bring the knee into full hyperextension. The burr should not impinge into the anterior notch. This defines the millimeters of the anterior and lateral aspect of the notch that are removed to prevent graft impingement. Normally, this is 3–4 mm; more is removed only when there is excessive hyperextension.
4. The anterior notch is gently curved, removing an A-shaped notch if present. Before graft passage, the arthroscope is placed within the tibial tunnel "worm's-eye view" and the knee taken to full hyperextension, observing whether any portion of the anterior notch comes into view that would require removal. This provides for direct arthroscopic confirmation that there is no ACL graft impingement, and intraoperative fluroscopy is not required.
5. Avoid use of a commercially available "tunnel smoother," because this is too aggressive. When placed in an intra-articular location within both femoral and tibial tunnels and moved proximally and distally, this instrument may remove the anterior aspect of the femoral tunnel and posterior aspect of the tibial tunnel, producing a vertical graft.
6. Once the anterior and lateral aspects of the femoral notch (shallow portion) are prepared, it is possible to completely view the deep portion of the notch, identify the appropriate place for the ACL graft on the lateral wall, and remove an anterior bone buttress in front of the ACL attachment (resident's ridge). Maintain the knee at 20°–30° flexion.
7. The deep roof portion of the notch represents Blumensaat's line, and it is important not to elevate the notch because this would change the anatomic reference points for the native femoral ACL attachment. In addition, the lateral deep wall of the notch is not changed or removed in order to maintain the native ACL attachment location for the ACL graft. Only in rare instances is there overgrowth in this region and insufficient clearance between the lateral notch and the PCL. The tissue in this region is gently removed, and the PCL synovium is protected. A sharp curet is used to remove soft tissues on the lateral wall to the femoral condyle articular cartilage edge, which is the required reference for ACL graft placement. The mistake is made not to go deep enough in the notch on the lateral wall to view "around the corner," because sometimes the notch wall will have a gentle deep lateral slope of a few degrees.

using a single pin transfixation is shown later in this chapter. The bone portion of the QT-PB or Achilles allograft is usually placed into the femoral tunnel, however, the graft can be reversed with the bone plug placed into the tibial tunnel and located appropriately to make up for an enlarged tibial tunnel that requires the bone portion of the graft.

A variety of techniques for femoral fixation (Fig. 7–34) and tibial fixation (Fig. 7–35) are available, based on the preference of the surgeon. The two-incision technique is preferred over the EndoButton technique. The tibial fixation is usually the weakest, and especially in revision surgery, a suture post is added. Interference screw fixation alone of an STG or soft tissue allograft is also not recommended. A suture post is commonly required to achieve adequate fixation.

Alternative Procedures

Outside-In "Flip-Drill" for Femoral Tunnel

An alternative approach is to use a two-incision technique with the proximal skin incision only of sufficient length to accommodate the guide pin "flip-drill" to locate and drill the tunnel from inside-out (Fig. 7–36). This procedure provides a long femoral tunnel for graft healing and incorporation. It also allows control of the guide pin for the femoral tunnel to be oriented into the

most ideal position to achieve good-quality bone for interference screw fixation and, in revision knees, to avoid prior tunnels. This technique avoids the necessity for tunnel drilling in a hyperflexed knee position, which is less ideal in revision knees when the femoral tunnel has to be controlled in an exact manner to avoid a prior misplaced tunnel.

The steps for this technique are shown in Figure 7–36. The steps already described for locating the central femoral ACL guide pin placement are performed. A 10-mm incision is made at the posterior one third of the thigh and at the proximal margin of the lateral femoral condyle. The drill guide is placed and the blunt proximal guide sleeve bluntly advanced to the femur. The guide pin flip drill is advanced and the position and entrance determined with the arthroscope in the AM portal. The drill socket is created. The tunnel joint entrance is chamfered to prevent graft abrasion. The graft is passed in a retrograde manner and fixed either endoscopically or retrograde with the tunnel extending proximally and using the second incision. When the bone quality on the femur is not ideal and a femoral suture post is desired, it is easy to enlarge the incision for visualization, extend the femoral tunnel to exit proximally, and provide a graft suture post.

Endoscopic ACL Reconstruction

Multiple endoscopic ACL reconstructive techniques have been described in the literature for B-PT-B and soft tissue grafts.

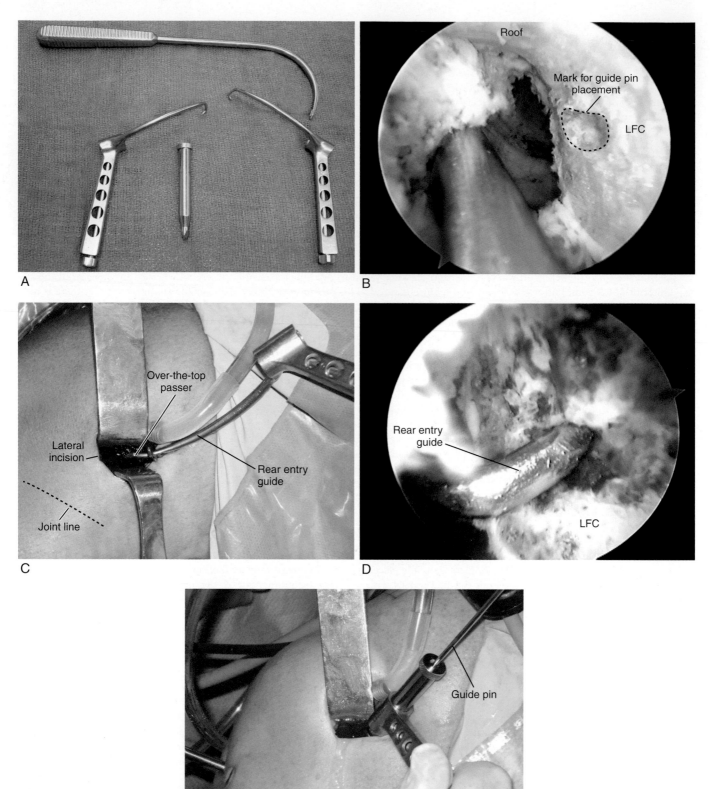

FIGURE 7–33. **A,** The rear-entry drill guide system (Smith-Nephew, Endoscopy, ACUFEX, Andover, MA). **B,** Central ACL femoral attachment location. **C,** Passage of the guide through the second incision. **D,** Guide pin location on the lateral femoral wall. **E,** Drilling of the femoral tunnel from outside-in.

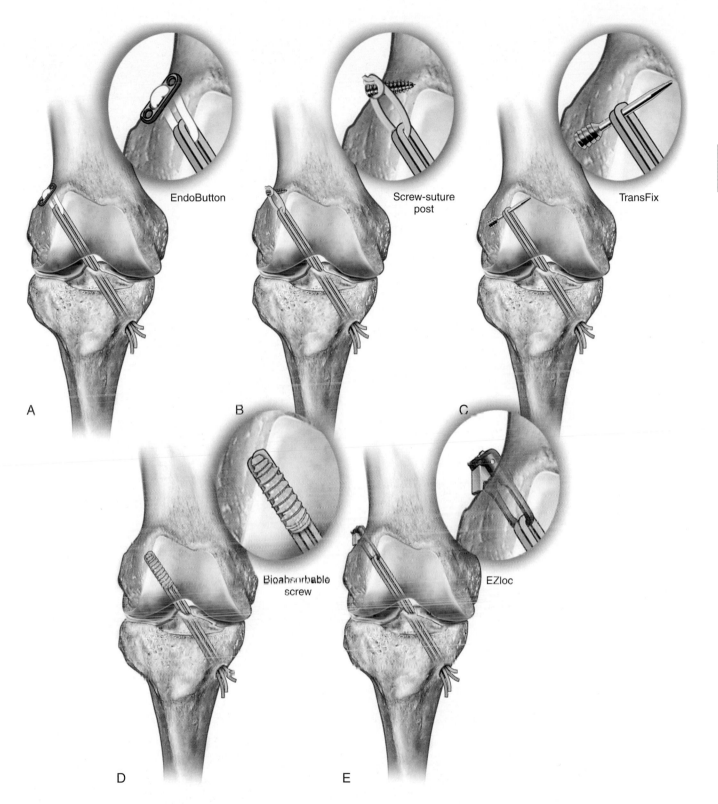

EndoButton

Screw-suture post

TransFix

A

B

C

Bioabsorbable screw

EZloc

D

E

FIGURE 7–34. A variety of ACL femoral fixation techniques. The interference screw alone is not recommended because it produces the lowest graft tensile strength to pull-out.

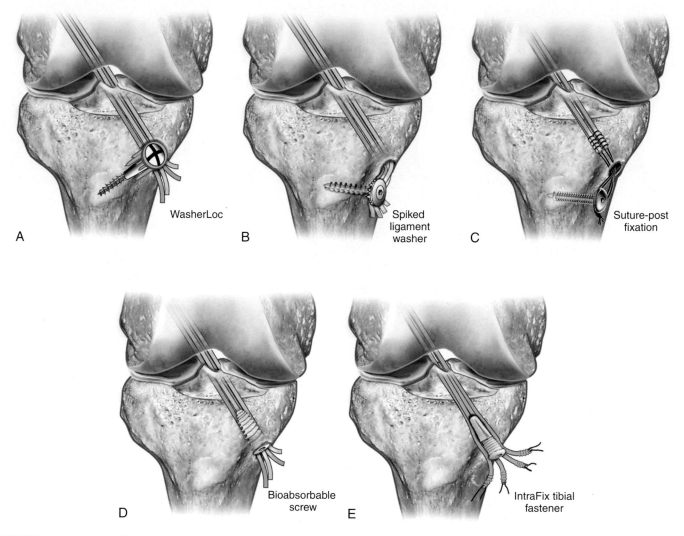

FIGURE 7–35. Various tibial fixation techniques. An interference screw alone is not recommended.

The approach taken in this chapter is to describe some of these techniques without specifically endorsing one over another. Regardless of the technique the surgeon selects, the anatomic placement of the tibial and femoral tunnels is exactly what has previously been described and illustrated. In Figure 7–37,

Critical Points OPERATIVE TECHNIQUES: ALTERNATIVE PROCEDURES

Outside-In "Flip Drill" for Femoral Tunnel

- Two-incision technique.
- 10-mm proximal skin incision to accommodate guide pin flip drill.
- Provides long femoral tunnel, avoids prior tunnels.
- Place drill guide, advance blunt guide sleeve to femur.
- Advance flip drill, create drill socket.
- Chamfer tunnel entrance, pass grade retrograde, fix either endoscopically or retrograde.

Endoscopic Procedures

- RetroConstruction procedure example provided.
- Cross-femoral pin for proximal graft fixation useful with semitendinosus-gracilis tendons grafts.

the all-inside B-PT-B ACL "RetroConstruction" procedure (Arthrex, Naples, FL) is shown as an example of an advanced endoscopic technique that the senior author has used. A complete description of this technique is available from the manufacturer. There is a learning curve for the tibial interference screw fixation. The femoral tunnel technique is the same as already described.

Endoscopic Transfix ACL Reconstruction

Numerous procedures are described in which a cross-femoral pin is used to provide proximal graft fixation. The author has found this represents an alternative technique to the two-incision procedure with the use of a four-strand STG graft. An example of this procedure is shown in Figure 7–38. A complete description of this technique and videotape demonstration are available from the manufacturer. It is recommended that this technique be performed in a bioskills setting prior to patient application, because there are specific steps to master. Placement of the cross-pin requires caution to ensure that the tunnel is on the lateral femoral wall and central ACL attachment location, similar to the outside-in two-incision technique previously described. This means that the cross-pin will be entering in a relatively distal position

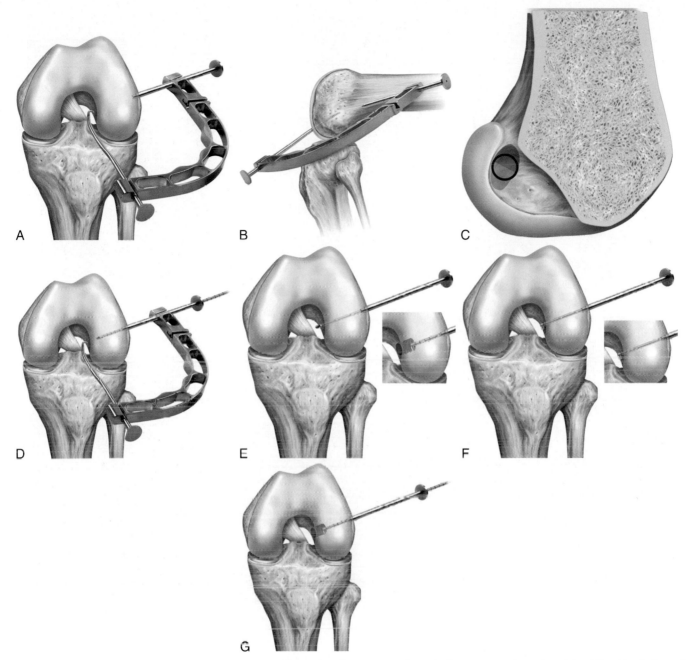

FIGURE 7–36. Demonstration of the flip drill technique for femoral socket or tunnel. **A** and **B,** Placement and location of the drill guide. **C,** Central ACL anatomic tunnel placement. **D,** Placement of the flip drill. **E,** The flip drill is advanced at the femoral attachment. **F,** The drill end is "flipped" at a right angle to the pin. **G,** Creation of a femoral socket that can extend completely as a tunnel if desired. (Courtesy of Arthrex, Naples, FL.)

on the femoral condyle and placed posteriorly to avoid damaging the FCL attachment. The common mistake is to locate the femoral tunnel high in the attachment, adjacent to the roof.

Management of Graft Malposition

It is important in the operative technique to recognize whether an improper graft position has occurred so that steps may be taken to address the problem. An excessive anterior femoral tunnel results when all of the soft tissues have not been removed from the lateral femoral wall and the "around-the-corner" view posteriorly of the femoral condyle has not been achieved. It is important that the AM portal be used to view the entire lateral sidewall in selecting the ideal femoral tunnel position. When an anterior tunnel is adjacent, but has no communication with the selected femoral tunnel, an allograft bone dowel or interference screw placed in the tunnel, maintaining the proper location of the tunnel more posteriorly, is usually possible. If the anterior tunnel is large, extending posteriorly, a bone-graft procedure is indicated and ACL revision delayed. Excessive posterior placement of a femoral tunnel with a back-wall blow-out would provide a compromise to interference screw fixation. In these cases, a two-incision reorientation of the femoral tunnel is indicated, and a suture post is usually added to provide a combined interference screw–suture fixation.

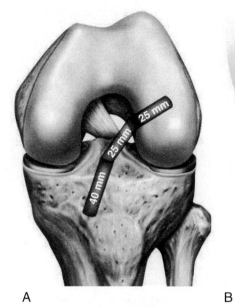

A

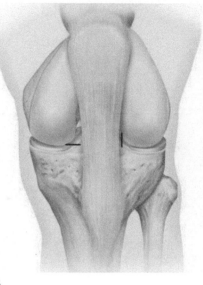

B

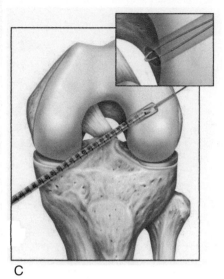

C

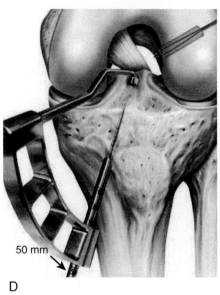

D

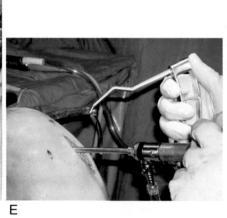

E

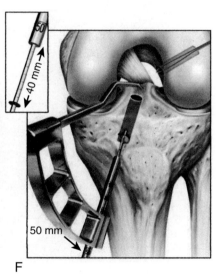

F

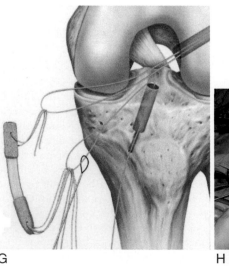

G

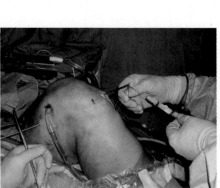

H

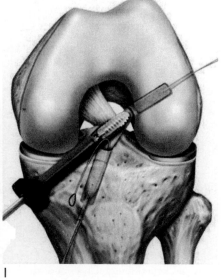

I

Legend continued on next page.

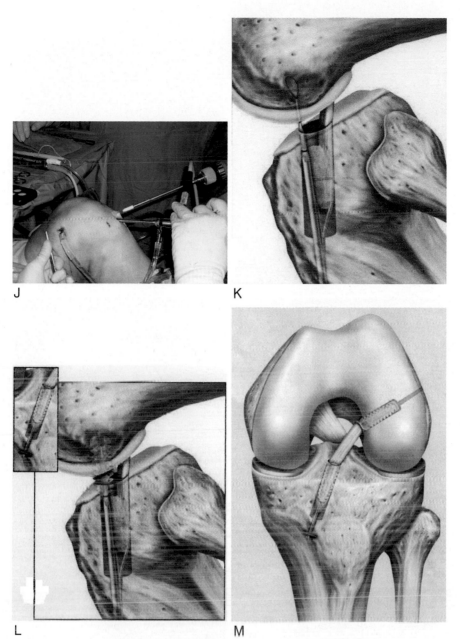

FIGURE 1-37—cont'd. Endoscopic ACL reconstruction: RetroReconstruction Procedure. The overall length of the graft must be at least 5 mm shorter than the combined length of the femoral socket, intra-articular space, and tibial socket. **A,** In this example, the total distance is 90 mm and the tunnels allow adequate space for tensioning of the graft. **B,** The lateral portal is placed in standard fashion along the lateral edge of the patellar tendon. The medial portal should be placed just medial to the patellar tendon and inferior to standard position to facilitate femoral socket preparation. Medial portal incisions may be oriented horizontally to allow instruments to be moved in the transverse plane. **C,** Bring the knee to 120° of hyperflexion and place the Beath pin through the medial portal into the 2 o'clock femoral position, already described. Ream the femoral socket to a 25-mm depth. Use a Beath pin to pass a graft-passing suture and dock the suture in the femoral socket for later use during graft passing. **D** and **E,** Place a RetroCutter that is 1 mm larger than the tibial graft diameter and drill the tibial socket as deep as possible without violating the distal cortex. **F,** Example: If the distance between the tibial plateau and the distal tibial cortex is 50 mm, as read off the drill sleeve, then drill the socket 40 mm deep. **G** and **H,** Retrieve both the femoral and the tibial graft-passing sutures out of the medial portal. A cannula may be used to avoid tissue bridges. Using the tibial-passing suture, tie a loop around a looped Nitinol wire. Place the graft sutures from the femoral end of the graft into the femoral-passing suture. Load the tibial graft sutures into the tibial-passing suture loop. **I** and **J,** Pass the tibial bone block into place while maintaining the wire anterior in the socket. Hyperflex the knee and fix the femoral side of the graft with a biointerference screw through the medial portal. Condition the graft under tension, as described previously. **K,** Pass the RetroScrew Driver over the Nitinol wire and into the joint. Remove the Nitinol wire and replace it with a FiberStick. Retrieve the FiberStick out the medial portal through a Shoehorn cannula. Attach the RetroScrew, 2 mm smaller than the socket diameter, to the FiberStick. **L,** Pass the RetroScrew into the joint and load on the RetroScrew Driver. This step requires practice. **M,** Keep tension on the graft while the screw is inserted into the tibial socket. A RetroScrew Tamp may be used to ease insertion of the screw and the tibial tunnel should be 2–3 mm larger at the anterior margin to facilitate the interference screw. Backup fixation may be accomplished by tying the tibial graft-passing sutures over a two-hole suture button on the anterior cortex with a sliding knot. (Courtesy of Arthrex, Naples, FL.)

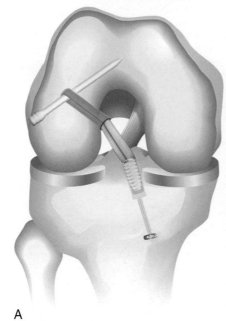

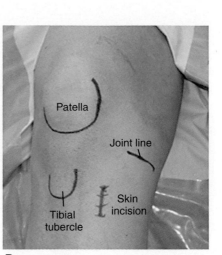

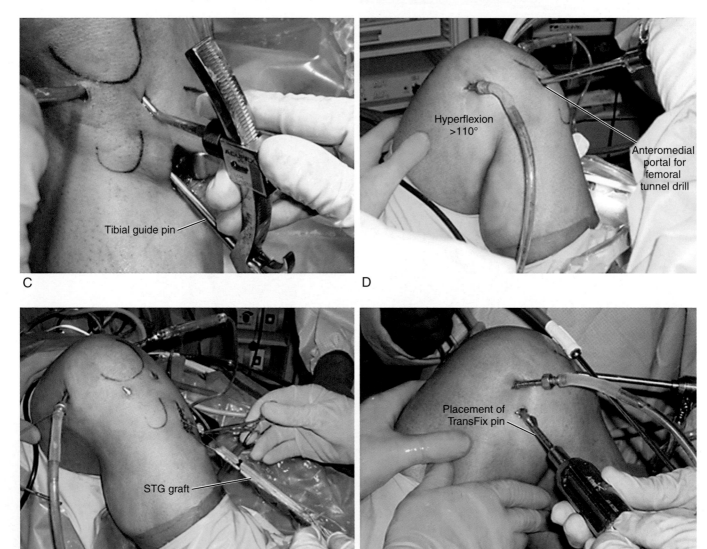

FIGURE 7–38. A, Endoscopic Transfix ACL reconstruction (Courtesy of Arthrex, Naples, FL). **B,** Placement of the AM incision. **C,** Placement of the tibial tunnel. **D,** A hyperflexion position and drilling through the AM portal are used for a central femoral ACL tunnel placement. **E,** Four-strand STG graft looped around the wire to be passed through the tibial tunnel. **F,** Placement of the TransFix implant is passed over the wire and into the lateral femoral condyle to secure the graft. Prior to placing the implant, the wire should move freely in a medial-to-lateral direction. The implant should be advanced gently into the femoral tunnel and seated with the end placed into the prepared lateral cortex. The tibial fixation is with a suture post and absorbable interference screw.

An excessively posterior femoral tunnel results in shortening of the graft in extension; this requires an anterior adjustment in the tunnel. When the guide pin is placed in the femoral ACL attachment from either an inside-out or an outside-in approach, it is possible to start with a 6-mm acorn-shaped reamer to readjust the tunnel and subsequent tunnel entrance with a stepwise progression in the reamers. In this manner, the most ideal placement of the femoral tunnel may be achieved. A distal femoral tunnel past the 9 o'clock position may result in a graft impinging on the lateral femoral condyle, requiring excessive notchplasty. The final graft length is short and not ideal.

A tibial tunnel malposition posteriorly produces a vertical graft. A tibial tunnel placed too far anteriorly may result in anterior graft impingement or loss of the anterior tibial cortex for adequate interference screw fixation. A tibial tunnel placed too far medially or laterally may impinge on the PCL or lateral femoral condyle, respectively. Small adjustments may be made in medial or lateral graft position by placement of the interference screw in a medial or lateral placement. A posterior bone dowel allograft may be used in a posteriorly placed tunnel to displace the graft to a more central tibial location. Additional sutures are added to the graft for a tibial post, expecting that added fixation is necessary. The principle is never to accept a misplaced tibial or femoral tunnel and risk of a graft failure and revision knee problem.

A fracture of the bone portion of the graft, in which 15 mm of bone remains, may be managed by placing two additional sutures in the tendon portion of the graft and two sutures in the bone portion. An interference screw is used along with a suture post. If there is disruption at the bone-tendon junction, the senior author prefers to harvest an STG autograft instead of adding sutures to the tendon portion because the diameter of the patellar tendon is not ideal in the absence of the bone ends.

In cases of an Osgood-Schlatter disease or an accessory ossification of the patellar tendon at the patella attachment (that is not appreciated until the graft is harvested), it is possible to remove the excess bone that will not affect the length or integrity of the graft. However, it is best to avoid a graft from these locations in these disease states and inform the patient that an alternative graft source will be used. The problem is that it may be necessary in a large Osgood-Schlatter lesion to dissect intact tendon adjacent to the graft harvest site to remove the bony lesion entirely, which results in weakening of the tendon attachment site. This problem requires added postoperative protection and modification of the immediate rehabilitation program. B-PT-B fixation problems with interference screws are usually solvable by upsizing the screw diameter and adding a suture fixation post. It is important never to compromise the final graft fixation strength and accept a less than ideal fixation because this would potentially result in graft loosening in the early postoperative period.

It is more difficult to manage an enlarged tibial or femoral tunnel with an STG graft because the technique requires that a snug-diameter tunnel be placed to achieve a graft-tunnel interface to allow graft incorporation and avoid excessive tunnel widening. An absorbable interference screw may be necessary to compress one side of the graft into the tunnel, which would require modification of the postoperative rehabilitation to protect the graft during the initial healing stages. EndoButton techniques are frequently used with STG grafts, and problems may be encountered with inadvertent reaming of the femoral cortex and loss of fixation strength. Fixation with an interference screw provides a weaker graft fixation, and consideration of a two-incision technique with a suture post is warranted. A cross-pin fixation technique may also be used. When the EndoButton does not adequately flip and provide seating against the femoral cortex, it is necessary to add a longer length of the synthetic loop to the graft end and repeat measurements of the graft tunnel.

Identification of Tibial Tunnel Problems in Revision Knees and Need for Staged Bone-Grafting

The arthroscopic procedure is done in a standard manner and appropriate meniscus and débridement procedures are performed. It is next important to determine that the tibial and femoral tunnels can be placed into the ideal position before the autograft or allograft is harvested and prepared. The selection and preparation of autografts is described in the prior section and this is performed only after the tibial and femoral tunnels have been determined to be adequate or have been bone-grafted previously.

It is usually not difficult to identify the prior tibial tunnel entrance into the joint after removal of the soft tissues and graft material at the ACL attachment location. The adjacent lateral meniscus attachment may be encased in scar tissue and is preserved. The PCL, posterior ridge, medial tibial spine, and medial articular cartilage are all identified. The farthest extent of the posterior ACL tibial attachment is approximately 8 mm anterior to the posterior ridge (RER), as already discussed. This is a critical measurement because many primary ACL operative procedures place the ACL graft into the posterior one third of the ACL attachment. It is often the case that during the drilling procedure for the posterior tibial tunnel, or in using this tunnel for the femoral tunnel placement, the tunnel is enlarged posteriorly out of the native ACL footprint and extends to the RER. This situation results in a vertical ACL graft. Often, the preoperative MRI will allow measurements of the tunnel location relative to the AP width, as already described, and the surgeon is aware preoperatively of this problem (Fig. 7–39).

It may initially appear that the tibial tunnel is acceptable; however, after removing all of the soft tissues or when the tibial tunnel drilling is performed, the surgeon may discover that a posterior tibial tunnel exists that extends all the way to or through the RER, which is not acceptable for the revision graft. These cases require staged bone-grafting (Fig. 7–40). On occasion, the posterior tibial tunnel is located in the posterior one third of the native ACL attachment, with only a 5-mm bridge between the tunnel and the RER. If the tibial tunnel is not dilated requiring grafting, it is possible to drill and relocate the tibial tunnel approximately 8 mm anteriorly into a more advantageous central ACL attachment position. A cortical allograft dowel is positioned to occupy and fill the posterior one third of the tunnel, maintaining the graft

in the ideal central position. Another technique is to fashion the bone plug of a revision allograft, maintaining an enlarged bone block to fill the posterior portion of the tibial tunnel and prevent the collagen portion of the graft displacing posteriorly. A third technique is to perform a double-bundle reconstruction with the posterior tibial tunnel used for the PL bundle (assuming the graft is placed into the native ACL tibial footprint and not located in an abnormal posterior position). A second anterior tibial tunnel is used for the AM bundle. Use of double-bundle grafts in a revision procedure requires that the femoral tunnel location also be ideal, which is often a problem. A misplaced femoral tunnel may prevent two additional tunnels to be adequately placed or the two additional tunnels could possibly weaken the femoral condyle.

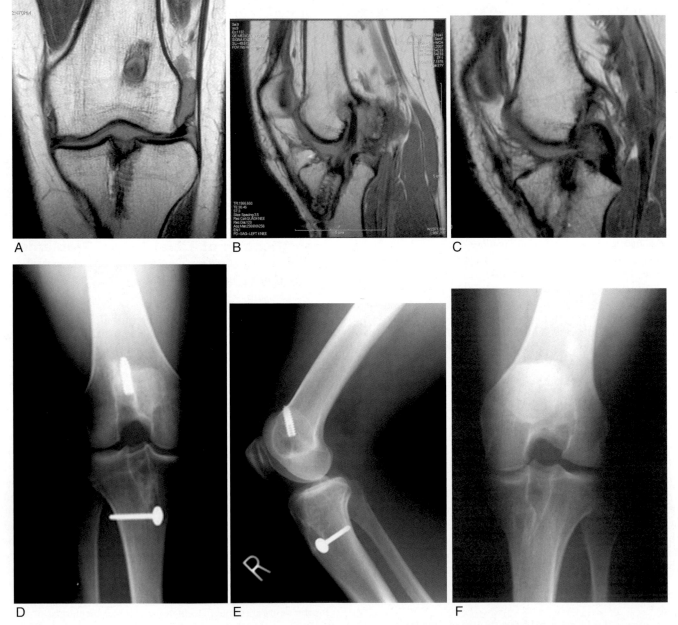

FIGURE 7–39. A series of four cases with enlarged tibial tunnels and vertical ACL graft orientation requiring staged bone grafting prior to ACL revision surgery. Often, the radiograph underestimates the extent of tunnel widening requiring bone grafting. If these tibial tunnels were accepted for a revision graft, the graft placement would remain too posterior, not in the ideal ACL central attachment, and a snug graft tunnel interface would not be established. Accordingly, bone grafting was required in all cases prior to revision surgery.

Continued

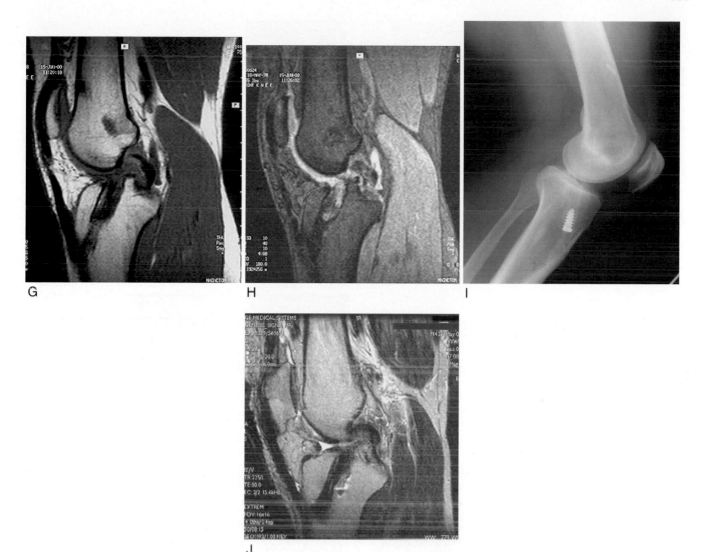

FIGURE 7–39—cont'd.

In the authors' opinion, the mistake that is possible at ACL revision is to accept a posterior tibial tunnel position for a single-graft procedure. If there is any question that the bone quality is not ideal and that the revision graft would be placed into the posterior one third of the native tibial attachment and result in a windshield effect on weakened bone posteriorly eroding through to the RER, it is preferable to proceed with the staged bone-grafting. The alternatives listed previously to relocate the graft tunnel are indicated only when good bone quality exists and the prior tibial tunnel does not extend beyond the native ACL attachment. In the authors' experience, in the majority of revision cases involving a posteriorly placed tibial tunnel, the tunnel is frequently dilated and expanded. This is not suitable for bone incorporation into the revision graft, and there is little question that a staged bone-grafting is necessary.

Identification of Prior Femoral Tunnel in Revision Knees and Need for Staged Bone-Grafting

The arthroscope is placed in the AM portal to view the entire lateral notch and notch roof, and all soft tissues and graft material are removed. An angled curet, suction cutting device, and occasionally a radiofrequency probe are used. Any spurs or overgrowth of the notch are removed and a limited notchplasty performed to view the farthest posterior aspect of the lateral notch. A mistake is to not remove all of the lateral soft tissues adjacent to the lateral femoral condyle articular cartilage edge because this is the landmark for identification of the correct location of the revision graft. With a prior vertical tunnel or anterior tunnel, it is often possible to outline the native ACL attachment, which provides important identification landmarks for graft location. The ACL footprint is mapped out and the determination is made whether an ideal anatomic tunnel is possible, as described.

In a majority of revision cases, the index graft is placed in a vertical nonanatomic position on the roof of the intercondylar notch (Fig. 7–41), and it is possible to place the revision tunnel in the ideal central ACL anatomic attachment. The author uses the two-incision approach to reorient the tibial tunnel entirely away from the index tunnel. It is sometimes possible to perform an endoscopic approach using an AM portal to drill the femoral tunnel with a hyperflexed knee; however, the two-incision technique is preferable in most revision procedures. In posterior wall femoral blow-out situations, a reoriented tunnel wall can often be used and the bone portion of the graft fashioned so that the bone

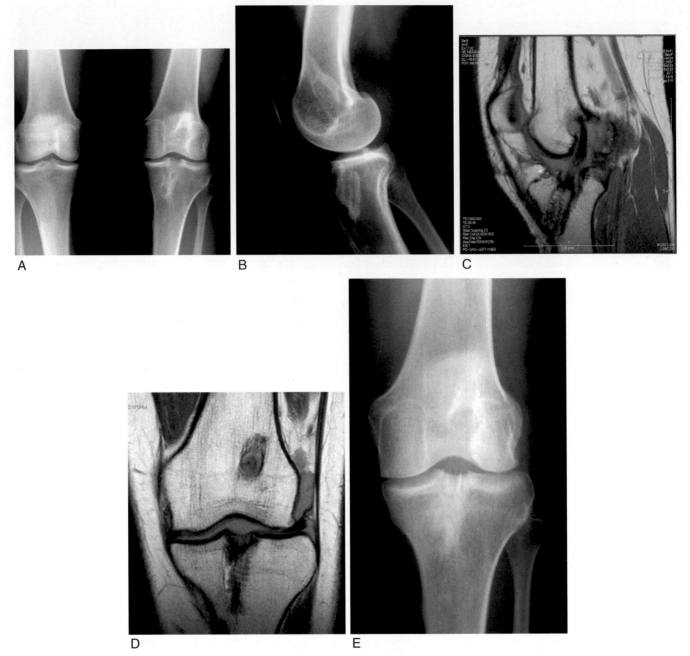

FIGURE 7–40. A, A 31-year-old woman with failure of a primary ACL STG autograft and revision anterior tibial allograft of the left knee. **B,** A bone graft of a large tibial tunnel was performed with allograft. **C** and **D,** The allograft procedure did not provide a restitution of the tibial tunnel and a residual widening was present. **E,** A repeat bone graft using autogenous iliac crest was required to obtain bone of sufficient quality for an ACL revision.

is placed in the posterior portion of the tunnel to maintain the collagen portion of the graft within the native ACL femoral footprint.

The more difficult problem is the management of a dilated and slightly misplaced femoral tunnel that is at the native ACL attachment or perhaps extends a few millimeters beyond the native ACL attachment. The new tunnel will overlap and produce an enlarged dilated tunnel with portions extending beyond the native ACL footprint. There is a technique in which two stacked interference screws (absorbable or metallic) are used to provide a buttress against one side of a dilated tunnel to locate the graft within the ideal femoral attachment. However, this technique is possible only when the femoral tunnel is close to ideal and the stacked interference screw is truly used as a buttress screw against one side

of the tunnel wall. The remainder of the femoral tunnel cannot be dilated or enlarged, and the bone quality about the femoral tunnel is not osteopenic and allows for graft fixation. The femoral tunnel does not extend to the roof of the notch or to the edge of the femoral articular cartilage.

As previously described for the tibial tunnel, the mistake that may be made is to accept a "slightly enlarged" femoral tunnel in which the graft placement is not ideal, such as too proximal or anterior on the lateral femoral wall. If there is any question, a bone-grafting procedure is performed and the revision procedure done 6 months later. Meniscus repairs may be done with the bone-grafting procedure to protect the meniscus, and a functional brace used until the revision procedure is performed.

Critical Points OPERATIVE TECHNIQUES: IDENTIFICATION PRIOR TUNNELS IN REVISION KNEES, NEED FOR STAGED BONE GRAFTING

Tibial Tunnel

- Identify prior tibial tunnel entrance after removal of soft tissues and graft material at the ACL attachment location.
- Identify lateral meniscus attachment, PCL, posterior ridge, medial tibial spine, medial articular cartilage.
- Posterior expanded tibial tunnel extending all the way to RER is not acceptable for revision graft, requires staged bone grafting with autogenous bone.
- Posterior tibial tunnel located in posterior one third of the native ACL attachment, with 5 mm bridge between the tunnel and the RER, if not dilated, may be relocated anteriorly.
- Use cortical allograft dowel to fill posterior one third of tunnel.
- Or perform double-bundle reconstruction. Posterior tibial tunnel used for PL bundle, second anterior tibial tunnel used for AM bundle when two femoral tunnels are possible.

Femoral Tunnel

- Place arthroscope in AM portal, view entire lateral notch and notch roof.
- Remove all soft tissues and graft material.
- Perform limited notchplasty to view farthest posterior aspect of lateral notch.
- Map out central anatomic ACL position knee in 20°–30° flexion.
- Majority knees will have vertical grafts on roof of notch, allowing new lateral wall tunnel to be placed.
- For dilated and slightly misplaced femoral tunnel, use two stacked interference screws to provide a buttress against one side of the tunnel. Only possible if tunnel is close to ideal anatomic position. Otherwise, staged bone graft required.

ACL, anterior cruciate ligament; AM, anteromedial; PCL, posterior cruciate ligament; PL, posterolateral; RER, retroeminence ridge.

Bone-Grafting Procedure for Tibial and Femoral Enlarged Tunnels

Principles are available to follow in performing bone-grafting of enlarged tunnels. The first is to adequately prepare the graft site by removing all soft tissues, curet, and place small drill holes into the cortical tunnel walls to provide the most ideal surface for bone graft healing. Cultures of the removed soft tissues are obtained. Rarely, a gram stain and frozen section are necessary to exclude an occult infectious process within a tibial or femoral

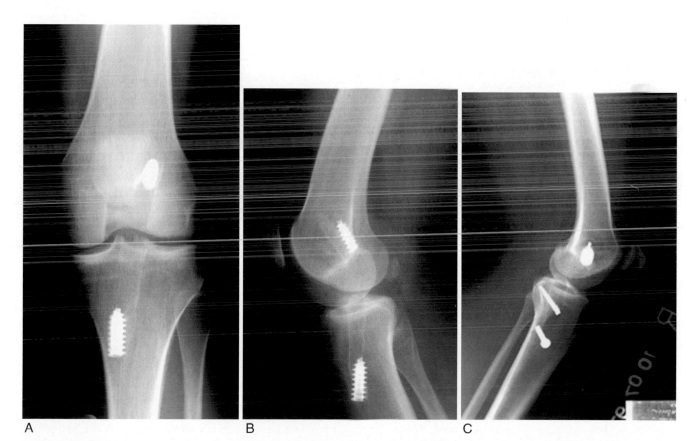

A   B   C

FIGURE 7–41. Patients who presented to the authors' center for ACL revision with a vertical ACL graft, easily detected on anteroposterior (AP) and lateral radiographs and magnetic resonance imaging. The femoral graft location is primarily on the notch roof. In the authors' experience, this vertical graft orientation is the primary cause for ACL failure.

Continued

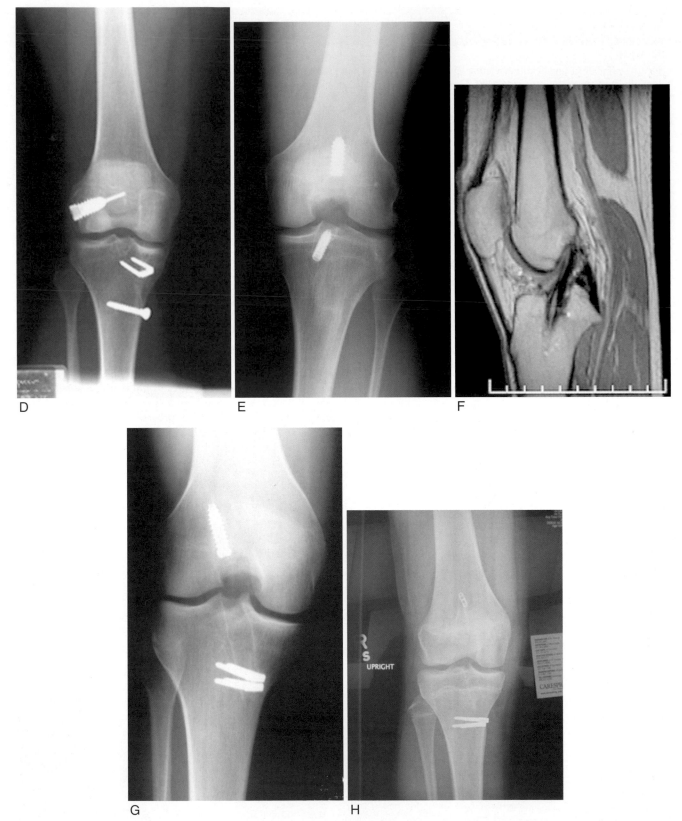

FIGURE 7–41—cont'd.

tunnel, particularly when an allograft was used. Second, it is ideal to use autogenous bone that is supplemented by allograft bone in larger defects. Third, the posterior tibial RER, when deficient, is replaced with good-integrity cortical-cancellous bone (such as a bicortical iliac crest autograft) and not cancellous bone, which is a weaker construct. The goal is to prevent the revision graft in the newly placed tunnel from enlarging the tunnel posteriorly by a windshield-wiper effect against poor-quality bone. The same situation applies to an enlarged dilated femoral tunnel in which the anterior shallow portion of the tunnel is grafted with a combined cortical-cancellous autograft to obtain a good-quality bone construct. The senior author prefers a "minimally invasive" iliac crest autograft procedure, removing only the superior and outer portions and not disturbing the inner table and muscle attachments. This procedure is described in detail in Chapter 31, Primary, Double, and Triple Varus Knee Syndromes: Diagnosis, Osteotomy Techniques, and Clinical Outcomes. The outer iliac crest can be fashioned into a rectangular or circular dowel that is wedged into the enlarged tibial or femoral tunnel, providing a near-complete filling of the expanded tunnel and likelihood of the revision procedure being performed in 3 to 5 months. Strips of cortical-cancellous bone are packed into any remaining defects and, if necessary, supplemented with allograft iliac crest bone. In major defects, cancellous bone in the range of 5 to 8 mm fragments are packed between the cortical-cancellous strips. The bone-grafting procedure is easily performed in an arthroscopically assisted manner, enlarging the portals as necessary to deliver the bone graft into the femoral tunnel. The tibial tunnel is packed in a retrograde manner, observing the final position of the graft from an appropriate arthroscopic portal.

Thomas and colleagues[181] performed staged ACL revision reconstruction in a series of 49 knees, all of which required bone-grafting of previous tibial tunnels to avoid overlap into correctly placed revision tunnels. The authors stressed the importance of ensuring good-quality bone stock to achieve anatomic ACL graft placement and adequate fixation. At follow-up a mean of 6 years postoperatively, only 2 of the revision knees had failed.

Bone-graft substitutes are commercially available; however, their role instead of autogenous or allograft bone has not been established in clinical studies. The authors recommend autogenous bone that is supplemented with allograft when necessary. It is probable that under certain circumstances, an allograft bone supplemented with a platelet gel or cancellous marrow cells will provide an equal alternative to autograft iliac bone. This procedure is being used for opening wedge osteotomy and may be applicable to enlarged tibial and femoral tunnels. There is a longer period of time for host replacement of an allograft in large expanded tunnels until the revision procedure is performed. With autogenous bone, the healing of the tunnels is prompt and predictable, and the

revision may be performed within a few months. A computed tomography scan may be necessary to confirm bone-graft incorporation in suspect cases.

The postoperative rehabilitation program is described in Chapter 13, Rehabilitation of Primary and Revision Anterior Cruciate Ligament Reconstructions. The authors do not administer preoperative or intraoperative intra-articular anesthetic injections or use pain pump catheters postoperatively owing to the possible complication of adverse effects on articular cartilage.[68,84,154]

AUTHORS' ACL PRIMARY RECONSTRUCTION CLINICAL STUDIES

The authors published a series of prospective clinical studies on ACL primary reconstruction in over 650 knees with acute, subacute, and chronic ruptures.* The data from these investigations provide information regarding the following variables on clinical outcome: type of graft, sterilization of allografts, gender, chronicity of injury, concomitant operative procedures, preexisting joint arthritis, varus osseous malalignment, the rehabilitation program, and type of insurance (workers' compensation vs. private). This chapter provides summaries of these investigations, and the reader is encouraged to refer to the original publications for further detail. The grafts studied included freeze-dried fascia lata and fresh-frozen or irradiated (2.5 mrad) B-PT-B allografts and B-PT-B autografts. An ACL reconstruction was considered failed if more than 5 mm of increased AP displacement was measured on knee arthrometer testing or if a grade II or III pivot shift was elicited on clinical examination (International Knee Documentation Committee [IKDC] categories of abnormal and severely abnormal combined).

Type of Graft

A higher rate of ACL graft failure was noted in knees with chronic ACL ruptures that received fresh-frozen or irradiated allografts (16%–30%[111,112]) compared with those that received autografts (3%–8%[115]; Table 7–6). The only exception was in a group of knees that underwent a combined allograft and ITB extra-articular procedure in which a failure rate of only 3% was found.[112]

In knees that underwent ACL reconstruction for acute or subacute ruptures, there was no difference in the overall failure rate between fascia lata or B-PT-B allografts (5%–7%[124]) and autografts (3%[115]). However, a greater percentage of knees that received allografts had 3 to 5 mm of increased AP displacement, indicating partial graft function, compared with autografts (Fig. 7–42). The knees in this category typically demonstrate a grade I pivot shift and may be at increased risk for progression to a fully positive pivot shift in the future. The authors prefer autogenous tissue whenever possible for all ACL reconstructions, as discussed previously.

*See references 6, 14–16, 28, 111–117, 120, 121, 123, 124, 129, 130, 137.

TABLE 7-6 Summary of Select Authors' Primary Anterior Cruciate Ligament Reconstruction Clinical Studies: Knee Arthrometer Data and Final Failure Rates

Graft Type, Study Citation, Follow-up	Patient Data	Allograft Sterilization	Knee Arthrometer Test Force Level	Preoperative Total AP Displacement (mean, range)	Follow-up Total AP Displacement (mean, range)	Knee Arthrometer Testing			Final Failure Rate* (%)
						Follow-up Total AP Displacement < 3 mm (I-N) (%)	Follow-up Total AP Displacement 3–5 mm (I-N) (%)	Follow-up Total AP Displacement > 5 mm (I-N) (%)	
Allograft[113]	N = 28 B-PT-B	Fresh-frozen	134 N	Not done	1.0 ± 3.1 (−2.5–+6.5)	77	20	3	7
F/U 5–9 yr Acutes	N = 40 fascia lata	Freeze-dried, ETO in 32			1.0 ± 2.9 (−7.0–+5.0)	75	20	5	5
Allograft[112] F/U 2–4.5 yr Chronics	N = 64 B-PT-B	Fresh-frozen in 54 knees, Irradiated in 10 knees	89 N	9.2 ± 3.0 (3.0–16.0)	2.6 ± 2.5 (−2.8–+8.0)	54	34	12	16
Subgroups:	Fresh-frozen only			9.0 ± 3.0 (3.0–16.0)	2.5 ± 2.3 −2.0–+7.5	53	31	16	16
	Irradiated only			10.0 ± 2.0 (7.0–13.5)	2.8 ± 3.2 (−2.0–+8.0)	60	10	30	30
Allograft[112] F/U 2–4.5 yr Chronics	N = 40 B-PT-B + ITB extra-articular	Fresh-frozen in 38, Irradiated in 2	89 N	8.3 ± 3.3 (3.0–15.5)	1.1 ± 2.5 (−4.0–+6.5)	74	23	3	3
Allograft[111] F/U 2–3.4 yr Chronics	N = 49 B-PT-B + LAD	Irradiated	134 N	9.5 ± 3.5 (5.0–18.0)	2.7 ± 3.5 (−3.0–+12.0)	53	30	17	20
B-PT-B Autograft[115] 2–3 yr	N = 57 chronic	NA	134 N	11.4 ± 4.5 (4.0–22.0)	0.4 ± 2.7 (−3.5–+10.0)	84	12	4	8
	N = 30 acute			9.0 ± 2.9 (3.5–14.0)	−0.3 ± 2.6 (−5.5–+7.0)	92	4	4	3
B-PT-B Autograft[15] 2–3 yr Acute & chronic	N = 47 men	NA	134 N	10.3 ± 4.0 (3.5–22.0)	0.2 ± 2.9 (−5.5–+8.0)	80	16	4	4
	N = 47 women			12.9 ± 4.5 (4.5–22.5)	0.7 ± 2.8 (−3.5–+10.0)	87	8	5	6
B-PT-B Autograft[116] 2–3.4 yr Acute & chronic	N = 19 workers' compensation	NA	134 N	11.2 ± 3.7 (6.5–15.0)	0.6 ± 3.1 (−3.0–+10.0)	87	13	0	0
	N = 19 private insurance			10.4 ± 2.3 (4.0–16.5)	0.5 ± 2.2 (−4.5–+4.0)	80	13	7	5

*Failed = >5 mm increase total AP displacement or grade 2 or grade 3 pivot shift.

AP, anteroposterior; B-PT-B, bone-patellar tendon-bone; ETO, ethylene oxide; F/U, follow-up; I-N, involved knee–noninvolved knee; ITB, iliotibial band; LAD, ligament augmentation device; NA, not applicable.

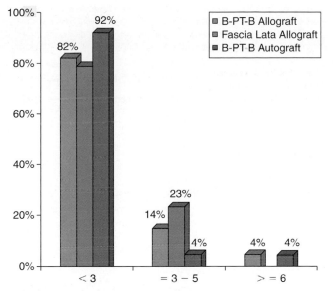

FIGURE 7–42. Knee arthrometer results from the authors' clinical studies in patients who received ACL reconstruction for acute or subacute ruptures with B-PT-B allograft, fascia lata allograft, or B-PT-B autograft tissue.

Augmentation Procedures for Allografts (ITB Extra-articular, Ligament Augmentation Device)

The authors conducted a prospective study (level II) on the use of an extra-articular ITB tenodesis procedure combined with a B-PT-B allograft for chronic ACL ruptures.[112] This was the first study that compared the outcomes of this combined procedure (64 patients) with those of an allograft alone (40 patients). The knees in this study had a high grade of instability before surgery because 50% or more had a grade III pivot shift, indicating deficiency of the extra-articular lateral restraints.

At follow-up, a mean of 35 months postoperatively, the rate of graft failure was 16% in the allograft-alone subgroup compared with 3% in the combined allograft-ITB subgroup (P < .05; see Table 7–6). The difference in AP displacements measured on KT-1000 testing was also significant (Fig. 7–43; P < .01). The difference in the rate of failure was not due to

an irradiation effect because only 10 patients in the allograft-alone group and 2 patients in the combined allograft-ITB group received irradiated grafts. The combined subgroup returned to significantly higher levels of sports activity (P < .05) and had higher overall rating scores on the CKRS (P < .01). There were no differences between the subgroups in isokinetic test scores, functional limitations, symptoms, or patellofemoral crepitus.

The authors hypothesized that the ITB tenodesis provided support to the intra-articular allograft by restoring the secondary lateral restraints to anterior translation and internal rotation. Therefore, the procedure may be useful in knees with a grade III pivot shift. However, the study cohort is not large enough to provide definitive recommendations and further study is indicated. The results of this study may have implications in the treatment of ACL revision knees in which an allograft approach is selected, to be discussed later.

The authors conducted a prospective, randomized clinical trial (level I) on the effect of a ligament augmentation device (LAD) combined with an irradiated B-PT-B allograft for chronic ACL ruptures.[111] The results of the combined procedure in 49 knees were compared with those of a fresh-frozen B-PT-B allograft used alone in 66 knees. At an average of 34 months postoperatively, there was no difference in overall graft failure rates (20% and 16%, respectively; see Table 7–6) or in the individual symptom, functional limitation, or overall rating scores. The LAD did not improve the efficacy of the reconstruction and was therefore not recommended for use with an allograft for ACL reconstruction.

Secondary Sterilization Process Used for Allografts

Based on the two studies in the chronic ACL groups shown in Table 7–6, a higher rate of ACL graft failure was measured in knees that received allografts sterilized with 2.5 Mrad of gamma irradiation (23%; 14 of 61 knees) compared with those that were fresh-frozen (11%; 10 of 92 knees, P < .05[111,112]). To the authors' knowledge, only one other study from another institution addressed the issue of the effect of irradiation on allograft failure rates. Rappe and colleagues[153] reported that irradiated Achilles tendon allografts (2.0–2.5 Mrad) had a significantly higher failure

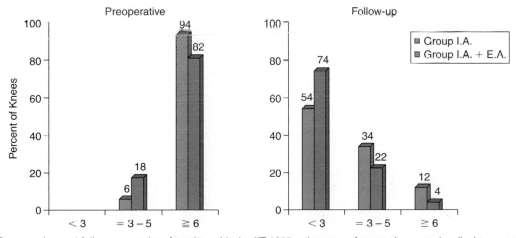

FIGURE 7–43. Preoperative and follow-up results of testing with the KT-1000 arthrometer for anterior-posterior displacement at 89 N of total force for group I.A. (allograft alone) and Group I.A. + E.A. (allograft and extra-articular procedure). At the latest follow-up evaluation, the difference in the displacement between the two groups was statistically significant (P < .01). *(From Noyes, F. R.; Barber, S. D.: The effect of an extra-articular procedure on allograft reconstructions for chronic ruptures of the anterior cruciate ligament. J Bone Joint Surg Am 73:882–892, 1991.)*

rate than those that were frozen (33% and 2.4%, respectively; $P < .01$). A meta-analysis of five investigations that compared B-PT-B allografts and autografts reported that, when irradiated and chemically processed allografts were removed (thereby comparing 82 and 230 patients in each group, respectively), no difference was found in outcome and knee stability for Lachman and pivot shift testing between these graft options.[87] That investigation did not analyze objective KT-2000 data that were reported in the five studies. Other methods of secondary sterilization are preferred and recommended by the authors and have been discussed in detail by others elsewhere.[100,185,186]

Gender

The authors conducted a prospective study (level II) on 94 patients (47 males, 47 females) who received B-PT-B autografts to determine whether a difference in outcome existed between men and women.[15] This was the first study of its kind to conduct this type of comparison. The patient groups were stratified according to chronicity of the injury to determine whether this factor affected the results. Patients in the acute subgroup received the operation within 14 weeks of the original injury; all others were placed in the chronic subgroup. The patients were matched for age, preoperative sports activity levels, condition of the articular cartilage, and months of follow-up.

At a mean of 26 months postoperatively, there were no significant differences in outcome between the men and the women. Although the women demonstrated greater mean AP displacements before surgery than the men (14.3 ± 5 and 11.2 ± 4, respectively; $P = .05$), these data were similar at follow-up (0.90 ± 2.69 for men, 0.70 ± 3.49 for women), as were the percentages of patients with less than 3 mm, 3 to 5.5 mm, and 6 mm or more of increased AP displacement (Fig. 7–44). The overall failure rate was 4% for men and 6% for women. There was no difference between genders for range of knee motion, patellofemoral crepitus, anterior knee pain, muscle strength deficits (Table 7–7), or complications. In addition, there was no significant difference between men and women for symptoms, functional limitations with daily or sports activities, or the overall rating scores. The conclusion was reached that equal consideration should be given to active patients for ACL reconstruction

TABLE 7–7   Results of Isometric Muscle Testing between Men and Women after Anterior Cruciate Ligament Bone–Patellar Tendon–Bone Autograft Reconstruction

Deficit of Reconstructed Limb Compared with Opposite Limb (%)	Knee Extensors (%)		Knee Flexors (%)	
	Men	Women	Men	Women
0–10	67	62	74	69
11–20	24	24	11	24
21–40	9	7	15	7
>40	0	7	0	0

regardless of gender. Subsequently, other authors conducted similar analyses and reached the same conclusions for men and women receiving B-PT-B autografts[48] and STG autografts with interference screw fixation.[162]

Chronicity of Injury

The authors prospectively followed 94 consecutive patients who received B-PT-B autografts to determine whether a difference existed in objective or subjective outcome between acute and chronic ACL ruptures.[115] Eighty-seven patients returned for follow-up evaluations from 22 to 44 months postoperatively. The acute subgroup comprised 30 patients who underwent reconstruction a mean of 6 weeks (range, 2–14 wk) after the injury. The chronic subgroup comprised 57 patients who underwent reconstruction a mean of 54 months (range, 3–348 mo) after the original knee injury. All of these patients had symptoms or functional limitations that failed to improve with rehabilitation or activity modification. A total of 94 operative procedures had been done in 34 of these patients before the ACL reconstruction, including 20 medial meniscectomies and 9 lateral meniscectomies (partial or total).

The results of the comparisons are shown in Table 7–8. There was no difference between the subgroups in mean AP displacements (chronic group, 0.4 ± 2.7 mm; acute group, –0.3 ± 2.6 mm), pivot shift testing, knee motion complications, or overall rating of graft failure (chronic group, 8%; acute subgroup, 3%). A total of 46 menisci had been repaired during the ACL reconstruction. At follow-up, there was no evidence of retears in 41 of these knees.

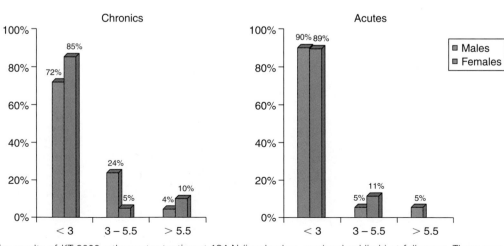

FIGURE 7–44. The results of KT-2000 arthrometer testing at 134 N (involved vs. noninvolved limb) at follow-up. There was no statistically significant difference found between men and women in the percentage of patients in the three AP displacement categories. Acutes, acute subgroup; Chronics, chronic subgroup. *(From Barber-Westin, S. D.; Noyes, F. R.; Andrews, M.: A rigorous comparison between the sexes of results and complications after anterior cruciate ligament reconstruction. Am J Sports Med 25:514–526, 1997.)*

TABLE 7–8 Summary of Data Comparison between Acute and Chronic Anterior Cruciate Ligament Bone–Patellar Tendon–Bone Autogenous Reconstructions

Outcome Factor	Result: Acute vs. Chronic*	Method
Postoperative stability	NS	KT-2000 arthrometer
Patellofemoral crepitus	NS	Knee examination
Patellofemoral pain	NS	Knee examination
Range of knee motion	NS	Goniometer
Knee motion complications	NS	Knee examination
Meniscal repair	NS	Knee examination
Tibial tunnel width	NS	Radiographs
Femoral tunnel width	NS	Radiographs
Patellar tendon height	NS	Radiographs
Articular cartilage	NS	Arthroscopy
Functional analysis	S: squatting, running, jumping, twisting NS: walking, stairs	Cincinnati Knee Rating System
Symptoms	S: pain NS: swelling, giving-way	Cincinnati Knee Rating System
Overall rating score	S	Cincinnati Knee Rating System
Patient rating outcome	S	Cincinnati Knee Rating System

*NS, difference not statistically significant; S, difference statistically significant; all S values, acute subgroup had better results than chronic subgroup.

TABLE 7–9 Reoperation Rates of Meniscus Repairs According to Anterior Cruciate Ligament Function*

ACL Function	Repaired Menisci that Required Follow-up Arthroscopy for Tibiofemoral Joint Symptoms
Functional (N = 166)	32 (19%)
Not functional (N = 32)	7 (22%)
Total (N = 198)	39

*Functional, <5 mm of increased AP displacement on arthrometer testing or pivot shift grade 0 or I; nonfunctional, >5 mm of increased AP displacement on arthrometer testing or pivot shift grade II or III.
ACL, anterior cruciate ligament; AP, anteroposterior.

There were significant differences between the subgroups for pain ($P = .04$), squatting/kneeling ($P = .03$), running ($P = .02$), jumping ($P = .04$), twisting/turning ($P = .01$), the patient rating of the overall condition of the knee ($P = .007$), and sports activity levels ($P = .05$). Patients in the acute subgroup had less pain and limitations with sports functions and returned to more strenuous activities than those with chronic deficiency. The conclusion was reached that joint stabilization should be performed early in active patients prior to reinjuries and loss of meniscus tissue. In addition, investigations that assess the results of ACL reconstruction should separately assess the outcome of acute/subacute and chronic ruptures with rigorous knee rating systems.

Concomitant Operative Procedures

Several studies were conducted by the authors on patients who received concomitant procedures with an ACL reconstruction, including complex meniscus repair for tears that extended into the central one third region,[28,119,120,158] HTO,[114,130] PL reconstructions,[122,123,127–129] MCL repairs,[129] and multiligament procedures.[123]

In a series of 177 patients who underwent repair of 198 meniscus tears that extended into the central one third region, the ACL was also reconstructed in 126 knees (71%) with either irradiated allografts (72 knees) or B-PT-B autografts (54

knees).[158] At a mean of 42 months postoperatively, the failure rates were 4% for the autografts and 15% for the allografts. The increased failure rate for the allografts may have been related to the irradiation sterilization process. The study found that 159 of the meniscus repairs (80%) were successful, with no tibiofemoral joint symptoms. Thirty-nine (20%) required repeat arthroscopy for symptoms. No statistical relationship was found between ACL function at follow-up and the reoperation rate for a symptomatic meniscus repair (Table 7–9).

A separate investigation was performed of 28 complex meniscus repairs for tears that extended into the avascular zone in 27 patients aged 40 to 58 years.[120] The ACL was reconstructed in 21 patients with B-PT-B autografts in all but 5 knees. At a mean of 34 months postoperatively, none of the ACL grafts had failed. Twenty-six of the meniscus repairs (87%) were asymptomatic and considered successful. Concomitant ACL reconstruction appeared to increase the healing rate of meniscus repairs. This older group of patients was physically active and the authors believed it was important to both stabilize the knee and preserve the meniscus, as all desired to return to athletics.

A third investigation followed 61 knees in 58 patients under the age of 20 who underwent a total of 71 complex meniscus repairs that extended into the avascular zone. Forty-seven had a concurrent ACL reconstruction with either irradiated B-PT-B allografts (20 knees) or B-PT-B autografts (27 knees).[119] At a mean of 51 months postoperatively, none of the autografts had failed, whereas 5 of the allografts (25%) had failed, which was most likely related to the irradiation sterilization process. Fifty-three of the meniscus repairs (75%) were asymptomatic and had not required further surgery. None of the patients in whom the allografts failed had tibiofemoral symptoms. The success rates of these three investigations warrant repair of complex meniscus tears that extend into the central one third region in active individuals, along with stabilization of ACL deficiency (see Chapter 28, Meniscus Tears: Diagnosis, Repair Techniques, and Clinical Outcomes).

In the authors' experience, the majority of patients who require PL reconstructions also require ACL or PCL reconstruction. Three investigations determined the outcome of a proximal advancement of the PLS,[178] a femoral-fibular allograft reconstruction,[127] and an anatomic B-PT-B FCL reconstruction[122]; all of which are described in detail in Chapter 22, Posterolateral Ligament Injuries: Diagnosis, Operative Techniques, and Clinical Outcomes. In the first study, 21 patients were followed who received a proximal advancement of the PLS; 12 patients also had an ACL B-PT-B reconstruction (allograft in 10, autograft in 2).[128]

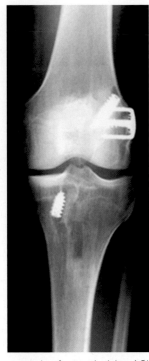

FIGURE 7–45. An example of a two-incision ACL B-PT-B autograft technique combined with a proximal advancement of the PL complex for abnormal lateral tibiofemoral joint opening. The PL insufficiency represented an interstitial stretching and not a traumatic rupture, which was an ideal indication for the proximal advancement, avoiding a more complex PL graft reconstruction.

These patients all had a definitive FCL, although lax, which did not require graft reconstruction (Fig. 7–45). At follow-up, a mean of 42 months postoperatively, only 1 of the ACL reconstructions had failed. The PL procedure was successful in restoring function or partial function in all but 2 knees.

In a second study, the authors followed 20 patients who received an allograft femoral-fibular PL reconstruction, of whom 13 also had a B-PT-B ACL reconstruction (11 allografts, 2 autografts).[127] All of the allograft tissues were irradiated. At follow-up a mean of 42 months postoperatively, only 1 ACL reconstruction had failed. The PL procedure restored function or partial function in all but 2 knees.

In a third investigation, 13 patients who underwent 14 anatomic FCL B-PT-B reconstructions were followed 2 to 13.7 years postoperatively.[122] In this group, 12 patients underwent concomitant ACL reconstruction with irradiated B-PT-B allografts, B-PT-B autografts, or QT-PB autografts. At follow-up, all but 2 of the ACL reconstructions were rated as normal or nearly normal (IKDC rating), and all but 1 of the PL reconstructions were rated normal or nearly normal. These studies emphasize the importance of surgically restoring all deficient knee ligamentous structures concomitantly. The selection criteria for the appropriate PL procedure are described in Chapter 22, Posterolateral Ligament Structures: Diagnosis, Operative Techniques, and Clinical Outcomes.

The authors followed a series of 46 patients who had combined ACL and MCL deficiency to determine the appropriate treatment (operative or conservative) for MCL ruptures, described in detail in Chapter 24, Medial and Posteromedial Ligament Injuries: Diagnosis, Operative Techniques, and Clinical Outcomes.[129] All patients

underwent ACL allograft reconstruction (fascia lata in 21, irradiated B-PT-B in 25 knees). In 34 patients in whom all of the medial structures were ruptured, an MCL repair was performed. In 12 patients, only the superficial MCL fibers were torn and these were not repaired. At follow-up, a mean of 5.3 years postoperatively, 7 of the ACL allografts (15%) had failed; 5 of which were fascia lata grafts. All of the knees had less than 3 mm of increased medial joint opening at 5° and 25° of flexion. The study found that knee motion problems and patellofemoral symptoms were more common in patients who received the MCL repair. Therefore, the recommendation was made in knees with combined ACL-MCL ruptures to treat the MCL injury with appropriate conservative measures first, followed by ACL reconstruction (see Chapter 25, Rehabilitation of Medial Ligament Injuries). An exception is a displaced medial meniscus tear, which requires early operative intervention.

The authors followed a series of 11 patients who presented with dislocated knees in whom all ligament ruptures were surgically restored.[123] Seven patients had acute injuries and 4 had chronic injuries in which previous surgical treatment had failed to restore knee stability. All required both ACL and PCL reconstructions, which were done with allograft tissues. Six knees had concurrent repair of the MCL and 6 had concurrent reconstruction of the PLS. The operative procedures allowed immediate knee motion in an effort to decrease the rate of postoperative arthrofibrosis in these complex knees. At follow-up a mean of 4.8 years postoperatively, the failure rates were 9%, ACL reconstructions; 18%, PCL reconstructions; 17%, PL reconstructions; and 0%, MCL procedures. These numbers are too small for definitive analyses to be conducted.

Preexisting Joint Arthritis and Prior Meniscectomy

The authors studied the effect of preexisting advanced articular cartilage damage in knees undergoing ACL reconstruction for giving-way symptoms to determine whether the operation was effective in improving the overall quality of life. In one investigation,[117] 53 patients received autogenous B-PT-B ACL reconstructions an average of 7.5 years after the original injury. A total of 90 prior operative procedures had been performed in these knees, including 10 ACL reconstructions that had failed, 27 medial meniscectomies, and 10 lateral meniscectomies (partial or total). During the reconstruction, a total of 84 advanced lesions were found; subchondral bone exposure was noted in 20 knees and extensive fissuring and fragmentation (extending greater than half of the depth of the surface) was found in 33 knees. Eight-seven percent of the knees that had lesions in the tibiofemoral compartment had undergone prior meniscectomy. At follow-up a mean of 27 months postoperatively, 40 ACL reconstructions (75%) were rated as normal; 10 (19%) as nearly normal; and 3 (6%) as failed. Statistically significant improvements were found for pain, swelling, giving-way (Table 7–10), functional limitations with daily and sports activities, the patient perception of the overall knee condition (Fig. 7–46), and the overall CKRS score.

In a second study, 40 patients with advanced articular cartilage deterioration underwent ACL B-PT-B allograft reconstruction an average of 7 years after the original knee injury. Thirty-two of the allografts (80%) had received 2.5 Mrad of gamma irradiation prior to implantation. A total of 102 prior operative procedures had been done, including 16 prior failed ACL procedures in 12

TABLE 7–10   Change in Symptom Scores from the Preoperative to the Follow-up Evaluation in 53 Patients with Advanced Joint Arthrosis after Anterior Cruciate Ligament Bone–Patellar Tendon–Bone Autograft Reconstruction

Symptom	Improved	Same	Worse
Pain	37 (70%)	14 (26%)	2 (4%)
Swelling	38 (72%)	14 (26%)	1 (2%)
Partial giving-way	47 (89%)	6 (11%)	0
Full giving-way	42 (79%)	8 (15%)	3 (6%)

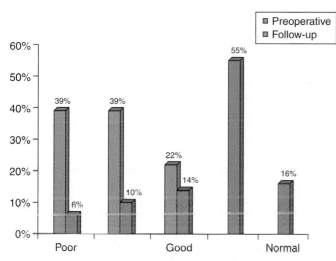

FIGURE 7–46. The patients' own ratings of the overall knee condition showed significant improvement from the preoperative condition to that recorded at the follow-up evaluation ($P = .0001$). *(From Noyes, F. R.; Barber-Westin, S. D.: Anterior cruciate ligament reconstruction with autogenous patellar tendon graft in patients with articular cartilage damage. Am J Sports Med 25:626–634, 1997.)*

patients, 24 medial meniscectomies, and 18 lateral meniscectomies. A total of 64 noteworthy articular cartilage lesions were identified at surgery, including subchondral bone exposure in 15 knees (38%) and extensive fissuring and fragmentation in 25 knees (62%). Seventy-nine percent of knees with damage in a tibiofemoral compartment had undergone a prior meniscectomy. At follow-up, a mean of 37 months postoperatively, 45% of the ACL reconstructions were rated as normal; 25% as nearly normal; and 30% as failed. The failure rate was most likely related to the irradiation of the grafts. Statistically significant improvements were found for pain, partial giving-way, and full giving-way ($P < .01$). Significant improvements were also found for squatting, running, jumping, twisting/turning, and the overall rating score. In the patient rating of the overall knee condition, 42% rated the knee as normal or very good, 24% as good, 21% as fair, and 13% as poor.

These investigations demonstrated that ACL reconstruction is effective in reducing symptoms and functional limitations and increasing activity levels in approximately two thirds of patients with advanced articular cartilage damage. Many patients return to low-impact activities based on the advice to avoid sports involving jumping, cutting, twisting, and pivoting. This is especially true in those in whom prior meniscectomy has been performed. It is important to note that these patients suffered giving-way symptoms and, therefore, the requirement for stabilization was justified. A trial of function is frequently attempted

in patients who have advanced arthritis, pain, and giving-way that includes muscle strengthening and a functional knee brace. If this trial is unsuccessful in resolving these symptoms, ACL surgery is warranted. These studies do not answer the question of the ability of an ACL reconstruction to prevent or delay worsening of the preexisting articular cartilage damage.

Varus Osseous Malalignment

Two investigations assessed the outcome of treatment of varus angulated, ACL-deficient knees[114,130]; both are described in detail in Chapter 31, Primary, Double, and Triple Varus Knee Syndromes: Diagnosis, Osteotomy Techniques, and Clinical Outcomes. In one study,[130] 41 patients were treated with HTO and an ACL reconstruction with a B-PT-B allograft or autograft, which was staged after the HTO in the majority a mean of 6 months later. In addition, PL reconstructions were done in 18 triple varus knees along with the ACL reconstruction, which were all staged after the HTO. At follow-up, a mean of 49 months after the ACL reconstruction, a decrease was noted in the mean AP displacement measurement of the autografts compared with the allografts (autograft mean preoperative, 12.8 ± 5.5 mm, and mean follow-up, 1.4 ± 54.4 mm; allograft mean preoperative, 12.2 ± 3.9, and mean follow-up, 4.1 ± 5.8 mm; $P =$ not significant). The failure rates were 43% for the allografts and 23% for the autografts. Owing to the small numbers in each graft subgroup (21 allografts [13% irradiated], and 20 autografts), no conclusion could be reached regarding the effect of each type of graft on the failure rate. However, prior to referral to our center, 15 of these patients had undergone ACL reconstructions that had failed, and there was a significant difference in the failure rate between the revision and the primary cases (67% and 33%, respectively; $P < .05$).

In a second investigation, 41 patients underwent HTO, 16 of whom also had a staged ACL allograft reconstruction.[114] This investigation demonstrated that not all varus-angulated, ACL-deficient knees require both procedures, but that ACL reconstruction is warranted when giving-way symptoms continue after osteotomy. Patients who do not experience such symptoms and who have advanced arthritis may avoid ACL surgery by activity modification. Staging these two operative procedures allows the patient and clinician to determine whether joint stabilization is required. Indications for concurrent ACL reconstruction or staged after HTO are discussed in detail in Chapter 31, Primary, Double, and Triple Varus Knee Syndromes: Diagnosis, Osteotomy Techniques, and Clinical Outcomes.

Rehabilitation Program

The authors' rehabilitation protocols are described in detail in Chapter 13, Rehabilitation of Primary and Revision Anterior Cruciate Ligament Reconstructions. Several investigations assessed the effects of these programs on knee motion complications and graft failure rates.[14,16,132,137,138] The use of immediate knee motion after both ACL allograft and autograft reconstruction was proved to be effective in reducing the risk of arthrofibrosis and was not deleterious to the healing graft (see Chapter 12, Scientific Basis of Rehabilitation after Anterior Cruciate Ligament Autogenous Reconstruction). In a series of 207 patients who received ACL allograft reconstruction, 189 (91%) achieved a full range of motion without additional treatment measures.[138] The remaining 19 patients were placed into a phased program that included serial extension casting (6 knees), early gentle manipulation under anesthesia (9 knees), and arthroscopic lysis of adhesions and scar tissue (3 knees). At follow-up, 2 patients had a loss of 5° of full extension and 2 others had a permanent and significant limitation of motion. The incidence of knee motion problems was 4% in patients who had only an ACL reconstruction, 10% in knees in which an ITB extra-articular procedure had also been done, 12% in knees in which a meniscus repair had been performed, and 23% in knees that also had a MCL repair.

In a second investigation, the authors followed 443 patients who had a B-PT-B autogenous reconstruction for either an isolated rupture (219 knees) or combined with other procedures (224 knees).[132] At follow-up, a normal range of motion was detected in 436 knees (98%) and a mild loss of extension (≤5°) was found in 7 knees. Twenty-three knees required a treatment intervention for an early postoperative limitation of knee motion, including extension casting (9 knees), gentle manipulation under anesthesia (9 knees), arthroscopic débridement (3 knees), and continuous epidural anesthetic and inpatient physical therapy (2 knees). At follow-up, 87% had less than 3 mm of increased AP displacement on arthrometer testing, 9% had 3 to 5.5 mm, and 4% had 6 mm or greater. There was no effect of gender, injury chronicity, articular cartilage condition, location of physical therapy, prior surgery performed, or prior ACL reconstruction performed on the risk of a motion problem (Table 7–11). Although not statistically significant owing to the small number present, a concurrent MCL repair was believed to be a clinically significant risk factor for a knee motion problem.

Two investigations were performed in which serial knee arthrometer measurements were done postoperatively to determine whether any phase of the rehabilitation program or the amount of time that elapsed after surgery was associated with increased AP displacement (>3 mm) or graft failure.[14,16] In the first study, 84 patients who received a fresh-frozen B-PT-B ACL allograft

reconstruction were followed a mean of 37 months postoperatively.[14] The clinical outcome of these patients had been described in another report on the effectiveness of an ITB extra-articular procedure with allograft tissue.[112] This study included 52 patients who had the allograft alone and 32 who also had the ITB extra-articular procedure. Knee arthrometer measurements were taken at postoperative weeks 4, 8, 12, 16, 24, 52, and 128 for the majority of patients. The rehabilitation program was divided into four phases: assisted ambulatory, early strength training, intensive strength training, and return to sports activities.

There were a total of 28 patients in the allograft-alone group and 9 patients in the allograft-ITB procedure group with abnormal displacements detected postoperatively. The abnormal displacements were first identified a mean of 83 weeks after surgery in both groups. The majority of abnormal displacements (86%) were detected during the intensive strength training or return to sports activities phases. The rehabilitation program did not result in early stretching of failure of the allografts in this cohort.

A similar investigation was done in a group of 142 patients who underwent ACL B-PT-B autograft reconstruction.[16] A total of 938 serial KT-2000 measurements were collected the first 2 years postoperatively. Twenty-one knees had abnormal displacements detected after surgery. No association was found between the initial onset of the abnormal displacements and either the amount of time after surgery or the rehabilitation program. The failure rate was an acceptable 5%.

Insurance (Workers' Compensation)

A study was conducted to determine whether differences existed after B-PT-B autograft ACL reconstruction between patients who received workers' compensation (WC) benefits and patients who received private insurance benefits (NoWC).[116] Nineteen patients from each group were matched for age, injury chronicity, number of prior operations, and months of follow-up. The only significant difference in outcome was the mean days of lost employment (Fig. 7–47) before surgery (WC, 122 days; NoWC, 3 days; P < .001) and after surgery (WC, 222 days; NoWC, 37 days; P < .001). At a mean of 27 months postoperatively, 17 patients in the WC group had returned to work (6 with symptoms) and 2 were disabled. In the NoWC group, all patients had returned to work, 2 with symptoms. There were no differences between the groups in AP displacements, functional limitations with sports or daily activities, patient perception of the knee condition, the overall rating score, or complications. None of the autografts failed in the WC group and only 1 graft failed in the NoWC group. In the WC group, 13 patients rated their knee condition as normal or very good, 3 as good, and 3 as fair. In the NoWC group, 15 rated their knee condition as normal or very good, 4 as good, and 1 as poor. The hypothesis proposed was that the difference in the days of lost employment was due to wage systems that support WC injuries for long periods of time, the lack of a case-management system that closely follows injured workers, the inability of workers to modify existing job requirements, or improper early diagnosis and treatment of the injury.

After this study, Wexler and coworkers[191] conducted an investigation on 22 WC patients who underwent ACL B-PT-B reconstruction. All patients returned to work and none of the grafts failed. The authors concluded that the outcomes were similar to historical controls and that WC did not compromise the results of ACL reconstruction.

TABLE 7–11   Assessment of Possible Risk Factors for Knee Motion Limitation after Anterior Cruciate Ligament Bone–Patellar Tendon–Bone Autogenous Reconstruction in 443 Knees

Risk Factor	Number in Study	Number (%) with Motion Limitations
Sex		
Male	293	15 (5%)
Female	150	15 (10%)
Injury chronicity		
Acute, subacute	161	10 (6%)
Chronic	282	20 (7%)
Articular cartilage condition at reconstruction		
Normal	236	21 (9%)
Damaged*	207	9 (4%)
Location of physical therapy		
Authors' center	259	20 (8%)
Outside authors' center	184	10 (5%)
Prior surgery performed		
Yes	193	13 (7%)
No	250	17 (7%)
Prior ACL reconstruction performed		
Yes	60	6 (10%)
No	383	24 (6%)

*Fissuring and fragmentation greater than half the depth of the surface or subchondral bone exposed.
ACL, anterior cruciate ligament.

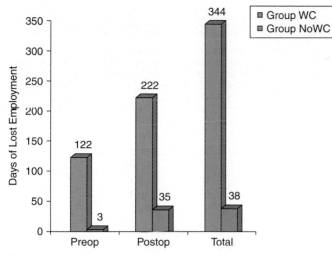

FIGURE 7–47. The mean number of days of lost employment are shown for patients who received workers' compensation (WC) benefits and those who did not receive such benefits before and after ACL reconstruction. The difference between the groups was statistically significant for all time periods analyzed (P < .001). *(From Noyes, F. R.; Barber-Westin, S. D.: A comparison of results of arthroscopic-assisted anterior cruciate ligament reconstruction between workers' compensation and noncompensation patients. Arthroscopy 13:474–484, 1997.)*

A summary of the outcomes from the authors' primary ACL reconstruction investigations is shown in Table 7–12. One additional analysis was conducted by the authors to determine whether the amount of preoperative anterior tibial translation and pivot shift grade affected the outcome. The hypothesis was

that knees that had greater than 10 mm of increased AP displacement on knee arthrometer testing and a grade III pivot shift test would have a higher rate of failure than those with less than 10 mm of increased AP displacement or a grade II pivot shift test. In reviewing select studies in both primary and revision populations, no clear trend was detected (Table 7–13).

AUTHORS' ACL REVISION CLINICAL STUDIES

The authors conducted three prospective studies on ACL revision reconstruction to determine the causes of failure of the previous operations and effects of revision graft type, concurrent ligament reconstructive procedures, and joint damage on patient outcome.[118,126,131] A total of 145 patients were entered into these investigations, of whom 141 (97%) were followed with formal research visits at the authors' center 2 to 7 years postoperatively. In all patients, the grafts were placed within the ACL anatomic footprint of the femur and the anterior-central portion of the ACL tibial footprint. Patient outcome was assessed using the CKRS and KT-2000 testing.

QT-PB Autografts

In 2006, the authors reported the results of a prospective study of 22 consecutive patients who received a QT-PB autograft ACL revision reconstruction.[118] Twenty-one patients (95% follow up) were followed a mean of 49 months (range, 25–83 mo) postoperatively. Sixty operative procedures had been done before the revision operation, including 32 ACL procedures.

TABLE 7–12   Summary of Conclusions from Authors' Primary Anterior Cruciate Ligament Reconstruction Clinical Studies

	Conclusion
Type of graft	B-PT-B autografts preferred whenever possible, decreased failure rate in chronic knees, more rapid graft healing. Autografts provide higher success rate in subjective, objective, and functional parameters. Allografts reserved for multiligament surgery, knee dislocations, special situations.
Augmentation procedures for allografts	ITB extra-articular procedure decreases allograft failure rate in chronic knees, recommended. LAD does not provide any benefit.
Secondary sterilization of allografts	Irradiation most likely deleterious with increase in failure rate, not recommended.
Gender	No difference in outcomes between males and females. No scientific basis to use gender as selection criteria for reconstruction.
Chronicity of injury	No difference in objective stability after B-PT-B autograft reconstruction. Significantly poorer results in chronic knees for symptoms, limitations with sports and daily activities, patient rating of knee condition for chronic owing to loss of meniscus tissue, preexisting joint damage. Reconstruct ACL early after injury in active patients.
Concomitant operative procedures	Meniscus repairs frequent, results may be improved by concomitant ACL reconstruction. High success rates, even in complex tears extending into central one third region, regardless of patient age. Posterolateral injuries frequently accompanied by ACL ruptures—reconstruct all ligamentous ruptures concurrently. MCL injuries usually do not require surgical treatment.
Preexisting joint arthrosis	Symptomatic unstable knees can be improved by ACL reconstruction. Advise return low-impact activities.
Varus osseous malalignment	ACL reconstruction usually staged after osteotomy in symptomatic unstable knees. ACL not required after osteotomy in knees that are asymptomatic, willing to modify activities.
Rehabilitation program	Immediate motion and rehabilitation safe, not deleterious to healing graft, low incidence (<1%) of arthrofibrosis. Identify and immediately treat limitation of knee motion with overpressure program. Full motion regained within weeks of surgery (with exception of PCL reconstructions in which hyperflexion is delayed).
Insurance	No difference in outcome between WC and privately insured patients except days of lost employment. Reconstruct WC patients earlier after injury.

ACL, anterior cruciate ligament; B-PT-B, bone–patellar tendon–bone; ITB, iliotibial band; LAD, ligament augmentation device; MCL, medial collateral ligament; PCL, posterior cruciate ligament; WC, workers' compensation.

TABLE 7–13   Select Authors' Anterior Cruciate Ligament Reconstruction Clinical Studies: Failure Rates According to Preoperative Pivot Shift, KT-1000 Testing*

Graft Type, Study Citation	Number of Patients, Subgroup, Follow-up	Allograft Sterilization	Knee Arthrometer Test Force Level	Failure Rate Preoperative Pivot Shift Grade 2	Failure Rate Preoperative Pivot Shift Grade 3	Failure Rate Preoperative KT < 10 mm (I-N)	Failure Rate Preoperative KT < 10 mm (I-N)
B-PT-B Allograft, Chronics[112] F/U 2–4.5 yr	N = 64	Fresh-frozen in 54 knees, irradiated in 10 knees	89 N	13% N = 30	22% N = 31	20% N = 30	22% N = 22
B-PT-B Allograft	N = 54	Fresh-frozen subgroup only		8% N = 26	24% N = 25	15% N = 26	22% N = 18
B-PT-B Allograft + LAD Chronics[111] F/U 2–3.4 yr	N = 49	Irradiated	134 N	17% N = 12	20% N = 34	4% N = 23	50% N = 16
B-PT-B Allograft	N = 40	Irradiated	134 N	31% N = 16	43% N = 23	37% N = 19	42% N = 12
Revision[131] F/U 2–6.5 yr	N = 26	Fresh-frozen		12% N = 16	0% N = 10	0% N = 11	12% N = 8
B-PT-B Autograft	N = 55	NA	134 N	28% N = 18	22% N = 36	30% N = 20	19% N = 26
Revision[126] F/U 2–6 yr	N = 32 Revision alone†			25% N = 12	11% N = 19	23% N = 13	0% N = 15
QT-PB Autograft Revision[118] F/U 2–7 yr	N = 21	NA	134 N	21% N = 14	14% N = 7	8% N = 12	20% N = 5

*Analysis not done in study populations with overall failure rate of 8% or less. KT > 5 mm, pivot shift grade II or III.
†No other ligament reconstructions or staged osteotomies.
B-PT-B, bone–patellar tendon–bone; F/U, follow-up; I-N, involved knee–noninvolved knee; LAD, ligament augmentation device; NA, not applicable; QT-PB, quadriceps tendon–patellar bone.

Six PL procedures had been done in 5 knees, of all but 1 of which had failed. A HTO was done in 4 knees at the authors' center and in 1 knee elsewhere a mean of 49 months (range, 4–156 mo) before the revision. Concomitant operative procedures were done in 15 knees, including a PL reconstructive procedure in 5 knees and a HTO in 2 knees. Ten knees had abnormal articular cartilage surfaces.

Multiple factors were involved in the failure of the prior ACL reconstructions, including misplaced femoral or tibial tunnels, vertical ACL graft placement, untreated or failed PL procedures, and untreated varus osseous malalignment. An endoscopic revision procedure was performed in 7 knees (Fig. 7–48) and a two-incision procedure in 14 knees (Fig. 7–49).

Statistically significant improvements were found in the mean scores for pain, swelling, and giving-way (Table 7–14; $P < .0001$). Before the revision, 14 knees (67%) had moderate or severe pain with activities of daily living, whereas only 4 knees (19%) had such pain at follow-up. The mean score of the patient rating of the overall knee condition improved from 2.7 ± 1.3 points before the operation to 6.2 ± 2.6 points (scale, 1–10 points) at follow-up ($P < .0001$). Eighteen patients (86%) rated the condition of the knee as improved and 3 rated the condition as the same as before the operation (Fig. 7–50).

The mean AP displacement value decreased from 8.4 ± 3.1 mm (range, 4.0–15.0 mm) preoperatively to 2.1 ± 2.2 mm (range, –4.0–+5.0 mm) at follow-up ($P < .001$). At follow-up, 8 of 21 grafts were rated as normal; 9 as nearly normal; and 4 as failed (Table 7–15).

This study contains too small a cohort to form definitive conclusions; however, these published data and the authors'

subsequent experience in other revision knees demonstrate that the QT-PB graft is an important autograft to consider for this operation. The QT-PB is a large cross-sectional area graft, nearly double that of a B-PT-B, and provides the surgeon with the ability to use the bone portion of the graft at either the femoral or the tibial site, based upon any perceived deficiency in bone at one of these sites. However, the overall results of these revision knees were inferior to those previously reported by the authors for primary ACL reconstructions.[115] Ninety percent of the knees had one or more compounding problems including articular cartilage damage, meniscectomy, varus malalignment, and additional ligamentous injuries, which affected the outcome.

B-PT-B Autografts

In 2001, the authors[126] reported a prospective consecutive study of 57 ACL revision reconstructions using a B-PT-B autograft. Fifty-five knees (96% follow-up) were followed a mean of 34 months (range, 24–74 mo) postoperatively. A total of 218 prior operative procedures had been done in these knees, including 60 ACL procedures. A two-incision technique was used for the revision procedure in 35 knees (64%). Concurrent operative procedures were common and included reconstructive procedures for PL or MCL deficiency in 17 knees (31%). During the revision operation, 28 knees (57%) had noteworthy damage of the articular cartilage.

There were significant improvements in pain (Fig. 7–51; $P = .0001$), functions of activities of daily living ($P < .05$) and sports ($P < .001$), patient perception of the overall knee condition ($P = .0001$), and the overall rating score ($P = .0001$). Preoperatively,

19 patients (39%) participated in sports activities, all with symptoms or limitations. At follow-up, 30 patients (61%) had returned to athletics without symptoms. Seven other patients were participating in sporting activities with symptoms against our advice.

The mean preoperative patient perception score of 4.2 ± 2.8 points significantly improved to 6.4 ± 2.0 points at follow-up (P = .0001). In 46 knees (94%), patients indicated that the overall condition had improved by circling at least one point higher on the scale at follow-up compared with the preoperative questionnaire (Fig. 7–52). Two patients rated the overall condition as the same, and 1 rated the knee condition as worse at follow-up.

AP displacements significantly decreased from a mean of 11.6 ± 3.9 mm preoperatively to a mean of 1.2 ± 4.0 mm at follow-up (P = .0001). At follow-up, 60% of the grafts were rated as normal, 16% as nearly normal, and 24% as failed.

The population was sorted according to concurrent operative procedures performed with the ACL revision reconstruction to determine the effect of these procedures on outcome (Table 7–16). In regard to graft failure, 5 of the 32 knees (16%) that had only the ACL revision reconstruction failed, 2 of the 9 knees (22%) that had an HTO before the revision procedure failed, and 6 of the 14 knees (43%) that had additional ligament procedures failed. There were statistically significant differences between the knees that had the revision reconstruction only and those that

had HTO before the revision procedure. Patients who underwent HTO had poorer mean patient perception scores and overall rating scores at follow-up (P < .05).

No complications were related to the graft harvest procedure. There was a statistically significant difference between the 31 knees (56%) that had abnormal articular cartilage surfaces and the knees with normal surfaces in the scores for twisting and turning activities and the ability to return to strenuous activities (P < .05). The study concluded that B-PT-B autograft knees, compared with historical ACL revision knees that received an irradiated allograft, had improved knee stability and avoided the added risk of infection, expense of the allograft, and other issues related to allografts, discussed previously. It is not possible on a statistical basis to determine in the authors' studies the benefit of an autogenous QT-PB over a B-PT-B graft owing to the small sample size of the cohorts.

B-PT-B Allografts

The authors[131] conducted a prospective study on 66 consecutive patients who received a B-PT-B allograft ACL revision reconstruction, of whom 65 (98% follow-up) were followed an average of 42 months (range, 23–78 mo) postoperatively. Concomitant procedures were common and included reconstruction of the FCL (7 knees), advancement of the PL complex (11 knees), reconstruction of the MCL (4 knees), and reconstruction of the PCL (2 knees). Forty of the allografts had been sterilized with gamma irradiation (25,000 grays) and 26 were fresh-frozen.

At follow-up, significant improvements were found for pain, swelling, giving-way, walking, stair climbing, kneeling, running, jumping, and twisting/turning (P < .0001). Forty-two patients (65%) returned to mostly low-impact sports without problems.

Thirty-seven knees (56%) had noteworthy deterioration of the articular cartilage surfaces. At follow-up, significant differences were found between these knees and those with normal cartilage surfaces for the variables of pain (Fig. 7–53), stair-climbing, kneeling, running, jumping, twisting/turning, sports activity level, and the overall rating score (Table 7–17; P < .05).

The preoperative CKRS overall rating score for all 65 knees of 54 ± 10 points significantly improved to 77 ± 13 points at follow-up (P < .0001). All patients except 1 had an improvement in this score; the average increase was 23 ± 11 points.

At follow-up, 43% of the grafts were rated as normal; 21% as nearly normal; and 36% failed. Table 7–13 shows an apparent effect of irradiation on the failure rate of this study, because 40 of the 66 allografts had undergone irradiation (2.5 Mrad). The increased failure rate in allograft studies (excluding irradiation effects), the cost of allograft tissue, and risk of disease transmission (even though rare) led the authors to consider autografts as the primary graft source for ACL reconstruction. Allografts are reserved for knees that do not have suitable autogenous tissues or knees that required multiple ligament reconstructive procedures.

OTHER AUTHORS' CLINICAL STUDIES

It is not the purpose of this chapter to conduct an exhaustive review of ACL primary and revision reconstructions. Rather, the reader is encouraged to review recent meta-analyses[23,24,63,87,103,150–152,182] and review articles* on this topic. A review of the objective stability

---

*See references 12, 21, 22, 27, 37, 39, 58, 59, 66, 147, 175, 180, 190, 206.

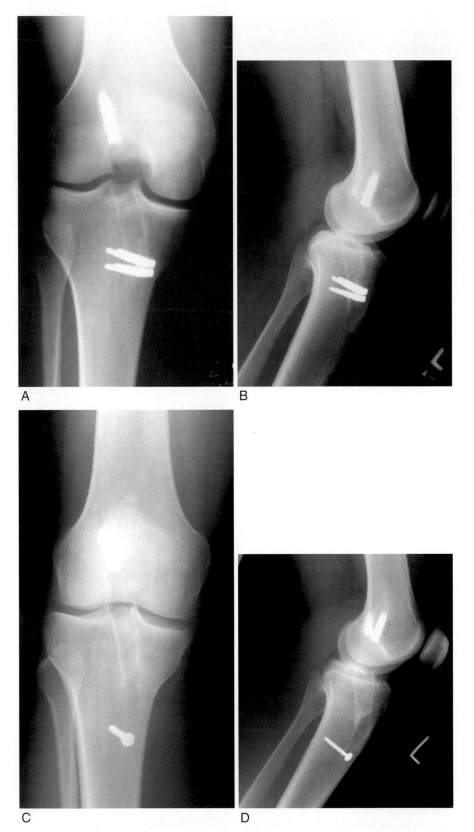

FIGURE 7–48. AP (**A**) and lateral (**B**) radiographs of the right knee of an 18-year-old woman 26 months after a failed ACL Achilles tendon allograft reconstruction. Note the anterior orientation of the femoral tunnel. AP (**C**) and lateral (**D**) radiographs 50 months postoperatively demonstrate the quadriceps tendon–patellar bone (QT-PB) autograft revision. The femoral cancellous screw was retained from the primary reconstruction to avoid creating an excessively large femoral tunnel. The placement of the new femoral tunnel was accomplished using an endoscopic technique. (**A–D,** *From Noyes, F. R.; Barber-Westin, S. D.: Anterior cruciate ligament revision reconstruction: results using a quadriceps tendon–patellar bone autograft.* Am J Sports Med *34:553–564, 2006.)*

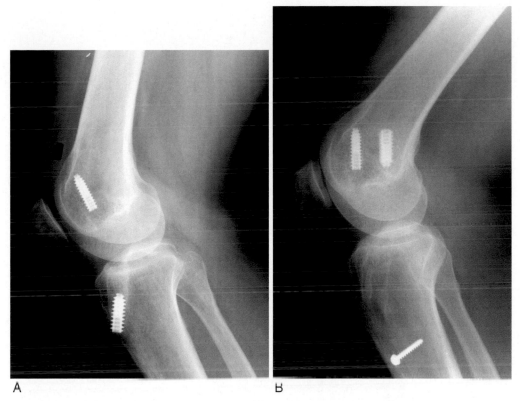

A   B

FIGURE 7–49. A, Lateral radiographs of the right knee of a 46-year-old man 12 months after a failed ACL reconstruction with a patellar tendon autograft demonstrates anterior placement of the femoral and tibial tunnels. **B,** Lateral radiograph 18 months after the QT-PB autograft revision that reestablished the correct anatomic placement of the tibial and femoral attachment sites. The patellar bone was placed in the femoral tunnel, and the quadriceps tendon was placed in a new tibial tunnel located in the central ACL attachment position. The femoral screw from the primary reconstruction was deeply placed and therefore not removed. *(A and B, From Noyes, F. R.; Barber-Westin, S. D.: Anterior cruciate ligament revision reconstruction: results using a quadriceps tendon–patellar bone autograft. Am J Sports Med 34:553–564, 2006.)*

TABLE 7–14 Symptoms and Functional Limitations before and after Quadriceps Tendon–Patellar Bone Anterior Cruciate Ligament Revision

Factor	Point Scale	Preoperative (mean ± SD)	Followup (mean ± SD)	P value
Pain	0–10	2.8 ± 1.5	5.6 ± 2.7	<.001
Swelling	0–10	2.9 ± 1.4	6.1 ± 2.7	<.001
Giving-way	0–10	4.3 ± 2.6	7.3 ± 2.9	<.001
Patient perception	1–10	2.7 ± 1.3	6.2 ± 2.6	<.001
Walking	0–40	30 ± 10	34 ± 10	.02
Stair-climbing	0–40	24 ± 14	31 ± 12	.002
Squatting	0–40	9 ± 15	19 ± 16	.05
Running	40–100	49 ± 14	70 ± 24	.003
Jumping	40–100	46 ± 11	59 ± 22	.007
Twisting	40–100	48 ± 13	65 ± 24	.003

SD, standard deviation.

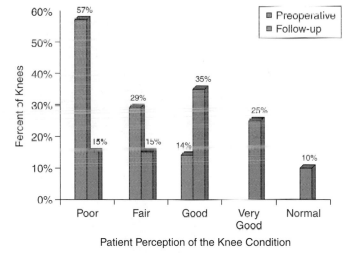

FIGURE 7–50. The distribution of patient ratings of the knee condition before surgery and at follow-up. The difference between evaluations was significant (P < .0001). *(From Noyes, F. R.; Barber-Westin, S. D.: Anterior cruciate ligament revision reconstruction: results using a quadriceps tendon–patellar bone autograft. Am J Sports Med 34:553–564, 2006.)*

results of double-bundle ACL reconstructions is provided in Table 7–18.* It should be noted in the studies comparing single- and anatomic double-bundle reconstructions that the single graft typically represented a vertical ACL graft placement (posterior tibial attachment, high femoral attachment). This single vertical graft placement has been shown in a number of in vivo and in vitro

*See references 1, 3, 11, 33, 53, 67, 80, 86, 109, 110, 170, 176, 198, 201, 202, 208.

studies previously discussed to result in an inferior control of rotatory loading of the knee joint and pivot shift phenomena. Meredick and associates[103] conducted a meta-analysis of level I–III clinical studies that compared single- and double-bundle reconstructions

TABLE 7–15 Summary of Authors' Revision Anterior Cruciate Ligament Reconstruction Clinical Studies: Knee Arthrometer Data and Final Failure Rates

Graft Type, Study Citation, Follow-up	Number of Patients, Subgroup	Allograft Sterilization	Knee Arthrometer Test Force Level	Preoperative Total AP Displacement (mean, range)	Follow-up Total AP Displacement (mean, range)	Knee Arthrometer Testing			Final Failure Rate* (%)
						Follow-up Total AP Displacement < 3 mm (I-N) (%)	Follow-up Total AP Displacement 3–5 mm (I-N) (%)	Follow-up Total AP Displacement >5 mm (I-N) (%)	
QT-PB Autograft[118] F/U 2–7 yr	N = 21	NA	134 N	8.4 ± 3.1 (4.0–15.0)	2.1 ± 2.2 (−4.0–+5.0)	42	37	21	19
B-PT-B Autograft[126] F/U 2–6 yr	N = 55	NA	134 N	11.2 ± 3.9 (5.0–21.0)	2.2 ± 4.9 (−6.0–+15.5)	64	15	21	24
	Subgroups: n = 32 revision only, no other operative procedures			10.9 ± 4.3 (5.0–21.0)	0.7 ± 3.6 (−3.5–+10.5)	82	7	11	16
	n = 9 revision after staged HTO			10.7 ± 2.1 (8.5–13.0)	4.8 ± 5.9 (−1.0–+15.0)	33	33	33	22
	n = 17 revision & other ligament procedures			11.9 ± 4.0 (6.0–18.5)	4.1 ± 5.8 (−6.0–+15.5)	38	23	38	35
B-PT-B Allograft[124] F/U 2–6.5 yr	N = 40	Irradiated	134 N	9.3 ± 3.1 (5.5–19.0)	4.1 ± 4.7 (−4.0–+17.5)	44	32	24	26
	N = 26	Fresh-Frozen		9.1 ± 2.8 (5.5–15.0)	1.8 ± 3.2 (−3.0–+5.0)	52	39	9	8

*KT > 5 mm, pivot shift grade II or III.

AP, anteroposterior; B-PT-B, bone-patellar tendon–bone; F/U, follow-up; HTO, high tibial osteotomy; I-N, involved knee–noninvolved knee; NA, not applicable; QT-PB, quadriceps tendon–patellar bone.

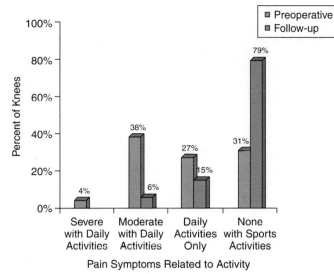

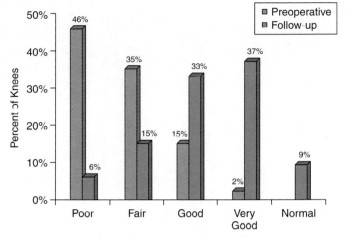

FIGURE 7–51. The preoperative and follow-up distribution of patient responses on the rating scale for pain. The improvement was significant ($P = .0001$). The scale shows the highest level of activity possible without the patient experiencing pain. *(From Noyes, F. R.; Barber-Westin, S. D.: Revision anterior cruciate surgery with use of bone–patellar tendon–bone autogenous grafts. J Bone Joint Surg Am 83:1131–1143, 2001.)*

FIGURE 7–52. The preoperative and follow-up distribution of patient responses on the rating scale for perception of the overall knee condition. The improvement was significant ($P = .0001$). *(From Noyes, F. R.; Barber-Westin, S. D.: Revision anterior cruciate surgery with use of bone–patellar tendon–bone autogenous grafts. J Bone Joint Surg Am 83:1131–1143, 2001.)*

TABLE 7–16 Effect of Additional Operative Procedures on Outcome of Anterior Cruciate Ligament Bone–Patellar Tendon–Bone Revision Reconstruction

	Pain (points)			Patient Perception (points)			Graft Failure Rate (%)	Overall Rating Score (points)		
	Preoperative	Follow-up	P Value	Preoperative	Follow-up	P Value	Follow-up	Preoperative	Follow-up	P Value
Revision with no other major operative procedures ($N = 32$)	4.1 ± 1.7	5.7 ± 0.7	.0001	3.2 ± 1.6	7.1 ± 1.6	.0001	16	64 ± 10	91 ± 8	.0001
Revision staged after HTO ($N = 9^\dagger$)	$2.9 \pm 1.4^*$	4.9 ± 2.0	.05	2.0 ± 1.4	$4.3 \pm 1.9^*$	.03	??	$53 \pm 9^*$	$81 \pm 10^*$	.0004
Revision and other ligament procedure ($N = 17^\dagger$)	3.5 ± 1.7	4.7 ± 2.3	.05	3.2 ± 1.9	4.8 ± 2.2	.02	35^*	$56 \pm 9^*$	$84 \pm 12^*$	.0001

*The value was significantly different from that in the subgroup with revision and no other major procedure ($P < .05$)
†Three knees had both a high tibial osteotomy (HTO) and another ligament procedure.

and reported no clinically relevant difference existed in KT-2000 and pivot shift test data. The mean difference between the reconstructed and the contralateral knee on KT-2000 testing was 0.5 mm and there was no difference in the odds of having a normal or nearly normal pivot shift result between reconstruction methods.

The outcome of ACL revision reconstruction using autogenous graft sources has been described by many investigators (Table 7–19). The most common autograft source is the B-PT-B,* followed by the STG tendons[49,54,144,161,177,181] and the quadriceps tendon.[57,193] The failure rates of these graft sources vary greatly, and most investigations followed patients an average of less than 5 years postoperatively. Authors agree that the outcomes of revision reconstruction remain inferior to that

of primary ACL procedures, usually owing to preexisting articular cartilage damage and loss of meniscal tissue.[58,195] Problems with published studies were recently reviewed by George and colleagues[58] who cited small cohorts, heterogeneous populations, and lack of concurrent control groups as issues preventing definitive conclusions on the optimal treatment for these knees.

Although authors of early studies[18,36] postulated that reharvest of the ipsilateral patellar tendon was feasible for revision reconstruction, others disagreed.[20,85,88,93] Kartus and coworkers[85] compared the results of 12 knees in which the ipsilateral patellar tendon was reharvested with 12 knees that received contralateral patellar tendon grafts for ACL revision reconstruction. Two years postoperatively, no differences were found between the subgroups on MRI for patellar ligament length, width, thickness, or donor site gap measurements. However, the knees

*See references 34, 41, 43, 44, 85, 111, 145, 168, 177, 181, 183, 193, 194.

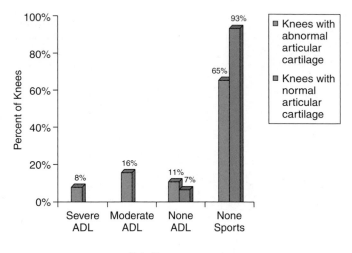

FIGURE 7–53. Comparison of the pain scores at the most recent follow-up evaluation between 28 knees with normal articular cartilage and 37 knees with abnormal articular cartilage. The difference between groups was significant ($P < .05$). Severe ADL, severe pain (constant, not relieved) with activities of daily living; moderate ADL, moderate pain (frequent, limiting) with activities of daily living; none ADL, no pain with activities of daily living but pain with any sports activity; and none sports, no pain with sports activity. *(From Noyes, F. R.; Barber-Westin, S. D.; Roberts, C. S.: Use of allografts after failed treatment of rupture of the anterior cruciate ligament. J Bone Joint Surg Am 76:1019–1031, 1994.)*

TABLE 7–17   Effect of the Condition of the Articular Cartilage at the Anterior Cruciate Ligament Allograft Revision Reconstruction on the Subjective Scores and Overall Rating at the Latest Follow-up Examination

Variable	Point Scale	Patients Who Had Normal Articular Cartilage* (mean ± SD)	Patients Who Had Abnormal Articular Cartilage (mean ± SD)	P Value
Pain	0–6	5.9 ± 0.5	4.6 ± 2.1	.03
Swelling	0–6	5.8 ± 0.6	5.2 ± 1.4	NS
Partial giving-way	0–6	5.9 ± 0.4	5.2 ± 1.5	NS
Full giving-way	0–6	6.0	5.5 ± 1.4	NS
Walking	0–40	38 ± 4	34 ± 8	NS
Stair-climbing	0–40	36 ± 5	29 ± 11	.01
Kneeling	0–40	28 ± 14	21 ± 14	.01
Running	40–100	84 ± 18	61 ± 21	.001
Jumping	40–100	78 ± 21	57 ± 22	.01
Twisting and turning	40–100	73 ± 21	55 ± 20	.01
Overall rating	0–100			
Follow-up		85 ± 9	71 ± 12	.0001
Improvement from preoperative		26 ± 10	21 ± 11	NS

*Abnormal was defined as fissuring and fragmentation of 15 mm or more in diameter that extended into more than one half of the involved surface or any exposed subchondral bone.
NS, not significant; SD, standard deviation.

that received the reharvested grafts had lower functional scores and a higher rate of complications including 1 patellar fracture and 1 patellar ligament rupture postoperatively. Three investigations involving small case series of patients (8–13) found no obvious deleterious effect of this procedure.[34,145,194] Only two authors[85,168] investigated the use of the contralateral patellar tendon after failure of knees in which the ipsilateral patellar tendon had previously been harvested.

Recently, reports have documented acceptable outcomes after STG revision reconstructions.[49,161,189] Ferretti and coworkers[49] followed a group of 30 knees that received an ACL revision STG autograft and an extra-articular ITB tenodesis. The failure rate was 10%. It should be noted that these authors used a procedure in which the strip of ITB was looped around the lateral structures including the FCL, which is not at the ideal "isometric" attachment site. The description of the ITB tenodesis procedure in this chapter specifically avoids placing the graft around the FCL for this reason. The ITB graft is secured to the proximal aspect of the lateral femoral condyle just distal to the lateral intramuscular septum to reproduce the posterior attachment of the ITB at this location.

Salmon and associates[161] followed 50 patients who received this operation and documented a 10% failure rate. However, only 56% of the knees were rated as normal or nearly normal according to the IKDC rating. The poor subjective and functional outcomes were related to the degree of joint (articular cartilage) damage. Weiler and colleagues[189] reported a 6.5% graft failure in 62 patients who underwent four-strand STG ACL revision. However, compared with a group of knees that had primary ACL STG reconstruction, the revision patients had inferior subjective knee function results. A greater percentage of the revision knees had undergone prior meniscectomy, which may have lead to the poorer outcome.

O'Neill[144] performed ACL revision using STG in 23 patients and B-PT-B autografts in 25 patients. The patients were followed from 2 to 13 years postoperatively, at which time 73% of the reconstructions were rated as functional, 21% were partially functional, and 6% (3 grafts) failed. The failed grafts were from the B-PT-B group, which the author attributed to a "steep learning curve." In addition, these patients were followed the longest amount of time from surgery.

Thomas and colleagues[181] reported the outcome of a staged ACL revision procedure in 49 patients who required bone-grafting of the tibial tunnel first in order to achieve an anatomic ACL reconstruction. Thirty-four patients received a STG autograft and 15 had a B-PT-B autograft; all were followed a mean of 6.2 years postoperatively. The results were compared with those of a group of patients who underwent primary ACL reconstruction matched for age, gender, type of graft used, and follow-up time period. The revision patients demonstrated a greater number of meniscus tears and a significantly greater number of chondral lesions in the patellofemoral ($P = .015$) and lateral tibiofemoral compartments ($P < .001$) and had significantly lower IKDC subjective ($P = .006$) and objective ($P = .035$) scores than the primary ACL reconstruction group. There was no difference in instrumented laxity measurements. The results demonstrated that revision ACL knees without major associated instability, with abnormal bone tunnels grafted and bone quality restored, have a good success rate in terms of achieving postoperative stability. There were 2 failures in the revision group and 1 in the primary ACL reconstruction group. The results apply to knees that have intact secondary restraints, because knees requiring an additional

TABLE 7-18 Published Failure Rates of Anterior Cruciate Ligament Semitendinosus-Gracilis Double-Bundle Reconstructions

Reference, Level of Evidence	Number of Patients DB, SB, Follow-up	Postoperative Pivot Shift	Postoperative Knee Arthrometer Mean ± SD (mm)	Failure Rate	Authors' Recommend Double-Bundle?
Fu et al.[53] Level 4	100 DB 17 STG 83 Tibialis anterior allograft F/U 2 yr in 73 patients	94% Grade 0 6% Grade I	1.0 ± 2.3 mm 59% <3 mm 37% 3–5 mm 4% >5 mm	11% (8/73 patients who returned for 2-yr evaluations)	Yes
Kondo et al.[86] Level 2	171 DB 157 SB F/U 24–60 mo	DB: 81% Grade 0 16% Grade I 3% Grade II–III SB: 51% Grade 0 37% Grade I 12% Grade II–III P < .0001	DB: 1.2 ± 1.9 3% >5 mm SB: 2.5 ± 2.5 12% >5 mm P < .0001	DB: 5% SB: 12% P < .05	Yes, but for objective stability only, no difference in subjective function.
Siebold et al.[170] Level 1	35 DB 35 SB F/U mean, 19 mo (range, 13–24 mo)	DB: 97% Grade 0 3% Grade I SB: 71% Grade 0 29% Grade I P < .01	DB: 1.0 (range, 0–4) SB: 1.6 (range, 0–5) P = .054	DB: 3% (traumatic rerupture) SB: 0%	Yes, but no difference in subjective function
Streich et al.[176] Level 1	24 DB 24 SB F/U 23–25 mo	DB: 96% Grade 0 4% Grade I SB: 76% Grade 0 24% Grade I P = NS	DB: 0.94 ± 1.76 79% <3 mm 21% 3–5 mm SB: 1.10 ± 1.57 80% <3 mm 20% 3–5 mm P = NS	0% both groups	No
Jarvela et al.[80] Level 1	23 DB 26 SBB 24 SBM F/U 24–35 mo	DB: 82% Grade 0 18% Grade I SBB: 76% Grade 0 19% Grade I 5% Grade II SBM: 50% Grade 0 50% Grade I P < .05 DB vs. SBM	DB: 1.3 ± 2.1 SBB: 2.2 ± 2.9 SBM: 2.1 ± 2.0 P = NS	DB: 4% (traumatic rerupture) SBB: 23% (5/6 traumatic rerupture) SBM: 4% (traumatic rerupture) P < .05 DB vs. SBB & SBM	Yes for rotational stability, no difference between groups in subjective knee functional scores.
Asagumo et al.[11] Level 3	71 DB 52 SB F/U 24–36 mo	DB: 87% Grade 0 10% Grade I 3% Grade II SB: 81% Grade 0 14% Grade I 5% Grade II P = NS	DB 1.7 ± 2.0 93% ≤3 mm SB: 1.9 ± 2.2 90% ≤3 mm	DB: 4% SB: 5%	No, extension deficit 26% DB, 10% SB 5 knees DB ruptured PL bundle

Continued

TABLE 7-18 Published Failure Rates of Anterior Cruciate Ligament Semitendinosus-Gracilis Double-Bundle Reconstructions—Cont'd

Reference, Level of Evidence	Number of Patients DB, SB, Follow-up	Postoperative Pivot Shift	Postoperative Knee Arthrometer Mean ± SD (mm)	Failure Rate^	Authors' Recommend Double-Bundle?
Muneta et al.[109] Level 1	34 DB 34 SB F/U 18–41 mo	DB: 85% Grade 0 15% Grade I SB: 59% Grade 0 41% Grade I $P < .05$	DB: 1.4 ± 1.4 (range, −2–+4 mm) SB: 2.4 ± 1.4 (range, −1–+6 mm) $P < .05$	0% both groups	Yes for objective stability only, no difference subjective knee function scores.
Aglietti et al.[3] Level 2	25 DBT 25 DB2 25 SB F/U 2 yr	DBT: 76% Grade 0 20% Grade I 4% Grade II DB2: 84% Grade 0 12% Grade I 4% Grade II SB: 58% Grade 0 34% Grade I 8% Grade II $P < .05$ DB2 vs. SB	DBT: 64% <3 mm 32% 3–5 mm 4% >5 mm DB2: 80% <3 mm 16% 3–5 mm 4% >5 mm SB: 58% <3 mm 34% 3–5 mm 8% >5 mm $P < .05$ DB2 vs. SB	DBT: 4% DB2: 4% SB: 8%	Yes for DBT technique
Yagi et al.[198] Level 2	20 DB 20 SBA 20 SBP F/U 1 yr	DB: 85% Grade 0 15% Grade I SBA: 75% Grade 0 15% Grade I 10% Grade II SBP: 80% Grade 0 5% Grade I 15% Grade II $P = NS$	DB: 1.3 ± 1.2 SBA: 1.9 ± 1.6 SBP: 1.7 ± 1.7 $P = NS$	DB: 0% SBA: 10% SBP: 15%	Yes, but more data required for definitive recommendation
Yasuda et al.[202] Level 2	24 DBA 24 DBN 24 SB F/U 2 yr	DBA: 100% Grade 0 DBN: 87% Grade 0 13% Grade I SB: 50% Grade 0 37% Grade I 13% Grade II $P = .025$ SB vs. DBA	DBA: 1.1 DBN: 2.2 SB: 2.8 $P = .002$ SB vs. DBA	DBA: 0% DBN: 12.5% SB: 12.5%	Yes for objective stability, no difference in subjective function scores.
Colombet et al.[33] Level 4	33 DB F/U 18–31 mo	84% Grade 0 9% Grade I 6% Grade II	0.9 ± 1.9 81% <3 mm 16% 3–5 mm 3% >5 mm	9%	Preliminary study, results encouraging

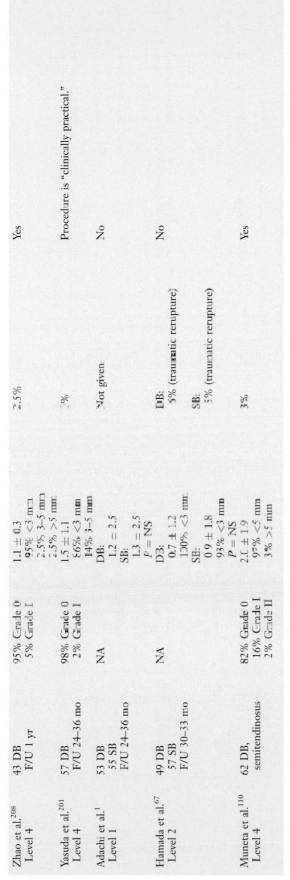

Study	Procedure / F/U	IKDC	Laxity	Failure	Anatomic
Zhao et al.[208] Level 4	43 DB F/U 1 yr	95% Grade 0 5% Grade I	1.1 ± 0.3 95% <3 mm 2.5% 3–5 mm 2.5% >5 mm	2.5%	Yes
Yasuda et al.[201] Level 4	57 DB F/U 24–36 mo	98% Grade 0 2% Grade I	1.5 ± 1.1 86% <3 mm 14% 3–5 mm	?%	Procedure is "clinically practical."
Adachi et al.[1] Level 1	53 DB 55 SB F/U 24–36 mo	NA	DB: 1.2 ± 2.5 SB: 1.3 ± 2.5 P = NS	Not given	No
Hamada et al.[67] Level 2	49 DB 57 SB F/U 30–33 mo	NA	DB: 0.7 ± 1.2 100% <3 mm SB: 0.9 ± 1.8 93% <3 mm P = NS	DB: 5% (traumatic rerupture) SB: 5% (traumatic rerupture)	No
Muneta et al.[110] Level 4	62 DB, semitendinosus	82% Grade 0 16% Grade I 2% Grade II	2.0 ± 1.9 97% <5 mm 3% >5 mm	3%	Yes

DB, double-burdle; DB2, double-bundle, two-incision; DBA, double-bundle, anatomic; DBI, double-bundle, transtibial; F/U, follow-up; NA, not applicable; NS, not significant; PL, posterolateral; SB, single-bundle; SBA, single-bundle, anatomic; DBN, double-bundle, nonanatomic; SBB, single-bundle, anteromedial bundle; SM, single-bundle, metallic screw; SBP, single-bundle, posterolateral bundle; SD, standard deviation; STG, semitendinosus-gracilis.

TABLE 7–19 Clinical Outcome Data of ACL Revision Reconstruction

Reference	Number Patients Seen/Entered into Study, Follow-up	Graft(s) Used	Other Ligament Instabilities, Procedures	KT-1000 Results	Pivot Shift Results	Subjective and Functional Results	Authors' Comments
Diamantopoulos et al.[41]	N = 107/148, Mean 72.9 ± 20.6 mo (range, 36–111 mo)	STG: 45, PT autograft: 41, QT autograft: 21	Not provided	Mean KT 0.93 ± 1.15 mm, 85% <3 mm, 8.4% 3–5 mm, 6.6% >5 mm	74% negative, 16% glide, 10% clunk	IKDC subjective: 65% NL, nearly NL, 35% abnormal; IKDC Symptoms: 80% NL, nearly NL, 20% abnormal	Early revisions better results, meniscal and chondral lesions correlated with poorer reults.
Weiler et al.[189]	N = 50/55, Mean 2.5 ± 1.8 yr	STG quadrupled	MCL 5 patients	Mean KT 2.1 ± 1.6 mm	36 negative, 12 glide, 2 clunk	Lysholm mean preoperative: 65 ± 17, F/U, 90 ± 9 points	Inferior subjective results compared with primary ACL STG; no difference in knee stability.
Ferretti et al.[49]	N = 28/30, Mean 5 yr (range, 2–8 yr)	STG (doubled) + EA	None	71% <3 mm, 21% 3–5 mm, 7% >5 mm	10% failed KT & pivot shift (grade II or III)	IKDC subjective: 93% NL, nearly NL, 7% abnormal; All patients satisfied	Fewer patients in IKDC normal category compared with primary STG ACL patients. STG & EA preferred revision technique.
Salmon et al.[161]	N = 50/57, Mean 7.4 yr (range, 5–9 yr)	STG four-strand	None	50% <3 mm, 50% 3–5 mm, 5 (10%) failed, no KT done	69% 0, 31% Grade I	IKDC overall: 50% NL, nearly NL, 50% abnormal; IKDC Symptoms: 37% abnormal	11 patients sustained contralateral ACL tear. Poor results correlated with articular cartilage damage.
Garofalo et al.[57]	N = 28/31, Mean 4.2 yr (range 3.3–5.6 yr)	QT autograft	None	65% <3 mm, 32% 3–5 mm, 3% >5 mm	75% negative, 25% Grade I+	93% returned to preinjury sports levels (IKDC), 93% rated knee NL or nearly NL	QT viable graft option for revision.
Grossman et al.[65]	N = 29/35, Mean 5.6 yr (range, 3–9 yr)	PT allograft: 22, AT allograft: 1, PT autograft: 6	None	Mean KT allograft: 3.21, autograft: 1.33 ($P <.05$)	1 failure (allograft)	100% satisfied, 68% returned to sports	Recommends early revision, results inferior to primary reconstruction.
Thomas et al.[181]	N = 49/49, Mean 6.2 yr (range, 3–11 yr)	STG: 34, PT autograft: 15, All two-stage tibial tunnel bone graft	None	Westminster cruciometer (89 N): 94% <3 mm, 2% 3–4 mm, 4% ≥5 mm	NA	IKDC subjective: Mean 61.2 ± 19.6 points	Staged procedure effective in restoration of stability. Subjective and functional results inferior to primary reconstruction.
O'Neill[144]	N = 48, Mean 7.5 yr (range, 2–13 yr)	All ipsilateral, no graft reharvested, PT autograft: 25, STG: 23	None	73% <3 mm, 21% 3–5 mm, 6% >5 mm (all PT)	KT-1000 & pivot shift tests used to determine graft function	IKDC ratings: 84% NL, nearly NL, 12% abnormal, 4% severely abnormal	PT failures endoscopic technique: high learning curve & also longest F/U.
Fox et al.[52]	N = 32/38, Mean 4.8 yr (range, 2–12 yr)	PT allograft: fresh-frozen	None	84% <3 mm, 9% 3–5 mm, 6% >5 mm	29% Grade I, 3% Grade II	87% Satisfied	Subjective results worse than primary reconstructions, correlated with arthrosis.
Taggart et al.[177]	N = 20/26, Mean 3.4 yr (range, 1.1–5.3 yr)	PT allograft: 7, PT autograft: 7, STG: 6	None	40% <3 mm, 25% 3–5 mm, 35% >5 mm	60% Grade 0, I, 40% Grade II, III	40% returned to preinjury sports, 90% would have surgery again	6/7 failures had either PT allograft or STG, recommend PT autograft.

Study	Patients / Follow-up	Graft	Associated Procedure	Laxity	Pivot Shift	Outcome	Comments
Fules et al.[?]	N = 29, Mean 4.1 yr (range, 1–8.1 yr)	STG: 26, QT autograft: 2, PT autograft: 1, Used polyester femoral fixation device with STG, OTT technique	None	65% <3 mm, 31% 3–5 mm, 4% >5 mm	NA	IKDC ratings: 76% Nearly NL, 17% abnormal, 7% severely abnormal	1 Medial OA, 1 arthrofibrosis, 1 transient RSD. Most revisions done for failed prosthetic ligaments.
Shelbourne & O'Shea[168]	N = 31/61 objective data, N = 51/61 subjective data, Mean 3.5 yr (range, 2–9.1 yr)	PT autograft: contralateral	None	84% <3 mm, 13% 3–5 mm, 3% >5 mm	NA	69% Level I sports competitive, 18% Level I sports recreational	Lower scores correlated with arthrosis
O'Shea & Shelbourne[145]	N = 8/11, Mean 4.1 yr (range, 2.1–5.6 yr)	PT autograft: reharvested	None	All <3 mm	NA	Means only given	
Colosimo et al.[34]	N = 13/15, Mean 3.2 yr (range, 2–5.4 yr)	PT autograft: reharvested	None	92% ≤3 mm, 8% 3–5 mm	15% Grade I	69% returned preinjury activity level	
Woods et al.[194]	N = 10/13, Mean 3.5 yr (range, 2–5.2 yr)	PT autograft: reharvested, lateral one third	None	7 ≤5 mm, 1 >5 mm	All negative	No problems ADL, 8 increased activity levels	
Eberhardt et al.[43]	N = 44/47, Mean 3.4 yr	PT autograft	None	41% <3 mm, 45% 3–5 mm, 14% >5 mm	5% Grade II	IKDC ratings: 75% NL, nearly NL	Progression arthrosis seen on x-ray.
Eberhardt et al.[4]	N = 24 semi-professional athletes, Mean 3.1 yr (range, 1–4.8 yr)	PT autograft	None	NA	3% positive	67% returned to sports, 63% pain with sports, 58% IKDC NL, nearly NL	63% progression arthrosis x-ray
Kartus et al.[85]	N = 24, Mean 2.1 yr (range, 1.6–2.7 yr)	PT autograft: Reharvest: 12, Contralateral: 12	None	63% <3 mm, 37% ≥3 mm	NA	IKDC ratings: 11 abnormal, 3 severely abnormal; reharvest group results inferior	MRI: no difference reharvest & contralateral PT
Johnson et al.[81]	N = 25, Mean 2.3 yr (range, 2–3 yr)	PT allograft: 13, AT allograft: 12, All irradiated	None	13% <3 mm, 48% 3–5 mm, 39% >5 mm	20% Grade II	IKDC ratings: 22 abnormal/severely abnormal, 76% satisfied, 90% no problems ADL	Patients improved, but results inferior to primary reconstruction.
Uribe et al.[183]	N = 54/64, Mean 2.5 yr (range, 1.6–6.5 yr)	PT autograft: 33 (no reharvest), STG: 2, PT allograft: 19	5 posteromedial or posterolateral reconstruction	Mean: PT autograft 2.2 = 1.3 mm, PT allograft 3.3 ± 1.5 mm	24% Grade I, 2% Grade II, 6% soft endpoint, possible failure	All satisfied, 54% returned to preinjury activity level	Results inferior to primary reconstruction.
Wirth & Kohn[193]	N = 87, Mean 8 yr (range, 2–18 yr)	PT autograft: 57, QT autograft: 30	AMRI: 42, AMRI + ALRI: 33, AMRI + ALRI + PLRI: 7	None	None, Lechman not given	60% satisfied, 75% symptomatic	Results inferior, correlated with arthrosis.

ACL, anterior cruciate ligament; ADL, activities of daily living; ALRI, anterolateral rotatory instability; AMRI, anteromedial rotatory instability; AT, Achilles tendon; EA, extra-articular; F/U, follow-up; IKDC, International Knee Documentations Committee; MCL, medial collateral ligament; MRI, magnetic resonance imaging; NA, not available; NL, normal; OA, osteoarthritis; OTT, over the top; PLRI, posterolateral rotatory instability; PT, patellar tendon; QT, quadriceps tendon; RSD, reflex sympathetic dystrophy; STG, semitendinosus-gracilis tendons.

medial or lateral ligament reconstruction were excluded and 9 of the 49 knees (18%) had only 3 to 4 mm of increased anterior tibial displacement before the operative procedure.

Only a few investigators[57,193] have reported outcome using the QT-PB autograft for ACL revision reconstruction. Garofalo and coworkers[57] followed 28 patients 3.3 to 5.6 years postoperatively at which time 25% had a grade 1+ pivot shift and only 1 graft failed. Patient satisfaction was high, with 93% grading their knee condition as normal or nearly normal.

Fewer reports have appeared on the outcome of ACL revision reconstruction using allograft tissue (see Table 7–19).[52,60,65,81,174,177,183] Grossman and associates[65] followed 29 patients, of whom 23 received allografts for the ACL revision and 6 had a B-PT-B autograft. The allograft knees had a significantly higher (P < .05) average KT-1000 value (3.21 mm) than the autografts (1.33 mm), and 1 allograft failed. All patients felt the knee condition was improved and would undergo the operation again. The condition of the articular cartilage had a significant effect on the subjective outcome. Fox and colleagues[52] followed 32 patients who received fresh-frozen B-PT-B allografts from 2 to 12 years postoperatively. The authors excluded patients who required other ligament reconstructions, HTOs, and meniscus transplants. Preoperatively, only 9% of these patients had greater than 5 mm increased anterior tibial translation on knee arthrometer testing. At follow-up, 84% had a functional reconstruction, 9% had partial function, and 6% failed.

Johnson and coworkers[81] reported the results of 25 consecutive patients who received fresh-frozen irradiated B-PT-B or Achilles tendon allograft revision ACL reconstructions. All patients were followed between 24 and 36 months postoperatively. Nine patients (36%) had failed grafts, with greater than 5 mm increased translation on KT-1000 testing. Seventeen patients (68%) could perform at least light sports activities without pain, swelling, or giving-way. Nineteen patients (76%) were satisfied with their results.

Getelman and associates[60] compared the results of 14 patients who had fresh-frozen B-PT-B allografts with those of 12 patients who had ipsilateral B-PT-B autogenous grafts. The patients were followed between 20 and 34 months postoperatively. The allograft group had poorer IKDC rating scores (normal or nearly normal, 29% allografts and 67% autografts; P < .05), which were related to patellofemoral crepitus and radiographic evidence of joint narrowing. There were 5 failures in the study; however, the authors did not indicate whether these were from the allograft or the autograft subgroup.

Uribe and colleagues[183] followed 54 patients between 2 and 6.5 years postoperatively. Nineteen received B-PT-B allografts and 35 had autogenous grafts (ipsilateral or contralateral patellar tendon or STG tendons). The allograft group had a significantly greater mean increase in KT-1000 test scores than the autograft group (3.3 ± 1.5 mm and 2.2 ± 1.3 mm, respectively; P < .005). Three knees (6%) had a soft endpoint; however, the authors did not indicate which type of graft these knees had received. Twenty-nine patients (54%) returned to their preinjury level of activity. All patients felt they had benefited from the surgery and none reported recurrent giving-way postoperatively.

PREVENTION AND MANAGEMENT OF COMPLICATIONS

Arthrofibrosis and Limitation of Knee Motion

The postoperative complications of arthrofibrosis (either primary or secondary) or a limitation of knee flexion and extension resulting from other factors such as a cyclops lesion are frequently reported problems after ACL reconstruction. The causes, risk factors, preventive measures, and effective treatment strategies for knee motion complications are discussed in detail in Chapter 41, Prevention and Treatment of Knee Arthrofibrosis. In addition, the reader is referred to the authors' postoperative rehabilitation protocols provided in Chapter 13, Rehabilitation of Primary and Revision Anterior Cruciate Ligament Reconstructions, for comprehensive exercises and modalities used after ACL reconstruction.

Infection

Deep joint infection after ACL reconstruction is a rare problem, occurring in approximately 0.14% to 1.70% of patients according to recent literature.[26,51,76,82,101,187,192] Matava and colleagues[99] conducted a survey in which 61 orthopaedic surgeons participated to determine the preferred treatment recommendations for postoperative infection. The infecting organism and systemic signs of sepsis were viewed as the most important factors in determining the initial treatment. Arthroscopic débridement and irrigation as early as possible was recommended by the majority; this protocol is also supported by several more recently published studies.[26,101,163,184,192] The majority of surgeons in Matava and colleagues' survey[99] (85%) used culture-specific intravenous antibiotics and attempted to retain the ACL graft when possible. Graft excision and hardware removal were reserved for resistant infections that required multiple débridement procedures. Immediate graft removal was recommended by only 6% of surgeons treating infected autografts and 33% of those treating infected allografts. Only one half of the surgeons surveyed routinely used a drain after ACL reconstruction. The infection rate was twice as high for these surgeons than for those who did not use a drain (0.27% and 0.10%, respectively; P = .04). The authors stressed that although obtaining a stable knee is the primary goal of ACL reconstruction, eradication of infection supersedes graft preservation in order to avoid the deleterious consequences of a chronic infection.

Critical Points PREVENTION AND MANAGEMENT OF COMPLICATIONS

- Rules to prevent and treat infection are summarized in Table 7–20.
- Graft contamination: Prefer harvest second autograft. In allograft procedure, discard and use second allograft.
- Fluid extravasation: Be constantly aware of joint pressure, fluid inflow and outflow, increased thigh tension, any lack of joint distention during arthroscopic procedures. Palpate popliteal and calf region during procedure.

TABLE 7–20   Rules to Prevent and Treat Postoperative Infection

1. Obtain a preoperative history of the patient's health and diet, perform a general assessment of nutritional status and the need for vitamin supplementation (including vitamin C). A history of prior infections, methicillin-resistant *Staphylococcus aureus* requires infectious disease consultation (e.g., preoperative nasal swab).
2. Preoperative preparation to avoid postoperative anemia with low hemoglobin values, menstruation issues. Consider appropriate serum iron, iron-binding capacity studies, and others.
3. Conduct a skin evaluation, avoid skin rashes or sores, have the patient conduct a preoperative antibacterial wash from the toes to groin the evening before and the morning of surgery, use hair clippers (instead of a razor) in the preanesthetic room.
4. Administer antibiotics 1 hr before surgery, confirm at "time-out" (when the limb to be reconstructed is signed by both patient and surgeon), repeat antibiotics for longer cases based on half-life (usually 4 hr for most cephalosporins). Repeat intravenous antibiotics in recovery room and over 24 hr if admitted.
5. Use skin preparation agent of choice in meticulous manner, occlusive skin dressing.
6. Careful planning of skin incision in knees with prior incisions to avoid flap necrosis or delayed healing. Perform a meticulous dissection of skin flaps beneath the fascial plane and not directly in the subcutaneous plane to protect the blood supply. Avoid undue skin tension and retraction, avoid grasping the skin with forceps, use blunt retractors instead of sharp rakes, and observe skin viability after the tourniquet has been deflated. Use tourniquet only as required. Perform a meticulous closure, do not place tension on skin Steri-Strips to prevent blister formation with postoperative edema.
7. Operative technique issues: Perform sharp dissection and a meticulous gentle handling of soft tissues, avoid a "blunt finger" or "sponge" dissection. Limit the number of times that fingers are "poked" into the wound by using instruments instead of fingers. Débride devitalized soft tissues, limit the dissection to only the operative site. Use meticulous hemostasis, maintain the blood supply to tissues, limit electrocoagulation to direct operative site. Use the least number of nonabsorbable sutures possible, limit suture load to that which is required, and close all dead spaces. Deflate the tourniquet prior to closure, and limit operative time with trained staff.
8. Operating room staff issues: Staff double-checks operative instrument pack sterility markers, avoid operating rooms used for general surgery and infectious cases (even though assured that clean room is reestablished in the "perfect world"). Conduct a monthly check of the incidence of infections or undue occurrence of infections within operating room. Document hospital procedures to detect remote infections, share information with surgeons and hospital infectious committee. Limit traffic in and out of the operating room. Cover all hair on head, use long operative gowns when the knee is flexed over bed, closely monitor for any break in sterility.
9. Postoperative dressing: Double cotton–double elastic bandage (Robert Jones dressing) to provide firm uniform compression, avoid rewrap unless a problem occurs. If the dressing becomes loose, rewrap, maintain for 48–72 hr, then replace with elastic stocking and supplemental elastic bandage for added compression. The goal is to prevent hematoma and soft tissue swelling without compromise of skin circulation. Use commercial ice delivery systems, maintain limb elevation, avoid limb-dependent conditions. Avoid use of drains unless specifically indicated. Frequently check wound and joint based on surgery performed, recheck for calf tenderness, perform deep venous thrombosis assessment.
10. First postoperative day: Patient performs active quadriceps co-contraction with hamstrings, must show active muscle contraction, which is repeated every hour. The patient places a hand on the thigh to monitor quadriceps firmness and turgor. Ankle pumps are performed every hour while awake.
11. Intraoperative meticulous coagulation of any intra-articular bleeding sites during procedure. Aspirate knee joint hematoma on first postoperative day, or subsequently if tense, painful, or over approximately 50 ml.
12. Patient takes oral temperature during day and importantly at night and records results. The surgeon is notified immediately if temperature reaches 101°F. The surgeon is also notified if the patient maintains a low-grade temperature or experiences persistent joint pain, redness, warmth, and increased swelling.
13. Conduct a careful weekly assessment of the wound for redness, swelling, or any other signs of infection. Maintain a low tolerance for knee joint aspiration and fluid analysis (cells, gram stain, sugar, cultures) for any abnormal signs suggesting infection such as low-grade temperature; persistent joint swelling, redness, or warmth; failure to achieve dry knee within first 2–3 wk of surgery. Repeat blood studies as necessary (use sedimentation rate, C-reactive protein studies, although often not helpful 4–6 wk postoperative owing to elevation from surgery). Clinical findings alone are sufficient to proceed with emergent arthroscopic washout and soft tissue cultures as described later.
14. Occurrence of postoperative infection

    a. Immediate emergent arthroscopic washout and arthroscopic débridement of devitalized tissues, intravenous antibiotics switched to culture specific antibiotics when tissue cultures and gram stain are available. Recognize tissue specimens for culture rather than fluid aspirate. Magnetic resonance imaging (MRI) obtained before washout to assess soft tissue abscess, sinus tracks, and Baker's cyst, which may represent a closed abscess.
    b. First-time washout and débridement: Grafts and hardware left in place, consider removal if subsequent arthroscopic washout is required.
    c. Recognize frequent need to repeat washout after 48 hr.
    d. Do not stop gentle flexion and extension overpressure program, including patellar mobilization, to maintain knee motion; otherwise, a joint fibrosis will rapidly develop.

Continued

TABLE 7–20   Rules to Prevent and Treat Postoperative Infection—Cont'd

e. Open graft harvest wound or meniscus repair wound: If any local signs of infection are noted, opening of these wounds is not required in the majority of cases.

f. Recognize that cause of recurrent infection may be presence of Baker's cyst or other soft tissue abscess requiring open drainage. Repeat MRI is beneficial in resistant cases.

g. When major concurrent medial or lateral reconstructive procedure is involved, open the wounds and perform débridement. Proceed with secondary closure rules, allow granulation tissue formation, consider skin tension sutures to prevent abnormal skin contracture.

h. Closely inspect any soft tissue areas that are involved that would allow open drainage into joint. These require urgent treatment and soft tissue joint closure, including necessary muscle flaps in severe cases.

i. Close follow-up of infectious disease team to monitor progress, use appropriate blood studies, repeat aspiration as necessary, monitor for recurrence. Monitor carefully for osteomyelitis with residual hardware in osseous tunnels as shown by increasing edema signal intensity on repeat MRI.

j. Length of time on intravenous antibiotics is usually 4–6 wk based on organism and cultures, with a subsequent 6 wk of oral antibiotics. These programs are often empirical and based on surgeon and infectious disease team assessments.

Schulz and coworkers[163] treated 24 patients who developed postoperative septic arthritis after ACL reconstruction. The treatment protocol was based on the classification of the grade of infection proposed by Gachter[56] and included arthroscopic débridement, irrigation, partial to total synovectomy, and placement of intra-articular gentamicin-containing polymethylmethacrylate (PMMA) beads. The mean time from the ACL reconstruction to the first arthroscopic débridement was 62 days (range, 5–196 days). The ACL grafts had autodigested in 8 knees and were removed in 9 others. The infection resolved in all cases. Van Tongel and associates[184] described a series of 15 patients who underwent arthroscopic management of this complication, followed by intravenous antibiotics and then oral antibiotics. The infection resolved in all patients and the ACL grafts were retained in all but 1 knee.

Burks and colleagues[26] described a small series of four knees in whom graft removal was required during arthroscopic débridement and irrigation for septic arthritis. The patients developed the infection an average of 24 days postoperatively. The autografts had a fibrinous coating that led the authors to be concerned about the potentially deleterious effects of persistent infection or a delay in resolving the joint infection. All four patients had a revision ACL reconstruction between 1 and 6 weeks after completion of 6 weeks of antibiotics. At an average of 21 months postrevision, the patients had a normal range of knee motion and a mean of 3.0 mm (range, 1.9–4.0 mm) of increased anterior tibial displacement on KT-1000 testing.

The senior author has followed a series of operative rules over many years to prevent and treat operative infections; these are summarized in Table 7–20.

Graft Contamination

In 2005, Izquierdo and coworkers[77] reported the results of a survey of orthopaedic surgeons on the management of contaminated ACL grafts. This represented the first report to describe the clinical experience, management, and outcome of this problem. Of the 196 surgeons who participated, 57 had managed at least one contaminated graft in their career. The majority (75%) cleaned the graft and proceeded with the reconstruction. Others (18%) harvested a different graft or used an allograft. No infections were reported. The grafts that underwent cleansing were cleaned with either Hibiclens (Regent Medical, Norcross, GA) or chlorhexidine gluconate, using different protocols. The authors cautioned that potential side effects of graft cleansing should be considered, including increased polymorphonuclear granulocyte toxicity and impaired phagocytic efficiency, intra-articular reactive synovitis and chondrolysis, and increased postoperative morbidity. Basic science studies support a combination of chlorhexidine and triple antibiotic solution.[62]

Molina and associates[105] measured the incidence of positive cultures resulting from ACL specimens that were dropped on the operating room floor and then treated by soaking in one of three antimicrobial solutions: an antibiotic solution of neomycin and polymyxin B, a 10% providone-iodine solution, or a chlorhexidine gluconate solution. Sixty percent of the dropped specimens cultured positive, although the majority grew nonvirulent species. The incidence of specimens that tested positive after the treatment protocols was 24% for providone-iodine solution; 6% for antibiotic solution; and 2% for chlorhexidine gluconate solution. The authors recommended sterilization with chlorhexidine gluconate, although there was no significant difference in the incidence of positive cultures with this method compared with the antibiotic solution.

In the authors' experience, harvest of a second autograft may be preferred to graft cleansing. With an allograft procedure, the contaminated allograft is always discarded and substituted with another allograft.

Fluid Extravasation

The senior author and Spievack[142] conducted a cadaver study many years ago that determined a subtle mechanism for extra-articular fluid extravasation during arthroscopy. Weak tissues in the suprapatellar pouch or semimembranosus bursa ruptured at only moderate intra-articular pressures, with flexion of the knee markedly increasing these pressures. The recommendation was made that the surgeon be constantly aware of the joint pressure, fluid inflow and outflow, increased thigh tension, and any lack of joint distention during arthroscopic procedures. Intermittent palpation of the popliteal and calf region is performed during the operative procedure to detect fluid extravasation caused by an inadvertent puncture of the suprapatellar posterior capsule.[142]

ILLUSTRATIVE CASES

Case 1. A 47-year-old man presented 6 weeks after a left knee injury sustained during skiing. Physical examination revealed a moderate effusion, a severe restriction in knee motion of 0° to 30°, and moderate quadriceps atrophy. Radiographs demonstrated moderate loss of lateral tibiofemoral joint space (Fig. 7–54A). The patient underwent 2 months of physical therapy to improve his knee motion and muscle strength. The patient desired to return to his active lifestyle and was treated with an ACL B-PT-B autograft reconstruction. Under anesthesia, he had 5 mm of increased medial joint opening at 25° of flexion, no increase of medial joint opening at 0°, and a grade III pivot shift. A repair of a complex double longitudinal lateral meniscus tear was also performed. The patient had an extensive area of grade 2B articular cartilage damage on the undersurface of the patella.

The patient recovered with no problems and resumed tennis, squash, and skiing. At 11 years postoperatively, physical examination revealed a normal range of motion, no lateral compartment pain, a negative pivot shift, 2 mm increase in medial joint opening at 25° of flexion, and no increase in AP displacement on KT-2000 testing. However, radiographs demonstrated severe loss of lateral tibiofemoral joint space (see Fig. 7–54B).

He did well until 14 years postoperatively, when he slipped and fell onto his left knee. MRI revealed bilateral meniscus tears, and the patient underwent a partial medial and lateral meniscectomy. At that time, extensive grade 2B damage was noted on the lateral femoral condyle.

Authors' comment: This patient required 2 months of rehabilitation owing to muscle atrophy and limitation of motion prior to the initial ACL surgery. Because he had a grade III pivot shift, a B-PT-B autograft was selected instead of an STG autograft or allograft. Unfortunately, the lateral meniscus repair did not provide a long-term chondroprotective effect.

Case 2. A 44-year-old woman presented 5 weeks after a twisting injury sustained to her right knee while playing badminton. She had a mild effusion, 0° to 120° of knee motion, severe medial joint line pain, a grade II pivot shift, and 8 mm of increase in AP displacement on KT-2000 testing. The patient was treated conservatively for 1 month and wished to remain active in recreational softball and volleyball. She underwent an endoscopic ACL B-PT-B autograft reconstruction. There were no meniscal tears; however, fissuring and fragmentation were noted on the undersurface of the patella.

One year postoperatively, the patient complained of pain over the tibial hardware and saphenous nerve. She underwent removal of the tibial interference screw and scar tissue resection. No neuroma was identified. This procedure successfully resolved her pain, and she returned to softball without problems.

At the most recent follow-up evaluation, 11 years postoperatively, the patient had a normal range of knee motion, no effusion, no joint line pain, a negative pivot shift, and 3 mm of increase in AP displacement on KT-2000 testing. Radiographs demonstrated preservation of the medial and lateral tibiofemoral joint spaces (Fig. 7–55). She had no symptoms with low-impact activities and rated the overall condition of her knee as good.

Authors' comment: This case, 11 years after ACL reconstruction with intact menisci and no evidence of arthritis, is in marked contrast to the frequent occurrence of arthritis that develops in the long term in patients who undergo meniscectomy.

Case 3. An 18-year-old male collegiate athlete presented 2 weeks after an acute twisting injury sustained to his right knee while playing basketball. He had a mild effusion, medial and lateral joint line pain, a grade II pivot shift, and 13.5 mm of increased AP displacement on KT-2000 testing. He was treated 4 months later with an ACL B-PT-B autograft and bilateral meniscus repairs

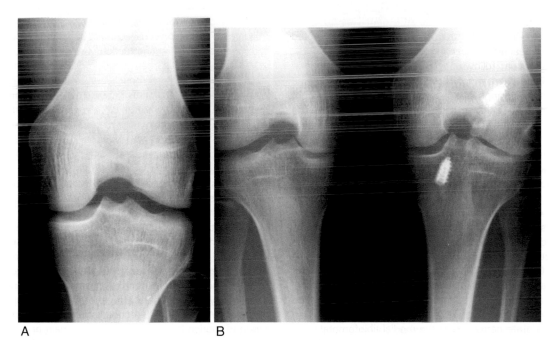

A   B

FIGURE 7–54. Case 1.

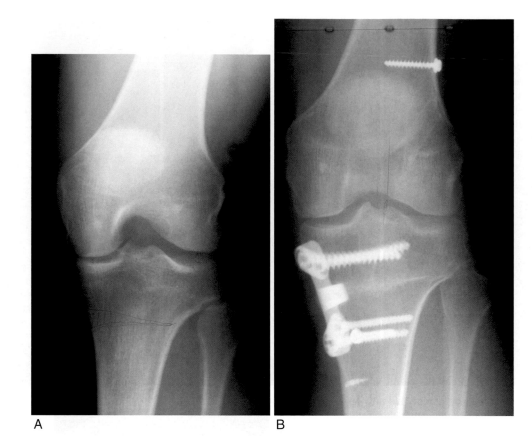

FIGURE 7–57. Case 4.

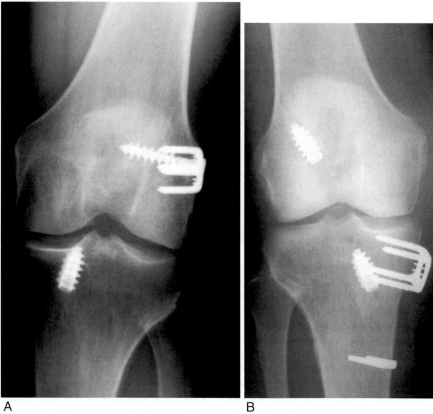

FIGURE 7–58. Case 5.

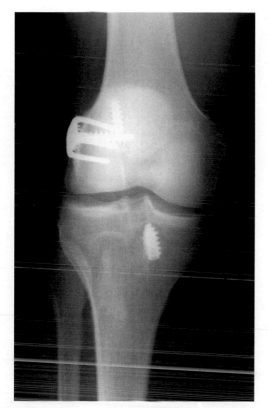

FIGURE 7–59. Case 6.

a recent hyperextension injury. Physical examination revealed no effusion, a mild loss of extension, a grade II pivot shift, and 7 mm of increase in lateral joint opening at 25° of flexion.

The patient was treated with an ACL B-PT-B reconstruction, a proximal advancement of the PL complex (Fig. 7–59), a repair of a complex medial meniscus tear, and a repair of a peripheral lateral meniscus tear. There was grade 2B articular cartilage damage noted on the medial femoral condyle and medial tibial plateau.

At follow-up, 3 years postoperatively, the patient had no effusion, a normal range of motion, no tibiofemoral compartment pain, no crepitus, a negative pivot shift, 2 mm of increase in lateral joint opening at 25° of flexion, and no increase in AP displacement on KT-2000 testing. He had no problems with basketball and rated the overall condition of his knee as normal.

Authors' comment: The treatment of a concurrent PL ligament injury with an ACL rupture requires different procedures, described in Chapter 22, Posterolateral Ligament Injuries: Diagnosis, Operative Techniques, and Clinical Outcomes. In this case, FCL and PLS appeared normal, representing a prior interstitial tear with subsequent healing. Therefore, a more simplified proximal advancement procedure restored PL stability.

Case 7. A 19-year-old male presented 2 years after a failed ACL B-PT-B autograft reconstruction. The procedure had been done for symptoms of full giving-way and pain 16 months after a left knee injury sustained during a hockey game. Although the patient completed a rigorous postoperative rehabilitation program, his giving-way symptoms persisted. He had given up all sports activities and noted generalized pain with daily activities. Physical examination demonstrated no effusion, a full range of

knee motion, a grade III pivot shift, and 16.5 mm of increased AP displacement on KT-2000 testing. The patient also had 5 mm of increased lateral joint opening at 25° of flexion, but no increase in external tibial rotation. He had a bilateral varus thrust on ambulation and increased recurvatum of the left knee. Full standing radiographs revealed bilateral varus malalignment, with a weight-bearing line of 20% on the involved left knee (Fig. 7–60A) and 40% on the contralateral right knee.

The patient underwent a closing wedge HTO, followed 4 months later with a two-incision ACL B-PT-B autogenous reconstruction. During the procedure, the lateral tibiofemoral gap test was normal, indicating that a PL procedure was not required. The B-PT-B graft was harvested from the contralateral knee. A new femoral tunnel, required to achieve anatomic graft placement on the lateral wall, was positioned adjacent to the previous tunnel. Fixation was achieved with interference screws proximally and distally. The patient had grade 2A articular cartilage damage on the medial femoral condyle, and a stable lateral meniscus tear that did not require treatment.

At the most recent follow-up evaluation, 10 years postoperatively, the patient had no effusion, a normal range of knee motion, a grade 0 pivot shift, and 1 mm of increase in AP displacement on KT-2000 testing. He had no symptoms with light recreational activities and rated the overall condition of his knee as good. Standing PA radiographs at 45° of flexion showed no difference between the noninvolved (see Fig. 7–60B) and the involved knees (see Fig. 7–60C), with only mild narrowing of the medial tibiofemoral joint space.

Authors' comment: In revision knees, the authors prefer autogenous grafts owing to the higher success rate compared with that of allografts. Contralateral graft harvest carries low postoperative morbidity, with careful attention to handling of soft tissue and bone-grafting of the patellar and tibial defects. In this case, a closing wedge osteotomy of the tibia and fibular neck was performed, protecting the proximal tibiofibular joint and proximal fibular ligament attachments. The authors favor opening wedge osteotomy, which does not require fibular osteotomy and is described in Chapter 31, Primary, Double, and Triple Varus Knee Syndromes: Diagnosis, Osteotomy Techniques, and Clinical Outcomes.

Case 8. A 40-year-old man presented 5 years after a failed ACL allograft reconstruction on the right knee. The operative procedure had included a LAD placed with the allograft, a primary repair of the MCL, a lateral meniscus repair, a medial meniscus repair, and a proximal patellar realignment. The patient had also undergone an ACL allograft reconstruction on the left knee 2 years after the right knee procedure. Upon the initial evaluation, he described a feeling of looseness in the right knee, which began gradually but had recently become more symptomatic, although he had not experienced full giving-way episodes. He had given up all sports activities and desired an active lifestyle. Physical examination demonstrated a full range of knee motion, a grade III pivot shift test, and moderate crepitus in the lateral tibiofemoral compartment. There was normal axial alignment and no valgus alignment, requiring corrective osteotomy.

The patient was treated with a revision ACL B-PT-B autogenous reconstruction of the right knee and a repair of a complex longitudinal medial meniscus tear located at the red-white junction. The allograft and LAD were removed and the autogenous graft placed in the previous bone tunnels, because they were in an anatomically correct position. Fixation was achieved with an

The patient was treated with an ACL B-PT-B autogenous reconstruction using the contralateral patellar tendon. New femoral and tibial tunnels were required to achieve anatomic graft placement. Fixation was accomplished with interference screws proximally and distally. In addition, an anatomic reconstruction of the PLS (see Chapter 22, Posterolateral Ligament Injuries: Diagnosis, Operative Techniques, and Clinical Outcomes) was done using a B-PT-B autograft to replace the FCL, a semitendinosus tendon autograft to replace the popliteus tendon and popliteofibular ligament, and a proximal advancement of the PL capsule (Fig. 7–64A and B). Advancement of the ITB and PM capsule were also required. The patient had noteworthy articular cartilage damage (grade 2B) on the undersurface of the patella, the trochlea, and the medial femoral condyle.

At the most recent follow-up evaluation, 10 years postoperatively, the patient reported no problems with low-impact activities. She rated the overall condition of her knee as very good and was able to ski with minimal complaints. Physical

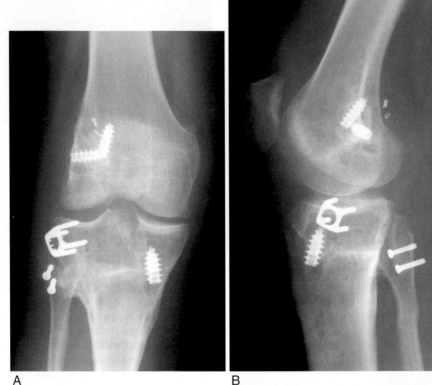

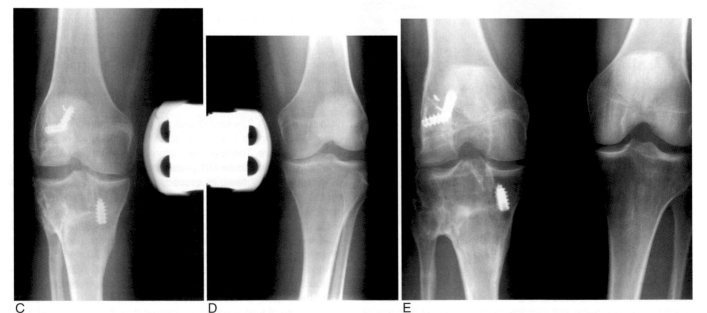

A   B   C   D   E

FIGURE 7–64. Case 11.

examination demonstrated a negative pivot shift, no increase in lateral joint opening on stress radiographs (see Fig. 7–64C and D), 5 mm of increased AP displacement on KT-2000 testing, no increase in external tibial rotation, and an overall valgus lower limb alignment. Weight-bearing PA radiographs at 45° of flexion demonstrated early narrowing of the lateral compartment (see Fig. 7–64E). Use of an unloader brace and continued avoidance of impact activities were advised.

Case 12. A 27-year-old man presented after three failed ACL reconstructions, including an ipsilateral B-PT-B autograft, a contralateral B-PT-B autograft, and an ipsilateral (reharvested) B-PT-B autograft. The patient had also undergone a total medial meniscectomy. The history and medical records revealed that the causes of failure of the reconstructions were anterior graft placement on the femur, uncorrected varus osseous malalignment, and uncorrected deficiency of the PLS. Physical examination demonstrated a grade III pivot shift, 15 mm of increased AP displacement on KT-2000 testing, 5 mm of increase in lateral joint opening, and a weight-bearing line of 15%. The patient complained of symptoms with all activities and ambulated with a varus thrust.

The patient underwent a closing wedge HTO and proximal advancement of the PLS, followed later with a QT-PB autogenous ACL reconstruction. A new femoral tunnel to achieve a central ACL graft placement was required, and the previously placed vertical femoral tunnel screw was left intact. Fixation was achieved with an interference screw proximally and an interference screw and graft suture post distally. Noteworthy articular cartilage damage (grade 2B) was evident on the undersurface of the patella and on the medial femoral condyle.

At the most recent follow-up evaluation, 6 years later, the patient had a grade I pivot shift bilaterally, 1.0 mm of increased AP displacement on KT-2000 testing, no increase in lateral joint opening or external tibial rotation, a normal range of knee motion, and correction to a valgus alignment. Radiographs demonstrated medial compartment joint space narrowing (Fig. 7–65). The patient declined further surgery such as a meniscus transplant. He was able to participate in low-impact activities and had only

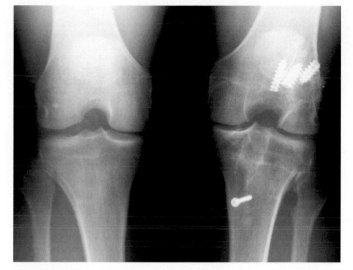

FIGURE 7–65. Case 12.

minimal problems in his occupation as a flooring installer. He rated the overall condition of the knee as good. The patient was advised that the long-term prognosis of the knee joint was poor.

Authors' comment: This case demonstrates a protracted course of treatment that included two prior ACL revision procedures that failed, in part, owing to vertical graft placement. In addition, the varus malalignment was not corrected, which produced pain and an obvious varus thrust with walking. After the valgus producing osteotomy and PL reconstruction, a QT-PB autograft was favored over an allograft to decrease the possibility of failure of the third ACL revision procedure. Tibial tunnel dilatation does occur in a small percentage of cases when the QT-PB graft is selected. In this case, the collagenous tendon portion was placed in the tibial tunnel and the patellar bone plug was placed in the femoral tunnel. The QT-PB graft provides the option of placing the bone plug at either the tibial or the femoral location, based on the best graft fit at surgery.

REFERENCES

1. Adachi, N.; Ochi, M.; Uchio, Y.; et al.: Reconstruction of the anterior cruciate ligament. Single- versus double-bundle multistranded hamstring tendons. *J Bone Joint Surg Br* 86:515–520, 2004.
2. Aglietti, P.; Giron, F.; Buzzi, R., et al.: Anterior cruciate ligament reconstruction: bone–patellar tendon–bone compared with double semitendinosus and gracilis tendon grafts. A prospective, randomized clinical trial. *J Bone Joint Surg Am* 86:2143–2155, 2004.
3. Aglietti, P.; Giron, F.; Cuomo, P.; et al.: Single-and double-incision double-bundle ACL reconstruction. *Clin Orthop Relat Res* 454:108–113, 2007.
4. Amis, A.; Dawkins, G.: Functional anatomy of the anterior cruciate ligament. Fibre bundle actions related to ligament replacements and injuries. *J Bone Joint Surg Br* 73:260–267, 1991.
5. Amis, A. A.; Jakob, R. P.: Anterior cruciate ligament graft positioning, tensioning and twisting. *Knee Surg Sports Traumatol Arthrosc* 6 (suppl 1):S2–S12, 1998.
6. Andrews, M.; Noyes, F. R.; Barber-Westin, S. D.: Anterior cruciate ligament allograft reconstruction in the skeletally immature athlete. *Am J Sports Med* 22:48–54, 1994.
7. Arciero, R. A.; Scoville, C. R.; Snyder, R. J.; et al.: Single- versus two-incision arthroscopic anterior cruciate ligament reconstruction. *Arthroscopy* 12:462–469, 1996.
8. Arnoczky, S. P.; Warren, R. F.; Ashlock, M. A.: Replacement of the anterior cruciate ligament using a patellar tendon allograft. An experimental study. *J Bone Joint Surg Am* 68:376–385, 1986.
9. Arnold, M. P.; Kooloos, J.; van Kampen, A.: Single-incision technique misses the anatomical femoral anterior cruciate ligament insertion: a cadaver study. *Knee Surg Sports Traumatol Arthrosc* 9:194–199, 2001.
10. Arnold, M. P.; Verdonschot, N.; van Kampen, A.: The normal anterior cruciate ligament as a model for tensioning strategies in anterior cruciate ligament grafts. *Am J Sports Med* 33:277–283, 2005.
11. Asagumo, H.; Kimura, M.; Kobayashi, Y.; et al.: Anatomic reconstruction of the anterior cruciate ligament using double-bundle hamstring tendons: surgical techniques, clinical outcomes, and complications. *Arthroscopy* 23:602–609, 2007.
12. Baer, G. S.; Harner, C. D.: Clinical outcomes of allograft versus autograft in anterior cruciate ligament reconstruction. *Clin Sports Med* 26:661–681, 2007.
13. Baer, G. S.; Shen, W.; Nozaki, M.; et al.: Anatomic double-bundle ACL reconstruction: effect of knee flexion angle during femoral tunnel preparation. In *AOSSM 2008 Annual Meeting.* Orlando, FL: 2008; pp. 108–109.

14. Barber-Westin, S. D.; Noyes, F. R.: The effect of rehabilitation and return to activity on anterior-posterior knee displacements after anterior cruciate ligament reconstruction. *Am J Sports Med* 21:264–270, 1993.

15. Barber-Westin, S. D.; Noyes, F. R.; Andrews, M.: A rigorous comparison between the sexes of results and complications after anterior cruciate ligament reconstruction. *Am J Sports Med* 25:514–526, 1997.

16. Barber-Westin, S. D.; Noyes, F. R.; Heckmann, T. P.; Shaffer, B. L.: The effect of exercise and rehabilitation on anterior-posterior knee displacements after anterior cruciate ligament autograft reconstruction. *Am J Sports Med* 27:84–93, 1999.

17. Barber-Westin, S. D.; Noyes, F. R.; McCloskey, J. W.: Rigorous statistical reliability, validity, and responsiveness testing of the Cincinnati Knee Rating System in 350 subjects with uninjured, injured, or anterior cruciate ligament–reconstructed knees. *Am J Sports Med* 27:402–416, 1999.

18. Benedetto, K. P.; Sperner, G.; Gloetzer, W.; et al.: Ultrasonographic follow-up of patellar tendon following graft dissection for ACL-replacement. *Am J Sports Med* 17:709, 1989.

19. Bernard, M.; Hertel, P.; Hornung, H.; Cierpinski, T.: Femoral insertion of the ACL. Radiographic quadrant method. *Am J Knee Surg* 10:14–21; discussion 21–22, 1997.

20. Bernicker, J. P.; Haddad, J. L.; Lintner, D. M.; et al.: Patellar tendon defect during the first year after anterior cruciate ligament reconstruction: appearance on serial magnetic resonance imaging. *Arthroscopy* 14:804–809, 1998.

21. Beynnon, B. D.; Johnson, R. J.; Abate, J. A.; et al.: Treatment of anterior cruciate ligament injuries, part 2. *Am J Sports Med* 33:1751–1767, 2005.

22. Beynnon, B. D.; Johnson, R. J.; Abate, J. A.; et al.: Treatment of anterior cruciate ligament injuries, part I. *Am J Sports Med* 33:1579–1602, 2005.

23. Biau, D. J.; Tournoux, C.; Katsahian, S.; et al.: ACL reconstruction: a meta-analysis of functional scores. *Clin Orthop Relat Res* 458:180–187, 2007.

24. Biau, D. J.; Tournoux, C.; Katsahian, S.; et al.: Bone–patellar tendon–bone autografts versus hamstring autografts for reconstruction of anterior cruciate ligament: meta-analysis. *BMJ* 332(7548):995–1001, 2006.

25. Bull, A. M.; Earnshaw, P. H.; Smith, A.; et al.: Intraoperative measurement of knee kinematics in reconstruction of the anterior cruciate ligament. *J Bone Joint Surg Br* 84:1075–1081, 2002.

26. Burks, R. T.; Friederichs, M. G.; Fink, B.; et al.: Treatment of postoperative anterior cruciate ligament infections with graft removal and early reimplantation. *Am J Sports Med* 31:414–418, 2003.

27. Busam, M. L.; Provencher, M. T.; Bach, B. R., Jr.: Complications of anterior cruciate ligament reconstruction with bone–patellar tendon–bone constructs: care and prevention. *Am J Sports Med* 36:379–394, 2008.

28. Buseck, M. S.; Noyes, F. R.: Arthroscopic evaluation of meniscal repairs after anterior cruciate ligament reconstruction and immediate motion. *Am J Sports Med* 19:489–494, 1991.

29. Butler, D. L.; Noyes, F. R.; Grood, E. S.: Ligamentous restraints to anterior-posterior drawer in the human knee. A biomechanical study. *J Bone Joint Surg Am* 62:259–270, 1980.

30. Carson, E. W.; Simonian, P. T.; Wickiewicz, T. L.; Warren, R. F.: Revision anterior cruciate ligament reconstruction. In Cannon, W. D. (ed.): *Instructional Course Lectures.* Rosemont, IL: American Academy of Orthopaedic Surgeons, 1998; pp. 361–368.

31. Clancy, W. G. J.; Nelson, D. A.; Reider, B.; Narechania, R. G.: Anterior cruciate ligament reconstruction using one-third of the patellar ligament, augmented by extra-articular tendon transfers. *J Bone Joint Surg Am* 64:352–359, 1982.

32. Colombet, P.; Robinson, J.; Christel, P.; et al.: Morphology of anterior cruciate ligament attachments for anatomic reconstruction: a cadaveric dissection and radiographic study. *Arthroscopy* 22:984–992, 2006.

33. Colombet, P.; Robinson, J.; Jambou, S.; et al.: Two-bundle, four-tunnel anterior cruciate ligament reconstruction. *Knee Surg Sports Traumatol Arthrosc* 14:629–636, 2006.

34. Colosimo, A. J.; Heidt, R. S.; Traub, J. A.; Carlonas, R. L.: Revision anterior cruciate ligament reconstruction with a reharvested ipsilateral patellar tendon. *Am J Sports Med* 29:746–750, 2001.

35. Corsetti, J. R.; Jackson, D. W.: Failure of anterior cruciate ligament reconstruction: the biologic basis. *Clin Orthop Relat Res* 325:42–49, 1996.

36. Coupens, S. D.; Yates, C. K.; Sheldon, C.; Ward, C.: Magnetic resonance imaging evaluation of the patellar tendon after use of its central one-third for anterior cruciate ligament reconstruction. *Am J Sports Med* 20:332–335, 1992.

37. Crawford, C.; Nyland, J.; Landes, S.; et al.: Anatomic double-bundle ACL reconstruction: a literature review. *Knee Surg Sports Traumatol Arthrosc* 15:946–964; discussion 945, 2007.

38. Cuomo, P.; Rama, K. R.; Bull, A. M.; Amis, A. A.: The effects of different tensioning strategies on knee laxity and graft tension after double-bundle anterior cruciate ligament reconstruction. *Am J Sports Med* 35:2083–2090, 2007.

39. DeAngelis, J. P.; Fulkerson, J. P.: Quadriceps tendon—a reliable alternative for reconstruction of the anterior cruciate ligament. *Clin Sports Med* 26:587–596, 2007.

40. DeHaven, K. E.; Lohrer, W. A.; Lovelock, J. E.: Long-term results of open meniscal repair. *Am J Sports Med* 23:524–530, 1995.

41. Diamantopoulos, A. P.; Lorbach, O.; Paessler, H. H.: Anterior cruciate ligament revision reconstruction: results in 107 patients. *Am J Sports Med* 36:851–860, 2008.

42. Drogset, J. O.; Grontvedt, T.; Robak, O. R.; et al.: A sixteen-year follow-up of three operative techniques for the treatment of acute ruptures of the anterior cruciate ligament. *J Bone Joint Surg Am* 88:944–952, 2006.

43. Eberhardt, C.; Kurth, A. H.; Hailer, N.; Jager, A.: Revision ACL reconstruction using autogenous patellar tendon graft. *Knee Surg Sports Traumatol Arthrosc* 8:290–295, 2000.

44. Eberhardt, C.; Wentz, S.; Leonhard, T.; Zichner, L.: Effects of revisional ACL surgery in semi-professional athletes in "high-risk pivoting sports" with chronic anterior instability of the knee. *J Orthop Sci* 5:205–209, 2000.

45. Edwards, A.; Bull, A. M.; Amis, A. A.: The attachments of the anteromedial and posterolateral fibre bundles of the anterior cruciate ligament: part 1: tibial attachment. *Knee Surg Sports Traumatol Arthrosc* 15:1414–1421, 2007.

46. Edwards, A.; Bull, A. M.; Amis, A. A.: The attachments of the anteromedial and posterolateral fibre bundles of the anterior cruciate ligament: part 2: femoral attachment. *Knee Surg Sports Traumatol Arthrosc* 16:29–36, 2008.

47. Edwards, A.; Bull, A. M.; Amis, A. A.: The attachments of the fiber bundles of the posterior cruciate ligament: an anatomic study. *Arthroscopy* 23:284–290, 2007.

48. Ferrari, J. D.; Bach, B. R., Jr.; Bush-Joseph, C. A.; et al.: Anterior cruciate ligament reconstruction in men and women: an outcome analysis comparing gender. *Arthroscopy* 17:588–596, 2001.

49. Ferretti, A.; Conteduca, F.; Monaco, E.; et al.: Revision anterior cruciate ligament reconstruction with doubled semitendinosus and gracilis tendons and lateral extra-articular reconstruction. *J Bone Joint Surg Am* 88:2373–2379, 2006.

50. Ferretti, M.; Levicoff, E. A.; Macpherson, T. A.; et al.: The fetal anterior cruciate ligament: an anatomic and histologic study. *Arthroscopy* 23:278–283, 2007.

51. Fong, S. Y.; Tan, J. L.: Septic arthritis after arthroscopic anterior cruciate ligament reconstruction. *Ann Acad Med Singapore* 33:228–234, 2004.

52. Fox, J. A.; Pierce, M.; Bojchuk, J.; et al.: Revision anterior cruciate ligament reconstruction with nonirradiated fresh-frozen patellar tendon allograft. *Arthroscopy* 20:787–794, 2004.

53. Fu, F. H.; Shen, W.; Starman, J. S.; et al.: Primary anatomic double-bundle anterior cruciate ligament reconstruction: a preliminary 2-year prospective study. *Am J Sports Med* 36:1263–1274, 2008.

54. Fules, P. J.; Madhav, R. T.; Goddard, R. K.; Mowbray, M. A.: Revision anterior cruciate ligament reconstruction using autografts with a polyester fixation device. *Knee* 10:335–340, 2003.

55. Gabriel, M. T.; Wong, E. K.; Woo, S. L.; et al.: Distribution of in situ forces in the anterior cruciate ligament in response to rotatory loads. *J Orthop Res* 22:85–89, 2004.

56. Gachter, A.: The joint infection. *Inform Arzt* 6:35–43, 1985.

57. Garofalo, R.; Djahangiri, A.; Siegrist, O.: Revision anterior cruciate ligament reconstruction with quadriceps tendon–patellar bone autograft. *Arthroscopy* 22:205–214, 2006.

58. George, M. S.; Dunn, W. R.; Spindler, K. P.: Current concepts review: revision anterior cruciate ligament reconstruction. *Am J Sports Med* 34:2026–2037, 2006.

59. George, M. S.; Huston, L. J.; Spindler, K. P.: Endoscopic versus rear-entry ACL reconstruction: a systematic review. *Clin Orthop Relat Res* 455:158–161, 2007.

60. Getelman, M. H.; Schepsis, A. A.; Zimmer, J.: Revision ACL reconstruction: autograft versus allograft. *Arthroscopy* 11:378, 1995.

61. Giron, F.; Buzzi, R.; Aglietti, P.: Femoral tunnel position in anterior cruciate ligament reconstruction using three techniques. A cadaver study. *Arthroscopy* 15:750–756, 1999.

62. Goebel, M. E.; Drez, D., Jr.; Heck, S. B.; Stoma, M. K.: Contaminated rabbit patellar tendon grafts. In vivo analysis of disinfecting methods. *Am J Sports Med* 22:387–391, 1994.

63. Goldblatt, J. P.; Fitzsimmons, S. E.; Balk, E.; Richmond, J. C.: Reconstruction of the anterior cruciate ligament: meta-analysis of patellar tendon versus hamstring tendon autograft. *Arthroscopy* 21:791–803, 2005.

64. Grood, E. S.; Hefzy, M. S.; Lindenfeld, T. N.: Factors affecting the region of most isometric femoral attachments. Part I: the posterior cruciate ligament. *Am J Sports Med* 17:197–207, 1989.

65. Grossman, M. G.; ElAttrache, N. S.; Shields, C. L.; Glousman, R. E.: Revision anterior cruciate ligament reconstruction: three- to nine-year follow-up. *Arthroscopy* 21:418–423, 2005.

66. Gulotta, L. V.; Rodeo, S. A.: Biology of autograft and allograft healing in anterior cruciate ligament reconstruction. *Clin Sports Med* 26:509–524, 2007.

67. Hamada, M.; Shino, K.; Horibe, S.; et al.: Single- versus bi-socket anterior cruciate ligament reconstruction using autogenous multiple-stranded hamstring tendons with EndoButton femoral fixation: a prospective study. *Arthroscopy* 17:801–807, 2001.

68. Hansen, B. P.; Beck, C. L.; Beck, E. P.; Townsley, R. W.: Postarthroscopic glenohumeral chondrolysis. *Am J Sports Med* 35:1628–1634, 2007.

69. Hart, A. J.; Buscombe, J.; Malone, A.; Dowd, G. S.: Assessment of osteoarthritis after reconstruction of the anterior cruciate ligament: a study using single-photon emission computed tomography at ten years. *J Bone Joint Surg Br* 87:1483–1487, 2005.

70. Hefzy, M. S.; Grood, E. S.; Noyes, F. R.: Factors affecting the region of most isometric femoral attachments. Part II: the anterior cruciate ligament. *Am J Sports Med* 17:208–216, 1989.

71. Heming, J. F.; Rand, J.; Steiner, M. E.: Anatomical limitations of transtibial drilling in anterior cruciate ligament reconstruction. *Am J Sports Med* 35:1708–1715, 2007.

72. Hertel, P.; Behrend, H.; Cierpinski, T.; et al.: ACL reconstruction using bone–patellar tendon–bone press-fit fixation: 10-year clinical results. *Knee Surg Sports Traumatol Arthrosc* 13:248–255, 2005.

73. Hewett, T. E.; Noyes, F. R.; Lee, M. D.: Diagnosis of complete and partial posterior cruciate ligament ruptures. Stress radiography compared with KT-1000 arthrometer and posterior drawer testing. *Am J Sports Med* 25:648–655, 1997.

74. Howell, S. M.: Principles for placing the tibial tunnel and avoiding roof impingement during reconstruction of a torn anterior cruciate ligament. *Knee Surg Sports Traumatol Arthrosc* 6(suppl 1).S49–S55, 1998.

75. Howell, S. M.; Clark, J. A.: Tibial tunnel placement in anterior cruciate ligament reconstructions and graft impingement. *Clin Orthop Relat Res* 283:187–195, 1992.

76. Indelli, P. F.; Dillingham, M.; Fanton, G.; Schurman, D. J.: Septic arthritis in postoperative anterior cruciate ligament reconstruction. *Clin Orthop Relat Res* 398:182–188, 2002.

77. Izquierdo, R., Jr.; Cadet, E. R.; Bauer, R.; et al.: A survey of sports medicine specialists investigating the preferred management of contaminated anterior cruciate ligament grafts. *Arthroscopy* 21:1348–1353, 2005.

78. Jackson, D. W.; Corsetti, J.; Simon, T. M.: Biologic incorporation of allograft anterior cruciate ligament replacements. *Clin Orthop Relat Res* 324:126–133, 1996.

79. Jackson, D. W.; Grood, E. S.; Cohn, B. R.; et al.: The effects of in situ freezing on the anterior cruciate ligament. An experimental study in goats. *J Bone Joint Surg Am* 73:201–213, 1991.

80. Jarvela, T.; Moisala, A. S.; Sihvonen, R.; et al.: Double-bundle anterior cruciate ligament reconstruction using hamstring autografts and bioabsorbable interference screw fixation: prospective, randomized, clinical study with 2-year results. *Am J Sports Med* 36:290–297, 2008.

81. Johnson, D. L.; Swenson, T. M.; Irrgang, J. J.; et al.: Revision anterior cruciate ligament surgery: experience from Pittsburgh. *Clin Orthop* 325:100–109, 1996.

82. Judd, D.; Bottoni, C.; Kim, D.; et al.: Infections following arthroscopic anterior cruciate ligament reconstruction. *Arthroscopy* 22:375–384, 2006.

83. Kaeding, C. C.; Pedroza, A.; Aros, B. C.; et al.: Independent predictors of ACL reconstruction failure from the MOON prospective longitudinal cohort. In *AOSSM 2008 Annual Meeting*. Orlando, FL: AOSSM, 2008; p. 121.

84. Karpie, J. C.; Chu, C. R.: Lidocaine exhibits dose- and time-dependent cytotoxic effects on bovine articular chondrocytes in vitro. *Am J Sports Med* 35:1621–1627, 2007.

85. Kartus, J.; Stener, S.; Lindahl, S.; et al.: Ipsi- or contralateral patellar tendon graft in anterior cruciate ligament revision surgery. A comparison of two methods. *Am J Sports Med* 26:499–504, 1998.

86. Kondo, E.; Yasuda, K.; Azuma, H.; et al.: Prospective clinical comparisons of anatomic double-bundle versus single-bundle anterior cruciate ligament reconstruction procedures in 328 consecutive patients. *Am J Sports Med* 36:1675–1687, 2008.

87. Krych, A. J.; Jackson, J. D.; Hoskin, T. L.; Dahm, D. L.: A meta-analysis of patellar tendon autograft versus patellar tendon allograft in anterior cruciate ligament reconstruction. *Arthroscopy* 24:292–298, 2008.

87a. Kurosawa, H.; Yasuda, K.; Yamakoshi, K.; et al.: An experimental evaluation of isometric placement for extraarticular reconstructions of the anterior cruciate ligament. *Am J Sports Med* 19:384–388, 1991.

88. LaPrade, R. F.; Hamilton, C. D.; Montgomery, R. D.; et al.: The reharvested central third of the patellar tendon. A histologic and biomechanical analysis. *Am J Sports Med* 25:779–785, 1997.

89. Lebel, B.; Hulet, C.; Galaud, B.; et al.: Arthroscopic reconstruction of the anterior cruciate ligament using bone–patellar tendon–bone autograft: a minimum 10-year follow-up. *Am J Sports Med* 36:1275–1282, 2008.

90. Li, G.; Defrate, L. E.; Rubash, H. E.; Gill, T. J.: In vivo kinematics of the ACL during weight-bearing knee flexion. *J Orthop Res* 23:340–344, 2005.

91. Liden, M.; Movin, T.; Ejerhed, L.; et al.: A histological and ultrastructural evaluation of the patellar tendon 10 years after reharvesting its central third. *Am J Sports Med* 36:781–788, 2008.

92. Linclau, L.: Measuring patellar height. *Acta Orthop Belg* 50:70–74, 1984.

93. Liu, S. H.; Hang, D. W.; Gentili, A.; Finerman, G. A.: MRI and morphology of the insertion of the patellar tendon after graft harvesting. *J Bone Joint Surg* 78:823–826, 1996.

94. Longo, U. G.; King, J. B.; Denaro, V.; Maffulli, N.: Double-bundle arthroscopic reconstruction of the anterior cruciate ligament: does the evidence add up? *J Bone Joint Surg Br* 90:995–999, 2008.

95. Luber, K. T.; Greene, P. Y.; Barrett, G.: Allograft anterior cruciate ligament reconstruction in the young, active patient (Tegner activity level and failure rate). In *AOSSM 2008 Annual Meeting*. Orlando, FL: AOSSM, 2008; p. 123.

96. Mae, T.; Shino, K.; Miyama, T.; et al.: Single- versus two-femoral socket anterior cruciate ligament reconstruction technique: biomechanical analysis using a robotic simulator. *Arthroscopy* 17:708–716, 2001.

97. Markolf, K. L.; Park, S.; Jackson, S. R.; McAllister, D. R.: Contributions of the posterolateral bundle of the anterior cruciate ligament to anterior-posterior knee laxity and ligament forces. *Arthroscopy* 24:805–809, 2008.

98. Markolf, K. L.; Park, S.; Jackson, S. R.; McAllister, D. R.: Simulated pivot-shift testing with single- and double-bundle anterior cruciate ligament reconstructions. *J Bone Joint Surg Am* 90:1681–1689, 2008.

99. Matava, M. J.; Evans, T. A.; Wright, R. W.; Shively, R. A.: Septic arthritis of the knee following anterior cruciate ligament reconstruction: results of a survey of sports medicine fellowship directors. *Arthroscopy* 14:717–725, 1998.

100. McAllister, D. R.; Joyce, M. J.; Mann, B. J.; Vangsness, C. T., Jr.: Allograft update: the current status of tissue regulation, procurement, processing, and sterilization. *Am J Sports Med* 35:2148–2158, 2007.

101. McAllister, D. R.; Parker, R. D.; Cooper, A. E.; et al.: Outcomes of postoperative septic arthritis after anterior cruciate ligament reconstruction. *Am J Sports Med* 27:562–570, 1999.

pathogens from allografts. Furthermore, some of these methods can alter the biomechanical properties of soft tissue grafts. Aseptic harvesting and processing alone preserve the strength of tendon grafts, but these do not eliminate bacteria, fungi, spores, or viruses. In addition, this method removes blood and lipids from only the surface of the graft. Chemical soaking can eliminate bacteria and fungi, but this process does not eradicate spores or viruses.

Two commonly employed methods for terminal sterilization are gamma irradiation (GI) and ethylene oxide (EO). GI is effective against bacteria at doses of 1.5 to 2.5 Mrad. However, as much as 4.0 Mrad is required to inactivate HIV, and even higher doses may be necessary to kill spores.[13] Unfortunately, higher doses of GI result in a substantial decrease of the strength of tendinous grafts. Fideler and colleagues[14] studied the effects of GI on B-PT-B allografts. These investigators noted a 15%, 24%, and 46% reduction in all biomechanical properties of the grafts after exposing them to doses of 2.0, 3.0, and 4.0 Mrad of irradiation, respectively. EO has successfully been used to sterilize surgical instruments. However, its use as a method to sterilize ACL allografts has been associated with intra-articular reactions with chronic synovitis, graft failure, and bone dissolution developed from the chemical residues that EO leaves in moist tissues.[19]

In an attempt to ameliorate the problems associated with each individual method of sterilization, several companies have developed proprietary techniques to process allografts that combine the methods previously discussed or introduce new ones.[50] Cryolife, Inc. (Kennisaw, GA) uses slow freezing combined with a dehydrating solvent, such as dimethyl sulfoxide or glycerol, to cryopreserve allografts. After desiccation, the grafts are treated for an extended period of time with an antimicrobial solution. No secondary sterilization technique is used. BioCleanse (Regeneration Technologies, Inc., Alachua, FL) uses a low-temperature chemical sterilization method, which allows better tissue penetration of the chemical and thus eliminates endogenous contamination from the allografts.

Allowash (Lifenet, Virginia Beach, VA) uses ultrasound, centrifugation, and negative pressure combined with biologic detergents, alcohols, and hydrogen peroxide to remove lipids, blood, and marrow cells from the allograft tissue that may act as reservoirs for potential pathogens. Clearant Process (Clearant, Inc., Los Angeles, CA) uses high doses of radiation (50 kGy). To prevent soft tissue damage, the technique is combined with freezing, water extraction, and addition of stabilizers and antioxidants that (according to the company) protect the grafts from biomechanical deterioration.

Healing of Allografts Postimplantation

Biologic integration and tissue compatibility merit consideration when allografts are used in primary or revision ACL reconstruction. Allografts follow the same healing process observed with autograft reconstruction of an initial period of avascular necrosis, followed by revascularization and cell proliferation.[4] However, several studies have documented that this integration occurs at a much slower rate. Jackson and coworkers[18] evaluated patellar tendon autografts and fresh frozen allografts 6 months after ACL reconstruction in a goat model. Compared with the allografts, the autografts demonstrated a smaller increase in AP displacement, two-times greater values of maximum force to failure, a significant increase in cross-sectional area, a more rapid loss of large-diameter collagen fibrils, and an increased density

and number of small-diameter collagen fibrils. The allografts had a greater decrease in structural properties, a slower rate of biologic incorporation, and a prolonged presence of an inflammatory response. The autografts demonstrated a more robust biologic response, improved stability, and increased strength to failure values.

More recently, Malinin and associates[28] studied nine ACL allografts and one autograft, retrieved at autopsy or at the time of revision surgery, to determine the rate and the extent of graft cellular replacement and remodeling. Examination of specimens from 20 days to 10 years after transplantation revealed a pattern of revascularization similar to that reported in previous biopsy studies. However, examination of entire allografts 2 years after transplantation revealed that the central portions of the grafts remained acellular and complete attachment was not present. One specimen retrieved 3.5 years post-transplantation did demonstrate complete attachment. The authors concluded that complete remodeling and cellular replacement of the entire graft may require 3 years or longer.

Similar findings were documented in a study by Beck and coworkers.[6] These authors obtained biopsies during arthroscopy from ACL allografts at various times after implantation. Histologic examination of the specimens showed that allografts remain largely avascular and acellular as late as 8 years postimplantation (Fig. 8–5).

ACL allograft antigenicity may be another factor that determines the fate of these tissues. In an animal study, transplantation of a serologically mismatched fresh patellar tendon allograft resulted in a marked inflammatory response and rejection of the graft.[4] Bugbee and colleagues[9] in a study of blood type in fresh osteochondral allograft transplantation suggested that ABO mismatch may adversely affect the clinical outcome of transplantation through an immune-mediated response. The inflammatory response to allograft tissue has been implicated in osteolysis and tunnel widening observed after ACL reconstruction.[11] However, it is difficult to distinguish the contribution of other parameters such as mechanical factors, fixation failure, and exposure to synovial fluid in this phenomenon. It must be noted that the preservation method affects the antigenicity of allografts. Freezing decreases cellular antigenicity, whereas freeze-drying produces grafts considered even less antigenic.

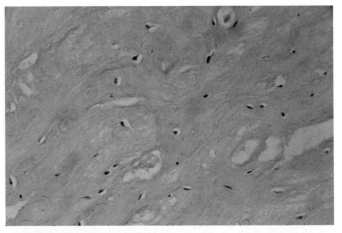

FIGURE 8–5. Histologic examination of specimens from Beck and coworkers[6] shows that allografts remain largely avascular and acellular as late as 8 years postimplantation.

Clinical outcome studies after revision ACL allograft reconstruction have shown satisfactory subjective results, although inferior to primary reconstructions. These investigations also reflect findings from basic science studies that have demonstrated slower biologic incorporation of the allografts and inferior biomechanical properties than those of autografts. Uribe and coworkers[52] reported the results of 54 patients who underwent revision ACL reconstruction. A fresh-frozen B-PT-B allograft was used in 35% of the cases and autogenous B-PT-B and hamstring grafts were used in 65%. The authors found no significant difference in the subjective outcomes between the two groups, but autografts provided greater objective stability during KT-1000 testing compared with allografts. In a prospective study of revision ACL reconstruction, Noyes and Barber-Westin[34] prospectively evaluated 65 patients who received B-PT-B allografts and 20 patients revised with autogenous B-PT-B grafts. The overall failure rate was 33% for the allografts and 27% for the autografts. Knee examination with KT-2000 showed that 53% of the patients in the allograft group and 67% in the autograft group had less than 3 mm increased displacement, although this difference was not statistically significant. Grossman and associates[17] reported on 29 revision ACL reconstructions in which B-PT-B allografts were used in 26 knees, B-PT-B autografts in 6, and AT allograft in 1. The allograft group demonstrated increased laxity during instrumented knee laxity testing compared with autografts (3.21 mm vs. 1.33 mm, respectively). Subjective scores were not significantly different between the two groups.

Smith and colleagues[49] reviewed retrospectively the results of 32 revision ACL reconstructions using nonirradiated B-PT-B allografts. The authors reported a 28% failure rate based on the presence of a pivot shift and/or greater than 5 mm side-to-side difference on KT-1000 testing. Similar findings were reported by Johnson and coworkers[21] in a review of 25 consecutive revision reconstructions with the use of fresh-frozen irradiated B-PT-B (13 patients) or AT (12 patients) allografts. At a mean follow-up of 28 months, 36% of the patients had greater than 5.5 mm side-to-side difference in anterior translation under manual maximum force on KT-1000 testing. Twenty percent of the patients had a grade II pivot shift.

In 1987, the senior author conducted a randomized, prospective study comparing 20 B-PT-B autograft patients with 20 B-PT-B fresh-frozen allograft patients. At 24 months postoperatively, manual maximum KT-1000 arthrometer testing revealed no significant difference in mean displacement values (autograft mean, 1.7 mm; allograft mean, 2.1 mm). There were fewer motion problems in the allograft group, but surprisingly, isokinetic muscle testing revealed no difference in the two groups. However, 2 individuals in the allograft group had suffered traumatic ruptures of their grafts when they returned to sports.

Based on the allograft rupture rate observed in the previously described prospective study,[39a] the senior author conducted a retrospective review of additional patients with longer follow-up evaluations. One hundred sixteen allograft patients with an average follow-up of 4.4 months were compared with 62 autograft patients with an average follow-up of 44.2 months. Patients in both groups were evenly divided between chronic and acute reconstructions. The results revealed that the allografts had significantly greater AP displacements ($P < .001$), according to manual maximum knee arthrometer testing (Table 8–1). When only acute reconstructions were compared, this difference was not significant (Table 8–2). However, comparison of chronic reconstruction groups showed significantly greater AP

TABLE 8–1 Results of Manual Maximum Knee Arthrometer Testing in Patients Receiving Allograft and Autograft Anterior Cruciate Ligament Reconstruction		
Difference between Reconstructed and Contralateral Knee (mm)	**Allografts (N = 116)**	**Autografts (N = 62)**
<3	67 (58%)*	44 (71%)
3–5	33 (28%)	16 (26%)
>5	16 (14%)*	2 (3%)

*$P < .001$.

TABLE 8–2 Results of Manual Maximum Knee Arthrometer Testing in Patients Receiving Acute Allograft and Autograft Anterior Cruciate Ligament Reconstruction		
Difference between Reconstructed and Contralateral Knee (mm)	**Allografts (%)**	**Autografts (%)**
<3	69	75
3–5	19	17
>5	12	8

TABLE 8–3 Results of Manual Maximum Knee Arthrometer Testing in Patients Receiving Chronic Allograft and Autograft Anterior Cruciate Ligament Reconstruction		
Difference between Reconstructed and Contralateral Knee (mm)	**Allografts (%)**	**Autografts (%)**
<3	48	65
3–5	37	35
>5	15*	0

*$P = .001$.

displacements in the allograft group (Table 8–3). In the allograft group, 1 acute reconstruction and 3 chronic reconstructions suffered traumatic ruptures at an average of 3.8 years after surgery. In the autograft group, only 1 patient (chronic) suffered a traumatic rupture.

Based on their experience, as well as other reports in the literature, the authors believe that allografts do not restore ACL function as reliably as autografts, especially in chronic cases in which healing and secondary restraints may be compromised.

AUTOGRAFTS

Similar to primary ACL reconstructions, autografts remain the graft of choice of many surgeons in the revision setting. Despite the morbidity associated with graft harvest, autografts carry no risk of disease transmission and there are no concerns for immunologic rejection. Autografts provide more reliable biologic integration, which has great significance in the often-compromised biologic environment of the multiple-operated knee. In addition, the use of an autograft reduces the cost of the procedure. However, because ipsilateral autograft(s) have usually already been used in the primary reconstruction, the surgeon may have to resort to harvesting the necessary graft in the opposite extremity. This tactic may be objectionable to some patients. Shelbourne and associates[45,46] studied the use of a contralateral B-PT-B graft in both primary and revision ACL reconstructions. The investigators reported low morbidity rates and expedited recovery in both the donor and the reconstructed knees. In addition, subjective scores were not significantly different from those obtained with primary reconstructions.

Ipsilateral unharvested autografts have been used in other series with good outcomes. In a prospective, nonrandomized study, O'Neil[36] reported the results of 48 patients who underwent revision ACL reconstruction using ipsilateral, previously unharvested hamstrings or B-PT-B autografts. At a mean follow-up of 90 months, 73% of the patients had International Knee Documentation Committee (IKDC) scores of normal (A) or nearly normal (B). Sixty-seven percent of the knees had a KT-2000 arthrometer side-to-side difference of 3 mm or less, and an additional 21% had a side-to-side difference of 3 to 5 mm. Therefore, 94% of the grafts were functional or partially functional. Six percent of grafts had more than 5 mm of laxity and were considered failures.

The ipsilateral QT has been used for revision ACL reconstruction.[33] In one study, the indications to use the QT included prior harvest of the patellar tendon in the ipsilateral knee, inability to harvest the contralateral patellar tendon (prior harvest, patient refusal), inability to consider the semitendinosus gracilis (STG) tendons because of expanded tunnels, and patient request for autogenous rather than allograft tissues. Persistent patellar bony defect from prior patellar tendon harvest was considered a contraindication to harvest the QT. Using IKDC rating, 17 of the 21 knees included in the study were rated as normal or nearly normal, 3 were graded as abnormal, and 1 was graded as severely abnormal at a mean follow-up of 49 months. During instrumented knee laxity testing, 8 knees had less than 3 mm, 7 knees had 3 to 5 mm, and 4 knees had more than 5 mm increased AP displacement. On physical examination, 10 knees had a grade 0 pivot shift; 7 knees, grade I; 3 knees, grade II; and 1 knee, grade III.

Hamstring autografts have been successfully used in revision ACL reconstruction.[15,44] Salmon and colleagues[44] reported on 57 consecutive revision ACL reconstructions with a four-strand hamstring tendon graft and interference screw fixation. Assessment included the IKDC knee ligament evaluation, instrumented laxity testing, and radiologic examination. The average length of follow-up was 89 months. Of the 50 knees reviewed, 5 (10%) had objective failure of the revision ACL reconstruction. Of the 45 patients with functional grafts, knee function was normal or nearly normal in 33 patients (73%). Thirty-four patients were evaluated with KT-1000. The mean side-to-side

difference on manual maximum testing was 2.5 mm. Fifty percent of the tested patients had translation of less than 3 mm, and 50% had between 3 and 5 mm. On pivot shift testing, 31 knees (69%) had grade 0 and 14 knees grade I test results.

Reharvested B-PT-B autografts have also been used in revision ACL reconstruction. Nixon and coworkers[31] evaluated the donor site in the patellar tendon at various time periods after a graft from the central third of the patellar tendon was harvested. Two groups of patients were evaluated, one with magnetic resonance imaging (MRI) of the knee and the other with an open biopsy from the donor site in the patellar tendon. On MRI, the size of the defect and the intensity of the signal in the central third of the tendon decreased with time from surgery. At 2 years, the defect was indistinguishable from normal tendon. Histologically, the scar in the defect progressively matured with time, becoming nearly identical to normal tendon at 2 years. However, Proctor and associates[42] showed in the goat model that even with restoration of the signal intensity, the biomechanical and histologic properties of the reconstituted tendon had not returned to normal. In this study, the maximum force to failure and ultimate stress of the reharvested tendons had decreased by 51% and 65%, respectively, compared with the contralateral side. Using a canine model, LaPrade and colleagues[25] demonstrated with biomechanical testing that average load to failure of the reharvested central third patellar tendon was 54% of that of the contralateral control tendons after 1 year.

Clinical studies on revision ACL reconstruction with reharvested B-PT-B grafts reflect the controversy surrounding this graft choice. Colosimo and coworkers[10] reported on 13 patients undergoing revision ACL reconstruction with a reharvested patellar tendon. At an average follow-up of 39.4 months, 11 patients had good or excellent results and 2 patients had fair results. Postoperative KT-1000 arthrometer results showed an average side-to-side difference of 1.92 mm. No patient demonstrated loss of range of knee motion and only 1 reported patellofemoral problems, which were moderate. The authors concluded that reharvesting the patellar tendon was a viable option in revision ACL reconstruction but advised against the use of this graft in any patient with patellofemoral disease or patella baja. Good subjective and objective results were also reported by O'Shea and Shelbourne[37] in a group of 11 patients with a mean objective follow-up of 49 months. In these two studies, the average length of time between primary B-PT-B harvest and reharvest of the tendon was 82.5 and 71 months, respectively. In contrast, Kartus and associates[22] found a higher rate of complications with the use of reharvested central-third patellar tendons, as well as poorer functional scores, when compared with the use of the contralateral patellar tendon. Of the 12 patients who had reconstruction with a reharvested tendon, 1 sustained a displaced patellar fracture 2 weeks after the index procedure, and another, a patellar tendon rupture 6 months postoperatively. In a more recent 10-year follow-up study, Liden and colleagues[27] reported on the clinical and radiographic results of 14 patients who had revision ACL reconstruction with reharvested patellar tendon. The average time between the primary and the revision reconstruction was 64 months. The patellar tendon at the donor site had not normalized 10 years after the reharvesting procedure, as evaluated on MRI. Clinical results in terms of the Lysholm score, IKDC evaluation system, single-leg hop test, KT-1000 test, and knee-walking test revealed no significant differences between the 2- and the 10-year assessments. In overall terms, the clinical results were considered to be poor on both occasions. Two major complications, 1 patellar fracture and 1 patellar tendon rupture, occurred in this series as well.

AUTHORS' APPROACH

Aside from knowledge of the performance of various grafts, the choice of revision graft material is predicated on a number of clinical factors that are inextricably related (Table 8–4). Each case must be evaluated and decisions made based on the unique presentation of the patient.

Cause of Failure

Determining the cause of failure is frequently very difficult because rarely there is just one factor; more often, several factors exist. Erroneous tunnel placement is the most common cause and includes both tibial and femoral malposition (Fig. 8–6). If the old tunnel position infringes on normal tunnel placement, graft/tunnel size mismatch will occur. This limits the choice of graft source, and if the surgeon's and the patient's desire is to avoid allografts, a two-stage procedure is required. This approach begins with arthroscopic bone grafting and ends approximately 12 weeks later with ACL reconstruction using ipsilateral or contralateral autograft material. In the authors' experience, which is supported by recent publications, a two-staged procedure results in more stable knees more frequently than a single-stage procedure, which compromises optimal tunnel placement or size and employs slower healing allograft tissues.[51]

On many occasions, the biologic environment of the knee may be compromised for a variety of reasons such as multiple knee operations, bone loss, prior infection, or chronic use of steroids or nonsteroidal anti-inflammatory medications. In this setting, the use of slower-healing allografts is risky. In the authors' opinion, patients with a connective tissue profile clinically demonstrated with joint hyperlaxity are also poor candidates for allografts.

Conversely, a poor surgical technique with grossly malpositioned tunnels, inadequate fixation (Fig. 8–7), failure to recognize and address complex instabilities, or prior traumatic

TABLE 8–4	Clinical Factors That Influence the Choice of Graft Material

Cause of failure of the previous reconstruction(s)
Previous graft selection
Type and location of hardware used in previous reconstruction(s)
Bone quality
Unrecognized concomitant ligament instability
Condition of the patellofemoral joint
Condition of the contralateral knee
Skin condition
Is staged reconstruction necessary?
Individual patient factors
    Age
    Activity level
    Personal preferences, religious beliefs

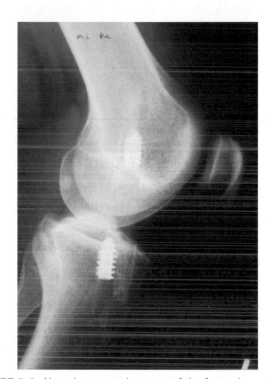

FIGURE 8–6. Note the errant placement of the femoral tunnel that is located too distal on the femur. This graft will fail as normal flexion is achieved.

rupture of the primary ACL graft generally allows the surgeon more latitude as to graft choice.

Previous Graft Selection

In the favorable scenario in which autograft tissue is still available in the same knee, this graft source should be selected. In patients in whom a B-PT-B graft has previously been harvested and there is a persistent bone defect in the patella, an ipsilateral QT graft is not harvested because this may increase the risk of postoperative patellar fracture. If autograft tissue from the same knee is unavailable or cannot be used, the authors favor harvesting an autograft from the opposite knee. If the patient opposes such a tactic, an allograft is used, preferably an AT or a B-PT-B. The bone segments of these allografts can help address bone loss from hardware removal or tunnel widening.

Critical Points AUTHORS' APPROACH

- The cause(s) of failure of the original reconstruction influences the choice of the revision graft.
- Autografts should be used as the first choice in revision ACL reconstruction.
- The biologic environment of the knee requiring a revision ACL reconstruction is often compromised. In this setting, slower-healing allografts may be a risky choice.
- The bone quality of knee should be carefully evaluated.
- With current fixation methods, tunnel widening is not a contraindication for tendinous grafts, especially if the bone loss is addressed in a staged approach.
- Staged reconstruction reduces the technical challenges of the procedure, more frequently allows the use of an autograft, and provides more stable knees.
- The condition of the ipsilateral patellofemoral joint should be scrutinized. In the presence of significant degenerative joint disease, ipsilateral quadriceps tendon or B-PT-B autografts should not be used.
- If a single-stage reconstruction is desired, or coexisting ligament injuries need to be addressed, allografts should be readily available.
- Older age or decreased activity levels do not by themselves constitute an indication for allograft use.

Chapter 9

Allografts: Graft Sterilization and Tissue Banking Safety Issues

C. Thomas Vangsness, Jr., MD

OVERVIEW OF CURRENT ALLOGRAFT TISSUE USE

Allografts are commonly used in the United States and their acceptance, availability, and safety profile have never been stronger. The numbers of grafts harvested and distributed by tissue banks in the United States have steadily increased. The American Association of Tissue Banks (AATB) recovered approximately 17,000 donor grafts in 1996, and this had increased to approximately 23,000 donor grafts in 2003.[14] Over 300,000 musculoskeletal tissues were distributed in 1996, and about 1.3 million musculoskeletal grafts were distributed in 2003. It has been estimated that there have been about 4 to 5 million tissue transplants between 2000 and 2005.[25] Issues relating to graft procurement, sterilization, and overall tissue banking safety continue to be a concern. A recent survey by the American Orthopaedic Sports Medicine Society of over 350 members documented a concern and widespread misunderstanding of the tissue banking industry.[14] Over 80% used allografts and almost 75% were concerned about safety and sterilization. Most surgeons reported not knowing much about sterilization processing and about half did not know whether their tissues were sterilized or which sterilization process was used.

Critical Points OVERVIEW OF CURRENT ALLOGRAFT TISSUE USE

- The numbers of grafts harvested and distributed by tissue banks in the United States have steadily increased.
- The American Association of Tissue Banks (AATB) recovered approximately 23,000 donors in 2003 and about 1.3 million musculoskeletal grafts were distributed.
- Issues relating to graft procurement, sterilization, and overall tissue banking safety continue to be a concern.
- Recent advancements from government agencies have made tissue banking and the use of allograft tissue safer than ever.

Recent advancements from government agencies have made tissue banking and the use of allograft tissue safer than ever. Improved standards and techniques of tissue handling have made allografts more appealing to both surgeons and patients. Evaluation with evidence-based medicine techniques will continue to confirm the safety and efficacy of soft tissue allografts in knee surgery. The safety records of this tissue transplantation were remarkable. This chapter reviews the issues relating to the tissue banking industry, graft sterilization, and allograft safety.

CURRENT TISSUE BANK REGULATION

The U.S. Food and Drug Administration (FDA) is the government authority that regulates musculoskeletal tissue. The FDA authorizes and enforces tissue regulation to prevent the introduction, transmission, or spread of communicable diseases between states or from foreign countries into the United States. In 2004, the FDA published the "Final Rule: eligibility and determination of donors of human cells tissues and cellular and tissue-based products."[20] Also published in 2004 was the Draft guidance for industry: eligibility to determination for donor of human cells, tissue and tissue-based products (HCT/Ps).[22] In 2005, the FDA implemented the industry requirements for good tissue practices (GTP) for all establishments that manufacture human cell and cellular tissue–based products. The purpose of these new government regulations was to set standards for tissue banking and prevent the potential introduction, transmission, and spread of communicable diseases by allograft tissues. These standards are also in place to prevent contamination during the process of screening, procuring, and processing of allograft tissue. All tissue establishments are required to register with the FDA.

Before these recent regulations, the federal government was not able to establish or register tissue banks in the United States.

- The purpose of this government regulation is to set standards for tissue banking and prevent the introduction, transmission, and spread of communicable diseases.
- The AATB, founded in 1976, is a nonprofit organization to establish voluntary standards.
- The AATB first published "the standards for tissue banking" in 1984.
- The U.S. Food and Drug Administration (FDA) is the ultimate enforcer of tissue banks, with powers of warning letters and the ultimate shutdown of tissue banks.
- 90% of musculoskeletal tissues are distributed through AATB-accredited tissue banks.
- The American Academy of Orthopaedic Surgery (AAOS) released an advisory statement urging all tissue banks to follow the AATB guidelines and standards.
- In 2005, the Joint Commission (JC) set standards for storage of tissues intended for transplantation for hospitals and outpatient surgery centers.

This registration and the GTP rule allow the FDA to inspect facilities anytime without notice. FDA regulations require donors to be screened and tested for human immunodeficiency virus (HIV) types 1 and 2, hepatitis B and C viruses (HBV, HCV), *Treponema pallidium*, and human transmissible spongiform encephalopathies.[23] In August 2007, the FDA increased screening standards by requiring recovery tissues to be negative for HIV 1 nucleic acid testing (NAT), HCV NAT, and hepatitis B core antibody (total). All tissue banks must keep a document of these tests.

The AATB, founded in 1976, is a nonprofit organization that establishes and sets voluntary standards for safe transmittal of cells and tissues.[3] This organization consists of both accredited tissue banks and individual members. It promotes education and research. The goal of the AATB is to educate and prevent disease transmission with cell and tissue allografts.

The AATB first published "the standards for tissue banking" in 1984 to give recommendations and guidelines to tissue banks. These safety guidelines are periodically reviewed and updated.[3] All members of the AATB must follow the published tissue bank standards for donor suitability determination (screening and testing), donor consent/authorization, tissue recovery, quality insurance/quality control, record keeping, processing, labeling, storage, distribution, and safety. The AATB has been doing on-site inspections and accreditations since 1986. Tissue banks are to be inspected every 3 years, and renewal of accreditation is granted after a formal review of any reinspection. It should be noted that membership in this trade organization is voluntary. The AATB does not have any formal disciplinary powers outside of restriction or exclusion from the organization itself. The FDA is the ultimate enforcer of tissue banks, with powers of warning letters and possibly the ultimate shutdown of the tissue banks itself.

It is currently estimated that 90% of musculoskeletal tissues are distributed through AATB-accredited tissue banks.[25] Through 2006 there were 95 accredited tissue banks with 70 banks involved in musculoskeletal, cardiovascular, and skin allograft tissues. The AATB requires infectious disease testing for HIV types 1 and 2 antibody, hepatitis B surface antigen, total antibody to hepatitis B core (immunoglobulin [Ig] G and IgM), human T-cell lymphotrophic virus (HTLV)–I/HTLV-II antibody, HCV antibody, NAT for HCV and HIV-1, and a syphilis assay. AATB also requires discarding allografts with cultures that are positive for

clostridium or *Streptococcus pyrogenes* (group A streptoccoccus). Any positive final culture requires discarding of that tissue.

The American Academy of Orthopaedic Surgeons (AAOS) first released an advisory statement regarding tissue allograft use in 1991 and updated this in 2001 and 2006.[1] The AAOS urged all tissue banks to follow the AATB guidelines and standards.

The Department of Health and Human Services, through the Centers for Disease Control and Prevention (CDC), has begun to improve communication within the tissue/organ community to identify and track tissues.[15] A single unique national identification number will be applied to donors and tissues that then can be tracked during the entire donation and transplantation process. This is an ongoing effort to help monitor individual tissues and ultimately improve our tissue knowledge base and increase safety standards.

In 2005, the Joint Commission (JC), which is formally known as the Joint Commission on Accreditation of Healthcare Organizations (JCAHO), also set standards for storage of tissues intended for transplantation for hospitals and outpatient surgery centers.[13] The JC is an independent organization separate from the FDA and is the nation's oldest and largest accrediting body in health care. Their standards will help ensure safety at hospitals and surgery centers that handle tissues through the monitoring and recording of the use and storage of allograft tissues.

Overall, donor safety issues have been refined with the advancement of these federal laws and the increased tissue bank involvement with the AATB and its critical standards. Very few infections or tissue problems are at present occurring with tissue banks that are compliant with the AATB. With newer processing techniques, safety issues will be better monitored than ever before.

ALLOGRAFT TISSUE PROCESSING

There are two ways to transmit disease with allograft tissue. The first is by direct transmission of an infection from an infected donor. Contamination can come from the bacteria of donors, their blood, body cavity, or blood organs. The second form of contamination occurs with tissue handling during its preparation. After tissue is donated, it goes through three steps before it is packaged and delivered for implantation. The first step is donor screening, the second is tissue processing, and the third step is packaging and terminal sterilization.

- There are two ways to transmit disease with allograft tissue. One is by direct transmission of the infection, which can come from an infected donor or through tissue handling or during procurement, processing, and packaging.
- The medical directors of each tissue bank have an important position to monitor and document all regulatory issues and quality control of tissue processing.
- Sterilization is defined as a process that kills all forms of life, especially microorganisms. The FDA has established a sterility insurance level (SAL) 10^{-3} (1 in 1000) as adequate for implantable medical biologic devices. The Association for the Advancement of Medical Instrumentation (AAMI) states that a SAL of 10^{-6} is appropriate for medical devices. The AATB requires a SAL of 10^{-6} as their standard.
- Tissue banks use a proprietary formula for tissue processing involving different biologic detergents, alcohol, antibiotics, or hydrogen peroxide.

Step One: Donor Screening

The screening process is critical to safely optimize donor selection. A health care professional interviews the family or any other knowledgeable historian of the donor to help identify risk factors for infectious diseases. Social and/or medical risk assessment is investigated to get a medical history from all potential sources including the donors' previous interfaces with hospitals, clinics, private donor offices, or surviving relatives. A history of blood donation is investigated. Autopsy reports can be reviewed to investigate ongoing medical problems of the donor, if this is available.

There is always a concern for the window period for viruses when the donor does not have any detectable viral antibodies or immunogens.[7] With NAT, this window period can be as low as 7 days for HIV and HCV and up to 20 days for HBV. The risk of transplant tissues from HIV-infected donors has been estimated to be 1 in 173,000 to 1 in 1,000,000.[5,11,27] Current estimates for Americans infected with HIV vary from 850,000 to 950,000. The risk of contracting HBV and HCV from an infected donor is much higher than that of HIV. The general population is estimated to have 1.2 million Americans infected with HBV and approximately 4 million with HCV.[11] Approximately 50% of these HCV patients do not know they are carriers and about 50% acknowledge no risk history associated with HCV. The current risk of transplanted tissues from HCV-infected donors is estimated to be 1 in 421,000.[27] In reality, the actual number of potential tissue donors who are infected with these viruses is not known. Blood donation data give a general indication of the inherent risk associated with the screening and processing of human blood. The risk of bacterial infection from screening and processing has been reported to be 1 in 3500 to 1 in 5000.[2,8,17]

The National Nosocomial Infection Surveillance System of the CDC has reported a postoperative orthopaedic infection rate ranging from 0.6% to 2%.[11] A recent government workshop documented 19 infection reports in a 5-year period when approximately 4 to 5 million tissues were distributed.[16] The risk of infection with all these transplanted tissues is very low; the precise number is difficult to evaluate. Overall, the current risk of allograft-transmitted infection in patients is much less than the overall risk of a generalized perioperative nosocomial infection. This is especially true with tissues used from certified AATB-associated banks.

There are several new pathogens on the horizon about which we have no information. This includes the West Nile virus, the severe acute respiratory syndrome (SARS) and the corona virus. There are no current screening tests for prion diseases associated with transmissible spongiform encephalopathies (TSE) like Creutzfeldt-Jakob disease and its variants.[21]

Step Two: Tissue Processing

After the donor has gone through the screening process, several steps are taken to ensure standardized processing of the allograft tissue. All tissues are processed with "aseptic" techniques, which incorporate standard operating room techniques. When tissues are obtained from the donor, the term *harvest* has been respectfully replaced with *recovery*. There are time limits for tissues to be recovered. A 24-hour window is established during which the body tissues must be recovered by AATB standards.

Recovery is done most often in an operating room theater or a designated recovery center. Occasionally, this can be done in a morgue. A team of technicians assist in this surgical procedure. Operating room techniques including preparing and draping the donor are similar to those of standard operating protocols. Sterile technique is used with drapes, gowns, gloves, and sterile instruments. Each tissue is procured, cultured, wrapped, labeled, sealed, and shipped in dedicated containers at freezing temperatures. The majority of these tissues are recovered with this aseptic technique of tissue recovery. Contamination can occur during this process or during the transfer to the containers before arriving at the tissue bank. This aseptic technique should not be considered a sterile process. Contamination has been documented to come from the donor's gastrointestinal or respiratory tract (agonal contamination).[10,12] Recent outbreaks have documented this contamination after death with the breakdown of the gastrointestinal system as well as recovery after asystole at late times outside tissue banking standards.[23]

Tissue banks examine the bioburden of the tissue surface and the accompanying tissue fluid of received tissues. *Bioburden* is defined as the number of contaminated organisms found in a given amount of material before undergoing a sterilizing procedure. Allograft tissue has a complex physical surface with cracks and fissures that make removal of all potential pathogens difficult. Surface swab cultures are documented to be only 70% to 92% sensitive.[26] The U.S. Pharmacopeial Convention,[18] the medical industry standard for sterility testing and other quality control procedures, has stated that swab cultures should not be used for definitive evidence of sterilization. Cultures should be used to monitor previously validated sterilizing processes. Some tissue banks will reject tissues if there is a large amount of bioburden when they initially receive the tissue.

When processing tissue, the tissue banks strive to clean and sterilize tissue for transplantation. *Sterilization* is defined as a process that kills all forms of life, especially microorganisms. Sterility has been expressed as a mathematical probability of risk. The FDA has established a sterility insurance level (SAL) 10^{-3} as adequate for implantable medical biologic devices. This means that there is a 1 in 1000 chance (probability) that a living viable microbe can exist in or on the implantable device. Conventional musculoskeletal allografts are routinely classified as HCT/P by the FDA/Center for Biologics Evaluation in Research (CBER). The Association for the Advancement of Medical Instrumentation (AAMI)[4] states that an SAL of 10^{-6} is appropriate for medical devices. Currently, the AATB requires an SAL of 10^{-6} as their standard, different from that of the FDA.[3]

Different sterilization and validated processing techniques are currently used by the major tissue banks across the United States. Newer processing techniques continue to be developed to improve tissue safety. Most sterilization processes are based on the treatment of tissues "spiked" with different pathogens or the tissues are emerged or dipped into fluids containing the pathogens of interest. Biologically, this is not the same as tissue that has been "systemically" infected. The validity of these testing techniques needs further study.

The FDA is the ultimate governing body over the tissue banking industry but does not specifically state which sterilization processing technique is the best or which should be used. Within the recent rules for GTP, the FDA requires that any tissue banking establishment that makes a written statement of allograft sterility with their labeling will be subject to surprise inspections and review by the FDA.[19,22] Each tissue bank must have validated data for their statements of sterility by their individual tissue processing method. Most tissue banks use a proprietary formula of different biologic detergents, alcohol, antibiotics, and hydrogen peroxide.

Table 9–1 lists examples of a few of the major tissue bank processes including formulas such as Allowash XG by Lifenet, which

TABLE 9–1 Major Tissue Banks and Their Current Sterilization Methods

Tissue Bank	Sterilization Method
AlloSource	SterileR: validated bioburden reduction cleansing system followed by low-dose terminal irradiation to provide SAL 10^{-6}. Package is labeled "sterile."
Bone Bank Allografts	GraftCleanse: proprietary blend of cleansing agents used to reduce bioburden and provide aesthetic white appearance. GraftCleanse: terminal low-dose gamma irradiation achieves package sterility.
Community Tissue Services (CTS)	Musculoskeletal grafts are soaked and rinsed in antibiotics, hydrogen peroxide, alcohol, sterile water, and AlloWash solutions. Low-dose terminal gamma irradiation is used to eliminate most bacteria.
LifeNet	AlloWash XG: rigorous cleansing removes blood elements, followed by decontamination and a scrubbing regimen to eliminate bacteria and viruses. Tissue is terminally irradiated at a low dose to reach SAL 10^{-6} and is labeled "sterile."
Musculoskeletal Tissue Foundation (MTF)	MTF processes soft tissue allografts aseptically and treats the grafts with an antibiotic cocktail of gentamicin, amphotericin B, and imipenem and cilastin sodium (Primaxin). Some incoming tissue is pretreated with low-dose gamma irradiation to reduce bioburden. No terminal irradiation is used.
OsteoTech	OsteoTech processes allograft tissue using aseptic technique in class 100 clean rooms. Isolators are used to prevent cross-contamination.
RTI Biologics, Inc.	BioCleanse: an automated chemical sterilization process that is validated to remove blood, marrow, and lipids and eliminate bacteria, fungi, spores, and viruses while maintaining biomechanical integrity and biocompatibility. No preprocessing or terminal irradiation is used on sports medicine allografts. All tissue reaches SAL 10^{-6} after BioCleanse.
Tissue Banks International (TBI)	Clearant Process: pathogen inactivation process involving high-dose gamma irradiation at (5.0 Mrad) combined with radioprotectant that sterilizes tissue in the final packaging and significantly inactivates infectious agents and maintains the function of the allograft. Process yields SAL 10^{-6} and package is labeled "sterile."

SAL, sterility insurance level.

uses a scrubbing technique and intensive decontamination steps with alcohol, antibiotics, and hydrogen peroxide. The BioCleanse tissue process from Regeneration Technologies, Inc. (RTI), uses a vacuum-pressure low-temperature automated process with hydrogen peroxide and alcohol. The Musculoskeletal Transplantation Foundation (MTF) uses an allograft tissue purification process (ATP), a nonconic detergent, hydrogen peroxide, and alcohol process with an antibiotic cocktail. Tissue Bank International (TBI) has TranZgraft, a proprietary sterilizing process used at low temperature. Allosource uses Validated Sterilizer as a disinfection process. These tissue banks have validated their individual proprietary sterilizing processes to an SAL level of 10^{-6}.

Any tissue processing method should be effective for inactivating viruses and killing bacteria. It should effectively penetrate into the tissue and be safely removed from the tissue while preserving the mechanical and biologic properties of the tissue.

No proven technique is more effective in processing or sterilizing allograft tissue for human use. Long-term studies are needed to evaluate the different processing techniques over time. Not all soft tissue musculoskeletal allografts can be safely sterilized. The chondrocytes in articular cartilage allografts can be irreparably damaged by different processing techniques.

Gamma radiation is a very effective sterilization agent that generates free radicals, which can adversely affect the structure of collagen. Higher doses of radiation have been documented to be deleterious to the tissue, and at this time, low-dose radiation is commonly used by tissue banks to remove surface contaminants.[6,9]

A few tissue banks use a freeze-drying process (lyophilization). This allows the allograft tissue to be stored at room temperature in a sealed package. This lyophilization process freezes the tissue and the water content is reduced to less than 6% of its initial weight. This is done by a primary drying process called *sublimation*, which is followed by a secondary drying process called *desorption*. This reduction of water content does not support any biologic activity or chemical reactions in the tissue. Generally, freeze-dried allografts are not commonly used for sports medicine

applications in the United States. They are widely used for non orthopaedic reconstruction procedures in the neurosurgical and urologic fields.

Step Three: Packaging and Terminal Sterilization

The last step of preparation before tissues are distributed for implantation involves packaging and terminal sterilization. All tissue banks are concerned with the handling of the graft after the tissue cleaning process. This packaging process can involve human contact in a clean room and can be a source of infection. To remove concerns about this contamination, terminal sterilization is the final processing step to prepare tissues for shipping in their prepared packages. Two methods are used to terminally sterilize tissue: (1) Ethylene oxide (ETO) gas has fallen out of favor because of documented host tissue reactions with ETO-treated grafts. (2) Gamma radiation is most commonly used at low doses. These lower doses of radiation are believed to not mechanically harm the tissue and are effective in removing any low-dose bioburden in or on the tissue. It is very easy to irradiate tissue after packaging, and this is done in the frozen state at two major centers in the United States.[24,26]

Tissue banks label their packaged allografts in different ways. Some put the age of the graft and some claim sterility on the packaging. With new GTP regulations, any label claims are subject to FDA scrutiny, and as noted previously, tissue banks must have validated justifications for any label claims.[19] The medical director of each tissue bank has a critically important position to monitor and document all regulatory issues. This director oversees the inspection of the tissues, quality control, and tissue processing at the tissue bank.[24]

After processing, packaging, and terminal sterilization are complete, most allograft tissues are stored frozen. All accredited tissue banks follow common storage guidelines specified by the AATB.[3] The tissue is also kept frozen during overnight shipping and delivering to the end user at the point of surgery. Hospitals, surgery centers, and other organizations continue to maintain the graft frozen in storage prior to implantation.

SUMMARY

Musculoskeletal allograft use continues to increase in the clinical practice of orthopaedic surgery and sports medicine. The risk of infection and disease transmission are at an all-time low. Regulation has improved, and standardized methods have been implemented to ensure graft safety and efficacy. Trade groups such as AATB have been instrumental in setting standards and policing tissue banks. The FDA will continue to randomly inspect tissue banks and to be the ultimate enforcer of tissue bank standards.

As newer sterilization processes for allograft human tissues are developed, their in vivo biologic and biomechanical effects need to be evaluated. The AAOS recommends that surgeons use AATB member banks.[1] Surgeons need to be familiar with the processing of allograft tissue and know the tissue banks with which they work. Routine culture of the allograft tissue out of the package in the operating room is not necessary because it has been documented that these swab

cultures are not only inaccurate but also a minor source of contamination compared with the operation itself. There is a growing emphasis on monitoring these individual tissues on a national website. Adverse events need to be reported to all health personnel, further emphasizing the importance of the relationship between the tissue banks and the health care providers.

Critical Points SUMMARY

- Musculoskeletal allograft use continues to increase in orthopaedic surgery and sports medicine.
- The risks of infection and disease transmission are at an all-time low.
- The AAOS recommends that surgeons use AATB member banks.
- Surgeons need to be familiar with the processing of allograft tissue and know the tissue banks they work with.
- Routine culture of the allograft tissue out of the package in the operating room is not necessary and is inaccurate.

REFERENCES

1. American Academy of Orthopaedic Surgeons: American Academy of Orthopaedic Surgeons Advisory Statement #1011: Use of musculoskeletal tissue allografts. Available at http://www.aaos.org/wordhtm/papers/advistm/allograf.htm
2. American Association of Blood Banks: Guidelines for managing tissues allografts in hospitals. Available at http://www.aabb.org
3. American Association of Tissue Banks: Standards for Tissue Banking, 11th ed. McLean, VA: AATB, 2006. Available at www.aatb.org
4. Association for the Advancement of Medical Instrumentation: Sterilization of health care products—radiation—part 1: requirements for the development, validation and routine control of a sterilization process for medical devices. AAMI/ISO 11137-12. Arlington, VA: Association for the Advancement of Medical Instrumentation, 2006.
5. Buck, B. E.; Malinin, T. I.: Human bone and tissue allografts. Preparation and safety. *Clin Orthop* 303:8–17, 1994.
6. Curran, A. R.; Adams, D. J.; Gill, J. L.; et al.: The biomechanical effects of low-dose irradiation on bone–patellar tendon–bone allografts. *Am J Sports Med* 32:1131–1135, 2004.
7. Dodd, R. Y.; Notari, E. P., 4th; Stramer, S. L.: Current prevalence and incidence of infectious disease markers and estimated window-period risk in the American Red Cross blood donor population. *Transfusion* 42:975–979, 2002.
8. Fang, C. T.; Chambers, L. A.; Kennedy, J.; et al.; and the American Red Cross Regional Blood Centers: Detection of bacterial contamination in apheresis platelet products: American Red Cross experience, 2004. *Transfusion* 45:1845–1852, 2005.
9. Fideler, B. M.; Vangsness, C. T., Jr.; Moore, T.; et al.: Effects of gamma irradiation on the human immunodeficiency virus. A study in frozen human bone–patellar ligament–bone grafts obtained from infected cadavers. *J Bone Joint Surg Am* 76:1032–1035, 1994.
10. Finegold, S. M.; Attebery, H. R.; Sutter, V; L.: Effect of diet on human fecal flora: comparison of Japanese and American diets. *Am J Clin Nutr* 27:1456–1469, 1974.
11. Gocke, D. J.: Tissue donor selection and safety. *Clin Orthop* 135:17–21, 2005.
12. Hirn, M. Y.; Salmela, P. M.; Vuento, R. E.: High-pressure saline washing of allografts reduces bacterial contamination. *Acta Orthop Scand* 72:83–85, 2001.
13. Joint Commission on Accreditation on Health Care Organizations. New Standards PC, 17, 20 and PC 17, 20. Available at http://www.jcaho.org (accessed September 9, 2006).
14. McAllister, D. R.; Joyce, M. J.; Mann, B. J., Vangsness, C. T., Jr.: Allograft update—the current status of tissue regulation, procurement, processing, and sterilization. *Am J Sports Med* 35:2148–2158, 2007.
15. NNIS System, Division of Healthcare Quality Promotion, National Center for Infectious Diseases, Centers for Disease Control and Prevention, Public Health Service: National Nosocomial Infections Surveillance (NNIS) System Report, data summary from January

1992 through June 2004. Atlanta: U.S. Department of Health and Human Services, 2004.
16. Srinivasan, A.: Epidemiology of organ- and tissue-transmitted infections. Presented at Workshop on Preventing Organ- and Tissue Allograft-Transmitted Infection: Priorities for Public Health Intervention. June 2, 2005, Atlanta. Proceedings available at http://www.cdc.gov/ncidod/dhqp/pdf/bbp/organ-tissueWorkshop_June2005.pdf
17. Strong, D. M.; Katz, L.: Blood-bank testing for infectious diseases: how safe is blood transfusion? *Trends Mol Med* 8:355–358, 2002.
18. United States Pharmacopeial Convention: Sterilization and sterility assurance of compendial articles, Chapter 1211. In *United States Pharmacopeia and National Formulary* (USP25-NF20). Rockville, MD: The United States Pharmacopeial Convention, Inc., 2002.
19. U.S. Food and Drug Administration: Current good tissue practice for manufacturers of human cellular- and tissue-based products establishments: inspection and enforcement: proposed rule. *Fed Reg* 2001 Jan 8;66:1508–1559. Available at http://www.fda.gov/cber/tiss/htm
20. U.S. Food and Drug Administration: Current good tissue practice for human cell, tissue, and cellular- and tissue-based product establishments: inspection and enforcement; Final Rule 21 CFR Parts 16, 1270, and 1271 (D,E,F) 69. Fed Reg:16-611-68688, November 24, 2004. Available at www.fda.gov/cber/tiss/htm
21. U.S. Food and Drug Administration: Draft document guidance for industry: preventive measures to reduce the possible risk of transmission of Creutzfeldt-Jakob Disease (CJD) and variant Creutzfeldt-Jakob Disease (vCJD) by human cells, tissues and cellular- and tissue-based products (HCT/Ps), June 14, 2002. Available at http://www.fda.gov/cber/tiss/htm
22. U.S. Food and Drug Administration: Draft guidance for industry: eligibility determination for donors of human cells, and tissues and tissue-based products (HCT/Ps), May 2004. Available at http://www.fda.gov/cber/tiss/htm
23. Vangsness, C. T., Jr.; Garcia, I. A.; Mills, C. R.; et al.: Allograft transplantation in the knee: tissue regulation, procurement, processing, and sterilization. *Am J Sports Med* 31:474–481, 2003.
24. Vangsness, C. T. Jr.; Wagner, P. P.; Moore, T. M.; Roberts, M. R.: Overview of safety issues concerning the preparation and processing of soft-tissue allografts. *J Arthroscopy* 22:1351–1358, 2006.
25. Vangsness, C. T., Jr.: Soft-tissue allograft processing controversies. *J Knee Surg* 19:215–219, 2006.
26. Veen, M. R.; Bloem, R. M.; Petit, P. L.: Sensitivity and negative predictive value of swab cultures in musculoskeletal allograft procurement. *Clin Orthop* 300:259–263, 1994.
27. Zou, S.; Dodd, R. Y.; Stramer, S. L.; Strong, D. M.; and the Tissue Safety Study Group: Probability of viremia with HBV, HCV, HIV, and HTLV among tissue donors in the United States. *N Engl J Med* 351:751–759, 2004.

Chapter 10

Scientific and Clinical Basis for Double-Bundle Anterior Cruciate Ligament Reconstruction in Primary and Revision Knees

Susan Jordan, MD ■ *Wei Shen*, MD, PhD ■ *Freddie Fu*, MD

INDICATIONS

Scientific Background: Anatomy and Biomechanics

The anterior cruciate ligament (ACL) consists of dense connective tissue enveloped in a synovial membrane, which places the ligament in an intra-articular but extrasynovial position.[2,5] It attaches proximally on the posterior aspect of the lateral femoral condyle (LFC) and runs in an oblique course distally through the intercondylar notch to insert between the medial and the lateral tibial spines. Many authors have studied the ACL bundle anatomy and reached a general consensus that the ACL consists of two bundles: an anteromedial (AM) bundle and a posterolateral (PL) bundle (Fig. 10–1A). The AM bundle is slightly larger in diameter than the PL bundle. The bundles are named for their relative positions on their tibial insertion sites[4] (see Fig. 10–1B). Recently, the two-bundle anatomy was also verified in a fetal study by Ferretti and coworkers.[6]

The authors have studied the bony topography of the femoral attachment of ACL extensively. Using fetal specimens, cadavers, and in vivo arthroscopic observation, we have identified two osseous ridges that define the origins of the AM and PL bundles. The lateral intercondylar ridge runs proximal to distal through the entire ACL femoral attachment. With the knee in extension, no fibers of the ACL are attached anterior to this ridge. A second osseous ridge, the lateral bifurcate ridge, divides the femoral attachments of the AM and the PL bundles. It is important to note that when the knee is in full extension (anatomic position), the femoral origin of the AM bundle is located at the posterior and proximal portion of the lateral intercondylar wall, whereas the origin of the PL bundle is located slightly distally. The two bundles are parallel in extension. As the knee is flexed to 90°, which is the typical position during ACL reconstruction, the origins of the two bundles change from a vertical alignment to a horizontal alignment and the bundles cross.[4] The lateral intercondylar ridge delineates the superior border of ACL femoral attachment (Fig. 10–2), whereas the lateral bifurcate ridge runs from superior to inferior and separates the femoral AM and PL attachments.

Biomechanically, the two bundles are not isometric throughout the range of knee motion. Generally, the AM bundle maintains at a constant level of tension throughout the range of motion, with some increase when the knee is flexed that reaches a maximum at 60°.[7] The tension of the PL bundle is more

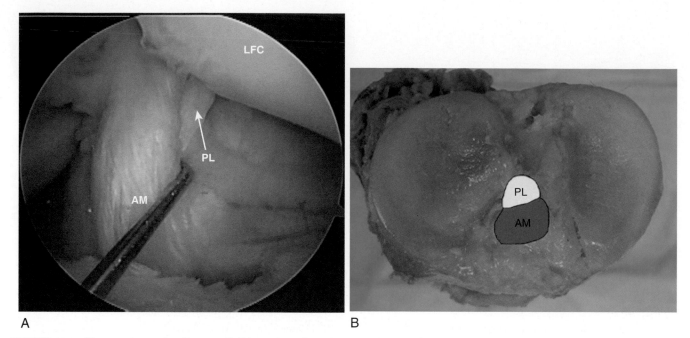

A   **B**

FIGURE 10–1. The anterior cruciate ligament (ACL) consists of two functional bundles, the anteromedial (AM) bundle and the posterolateral (PL) bundle. **A,** Arthroscopic view of the AM and PL bundle. **B,** Cadaveric dissection of tibial AM and PL insertion site.

variable because it tightens in knee extension and slackens in flexion past 30°. Thus, the AM and PL bundles have varying contributions to knee stability at different flexion angles. The AM bundle limits anteroposterior (AP) translation throughout knee motion, whereas the PL bundle plays an important role in limiting not only anterior tibial translation but also rotation.[3,7,10]

Biomechanical studies have emphasized the importance of both bundles in knee stability. Yagi and associates[13] showed that double-bundle (DB) ACL reconstruction better restores knee biomechanics than single-bundle (SB) ACL reconstruction. The addition of a PL bundle produces in situ forces within each bundle that closely

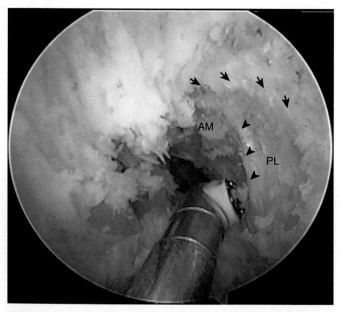

FIGURE 10–2. The lateral intercondylar ridge (*arrows*) marks the superior aspect of the femoral insertion sites of the AM and PL bundles when the knee is in 90° of flexion. The lateral bifurcate ridge (*arrowheads*) separates the insertions between the two bundles.

match the in situ forces found in a native ACL ligament. Tashman and colleagues[11] studied the in vivo kinematics after ACL reconstruction with the use of high-speed stereoradiography. This study demonstrated that SB ACL reconstruction sufficiently restored AP tibial stability. An unexplained increase of 3° to 4° in adduction and external tibial rotation was reported. Zantop and coworkers[15] showed that isolated transection of the AM bundle increased anterior tibial translation at 60° and 90° of knee flexion significantly, whereas isolated transection of the PL bundle significantly increased anterior tibial translation at 30° of flexion. In addition, PL bundle transection led to significantly increased rotation at 0° and 30° in response to a combined rotatory load when compared with the intact knee and the AM bundle–deficient knees. This study supports the concept that SB (AM bundle) reconstruction cannot restore native knee stability, particularly rotatory stability.

Primary Knees

DB ACL reconstruction is indicated for acute or chronic ACL ruptures that cause symptomatic instability. The criteria for DB ACL reconstruction are (1) a history of instability, shifting, or giving-way with activities; (2) positive Lachman and pivot shift tests; (3) increased KT-1000 measurement compared with the contralateral knee; and (4) patient desires to undergo ACL reconstruction. Whereas some surgeons reserve the DB procedure for patients with global ligamentous laxity or very large pivot shifts, the authors currently advocate the procedure for most patients with clinical instability from an ACL tear.

Revision Knees

DB ACL reconstruction as a revision procedure may be indicated when an SB ACL reconstruction has failed owing to graft rupture or when an SB graft is intact but does not provide adequate stability. In the latter case, depending on the position of the original tunnels, the surgeon may either augment the intact SB graft

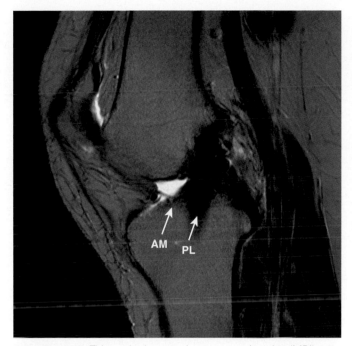

FIGURE 10–3. This sagittal magnetic resonance imaging (MRI) scan shows an example of tunnel mismatch. The tibial tunnel occupies the position of the PL bundle. The femoral tunnel is closer to the attachment of the AM bundle.

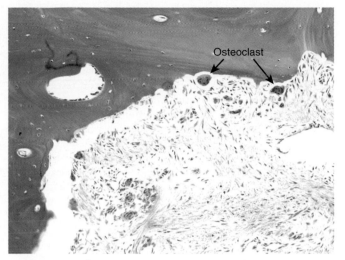

FIGURE 10–4. Osteoclasts are shown at the graft–bone tunnel interface. We have observed increased osteoclastic activity at the graft-bone interface in cases of tunnel mismatch.

with an additional graft or implant two new grafts. In the authors' practice, patients frequently present with an intact SB graft but complain of clinical symptoms of instability and demonstrate a positive pivot shift on examination. In these cases, there is often a mismatch in the femoral and tibial tunnel placements. For example, the tibial tunnel occupies the position of the PL bundle and the femoral tunnel is located in a high position in the notch above the AM bundle attachment (Fig. 10–3). This pattern of mismatch is often a result of the transtibial technique for femoral tunnel preparation, in which the femoral tunnel position is dictated by the tibial tunnel position. The graft in this case may provide stability in the AP plane but does not provide adequate rotational stability and results in symptomatic instability.

A nonanatomic tunnel placement, or tunnel mismatch, may lead to graft laxity and ultimate failure. In the laboratory, increased osteoclastic activity has been observed at the graft-bone interface in such mismatched tunnels (Fig. 10–4). When a graft is placed at a nonanatomic position relative to the native ACL, it experiences large tensile forces secondary to this abnormal position. These abnormal forces compromise biologic healing and ultimately may contribute to graft laxity and failure.

CONTRAINDICATIONS

Primary Knees

There are certain contraindications to DB ACL reconstruction. Patients with ACL rupture who do not have symptomatic instability and do not participate in cutting and pivoting sports may choose not to undergo ACL surgery, because they can function well without an intact ligament. Patients with a limitation of knee motion and flexion contractures must first be rehabilitated appropriately with aggressive physical therapy before consideration of DB ACL reconstruction. Patients with active infection are not candidates

for reconstructive surgery. Skeletally immature patients are not candidates for DB ACL reconstruction owing to the risk of growth arrest from transphyseal tunnel drilling.

Revision Knees

Contraindications to DB ACL reconstruction in the revision setting include active infection and skeletal immaturity. Excessive tunnel widening and bone loss from prior ACL reconstruction surgery necessitates staging of the revision procedure. In these cases, bone-grafting of the femoral and tibial tunnels is first performed. After the bone graft has healed, revision DB ACL surgery is accomplished.

CLINICAL EVALUATION

Primary Knees

The first portion of the clinical evaluation consists of obtaining a thorough history from the patient. The timing and description of the injury mechanism should be reviewed carefully because this information may raise suspicion of injury to particular structures depending on the direction of force to the knee. The patient should be asked if he or she felt or heard a pop at the time of the injury. In addition, the development of an effusion and difficulty with weight-bearing should be noted. Episodes of recurrent shifting or instability are important to document, including the situations in which they occurred. Any previous treatment of the injury such as physical therapy or bracing should be documented. The patient's preinjury activity level should be determined to assess if he or she engages in activities, such as soccer or basketball, that require cutting and pivoting motions. Any previous history of knee injury or knee surgery should be explored.

The second portion of the clinical evaluation is a comprehensive physical examination. Weight-bearing alignment is evaluated for any valgus or varus deformity. Before the patient sits or lies on the examining table, it is important to assess her or his gait for the presence of a limp and note whether any assistive devices are required for ambulation. With the patient supine, the presence and size of an effusion is noted. Quadriceps function and atrophy are assessed, including the patient's ability to perform a straight leg raise without an extensor lag. Joint range of motion is measured and compared with that of the contralateral knee. The patellofemoral joint is examined for apprehension, crepitation, and facet tenderness. The ligament examination includes the Lachman, pivot shift, anterior drawer, posterior drawer, and valgus and varus laxity tests. The ligament examination is performed bilaterally for comparison. Joint line tenderness and the McMurray flexion test are done to detect meniscal pathology. KT-1000 testing of both knees is performed and the difference in millimeters recorded.

When an ACL injury is suspected, diagnostic studies are ordered. Radiographs include a weight-bearing posteroanterior flexion view, a lateral view of the injured knee, and a Merchant view of both knees. In patients with abnormal alignment or previous surgery or who are older, long-leg cassette films are obtained to quantify malalignment. Radiographs are scrutinized for joint space narrowing, osteochondral lesions, fractures, and alignment abnormalities.

The other diagnostic study of importance is magnetic resonance imaging (MRI). At the authors' center, a special protocol to study the ACL consists of a series of images in the plane of the two bundles of the ACL (Fig. 10–5A) in addition to the usual coronal, axial, and sagittal images. This provides improved visualization of the individual AM and PL bundles, allowing identification of individual bundle ruptures (see Fig. 10–5B) and the location of the rupture as either off the femur or the tibia or in mid-substance. In addition, assessment is performed of the condition of the other knee ligaments, menisci, cartilage, and bony structures.

Revision Knees

Clinical evaluation of a patient with a failed previous ACL reconstruction is identical to that of a patient with a primary

ACL rupture, including a complete history and comprehensive physical examination. It is important to ascertain the mechanism of graft failure as well as the timing in relation to the primary procedure. Some patients will recall a specific episode in which the knee was reinjured. Others will not recall a reinjury but will state that the knee never felt stable even after the initial ACL reconstruction. Another important component of the history includes the operative report from the primary surgeon to identify the type of graft used, fixation methods, and tunnel widths.

A complete physical examination is performed, as previously described. The surgeon must pay specific attention to previous incisions and sites of graft harvest in order to plan the revision appropriately. In some cases, the Lachman and KT-1000 measurements are not as impressive as the pivot shift, indicating the presence of a nonanatomic graft that provides AP stability but not rotational stability.

Radiographs are required to determine fixation methods used in the primary procedure (Fig. 10–6A). Joint space narrowing, osteochondral lesions, and tunnel width are identified. MRI is performed to determine whether the original graft is intact or ruptured, assess tunnel location and width (see Fig. 10–6B and C), and identify additional pathology involving the cartilage or menisci.

PREOPERATIVE PLANNING

Primary Knees

Once the ACL rupture has been diagnosed and DB ACL reconstruction selected, preoperative planning is conducted that includes a careful review of any associated injuries, such as

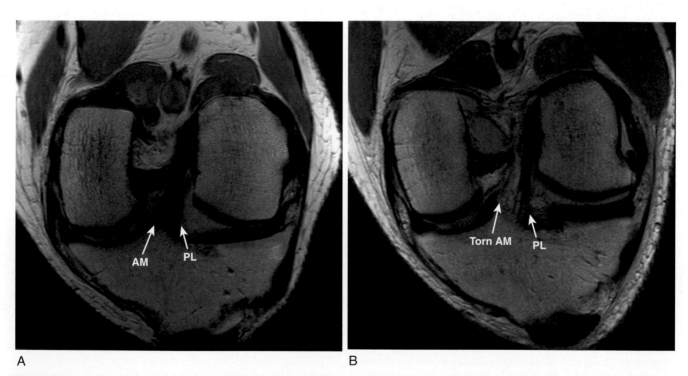

A   B

FIGURE 10–5. A, An example of the special MRI scan in the oblique plane of the ACL clearly demonstrates the presence of intact AM and PL bundles. **B,** MRI scans in the plane of the ACL allow identification of individual bundle rupture. In this case, the PL bundle is intact and the AM bundle is torn.

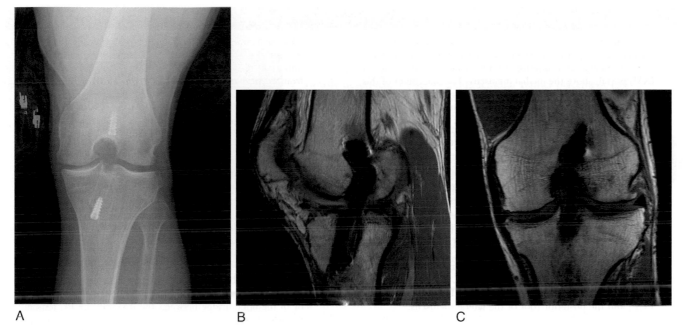

A   B   C

FIGURE 10–6. Anteroposterior (AP) radiograph (**A**), sagittal (**B**) and coronal images (**C**) from a patient with a failed single-bundle ACL reconstruction. **A** and **C**, Vertical femoral tunnel placement is noted. **B**, The graft is shown to insert in the area of PL bundle insertion on the tibia. On the femoral side, the graft inserts anteriorly and superiorly to the AM bundle femoral insertion. A revision ACL reconstruction using the double-bundle technique was performed in a single stage procedure.

meniscal tears, and plan for treatment of these associated injuries. Graft options are reviewed and discussed with the patient. The authors routinely use two tibialis anterior allografts for this procedure. The operation and postoperative rehabilitation are reviewed with the patient prior to surgery.

Revision Knees

Preoperative planning takes on special importance in the case of revision DB ACL surgery. The surgeon must review the patient's prior operative report and arthroscopic images, if available. From the physical examination and imaging, the integrity of the graft and the location of the femoral and tibial tunnel positions in relation to the anatomic attachments of the AM and PL bundles are determined. Tunnel mismatch is assessed. The overall orientation of the graft (e.g., vertical) is determined from the coronal and sagittal images of the MRI. If tunnel widening is severe, the surgeon should stage the revision ACL surgery by first bone grafting the old tunnels.

If the graft is intact and there is no tunnel mismatch, an appropriate plan may entail augmentation of the old graft with a new graft. If the graft is ruptured, or the tunnels are nonanatomic, the graft is removed and new femoral and tibial tunnels drilled. The surgeon must be aware of the limited space available for creation of new tunnels and try to determine preoperatively whether the previous tunnel will interfere with anatomic tunnel placement. In some cases, an over-the-top location for the femoral AM graft is required owing to limited space on the femoral side. However, use of the transtibial technique in the primary procedure frequently results in an excessively high femoral tunnel. This tunnel is usually well superior to the anatomic AM bundle attachment site and does not preclude placement of new anatomic AM and PL femoral tunnels during revision DB ACL surgery.

INTRAOPERATIVE EVALUATION

Once the patient is anesthetized with either a general or a spinal anesthetic, an examination under anesthesia is performed. Range of motion of both the injured and the noninjured knee is compared. The Lachman, pivot shift, and anterior drawer tests are performed to assess laxity under anesthesia. The operative limb is elevated for 3 minutes to allow exsanguination, and a tourniquet is then inflated to 350 mm Hg. The thigh is placed in a thigh holder and the bed is positioned with the distal portion flexed. The nonoperative leg is placed in a well-padded leg holder in the abducted position (Fig. 10–7). At this point, the operative lower extremity is prepared and draped with alcohol and povidone-iodine (Betadine).

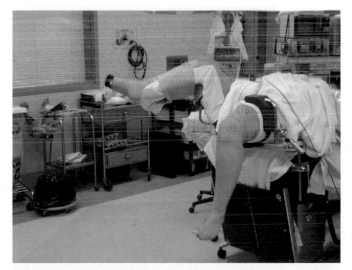

FIGURE 10–7. The set-up for a double-bundle ACL reconstruction, using a thigh-holder, allows knee range of motion from full extension to 120° of flexion. Hyperflexion is critical when performing the double-bundle ACL reconstruction procedure.

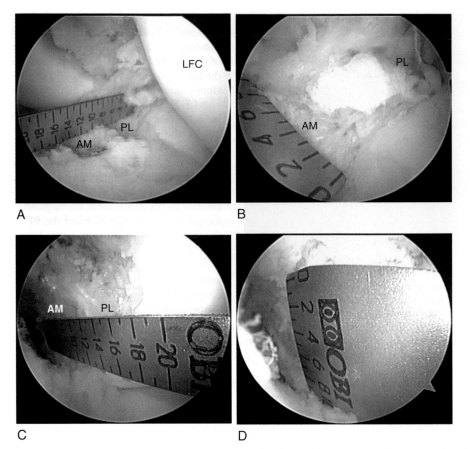

FIGURE 10–11. The tibial footprints are measured for length (**A**) and width (**B**). The femoral footprints are also measured for length (**C**) and width (**D**).

Next, the AM and PL tibial tunnels are prepared. A 3- to 4-cm skin incision is made over the AM surface of the tibia at the level of the tibial tubercle. The PL tibial tunnel is drilled first. With the arthroscope in the AL portal, the elbow ACL tibial drill guide is set at 45° and the tip of the drill guide is placed on the tibial footprint of the PL bundle via the AAM portal. The tibial PL bundle footprint is adjacent to the posterior root of the lateral meniscus and posterolateral to the AM bundle of the ACL (Fig. 10–12). On the tibial cortex, the tibial drill for the PL tunnel starts just anterior to the superficial medial collateral ligament fibers. Once the tibial drill guide is set, a 3.2-mm guidewire is passed into the base of the PL tibial footprint. The AM tibial tunnel is similarly drilled with the elbow ACL tibial drill guide set at 45° inserted through the AM portal. On the tibial cortex, the starting point for the AM bundle is midway between the PL starting point and the tibial tuberosity. There should be an adequate distance between these two pins to ensure sufficient bony bridge between the tunnels (Fig. 10–13). The AM and PL tibial tunnels are then overdrilled using a cannulated drill. The PL tunnel is usually accomplished with a 6-mm drill and the AM with a 7-mm drill. A curette is placed over the tip of the guidewire during reaming to protect the femoral articular cartilage. A dilator is used to widen the tunnels to the specific diameters, which are most commonly 8 mm for the AM tunnel and 7 mm for the PL tunnel.

The femoral AM tunnel is the last tunnel to be drilled. The arthroscope is placed in the AM portal for this part of the procedure. First, a transtibial approach is attempted with a guidewire placed through the AM tibial tunnel (Fig. 10–14A). However, in

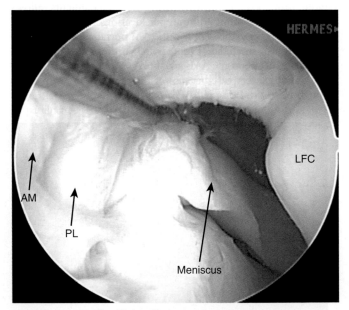

FIGURE 10–12. The PL bundle inserts on the tibia adjacent to the posterior horn attachment of the lateral meniscus.

some cases, the correct position for the AM femoral tunnel cannot be reached with this technique. Often, this places the guidewire too high and too far anterior on the medial wall of the lateral femoral condyle, outside of the anatomic footprint. In these cases, a transtibial technique through the PL tibial tunnel is attempted (see Fig. 10–14B). In some cases, the trajectory of

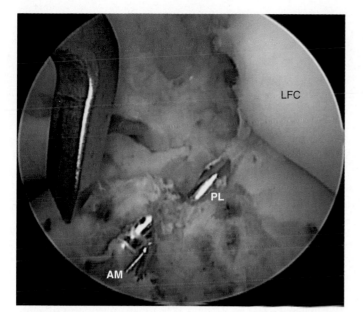

FIGURE 10–13. Guidewires for the AM and PL tibial tunnels are placed, centered in the insertions of the AM and PL bundles.

the guidewire is still too high. When the center of the AM femoral footprint cannot be reached through either the AM or the PL tibial tunnel, the guidewire is placed through the AAM portal (see Fig. 10–14C). Usually, the knee must be flexed greater than 90° to position the pin appropriately in the center of the AM bundle attachment.

With the tip of the guidewire in place at the center of the AM femoral footprint, a cannulated acorn drill is inserted over the guidewire, drilling to a depth of 20 to 30 mm. A smaller depth is used when drilling through the AAM portal than transtibially owing to the shorter distance to the femoral cortex. The far cortex of the AM femoral tunnel is breached with a 4.5-mm EndoButton drill, and the depth gauge is used to measure the distance to the far cortex. The appropriate depth for the EndoButton to flip is calculated (the tunnel length minus 7 mm if a 15-mm loop is used), and the tunnel is reamed by hand to this depth with an 8-mm reamer. An assistant marks both the AM and the PL grafts with a marking pen at the appropriate distance from the EndoButton for the tunnel

length. The final appearance of the tunnels after completion of preparation is shown in Figure 10–15.

The next step is graft passage, beginning with the PL graft. A Beath pin with a very long looped suture in the eyelet is passed through the AAM portal and out through the PL femoral tunnel. The looped suture is visualized intra-articularly and retrieved with an arthroscopic suture grasper through the PL tibial tunnel. This process is repeated for the AM graft, passing the Beath pin through whichever tunnel or portal was used to drill the AM femoral tunnel, and retrieving it through the AM tibial tunnel. The sutures from the Beath pin cross over each other with the knee in flexion (Fig. 10–16). Both Beath pins are passed before inserting the PL graft into the joint to protect it from injury. Subsequently, the PL graft is passed through the PL tibial tunnel into the PL femoral tunnel. Once the graft markings are seen, the EndoButton is flipped. During PL graft passage, the knee must be hyperflexed, just as it was during PL femoral tunnel preparation.

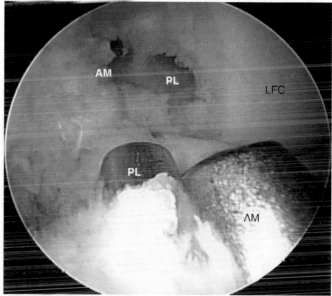

FIGURE 10–15. The final appearance of the tunnels prior to graft passage, with dilators protruding from the AM and PL tibial tunnels.

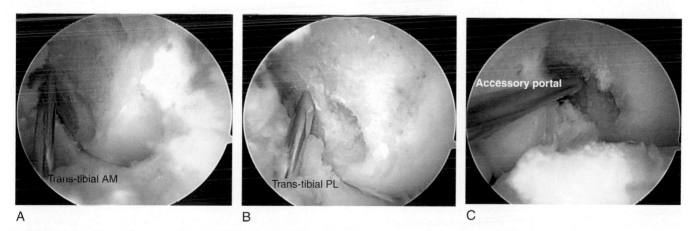

A   **B**   **C**

FIGURE 10–14. The guidewire can be inserted in one of three ways to reach the AM femoral attachment site for AM femoral tunnel preparation: transtibially through the AM tibial tunnel (**A**), transtibially through the PL tibial tunnel (**B**), or through the accessory anteromedial (AAM) portal (**C**).

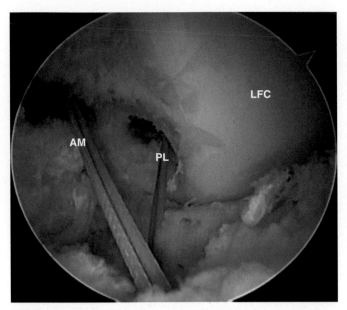

FIGURE 10–16. When both Beath pins have been passed into the AM and PL tunnels, the suture loops from the Beath pins cross over each other at 90° of knee flexion.

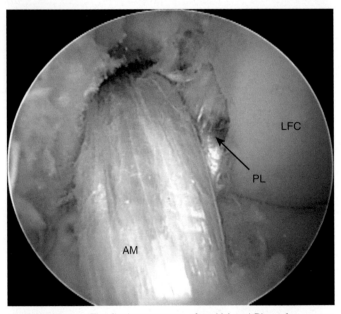

FIGURE 10–17. The final appearance after AM and PL graft passage shows a crossing pattern when in flexion. Also, the PL bundle is mostly covered by the AM bundle.

After passing the PL graft, the AM graft is passed retrograde and the EndoButton is flipped onto the lateral femoral cortex (Fig. 10–17). Preconditioning of the grafts is performed by flexing and extending the knee from 0° to 120°, approximately 20 to 30 times. Fixation on the tibial side is performed with bioabsorbable screws that are the same size in diameter as the grafts. We don't actually measure the tension, but manually tension the graft and then confirm adequate tension by checking Lachman test and graft tension intraoperatively after fixation. The PL graft is fixed with the knee in extension, and the AM graft is fixed at 60° of

flexion. After tibial fixation, a final arthroscopic inspection is performed to confirm the correct position and tension of the grafts. The surgeon verifies that there is no roof impingement or posterior cruciate ligament (PCL) impingement. Interestingly, these phenomena have not been observed in the setting of an anatomic DB ACL reconstruction.

Subcutaneous tissue and skin are closed in layers. A dry sterile dressing is applied. A Cryo-Cuff (Aircast, Vista, CA) is used for cold therapy and compression. A hinged knee brace is applied and locked in extension for ambulation.

Rehabilitation for anatomic DB ACL reconstruction is the same as that used for SB ACL reconstruction. Weight-bearing with crutches is allowed immediately after surgery, progressing from partial to full. During the first 1 to 3 months postoperatively, restoration of normal range of knee motion and recovery of muscle strength are emphasized. Closed-chain and functional exercises are incorporated, as well as balance and neuromuscular training. Plyometric and sports-specific exercises are begun 3 months postoperatively. The patient is allowed to gradually return to sports activities at approximately 6 months postoperatively. The individual should have no pain or swelling, 80% to 90% quadriceps strength, a normal single-leg hop test, and adequate proprioception and neuromuscular control before being fully released back to sports.

Revision Knees

The AL, AM, and AAM portals are established as previously described. A careful arthroscopic examination is performed to assess the position and integrity of the graft. The graft may be intact but quite lax and stretched out, rendering it nonfunctional. If the graft is intact and functional, the location of the femoral and tibial tunnels must be judged. If the intact, functional graft is in an acceptable position for an AM or PL bundle, an augmentation procedure is performed in which the absent bundle is reconstructed, leaving the intact graft alone. Commonly, the tunnels for the intact graft are mismatched. Most often, the tibial tunnel is located in the area of the PL bundle attachment, and the femoral tunnel is placed anterior and superior to the AM bundle attachment (Fig. 10–18). In this case, the graft must be resected and new femoral tunnels established. Depending on the size of the original tibial tunnel, either one large tunnel for both AM and PL bundles or two separate tunnels may be used. If tunnel widening is excessive, the surgeon should consider bone-grafting the tunnel and staging the revision DB ACL reconstruction.

Once the surgeon has determined that the graft is either incompetent or nonanatomic, the fixation devices on the tibial and femoral side are addressed. Staples and screws may be removed from the tibial side through the old incision to facilitate tibial tunnel preparation. On the femoral side, if the tunnel is nonanatomic and does not interfere anatomically with the creation of two new tunnels, the fixation device is left alone.

If the graft is incompetent or nonanatomic, it is resected with a thermal device. The thermal device is used to perform a gentle dissection of any remaining soft tissue to identify locations for the new femoral tunnels. In primary DB ACL surgery, the lateral intercondylar ridge and lateral bifurcate ridge are helpful bony landmarks to guide AM and PL femoral tunnel placement. In revision DB ACL surgery, these landmarks are often not easily identified. Frequently, a notchplasty was performed at the time of the primary ACL reconstruction, removing these

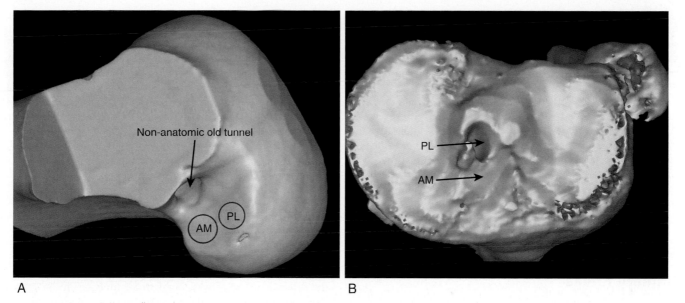

FIGURE 10–18. **A,** A three-dimensional computed tomographic rendering of the distal femur in a failed single-bundle ACL reconstruction. The rendering demonstrates the nonanatomic position of the previous femoral tunnel, well superior to the native AM bundle attachment. **B,** A similar rendering of the proximal tibia in the same case of failed single-bundle ACL reconstruction. The tibial tunnel occupies the PL tibial insertion site, thus creating femoral and tibial tunnel mismatch.

landmarks and distorting the anatomy. In these cases, the surgeon must rely on his or her knowledge of ACL insertional anatomy to guide tunnel placement in the revision procedure.

As described for primary DB ACL reconstruction, a Steadman awl is used to mark the center of the eventual AM and PL tunnels on the lateral femoral wall. Placing the arthroscope in the AM portal facilitates visualization of the wall and allows accurate tunnel markings. Attention is turned first to preparation of the PL femoral tunnel, which is done in the same manner as previously described.

Next, attention is turned to tibial tunnel preparation. If the original tibial tunnel is small enough in relation to the size of the knee and placed near the insertion of either the AM or the PL bundle, it is theoretically possible to drill a separate new tibial tunnel. However, in many revision cases, the original tibial tunnel is enlarged, occupying the area of both AM and PL bundle attachments. Therefore, two separate tibial tunnels cannot be used because both AM and PL grafts will traverse a single tibial tunnel. The old tibial tunnel is reamed and all remaining soft tissue removed from the walls of the tunnel. The tunnel is then expanded to accommodate both the AM and the PL grafts, attempting to create a figure-of-eight–type aperture that allows an anterior recess for the AM graft and a posterior recess for the PL graft. If the position of the original tibial tunnel is completely unsatisfactory, the surgeon should strongly consider bone-grafting the tunnel and staging the revision DB ACL procedure.

The AM femoral tunnel is prepared. In many cases, the original femoral tunnel is superior to the AM femoral insertion and, therefore, does not interfere with drilling a new, anatomic AM femoral tunnel. In this case, the AM femoral tunnel is prepared as described for a primary DB ACL procedure. Upon completion of tunnel preparation, the grafts are passed as described for a primary DB ACL reconstruction. If a single tibial tunnel is used, the surgeon must use a probe during graft passage to maintain the relative anterior and posterior positions of the AM and PL grafts.

In some cases, the original tunnel encroaches upon the AM femoral insertion and there may not be enough room to drill a new AM femoral tunnel. An over-the-top procedure will circumvent this problem and allow near-anatomic graft placement. For the over-the-top procedure, the back wall of the lateral femoral condyle is rasped to create a healing surface for the graft. Next, an incision is made along the lateral aspect of the thigh near the lateral femoral condyle. Dissection is carried down to the level of the vastus lateralis, which is elevated superiorly with a retractor to expose the over-the-top position on the posterior aspect of the lateral femoral condyle. Next, a looped 18-gauge wire is passed on a curved clamp from the intercondylar notch around to the over-the-top position. This wire is retrieved through the lateral incision. Another looped wire is placed through the original wire, and the original wire is retrieved through the notch, thereby pulling the looped wire anterograde into the notch. The loop is retrieved with an arthroscopic grasper through the tibial tunnel.

Once the wire loop is positioned in the tibial tunnel, the Beath pin for the PL tunnel is passed as previously described. The PL graft is passed first, and the EndoButton deployed on the outer femoral cortex. Next, the sutures on the AM graft are passed through the wire loop, and the wire is pulled out of the lateral incision, bringing the AM graft into the tibial tunnel and into the over-the-top position on the femur. The graft is secured with staples, a screw, and a spiked washer or tied around a post on the distal femur.

If two separate tibial tunnels are used, the grafts are tensioned separately as described for a primary DB ACL procedure. In the revision setting, supplementary fixation with staples or a post is used in addition to a biointerference screw. If a single tibial tunnel is used for both grafts, tensioning of the grafts becomes more complex. Both bundles are manually tensioned at 20° of flexion and fixed with an interference screw in the single tibial tunnel. We don't actually measure the tension of the graft. But the graft is manually tensioned and then adequate tension is confirmed by checking Lachman test and graft tension intraoperatively after fixation. Alternatively, the surgeon can tension and fix each graft separately, using either staples or sutures tied around a post. An interference screw may be added to the single tibial tunnel after individual bundle fixation if supplementary fixation is required.

Graft preparation for a revision DB ACL reconstruction is the same as that described for a primary DB ACL reconstruction. The authors commonly use two tibialis anterior allografts and EndoButtons for fixation on the femoral side. If an over-the-top procedure is performed, a long graft is required. For the over-the-top procedure, a 40- to 50-mm Endoloop may be placed on the doubled-over tibialis anterior allograft and the Endoloop fixed to the distal lateral femur around a screw and washer.

AUTHORS' OUTCOMES

Primary Knees

From November 2003 to October 2007, one of the authors (F.F.) performed 489 anatomic DB ACL reconstructions. In a total of 393 primary cases, 374 patients (95%) underwent primary DB reconstruction and 19 patients (5%) underwent primary SB augmentation. Primary SB augmentation was performed when one of the bundles was found to be intact. In these cases, the intact bundle was augmented by reconstruction of the ruptured bundle.

A prospective study was done to evaluate the outcomes of anatomic DB ACL reconstruction. Lachman and pivot shift tests, KT-2000 testing, range of knee motion, and overall International Knee Documentations Committee (IKDC) rating were accomplished. Compared with primary SB ACL reconstruction,[6a] knees that had primary DB ACL reconstruction demonstrated superior range of knee motion at 1, 4, and 12 weeks postoperatively. All patients who undergo DB ACL reconstruction will be followed prospectively for long-term results to document range of knee motion, ligamentous laxity, functional strength, and activity and sports participation.

At the time of writing, the initial 100 consecutive patients who underwent primary DB ACL reconstruction had been followed an average of 2.1 ± 0.5 years postoperatively. None of these patients had undergone concomitant ligament or cartilage restorative procedures. Fifteen had a concomitant medial meniscus repair, 14 had a partial lateral meniscectomy, 9 had a partial medial meniscectomy, and 1 had a lateral meniscus repair.

Evaluation revealed a mean side-to-side difference in range of motion of 2° ± 3° for extension and 2° ± 5° for flexion. One patient lacked 15° of extension and another lacked 13° of extension compared with the opposite knee. In both, the contralateral knee had a large amount of hyperextension (−10° and −13°) and a manipulation under anesthesia was required to restore hyperextension.

The Lachman test was normal in 65% and nearly normal in 33%. The pivot shift test was normal in 94% and nearly normal in 6%. KT-2000 testing had been done in 87 patients at the time of writing. The mean side-to-side difference was 1.0 ± 2.3 mm. Fifty-one patients had less than 3 mm of increased anterior translation, 32 patients had 3 to 5 mm of increased translation, and 4 patients had greater than 5 mm of increased translation. There were 8 graft failures, 7 of which underwent subsequent revision surgery.

No patient had complaints of pain, swelling, or instability during activities of daily living, and 73% to 78% had no symptoms during very strenuous or strenuous sports activities. The IKDC

Subjective Knee Form and Knee Osteoarthritis Outcome Score Activities of Daily Living and Sports Activity scores were 85.0, 91.8, and 87.0, respectively. These scores were similar in comparison with patients undergoing SB ACL reconstruction previously reported. Fifty-one percent of the patients described their current activity level as normal and 35% as nearly normal. From these initial results, the conclusion was reached that anatomic DB ACL reconstruction results in good restoration of joint stability and patient-reported outcomes when evaluated 2 years after surgery.

Revision Knees

In a total of 100 revision cases, 73 patients underwent DB ACL revision and 27 patients had secondary SB augmentation. For secondary augmentation cases,[4a] 23 patients had previous SB reconstruction and complained of instability. In spite of good range of motion and minimal side-to-side differences on KT-2000 testing, they were unstable during pivot shift testing. During surgery, the original AM graft was found to be functionally intact, and therefore, only PL bundle reconstruction was performed. The other 4 secondary augmentation patients had previous DB ACL reconstruction. The AM graft was shown to be stretched, and the PL graft remained functional. Therefore, only the AM graft was reconstructed; the PL graft was left intact.

Clinical and surgical data were prospectively collected on 16 patients with a failed SB ACL reconstruction that was revised to a DB reconstruction with a minimum 1 year follow-up.[4a] All patients were clinically unstable preoperatively. The AM graft was placed either in the original femoral tunnel, in a new femoral tunnel, or in an over-the-top position on the femur. At latest follow-up of an average of 1.1 years, 14 patients had a grade I Lachman and all 16 patients had a grade I pivot shift test.

OTHER AUTHORS' OUTCOMES

The literature contains few studies of outcomes after DB ACL reconstruction with techniques similar to those reported in this chapter. Most studies have short-term follow-up and employed different surgical techniques (e.g., use of a single tibial tunnel for both grafts along with two femoral tunnels). A few studies in the literature suggest improved rotational stability with DB techniques,[1,8,9,12,14] but well-designed outcome studies with long-term follow-up are lacking.

PREVENTION AND MANAGEMENT OF COMPLICATIONS

General complications after knee surgery include deep venous thrombosis, pulmonary embolus, neurovascular injury, and wound infection. Tunnel widening is a known complication after SB reconstruction and is also seen after anatomic DB ACL reconstruction. The authors studied tunnel widening after DB ACL reconstruction and found no correlation between tunnel size and clinical outcome. Fracture is a theoretical risk; however, the authors performed a study that found the probability of fracture to be exceedingly low and have not experienced this complication clinically. Intra-articular tunnel convergence may occur on the tibial side if the tunnels are not appropriately spaced. If the knee is not hyperflexed during PL femoral tunnel placement, the guidewire may exit near the common peroneal nerve or violate the articular cartilage of the LFC. The authors performed a cadaveric anatomic study and demonstrated that these structures are protected if the knee is flexed beyond 110°. When performing the tibial incision,[2a] the infrapatellar branch of the saphenous nerve may be damaged, leaving a small numb area along the anterolateral aspect of the knee and, rarely, a painful neuroma. The incidence of other complications such as impingement on the notch roof or on the PCL may be avoided or significantly reduced by performing anatomic DB ACL reconstruction because the anatomic placement of insertion sites closely restores the normal anatomy.

Complications of DB ACL revision reconstruction are similar to those in any revision setting. If tunnel widening is excessive, the surgeon should stage the procedure and bone-graft the tunnels to avoid compromising the outcome of the revision procedure. In the revision procedure, fixation may be suboptimal, and back-up methods should be employed as required. The rehabilitation should be tailored to the individual case and may require more gradual progression than a primary DB ACL to protect the healing grafts.

REFERENCES

1. Aglietti, P.; Giron, F.; Cuomo, P.; et al.: Single- and double-incision double-bundle ACL reconstruction. *Clin Orthop Relat Res* 454:108–113, 2007.
2. Arnoczky, S. P.: Anatomy of the anterior cruciate ligament. *Clin Orthop Relat Res* 172:19–25, 1983.
2a.Baer, G. S.; Shen, W.; Nozaki, N.; et al.: Effect of knee flexion angle on tunnel length and articular cartilage damage during anatomic double-bundle ACL reconstruction. AANA Annual Meeting, 2008, Washington, DC.
3. Buoncristiani, A. M.; Tjoumakaris, F. P.; Starman, J. S.; et al.: Anatomic double-bundle anterior cruciate ligament reconstruction. *Arthroscopy* 22:1000–1006, 2006.
4. Chhabra, A.; Starman, J. S.; Ferretti, M.; et al.: Anatomic, radiographic, biomechanical, and kinematic evaluation of the anterior cruciate ligament and its two functional bundles. *J Bone Joint Surg Am* 88(suppl 4):2–10, 2006.
4a.Colvin, A.; Shen, W.; Irrgang, J.: The double bundle concept application for revision ACL surgery. AAOS, 2009, Las Vegas.
5. Dienst, M.; Burks, R. T.; Greis, P. E.: Anatomy and biomechanics of the anterior cruciate ligament. *Orthop Clin North Am* 33:605–620, v, 2002.
6. Ferretti, M.; Levicoff, E. A.; Macpherson, T. A.; et al.: The fetal anterior cruciate ligament: an anatomic and histologic study. *Arthroscopy* 23:278–283, 2007.
6a.Fu, F.; Shen, W.; Okeke, N.; et al.: Primary anatomic ACL double bundle reconstruction. 2 years follow-up of first 100 consecutive patients. *Am J Sports Med* 90:249–255, 2008.
7 Gabriel, M. T.; Wong, E. K.; Woo, S. L.; et al.: Distribution of in situ forces in the anterior cruciate ligament in response to rotatory loads. *J Orthop Res* 22:85–89, 2004.

8. Jarvela, T.: Double-bundle versus single-bundle anterior cruciate ligament reconstruction: a prospective, randomized clinical study. *Knee Surg Sports Traumatol Arthrosc* 15:500–507, 2007.
9. Muneta, T.; Koga, H.; Mochizuki, T.; et al.: A prospective randomized study of 4-strand semitendinosus tendon anterior cruciate ligament reconstruction comparing single-bundle and double-bundle techniques. *Arthroscopy* 23:618–628, 2007.
10. Sakane, M.; Fox, R. J.; Woo, S. L.; et al.: In situ forces in the anterior cruciate ligament and its bundles in response to anterior tibial loads. *J Orthop Res* 15:285–293, 1997.
11. Tashman, S.; Collon, D.; Anderson, K.; et al.: Abnormal rotational knee motion during running after anterior cruciate ligament reconstruction. *Am J Sports Med* 32:975–983, 2004.
12. Yagi, M.; Kuroda, R.; Nagamune, K.; et al.: Double-bundle ACL reconstruction can improve rotational stability. *Clin Orthop Relat Res* 454:100–107, 2007.
13. Yagi, M.; Wong, E. K.; Kanamori, A.; et al.: Biomechanical analysis of an anatomic anterior cruciate ligament reconstruction. *Am J Sports Med* 30:660–666, 2002.
14. Yasuda, K.; Kondo, E.; Ichiyama, H.; et al.: Clinical evaluation of anatomic double-bundle anterior cruciate ligament reconstruction procedure using hamstring tendon grafts: comparisons among 3 different procedures. *Arthroscopy* 22:240–251, 2006.
15. Zantop, T.; Herbort, M.; Raschke, M. J.; et al.: The role of the anteromedial and posterolateral bundles of the anterior cruciate ligament in anterior tibial translation and internal rotation. *Am J Sports Med* 35:223–227, 2007.

Chapter 11

Anterior Cruciate Ligament Reconstruction in Skeletally Immature Patients

Kelly L. Vander Have, MD ■ *Edward M. Wojtys*, MD

INTRODUCTION

Prior to the mid-1980s, mid-substance anterior cruciate ligament (ACL) injuries in the skeletally immature athlete were believed to be rare.[25] More recently, ACL injury has been reported in 10% to 65% of pediatric knees with acute hemarthroses.[19,42] Although the true incidence and prevalence of ACL tears in the pediatric population have not been established, these injuries are now being recognized with increasing frequency.[42,44] Explanations for this apparent change may include improved ability to diagnose injury by physical examination and magnetic resonance imaging (MRI) as well as changes in the activity patterns of young athletes. The puzzling question facing clinicians centers on whether youngsters of today are training and conditioning to the point that the ACL has become more susceptible to injury.

Controversy exists regarding the initial management, indications for operative treatment, and the effect of age and maturity on management. In addition, there is a large practice variation in operative techniques to treat ACL injuries in these patients.

Previously, the concern for iatrogenic growth disturbance in children prevented the routine use of anatomic ACL reconstruction that has proved successful in adults. Alternative surgical treatment options include primary repair, extra-articular reconstruction, and transepiphyseal intra-articular reconstruction. Even though these injuries are occurring with increasing frequency, no unanimity exists concerning the appropriate and safest treatment. There are no long-term studies to help determine the optimal management approach. The few studies that have followed skeletally immature patients to physeal closure after transphyseal ACL reconstruction have documented growth comparable with that of age-matched controls without surgery.[1,27,39]

INDICATIONS

Historical recommendations for nonsurgical management of ACL insufficiency in the skeletally immature patient were based primarily on the concern for complications related to physeal injury. However, the majority of active patients treated nonsurgically were unable to return to sports, developed symptomatic instability, sustained meniscal tears, and suffered from long-term sequelae of articular cartilage damage. Unfortunately, the options for the young patient who develops traumatic osteoarthritis are very limited. Therefore, instability (giving-way) must be controlled. If activity modification is successful in limiting episodes of instability, nonoperative treatment is an option. If instability persists, the permanent sequelae from nonoperative treatment are seemingly more difficult to deal with than growth plate injury. For these reasons, ACL reconstruction should be considered.

Graf and associates[11] reported poor results at 15 months after injury, with new meniscal tears and episodes of instability in seven of eight skeletally immature patients who did not undergo reconstruction or activity limitations after ACL injury. Similarly, in a series of 18 skeletally immature patients examined an average of 51 months after complete ACL tear, Mizuta and colleagues[35] found that all patients had symptoms, 6 had meniscal tears, and 11 had developed radiographic changes. Janarv and coworkers[16] found that 10 of 23 skeletally immature patients treated with rehabilitation eventually needed reconstruction. McCarroll and associates[29] reported superior results with surgical management of complete ACL tears in prepubescent and junior high school patients compared with patients receiving conservative treatment. Of 16 prepubescent patients treated nonoperatively, 9 ceased sports participation, 4 sustained at least one reinjury, and only 3 were able to return to sport. In a separate group of 75 junior high school athletes with mid-substance tears, McCarroll and colleagues[30] reported that 37 of 38 patients who were initially treated nonoperatively had instability and 27 (71%) developed meniscal tears. Overall, 92% (55 of 60) of those treated with reconstruction returned to play.

CONTRAINDICATIONS

Nonoperative treatment is contraindicated in patients with giving-way episodes that produce meniscal tears or articular cartilage damage. If surgical repair is chosen, the patellar tendon autograft should not be harvested in a skeletally immature individual because it violates the proximal tibial apophysis and may result in tibial recurvatum. The placement of bone blocks into tunnels drilled across the femoral or tibial physis reliably causes growth arrest and must be avoided. Similarly, disruption of the periosteum over a growth plate can alter growth.

In the pubescent patient in whom a final growth spurt is anticipated, a soft tissue graft can be used. The exact risk of growth plate injury is unknown but can be extrapolated from the literature on trauma and fractures involving the growth plates around the knee.[8] If parents are unwilling to accept the risk of growth plate injury, reconstruction should be delayed until the physes are closed.

CLINICAL EVALUATION

History

A tear of the ACL can result from an impact to the knee or, more commonly, a noncontact twisting or landing injury. The timing of injury, either acute or chronic, should be noted. Knee effusion, pain, and ability to bear weight are important factors in diagnosing an ACL tear. An audible pop heard at the time of injury may be reported. An acute hemarthrosis, particularly in

the first 6 to 12 hours after injury, should raise concern for ACL injury. Stanitski and coworkers[42] found that 47% of preadolescents with a knee effusion had an ACL injury.

Children with congenital limb deficiencies, such as tibial and fibular hemimelia, congenital short femur, or proximal femoral focal deficiencies are other subsets of patients with ACL insufficiency. These children may develop instability at a much younger age and without any history of trauma to the knee. These cases are more complex and must be evaluated on an individual basis.

Physical Examination

The most important component in diagnosing pediatric knee injuries is the physical examination.[41] The presence of an effusion should be noted. Palpation of the joint line and physeal plates should be performed. Active and passive motion should be documented. Varus and valgus laxity should be checked in full extension and at 30° of flexion. Lachman testing should be assessed for magnitude. Pivot shifting may be quite uncomfortable in the acute setting and is not recommended. If the Lachman examination is positive acutely, the pivot shift test can be deferred until the examination under anesthesia if surgical intervention is chosen. Findings should always be compared with those in the contralateral knee. The patient should be assessed for generalized laxity with the degree of knee hyperextension noted.

Diagnostic Tests

A routine four-view radiographic series should be obtained. The formation of the tibial spine and femoral notch should be assessed. Children with congenital limb deficiencies often have a deficient tibial spine and lateral femoral condyle. Comparison views and stress views may be selectively needed if physeal injury is suspected. Magnetic resonance imaging (MRI) can assist in detecting ACL tears as well as associated meniscal pathology and chondral injury in those individuals who are difficult to examine. However, physical examination has been found to be more sensitive and specific than MRI in the evaluation of these patients. In reality, MRI can localize areas of injury but cannot determine degrees of laxity. MRI may be helpful in assessing other causes of anterior knee instability in the young patient, including tibial eminence fractures, periarticular (physeal) fractures, and congenital absence of the ACL. As in adults, arthrometric measurements can be done to support the diagnosis.

PREOPERATIVE PLANNING

Skeletal Maturity

The patient's level of skeletal maturity should be defined preoperatively. It is generally assumed that girls grow until age 14 ± 1 years and boys until age 16 ± 1 years[2]; however, age may not be the best indicator of potential growth. Peak growth velocity occurs between the ages of 10 to 11 years for girls and 13 to 14 years for boys. Closure of the triradiate cartilage, which can be seen on a standard radiograph of the pelvis, typically marks the end of peak growth velocity.[26] The patient can be assessed physiologically for signs of development, as noted by Tanner and Davies.[43] Age at onset of menses can be useful in females. After menarche, girls enter a deceleration phase of growth and typically reach skeletal maturity 18 months later. Family height can be used as an approximate estimate of growth potential as well. The patient can be assessed radiographically to determine skeletal maturity using the Risser sign on the pelvis.[37] The Risser sign is a radiographic measurement based on ossification of the iliac apophysis, beginning on the lateral aspect and progressing medially. Divided into four quadrants, the Risser sign proceeds from 0 (no ossification) to Risser 4, in which all four quadrants show ossification of the apophysis. Patients with Risser 0 or 1 have a significant amount of growth remaining, and the Risser 4 patient is skeletally mature. Bone age is another method to determine skeletal maturity by obtaining a radiograph of the hand and wrist and comparing it with the standards in the Gruelich and Pyle atlas.[12] The "rule of thirds" suggests that the distal femur and proximal tibia grow an average of 0.9 cm and 0.6 cm, respectively, per year of growth remaining.[32] Limb lengths and bilateral lower extremity alignment should be measured and any differences noted.

Associated Intra–articular Pathology

Previous studies have shown that 20% to 100% of pediatric patients who sustain ACL injuries have a concomitant meniscal injury.[11,34] Millett and associates[34] found that the incidence of medial meniscus tears increases significantly with chronic ACL insufficiency. Of the 22 patients who underwent surgery more than 6 weeks after injury, 72% had associated meniscal tears. If unstable meniscus tears exist, aggressive management is indicated. Every attempt should be made to salvage the meniscus in children and adolescents. Meniscectomy in this age group carries an even more ominous prognosis.[18] Manzione and colleagues[28] evaluated the results of partial and total meniscectomy in 20 patients with a mean age of 15 years (range, 5–15 yr). At 6-year follow-up, 16 knees had grade I osteoarthritis and 4 had grade II or III changes. Osteochondral injuries may require débridement, drilling, and/or stabilization at the time of ACL reconstruction.

INTRAOPERATIVE EVALUATION

A complete physical examination of the affected knee should be repeated under anesthesia for laxity, including Lachman and pivot shift tests, and again compared with the contralateral side. Prior to ligament reconstruction, arthroscopic visualization of the knee may be needed to assess for the partial or complete nature of the ACL tear if the examination under anesthesia is inconclusive. Partial-tear decisions should be based on the function of the remaining intact ligament and the degree of instability.

OPERATIVE TECHNIQUES AND CLINICAL OUTCOMES

Conventional surgical ACL reconstruction techniques used in adults risk potential iatrogenic growth disturbances in children owing to physeal injury. The spectrum of surgical techniques used in skeletally immature patients has included primary repair, extra-articular tenodesis, physeal sparing, and partial or complete transphyseal reconstruction. Skeletal age, activity level, associated injuries, reported success, and expected graft longevity are among the factors to consider when selecting a technique.

Primary Repair

DeLee and Curtis[7] reported on three patients who underwent primary ACL repair through sutures tied across the physis. At 21 months follow-up, all had clinical laxity and two of the three had episodes of giving-way. Engebretsen and coworkers[10] reviewed eight patients 3 to 8 years after primary repair and found that all experienced a decrease in activity level and five of the eight demonstrated instability on clinical examination. Grontvedt and associates[13] also noted that primary repair of the ACL in the skeletally immature patient had poor results, similar to those found in adults.

Physeal–Sparing Techniques

Early reports of physeal-sparing intra-articular reconstruction describe using a hamstring autograft left attached distally, passed into the knee under the anterior portion of the medial meniscus, and fixed to the lateral femoral condyle with staples in the over-the-top position on the femur[6] (Fig. 11–1). This technique is nonanatomic and does not reproduce the normal knee ligament kinematics. In a report of nine patients at 36.5 years follow-up, all had a 1+ Lachman and 1+ anterior drawer test. Six of nine patients returned to sports, but with bracing and precautions. No growth disturbances were reported.[6]

More recently, Kocher and colleagues[21] described Micheli and coworkers' technique,[33] which uses a combined intra- and extra-articular reconstruction and an autogenous iliotibial band (ITB) without violation of the physes. An incision is made obliquely from the lateral joint line to the superior border of the ITB. The ITB graft is harvested free proximally and left attached to Gerdy's tubercle distally and tubularized with a whipstitch. Arthroscopy of the knee is then performed through standard portals. The free end of the graft is brought into the knee in the over-the-top position posteriorly. A second incision

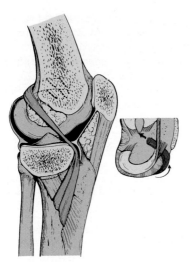

FIGURE 11–1. Cross-section of the left knee shows the trajectory of the graft. The *inset* shows the tibial plateau with the graft coursing under the anterior horn of the medial meniscus. *(Modified from Brief, L. P.: Anterior cruciate ligament reconstruction without drill holes. Arthroscopy 7:350–357, 1991. Used with permission from Elsevier.)*

is made over the proximal medial tibia. Dissection is carried down to the periosteum, and a curved clamp is passed from this incision into the joint under the intermeniscal ligament. The graft is then brought through the knee, under the intermeniscal ligament anteriorly, and out through the tibial incision. The graft is fixed to the femur with the use of sutures to the lateral femoral condyle at the insertion of the lateral intermuscular septum with the knee in 90° of flexion and external rotation. On the tibial side, the graft is sutured to the periosteum of the proximal tibia just distal to the physis with the knee flexed 20°, and tension is applied to the graft (Fig. 11–2).

Postoperatively, the patient ambulates with crutches and toe-touch weight-bearing for 6 weeks. Mobilization from 0° to 90° in a hinged knee brace is used initially, followed by progression to full motion after 2 more weeks.

Micheli and coworkers[33] reported the results of 17 patients with an average chronologic age of 11 years and a mean bone age of 10 years (range, 2–13 yr) who underwent the physeal-sparing reconstruction described previously. The mean follow-up was 66 months. All knees were subjectively and objectively stable by KT-1000 testing. No child developed a growth disturbance.

A study of Micheli and coworkers' technique[33] by Kocher and associates[20] reported on 44 skeletally immature patients (Tanner stage 1 or 2) with a mean chronologic age of 10.3 years and a mean skeletal age of 10.1 years. Functional outcome, graft survival, and growth disturbance were evaluated at a mean of 5.3 years (range, 2–15.1 yr) after surgery. Lachman examination was normal in 23 patients, nearly normal in 18 patients, and abnormal in 1. Two patients required revision reconstruction for graft failure at 4.7 and 8.3 years postoperatively. No patient had an angular deformity or limb length discrepancy clinically or radiographically. The authors strongly recommend this technique for Tanner stage 1 and 2 patients requiring ACL reconstruction.

Transepiphyseal Reconstruction

The nonanatomic, nonisometric positioning of physeal-sparing ACL reconstruction techniques creates concern for the biomechanics of the graft and, consequently, its longevity.

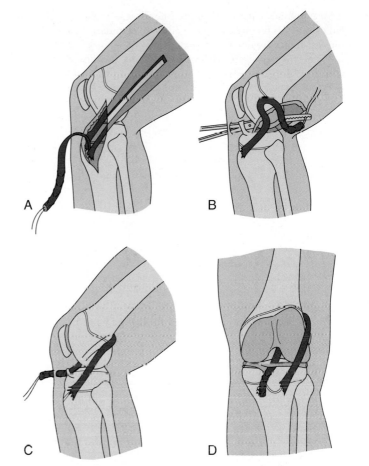

FIGURE 11–2. Physeal-sparing combined intra-articular and extra-articular reconstruction using an autogenous iliotibial band for prepubescent patients. **A,** The iliotibial band graft is harvested free proximally and left attached to Gerdy's tubercle distally. **B,** The graft is brought through the knee in the over-the-top position posteriorly. **C,** The graft is brought through the knee and under the intermeniscal ligament anteriorly. **D,** The graft is fixed to the intermuscular septum on the femoral side and to the periosteum of the proximal part of the tibia on the tibial side. *(A–D, Modified from Kocher, M. S.; Garg, S.; Micheli, L. J.: Physeal sparing reconstruction of the anterior cruciate ligament in skeletally immature prepubescent children and adolescents. Surgical technique. J Bone Joint Surg Am 88(suppl 1 pt 2):283–293, 2006. Used with permission from the Journal of Bone and Joint Surgery.)*

Critical Points AUTHORS' PREFERRED TECHNIQUES

- For prepubescent patients (Tanner 1 and 2), do an intra-articular extraphyseal reconstruction of the ACL using iliotibial band autograft as described by Micheli and coworkers.[33]
- In the pubescent patient with open growth plates and more than 1 year of growth remaining, a partial transphyseal reconstruction (vertical tunnel across the tibial physis, over-the-top on the femur) using either allograft or hamstring or quadriceps tendon autograft.
- Bone–patellar tendon–bone autograft when the physes are closed.

Transepiphyseal ACL reconstruction generally follows the principles of ACL reconstruction in adults but minimizes the risk of physeal injury by not crossing the tibial or femoral physis.

The affected leg is positioned with the hip flexed approximately 20°. Fluoroscopy is positioned on the side of the operating room table opposite the injured knee, and the femoral and tibial growth plates are visualized in both planes prior to preparing and draping. An oblique incision is made over the hamstring tendons. The semitendinosus and gracilis tendons are harvested and then doubled. Arthroscopy of the knee is accomplished in a standard fashion. With the C-arm in the lateral position, the point of the guidewire is positioned on the skin over the lateral femoral condyle, corresponding to the location of the footprint of the ACL. A small lateral incision is made, and the ITB is split longitudinally. The guidewire is advanced across the femoral epiphysis; the C-arm is used to confirm that the guidewire is not angulated in the anteroposterior or inferosuperior planes. The guidewire is visualized in the intercondylar notch arthroscopically, entering the joint at the proximal femoral footprint. A second guidewire is then inserted into the anteromedial tibia at the level of the epiphysis. The guidewire is advanced, clearing the tubercle anteriorly and entering the joint at the free edge of the lateral meniscus on the tibia (center of the footprint of the ACL). Tendon sizers are used to measure the diameter of the tendon graft, and the smallest appropriate reamer and EndoButton are chosen. The EndoButton and tendons are pulled up through the tibia and out the femoral hole with a suture. An EndoButton washer is placed over the Endo-Button and the graft is placed under tension, pulling the Endo-Button and washer to the surface of the lateral femoral condyle. With the knee in 10° of flexion, the graft is secured distally over a screw and post placed medial to the tubercle and distal to the tibial physis (Fig. 11–3).

Two series have been reported using transepiphyseal ACL reconstruction in skeletally immature patients. Guzzanti and coworkers[15] reported the results of this technique in five preadolescent patients (Tanner stage 1) with ACL injuries. The hamstring graft was left attached to the tibia, a transepiphyseal tibial

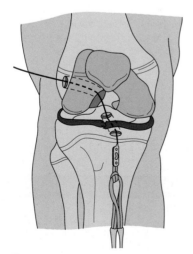

FIGURE 11–3. The semitendinosus and gracilis tendons are pulled up through the tibia and out the lateral femoral condyle with use of No. 5 suture in the EndoButton. *(Modified from Anderson, A. F.: Transepiphyseal replacement of the anterior cruciate ligament in skeletally immature patients. A preliminary report.* J Bone Joint Surg Am *85:1255–1263, 2003. Used with permission from the* Journal of Bone and Joint Surgery.)

tunnel was used, and the graft was looped over a staple placed at the femoral attachment of the ACL. At a minimum follow-up of 4 years, KT-1000 testing revealed an average side-to-side difference of 1.8 mm. Anderson[1] reported his results using the technique described previously in a series of 12 patients (Tanner stage 1–3). At a mean follow-up of 4.1 years (range, 2–8.2 yr), KT-1000 testing revealed a mean side-to-side difference of 1.5 mm. In both series, there were no reported growth abnormalities and no subjective or objective evidence of recurrent instability at a minimum of 4 years follow-up.

Partial Transphyseal Reconstruction

The partial transphyseal technique is a hybrid technique in which the graft is placed through a transphyseal tibia tunnel and fixed to the femur in the over-the-top position. A soft tissue graft is passed through a 6- to 8-mm drill hole that crosses the physis. The drill hole is placed more vertically to decrease the risk of damage to the physis. The graft is secured in the over-the-top position on the femur with care taken not to damage the distal femoral physis during fixation.

Lipscomb and Anderson[25] reported a series of 24 (21 males and 3 females) patients aged 12 to 15 years who underwent partial transphyseal reconstruction. Eleven patients had a completely open physis and 13 had a partially open physis. Skeletal age was not recorded. A hamstring autograft was placed across the tibial physis (6.4-mm tunnel) and exited out through the femoral epiphysis. In addition, an extra-articular reconstruction of the lateral side was routinely added to prevent rotational instability. At an average follow-up of 35 months, the side-to-side difference on Lachman testing averaged 1.8 mm and all patients denied swelling or giving-way. One patient developed a 2.0-cm limb length inequality as a result of stapling across the femoral and tibial physes.

Andrews and colleagues[3] performed an ACL reconstruction in eight adolescents using either a (7-mm) fascia lata or Achilles tendon allograft placed centrally across the tibial physis and secured to the femur in the over-the-top position. At skeletal maturity, there were no detected limb length discrepancies (Figs. 11–4 and 11–5).

Lo and coworkers[27] reported on five patients with an average age of 12.9 years (range, 8–14 yr) who underwent partial transphyseal reconstruction using either a hamstring or a patella tendon autograft passed centrally through the tibial physis (6 mm) to an over-the-top position on the femur. At an average follow-up of 7.4 years, scanograms revealed no angular deformities or leg length discrepancies.

Transphyseal Reconstruction

Complete transphyseal reconstruction is performed with standard bone tunnels that traverse the physes of both the tibia and the femur. This technique is equivalent to conventional ACL reconstruction in adults, with the use of either autograft or allograft.

Aronowitz and associates[5] reported on 19 skeletally immature patients ages 11 to 15 years who underwent allograft reconstruction through drill holes in the distal femur and proximal tibia (Fig. 11–6). All patients had a skeletal age of at least 14 years. At an average of 25 months after surgery (range, 12–60 mo), there were no significant leg length discrepancies or angular deformities

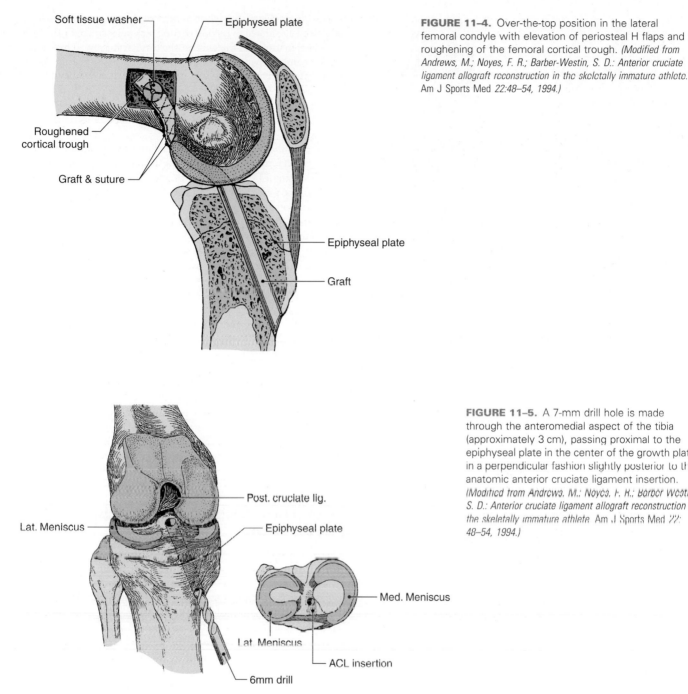

FIGURE 11–4. Over-the-top position in the lateral femoral condyle with elevation of periosteal H flaps and roughening of the femoral cortical trough. *(Modified from Andrews, M.; Noyes, F. R.; Barber-Westin, S. D.: Anterior cruciate ligament allograft reconstruction in the skeletally immature athlete. Am J Sports Med 22:48–54, 1994.)*

FIGURE 11–5. A 7-mm drill hole is made through the anteromedial aspect of the tibia (approximately 3 cm), passing proximal to the epiphyseal plate in the center of the growth plate in a perpendicular fashion slightly posterior to the anatomic anterior cruciate ligament insertion. *(Modified from Andrews, M.; Noyes, F. R.; Barber-Westin, S. D.: Anterior cruciate ligament allograft reconstruction in the skeletally immature athlete. Am J Sports Med 22:48–54, 1994.)*

determined by scanogram and anteroposterior and lateral radiographs of the femur and tibia. The mean Lysholm knee score was 97 (range, 94–100) and the mean KT-1000 arthrometer side-to-side difference was 1.7 mm (range, 0.0–3.0). All patients were satisfied with the results of surgery, and 16 of 19 patients returned to the same sport they were participating in before the injury.

McIntosh and colleagues[31] reported on 16 patients (11 males and 5 females) who underwent transphyseal ACL reconstruction. Each patient was followed until skeletal maturity, with a mean clinical follow-up of 41.1 months (range, 24–112 mo). At last follow-up, the mean leg length discrepancy measured 0.62 cm (range, 0.2–1.5 cm). Clinical or radiographic evidence of malalignment was not present in any patient. At follow-up, the mean

modified Lysholm score was 98.8 (range, 94–100) and the majority of patients (87.5%) had returned to their previous level of activity.

Shelbourne and coworkers[39] reported a series of 16 patients with open growth plates who underwent transphyseal ACL reconstruction using a patellar tendon autograft. At the time of surgery, 7 patients were Tanner stage 3 and 9 were Tanner stage 4. The authors noted that the surgical technique was meticulous for placing the bone plugs proximal to the physes and not over-tensioning the graft. Clinical follow-up (mean, 3.4 yr after surgery) showed that no patients had growth plate disturbances, angular deformities, or leg length discrepancies. All patients returned to competitive sports after surgery.

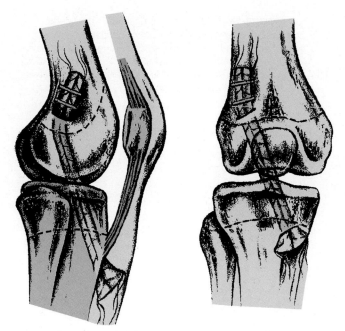

FIGURE 11–6. Lateral (**left**) and anteroposterior (**right**) views of the technique of passing an Achilles tendon allograft through drill holes across the open physis of both the proximal tibia and the distal femur. The graft is press-fitted on the tibial side before fixation with two staples on the femoral side. (*Left and right, From Aronowitz, E. R.; Ganley, T. J.; Goode, J. R.; et al.: Anterior cruciate ligament reconstruction in adolescents with open physes. Am J Sports Med 28:168–175, 2000.*)

Most recently, Kocher and associates[23] reported on 61 knees in 59 skeletally immature pubescent adolescents (Tanner stage 3) who underwent transphyseal ACL reconstruction using hamstring autograft and metaphyseal fixation. Functional outcome, graft survival, and growth disturbances were evaluated at a mean of 3.6 years after surgery. Two patients required revision for graft failure. The Lachman was normal in 51 knees and nearly normal in 8 knees and no patient had an abnormal pivot shift test. The mean increase in height was 8.2 cm (range, 1.2–25.4 cm) from the time of surgery and no angular deformities or limb length inequalities were detected clinically.

These and other reports consistently support the use of transphyseal ACL reconstruction in Tanner stage 3 and 4 adolescents. Overall, few growth disturbances have been reported after transphyseal reconstruction. Koman and Sanders[24] reported a case of a 14-year-old male who developed a distal femoral valgus deformity requiring osteotomy and contralateral epiphysiodesis after transphyseal reconstruction with a semitendinosus autograft. The skeletal age of the patient was unknown. The tibial tunnel diameter was unknown, but a 9-mm femoral tunnel was drilled. Cancellous bone plugs were inserted into both tunnels and the tendon was fixed with a cannulated screw across the lateral femoral condyle.

Despite the numerous reports describing ACL reconstruction using extra-articular techniques, intra-articular physeal-sparing surgery, and transphyseal reconstruction of the ACL, there are no prospective, randomized studies comparing the clinical success of graft type, graft placement, or graft fixation in skeletally immature patients. The existing literature includes studies with small sample sizes that use a variety of outcome measures, making comparisons between studies difficult. Unfortunately, some of these reports do not clearly state the gender of the patient, chronologic or skeletal age at which reconstruction was performed, or the level of skeletal maturity of the child at the time of surgery. These studies also combine patients from various age groups, making assessment difficult. Despite these limitations, the data available in the literature have not supported any trend or significant pattern of leg length inequality or angular deformity caused by reconstruction with or without physeal violation in patients with open physes.

For prepubescent patients (Tanner 1 and 2), the authors' preference is to perform an intra-articular extraphyseal reconstruction of the ACL using ITB autograft as described by Micheli and coworkers.[33] In the pubescent patient with open growth plates and more than 1 year of growth remaining, a partial transphyseal reconstruction (vertical tunnel across the tibial physis, over-the-top on the femur) using either allograft or hamstring or quadriceps tendon autograft is the authors' preferred technique. Transphyseal (tibial and femoral) reconstruction using hamstring allograft is reserved for patients with less than 1 year of growth remaining, and bone–patellar tendon–bone autograft is the preferred reconstruction when the physes are closed.

A careful assessment of the patient is required to determine the best treatment option. Nonoperative treatment has been used in the very young patient (<10 yr) because of the risk of iatrogenic growth disturbance. It is critical to determine the willingness of the patient and the family to give up sports and accept the risks of nonsurgical treatment. Activity modification, quadriceps and hamstring rehabilitation, and functional bracing are components of conservative treatment. If instability episodes persist, subsequent meniscal and chondral injuries have important implications in terms of prognosis for the knee and risk for degenerative joint disease.

COMPLICATIONS: CAUSES AND PREVENTION

The management of ACL injuries in the prepubescent child is particularly challenging, given the potential for remaining growth. However, the decision to delay reconstruction must be weighed against concerns for the development of chondral and meniscal injuries and their long-term consequences in the unstable knee. The physes of the distal femur and proximal tibia are both at risk during ACL reconstruction, with the risk of damage directly related to the immaturity of the physes at the time of surgery. The undulating nature of the distal femoral physis has been suggested as an explanation for the higher rates of growth arrest associated with injury to the distal femur.

Critical Points COMPLICATIONS

- The long-term implications of meniscal damage or chondral injury as a result of nonoperative treatment are much more vexing than the infrequent correctable growth disturbances after ACL reconstruction.
- The exact amount of physeal plate disruption before a growth plate arrest occurs remains unknown, emphasizing the need for caution and smaller tunnels whenever feasible.
- Patients who undergo ACL reconstruction should be observed until skeletal growth is complete.

Growth disturbance from physeal injury is usually evident at 2 to 6 months after injury but may not be evident for up to 1 year. Growth disturbance may result from formation of a bony bridge or bar across the physeal cartilage but can also occur without the formation of a bony bridge when injury to the physis slows rather than completely stops growth, resulting in angular deformity. Lipscomb and Anderson[25] reported one case of 20 mm of shortening in an immature patient associated with staple fixation of the graft across the physis.

The consequences of violating an active growth plate have been documented in both clinical and experimental reports. Stadelmaier and colleagues[40] examined the ability of a soft tissue graft to inhibit formation of a bony bridge within 4.0-mm tunnels drilled across open femoral and tibial growth plates in a canine model using a nontensioned graft. The growth plates were evaluated at 2 weeks and 4 months postoperatively. A bony bridge spanned the growth plate in all nongrafted animals as early as 2 weeks postoperatively (Figs. 11–7 and 11–8), whereas a fascia lata autograft prevented bone formation within the tunnels of all grafted animals and normal growth was maintained (Figs. 11–9 to 11–11). These results have been clinically supported by Andrews and colleagues[3] who used a 7-mm allograft centrally placed across the tibial physis and in the over-the-top femoral position in eight patients.

Guzzanti and coworkers[14] performed 21 semitendinosus reconstructions in a rabbit model using 2 mm tibial and femoral tunnels. This resulted in damage to 3% of the cross-sectional area of the femoral physis and 4% of the tibial physis. No alteration in growth of the femur was noted; however, 2 tibias developed valgus deformity and 1 tibia became shortened.

Factors such as size and location of the tibial and femoral tunnels have been shown to be important in determining the extent of growth plate damage. However, a safe threshold for physeal tunnels has yet to be determined. A study by Janarv and associates[17] concluded that physeal injuries involving 7%

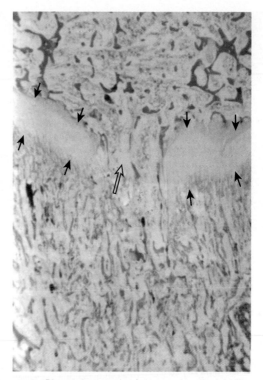

FIGURE 11–8. Photomicrograph of the section seen in Figure 11–7. Note the bony bridge (*open arrow*) that spans the growth plate (*small arrows*). (Hematoxylin and eosin x40.) *(From Stadelmaier, D. M.; Arnoczky, S. P.; Dodds, J.; et al.: The effect of drilling and soft tissue grafting across open growth plates. A histologic study. Am J Sports Med 23:431–435, 1995.)*

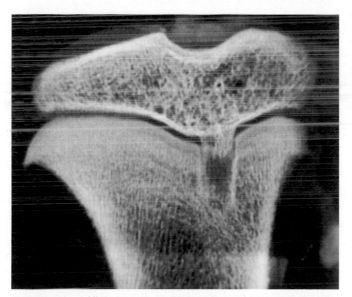

FIGURE 11–7. High-resolution radiograph of a proximal tibia of a dog 2 weeks after drilling across the growth plate shows the formation of a bony bridge. The longitudinal arrangement of the trabecular bone in the rapidly distracting metaphyseal bone is similar to that observed during distraction osteogenesis. *(From Stadelmaier, D. M.; Arnoczky, S. P.; Dodds, J.; et al.: The effect of drilling and soft tissue grafting across open growth plates. A histologic study. Am J Sports Med 23:431–435, 1995.)*

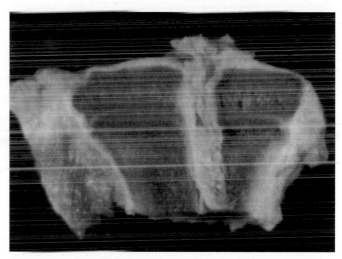

FIGURE 11–9. Coronal section of a proximal tibia of a dog 4 months after placement of a fascia lata graft through a drill hole made across the open growth plate. The graft has hypertrophied, but there is no evidence of any bone spanning the growth plate. *(From Stadelmaier, D. M.; Arnoczky, S. P.; Dodds, J.; et al.: The effect of drilling and soft tissue grafting across open growth plates. A histologic study. Am J Sports Med 23:431–435, 1995.)*

to 9% of the cross-sectional area of the physeal plate are enough to cause growth disturbance. For example, in an 8-year-old girl, an 8-mm tunnel would be 3% to 4% of the cross-sectional area of the physis and should not cause growth arrest.

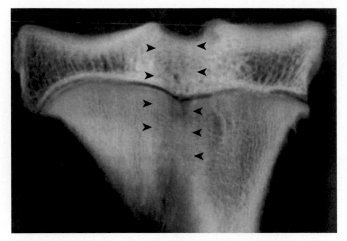

FIGURE 11–10. High-resolution radiograph of the section seen in Figure 11–9. There is no evidence of bony formation across the growth plate in the area of the bone tunnel (*outlined by small arrows*). *(From Stadelmaier, D. M.; Arnoczky, S. P.; Dodds, J.; et al.: The effect of drilling and soft tissue grafting across open growth plates. A histologic study. Am J Sports Med 23:431–435, 1995.)*

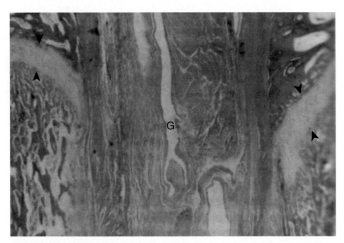

FIGURE 11–11. Photomicrograph of the section seen in Figure 11–9. The graft (G) crosses the growth plate, and there is no evidence of any bony formation across the physis (*arrows*). Note that the growth plate immediately adjacent to the graft-filled tunnel appears normal. (Hematoxylin and eosin x40.) *(From Stadelmaier, D. M.; Arnoczky, S. P.; Dodds, J.; et al.: The effect of drilling and soft tissue grafting across open growth plates. A histologic study. Am J Sports Med 23:431–435, 1995.)*

Care should be taken to avoid damage to the tibial tubercle and/or notching and dissection around the distal femoral physis when placing the graft in the over-the-top position. As evidenced by Seil and colleagues,[38] damage to the vulnerable perichondral ring is sufficient to cause growth arrest.

In a canine model, Edwards and coworkers[9] examined the effect of tensioned soft tissue grafts across the physis and found a substantial rate of distal femoral valgus and proximal tibia varus deformity despite no evidence of a bony bar. Excessive tension (80 N in dogs) across the physis may lead to angular deformities and should be avoided.[9] Pressure applied parallel to the direction of growth, such as when tensioning a graft, has also been shown to inhibit longitudinal growth.[4]

In 2002, the Herodicus Society and the ACL Study Group[22] surveyed their members on pediatric ACL reconstruction and complications. Fifteen cases of growth disturbance were reported. There were 8 cases of distal femoral valgus deformity with a physeal bar: 3 cases were associated with hardware crossing the distal physis, 4 with patella tendon–bone plugs crossing the distal femoral physis, and 1 with over-the-top graft placement. There were 2 cases of genu valgum without a physeal bar after lateral extra-articular tenodesis procedures. There were 2 cases of limb length discrepancy: 1 patient developed 2.5 cm of shortening and valgus of the distal femur associated with a 12-mm femoral tunnel and a patellar tendon–bone plug and required contralateral epiphysiodesis. The other case was an 11-year-old girl who underwent transphyseal reconstruction with hamstring autograft through 6-mm tunnels and developed 3.0 cm of overgrowth. There were 3 cases of genu recurvatum after closure of the tibial tubercle apophysis related to either a staple across the physis (2 cases) or a suture to the tibial periosteum (1 case).

If pediatric patients with complete ACL tears remain active in sports and childhood activities, there is a great probability that they will sustain functional instability and progressive damage to the knee, resulting in poor function in the long term. Guidelines for treatment should incorporate an assessment of skeletal maturity (bone age, Tanner stage, and growth spurt) into the decision before a treatment option is chosen. Although extraphyseal reconstruction is nonanatomic and nonisometric, the longevity of the graft and lack of growth disturbance support its use in the very young patient.

Transepiphyseal reconstruction reproduces the anatomy of the ACL more accurately, but it is technically more difficult, making results less predictable. If intra-articular reconstruction with transphyseal drill holes is planned, efforts should be made to minimize the risk of growth abnormality. Transphyseal tunnels should be kept small and centralized in the physis. In younger patients, crossing the growth plate with bone plugs or hardware must be avoided. Animal studies and clinical experience have shown that resection of physeal bars with interposition of soft tissue prevents the reformation of a bony bridge. This lends additional evidence that drill holes filled with tendon graft are less likely to cause growth deformity.[36]

The long-term implications of meniscal damage or chondral injury as a result of nonoperative treatment are much more vexing than the infrequent correctable growth disturbances after ACL reconstruction. The exact amount of physeal plate disruption before a growth plate arrest occurs remains unknown, emphasizing the need for caution and smaller tunnels whenever feasible. Overgrowth of the physis can occur owing to the penetration of the growth plate but appears to be rare and unpredictable. Patients who undergo ACL reconstruction should be observed until skeletal growth is complete. A growth chart should be maintained. A standing lower extremity radiograph and/or scanogram are obtained if malalignment or limb length discrepancy is suspected clinically. Additional imaging with computed tomography or MRI can be obtained to confirm and quantify physeal arrest. Leg length discrepancies under 2.0 cm are generally asymptomatic and can be managed with observation or a shoe lift. Larger differences can be treated with contralateral epiphysiodesis at the appropriate time. Angular deformities can be corrected with completion of epiphysiodesis or osteotomy.

REFERENCES

1. Anderson, A. F.: Transepiphyseal replacement of the anterior cruciate ligament in skeletally immature patients. A preliminary report. *J Bone Joint Surg Am* 85:1255–1263, 2003.
2. Anderson, M.; Messner, M. B.; Green, W. T.: Distribution of lengths of the normal femur and tibia in children from one to eighteen years of age. *J Bone Joint Surg Am* 46:1197–1202, 1964.
3. Andrews, M.; Noyes, F; R.; Barber-Westin, S. D.: Anterior cruciate ligament allograft reconstruction in the skeletally immature athlete. *Am J Sports Med* 22:48–54, 1994.
4. Arkin, A. M.; Katz, J. F.: The effects of pressure on epiphyseal growth; the mechanism of plasticity of growing bone. *J Bone Joint Surg Am* 38:1056–1076, 1956.
5. Aronowitz, E. R.; Ganley, T. J.; Goode, J. R.; et al.: Anterior cruciate ligament reconstruction in adolescents with open physes. *Am J Sports Med* 28:168–175, 2000.
6. Brief, L. P.: Anterior cruciate ligament reconstruction without drill holes. *Arthroscopy* 7:350–357, 1991.
7. DeLee, J. C.; Curtis, R.: Anterior cruciate ligament insufficiency in children. *Clin Orthop Relat Res* 172:112–118, 1983.
8. Edwards, P. H., Jr.; Grana, W. A.: Physeal fractures about the knee. *J Am Acad Orthop Surg* 3:63–69, 1995.
9. Edwards, T. B.; Greene, C. C.; Baratta, R. V.; et al.: The effect of placing a tensioned graft across open growth plates. A gross and histological analysis. *J Bone Joint Surg Am* 83:725–734, 2001.
10. Engebretsen, L.; Svenningsen, S.; Benum, P.: Poor results of anterior cruciate ligament repair in adolescence. *Acta Orthop Scand* 59:684–686, 1988.
11. Graf, B. K.; Lange, R. H.; Fujisaki, C. K.; et al.: Anterior cruciate ligament tears in skeletally immature patients: meniscal pathology at presentation and after attempted conservative treatment. *Arthroscopy* 8:229–233, 1992.
12. Greulich, W.; Pyle, S. (eds.): *Radiographic Atlas of Skeletal Development of the Hand and Wrist*, 2nd ed. Stanford, CA: Stanford University Press, 1959.
13. Grontvedt, T.; Engebretsen, L.; Benum, P.; et al.: A prospective, randomized study of three operations for acute rupture of the anterior cruciate ligament. Five-year follow-up of one hundred and thirty-one patients. *J Bone Joint Surg Am* 78:159–168, 1996.
14. Guzzanti, V.; Falciglia, F; Gigante, A.; et al.: The effect of intra-articular reconstruction on the growth plates of rabbits. *J Bone Joint Surg Br* 76:960–963, 1994.
15. Guzzanti, V.; Falciglia, F.; Stanitski, C. L.: Physeal sparing intra-articular anterior cruciate ligament reconstruction in preadolescents. *Am J Sports Med* 31:949–953, 2003.
16. Janary, P. M.; Nystrom, A.; Werner, S.; et al.: Anterior cruciate ligament injuries in skeletally immature patients. *J Pediatr Orthop* 16:673–677, 1996.
17. Janary, P. M.; Wikstrom, B.; Hirsch, G.: The influence of transphyseal drilling and tendon grafting on bone growth: an experimental study in the rabbit. *J Pediatr Orthop* 18:149–154, 1998.
18. Johnson, R. J.; Beynnon, B. D.; Nichols, C. E.; et al.: The treatment of injuries of the anterior cruciate ligament. *J Bone Joint Surg Am* 74:140–151, 1992.
19. Kloeppel-Wirth, S.; Kolel, J. L.; Dittmer, H.: Significance of arthroscopy in children with knee joint injuries. *Eur J Pediatr Surg* 2:169–172, 1992.
20. Kocher, M. S.; Garg, S.; Micheli, L. J.: Physeal sparing reconstruction of the anterior cruciate ligament in skeletally immature prepubescent children and adolescents. *J Bone Joint Surg Am* 87:2371–2379, 2005.
21. Kocher, M. S.; Garg, S.; Micheli, L. J.: Physeal sparing reconstruction of the anterior cruciate ligament in skeletally immature prepubescent children and adolescents. Surgical technique. *J Bone Joint Surg Am* 88(suppl 1 pt 2):283–293, 2006.
22. Kocher, M. S.; Saxon, H. S.; Hovis, W. D.; et al.: Management and complications of anterior cruciate ligament injuries in skeletally immature patients: survey of the Herodicus Society and The ACL Study Group. *J Pediatr Orthop* 22:452–457, 2002.
23. Kocher, M. S.; Smith, J. T.; Zoric, B. J.; et al.: Transphyseal anterior cruciate ligament reconstruction in skeletally immature pubescent adolescents. *J Bone Joint Surg Am* 89:2632–2639, 2007.
24. Koman, J. D.; Sanders, J. O.: Valgus deformity after reconstruction of the anterior cruciate ligament in a skeletally immature patient. A case report. *J Bone Joint Surg Am* 81:711–715, 1999.
25. Lipscomb, A. B.; Anderson, A. F.: Tears of the anterior cruciate ligament in adolescents. *J Bone Joint Surg Am* 68:19–28, 1986.
26. Little, D. G.; Song, K. M.; Katz, D.; et al.: Relationship of peak height velocity to other maturity indicators in idiopathic scoliosis in girls. *J Bone Joint Surg Am* 82:685–693, 2000.
27. Lo, I. K.; Kirkley, A.; Fowler, P. J.; et al.: The outcome of operatively treated anterior cruciate ligament disruptions in the skeletally immature child. *Arthroscopy* 13:627–634, 1997.
28. Manzione, M.; Pizzutillo, P. D.; Peoples, A. B.; et al.: Meniscectomy in children: a long-term follow-up study. *Am J Sports Med* 11:111–115, 1983.
29. McCarroll, J. R.; Rettig, A. C.; Shelbourne, K. D.: Anterior cruciate ligament injuries in the young athlete with open physes. *Am J Sports Med* 16:44–47, 1988.
30. McCarroll, J. R.; Shelbourne, K. D.; Porter, D. A.; et al.: Patellar tendon graft reconstruction for midsubstance anterior cruciate ligament rupture in junior high school athletes. An algorithm for management. *Am J Sports Med* 22:478–484, 1994.
31. McIntosh, A. L.; Dahm, D. L.; Stuart, M. J.: Anterior cruciate ligament reconstruction in the skeletally immature patient. *Arthroscopy* 22:1325–1330, 2006.
32. Menelaus, M. B.: Correction of leg length discrepancy by epiphyseal arrest. *J Bone Joint Surg Br* 48:336–339, 1966.
33. Micheli, L. J.; Rask, B.; Gerberg, L.: Anterior cruciate ligament reconstruction in patients who are prepubescent. *Clin Orthop Relat Res* 364:40–47, 1999.
34. Millett, P. J.; Willis, A. A.; Warren, R. F.: Associated injuries in pediatric and adolescent anterior cruciate ligament tears: does a delay in treatment increase the risk of meniscal tear? *Arthroscopy* 18:955–959, 2002.
35. Mizuta, H.; Kubota, K.; Shiraishi, M.; et al.: The conservative treatment of complete tears of the anterior cruciate ligament in skeletally immature patients. *J Bone Joint Surg Br* 77:890–894, 1995.
36. Peterson, H. A.: Partial growth plate arrest and its treatment. *J Pediatr Orthop* 4:246–258, 1984.
37. Risser, J. C.: The iliac apophysis; an invaluable sign in the management of scoliosis. *Clin Orthop* 11:111–119, 1958.
38. Seil, R.; Pape, D.; Kohn, D.: *ACL Replacement in Sheep with Open Physes: An Evaluation of Risk Factors.* Sardinia, Italy: ACL Study Group, 2004.
39. Shelbourne, K. D.; Gray, T.; Wiley, B. V.: Results of transphyseal anterior cruciate ligament reconstruction using patellar tendon autograft in tanner stage 3 or 4 adolescents with clearly open growth plates. *Am J Sports Med* 32:1218–1222, 2004.
40. Stadelmaier, D. M.; Arnoczky, S. P.; Dodds, J.; et al.: The effect of drilling and soft tissue grafting across open growth plates. A histologic study. *Am J Sports Med* 23:431–435, 1995.
41. Stanitski, C. L.: Correlation of arthroscopic and clinical examinations with magnetic resonance imaging findings of injured knees in children and adolescents. *Am J Sports Med* 26:2–6, 1998.
42. Stanitski, C. L.; Harvell, J. C.; Fu, F.: Observations on acute knee hemarthrosis in children and adolescents. *J Pediatr Orthop* 13:506–510, 1993.
43. Tanner, J. M.; Davies, P. S.: Clinical longitudinal standards for height and height velocity for North American children. *J Pediatr* 107:317–329, 1985.
44. Vahasarja, V.; Kinnuen, P.; Serlo, W.: Arthroscopy of the acute traumatic knee in children. Prospective study of 138 cases. *Acta Orthop Scand* 64:580–582, 1993.

Chapter 12

Scientific Basis of Rehabilitation after Anterior Cruciate Ligament Autogenous Reconstruction

Sue D. Barber-Westin, BS ■ *Timothy P. Heckmann*, PT, ATC ■ *Frank R. Noyes*, MD

FACTORS THAT AFFECT POSTOPERATIVE REHABILITATION AND OUTCOMES

Considerable advances have been made in the treatment of complete anterior cruciate ligament (ACL) ruptures and reconstruction methods since the mid 1980s. These include the appropriate selection of patient candidates and criteria that should be achieved before surgery, such as resolving limitations of knee motion, muscle atrophy, gait abnormalities, pain, and joint effusion. Appropriate graft selection, harvest, implantation, tensioning, and fixation are all paramount to achieving a reliable and desirable outcome, and considerable attention has been devoted to these principles in the orthopaedic literature.[18,19,62]

Appropriate postoperative rehabilitation after ACL reconstruction is critical to achieve normal knee function and prevent complications such as arthrofibrosis and reinjury. The goals of postoperative therapy are to regain normal knee motion, gait mechanics, lower extremity muscle strength, coordination, proprioception, and neuromuscular indices using exercises and modalities that are not deleterious to the healing graft. Dye introduced the concept of restoring normal knee osseous and soft tissue homeostasis after ACL injury and reconstruction using an appropriate combination of medical and therapeutic measures.[45,46] The exercise program should not produce undue forces on the patellofemoral or tibiofemoral compartments or result in chronic joint effusions. Unfortunately, few investigations have studied the effect of specific exercises and treatment modalities commonly used after ACL reconstruction. In fact, entire protocols have appeared and been used extensively based on clinical observations and retrospective analyses instead of prospective, randomized, controlled clinical trials.[83,179]

One of the difficulties in conducting rehabilitation investigations is the multitude of factors that may affect both the initial and the long-term recovery after ACL reconstruction. In addition, few ACL ruptures are truly isolated in nature, because approximately 80% of patients sustain concomitant bone bruises[52,93] and 60% suffer meniscus tears.[130,136] The factors that affect recovery include

- Timing of the reconstruction.
- Regaining normal knee motion and muscle strength before surgery
- ACL graft selection, placement, fixation, healing, and remodeling.
- Initial patient response to the trauma of surgery including pain, effusion, and muscle inhibition.
- Patient age, motivation, and compliance.
- The condition of the articular cartilage.
- The presence and severity of bone bruising.
- Concomitant major operative procedures including meniscus repairs or transplants, other ligament reconstructions, patellofemoral realignment procedures, and articular cartilage restorative procedures.
- Lingering postoperative deficits in neuromuscular indices and proprioception.
- Postoperative development of patellofemoral pain or tendinitis.
- Restoration of normal knee stability.

Authors have noted no benefit[28,117] and, in some cases, deleterious outcomes[120,176,182,205] when ACL reconstruction is performed early after injury before the resolution of limitations in knee motion, muscle atrophy, swelling, and pain. Meighan and coworkers[117] conducted one of the few prospective, randomized investigations regarding this issue. These investigators followed 31 patients who received either an early ACL hamstring reconstruction (within 2 wk of the injury) or a delayed reconstruction (8–12 wk) to determine outcomes up to 1 year postoperatively.

The early reconstruction group had significantly less knee extension and flexion at 2 weeks postoperatively, and greater deficits in quadriceps isokinetic work and power at 12 weeks postoperatively, than the delayed group. No other differences were noted in outcome throughout the study period. The authors concluded that early reconstruction did not provide any benefit to athletic individuals. Shelbourne and associates[182] noted an increased rate of arthrofibrosis in patients who underwent acute ACL reconstruction (within 1 wk of the injury) compared with those in whom the reconstruction was delayed for 21 days or more. Shelbourne and colleagues[166,177] have heavily emphasized the need to restore normal knee motion when possible before surgical intervention. The exception is the presence of a mechanical block to extension, such as a bucket-handle meniscus tear or ruptured ACL that is impinged in the intercondylar notch. In these cases, early surgical intervention is warranted to repair the meniscus tear or remove the ACL, regain full knee extension and flexion, and then proceed later with ACL reconstruction.

An important issue is whether the postoperative rehabilitation process should be governed and progressed according to the amount of time that has elapsed or by well-defined and measurable criteria. Although some programs allow a return to full activities according to a certain amount of time, such as 6 months postoperative, others will not release patients until specific muscle and function objectives have been achieved regardless of the amount of time that has passed since surgery. There is no consensus among investigators regarding which factors are the most important to measure to determine whether a rehabilitation program has been successful in allowing patients to return to activities safely.

Modern studies of ACL bone–patellar tendon–bone (B-PT-B) autograft reconstruction typically report low failure rates of approximately 5% to 10%.[10,67,129,143,161] Failure is defined as an increase in anteroposterior (AP) displacement of 6 mm or greater compared with the normal contralateral limb or a fully positive (grade II or III) pivot shift test. However, the percentage of grafts that undergo some amount of elongation, resulting in 3 to 5 mm of increased AP displacement or a mildly positive (grade I) pivot shift test, is quite variable and ranges from 5% to 50%.[1,7,72,129,143,173,174,206] Therefore, although the overall rate of failure is low, some authors express concern that any amount of abnormal anterior tibial translation may be detrimental to the knee joint over the long term.[20,148] Whether graft elongation occurs as a result of technical aspects of the operative procedure, inconsistencies in maturation of the collagenous and bony components of the construct, the rehabilitation program, or a combination of these controllable and uncontrollable factors is unknown. Only one study has been conducted, to our knowledge, that followed knees reconstructed with ACL B-PT-B autografts with serial KT-2000 testing throughout the postoperative period (2 yr), discussed in detail later in this chapter.[10]

The purpose of this chapter is to review the current knowledge surrounding rehabilitation after ACL autogenous reconstruction. The scientific basis for immediate knee motion, early weight-bearing, specific exercises, and evaluation criteria for return to activity are reviewed. The authors' ACL postoperative rehabilitation programs formulated from the scientific literature and nearly 3 decades of empirical clinical experience are detailed in Chapter 13, Rehabilitation of Primary and Revision Anterior Cruciate Ligament Reconstruction.

AUTOGENOUS ACL GRAFT MATURATION IN HUMANS

More than 100,000 ACL reconstructions are performed in the United States each year.[146] Few studies have been conducted on the maturation process of ligament grafts in humans; only a minuscule sampling (<1%) of B-PT-B and semitendinosus-gracilis (STG) grafts have undergone histologic analysis after implantation. The strong potential for sampling error prevents conclusions on when graft maturation is complete, indicated by when the transplanted tissue resembles a normal ACL's histologic, structural, biomechanical, and material properties.

Rougraff and coworkers[164] performed biopsies on 23 B-PT-B autografts 3 weeks to 6.5 years after implantation. The authors reported that all patients had "clinically stable" knees; however, Lachman, pivot shift, and knee arthrometer data were not provided. The patients were allowed full weight-bearing immediately postoperatively and returned to sports between 3 and 6 months after surgery. The authors described four stages of ligamentization. The first stage occurred during the first 2 postoperative months and was characterized by an increased number of fibroblasts compared with time zero, preservation of mature collagen, and early neovascular ingrowth. The second stage, composed of rapid remodeling, occurred from 2 to 10 months postoperatively. A rapid increase in the number of metabolically active fibroblasts and replacement of approximately two thirds of mature collagen with immature matrix was noted. The third stage, in which the fibroblast count slowly decreased, collagen matrix matured, and vascularity decreased, occurred from 1 to

---

Critical Points AUTOGENOUS ACL GRAFT MATURATION IN HUMANS

Small sample size of examined grafts and number of intrinsic and extrinsic variables that may affect graft maturation prevent definitive conclusions.

B-PT-B Autografts: Four Stages of Ligamentization

1. One to 2 months postoperative: increased number of fibroblasts compared with time zero, preservation of mature collagen, and early neovascular ingrowth.
2. Two to 10 months postoperative: rapid remodeling, rapid increase in number of metabolically active fibroblasts, and replacement of two thirds of mature collagen with immature matrix.
3. One to 3 years postoperatively: fibroblast count slowly decreases, collagen matrix matures, and vascularity decreases.
4. Grafts less cellular and vascular; appear similar to control ACLs.

B-PT-B specimens show evidence of survival of portions of the original tendon 3 to 8 weeks postoperative.

B-PT-B and STG Autografts

- Significant differences in vascularity, cellularity, and fiber pattern between grafts examined 3 to 6 months postoperative and grafts observed greater than 12 months after implantation.
- Seven to 12 months postoperative: transitional for vascular maturity.
- Graft maturity occurs over a 12-month period, most likely never recovers to normal strength, material properties, and microfiber geometry.

B-PT-B, bone–patellar tendon–bone; STG, semitendinosus-gracilis.

---

3 years postoperatively. In the final stage, the grafts were noted to be less cellular and vascular and appeared similar to those of control ACLs. The study did not include electron microscopy to evaluate the pattern of collagen fibril diameters in the grafts.

Rougraff and Shelbourne[165] performed biopsies on nine B-PT-B autografts between 3 and 8 weeks after implantation. All patients followed an accelerated rehabilitation protocol[179] and agreed to the biopsy for investigational purposes. All specimens showed evidence of survival of portions of the original tendon. Vascular invasion was present at 3 weeks postoperative, with increased cell counts compared with controls found in all samples. All specimens had areas of acellularity and degeneration; however, these were small (no more than 30% of the biopsied area) in comparison with the areas of vascularity and normal-appearing tendon tissue.

Petersen and Laprell[153] examined the insertion of B-PT-B and STG autografts to bone in 14 knees that required revision ACL reconstruction. The time from the primary ACL reconstruction to revision ranged from 6 to 37 months. The hamstring specimens revealed a fibrous insertion of the graft into the periphery of the tibial bone tunnel. The patellar tendon (PT) specimens taken from the femoral tunnel showed fibrocartilage at the bone-tendon interface and resembled the chondral insertion of a normal ACL.

Johnson[94] performed biopsies on 20 STG ACL grafts between 20 days and 44 months postoperative. All patients required follow-up arthroscopy for various symptoms, at which time biopsy samples were taken from the tendon graft and surrounding fibrous tissue. The reconstructed ACL was a composite of these two distinctly different tissues, which had diverse histologic properties. The 3-month postoperative tendon samples appeared normal histologically, with no signs of inflammation and organized collagen bundles. Specimens taken beyond 3 months showed continued tissue maturation and crimping of collagen bundles similar to those of the native ACL. Specimens taken from the fibrous tissue had a disorganized cellular pattern and hypervascularity at 3 months postoperative and, although with time they developed increasing amounts of collagen, never resembled a normal tendon.

Beynnon and associates[23] examined the knees of a B-PT-B autograft recipient 8 months after implantation after the patient had died of causes unrelated to the knee joint. The patient's rehabilitation program included immediate continuous passive motion (CPM) from 0° to 90°; however, he underwent a prolonged period of partial weight-bearing for 12 weeks for unknown reasons. At 4 months postoperative, he was examined clinically and had a stable reconstruction. The postmortem examination revealed 6 mm of increased AP displacement, a 13% reduction in ultimate failure loads, and a 53% reduction in energy absorbed at failure compared with the contralateral native ACL. Histologic analyses were not conducted. Interestingly, the ultimate failure load of the patient's contralateral native ACL of 1015.6 N was well below the expected value of 1725 ± 269 N.[132]

Delay and colleagues[40] inspected a retrieved whole B-PT-B autograft 18 months after implantation in a patient who died from a traumatic injury. Whereas the graft was mainly cellular and resembled a normal ACL morphologically, there were areas of acellularity deep within the tendinosis portion and also in the femoral intra-articular region where the autograft emerged from the tibial tunnel. The graft had been placed in an over-the-top position that the authors speculated could have caused increased stresses, resulting in inconsistent remodeling.

Falconiero and coworkers[53] obtained biopsies of 35 B-PT-B and 8 STG autografts in 48 patients from 3 to 120 months after implantation. The rehabilitation program the patients followed was not described. Significant differences were noted in vascularity, cellularity, and fiber pattern between grafts that were examined 3 to 6 months postoperative and those that were observed greater than 12 months after implantation. Grafts that were biopsied 7 to 12 months postoperatively were described as transitional in terms of vascular maturity. No difference was found between fiber patterns and vascularity in grafts that had been implanted 7 to 12 months before the biopsy and those that had been implanted more than 12 months before the biopsy. The authors concluded that whereas graft maturity generally occurs over a 12-month period, some autografts may reach full maturation even earlier.

Although it appears from the literature reviewed that ACL autografts undergo increasing maturation postoperatively, the small sample size of examined grafts and the host of both intrinsic and extrinsic variables affects this process and prevents definitive conclusions. Questions remain regarding whether the healing process produces a graft that has histologic, ultrastructural, and biomechanical characteristics equivalent to those of a native ACL. It is probable that the delicate nature and microgeometry of native ligament fibers is never regained, but that the ligament functions more as a checkrein to resist gross knee displacements rather than replicating normal kinematics.[89] Recent studies have demonstrated that even though B-PT-B and STG autograft reconstructions frequently restore normal AP displacements as measured with a KT-2000 arthrometer (<3 mm side-to-side difference), normal knee kinematics may not be restored, causing abnormal joint motions when the knee is subjected to weight-bearing activities.[148] The delay in maturation of ACL allografts and the potential effects on postoperative recovery are discussed in Chapter 5, Biology of ACL Graft Healing.

IMMEDIATE KNEE MOTION

The scientific basis supporting immediate knee motion after ACL reconstruction is well established.[18,78,87,131,134,135,158,163] Early knee joint motion decreases pain and postoperative joint effusions, aids in the prevention of scar tissue formation and capsular contractions that can limit normal knee flexion and extension, decreases muscle disuse effects (Fig. 12–1), maintains articular cartilage nutrition, and benefits the healing ACL graft.* There is a consensus in the medical community that immobilization is detrimental to the knee joint structures and may result in a permanent limitation of knee motion, prolonged muscle atrophy, patella infera, and articular cartilage deterioration.[33,70,95,139–141,150,170]

In 1983, Noyes and associates[133] first published recommendations for immediate knee motion after ACL B-PT-B autograft reconstruction after a successful 4-year experience with this program. Advances in knee ligament reconstructive and fixation techniques allowed the controlled movement of the knee from 0° to 90° and did not disrupt the healing graft. In 1987, these authors[134] published one of the first clinical studies that assessed joint effusion, joint motion, muscle atrophy, and the integrity of

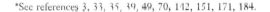

Critical Points IMMEDIATE KNEE MOTION

Scientific basis well established.

Immediate motion decreases pain and postoperative joint effusions, aids in the prevention of scar tissue formation and capsular contraction, decreases muscle disuse effects, maintains articular cartilage nutrition, benefits the healing ACL graft.

Immobilization is detrimental to the knee joint structures and may result in a permanent limitation of knee motion, prolonged muscle atrophy, patella infera, and articular cartilage deterioration.

No benefit of continuous passive motion (CPM) demonstrated in several studies, although useful in select cases.

---

*See references 3, 33, 35, 39, 49, 70, 142, 151, 171, 184.

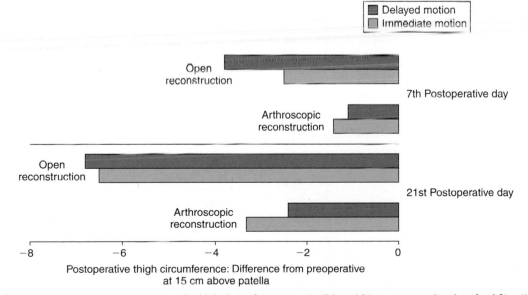

FIGURE 12–1. The graph demonstrates the decrease in thigh circumference on the 7th and 21st postoperative days for ACL arthroscopic versus open reconstruction. The difference between open and arthroscopic reconstructions is statistically significant ($P < .05$). *(Redrawn from Noyes, F. R.; Mangine, R. E.; Barber, S.: Early knee motion after open and arthroscopic anterior cruciate ligament reconstruction. Am J Sports Med 15:149–160, 1987.)*

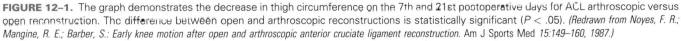

ACL grafts in a series of 18 patients who underwent ACL allograft reconstruction. Patients were randomly placed into either an immediate motion group that began CPM on the 2nd postoperative day or a delayed motion group that initiated passive and active-assisted flexion and extension exercises on the 7th postoperative day. All other parameters of the postoperative rehabilitation program were identical for the two groups, including exercises, bracing, and modalities. The results showed no differences between groups for knee joint effusion, the amount of knee flexion and extension achieved by 3 months postoperative, decrease in thigh circumference loss (Fig. 12–2), and frequency and type of pain medication used while in the hospital. There was no difference between groups in AP displacements at 12 months postoperative. Patients in whom the ACL graft had been implanted through an arthrotomy had significantly greater thigh circumference loss compared with those who had an arthroscopic-assisted technique, noted by the 7th postoperative day.

Richmond and colleagues in 1991[158] compared the effectiveness of CPM when used for the first 4 postoperative days to utilization during the first 14 days in 19 patients who underwent ACL B-PT-B autograft reconstruction. CPM was used for at least 6 hours a day. All patients also performed passive motion exercises from 0° to 90° three times daily. There were no differences between the groups at 6 weeks postoperative for swelling, thigh girth measurements, knee flexion and extension, time to regain full motion, or AP displacements. Immediate motion was concluded to be safe and not deleterious to the healing grafts in the initial postoperative period. No long-term benefit of CPM was demonstrated.

Rosen and coworkers[163] followed 75 patients who had ACL B-PT-B autogenous reconstruction and were sorted into three groups based on a knee motion and rehabilitation program. Patients who began active-assisted early knee motion exercises had similar results in regard to knee motion achieved at week 1 and at monthly intervals for the first 6 postoperative months as those who used CPM an average of 7 hours a day for 4 weeks postoperatively. There were no deleterious effects of early motion on AP displacements at the final follow-up evaluation, 6 months postoperative. The authors concluded that the CPM device offered no advantage and increased the cost of physical therapy by $1,800.

Beynnon and associates[21] conducted in vivo measurements of the elongation of B-PT-B autografts in 20 patients immediately after implantation. In 11 knees, the length of the graft increased after 14 knee flexion-extension motion cycles, and in 9 patients, the graft length decreased. The predicted maximum increase in anterior tibial translation after 20 knee motion cycles was only 1 mm.

The current authors[135] followed 207 knees that underwent arthroscopically assisted ACL allograft reconstruction and immediate knee motion. All patients began CPM for 8 to 10 hours a day immediately after surgery. In addition, passive and active-assisted motion exercises were initiated on the 2nd postoperative day. Partial weight-bearing was allowed immediately postoperative and was gradually progressed to full by 4 to 6 weeks based on resumption of normal gait mechanics. Any patient who demonstrated a limitation of knee flexion or extension from predetermined goals was placed into a specific treatment program as early as the 7th postoperative day.

FIGURE 12–2. The graphs show the circumference results after initiating intermittent passive motion on the 2nd postoperative day (motion group) versus the 7th postoperative day (delayed motion group). The change in thigh circumference from the preoperative value is shown. There was a nearly identical decrease in the joint circumference measurements in both groups. Note the marked loss of thigh circumference in both groups. *(From Noyes, F. R.; Mangine, R. E.; Barber, S.: Early knee motion after open and arthroscopic anterior cruciate ligament reconstruction. Am J Sports Med 15:149–160, 1987.)*

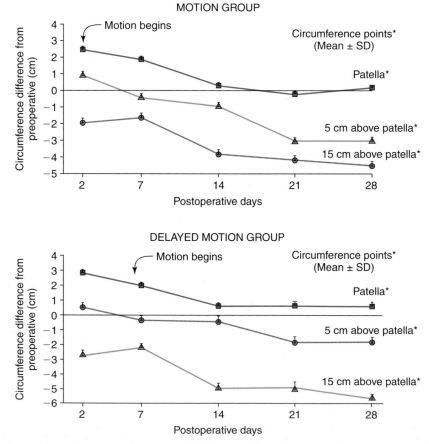

The program included overpressure exercises and modalities initially (Fig. 12–3), followed, if required, by a serial extension cast program (Fig. 12–4) and in rare instances, arthroscopic débridement of scar tissues (Fig. 12–5). Of the 207 knees, 189 (91%) regained at least 0° to 135° of motion without additional intervention. Eighteen knees were placed into the phased treatment program, of which 14 regained normal motion and 2 lacked 5° of full extension. Two other patients who had not complied with the rehabilitation program had a permanent significant limitation of motion. The incidence of postoperative motion problems was related to concomitant surgical procedures: medial collateral ligament (MCL), 23%; meniscus repair, 12%; iliotibial band extra-articular procedure, 10%; and isolated ACL, 4%.

In a second study from the authors' center,[131] 443 knees that had an arthroscopic-assisted ACL B-PT-B autograft reconstruction were followed to determine the effectiveness of an immediate knee motion program and treatment protocol for limitations of flexion and extension. A CPM device was not used in this group of patients. A normal range of motion (ROM) was achieved in 436 knees (98%) and a mild limitation of extension of 5° was detected in 7. Treatment intervention was required in 23 knees, all of which achieved normal knee motion. The 7 patients whose knees had mild losses of extension refused additional treatment. Only 3 knees (<1%) required an arthroscopic lysis of adhesions that, combined with an in-patient epidural program, resulted in successful resolution of the motion limitations. The incidence of knee motion problems based on

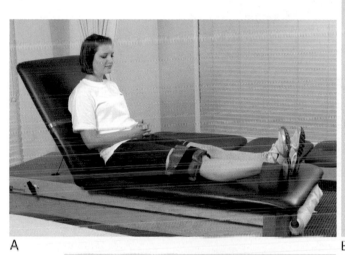

A

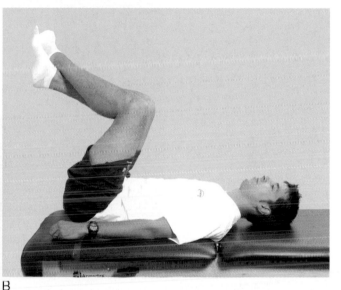

B

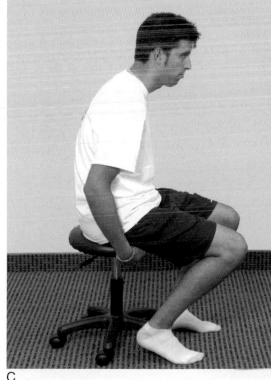

C

D

FIGURE 12–3. Knee overpressure exercises for limitation of extension (**A**) and flexion (**B–D**).

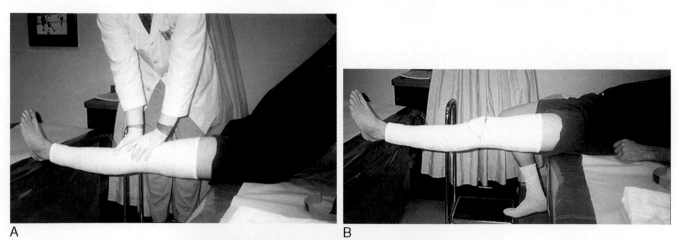

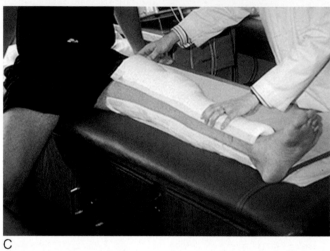

FIGURE 12–4. Extension cast application requires overpressure initially (**A**). The cast is worn for 48 hours (**B**) and is then split (**C**) and converted into a night splint.

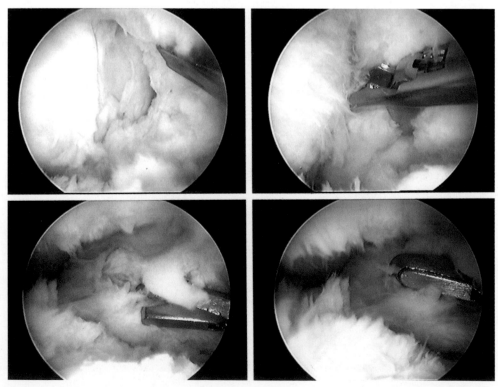

FIGURE 12–5. Arthroscopic débridement of scar tissues.

concomitant surgical procedures was 22% for MCL repairs, 18% for patellar realignment procedures, 8% for meniscus repairs, and 6% for isolated ACL reconstructions.

In 2002, Henriksson and coworkers[78] compared the outcome of 5 weeks of immobilization with early knee ROM exercises in 45 patients after ACL B-PT-B autograft reconstruction. Patients in the early ROM group began motion exercises from 0° to 90° from the 7th postoperative day. The early ROM group demonstrated greater extension and flexion for the first 20 weeks. Patients in the immobilization group generally required more physical therapy visits to achieve full knee motion.

EARLY WEIGHT-BEARING

Whereas many authors have recommended early partial or full weight-bearing immediately after ACL reconstruction, few studies have examined this factor and its potential effect on both short- and long-term recovery. The effect of immediate full weight-bearing on the outcome in knees with noteworthy articular cartilage damage or those in which major concomitant operative procedures were required is unknown. In addition, gait abnormalities that may ensue from immediate full weight-bearing due to pain, knee joint effusion, and muscle weakness have not been examined. It does appear from the literature and the authors' experience that immediate partial weight bearing is safe and not deleterious to the healing graft.[10]

In 1991, Ohkoshi and associates[144] recommended early weight-bearing exercises after ACL reconstruction based on results of a study in which shear forces on the tibia during standing were predicted from an analytical model at various trunk and knee flexion angles (Fig. 12–6). Although weight-bearing was normally prohibited in the initial postoperative period at the time of this publication, these investigators reported that the calculated shear forces were negative in all positions, with increasing posterior drawer forces found as trunk flexion angles increased (at knee flexion angles of 30° and 60°). Co-contraction of the quadriceps and hamstrings was observed at

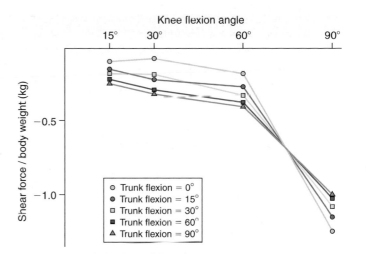

FIGURE 12–6. Shear force (kilograms) per body weight (kilograms) while standing on both legs at various flexion angles of the knee and the trunk. *(From Ohkoshi Y, Yasuda, K.; Kanoda, K.; et al.: Biomechanical analysis of rehabilitation in the standing position.* Am J Sports Med *19:605–611, 1991.)*

all knee and trunk flexion angle positions, with increasing hamstrings activity measured with increasing trunk flexion angles. Exercises performed in the standing position with the knees flexed and the trunk anteriorly flexed, such as half-squatting, were believed not only to be safe but also to have the potential advantages of increasing muscle strength, endurance, and proprioception and decreasing bone atrophy.

Tyler and colleagues in 1998[203] evaluated the effect of immediate full weight-bearing after ACL B-PT-B autograft reconstruction on ROM, patellofemoral pain, and AP displacement in a randomized, controlled trial. The results of 25 patients who were allowed immediate full weight-bearing were compared with those of 20 patients in whom no weight-bearing was allowed for 2 weeks postoperative. All patients performed immediate ROM exercises and followed an identical rehabilitation protocol (which was not detailed). There was no difference between groups for AP displacement, ROM, and vastus medialis obliquus (VMO) electromyographic activity at follow-up an average of 7 months postoperatively. Patients in the delayed weight-bearing group had a higher incidence of anterior knee pain than those in the immediate weight-bearing group (35% and 8%, respectively). Extension deficits of 5° or greater were reported in 14% of patients in the delayed weight-bearing group and in 20% in the immediate weight-bearing group. There was no correlation between loss of knee extension and anterior knee pain. Patients in the immediate weight-bearing group had significantly greater VMO electromyographic activity at 2 weeks postoperative compared with those in the delayed weight-bearing group, and the authors hypothesized that this aided in lowering the incidence of anterior knee pain by preventing the reflex inhibition of the VMO. Approximately 15% in each group had greater than 5 mm of increased AP displacement at follow-up.

POSTOPERATIVE BRACING

The effects of postoperative and functional braces on pain, return of normal knee motion, complications, sports activity performance, balance, and proprioception have been assessed by many investigators (Table 12–1). Most studies report that postoperative braces do not provide significant benefit in the

---

Critical Points EARLY WEIGHT-BEARING

Few studies have examined early weight-bearing and its potential effect on both short- and long-term recovery.

Ohkoshi et al.[144]

- Predicted shear forces on tibia during standing, analytical model, and various trunk and knee flexion angles.
- Calculated posterior drawer forces increased as trunk flexion angles increased.
- Co-contraction quadriceps and hamstrings observed all knee and trunk flexion angle positions.
- Hamstrings activity increased as trunk flexion angles increased.
- Recommended early weight-bearing exercises.

Tyler et al.[203]

- Compared 25 patients allowed immediate full weight-bearing with 20 patients on no weight-bearing for 2 weeks postoperative. B-PT-B autografts.
- No difference: AP displacement, range of knee motion, or vastus medialis oblique electromyographic activity.
- Patients in delayed weight-bearing group: higher incidence of anterior knee pain (35%) than those in the immediate weight-bearing group (8%). Lower incidence of extension deficits (≥5°).

Critical Points POSTOPERATIVE BRACING

Most studies: postoperative braces do not provide significant benefit:
- Time postoperatively normal range of knee motion is achieved.
- Isokinetic lower extremity muscle strength.
- Anteroposterior displacements.
- Lower limb symmetry assessed by single-leg hop tests.
- Functional knee rating and activity level scores.

Significant variation among surgeons surveyed on the use of braces postoperatively.

Authors recommend postoperative braces in complex multiligament reconstructions.

Unloading braces are advantageous in medial or posterolateral reconstructions to allow early weight-bearing.

amount of time postoperatively that normal range of knee motion is achieved, isokinetic lower extremity muscle strength, AP displacements, lower limb symmetry assessed by single-leg hop tests, and functional knee rating and activity level scores.* Negative effects of braces have been reported regarding quadriceps strength,[160] running and turning times,[218] and hamstrings isokinetic peak torque.[26] One study reported that a functional brace improved standing balance, but not more difficult tasks such as balance after a forward hop.[26] In regard to proprioception, two investigations reported significant, although small, improvements in static joint sense of 1° to 2° with brace utilization (Table 12–2).[26,219] The clinical impact of these improvements

*See references 25, 29, 73, 98, 116, 118, 121, 124, 160, 217, 219.

TABLE 12–1 Effects of Bracing after Anterior Cruciate Ligament Reconstruction

Reference	Type of ACL Reconstruction; Number of Subjects; Follow-up	Brace(s)	Protocol	Findings
Birmingham et al., 2008[25]	STG Randomized $N = 62$ brace $N = 65$ sleeve 24 mo PO	DonJoy Legend (dj Orthopedics, Vista, CA) Neoprene Knee Sleeve (dj Orthopedics, Vista, CA)	All patients received brace or sleeve 6 wk PO, instructed to wear for all physical activities.	No difference ACL quality of life scores, AP displacement, hop limb symmetry index, Tegner Activity score. Braced group higher ratings for confidence in the knee provided by brace/sleeve at 6 and 12 mo PO. Functional knee brace not recommended after ACL reconstruction.
McDevitt et al., 2004[116]	PT autograft Randomized $N = 47$ brace $N = 48$ no brace 24–42 mo PO	DonJoy IROM (dj Orthopedics, Vista, CA)	Brace group: DonJoy for 6 wk, then off-shelf functional brace for 1 yr for rigorous activity. No brace group: immobilizer used first 3 wk in full extension.	No difference ROM, isokinetic strength, hop test, AP displacement, IKDC score, x-rays. Authors use immobilizer 2–3 wk PO.
Mikkelsen et al., 2003[119a]	PT autograft Randomized $N = 22$ brace set 0° $N = 22$ brace set −5° hyperextension $N = 10$ controls 3 mo PO	Hypex (Aircast Europa, Neubeuern, Germany)	Brace used first 3 wk PO.	Control knees: lateral x-ray revealed when brace set to 0°, no knees were at 0°, range 1.5°–4.0°. ACL brace set 0°: 12 knees (55%) had extension limitations (2°–3° in 7; 5° in 4; 7° in 1) ACL brace set −5°: 2 knees had extension limitations (5°). No difference flexion, AP displacement, pain. Brace used in study not effective if set to 0°.
Melegati et al., 2003[118]	PT autograft $N = 18$ brace set 0°–90° $N = 18$ brace locked 0° 4 mo PO	Brace manufacturer not provided	Brace settings used 1st wk PO. Brace unlocked during 2nd wk, removed during 3rd wk.	Heel height: significant difference 4 and 8 wk PO. Brace locked 0° better extension, but mean difference was only 1° (1.6° ± 11.3° and 0.1° ± 13.9°). No difference in AP displacement.
Wu et al., 2001[218]	$N = 31$ ST autograft ≥5 mo PO	DonJoy Legend (dj Orthopedics, Vista, CA), placebo	Tested running, turning, jumping with brace, placebo, and unbraced conditions	Slower running, turning times with both braces compared with unbraced condition. Use of brace may be detrimental to sports performance.
Birmingham et al, 2001[26a]	$N = 27$ STG autograft 6–48 mo PO	DonJoy Defiance (dj Orthopedics, Vista, CA), worn by all during sports	Tested isokinetically with and without brace, SF-36 questionnaire	Significantly lower flexion peak torque with brace, no effect on extension peak torque. No association with SF-36 scores.
Brandsson et al., 2001[29]	PT autograft $N = 25$ braced $N = 25$ no brace 2 yr PO	DonJoy (dj Orthopedics, Vista, CA), worn for first 3 wk PO	Same both groups, CKC immediately, running at 3 mo, sports at 6 mo.	Braced group less pain first 2 wk PO. No difference IKDC, hop tests, AP displacement, isokinetic strength, complications.
Moller et al., 2001[121]	PT autograft $N = 29$ braced $N = 27$ no brace 2 yr PO	DonJoy ELS (dj Orthopedics, Vista, CA)	Brace used first 6 weeks PO, locked 0°.	No difference ROM, isokinetic strength, AP displacement. No benefit from brace wear.

TABLE 12–1   Effects of Bracing after Anterior Cruciate Ligament Reconstruction—Cont'd

Reference	Type of ACL Reconstruction; Number of Subjects; Follow-up	Brace(s)	Protocol	Findings
Risberg et al., 1999[160]	PT autograft Randomized N = 30 brace N = 30 no brace 2 yr PO	DonJoy IROM, DonJoy Functional (dj Orthopedics, Vista, CA)	Brace set 0°–90° first 6 wk. Used for 3 mo, then for strenuous activities only for 2 yr. Full ROM allowed both groups early PO.	No difference ROM, isokinetic strength, AP displacement, hop tests, subjective and functional scores. Braced group significantly greater thigh atrophy at 3 mo PO. Patients who wore brace for 1–2 yr had significantly lower quadriceps strength compared with those who wore brace for only 3 mo.
Muellner et al., 1998[124]	PT autograft Randomized N = 20 brace N = 20 bandage 1 yr PO	DonJoy (dj Orthopedics, Vista, CA)	Brace initially full extension, gradually increased. CPM, full weight-bearing as tolerated. Sports 6 mo.	No difference in isokinetic strength, hop tests, AP displacement. ROM significantly better in bandage patients during first 12 wk PO. No benefit from brace wear.
Kartus et al., 1997[98]	PT autograft Not randomized N = 39 brace N = 39 no brace 2 yr PO	Genu Syncro Quick-lock S 2300	Brace 3–6 wk PO, locked 0° for weight-bearing and sleep, otherwise unlocked.	No difference in AP displacement, hop tests, ROM, complications. No benefit from brace wear.
Harilainen et al., 1997[73]	PT autograft Randomized N = 30 brace N = 30 no brace 2 yr PO	DonJoy IROM (dj Orthopedics, Vista, CA)	Brace used 3 mo PO, unlocked.	No difference in AP displacement, isokinetic strength. No benefit from brace wear.

ACL, anterior cruciate ligament; AP, anteroposterior; CKC, closed kinetic chain; CPM, continuous passive motion; IKDC, International Knee Documentations Committee; PO, postoperative; PT, patellar tendon; ROM, range of motion; SF-36, Short-Form 36-item questionnaire (Medical Outcomes Study); ST, semitendinosus; STG, semitendinosus-gracilis.

TABLE 12–2   Effect of Knee Braces on Joint Proprioception

Reference	Type of ACL Reconstruction; Number of Subjects; Follow-up	Brace(s)	Protocol	Findings
Wu et al., 2001[219]	N = 31 ST autograft >5 mo PO.	DonJoy Legend (dj Orthopedics, Vista, CA), placebo	Proprioception and isokinetic testing three conditions: braced, placebo, unbraced.	No difference in isokinetic tests all three conditions. Proprioception: no difference in brace versus placebo, difference in both braces and unbraced in proprioception (1°–2°). Proprioception test measured only accuracy of static joint sense.
Rebel et al., 2001[154a]	Test 1: N = 25 ACL-reconstructed patients 7.4 wk PO N = 30 controls Test 2: N = 10 ACL-reconstructed patients 12.4 wk PO N = 10 controls	Hypex (Aircast Europa, Neubeuern, Germany)	Test 1: proprioception & balance (double-legged and single-legged on KAT) Test 2: double-legged drop jump, EMG, 50% body weight	Test 1: no difference in static balance index controls and patients without brace. Significant difference in patients braced versus unbraced—brace improved double-legged static and dynamic tests and single-legged static test. Test 2: brace improved jump height, knee flexion angle on ground contact versus no brace. Mean activity vastus lateralis, biceps femoris, gastrocnemius significantly lower with brace wear, but high variability in data. Brace enhanced coordination.
Birmingham et al., 2001[26]	N = 30 STG autograft ≥6 mo PO	DonJoy Defiance (dj Orthopedics, Vista, CA)	Proprioception, single-leg balance tests, braced versus unbraced.	Small but significant improvement in proprioception with brace (mean, 0.64° difference in target and reproduced knee flexion angles). Brace improved basic single-leg standing balance test, but not more difficult tasks (forward hop).
Risberg et al., 1999[159]	N = 20 PT autograft 24 mo PO (range, 11–32 mo) N = 10 controls	DonJoy Legend (dj Orthopedics, Vista, CA)	Proprioception (threshold to detection passive motion), braced versus unbraced	No difference in ACL-reconstructed knees and contralateral knees. No difference ACL-reconstructed knees and controls. No improvement with brace utilization. No impairment in proprioception in ACL-reconstructed knees mean 24 mo PO.

ACL, anterior cruciate ligament; EMG, electromyography; KAT, Kinaesthetic Ability Trainer; PO, postoperative; PT, patellar tendon; ST, semitendinosus; STG, semitendinosus-gracilis.

remains questionable. Risberg and coworkers[159] reported no improvement in the threshold to detect passive motion with application of a functional brace an average of 24 months after ACL B-PT-B autograft reconstruction. These investigators also found no impairment in proprioception in the ACL-reconstructed knees compared with those of controls.

Marx and associates[114] published a survey of data collected from 1998 to 1999 conducted by the American Academy of Orthopaedic Surgeons. Significant variation was reported among surgeons on the use of braces in the postoperative period, with half of the surgeons indicating they prescribed a brace for the first 6 postoperative weeks and the remaining half indicating no brace utilization. Surgeons who performed more ACL reconstructions reported less brace use. Approximately 60% of all surgeons responded that they recommended a brace for sports participation.

Beynnon and colleagues[18] concluded from a review of this topic that there "appears to be a consensus among investigators that, during the early phase of recovery, the use of a rehabilitation brace results in fewer problems with swelling, lower prevalence of hemarthrosis and wound drainage, and less pain compared to rehabilitation without a brace; however, at longer-term follow-up, rehabilitation bracing does not appear to have an effect on clinical outcome." The authors recommended postoperative bracing in complex multiligament reconstructions for protection of healing grafts and unloading braces in medial and posterolateral reconstructions to allow early partial weight-bearing.

LOWER EXTREMITY MUSCLE STRENGTH ATROPHY AND RECOVERY AFTER SURGERY

Lower extremity muscle weakness represents an unresolved problem after ACL reconstruction.* Studies have reported that the magnitude of quadriceps atrophy and strength loss exceeds

---

Critical Points LOWER EXTREMITY MUSCLE STRENGTH RECOVERY AFTER SURGERY

Lower extremity muscle weakness is an unresolved problem after ACL reconstruction.

Pathophysiology of the loss of muscle size and strength after major knee surgery is unknown.

Proposals

- Abnormal gamma loop function in quadriceps muscles from lack of normal sensory function (loss native ACL mechanoreceptors) in the reconstructed ACL.
- Reduction fast-twitch muscle fiber size.
- Residual abnormal anterior tibial displacement.
- Magnitude of preoperative muscle weakness.
- Nonoptimal activation of muscles during voluntary contraction in ACL-deficient knees.

High-intensity electrical muscle stimulation (EMS) significantly increases rectus femoris strength recovery (compared with the opposite limb) compared with the low-intensity EMS, effect not as pronounced for B-PT-B autogenous reconstructions.

Progressive eccentric resistance training effectively increases volume and cross-sectional area of the quadriceps STG and B-PT-B autogenous reconstructions.

---

*See references 6, 14, 38, 100, 101, 107, 115, 119, 176, 180, 188, 189, 214, 223.

20% and 30%, respectively, in the first few months postoperatively.[54,55,68,117,160] Deficits in semitendinosus and gracilis muscle volume of 10% and 30%, respectively, have been noted after STG reconstructions.[86,211] Conflicting data have been published regarding the return of normal quadriceps and hamstrings muscle strength 6 months or longer postoperatively.

The pathophysiology of the loss of muscle size and strength after major knee surgery remains speculative. Konishi and coworkers[101] proposed abnormal gamma loop function in the quadriceps muscles due to the lack of normal sensory function in the reconstructed ACL as a potential explanation. Other authors advocated that the loss of native ACL mechanoreceptors, which have an important role in enhancing normal activity of gamma motoneurons, was a potential cause of this problem.[90–92,187,192,193] Young and associates[224] attributed quadriceps atrophy to a reduction in muscle fiber size from histologic findings in 14 patients. Indeed, some clinical investigators have suggested that fast-twitch muscle fibers (accounting for ~60% of the rectus femoris muscle[187]) become hypotrophic after ACL injury and reconstruction.[13,48] Residual abnormal anterior tibial displacement after reconstruction may play a role in persistent quadriceps weakness.[84] Finally, the magnitude of preoperative muscle weakness may inhibit the ability of a patient to regain normal strength and endurance after surgery.

The question of whether differential atrophy exists between type I and II muscle fibers in the quadriceps remains unclear. Haggmark and colleagues[71] obtained muscle biopsies before surgery and after 5 weeks of postoperative immobilization in nine patients who underwent ACL reconstruction. A decrease in the cross-sectional area (CSA) of type 1 fibers and a reduction in the oxidative capacity of quadriceps muscle were noted, indicating a rapid fall in aerobic capacity. The authors concluded that selective atrophy of type 1 fibers occurred and that type 2 fibers were not significantly affected. In contrast, Gerber and coworkers[63] studied the changes in the quadriceps muscles of 41 chronic ACL-deficient knees and reported that neither histologic nor electron microscopy showed any selective loss of muscle fiber type. These authors concluded that there was no scientific rationale for selective rehabilitation of type 1 or type 2 fibers and that vigorous training of quadriceps muscles was essential after ACL injuries. Lorentzon and associates[109] studied the morphology of muscle types with biopsy and isokinetic testing of 18 male subjects with chronic ACL deficiency. These authors did not find any evidence of selective type 1 or type 2 fiber atrophy. In addition, there was no correlation between isokinetic test data and muscle size or morphologic changes. These authors concluded that decreases in muscle strength cannot be explained by muscle atrophy or structural change. They speculated that nonoptimal activation of muscles during voluntary contractions is the most causative mechanism of strength decrease found in patients with chronic ACL deficiency.

A comparison of high- and low-intensity electrical muscle stimulation (EMS), combined with an intensive rehabilitation program, on recovery of quadriceps strength and gait mechanics was conducted in two investigations.[189,191] A variety of ACL grafts implanted among 110 patients were included in these studies, including Achilles tendon allografts, B-PT-B allografts, STG autografts, and B-PT-B autografts. Although high-intensity EMS significantly increased rectus femoris strength recovery (compared with the opposite limb) compared with the low-intensity EMS protocol, this effect was not as pronounced for patients who underwent ACL PT autogenous reconstruction.

The strength of the quadriceps correlated with flexion and extension excursions of the knee during stance. Patients who were treated with high-intensity EMS walked with more normal excursions, which the authors attributed to the gains in quadriceps strength. Low-intensity EMS, delivered via portable units for home use, was ineffective in promoting return of normal quadriceps strength.

Fitzgerald and colleagues[58] reported modest (effect size, 0.48) improvements in quadriceps isometric peak torque 16 weeks after ACL reconstruction when a "modified" EMS-training protocol was incorporated into the postoperative rehabilitation program of 21 patients. EMS was delivered with the patient positioned supine, lying passively with the knee in full extension. This protocol was modified from previously reported training methods, in which high-intensity EMS was delivered with the patient seated in an isokinetic dynamometer, the knee positioned in approximately 60° of flexion, and the patient actively contracting the quadriceps during application of the electrical current.[41,189,190] The EMS protocol was modified for patients who experienced patellofemoral pain during the training sessions. The protocol involved 10 contractions to maximum patient tolerance, conducted twice weekly for 16 weeks. At 12 weeks postoperative, the experimental group demonstrated significantly greater quadriceps isometric peak torque compared with that of a matched group of patients who did not receive EMS training (75.9 ± 16.8 and 67.0 ± 19.9, respectively; $P < .05$). However, no significant differences were measured at 16 weeks postoperative between these groups. A greater proportion of the EMS-trained subjects initiated agility training at 16 weeks compared with the control group (62% and 32%, respectively; $P < .05$). Still, the authors concluded that the original high-intensity EMS training protocol was preferred when possible based on patient tolerance and equipment availability.

Investigators and clinicians have recently questioned whether rehabilitation programs should focus more efforts on eccentric training to reduce the early postoperative loss of muscle CSA, volume, and strength following ACL reconstruction.[61,66,105] In an exhaustive review of the literature on the effectiveness of concentric, eccentric, or combined concentric-eccentric training in normal, uninjured subjects, Wernbom and coworkers[207] concluded that there was no evidence to support one mode of training over another with regard to achieving superior muscle hypertrophy. These authors assessed published training programs according to frequency, intensity, and duration of work on CSA and volume of the quadriceps and elbow flexor muscle groups. The observation was made that training protocols to induce muscle hypertrophy may differ from those designed to produce maximum strength.

Eccentric training is believed by some authors to be superior to concentric training owing to its potential to overload the muscle and produce greater increases in muscle size and strength.[64,66] There are concerns with high-force eccentric training after ACL reconstruction, including the potential for inducing damage to the muscle and healing graft. A repeated, gradual, and progressive exposure to this type of training was successfully accomplished by Gerber and associates[64] who conducted eccentric training in patients who had either ACL B-PT-B autograft ($N = 20$) or STG autograft ($N = 20$) reconstruction. The patients were randomly assigned to either a 12-week program of eccentric exercises or a standard rehabilitation program. All patients followed a similar protocol for the first 3 postoperative weeks that emphasized regaining full knee motion and basic quadriceps function. Then, patients in the eccentric exercise group initiated progressive exercises using a recumbent eccentric ergometer. The duration and intensity of the negative-work training gradually increased throughout the 12-week period. The patients underwent magnetic resonance imaging (MRI) 3 and 15 weeks postoperative.

The volume and CSA measurements of the quadriceps in the reconstructed knees improved significantly ($P < .001$) in both groups (Fig. 12-7) between the pre- and the post-training time periods. The increases in these measurements were significantly greater ($P < .001$), by more than twofold, in the eccentrically trained patients than in the standard rehabilitation group. In the eccentric group, quadriceps volume increased 23.1 ± 12.9% and peak CSA increased 24.2 ± 12.6%. In comparison,

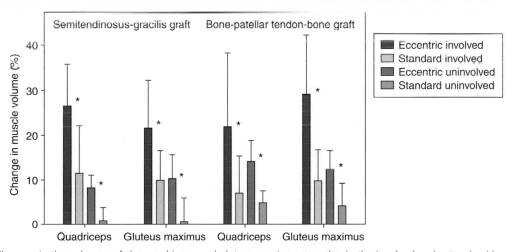

FIGURE 12–7. Changes in the volumes of the quadriceps and gluteus maximus muscles in the involved and uninvolved lower extremities during the 12-week training period after treatment with a semitendinosus-gracilis or bone–patellar tendon–bone graft. The *asterisks* indicate a significant difference in muscle-volume improvement between the eccentric and the standard rehabilitation groups ($P < .005$). *(From Gerber, J. P.; Marcus, R. L.; Dibble, L. E.; et al.: Effects of early progressive eccentric exercise on muscle structure after anterior cruciate ligament reconstruction. J Bone Joint Surg Am 89:559–570, 2007.)*

in the standard rehabilitation group, quadriceps volume increased 8.8 ± 9.3% and peak CSA increased 9.3 ± 9.4%. The increase was not related to the type of graft used for the ACL reconstruction. Significant increases in these measurements were also found in the quadriceps in the noninvolved side.

There were no significant differences between the training groups in the improvement in volume and CSA of the hamstring muscles (Fig. 12–8). When analyzed according to graft type, significant improvements were noted in these measurements in the B-PT-B autograft patients ($P \leq .006$), but not in the STG autograft patients. A reduction in gracilis muscle volume of nearly 20% was found 3 weeks postoperative in the STG group, which increased to a deficit of 35% by 15 weeks postoperative. The authors concluded that the gradual progressive eccentric exercise program safely and effectively improved quadriceps structure in comparison with a standard rehabilitation program. Whether the short-term results of this investigation will demonstrate longer-term benefits are unknown.

Shaw and colleagues[175] conducted a prospective, blinded, randomized trial to determine the effectiveness of instituting quadriceps exercises immediately after ACL reconstruction on a number of parameters. A total of 91 patients who underwent either a B-PT-B or an STG autograft reconstruction were randomized into either the quadriceps exercise–training group or the no-quadriceps exercise–training group. The quadriceps training included straight leg raises and isometric quadriceps contractions performed three times daily for the first 2 postoperative weeks. After 2 weeks, all patients were entered into a similar rehabilitation program. At 6 months postoperative, no difference was found between groups for isokinetic quadriceps strength or lower limb symmetry on functional hop testing.

It is important to note that several authors have documented quadriceps muscle inhibition from an experimentally induced knee joint effusion.[147,194,199,200] This problem has been documented in separate studies during walking, jogging, and landing from a jump. Therefore, it is imperative that knee joint effusion be avoided and, if noted, treated immediately to lessen its deleterious impact on quadriceps function.

OPEN VERSUS CLOSED KINETIC CHAIN EXERCISES: BIOMECHANICAL, IN VIVO, AND CLINICAL STUDIES

The process of graft maturation and healing is assumed to be influenced by strains and forces applied to the ACL during weight-bearing and exercises. Whereas a general consensus exists that some strain is necessary to promote the process of ligamentization,[20] questions remain regarding the amount of load that is safe and the amount that may produce graft elongation. In addition, ligamentization (the return to normal native ACL characteristics) has never actually been shown to occur with graft remodeling and healing. Since the mid 1980s, investigations have attempted to measure, through either analytical or direct means, force and strain incurred on the ACL during common exercises used in rehabilitation. These exercises are typically referred to as either *closed kinetic chain* (CKC) or *open kinetic chain* (OKC). During CKC exercises, the foot is fixed to a platform or surface, the motion at the knee joint is accompanied by predictable motions at the hip and ankle joints, and the entire limb is loaded such as during a leg press or squat. In OKC exercises, the foot is mobile and not fixed to a surface, and motion at the knee joint occurs independent of motion at the hip and ankle joints. Common examples include the leg extension and hamstring curl exercises.

Cadaver Studies

Grood and coworkers[69] biomechanically examined the knee extension exercise in cadavers to determine the conditions in which the ACL was loaded, the quadriceps force that developed during knee flexion-extension, and the forces that were incurred on the extensor mechanism as the knee was extended. Both ACL-intact and ACL-sectioned conditions were created, and the OKC knee extension exercise was simulated both without resistance and with 31 N (7 lb) of resistance applied with an ankle weight at the foot. Although the quadriceps force required

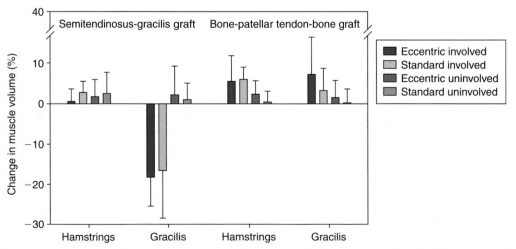

FIGURE 12–8. Changes in the volumes of the hamstrings and gracilis muscle in the involved and uninvolved lower extremities during the 12-week training period after treatment with a semitendinosus-gracilis or bone–patellar tendon–bone graft. There was no significant difference in muscle-volume changes between the eccentric and the standard rehabilitation groups. *(From Gerber, J. P.; Marcus, R. L.; Dibble, L. E.; et al.: Effects of early progressive eccentric exercise on muscle structure after anterior cruciate ligament reconstruction. J Bone Joint Surg Am 89:559–570, 2007.)*

Critical Points OPEN VERSUS CLOSED KINETIC CHAIN EXERCISES

Cadaver Studies

- Quadriceps force required to extend the knee remains at a constant value of 177 N between 50° and 15°, then rises rapidly to 350 N at 0°.
- Addition of 7-pound weight at the ankle doubles the quadriceps force required to extend the knee.
- Avoid 0° to 30° of flexion open kinetic chain (OKC) during rehabilitation of ACL-deficient or ACL-reconstructed knees or in patients with patellofemoral symptoms.
- Isolated hamstring contractions decrease ACL strain relative to normal passive strain from 0° to 120°.
- Isolated quadriceps isometric and isotonic contractions increase ACL strain from 0° to 45°.
- Isometric co-contractions of quadriceps and hamstrings increase ACL strain from 0° to 30°.
- During the squat exercise, the addition of a hamstrings load causes significant decrease in ACL graft load, most evident between 15° and 45°.

Effect of Open and Closed Kinetic Chain Exercises on Anterior Tibial Displacement in Intact and ACL-deficient Knees

- Overall, significantly greater anterior tibial displacements found in ACL-deficient knees during OKC activities than during closed kinetic chain (CKC) exercises.
- CKC squat exercises produce less anterior tibial translation than knee extension in ACL-deficient knees.
- Anterior tibial translation is significantly less during weight-bearing conditions than that measured during Lachman test and non–weight-bearing conditions.
- CKC exercises cause increased joint compression forces and co-activation of the gastrocnemius and quadriceps muscles and result in decreased anterior tibial displacements in ACL-deficient knees.

Calculated ACL Forces, Tibiofemoral Compressive Forces, and Muscle Forces in Human Subjects

- Three-dimensional models used to predict internal muscle forces, tibiofemoral compressive forces, tension in the ACL and posterior cruciate ligament (PCL), and patellofemoral compressive forces during OKC and CKC exercises.
- Greater tibiofemoral compressive forces occur during CKC exercises than during OKC knee extension and are greatest when the knee is fully flexed.
- CKC exercises produce greater co-contraction between quadriceps and hamstrings compared with knee extension; magnitude is dependent on trunk position and knee flexion angle.
- CKC squat produces double the amount of hamstring activity as the leg press and knee extension exercises.

Measurement of In Vivo ACL Strain in ACL-deficient and Intact Knees during Common Open and Closed Kinetic Chain Exercises

- Beynnon et al.[17,22,59,61,76]: series of studies, arthroscopically implanted a Hall effect transducer into the anteromedial fibers of the normal ACL
- Magnitude of ACL strain lowest in isometric contractions of hamstring muscles; contractions quadriceps and hamstrings 30°, 60° and 90°; isometric quadriceps contractions 60° and 90°; passive knee flexion and extension.
- Highest ACL strain in isometric quadriceps contractions 15° flexion with 30 Nm of extension torque, squatting without and with resistance, active knee flexion and extension with 45 N weight boot.

Muscle Recruitment Patterns during Common Open and Closed Kinetic Chain Exercises

- Onset activity for all quadriceps muscles simultaneous during CKC leg press
- During OKC knee extension, onset of vastus lateralis, vastus medialis longus, and rectus femoris occurs before vastus medialis obliquus.
- Peak levels quadriceps activation 201% and 207% of a maximum voluntary isometric contraction (MVIC) for single-leg squats and step-ups, respectively.
- Hamstring activity (biceps femoris muscle only) approximately 20% to 40% MVIC, could have been influenced by trunk flexion angle.

Comparative Clinical Studies

Bynum et al.[31]: Prospective, Randomized Study: OKC or CKC Program after ACL B-PT-B Autograft

- Significantly lower values mean anterior tibial translation and patellofemoral pain severe enough to restrict activities in CKC group.
- Significantly higher values patient rating of the end result of the operation in the CKC group.
- Authors recommended the exclusive use of CKC protocols after ACL reconstruction.

Mikkelsen et al.[119]: Prospective, Randomized Study: CKC or Combined CKC-OKC Program (Began OKC Exercises Week 6) after ACL B-PT-B Autograft

- Higher percentage of patients in combined OKC-CKC group returned to pre-injury sports levels than those in the CKC group.
- Authors recommended combined protocol under carefully supervised conditions.

  Three investigations same laboratory: No benefit from OKC short-term postoperative period.

Beynnon et al.[24]: Prospective, Randomized Double-Blind Study of Two Rehabilitation Programs ("Accelerated" Weight-Bearing, OKC, and Traditional) after ACL B-PT-B Autograft

- No differences between groups for anteroposterior (AP) displacement, International Knee Documentation Committee grading, activity levels, subjective function and patient satisfaction, or single-leg hop tests.
- Authors concluded that rehabilitation programs that allow early weight-bearing and early use of significant quadriceps contractions have the same effect as programs that delay weight-bearing and use of the quadriceps muscles.

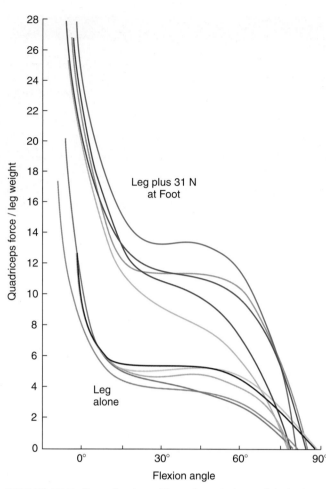

FIGURE 12–9. The ratio of quadriceps force to leg weight is shown for five specimens as a function of flexion angle. The *lower group of curves* shows the force measured when extending the leg against its own weight. The *upper group of curves* shows the forces measured when 31 N was placed at the foot. *(From Grood, E. S.; Suntay, W. J.; Noyes, F. R.; Butler, D. L.: Biomechanics of the knee-extension exercise. Effect of cutting the anterior cruciate ligament. J Bone Joint Surg Am 66:725–734, 1984.)*

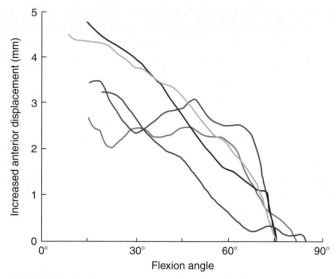

FIGURE 12–10. The increased anterior tibial displacement, relative to the intact knee, that resulted when the anterior cruciate ligament was removed and 31 N was placed at the foot is shown for five specimens. There is an increased displacement in the range of 30° to full extension compared with the intact knee with weights at the foot. *(From Grood, E. S.; Suntay, W. J.; Noyes, F. R.; Butler, D. L.: Biomechanics of the knee-extension exercise. Effect of cutting the anterior cruciate ligament. J Bone Joint Surg Am 66:725–734, 1984.)*

to extend the knee remained at a constant value of 177 N between 50° and 15°, it rose rapidly to 350 N at 0° (Fig. 12–9). The addition of resistance doubled the quadriceps force that was required to extend the knee, resulting in large muscle forces on the patellofemoral joint. There was no change in the quadriceps force required to extend the knee when the ACL was removed. However, loss of the ACL resulted in an increase in anterior tibial displacement from 0° to 30° of extension without resistance. The addition of 31 N of resistance resulted in further increases in anterior tibial displacement throughout the range of extension, with a mean increase of 3.8 mm at 15° (Fig. 12–10). The authors concluded that the range of 0° to 30° of flexion should be avoided during rehabilitation of ACL-deficient or ACL-reconstructed knees and in patients with patellofemoral symptoms.

Renstrom and associates[157] measured the strain of cadaver ACL specimens under simulated isometric contractions of various muscle groups. The authors reported that isolated hamstring contractions decreased ACL strain relative to normal passive strain at all knee flexion angles tested (0°–120°). Isolated quadriceps isometric and isotonic contractions increased ACL strain from 0° to 45° of flexion (Fig. 12–11); the greatest magnitude (5% above the normal passive strain) was measured at full knee extension. Isometric co-contractions of the quadriceps and hamstrings also increased ACL strain from 0° to 30°, with the maximum increase of 5% measured at 0° and 15° of flexion. The authors concluded that isolated quadriceps isometric and isotonic exercises, and isometric co-contraction exercises, could produce potentially harmful forces on healing ACL grafts.

More and colleagues[122] used a cadaver model that incorporated quadriceps and hamstrings muscle loads to examine knee kinematics and ACL loads during the squat exercise. In the intact knees, the addition of a hamstrings load resulted in a significant reduction of anterior tibial translation and internal tibial rotation during flexion. After the ACL was sectioned, the amount of anterior tibial translation increased significantly between 15° and 45° during the squat compared with the intact knee. After ACL reconstruction, maximal graft tension was measured at full extension. During the squat exercise, the addition of a hamstrings load caused a significant decrease in graft load that was most evident between 15° and 45°. The authors concluded that the squat exercise may be safe in the early postoperative period after ACL reconstruction.

Effect of OKC and CKC Exercises on Anterior Tibial Displacement in Intact and ACL-deficient Knees

Several investigators measured AP tibial displacements in ACL-intact and ACL-deficient knees during various OKC and CKC exercises, including active knee extension and squatting.[97,104,220] It is important to note that the amount of AP displacement is influenced by many factors including muscle activation, joint compression forces, geometry, and ligament restraints, primarily

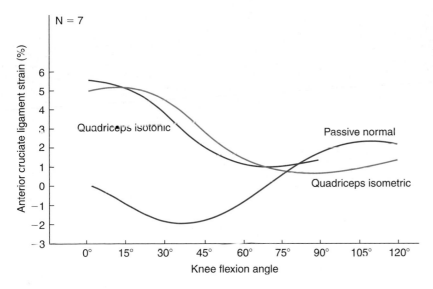

FIGURE 12–11. Mean passive normal, simulated quadriceps isometric, and simulated quadriceps isotonic strain patterns. *(From Renstrom, P.; Arms, S. W.; Stanwyck, T. S.; et al.: Strain within the anterior cruciate ligament during hamstring and quadriceps activity.* Am J Sports Med *14:83–87, 1986.)*

the ACL. Overall, significantly greater anterior tibial displacements were found in the ACL-deficient knees during OKC activities than during CKC exercises.

Yack and coworkers[220] measured the amount of anterior tibial displacement in 11 patients with unilateral ACL-deficient knees during an OKC exercise (resisted knee extension) and a CKC exercise (parallel squat). The average anterior tibial displacement during the squatting exercise (~7.5 mm) was significantly less in the ACL deficient knees than that measured in the knee extension exercise from 66° to 10° (~14 mm). There was no difference in anterior tibial displacement between these exercises in the contralateral normal knees. The conclusion was reached that CKC exercises produced significantly less stress to the ruptured ACL.

In a second study, Yack and associates[221] measured anterior tibial displacement in 14 patients with unilateral ACL-deficient knees during an OKC position and during progressive weight-bearing CKC positions. The progressive weight-bearing protocol included 25%, 50%, 75%, and 100% of each subject's body weight (BW) placed on the foot during a squat held at 20° of flexion. Hamstring muscle activation was controlled to be less than 10% of its maximum activation level during all test conditions. The amount of anterior tibial translation induced during an 89-N Lachman test was measured and compared with that produced during the weight-bearing and non–weight-bearing conditions. The authors reported that anterior tibial translation was significantly less during all weight-bearing conditions than that measured during the Lachman test and the non–weight-bearing conditions. The clinical implication was that rehabilitation after ACL reconstruction could institute weight-bearing exercises without causing excessive strain to the passive restraints. Progressive loading during non–weight-bearing activities should be delayed until the later stages of rehabilitation.

Similar findings were reported by Kvist and Gillquist,[104] who measured anterior tibial translation and lower limb muscle activation in patients with ACL-intact and ACL-ruptured knees during active knee extension (with and without resistance) and squatting exercises in which the center of gravity was placed either over, behind, or in front of the feet. The CKC squat exercises produced less anterior tibial translation than the knee extension in the ACL-deficient knees. In the normal knees,

anterior tibial translation increased with increasing loads in all of the exercises except during the squats with the center of gravity behind the feet. This activity produced less translation than did all of the other exercises in both the normal and the ACL-deficient knees. Overall, hamstring muscle activity was low in all knees during both the OKC and the CKC exercises, but co-activation of the gastrocnemius and quadriceps muscles was noted. The authors concluded that the CKC exercises caused increased joint compression forces and co-activation of the gastrocnemius and quadriceps muscles, thereby resulting in decreased anterior tibial displacements in ACL-deficient knees.

Jurist and Otis[97] measured anterior and posterior tibial displacement in five knees with intact ACLs to determine the effects of knee flexion angle (30°, 60°, and 90°) and the position of external resistance (proximal, middle, or distal on the long axis of the tibia) during isometric contractions. The results demonstrated that a proximal position of external load produced posterior displacement of the tibia. The authors concluded that quadriceps muscle strengthening could be safely initiated between 90° and 30° of flexion in ACL-reconstructed knees early postoperatively.

Calculated ACL Forces, Tibiofemoral Compressive Forces, and Muscle Forces in Human Subjects

Several investigators used two-dimensional mathematical models from in vivo experimental measures to calculate muscle forces, tibiofemoral shear, and compressive forces during isometric and isokinetic exercises.* The analytical models did not allow for the authors to determine the magnitude of the ligament forces incurred during various exercises.

Yasuda and Sasaki[222] calculated anterior and posterior drawer forces exerted on the tibia in 20 healthy adult males during isometric contractions of the quadriceps and hamstrings at knee flexion angles ranging from 5° to 90° (Fig. 12–12). During the quadriceps isometric contractions, maximum anterior shear

---

*See references 8, 36, 85, 99, 110, 126, 127, 144, 185, 222.

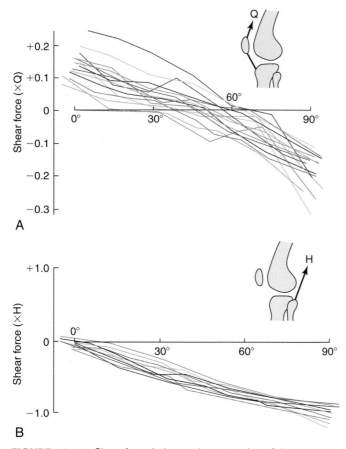

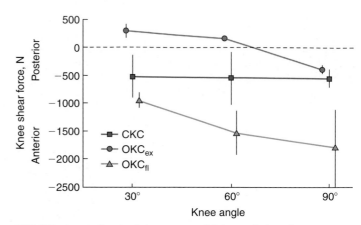

FIGURE 12–13. Graph of the average tibiofemoral shear forces observed during the closed kinetic chain (CKC) leg press, the open kinetic chain extension exercise (OKC$_{ex}$), and the open kinetic chain flexion exercise (OKC$_{fl}$). *(From Lutz, G. E.; Palmitier, R. A.; An, K. N.; Chao, E. Y.: Comparison of tibiofemoral joint forces during open-kinetic-chain and closed-kinetic-chain exercises.* J Bone Joint Surg Am *75:732–739, 1993.)*

FIGURE 12–12. Shear force in isometric contraction of the quadriceps (**A**) or hamstrings (**B**) at various flexion angles of the knee. The abscissa shows the flexion angle of the knee, and the ordinate shows the coefficient of a linear function that gives the shear force in proportion to tension of the quadriceps (**A**) or the hamstrings (**B**). Plus and minus values of the coefficient mean the anterior and posterior drawer force to the tibia. Each *polygonal line* shows a different subject. (**A**) The anterior drawer force is given to the tibia in the area of small flexion angle of the knee, and the posterior drawer force is given in the area of large flexion angle. (**B**) The posterior drawer force is given to the tibia at every flexion angle of the knee. *(A and B, From Yasuda, K.; Sasaki, T.: Exercise after anterior cruciate ligament reconstruction. The forces exerted on the tibia by the separate isometric contractions of the quadriceps or the hamstrings.* Clin Orthop Relat Res *220:275–283, 1987.)*

forces were measured at 5° of knee flexion. As the angle of knee flexion increased, the calculated anterior shear force decreased. The mean knee flexion angle at which the anterior drawer force changed to a posterior drawer force during this exercise was 45.3° ± 12.5°. During isometric hamstring contractions, posterior shear forces were measured at all knee flexion angles. The authors concluded that early postoperative rehabilitation should include quadriceps isometrics exercises with knee flexion greater than 70° and hamstrings isometric exercises at all flexion angles. The question was raised of the efficacy of quadriceps isometric training at high knee flexion angles for adequate muscle training.

Lutz and colleagues[110] analyzed forces at the tibiofemoral joint during OKC and CKC exercises in five healthy subjects. A two-dimensional model was used to calculate tibiofemoral shear and compression forces during maximal isometric contractions at 30°, 60°, and 90° of knee flexion. The OKC knee extension contraction produced the greatest amount of anterior shear

force (Fig. 12–13; 285 ± 120 N at 30° of flexion). CKC exercises produced significantly less anterior shear force at all flexion angles. In addition, CKC exercises produced significantly greater compressive forces and muscular co-contraction at the same knee flexion angles at which the OKC exercises produced maximum shear forces and minimum muscular co-contraction. The authors recommended CKC exercises after ACL injury or reconstruction.

Ohkoshi and associates[144] used a two-dimensional model derived from radiographs and electromyographic analyses to predict shear forces on the tibia during standing at various trunk and knee flexion angles in 21 normal male subjects. Co-contraction of the quadriceps and hamstrings was observed at all knee and trunk flexion angle positions. Hamstrings activity increased with increasing trunk flexion angles. The calculated shear forces were negative in all positions, with increasing posterior drawer forces found as trunk flexion angles increased (at knee flexion angles of 30° and 60°). The authors concluded that exercises done in the standing position with the knees flexed and the trunk anteriorly flexed (such as half-squatting) could be performed safely in the early stages after ACL reconstruction.

Other investigators used three-dimensional models to predict internal muscle forces, tibiofemoral compressive forces, tension in the ACL and posterior cruciate ligament, and patellofemoral compressive forces during OKC and CKC exercises.[51,99,201,210] Kaufman and coworkers[99] reported that an isokinetic OKC knee extension exercise produced mean tibiofemoral compressive forces of 4.0 ± 0.7 times BW at 60°/sec and 3.8 ± 0.9 BW at 180°/sec; however, these were calculated at 55° of knee flexion. Anterior shear forces existed between 40° and full extension, potentially loading the ACL.

Escamilla and coworkers[51] and Wilk and associates[210] reported that greater tibiofemoral compressive forces occurred during CKC exercises than during OKC knee extension (Fig. 12–14) and that these compressive forces were greatest when the knee was fully flexed. The calculated joint compression forces were dependent on the position of the trunk relative to the knee and ankle joints, with greater forces generated when the body was positioned directly over the knee. Peak ACL tensile forces occurred only during OKC exercises near full

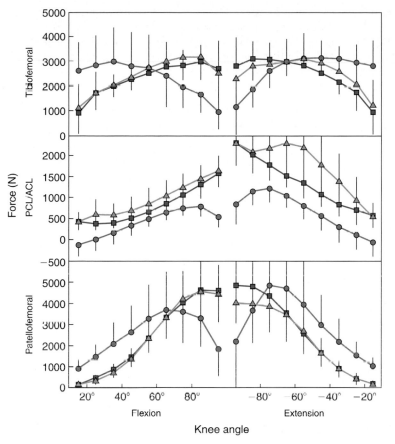

FIGURE 12–14. Mean and standard deviation of forces during squat (*triangle*), leg press (*square*), and knee extension (*circle*). Tibiofemoral compressive force, posterior cruciate ligament (PCL; +), anterior cruciate ligament (ACL; –) tensile force, and patellofemoral compressive force are shown. *(From Escamilla, R. F.; Fleisig, G. S.; Zheng, N.; et al.: Biomechanics of the knee during closed kinetic chain and open kinetic chain exercises. Med Sci Sports Exerc 30:556–569, 1998.)*

extension and were calculated as 0.20 × BW. CKC exercises produced greater co-contraction between the quadriceps and the hamstrings compared with knee extension; however, the magnitude was dependent on the trunk position and knee flexion angle. In addition, the squat produced approximately double the amount of hamstring activity as the leg press and knee extension exercises. Knee extension produced greater quadriceps activity, leading the investigators to conclude that the ACL could be loaded from 0° to 60° during this exercise.

Toutoungi and colleagues[201] determined cruciate ligament forces from analytical modeling in normal knees during OKC isokinetic and isometric exercises and during CKC double-leg and single-leg squatting. During isokinetic and isometric extension, peak ACL forces occurred from 35° to 40° of nearly 400 N, or 0.55 × BW. However, during isokinetic extension, ACL forces decreased significantly with increasing dynamometer speed, from 349 N at 60°/sec to 254 N at 180°/sec. Small forces were incurred on the ACL during squats at knee flexion angles less than 50°. The authors concluded that isokinetic flexion and squats were safe to perform in the early postoperative period after ACL reconstruction, but that isokinetic knee extension should be avoided until graft healing is well advanced.

Shields and coworkers[183] examined the single-leg squat in normal subjects to determine the effect of resistance to both flexion and extension and knee flexion angle on lower extremity muscle activity. Resistance to flexion and extension was set as a percentage of BW, being either 0%, 4%, or 8%. The results revealed that co-contraction of the quadriceps and hamstrings occurred throughout the squatting exercise (0°–40°). Although the quadriceps had greater activity than the hamstrings at all

levels of resistance, the quadriceps-to-hamstrings ratio decreased with higher levels of resistance. Biceps femoris activity increased during knee flexion with resistance from approximately 12% of that of a maximum voluntary isometric contraction (MVIC) during low resistance (0% BW) to 27% of that of a MVIC during high resistance (8% BW). The authors suggested that this CKC exercise done under controlled conditions with resistance to both flexion and extension was effective in increasing the dynamic control of the knee joint.

Measurement of In Vivo ACL Strain in ACL-deficient and Intact Knees during Common OKC and CKC Exercises

Henning and associates[77] were the first to measure the in vivo ACL strain in human subjects. The authors applied a strain gauge to two subjects with partially disrupted ACLs and measured ACL strain and elongation during OKC and CKC activities, which were compared with loads induced by an 356-N (80-lb) Lachman test. The sample size did not allow for statistical comparisons or analyses. The authors noted that activities such as partial weight-bearing with crutches and stationary bicycling produced only 7% as much elongation as the Lachman test. Knee extension exercises with 89 N (20 lb) of resistance produced 87% to 121% from 22° to 0°, but produced only 50% as much elongation as the Lachman test. The authors recommended avoidance of quadriceps exercises and testing by knee extension for the first year after ACL injury or reconstruction.

Beynnon and colleagues[17,22,59,61,76] conducted a series of studies in which a Hall effect transducer was arthroscopically implanted into the anteromedial fibers of the normal ACL in volunteers undergoing surgical procedures under local anesthesia. Patients performed a variety of OKC and CKC exercises at different knee flexion angles, including isometric contractions,[17] squatting,[22] bicycling,[60] stair climbing,[59] and lunging.[76] The mean peak ACL strains reported in these studies are shown in Table 12–3.[20] The magnitude of ACL strain produced by the exercises assessed in these studies was lowest in those that involved isometric contractions of the hamstring muscles; simultaneous contractions of the quadriceps and hamstrings at 30°, 60°, and 90° of knee flexion; isometric quadriceps contractions at 60° and 90° of knee flexion; and passive flexion and extension of the knee. The activities that produced the highest ACL strain included isometric quadriceps contractions at 15° of knee flexion with 30 Nm of extension torque, squatting without and with resistance, and active flexion and extension of the knee with a

45-N weight boot. The authors emphasized that the limits of ACL strain that are safe and not deleterious to healing ACL grafts remain unknown. Although excessive loading must be avoided early postoperatively, controlled loading is required to enhance graft healing and ligamentization.

Muscle Recruitment Patterns during Common OKC and CKC Exercises

Stensdotter and coworkers[197] studied onset time and amplitude of the quadriceps muscles during a knee extension and simulated leg press isometric contraction in 10 healthy subjects. The onset of activity for all of the quadriceps muscles was simultaneous during the CKC activity (Fig. 12–15). During the OKC task, the onset of vastus lateralis, vastus medialis longus, and rectus femoris occurred before that of VMO. The mean amplitude for rectus femoris was significantly greater during the OKC exercise, whereas the mean amplitude for VMO was significantly larger during the CKC exercise.

Beutler and associates[16] measured quadriceps and hamstring activation in healthy subjects during two CKC activities. The peak levels of quadriceps activation were 201% and 207% of a MVIC for single-leg squats and step-ups, respectively. Hamstring activity (biceps femoris muscle only) was approximately 20% to 40% MVIC, which could have been influenced by trunk flexion angle, which was not controlled for in this study. The authors concluded that both of these CKC exercises were effective for males and females for achieving maximal quadriceps contraction for strength training or rehabilitation.

Salem and colleagues[168] evaluated the kinematics and kinetics of the ankle, knee, and hip in eight ACL-reconstructed and contralateral knees during a two-legged squat. The patients were tested a mean of 30 ± 12 weeks postoperative; all had implemented the two-legged squat into their rehabilitation at least 6 weeks prior to testing. Two distinctly different strategies were noted for generating the joint torques required to perform the exercise.

Exercise	OKC or CKC	Peak ACL Strain (%)
TABLE 12–3 Rank Comparison of Mean Peak Anterior Cruciate Ligament Strain Values Measured In Vivo in Subjects with Uninjured Knees		
Isometric quadriceps contraction at 15° (30 Nm extension torque)	OKC	4.4
Squat with Sport Cord	CKC	4.0
Active flexion and extension (45-N weight boot)	OKC	3.8
Lachman test at 30° (150 N anterior shear load)		3.7
Squat, no resistance	CKC	3.6
Isometric gastrocnemius contraction at 15° (15 Nm plantar flexion torque)	OKC	3.5
Active flexion and extension, no resistance	OKC	2.8
Co-contraction quadriceps and hamstrings at 15°	OKC	2.8
Isometric gastrocnemius contraction at 5° (15 Nm plantar flexion torque)	OKC	2.8
Single-legged sit-to-stand exercise	CKC	2.8
Isometric quadriceps contraction at 30° (30 Nm extension torque)	OKC	2.7
Stair climbing	CKC	2.7
Step-up and step-down	CKC	2.5
Weight-bearing at 20°		2.1
Leg press at 20° (40% body weight)	CKC	2.1
Anterior drawer test at 90° (150 N anterior shear load)		1.8
Lunge	CKC	1.8
Stationary bicycling	CKC	1.7
Isometric hamstrings contraction at 15° (10 Nm flexion torque)	OKC	<1.0
Co-contraction quadriceps and hamstrings at 30°	OKC	<1.0
Isometric gastrocnemius contraction at 30° (15 Nm plantar flexion torque)	OKC	<1.0
Passive flexion and extension	OKC	<1.0
Isometric quadriceps contraction at 60° and 90° (30 Nm extension torque)	OKC	0
Isometric gastrocnemius contraction at 45° (15 Nm plantar flexion torque)	OKC	0
Co-contraction quadriceps and hamstrings at 60° and 90°	OKC	0
Isometric hamstrings contraction at 30°, 60°, and 90° (10 Nm flexion torque)	OKC	0

ACL, anterior cruciate ligament; CKC, closed kinetic chain; OKC, open kinetic chain.

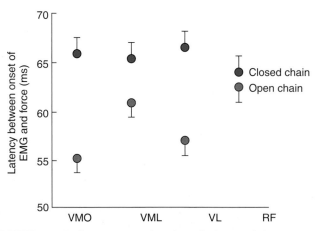

FIGURE 12–15. Group mean values (standard error of the mean [SEM]) for onsets of activity relative to onset of force increase. There was no difference in electromyographic onset time between muscle portions relative to force in CKC. In OKC, the latency between onset of activity and onset of force was shorter for the vastus medialis obliquus than for all other muscle portions, whereas the latency between onset of activity in rectus femoris relative to onset of force was longer than all others. *(From Stensdotter, A. K.; Hodges, P. W.; Mellor, R.; et al.: Quadriceps activation in closed and in open kinetic chain exercise. Med Sci Sports Exerc 35:2043–2047, 2003.)*

In the noninvolved limb, equal distribution of hip and knee muscular effort was noted. However, in the reconstructed limb, patients used a more hip-dominant strategy, thereby reducing the knee extension peak torque effort. The authors cautioned that patients may use substitution methods during bilateral CKC activities by either shifting the effort from the reconstructed limb to the contralateral limb or adopting a hip-dominant strategy, limiting the potential effectiveness of these exercises.

Comparative Rehabilitation Studies after ACL Reconstruction

Few investigators have prospectively compared the outcome of rehabilitation programs of OKC and CKC exercises. Bynum and coworkers[31] were the first to report a prospective, randomized study in which patients were placed into either an OKC or a CKC program after ACL B-PT-B autogenous reconstruction. Forty-seven patients performed OKC exercises beginning with hamstring isotonics immediately postoperatively, straight leg raises at 3 weeks, and quadriceps isotonics with low resistance at 6 weeks that progressed to unrestricted at 12 weeks. Knee motion restrictions for the OKC exercises were not detailed. Fifty patients performed CKC exercises including double-leg partial squats, leg press, and stationary bicycling initially. All 97 patients were entered into an immediate knee motion program (0°–90°) and allowed partial weight-bearing, progressing to full as tolerated. Only 64 patients (66%) returned for evaluation from 12 to 36 months postoperatively; 85 completed a subjective analysis by phone interview. At follow-up, significantly lower values were reported in mean anterior tibial translation and patellofemoral pain restricting activities in the CKC group. Significantly higher values were found in the patient rating of the end result of the operation in the CKC group as well. The authors recommended the exclusive use of CKC protocols after ACL reconstruction.

Mikkelsen and associates[119] followed 44 patients who underwent ACL B-PT-B autogenous reconstruction and who were randomized into either a CKC program or a combined CKC-OKC program that initiated OKC exercises at postoperative week 6. The OKC exercises consisted of quadriceps isokinetic training done under supervised conditions in the range of 90° to 40°, which gradually progressed during the next 6 weeks to 90° to 10°. The patients were reviewed at 6 months postoperative with knee arthrometer and muscle strength testing and at an average of 31 months postoperative with a questionnaire. There was no difference between groups in the mean anterior tibial displacement. Patients in the combined OKC-CKC group had significantly greater quadriceps peak torque values than those in the CKC group at 6 months postoperative; however, this difference was not observed after this time period. In addition, the peak torque values were not normalized for BW, so direct comparisons are susceptible to error. A higher percentage of patients (55%) in the combined OKC-CKC group returned to preinjury sports activities levels than those in the CKC group (23%). The authors recommended the combined protocol under carefully supervised conditions.

Three prospective trials were conducted from a group of surgeons in London, U.K., that compared OKC and CKC for hip and knee extensor training after ACL reconstruction.[81,123,152] The first study comprised 36 patients who underwent ACL

B-PT-B autogenous reconstruction; in 9, a ligament augmentation device (LAD) was implanted along with a small strip of the PT, and in 27, the central third of the PT was harvested.[123] At 2 weeks postoperative, patients were randomized into either a CKC program or an OKC program; the patients were trained and followed for the next 4 weeks. The CKC patients performed unilateral leg press exercises in the range of 90° to 0°, and the OKC patients performed hip and knee extension isotonic exercises through the range of 90° to 0° three times a week (for a total of 60 cycles of concentric and eccentric contractions). Neither group performed squats or step-ups, but all were allowed to use the stationary bicycle. The only outcome measure in this study was anterior tibial displacement, which was not significantly different at the conclusion of the 4-week training period. The authors concluded that because the OKC offered no benefit, only CKC should be used for rehabilitation after ACL reconstruction.

In the second investigation, gait analyses were conducted on the population described by Morrissey and colleagues before[123] and after training.[81] No statistically significant differences were found after training between the OKC and the CKC groups for 16 variables assessed during level walking and ascending and descending stairs. The authors were unable to provide a definitive recommendation for rehabilitation based on the study's findings.

The third study involved 49 patients from 12 surgeons who performed a variety of ACL reconstructive methods, including B-PT-B autograft and LAD, arthroscopic-assisted or open central third PT, and semitendinosus and/or gracilis tendons.[152] CKC and OKC training was initiated 8 weeks postoperative for hip and knee extensors as described by Morrissey and colleagues.[123] Training was conducted three times a week for 6 weeks, and all patients also performed stationary bicycling, lunges, single-leg exercises on a minitrampoline and a balance board, lateral plyometric hopping, and hamstring isotonic exercises. Post-training testing performed at 14 weeks postoperative revealed no significant differences between the groups for anterior tibial displacement, subjective function as measured by visual analog scales, or single-leg hop tests. The authors recommended only CKC after ACL reconstruction, citing no benefit of OKC.

Beynnon and coworkers[24] conducted a prospective, randomized, double-blind study of two rehabilitation programs after ACL arthroscopic-assisted B-PT-B autogenous reconstruction. The programs differed according to the time of supervised physical therapy patients were requested to participate in postoperatively and the amount of strain believed to be incurred on the graft based on the authors' prior in vivo studies. The "accelerated" program lasted 19 weeks and allowed exercises that produced high ACL strain to be initiated sooner than the nonaccelerated program, which lasted 32 weeks. For example, OKC exercises were initiated as early as week 2 (straight leg raises) in the accelerated group, as well as allowance of full weight-bearing without crutch support. Knee extensions from 0° to 90° were begun at week 6 in the accelerated group, compared with week 12 in the nonaccelerated group. The patients (10 in the accelerated group and 12 in the nonaccelerated group) were followed for 2 years postoperatively.

The results revealed no differences between the groups for AP displacement, International Knee Documentation Committee (IKDC) grading, activity levels, subjective function, patient satisfaction, and single-leg hop tests. The authors concluded that rehabilitation programs that allow early weight-bearing and early use of significant quadriceps contractions had the same effect as programs that delay weight-bearing and use of the quadriceps muscles. Cartilage biomarkers obtained shortly after the injury demonstrated elevated cleavage and synthesis of type II collagen and turnover of aggrecan compared with control values. After 1 year, cleavage of type II collagen was restored to normal levels; however, an excess of 2 years was required for synthesis of type II collagen and turnover of aggrecan to begin to reach normal limits. The authors concluded that the injury, surgery, and rehabilitation had a dramatic effect on the metabolism of articular cartilage and that further work was required to determine other measures of the progression of arthritis.

It appears from the literature that the incorporation of OKC exercises after the 6th postoperative week after ACL B-PT-B autogenous reconstruction, under carefully supervised conditions and in the range of 90° to 30° of knee flexion, may be advantageous. However, further randomized clinical studies are required to determine whether a combined OKC-CKC protocol will enhance earlier muscle strength recovery and return to activities.

PATELLOFEMORAL JOINT CONSIDERATIONS

As previously discussed, the quadriceps force that develops during knee flexion-extension and the forces incurred on the extensor mechanism as the knee extends were experimentally measured in the authors' laboratory.[69] The investigation demonstrated that the quadriceps force required to extend the knee remained at a constant value of 177 N between 50° and 15° of knee flexion, and then rose rapidly to 350 N at 0°. The addition of a small amount of resistance (31 N) doubled the quadriceps force that was required to extend the knee, resulting in large forces on the patellofemoral joint. This was the first investigation to recommend avoidance of quadriceps exercises in the

range of 0° to 30° of flexion during rehabilitation of the ACL-deficient or ACL-reconstructed knee and in knees with patellofemoral symptoms.

Doucette and Child[43] used computed tomography to measure the patellar congruence angle in patients with symptomatic lateral patellar compression syndrome under three conditions: with the lower extremity relaxed, holding an OKC (knee extension) position, and holding a CKC exercise position. Measurements were made in 10° increments from 0° to 40° of flexion. There were significant differences at 0°, 10°, and 20° of flexion between the OKC position and both the CKC and the relaxed conditions. At each flexion angle, significantly greater lateral patellar tracking occurred during the OKC exercise. During all three conditions, patellar congruence progressively improved from 0° to 40° of flexion. The authors concluded that a quadriceps contraction has less influence on patellar tracking at 30° of flexion than at 0° of flexion owing to the increased stability of the patella as it moves into the intercondylar groove as the knee is flexed. In low, functional knee ROMs, CKC exercises were recommended owing to the improved patellar positioning and decreased joint irritation in symptomatic patellofemoral patients.

Steinkamp and associates[196] calculated knee moments, patellofemoral joint reaction forces, and patellofemoral joint stresses in 20 normal subjects at four knee flexion angles (0°, 30°, 60°, and 90°) during the leg press and knee extension exercises. All three parameters were significantly greater at 0° and 30° in the leg extension exercises than during the leg press exercise (Fig. 12–16). The opposite was true at the high knee flexion angles, for which all parameters were significantly greater in

Critical Points PATELLOFEMORAL JOINT CONSIDERATIONS

- Quadriceps force required to extend the knee remains at a constant value (177 N) between 50° and 15° of knee flexion, then rises rapidly to 350 N at 0°.
- The addition of a small amount of resistance (7 lb) doubles the quadriceps force required to extend the knee, resulting in large forces on the patellofemoral joint.
- Avoid quadriceps exercises in the range of 0° to 30° of flexion.
- Significantly greater lateral patellar tracking occurs during OKC knee extension than during CKC at 0°, 10°, and 20° of flexion.
- Quadriceps contraction has less influence on patellar tracking at 30° of flexion than at 0° of flexion owing to the increased stability of the patella as it moves into the intercondylar groove as the knee is flexed.
- Knee moments, patellofemoral joint reaction forces, and patellofemoral joint stresses are significantly greater at 0° and 30° in the leg extension exercises than in the leg press exercise. The opposite occurs at high knee flexion angles.
- During the leg press exercise, compressive forces are high but distributed over a larger contact area.
- During the leg extension exercise, compressive forces are low but concentrated over a smaller contact area.
- Estimated loads on patellofemoral joint with weight-bearing activities: stair climbing 3.3 × body weight (BW); squatting 7.6 × BW; jumping 20 × BW.

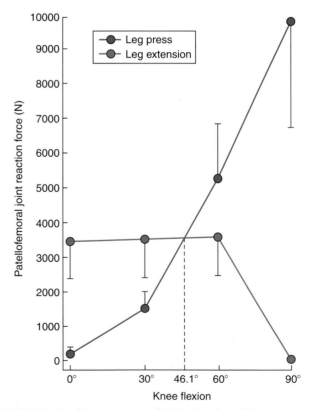

FIGURE 12–16. Mean ± standard deviation of patellofemoral joint reaction force at four flexion angles. *(From Steinkamp, L. A.; Dillingham, M. F.; Markel, M. D.; et al.: Biomechanical considerations in patellofemoral joint rehabilitation. Am J Sports Med 21:438–444, 1993.)*

the leg press exercise. The authors concluded that the leg press placed minimal stress on the patellofemoral joint in the functional ROM (low knee flexion angles) and noted empirically that patients with patellofemoral disorders frequently complained of pain with the knee extension exercise. During the leg press exercise, compressive forces were higher but distributed over a larger contact area, whereas during the leg extension exercise, compressive forces were lower but concentrated over a smaller contact area.

Witvrouw and colleagues[212,213] conducted investigations on 51 patients with isolated patellofemoral pain who were randomly assigned to either an OKC or a CKC 5-week exercise program. The OKC exercises consisted of maximal static quadriceps contractions with the knee in full extension, straight leg raises in the supine position, leg adduction exercises in the lateral decubitus position, and short arc movements from 10° of flexion to terminal extension. The CKC exercises included seated leg press, double or single one third knee bend, stationary biking, rowing machine, step-up and step-down exercises, and jumping on a minitrampoline. The patients were evaluated upon completion of the program and then 5 years later. There were no significant differences between the two treatment groups for the majority of parameters evaluated. At the 5-year evaluation, 92% of the OKC group was participating in sports compared with 60% of those in the CKC group. The OKC group demonstrated, on visual analog scales, less swelling, pain on descending stairs, and pain at night compared with the CKC group. Owing to the overall lack of differences between the groups in the majority of parameters studied, the authors recommended a combination of both OKC and CKC exercises in patients with patellofemoral symptoms.

Dye[45] reviewed the role of loading in patellofemoral pain, including the amount sustained by a single blow (such as during a fall onto the pavement) and the amount sustained with repeated smaller loads that disrupt normal tissue homeostasis (such as climbing up or down stairs, kneeling, squatting, or jumping). The stress on the patellofemoral joint depends not only on the load applied but also on the surface areas of the patella and femur that may be in contact at any given point in time. Estimated loads on the patellofemoral joint with weight-bearing activities ranged from 3.3 times BW with stair climbing to 7.6 times BW with squatting to up to 20 times BW with jumping.[156,186] The ability of the entire knee joint to absorb and distribute these forces is dependent on what Dye[45] termed the *envelope of function*, or "that range of loading applied across the joint that is compatible with and probably inductive of maintenance of tissue homeostasis." The envelope includes three zones. The first is the zone of subphysiologic underload, or diminished loads (e.g., prolonged bedrest), that cause muscle atrophy or calcium loss. The second zone, that of homeostatic loading, represents the range of acceptable loading in which tissue homeostasis is maintained. This zone is highly variable between individuals, because knee joints accept loads that range from less than 1 to nearly 8 times BW.[45] The third zone, supraphysiologic overload, represents loads that exceed the knee joint's ability to accept and distribute forces in a manner that maintains homeostasis. The author expressed that patellofemoral pain could frequently be diminished by simply lowering the forces to the patient's asymptomatic envelope of function.

The authors recommend avoidance of exercises that place large forces on the patellofemoral joint after ACL reconstruction, especially the leg extension exercise in the range of 30° to 0° of knee flexion. Patients who develop patellofemoral symptoms postoperatively must be carefully followed and the rehabilitation program altered as required to avoid activities, such as deep squatting and jumping, that place high forces on the patella.

ALTERATIONS IN GAIT, NEUROMUSCULAR FUNCTION, AND PROPRIOCEPTION AFTER ACL RECONSTRUCTION

Chronic ACL deficiency produces marked alterations in gait during a variety of activities.[4,5,15,137,149,208] During level walking, ACL-deficient subjects demonstrate significantly decreased external knee flexion moments and increased external knee extension moments compared with healthy control subjects.[208] The resultant quadriceps avoidance gait pattern has been identified in these knees in several investigations: in 16 of 32 knees that also had varus malalignment in the authors' laboratory,[137] in 7 of 8 subjects who were greater than 7 years postinjury by Wexler and coworkers,[208] and in 12 of 16 (75%) subjects by Berchuck and associates.[15] Wexler and coworkers[208] found that changes in sagittal plane knee moments were more pronounced as the amount of time after the injury increased. Berchuck and associates[15] reported that gait adaptations were present in both the injured and the contralateral limbs owing to the symmetrical function required for weight-bearing activities. Patel and colleagues[149] found that patients with ACL deficiency had a significantly reduced peak external flexion moment during jogging and stair climbing that correlated with significantly reduced quadriceps strength. Andriacchi and coworkers[5] used a finite-element model from three-dimensional cartilage volumes created from MRI to predict progression of osteoarthritis (OA) in normal and ACL-deficient knees. The model predicted a more rapid rate of cartilage thinning in the ACL-deficient knees, especially in the medial tibiofemoral compartment. The investigators concluded that this was due to a shift in the normal load-bearing regions of the knee joint during weight-bearing activities and stressed the importance of restoring proper gait mechanics after ACL reconstruction.

Several investigations have documented altered gait biomechanics, neuromuscular function, and proprioception many months or years after ACL reconstruction.[27,30,42,50,106,214] Unfortunately, the majority of these investigations did not provide detailed information regarding the postoperative rehabilitation program. Timoney and associates[198] were among the first investigators to document altered gait kinematics in a study conducted on 10 male patients an average of 10 months (range, 9–12 mo) after ACL B-PT-B autograft reconstruction. Compared with a control group, the patients had a significantly lower mean external knee flexion moment at midstance (3.74% and 2.02%, respectively) and a significantly lower mean heel-strike transient value (66.6 and 44.3 BW/sec, respectively). The patients' reconstructed limb had a significantly lower mean midstance external knee flexion moment than the uninvolved limb (2.02% and 3.10%, respectively). The patients did not demonstrate a quadriceps-avoidance gait, because a net external flexion moment was present throughout most of the stance phase.

Devita and colleagues[42] conducted gait analysis testing in eight patients who had a B-PT-B autograft ACL reconstruction 3 weeks and 6 months after surgery and an "accelerated"

Critical Points ALTERATIONS IN GAIT, NEUROMUSCULAR FUNCTION, AND PROPRIOCEPTION AFTER ACL RECONSTRUCTION

Altered Gait Biomechanics

- Timoney et al.[198]: Walking: Patients had significantly lower mean external knee flexion moment at midstance, significantly lower mean heel-strike transient value, significantly lower mean midstance external knee flexion moment compared with the uninvolved limb.
- DeVita et al.[42]: Walking: Although ACL-reconstructed patients walked with normal kinematic patterns 6 months postoperative, they demonstrated altered joint torque and power patterns at the hip and knee.
- Kowalk et al.[102]: Stair climbing: Significant reductions in peak moment, power, and work in reconstructed knees. Significant increases in excursion, moment, and power in the contralateral ankle joint.
- Ernst et al.[50]: Single-leg vertical jump, lateral step-up: Knee extension moment in ACL-reconstructed knees is less than the contralateral lower extremity and lower extremities of controls during take-off and landing.
- Bush-Joseph et al.[30]: Walking, stair climbing, jogging, jog-and-cut maneuver: Peak external flexion moment in ACL-reconstructed knees during jogging and a jog-and-cut maneuver was decreased compared with controls. Correlation existed between quadriceps muscle strength and decreased external flexion moment during jogging, but not during the jog-and-cut task.

Altered Neuromuscular Function

- Wojtys and Huston[214]: Quadriceps endurance in ACL-reconstructed knees was lower than in the opposite limb 18 months postoperative. Time to reach peak torque of quadriceps and hamstrings was significantly slower than in the uninvolved limb.

Altered Proprioception

- Literature is mixed regarding proprioceptive deficits after ACL reconstruction. Differences in findings are due to variability in test procedures, time from injury to ACL reconstruction, associated injuries to the menisci and articular cartilage, the rehabilitation program, and the use of internal versus external control limbs.
- Two most common tests for proprioception are threshold for detection of passive motion and joint position sense. Differences in the magnitude of error in the patients' ability to reproduce a specific joint position (flexion angle) postoperatively during these tests are frequently less than 1° to 2° when compared with either internal or external control data. Clinical significance is not clear. Studies have not assessed whether specific rehabilitation exercises (such as OKC vs. CKC) influence knee joint proprioception postoperatively.

---

rehabilitation program. The data were compared with those collected from 22 healthy subjects. Although the ACL-reconstructed patients walked with normal kinematic patterns 6 months postoperatively, they demonstrated altered joint torque and power patterns at the hip and knee. The hip extensors provided more vertical support and forward progression during the first half of stance compared with the contribution measured in the normal subjects. There was also a decrease in the magnitude of extensor torque at the knee in early stance compared with that in the healthy subjects.

Kowalk and coworkers[102] conducted gait analyses on 7 patients who had a B-PT-B autograft reconstruction (mean, 6 mo postoperative; range, 3.2–11.3 mo) and on 10 healthy subjects. The analysis consisted of ascending three steps that were attached to two force plates. The authors reported statistically significant reductions for peak moment, power, and work in the reconstructed knees along with significant increases in excursion, moment, and power at the contralateral ankle joint. The patients compensated during the stair ascent task by generating increased power at the contralateral ankle.

Ernst and associates[50] measured lower extremity kinematics in 20 patients who underwent a B-PT-B autograft reconstruction (mean, 9.8 mo postoperative; range, 8–15 mo) and in 20 matched normal subjects. The subjects performed a single-leg vertical jump and a lateral step-up. The knee extension moment of the ACL-reconstructed subjects was less than that of their contralateral lower extremity and those of the lower extremities of the controls during take-off and landing on the vertical jump and the lateral step-up exercise. The authors suggested that this finding was related to either weakness of the quadriceps femoris muscle or some alteration of the neuromuscular system in which hip or ankle extensors were recruited. Patients may compensate during these activities and not adequately recruit the quadriceps musculature, thereby reducing the potential effectiveness of the exercises.

Bush-Joseph and colleagues[30] measured knee kinematics and kinetics in 22 patients who had ACL B-PT-B autograft reconstruction 22 ± 12 months postoperative. The data were compared with a control group of 22 subjects. All patients were satisfied with the results of the reconstruction and all had negative Lachman and pivot shift tests. Quadriceps and hamstrings isokinetic peak torques were similar to those of the control group and the contralateral limbs. Peak external moments were similar between the ACL and the control subjects for light activities such as walking and stair climbing. However, a decrease was noted in the peak external flexion moment (net quadriceps moment) in the ACL-reconstructed knees compared with that of controls during jogging and a jog-and-cut maneuver (13.3 $\pm$ 3.9% BW $\times$ height [Ht] and 16.1 $\pm$ 4.2% BW $\times$ Ht, respectively; $P = .024$). The decrease in the peak external flexion moment during jogging significantly correlated with quadriceps muscle strength at 60°/sec ($R^2 = 0.464$, $P < .001$) and at 180°/sec and 240°/sec ($P < .02$). This correlation between quadriceps muscle strength and decreased external flexion moment was not found during the jog-and-cut task. Subjects in the ACL-reconstructed group with the weakest quadriceps muscles had the greatest reductions in the peak flexion moment during jogging. The investigators concluded that functional adaptations during more demanding athletic activities were present in patients who had well-functioning ACL reconstructions and minimal decreases in quadriceps strength compared with controls. The authors speculated that further improvements in lower extremity strength may improve these adaptations and reinforced the value of ensuring comprehensive quadriceps training after ACL reconstruction.

Wojtys and Huston[214] measured lower extremity muscle strength, endurance, reaction time, and time to reach peak torque in a group of 25 patients who received a B-PT-B autograft reconstruction at 6, 12, and 18 months postoperative. A group of 40 healthy subjects served as controls. At 18 months postoperative, 88% of the reconstructed knees were within 3 mm of increased AP displacement compared with the opposite limb and 80% of the patients believed they had regained their preinjury sports activity level. However, quadriceps peak torque of the reconstructed limbs was equal to that of the opposite limbs in only 72% (Fig. 12–17). Quadriceps endurance failed to reach the level of the opposite limb throughout the study period. Time to reach peak torque of both the quadriceps (Fig. 12–18) and the hamstrings (Fig. 12–19) was significantly slower than the uninvolved limb at all test sessions.

Although deficits in proprioception after ACL reconstruction have been documented by several investigators,[12,27,106,112] others have shown that no significant difference exists after surgery.[32,82,88,155,159] The differences in findings are based on variability in test procedures, time from injury to ACL reconstruction, the presence of associated injuries to the menisci and articular cartilage, the rehabilitation program, and the use of internal versus external control limbs.[155] It is also difficult to understand whether statistically significant differences reported by authors represent clinically relevant findings. The two most common tests for proprioception are threshold for detection of passive motion (TDPM) and joint position sense (JPS). Differences in the magnitude of error in the patients' ability to reproduce a specific joint position (flexion angle) postoperatively during these tests are frequently less than 1° to 2° compared with either internal or external control data.

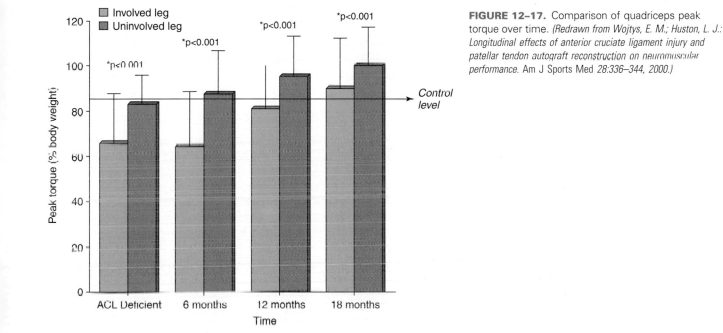

FIGURE 12–17. Comparison of quadriceps peak torque over time. *(Redrawn from Wojtys, E. M.; Huston, L. J.: Longitudinal effects of anterior cruciate ligament injury and patellar tendon autograft reconstruction on neuromuscular performance. Am J Sports Med 28:336–344, 2000.)*

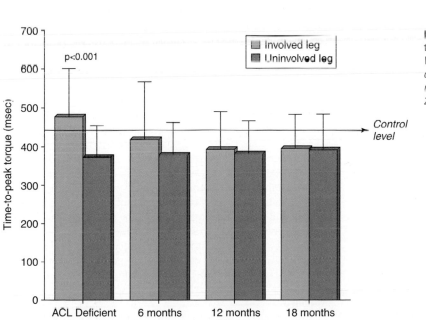

FIGURE 12–18. Comparison of the time to peak torque of the quadriceps over time. *(Redrawn from Wojtys, E. M.; Huston, L. J.: Longitudinal effects of anterior cruciate ligament injury and patellar tendon autograft reconstruction on neuromuscular performance. Am J Sports Med 28:336–344, 2000.)*

FIGURE 12-19. Comparison of the time to peak torque of the hamstring muscles over time. *(Redrawn from Wojtys, E. M.; Huston, L. J.: Longitudinal effects of anterior cruciate ligament injury and patellar tendon autograft reconstruction on neuromuscular performance. Am J Sports Med 28:336–344, 2000.)*

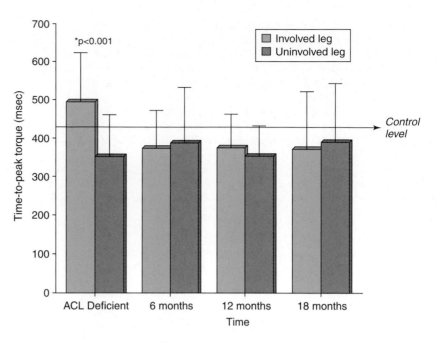

Lephart and coworkers[106] reported significantly decreased kinesthetic awareness in 12 ACL-reconstructed knees compared with the uninvolved limb near the terminal end of knee motion. The ACL-reconstructed knees demonstrated a longer TDPM at 15° of knee flexion (mean difference, ~1.5°, moving from 15° of flexion to full extension). However, no significant difference was found between limbs in kinesthetic awareness at higher knee flexion angles (≥45°). MacDonald and associates[112] reported a significant difference in the mean TDPM in ACL-reconstructed (0.17°–0.22°) as well as ACL-deficient (0.14°) knees when the mean values were compared with those of internal controls (uninvolved knees). However, this study found no difference in mean TDPM values when ACL-deficient and ACL-reconstructed knee data were compared with external control knee values. Neither of these studies conducted JPS testing.

Risberg and coworkers[159] found no significant difference in mean TDPM between ACL-reconstructed knees and internal or external controls. The patients were tested a mean of 24 months (range, 11–32 mo) after B-PT-B autogenous ACL reconstruction and a supervised rehabilitation program. No effects were found in TDPM values when a functional knee brace was applied to the reconstructed knees. Fischer-Rasmussen and Jensen[57] also found no difference in mean TDPM between ACL-reconstructed and ACL-deficient knees compared with external controls. These authors did find a significant difference in JPS at 60° of flexion between ACL-reconstructed and external controls and between ACL-deficient and external controls. No difference was found between the three groups in JPS at full extension.

Co and coworkers[32] measured TDPM and JPS in 10 patients a mean of 31.6 months after ACL B-PT-B autogenous reconstruction. All of the knees had less than 3 mm of increased AP displacement and a significantly decreased quadriceps isokinetic peak torque of the reconstructed limb compared with the opposite limb (84 ± 24 Nm and 98 ± 24 Nm, respectively; $P = .005$). An external control group of 10 subjects was included in the investigation. No significant differences were found between the ACL-reconstructed limbs and both the internal control (contralateral) and the external control limbs for JPS. However,

a significant difference was found for TDPM between the ACL-reconstructed limbs and both the internal control (contralateral) and the external control limbs. The ACL-reconstructed limbs had a more accurate response than the external controls. The authors concluded that, in successfully ACL reconstructed knees (demonstrating <3 mm of increased AP displacement), proper rehabilitation and training may help overcome loss of proprioception usually demonstrated in chronic ACL-deficient knees. The authors did not measure proprioception in ACL-reconstructed knees with less optimal results for AP displacement or poorer rehabilitation training methods.

Roberts and associates[161] reported that bilateral proprioception deficits were found in 20 patients who had a B-PT-B autogenous ACL reconstruction for chronic ruptures compared with an external control group. The patients were tested an average of 2 years postoperatively; however, no data were given regarding AP displacement or their overall functional status. The patients had a significantly higher TDPM in the reconstructed limb compared with external controls from starting positions of 20° and 40° for both extension (1.0° and 0.75°, respectively) and flexion. The differences between the reconstructed and the external control limbs for flexion were 1.0° at the starting position of 20° and 0.5° at 40°. Patients also had a higher TDPM in their contralateral limb compared with external controls from starting positions of 20° and 40° for both extension and flexion. However, there was high variability in the data, which could influence the significance of these findings. For instance, the range of values for threshold toward extension at the 20° flexion starting position in the patients' reconstructed limbs was 1.0° to 6.0°, with a median of 1.0°. The range of values for this test in the external control group was 0.5° to 2.25°, with a median of 0.75°. Further, the authors indicated that although some patients in their series demonstrated a marked "decrease in proprioception ability," others had small deviations from the group median. The number of patients with the marked proprioception deficits was not provided.

Bonfim and colleagues[27] conducted an investigation to detect sensory and motor deficits in 10 controls and 10 patients who had B-PT-B autogenous ACL reconstruction. The authors measured JPS, TDPM, latency of hamstring muscles, and maintenance of an upright stance position. The patients were tested an average of 18 months (range, 12–30 mo) postoperatively. The ACL-reconstructed knees demonstrated significantly decreased JPS (at 0°, 15°, 30°, 45°, and 60° of flexion) and significantly higher TDPM for both flexion and extension compared with the noninvolved side. The patients also showed longer latency of the hamstring muscles, and increased body sway during single-leg stance, in the reconstructed limb compared with the noninvolved side. The authors concluded that these findings were due to the disrupted ACL mechanoreceptors that were not restored by the reconstruction.

Hopper and coworkers[82] reported no significant differences in JPS measured during full weight-bearing in nine patients who underwent STG ACL reconstruction. No external control group was incorporated into this investigation. Reider and associates[155] found no significant differences in JPS or TDPM between ACL-reconstructed knees and external controls at 3 weeks, 6 weeks, and 3 months after surgery. At 6 months postoperative, the ACL-reconstructed knees had significantly better JPS mean values compared with the external control group (5.67° and 7.53°, respectively; mean difference, −1.86°). There was no difference between ACL-reconstructed knees and external controls in TDPM mean values 6 months postoperatively.

The differences in test methodology and populations studied do not allow definitive conclusions to be reached regarding the effect of ACL reconstruction on knee joint proprioception. Whether the finding of less than 1° to 2° of difference in JPS or TDPM between ACL-reconstructed knees and external controls is clinically relevant remains to be determined. Studies have not assessed whether specific rehabilitation exercises (such as OKC vs. CKC) influence knee joint proprioception postoperatively.

CLINICAL STUDIES AND OUTCOME OF ACL REHABILITATION PROGRAMS

Effect of Postoperative Exercises on AP Knee Displacements

The authors conducted a study to determine the effect of rehabilitation exercises and time elapsed postoperatively on AP knee displacements after ACL B-PT-B autograft reconstruction performed by a single surgeon.[10] A total of 142 patients were followed a minimum of 2 years postoperatively; 90 had the operation for chronic ACL ruptures and 52, for acute ruptures (reconstruction performed within 12 wk of the injury). One experienced examiner conducted KT-2000 testing throughout the study period (134 N) at 8, 12, 16, 20, 24, 52, and 128 weeks after surgery. A total of 938 arthrometer measurements were collected, for an average of 7 per patient.

The rehabilitation program was divided into four phases. The assisted ambulatory phase represented the length of time patients spend using crutch or cane support, which lasted until approximately the 4th to 8th week postoperative. During this phase, ROM exercises, straight leg raises (in all four planes), quadriceps muscle isometrics, EMS, and CKC exercises (minisquats, toe raises) were performed. The early strength-training phase lasted from between approximately the 4th to 8th week to the 12th to 16th week and added balance, proprioceptive, and gait-training exercises. The intensive strength-training

Critical Points   CLINICAL STUDIES AND OUTCOME OF ACL REHABILITATION PROGRAMS

Effect of Postoperative Exercises on Anteroposterior Knee Displacements

Barber-Westin et al.[10]: Studied effect of rehabilitation exercises and time elapsed postoperatively on AP knee displacements after ACL B-PT-B autograft reconstruction performed by a single surgeon.

- 142 patients followed minimum 2 years postoperatively.
- One experienced examiner conducted KT-2000 testing: total 938 arthrometer measurements were collected, average of 7 per patient.
- Most recent follow-up: 121 (85%) had normal displacements (<3 mm of increased AP displacement compared with the contralateral side) and 21 (15%) had abnormal displacements.
- 14 patients had 3 to 5.5 mm of increased displacement, 7 patients had 6 mm or more.
- No association between the initial onset of the abnormal displacements and the amount of time that had elapsed since surgery or the phase of rehabilitation in which they were detected.

Home- versus Clinically Based Supervised Physical Therapy Programs

- Four randomized investigations compared home-based rehabilitation with supervised clinically based physical therapy programs.
- All concluded similar outcomes between these programs. Did not provide data on the sports activities patients returned to (asymptomatically vs. symptomatically), details on end-stage functional progression of programs (e.g., plyometric training), long term outcome.
- Essential components for home-based program: preoperative patient education sessions, a comprehensive written description of the postoperative program, periodic monitoring of patient progress by a therapist.

phase focused on progressive resistive exercises, swimming, bicycling, ski machines, stair climbing machines, and running programs. This phase varied between patients, but typically lasted from approximately the 12th to 16th week to the 24th and 52nd postoperative week. The final phase, return to sports, was entered when patients successfully completed the intensive strength-training program. Return to running and light sports was allowed at 6 months postoperative, and full competitive sports, at approximately the 8th postoperative month in this group of patients.

At the most recent follow-up evaluation, 121 (85%) of the patients had normal displacement values (<3 mm of increased AP displacement compared with the contralateral side) and 21 (15%) had abnormal displacements. Fourteen patients had 3 to 5.5 mm of increased displacement and 7 patients had 6 mm or more, indicating graft failure. There was no significant difference in these measurements between the knees operated on for acute ACL ruptures and those with chronic ruptures.

There was no association between the initial onset of the abnormal displacements and the amount of time that had elapsed since surgery. The abnormal displacements were first detected a mean of 46 ± 51 weeks and a median of 24 weeks (range, 6–208 wk) postoperatively. In 7 patients, the abnormal displacements were detected less than 20 weeks postoperatively; in 9 patients, these were detected between 20 and 52 weeks; and in 5 patients, these were detected longer than 1 year postoperatively.

There was also no association between the initial onset of abnormal displacements and the phase of rehabilitation in which

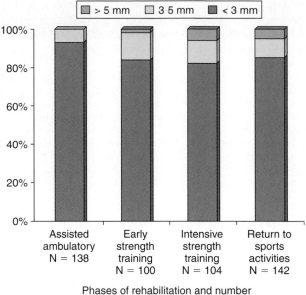

FIGURE 12–20. The percentage of knees distributed in the three arthrometer categories according to the phases of rehabilitation. *(Redrawn from Barber-Westin, S. D.; Noyes, F. R.; Heckmann, T. P.; Shaffer, B. L.: The effect of exercise and rehabilitation on anterior-posterior knee displacements after anterior cruciate ligament autograft reconstruction. Am J Sports Med 27:84–93, 1999.)*

they were detected. The percentage of knees with less than 3 mm, 3 to 5 mm, and greater than 5 mm during each phase of rehabilitation is shown in Figure 12–20. In 8 patients, the abnormal displacements were first detected during the early strength-training phase; in 6 patients, during the intensive strength-training phase; and in 7 patients, after return to sports. There was no relationship between the type of sports activity patients had returned to and the presence of abnormal AP displacements.

The study demonstrated that the operation and the rehabilitation program were effective and resulted in an acceptable failure rate of 5%. It is important to note that the patients in this investigation were widely varied with regard to the goals of the operation, age, injury chronicity, prior treatment of the injury, and condition of the menisci and articular cartilage. The rehabilitation program was individualized as required and was based on patient symptoms and functional testing.

Home- versus Clinically Based Supervised Physical Therapy Programs

Four randomized investigations[14,56,68,172] have been published to date that compared home-based rehabilitation to supervised clinically based physical therapy programs. All essentially concluded that similar outcomes are feasible between these programs. The authors described the essential components required for a successful home-based program: preoperative patient education sessions, a comprehensive written description of the postoperative program, and periodic monitoring of the patient's progress by a therapist.

Schenck and colleagues[172] conducted a randomized study in which the outcomes of a clinic-based program (average, 14.2

physical therapy clinic visits) were compared with those of a home-based rehabilitation program (average, 2.85 clinic visits) in a series of 37 patients who were 18 to 32 years old. The home-based program was monitored by a physical therapist and involved periodic postoperative visits to assess for potential problems and provide instruction on progression of activities. All patients also had preoperative instruction before the B-PT-B autograft reconstruction. Return to full activities was allowed at approximately 4 to 5 months postoperatively and was based on functional testing and symptoms.

At 1 year postoperative, no difference was reported between the two groups for patient satisfaction, AP displacement on KT-1000 testing (mean, 2.1 mm side-to-side difference for both groups), quadriceps atrophy (mean thigh circumference difference of 0.75 inches for both groups), or subjective questionnaire responses. There were no cases of arthrofibrosis. No data were provided regarding return to athletics. The authors stressed that the home-based program was not intended for patients younger than 18 years of age and may also not be appropriate for high-performance athletes. This program was monitored by an experienced surgeon-therapist team, which the authors stressed was essential to recognize potential and existing problems.

Beard and Dodd[14] conducted a randomized trial to compare the short-term outcome of a home-based rehabilitation program with that of a protocol that combined home exercises with a formal supervised program. Patients in the supervised program were asked to attend therapy classes twice a week from weeks 4 to 6 to weeks 16 to 18. Patients in the home-based program were evaluated and progressed based on the therapist's discretion. A total of 13 patients who all had a B-PT-B autogenous ACL reconstruction were enrolled in each group and followed for 6 months. There were no significant differences between the groups for all parameters examined, including IKDC grade and isokinetic quadriceps and hamstrings peak torque. Although a difference was found between groups for AP displacement (mean home-based, 3.3 ± 3.2 mm; mean supervised, 0.8 ± 4.3 mm), the sample size precluded statistical significance. In addition, although no difference was noted in IKDC grades, there was also insufficient statistical power to avoid a type II error. Attempts at measuring patient compliance were unsuccessful. The authors concluded that a home-based program was appropriate, but the recommendation was stressed for "regular physical therapy outpatient assessment."

Fischer and coworkers[56] randomly assigned 54 patients who underwent a B-PT-B autogenous ACL reconstruction to a home-based or a supervised therapy program. The patients in the home-based group averaged 5 therapy visits (range, 3–7) within the first 12 weeks, and those in the supervised group averaged 20 visits (range, 10–28). The home-based group was provided with formal written descriptions and diagrams of exercises and timing of progression. At 6 months postoperative, there were no significant differences between the groups for range of knee motion, thigh circumference, AP displacement, functional hop tests, and Lysholm scores. No data were provided regarding return to athletics. The authors stressed that in order to be successful, a home-based program must include careful patient selection for compliance, periodic monitoring of patient progress by a therapist, and formal written instructions.

A randomized investigation was performed by Grant and associates[68] to determine the initial (12-wk) outcome of home-based and supervised physical therapy programs. All patients underwent a B-PT-B autogenous ACL reconstruction; 66 patients in the supervised and 63 patients in the home-based programs were followed to the study endpoint assessment. The home-based group averaged 3 formal physical therapy sessions (range, 0–8) and the supervised group attended an average of 14 sessions (range, 2–20). All had preoperative patient education and received detailed written instructions regarding the four-phase therapy program. No differences were reported between the groups for AP displacement (mean 2.0 side-to-side difference in both groups) and isokinetic strength (mean quadriceps peak torque compared with the contralateral side, 61% home-based group and 60% supervised group). The home-based patients regained significantly more motion; however, the authors noted that the median differences between the groups (–2° and –3° for extension; 3° and 6° for flexion) were of questionable clinical relevance. The study concluded that the home-based program was effective in recreational athletes undergoing nonacute ACL reconstruction.

Retrospective studies were conducted by DeCarlo and Sell[37] and Treacy and colleagues[202] to determine whether the number of supervised physical therapy visits affected outcome after ACL reconstruction. In one investigation, patients were randomly selected and grouped based on the number of miles they lived from the authors' clinic and only those with "consistent follow-up" were included.[37] There was no difference in isokinetic muscle strength or subjective measures 12 months postoperative between those who lived in close proximity to the clinic (average, 7 therapy visits) and those who attended therapy elsewhere (average, 20 therapy visits).

In conclusion, the few studies that have assessed home-based versus supervised rehabilitation programs agree on the essential components required for a successful home-based program: preoperative patient education sessions, a comprehensive written description of the postoperative program, and periodic monitoring of patient progress by a therapist. However, the investigations did not provide a rigorous analysis of the sports activities patients returned to (both asymptomatically and symptomatically), details regarding the end-stage functional progression of their programs (e.g., plyometric training), or long-term outcome. Therefore, it remains unclear whether patients participating in a home-based program are able to achieve the same final goals as those in a supervised situation. In addition, the term *home-based* may be misleading, because the therapists in these investigations were actively involved in the patients' care and in fact stressed that this was an essential condition of this protocol.

ACCELERATED REHABILITATION: INDICATIONS, CONTRAINDICATIONS, AND OUTCOME

The phrase *accelerated rehabilitation* was introduced by Shelbourne and Nitz in 1990[179] to describe a program that incorporated rapid allotments for strength and functional training and return to full activities after B-PT-B autogenous ACL reconstruction. Light sports were permitted by 2 months and full activity by 4 to 6 months postoperative. Since then, many authors have used this term to describe other facets of rehabilitation and the authors agree with Beynnon and colleagues' assessment[18] that "there is little consensus in the literature about what composes an accelerated versus a more conservative rehabilitation program." Shelbourne and Nitz's report[179] provided

Critical Points ACCELERATED REHABILITATION: INDICATIONS, CONTRAINDICATIONS, AND OUTCOME

Definition accelerated rehabilitation: a program that incorporates rapid allotments for strength and functional training and return to full activities after B-PT-B autogenous ACL reconstruction. Light sports permitted by 2 months and full activity by 4 to 6 months postoperative.

Long-term effects: return to strenuous training early postoperatively on articular cartilage and future joint arthrosis unclear, no randomized studies performed to date.

One author reported a significant increase in the incidence of joint effusions in knees in accelerated program.[113]

Authors' Opinion: Contraindications
- Noteworthy bone bruising on MRI or articular cartilage damage on arthroscopy.
- Concomitant procedures including complex meniscus repair, reconstruction of other knee ligaments, patellar realignment procedures, or articular cartilage restorative procedures.
- Postoperative joint effusion and/or pain.
- Inability of the patient to regain normal gait, neuromuscular control, and muscle strength.

Authors' Opinion: Indications
- B-PT-B autograft with secure internal fixation.
- Serial evaluation of AP displacement postoperatively.
- Return of normal gait and muscle strength.
- Compliant patient.
- Carefully supervised environment.

outcome data on 73 of 237 (30%) patients who participated in the accelerated program. The results of these patients were compared retrospectively with those of others who had participated in a more conservative program. The authors reported that the accelerated program was more effective in restoring knee motion and preventing complications related to arthrofibrosis. There was no difference between programs in quadriceps strength at 1 year postoperative, patient perception of the results of surgery, or AP displacements on KT-1000 testing.

Subsequent reports by Shelbourne and coworkers[176,177] emphasized the need for preoperative rehabilitation to restore full ROM, decrease swelling, and resume normal gait and leg control. The longest postoperative follow-up of this program reported by these investigators to date (mean, 4 yr; range, 2–9.1) showed a low failure rate of 3%, a low arthrofibrosis rate of 1%, and an average time to return to sports of 6.2 ± 2.3 months. The authors did not report what types of athletic activities patients participated in before their injury or at the most recent follow-up evaluation. As well, the authors noted that some patients had problems with the accelerated program in terms of pain and chronic joint effusion, especially those whose quadriceps strength was less than 65% of that of the opposite limb. The long-term effects of the return to strenuous training in the early postoperative period (5 wk on average) on articular cartilage and future joint arthrosis are unclear.

Majima and associates[113] reported that accelerated rehabilitation (as described by Shelbourne[179]) produced a significant increase in the incidence of joint effusions in 32 patients who underwent STG reconstruction compared with 18 patients who were treated with a conservative protocol. Within the first 8 postoperative weeks, a total of 15 aspirations (in 3 patients) had been done in the conservative group compared with a total of 60 aspirations (in 13 patients) in the accelerated group ($P < .01$). No difference was found between the two protocols in regard to return of muscle strength (after 9 mo postoperative), IKDC scores, or knee function. Patients in the accelerated group had a trend toward greater AP displacement, as 20% had greater than 3 mm of increased displacement compared with 13% in the conservative group.

Roi and colleagues[162] published a detailed accelerated rehabilitation program that was used to return a professional soccer player to his sport 90 days after an ACL STG reconstruction. The athlete did not sustain concomitant ligament or meniscus injuries and had minimal pain and limitations with daily activities after the injury, all of which allowed surgery to be performed just 4 days later. Although the treatment protocol was successful in this case, the authors qualified their aggressive program as one that "may only be possible with an individual who has the resources (time and money) to invest in unlimited access to rehabilitation facilities and personnel."[162] The authors used objective criteria to advance the program including ROM, KT-2000, functional, isokinetic, aerobic, and anaerobic testing.

Wilk[209] questioned the applicability and indications of accelerated rehabilitation. Citing the ultimate goal of ACL reconstruction and postoperative rehabilitation as the return of normal homeostasis to the knee joint[47] over the long term, he cautioned that aggressive rehabilitation may have more risks than benefits, especially in regard to its impact on preexisting articular cartilage damage and bone bruising.

Yu and Paessler[225] investigated the influence of an aggressive rehabilitation protocol on tunnel widening after four-strand STG reconstruction. At 6 months postoperative, patients who followed the aggressive protocol (immediate full weight-bearing, OKC exercises begun at the 6th week, running allowed from the 8th to the 10th week) had significantly greater tibial tunnel widening on posteroanterior (PA) and lateral radiographs compared with a group of patients who followed a more conservative protocol. There was no difference between groups in mean KT-1000 arthrometer values.

Owing to the lack of randomized, prospective studies on the return to high-impact loading activities in the early postoperative period after ACL reconstruction, there remain unanswered questions regarding appropriate patient candidates, indications, and contraindications for this program. In the authors' opinion, contraindications include (1) noteworthy bone bruising on MRI or articular cartilage damage visualized on arthroscopy, (2) concomitant complex meniscus repairs, reconstructions of other knee ligaments, patellar realignment procedures, or articular cartilage restorative procedures, (3) postoperative joint effusion, pain, and (4) inability of the patient to regain normal gait, neuromuscular control, and muscle strength. Indications include use of a B-PT-B autograft with secure internal fixation, serial evaluation of AP displacement postoperatively, return of normal gait and muscle strength, a compliant patient, a carefully supervised environment, and completion of a neuromuscular-retraining program in all athletes prior to return to full competition.

CRITERIA FOR PATIENT RELEASE AND RETURN TO SPORTS ACTIVITIES

Different authors have described objective and subjective criteria that patients must achieve before clearance is given to return to strenuous sports activities. These include assessment of lower limb symmetry on single-leg functional tests, lower extremity

---

Critical Points CRITERIA FOR PATIENT RELEASE AND RETURN TO SPORTS ACTIVITIES

Kvist's[103] Criteria for Patient Release for Sports

- Less than 15% deficit on isokinetic testing and single-leg hop tests.
- No pain or effusion.
- Full range of motion (ROM).
- Functional knee stability.
- Static knee stability (normal AP displacement) on KT-1000 testing.

Authors' Criteria for Return to Athletics

- Patient activity level determined.
- Trial of function shows no symptoms with desired activity.
- Normal AP displacement on knee arthrometer testing.
- Less than 15% deficit on isokinetic testing and single-leg hop tests for jumping, pivoting, cutting, twisting, and turning sports.
- Completion of neuromuscular-retraining program for high-risk sports.

Patients with articular cartilage damage or majority of function of one or both menisci lost are encouraged to return to low-impact activities to preserve the knee joint.

---

muscle strength on an isokinetic dynamometer, AP displacement on knee arthrometer testing, trials-of-function of activities of increasing demand, and ROM.

Kvist[103] detailed multiple criteria to be fulfilled before release to full sports activities that included rehabilitation, surgical, and other factors. The assessment included objective muscle strength and performance, pain, effusion, ROM, functional knee stability, static knee stability, associated injuries, and psychological and social aspects. The patient had to demonstrate less than 15% deficit on isokinetic and single-leg hop tests, no pain or effusion, full ROM, functional knee stability, and static knee stability on KT-1000 testing. The influence of associated meniscal, cartilage, or other ligamentous injuries; psychological issues such as motivation or fear of reinjury; and social factors such as lost time owing to occupational demands could not be predicted on the ability to return to sports successfully after ACL reconstruction.

Discharge criteria at the authors' center after ACL reconstruction based on patient goals for athletics and occupations, the rating of symptoms, KT-1000 testing, muscle strength testing, and function testing have been previously described (Table 12–4).[75] First, patients complete the Cincinnati Sports Activity Scale[11] and the Occupational Rating Scale[11] in order to document sports and occupational levels that are desired after surgery (see Chapter 44, The Cincinnati Knee Rating System). Upon completion of the rehabilitation program, pain, swelling, and giving-way are rated on the Cincinnati Symptom Rating Scale.[11] The patient must not experience symptoms at the level of activity that she or he wishes to participate in prior to discharge. KT-2000 testing is performed at 134 N of total 'AP force and must be within normal limits (<3 mm difference between limbs) prior to allowance of return to strenuous activities. Muscle strength testing is performed with an isokinetic dynamometer to ensure that adequate strength exists prior to the initiation of the running and cutting programs. At least two single-leg hop function tests are completed and limb symmetry calculated as described previously.[9,128] Patients desiring to return to high-risk activities complete a neuromuscular-retraining program

TABLE 12–4 Discharge Criteria after Anterior Cruciate Ligament Reconstruction				
Sport/Occupation Level	Symptom Rating for Pain, Swelling, Giving-way*	KT-2000 Total AP (Involved–Noninvolved, 134 N, mm)	Biodex Isokinetic Test (% Deficit from Noninv)	Function Testing (Limb Symmetry, %)
Sports: I (jumping, pivoting, cutting) Occupation: heavy, very heavy	None, level 10	<3	≤15	≥85
Sports: II (running, turning, twisting) Occupation: moderate	None, level 8	<3	≤20	≥85
Sports: III (swimming, bicycling) Occupation: light	None, level 6	3–5	≤30	≥75
Sports: IV (none) Occupation: very light	None, level 4	3–5	≤30	≥75

*Level 10, normal knee, no symptoms with strenuous work/sports with jumping, hard pivoting; level 8, no symptoms with moderate work/sports with running, turning, twisting; level 6, no symptoms with light work/sports with no running, twisting or jumping; level 4, no symptoms with activities of daily living.
AP, anteroposterior.

before release to full competition. Recommendations for the types of activities that patients should consider resuming are made based on the results of these criteria and the condition of the articular cartilage and menisci. Patients in whom articular cartilage damage was visualized during the ACL reconstruction (especially those with grade 2B or 3; see Chapter 47[138]), or those in whom the majority of function of one or both menisci has been compromised are encouraged to return to low-impact activities to preserve the knee joint for as long as possible.

RISKS FOR REINJURY AND FUTURE JOINT ARTHROSIS

An important component of the surgery and rehabilitation decision making process is an understanding of the risks of reinjury to either the reconstructed or the contralateral knee and the chance of developing future joint arthrosis. A few studies have reported high rates of reinjury upon return to sports.[115,154,169,204] Salmon and coworkers[169] followed 67 patients for 7 to 13 years postoperatively after ACL B-PT-B autogenous reconstruction and a conservative rehabilitation program. Patients were kept non–weight-bearing for the first 4 postoperative weeks, with ROM permitted only from 30° to 90°. Competitive sports were not allowed until 9 months after surgery. A total of 23 patients (34%) sustained an ACL injury after return to sports; 9 (13%) patients reinjured the reconstructed ACL and 15 (22%) ruptured the contralateral ACL. The authors related that their patients had not participated in a neuromuscular-retraining program, which may have been at least partially responsible for the high reinjury rate. At 13 years postoperative, 37% of the patients reported swelling after moderate activity and 44% had a limitation in knee extension.

Orchard and associates[145] followed Australian football players over eight seasons to determine the occurrence of ACL injuries. The overall ACL injury incidence was 0.82/1000 athlete exposures. The incidence for noncontact ACL injuries was 0.62/1000 athlete exposures. All ACL injuries in this study were treated with reconstruction. The players who sustained an ACL

Critical Points RISKS FOR REINJURY AND FUTURE JOINT ARTHROSIS

Salmon et al.[169]

- 67 patients followed 7 to 13 years after ACL B-PT-B autograft and conservative rehabilitation.
- Patients did not participate in a neuromuscular-retraining program in rehabilitation.
- 9 (13%) patients reinjured reconstructed ACL, 15 (22%) ruptured contralateral ACL.

Pinczewski et al.[154]

- 90 patients ACL B-PT-B autograft, 90 patients STG autograft followed 10 years, sports allowed at 6 months.
- 19 patients (11%) ruptured ACL graft: 8% in the B-PT-B group, 13% in the STG group.
- 29 patients (16%) sustained contralateral ACL ruptures: 22% in the B-PT-B group and 10% in the STG group

Published rates of radiographically documented osteoarthritis (OA) after ACL reconstruction vary.

Whether mild OA changes on standing radiographs represent actual articular cartilage deterioration is questionable; two studies reported standing radiographs have low sensitivity rates in detecting mild articular cartilage damage.

Factors Influencing Development of Articular Cartilage Deterioration Postoperatively

- Effects of the initial impact injury on the subchondral bone (bone bruising).
- Loss of meniscus tissue.
- Age.
- Time from injury to reconstruction.
- Number of reinjuries prior to reconstruction.
- Failure of the reconstruction to restore normal AP displacement and knee kinematics.
- Rehabilitation program.
- Complications such as arthrofibrosis.
- Final knee motion achieved.
- Activity level patient resumes after surgery.

One conclusive association with future joint OA is loss of meniscus tissue.

ACL reconstruction appears to provide a protective effect in knees that have normal menisci and no articular cartilage damage.

79. Hertel, P.; Behrend, H.; Cierpinski, T.; et al.: ACL reconstruction using bone–patellar tendon–bone press-fit fixation: 10-year clinical results. *Knee Surg Sports Traumatol Arthrosc* 13:248–255, 2005.

80. Hogervorst, T.; Pels Rijcken, T. H.; Rucker, D.; et al.: Changes in bone scans after anterior cruciate ligament reconstruction: a prospective study. *Am J Sports Med* 30:823–833, 2002.

81. Hooper, D. M.; Morrissey, M. C.; Drechsler, W.; et al.: Open and closed kinetic chain exercises in the early period after anterior cruciate ligament reconstruction. Improvements in level walking, stair ascent, and stair descent. *Am J Sports Med* 29:167–174, 2001.

82. Hopper, D. M.; Creagh, M. J.; Formby, P. A.; et al.: Functional measurement of knee joint position sense after anterior cruciate ligament reconstruction. *Arch Phys Med Rehabil* 84:868–872, 2003.

83. Howell, S. M.; Taylor, M. A.: Brace-free rehabilitation, with early return to activity, for knees reconstructed with a double-looped semitendinosus and gracilis graft. *J Bone Joint Surg Am* 78:814–825, 1996.

84. Ikeda, H.: Isokinetic torque of quadriceps in patients with untreated anterior cruciate ligament injury of the knee joint. *J Jpn Orthop Assoc* 67:826–835, 1993.

85. Imran, A.; O'Connor, J. J.: Control of knee stability after ACL injury or repair: interaction between hamstrings contraction and tibial translation. *Clin Biomech (Bristol, Avon)* 13:153–162, 1998.

86. Irie, K.; Tomatsu, T.: Atrophy of semitendinosus and gracilis and flexor mechanism function after hamstring tendon harvest for anterior cruciate ligament reconstruction. *Orthopedics* 25:491–495, 2002.

87. Isberg, J.; Faxen, E.; Brandsson, S.; et al.: Early active extension after anterior cruciate ligament reconstruction does not result in increased laxity of the knee. *Knee Surg Sports Traumatol Arthrosc* 14:1108–1115, 2006.

88. Iwasa, J.; Ochi, M.; Adachi, N.; et al.: Proprioceptive improvement in knees with anterior cruciate ligament reconstruction. *Clin Orthop Relat Res* 381:168–176, 2000.

89. Jackson, D. W.; Grood, E. S.; Goldstein, J. D.; et al.: A comparison of patellar tendon autograft and allograft used for anterior cruciate ligament reconstruction in the goat model. *Am J Sports Med* 21:176–185, 1993.

90. Johansson, H.; Sjolander, P.; Sojka, P.: A sensory role for the cruciate ligaments. *Clin Orthop Relat Res* 268:161–178, 1991.

91. Johansson, H.; Sjolander, P.; Sojka, P.: Activity in receptor afferents from the anterior cruciate ligament evokes reflex effects on fusimotor neurones. *Neurosci Res* 8:54–59, 1990.

92. Johansson, H.; Sjolander, P.; Sojka, P.: Receptors in the knee joint ligaments and their role in the biomechanics of the joint. *Crit Rev Biomed Eng* 18:341–368, 1991.

93. Johnson, D. L.; Urban, W. P.; Caborn, D. N. M.; et al.: Articular cartilage changes seen with magnetic resonance imaging–detected bone bruises associated with acute anterior cruciate ligament rupture. *Am J Sports Med* 26:409–414, 1998.

94. Johnson, L. L.: The outcome of a free autogenous semitendinosus tendon graft in human anterior cruciate reconstructive surgery: a histological study. *Arthroscopy* 9:131–142, 1993.

95. Johnson, R. J.; Eriksson, E.; Haggmark, T.; Pope, M. H.: Five- to ten-year follow-up evaluation after reconstruction of the anterior cruciate ligament. *Clin Orthop Relat Res* 183:122–140, 1984.

96. Jomha, N. M.; Borton, D. C.; Clingeleffer, A. J.; Pinczewski, L. A.: Long-term osteoarthritic changes in anterior cruciate ligament reconstructed knees. *Clin Orthop Relat Res* 358:188–193, 1999.

97. Jurist, K. A.; Otis, J. C.: Anteroposterior tibiofemoral displacements during isometric extension efforts. The roles of external load and knee flexion angle. *Am J Sports Med* 13:254–258, 1985.

98. Kartus, J.; Stener, S.; Kohler, K.; et al.: Is bracing after anterior cruciate ligament reconstruction necessary? A 2-year follow-up of 78 consecutive patients rehabilitated with or without a brace. *Knee Surgery Sports Traumatol Arthrosc* 5:157–161, 1997.

99. Kaufman, K. R.; An, K. N.; Litchy, W. J.; et al.: Dynamic joint forces during knee isokinetic exercise. *Am J Sports Med* 19:305–316, 1991.

100. Keays, S. L.; Bullock-Saxton, J. E.; Keays, A. C.; et al.: A 6-year follow-up of the effect of graft site on strength, stability, range of motion, function, and joint degeneration after anterior cruciate ligament reconstruction: patellar tendon versus semitendinosus and gracilis tendon graft. *Am J Sports Med* 35:729–739, 2007.

101. Konishi, Y.; Fukubayashi, T.; Takeshita, D.: Mechanism of quadriceps femoris muscle weakness in patients with anterior cruciate ligament reconstruction. *Scand J Med Sci Sports* 12:371–375, 2002.

102. Kowalk, D. L.; Duncan, J. A.; McCue, F. C., 3rd; Vaughan, C. L.: Anterior cruciate ligament reconstruction and joint dynamics during stair climbing. *Med Sci Sports Exerc* 29:1406–1413, 1997.

103. Kvist, J.: Rehabilitation following anterior cruciate ligament injury: current recommendations for sports participation. *Sports Med* 34:269–280, 2004.

104. Kvist, J.; Gillquist, J.: Sagittal plane knee translation and electromyographic activity during closed and open kinetic chain exercises in anterior cruciate ligament–deficient patients and control subjects. *Am J Sports Med* 29:72–82, 2001.

105. LaStayo, P. C.; Woolf, J. M.; Lewek, M. D.; et al.: Eccentric muscle contractions: their contribution to injury, prevention, rehabilitation, and sport. *J Orthop Sports Phys Ther* 33:557–571, 2003.

106. Lephart, S.; Kocher, M. S.; Fu, F.; et al.: Proprioception following anterior cruciate ligament reconstruction. *J Sport Rehabil* 1:188–196, 1992.

107. Lephart, S. M.; Kocher, M. S.; Harner, C. D.; Fu, F. H.: Quadriceps strength and functional capacity after anterior cruciate ligament reconstruction. Patellar tendon autograft versus allograft. *Am J Sports Med* 21:738–743, 1993.

108. Lohmander, L. S.; Englund, P. M.; Dahl, L. L.; Roos, E. M.: The long-term consequence of anterior cruciate ligament and meniscus injuries: osteoarthritis. *Am J Sports Med* 35:1756–1769, 2007.

109. Lorentzon, R.; Elmqvist, L. G.; Sjostrom, M.; et al.: Thigh musculature in relation to chronic anterior cruciate ligament tear: muscle size, morphology, and mechanical output before reconstruction. *Am J Sports Med* 17:423–429, 1989.

110. Lutz, G. E.; Palmitier, R. A.; An, K. N.; Chao, E. Y.: Comparison of tibiofemoral joint forces during open-kinetic-chain and closed-kinetic-chain exercises. *J Bone Joint Surg Am* 75:732–739, 1993.

111. Lysholm, J.; Hamberg, P.; Gillquist, J.: The correlation between osteoarthrosis as seen on radiographs and on arthroscopy. *Arthroscopy* 3:161–165, 1987.

112. MacDonald, P. B.; Heeden, D.; Pacin, O.; Sutherland, K.: Proprioception in anterior cruciate ligament–deficient and reconstructed knees. *Am J Sports Med* 24:774–778, 1996.

113. Majima, T.; Yasuda, K.; Tago, H.; et al.: Rehabilitation after hamstring anterior cruciate ligament reconstruction. *Clin Orthop Relat Res* 397:370–380, 2002.

114. Marx, R. G.; Jones, E. C.; Angel, M.; et al.: Beliefs and attitudes of members of the American Academy of Orthopaedic Surgeons regarding the treatment of anterior cruciate ligament injury. *Arthroscopy* 19:762–770, 2003.

115. Mattacola, C. G.; Perrin, D. H.; Gansneder, B. M.; et al.: Strength, functional outcome, and postural stability after anterior cruciate ligament reconstruction. *J Athl Train* 37:262–268, 2002.

116. McDevitt, E. R.; Taylor, D. C.; Miller, M. D.; et al.: Functional bracing after anterior cruciate ligament reconstruction: a prospective, randomized, multicenter study. *Am J Sports Med* 32:1887–1892, 2004.

117. Meighan, A. A.; Keating, J. F.; Will, E.: Outcome after reconstruction of the anterior cruciate ligament in athletic patients. A comparison of early versus delayed surgery. *J Bone Joint Surg Br* 85:521–524, 2003.

118. Melegati, G.; Tornese, D.; Bandi, M.; et al.: The role of the rehabilitation brace in restoring knee extension after anterior cruciate ligament reconstruction: a prospective controlled study. *Knee Surg Sports Traumatol Arthrosc* 11:322–326, 2003.

119. Mikkelsen, C.; Werner, S.; Eriksson, E.: Closed kinetic chain alone compared to combined open and closed kinetic chain exercises for quadriceps strengthening after anterior cruciate ligament reconstruction with respect to return to sports: a prospective matched follow-up study. *Knee Surg Sports Traumatol Arthrosc* 8:337–342, 2000.

119a. Mikkelsen, C.; Cerulli, G.; Lorenzini, M.; et al.: Can a postoperative brace in slight hyperextension prevent extension deficit after anterior cruciate ligament reconstruction? A prospective randomised study. *Knee Surg Sports Traumatol Arthrosc* 11:318–321, 2003.

120. Mohtadi, N. G.; Webster-Bogaert, S.; Fowler, P. J.: Limitation of motion following anterior cruciate ligament reconstruction. A case-control study. *Am J Sports Med* 19:620–624; discussion 624–625, 1991.

121. Moller, E.; Forssblad, M.; Hansson, L.; et al.: Bracing versus nonbracing in rehabilitation after anterior cruciate ligament reconstruction: a randomized prospective study with 2-year follow-up. *Knee Surg Sports Traumatol Arthrosc* 9:102–108, 2001.

122. More, R. C.; Karras, B. T.; Neiman, F.; et al.: Hamstrings—an anterior cruciate ligament protagonist: an in vitro study. *Am J Sports Med* 21:231–237, 1993.

123. Morrissey, M. C.; Hudson, Z. L.; Drechsler, W. I.; et al.: Effects of open versus closed kinetic chain training on knee laxity in the early period after anterior cruciate ligament reconstruction. *Knee Surg Sports Traumatol Arthrosc* 8:343–348, 2000.

124. Muellner, T.; Alacamlioglu, Y.; Nikolic, A.; Schabus, R.: No benefit of bracing on the early outcome after anterior cruciate ligament reconstruction. *Knee Surg Sports Traumatol Arthrosc* 6:88–92, 1998.

125. Myklebust, G.; Holm, I.; Maehlum, S.; et al.: Clinical, functional, and radiologic outcome in team handball players 6 to 11 years after anterior cruciate ligament injury: a follow-up study. *Am J Sports Med* 31:981–989, 2003.

126. Nisell, R.; Ericson, M. O.; Nemeth, G.; Ekholm, J.: Tibiofemoral joint forces during isokinetic knee extension. *Am J Sports Med* 17:49–54, 1989.

127. Nisell, R.; Nemeth, G.; Ohlsen, H.: Joint forces in extension of the knee. Analysis of a mechanical model. *Acta Orthop Scand* 57:41–46, 1986.

128. Noyes, F. R.; Barber, S. D.; Mangine, R. E.: Abnormal lower limb symmetry determined by function hop tests after anterior cruciate ligament rupture. *Am J Sports Med* 19:513–518, 1991.

129. Noyes, F. R.; Barber-Westin, S. D.: A comparison of results in acute and chronic anterior cruciate ligament ruptures of arthroscopically assisted autogenous patellar tendon reconstruction. *Am J Sports Med* 25:460–471, 1997.

130. Noyes, F. R.; Bassett, R. W.; Grood, E. S.; Butler, D. L.: Arthroscopy in acute traumatic hemarthrosis of the knee. Incidence of anterior cruciate tears and other injuries. *J Bone Joint Surg Am* 62:687–695, 757, 1980.

131. Noyes, F. R.; Berrios-Torres, S.; Barber-Westin, S. D.; Heckmann, T. P.: Prevention of permanent arthrofibrosis after anterior cruciate ligament reconstruction alone or combined with associated procedures: a prospective study in 443 knees. *Knee Surg Sports Traumatol Arthrosc* 8:196–206, 2000.

132. Noyes, F. R.; Butler, D. L.; Grood, E. S.; et al.: Biomechanical analysis of human ligament grafts used in knee-ligament repairs and reconstructions. *J Bone Joint Surg Am* 66:344–352, 1984.

133. Noyes, F. R.; Butler, D. L.; Paulos, L. E.; Grood, E. S.: Intra-articular cruciate reconstruction. I: perspectives on graft strength, vascularization, and immediate motion after replacement. *Clin Orthop* 172:71–77, 1983.

134. Noyes, F. R.; Mangine, R. E.; Barber, S.: Early knee motion after open and arthroscopic anterior cruciate ligament reconstruction. *Am J Sports Med* 15:149–160, 1987.

135. Noyes, F. R.; Mangine, R. E.; Barber, S. D.: The early treatment of motion complications after reconstruction of the anterior cruciate ligament. *Clin Orthop* 277:217–228, 1992.

136. Noyes, F. R.; Mooar, P. A.; Matthews, D. S.; Butler, D. L.: The symptomatic anterior cruciate-deficient knee. Part I: the long-term functional disability in athletically active individuals. *J Bone Joint Surg Am* 65:154–162, 1983.

137. Noyes, F. R.; Schipplein, O. D.; Andriacchi, T. P.; et al.: The anterior cruciate ligament–deficient knee with varus alignment. An analysis of gait adaptations and dynamic joint loadings. *Am J Sports Med* 20:707–716, 1992.

138. Noyes, F. R.; Stabler, C. L.: A system for grading articular cartilage lesions at arthroscopy. *Am J Sports Med* 17:505–513, 1989.

139. Noyes, F. R.; Torvik, P. J.; Hyde, W. B.; DeLucas, J. L.: Biomechanics of ligament failure. II. An analysis of immobilization, exercise, and reconditioning effects in primates. *J Bone Joint Surg Am* 56:1406–1418, 1974.

140. Noyes, F. R.; Wojtys, E. M.: The early recognition, diagnosis and treatment of the patella infera syndrome. In Tullos, H. S. (ed.): *Instructional Course Lectures*. Rosemont, IL: AAOS, 1991; pp. 233–247.

141. Noyes, F. R.; Wojtys, E. M.; Marshall, M. T.: The early diagnosis and treatment of developmental patella infera syndrome. *Clin Orthop* 265:241–252, 1991.

142. O'Driscoll, S. W.; Kumar, A.; Salter, R. B.: The effect of continuous passive motion on the clearance of a hemarthrosis from a synovial joint. An experimental investigation in the rabbit. *Clin Orthop Relat Res* 176:305–311, 1983.

143. O'Neill, D. B.: Arthroscopically assisted reconstruction of the anterior cruciate ligament. A prospective randomized analysis of three techniques. *J Bone Joint Surg Am* 78:803–813, 1996.

144. Ohkoshi, Y.; Yasuda, K.; Kaneda, K.; et al.: Biomechanical analysis of rehabilitation in the standing position. *Am J Sports Med* 19:605–611, 1991.

145. Orchard, J.; Seward, H.; McGivern, J.; Hood, S.: Intrinsic and extrinsic risk factors for anterior cruciate ligament injury in Australian footballers. *Am J Sports Med* 29:196–200, 2001.

146. Owings, M. F.; Kozak, L. J.: Ambulatory and inpatient procedures in the United States, 1996. *Vital Health Stat 13* (139):1–119, 1998.

147. Palmieri-Smith, R. M.; Kreinbrink, J.; Ashton-Miller, J. A.; Wojtys, E. M.: Quadriceps inhibition induced by an experimental knee joint effusion affects knee joint mechanics during a single-legged drop landing. *Am J Sports Med* 35:1269–1275, 2007.

148. Papannagari, R.; Gill, T. J.; Defrate, L. E.; et al.: In vivo kinematics of the knee after anterior cruciate ligament reconstruction: a clinical and functional evaluation. *Am J Sports Med* 34:2006–2012, 2006.

149. Patel, R. R.; Hurwitz, D. E.; Bush-Joseph, C. A.; et al.: Comparison of clinical and dynamic knee function in patients with anterior cruciate ligament deficiency. *Am J Sports Med* 31:68–74, 2003.

150. Paulos, L. E.; Wnorowski, D. C.; Greenwald, A. E.: Infrapatellar contracture syndrome. Diagnosis, treatment, and long-term follow-up. *Am J Sports Med* 22:440–449, 1994.

151. Perkins, G.: Rest and movement. *J Bone Joint Surg Br* 35:521–539, 1953.

152. Perry, M. C.; Morrissey, M. C.; King, J. B.; et al.: Effects of closed versus open kinetic chain knee extensor resistance training on knee laxity and leg function in patients during the 8- to 14-week postoperative period after anterior cruciate ligament reconstruction. *Knee Surg Sports Traumatol Arthrosc* 13:357–369, 2005.

153. Petersen, W.; Laprell, H.: Insertion of autologous tendon grafts to the bone: a histological and immunohistochemical study of hamstring and patellar tendon grafts. *Knee Surg Sports Traumatol Arthrosc* 8:26–31, 2000.

154. Pinczewski, L. A.; Lyman, J.; Salmon, L. J.; et al.: A 10-year comparison of anterior cruciate ligament reconstructions with hamstring tendon and patellar tendon autograft. a controlled, prospective trial. *Am J Sports Med* 35:564–574, 2007.

154a. Rebel, M.; Paessler, H. H.: The effect of knee brace on coordination and neuronal leg muscle control: an early postoperative functional study in anterior cruciate ligament reconstructed patients. *Knee Surg Sports Traumatol Arthrosc* 9:272–281, 2001.

155. Reider, B.; Arcand, M. A.; Diehl, L. H.; et al.: Proprioception of the knee before and after anterior cruciate ligament reconstruction. *Arthroscopy* 19:2–12, 2003.

156. Reilly, D. T.; Martens, M.: Experimental analysis of the quadriceps muscle force and patello-femoral joint reaction force for various activities. *Acta Orthop Scand* 43:126–137, 1972.

157. Renstrom, P.; Arms, S. W.; Stanwyck, T. S.; et al.: Strain within the anterior cruciate ligament during hamstring and quadriceps activity. *Am J Sports Med* 14:83–87, 1986.

158. Richmond, J. C.; Gladstone, J.; MacGillivray, J.: Continuous passive motion after arthroscopically assisted anterior cruciate ligament reconstruction: comparison of short- versus long-term use. *Arthroscopy* 7:39–44, 1991.

159. Risberg, M. A.; Beynnon, B. D.; Peura, G. D.; Uh, B. S.: Proprioception after anterior cruciate ligament reconstruction with and without bracing. *Knee Surg Sports Traumatol Arthrosc* 7:303–309, 1999.

160. Risberg, M. A.; Holm, I.; Steen, H.; et al.: The effect of knee bracing after anterior cruciate ligament reconstruction. A prospective, randomized study with two years' follow-up. *Am J Sports Med* 27:76–83, 1999.

PHASE 7. WEEKS 27 TO 52—Cont'd

3 x/wk 20–30 min	**Aerobic conditioning** (patellofemoral precautions) Stationary bicycling Water walking Swimming (kicking) Walking Stair machine (low resistance, low stroke) Ski machine (short stride, level, low resistance) Elliptical (low resistance)
3 x/wk 20 min	**Running program** (straight) Interval training (20, 40, 60, 100 yd) Walk/rest phase (3:1 rest:work) Backward run
3 x/wk	**Cutting program**—lateral, carioca, figure-eights
3 x/wk	**Functional training** Plyometric training: box hops, level, double-leg Sports-specific drills
As required	**Modalities** Cryotherapy
Goals	Increase function, strength, endurance Return to previous activity level

Right column values:
- Backward run — 20 yards
- Cutting program — 20 yd
- Plyometric training — 15 sec, 4–6 sets
- Cryotherapy — 20 min

AP, anteroposterior; BAPS, Biomechanical Ankle Platform System (Camp, Jackson, MI); BBS, Biodex Balance System (Biodex Medical Systems, Inc., Shirley, NY); EMS, electrical muscle stimulation; ITB, iliotibial band; ROM, range of motion; RSD, reflex sympathetic dystrophy; UBC, upper body cycle (Biodex Medical Systems, Inc., Shirley, NY); X, when exercise is performed.

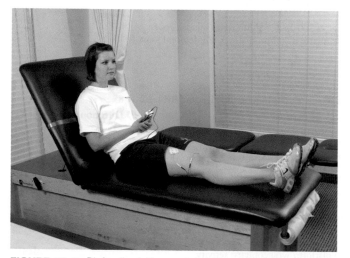

FIGURE 13–1. Electrical muscle stimulation is used to facilitate and enhance an adequate quadriceps contraction early postoperatively.

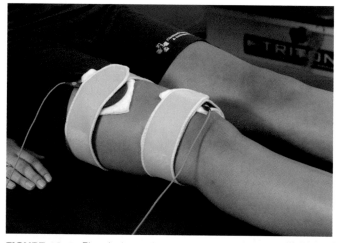

FIGURE 13–2. Biofeedback therapy is implemented to facilitate an adequate quadriceps muscle contraction early postoperatively.

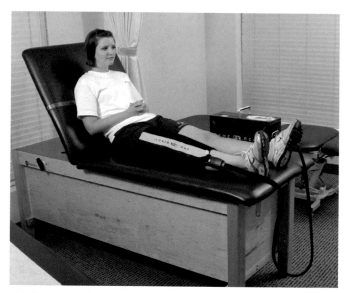

FIGURE 13–3. A motorized cooler unit used to provide cryotherapy.

controlled by using gravity to backflow and drain the water, refilling the cuff with fresh ice water as required. Cryotherapy is used for 20 minutes at a time from three times a day to every waking hour depending upon the extent of pain and swelling. In some cases, the treatment time is extended owing to the thickness of the buffer used between the skin and the device. The motorized units contain a thermostat, which is helpful when cold therapy is used for an extended treatment time. Vasopneumatic devices offer another option for cold therapy. The Game Ready device (Game Ready, Berkeley, CA) allows the clinician to set the temperature and, as well, one of four different compression levels depending on patient tolerance. Although this is primarily a clinical treatment tool, it may be used at home as well. Cryotherapy is typically done after exercise or when required for pain and swelling control and is maintained throughout the entire postoperative rehabilitation protocol.

Postoperative Bracing

The use of postoperative braces after ACL reconstruction represents a controversial area. Screening patients for personality type, pain tolerance, and program compliance may provide insight into the individual who will require brace protection postoperatively. The primary indication for the use of a brace is protection of the patient during weight-bearing in the event of a fall and to initiate early, more comfortable weight-bearing during the first few postoperative weeks. The brace should be rigid in nature and the knee held initially at 0° (Fig. 13–4). The brace is opened based on the protocol to allow normal knee flexion during ambulation. Periodic evaluation of the brace and its position on the leg must be done to ensure maximal benefit is achieved. The authors do not routinely prescribe a derotation or functional knee brace upon return to full activities after ACL reconstruction for patients in this protocol.

Range of Knee Motion

The goal in the 1st postoperative week is to obtain a ROM of 0° to 90°. A continuous passive motion machine is not required or routinely used by the authors. Patients perform passive and active ROM exercises in a seated position for 10 minutes a session, approximately four to six times per day (Fig. 13–5).

Full passive knee extension must be obtained immediately to avoid excessive scarring in the intercondylar notch and posterior capsular tissues. If the patient has difficulty regaining at least 0° by the 7th

postoperative day, he or she begins an overpressure program. The foot and ankle are propped on a towel or other device to elevate the hamstrings and gastrocnemius that allows the knee to drop into full extension (Fig. 13–6A). This position is maintained for 10 minutes and repeated four to six times per day. A 10-pound weight may be added to the distal thigh and knee to provide overpressure to stretch the posterior capsule. Full knee extension should be obtained by the 2nd postoperative week. If this is not accomplished, or if the clinician

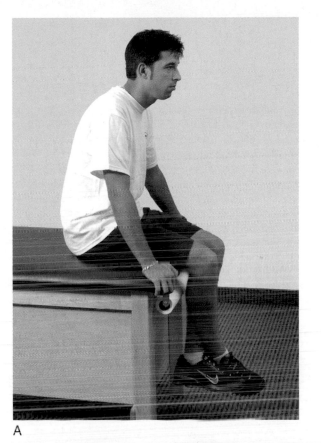

A

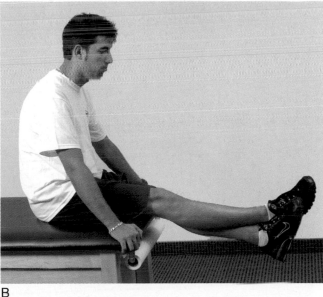

B

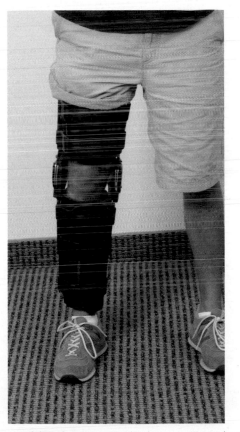

FIGURE 13–4. A long-leg postoperative brace protects the patient during weight-bearing in the event of a fall and promotes early, comfortable weight-bearing during the first few postoperative weeks.

FIGURE 13–5. Passive (**A** and **B**) and active range of motion exercises in a seated position.

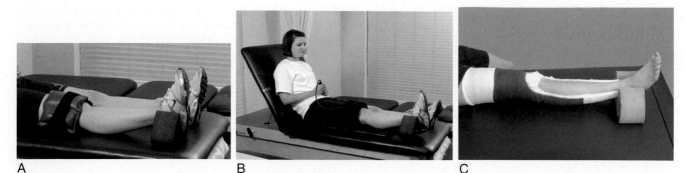

FIGURE 13–6. Overpressure program for extension. **A,** Hanging weight exercise. **B,** Extension board. **C,** Drop-out cast.

notes a firm end feel, then an extension board (see Fig. 13–6B) or additional weight of 15 to 20 pounds is used six times a day. If this is still not effective, a drop-out cast (see Fig. 13–6C) is implemented for 24 to 36 hours for continuous extension overpressure. The goal is to obtain 0° to 2° to 3° of hyperextension, which is in the normal knee motion limit. In patients with physiologic bilateral knee hyperextension, the authors recommend the gradual return of 3° to 5° of hyperextension in the reconstructed knee to more closely resemble the amount of hyperextension present in the contralateral knee. However, the authors do not recommend that the patient regain more than 5° of hyperextension owing to potentially deleterious forces that may be placed on the healing graft.

Knee flexion is gradually increased to 120° by the 3rd to 4th postoperative week and 135° by the 5th to 6th postoperative week. Passive knee flexion exercises are performed initially in the traditional seated position, using the opposite lower extremity to provide overpressure. Other methods to assist in achieving flexion greater than 90° include chair rolling (Fig. 13–7A), wall slides (see Fig. 13–7B and C), knee flexion devices (see Fig. 13–7D),

and passive quadriceps stretching exercises. Patients who have difficulty achieving 90° by the 4th week require a gentle ranging of the knee under anesthesia (not a forceful manipulation) as described in Chapter 41, Prevention and Treatment of Knee Arthrofibrosis.

Patellar Mobilization

Maintaining normal patellar mobility is critical to regain a normal range of knee motion. The loss of patellar mobility is often associated with arthrofibrosis and, in extreme cases, the development of patella infera.[18–20] Patellar glides are performed beginning the 1st postoperative day in all four planes (superior, inferior, medial, and lateral) with sustained pressure applied to the appropriate patellar border for at least 10 seconds (Fig. 13–8). This exercise is performed for 5 minutes before ROM exercises. Caution is warranted if an extensor lag is detected, because this may be associated with poor superior migration of the patella, indicating the

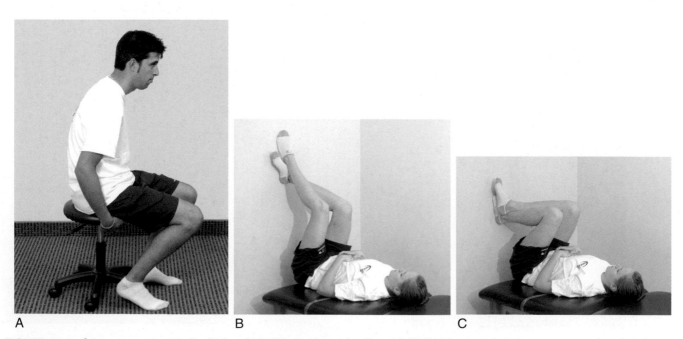

FIGURE 13–7. Overpressure program for flexion. **A,** Rolling stool exercise. **B** and **C,** Wall slides.

Continued

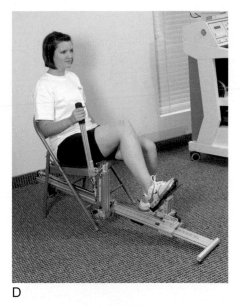

D

FIGURE 13-7—cont'd D, Overpressure flexion device.

need for additional emphasis on this exercise. Patellar mobilization is performed for approximately 6 weeks postoperatively.

Weight-Bearing

Partial weight-bearing is permitted immediately postoperatively as long as pain and swelling are controlled and a voluntary quadriceps contraction is demonstrated. Initially, bilateral crutches may be used and 50% body weight is placed on the involved foot. The amount of weight the patient is allowed to place on the involved limb is progressed as tolerated to allow full weight-bearing by the 3rd to 4th postoperative week. Importantly, a normal gait pattern is advocated that avoids a locked knee position and encourages normal knee flexion throughout the gait cycle. This technique allows for normal patterning of heel-to-toe ambulation, quadriceps contraction during midstance, and hip and knee flexion during the gait cycle. The locked-knee position

is avoided owing to the potential for the development of a quadriceps-avoidance gait pattern.

Flexibility

Hamstring and gastrocnemius-soleus flexibility exercises are begun the 1st day after ACL reconstruction. A sustained static stretch is held for 30 seconds and repeated five times. The most common hamstring stretch is the modified hurdler stretch (Fig. 13-9), and the most common gastrocnemius-soleus stretch is the towel pull (Fig. 13-10). These exercises help control pain owing to the reflex response created in the hamstrings when the knee is kept in the flexed position. As well, the towel-pulling exercise can help lessen discomfort in the calf, Achilles tendon, and ankle. These stretches represent critical components of the knee extension ROM program, because the ability to relax these two muscle groups is imperative to achieve full passive knee extension.

Quadriceps (Fig. 13-11) and iliotibial band (Fig. 13-12) flexibility exercises are performed to assist in achieving full knee flexion and controlling lateral hip and thigh tightness. A complete evaluation of the lower extremity will reveal deficit areas in flexibility that should be corrected. When designing a flexibility program, the therapist should take into account the particular sport or activity the patient wishes to return to as well as the position or physical requirements of that activity. Flexibility is incorporated in the maintenance program the patient performs once discharged.

Strengthening

The strengthening program is begun on the first postoperative visit. Early emphasis on the generation of a good voluntary quadriceps contraction is critical for a successful and safe return to functional activity. Isometric quadriceps contractions are completed on an hourly basis following the repetition rules of 10-second holds, 10 repetitions, 10 times per day. Adequate evaluation of the quadriceps contraction by both the therapist and the patient is critical. The patient can monitor contractions by visual or manual means, comparing the quality of the contractions with those achieved by the

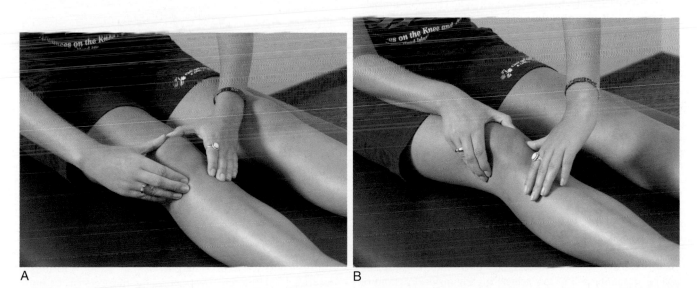

A   **B**

FIGURE 13-8. Patellar glides are begun the first postoperative day in all four planes: **A,** Superior and inferior. **B,** Medial and lateral.

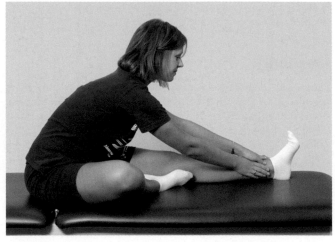

FIGURE 13–9. Hamstring modified hurdler stretch.

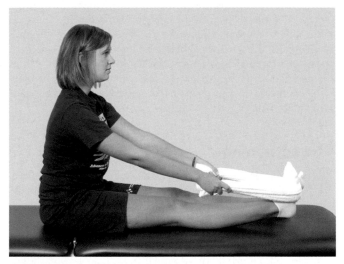

FIGURE 13–10. Gastrocnemius-soleus towel pull stretch.

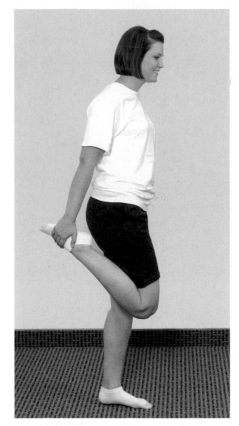

FIGURE 13–11. Quadriceps stretch.

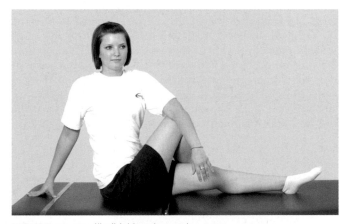

FIGURE 13–12. Iliotibial band stretch.

contralateral limb. The patient can also assess the superior migration of the patella during the contraction, which should be approximately 1 cm, and the inferior migration of the patella during the initial relaxation of the contraction. The patient must not let the knee go into hyperextension during isometric contractions, but hold the knee flexion position throughout the exercise. If necessary, biofeedback can also be used to reinforce a good quadriceps contraction.

Straight leg raises are initiated the 1st postoperative day in the four planes of hip movement. The adduction straight leg raise has a beneficial effect on the VMO. Supine straight leg raises must include a sufficient isometric quadriceps contraction to benefit the quadriceps. Straight leg raises in the other two planes are also important for proximal stabilization. As these exercises become easy to perform, ankle weights are added to progress muscle strengthening. Initially, 1 to 2 pounds of weight is used, and eventually, up to 10 pounds is added as long as this is not more than 10% of the patient's body weight. Active-assisted ROM can also be used to facilitate the quadriceps muscle if poor tone is observed during isometric contractions. These exercises are primarily used during the first 8 postoperative weeks in which emphasis is placed on controlling pain and swelling, regaining full ROM, achieving early quadriceps control and proximal stabilization, and resuming a normal gait pattern.

Closed kinetic chain exercises are initiated the 1st postoperative week. Mini-squats from 0° to 45° (Fig. 13–13A) are begun when tolerated by the patient. Initially, the patient's body weight is used as resistance and gradually, TheraBand (see Fig. 13–13B) or surgical tubing is employed as a resistance mechanism. Quick, smooth, rhythmic squats are performed to a high-set/high-repetition cadence to promote muscle fatigue. Hip position is important to monitor in order to promote a quadriceps contraction.

Toe-raises for gastrocnemius-/soleus strengthening and wall-sitting isometrics for quadriceps control are begun the 2nd postoperative week. The goal of wall-sitting is to improve quadriceps contraction by performing the exercise to muscle exhaustion (Fig. 13–14A). If anterior knee pain is experienced,

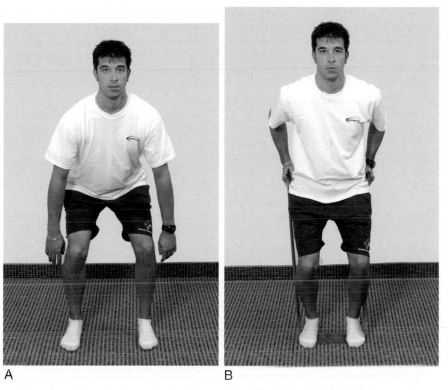

A   B

FIGURE 13–13. Minisquats from 0° to 45° using the patient's body weight (**A**) and TheraBand (**B**) for increased resistance.

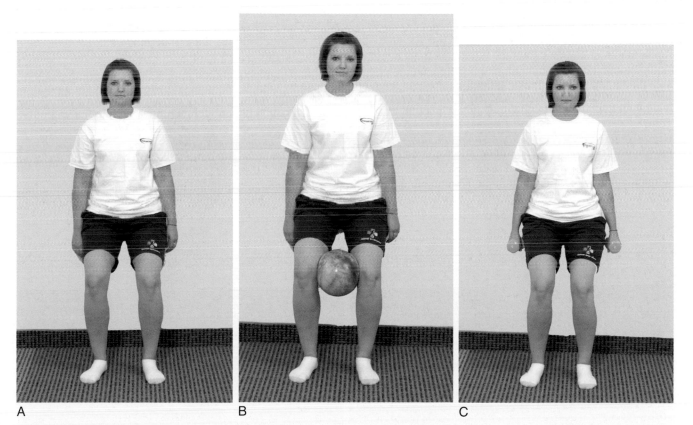

A   B   C

FIGURE 13–14. A, Wall sitting to muscle exhaustion. **B,** Squeezing a ball between the distal thighs induces a hip adduction contraction and a stronger vastus medialis obliquus contraction. **C,** Use of dumbbell weights to increase body weight promotes an even stronger quadriceps contraction.

it may be decreased by either altering the knee flexion angle of the sit or subtly changing the toe-out/toe-in angle by no more than 10°. The exercise may also be modified to produce greater challenge to the quadriceps. The patient may voluntarily set the quadriceps muscle once she or he reaches the maximum knee flexion angle, which is typically between 30° and 45°. This contraction and knee flexion position are held until muscle fatigue occurs and the exercise is repeated three to five times. The patient may squeeze a ball between the distal thighs, inducing a hip adduction contraction and a stronger VMO contraction (see Fig. 13–14B). In a third variation, the patient holds dumbbell weights in the hands to increase body weight, which promotes an even stronger quadriceps contraction (see Fig. 13–14C). Finally, the patient can shift the body weight over the involved side to stimulate a single-leg contraction. This exercise is promoted as an excellent one for the patient to perform at home four to six times a day to achieve quadriceps fatigue in a safe knee flexion angle that does not induce an abnormal anterior tibial translation.

Lateral step-ups are begun when the patient has achieved full weight-bearing (Fig. 13–15). The height of the step is gradually increased based on patient tolerance.

Hamstring curls are begun with Velcro ankle weights within the first few weeks and eventually advanced to weight machines (Fig. 13–16). Weight machines are advantageous owing to the muscle isolation obtained as the machine provides stability to the knee joint. The patient exercises the involved limb alone as well as both limbs together. If the lightest amount of weight on the machine is too heavy to be lifted by the involved limb alone, the exercise may be performed as an eccentric contraction in which the patient lifts the weight with both legs and lowers the weight with the involved side. Eccentric contractions may also be used in the advanced stages of strength training. Hamstring strength is critical to the overall success of the rehabilitation program because of the role that this musculature plays in the dynamic stabilization of the knee joint. Weight training is used throughout the advanced program and continues in the return-to-activity and maintenance phases of rehabilitation.

Open kinetic chain extension exercises are incorporated within the first few weeks to further develop quadriceps muscle strength. Caution is warranted because of the potential problems these exercises may create for the healing graft and the patellofemoral joint. Resisted knee extension is begun with Velcro ankle weights in the 1st week from 90° to 30°. The terminal phase of extension is avoided because of the forces placed on the patellofemoral joint and ACL graft. The patellofemoral joint must be monitored for changes in pain, swelling, and crepitus to avoid a patellar conversion in which painful patellofemoral crepitus develops with articular cartilage damage. The surgeon should advise the therapist if there are abnormal patellofemoral findings of joint damage.

A full lower extremity–strengthening program is critical for early and long-term success of the rehabilitation program. Other muscle groups included in this routine are the hip abductors, hip adductors, hip flexors, and hip extensors. These muscle groups can be exercised on either a multi-hip or cable system machine (Fig. 13–17) or a hip abductor-adductor machine. Gastrocnemius-soleus strength is a key component for both early ambulation and the running program. In addition, upper extremity and core strengthening are important for a safe and effective return to work or sports. Sport and position specificity are taken into account when devising the strengthening program to maximize its benefits. Kraemer and Ratamess[6] provided the recommendations for progression of muscle strength, hypertrophy, power, and endurance training according to the American College of Sports Medicine[1] (Tables 13–3 to 13–6). Specific strengthening and sports-specific timing drills are beyond the scope of this chapter; however, the therapist should work with the patient and appropriate coaches to determine the individual patient's program.

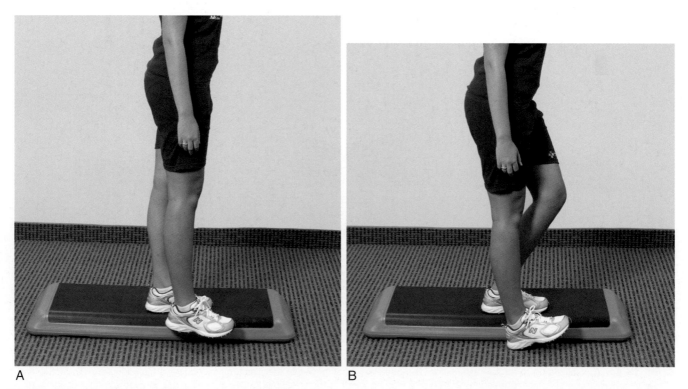

A   B

FIGURE 13–15. The step-up exercise.

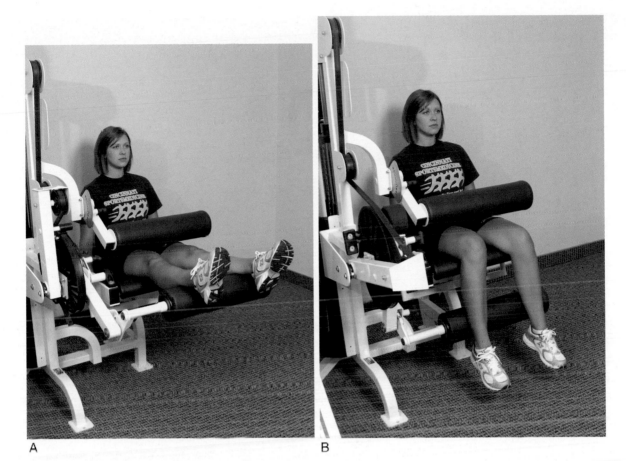

FIGURE 13–16. A and **B,** Hamstring curls.

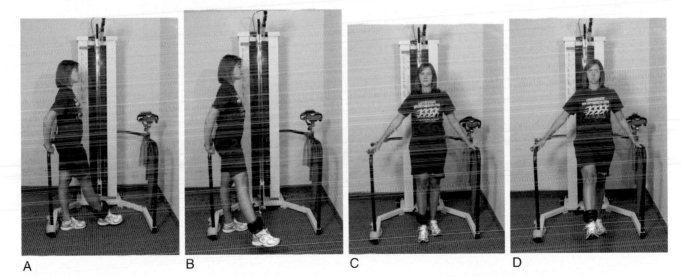

FIGURE 13–17. A–D, Multi-hip cable system machine.

Balance, Proprioceptive, and Perturbation Training

Balance and proprioceptive training are initiated the 1st postoperative week. Initially, the patient simply stands and shifts weight from side-to-side and front-to-back. This activity encourages confidence in the leg's ability to withstand the pressures of

weight-bearing and initiates the stimulus to knee joint position sense.

Cup-walking is begun when the patient achieves full weight-bearing (Fig. 13–18) to promote symmetry between the surgical and the uninvolved limbs. This exercise helps develop hip and knee flexion and quadriceps control during midstance of gait to prevent knee hyperextension. In addition, cup-walking

TABLE 13–3   American College of Sports Medicine Recommendations for Progression during Strength Training

	Novice	Intermediate	Advanced
Muscle action	Eccentric & concentric	Eccentric & concentric	Eccentric & concentric
Exercise selection	Single & multiple joint	Single & multiple joint	Single & multiple joint with emphasis on multiple
Exercise order	Large < small muscles Multiple < single High < low intensity	Large < small muscles Multiple < single High < low intensity	Large < small muscles Multiple < single High < low intensity
Loading	60%–70% 1 RM	70%–80% 1 RM	70%–100% 1 RM
Volume	1–3 sets x 8–12 reps	Multiple sets x 6–12 reps	Multiple sets x 1–12 reps
Rest intervals	1–2 min	2–3 min for core 1–2 minutes for others	3 min for core 1–2 min for others
Velocity	Slow to moderate	Moderate	Unintentional slow to fast
Frequency	2–3 day/wk	2–4 day/wk	4–6 day/wk

< Indicates that the preceding exercise is to be performed before the succeeding exercise.
1 RM, 1 repetition maximum.
Reprinted with permission from Kraemer, W. J.; Ratamess, N. A.: Fundamentals of resistance training: progression and exercise prescription. *Med Sci Sports Exerc* 36:674–688, 2004.

TABLE 13–4   American College of Sports Medicine Recommendations for Progression during Hypertrophy Training

	Novice	Intermediate	Advanced
Muscle action	Eccentric & concentric	Eccentric & concentric	Eccentric & concentric
Exercise selection	Single & multiple joint	Single & multiple joint	Single & multiple joint
Exercise order	Large < small muscles Multiple < single High < low intensity	Large < small muscles Multiple < single High < low intensity	Large < small muscles Multiple < single High < low intensity
Loading	60%–70% 1 RM	70%–80% 1 RM	70%–100% 1 RM with emphasis on 70%–85%
Volume	1–3 sets x 8–12 reps	Multiple sets x 6–12 reps	Multiple sets x 1–12 reps with emphasis on 6–12
Rest intervals	1–2 min	1–2 min	2–3 min for heavy ≤1–2 min for others
Velocity	Slow to moderate	Slow to moderate	Slow, moderate, and fast
Frequency	2–3 day/wk	2–4 day/wk	4–6 day/wk

< Indicates that the preceding exercise is to be performed before the succeeding exercise.
1 RM, 1 repetition maximum.
Reprinted with permission from Kraemer, W. J.; Ratamess, N. A.: Fundamentals of resistance training: progression and exercise prescription. *Med Sci Sports Exerc* 36:674–688, 2004.

TABLE 13–5   American College of Sports Medicine Recommendations for Progression during Power Training

	Novice	Intermediate	Advanced
Muscle action	Eccentric & concentric	Eccentric & concentric	Eccentric & concentric
Exercise selection	Multiple joint	Multiple joint	Multiple joint
Exercise order	Large < small muscles Most < least complete High < low intensity	Large < small muscles Most < least complete High < low intensity	Large < small muscles Most < least complete High < low intensity
Loading	60%–70% for strength 30%–60% for velocity/technique	70%–80% for strength 30%–60% for velocity/technique	>80% for strength 30%–60% for velocity
Volume	Similar to strength	1–3 sets x 3–6 reps	3–6 sets x 1–6 reps
Rest intervals	2–3 min for core 1–2 min for others	2–3 min for core 1–2 min for others	>3 min for heavy 1–2 min for moderate
Velocity	Moderate	Fast	Fast
Frequency	2–3 day/wk	2–4 day/wk	4–6 day/wk

< Indicates that the preceding exercise is to be performed before the succeeding exercise.
Reprinted with permission from Kraemer, W. J.; Ratamess, N. A.: Fundamentals of resistance training: progression and exercise prescription. *Med Sci Sports Exerc* 36:674–688, 2004.

TABLE 13-6   American College of Sports Medicine Recommendations for Progression during Endurance Training

	Novice	Intermediate	Advanced
Muscle action	Eccentric & concentric	Eccentric & concentric	Eccentric & concentric
Exercise selection	Single and multiple joint	Single and multiple joint	Single and multiple joint
Exercise order	Variety	Variety	Variety
Loading	50%–70% 1 RM	50%–70% 1 RM	30%–80% 1 RM
Volume	1–3 sets x 10–15 reps	Multiple sets x 10–15 reps or more	Multiple sets x 10–25 reps or more
Rest intervals	1–2 min for high reps <1 min for moderate reps	1–2 min for high reps <1 min for moderate reps	1–2 min for high reps <1 min for moderate reps
Velocity	Slow-to-moderate reps Moderate-to-high reps	Slow-to-moderate reps Moderate-to-high reps	Slow-to-moderate reps Moderate-to-high reps
Frequency	2–3 day/wk	2–4 day/wk	4–6 day/wk

1 RM, 1 repetition maximum.

Reprinted with permission from Kraemer, W. J.; Ratamess, N. A.: Fundamentals of resistance training: progression and exercise prescription. *Med Sci Sports Exerc* 36:674–688, 2004.

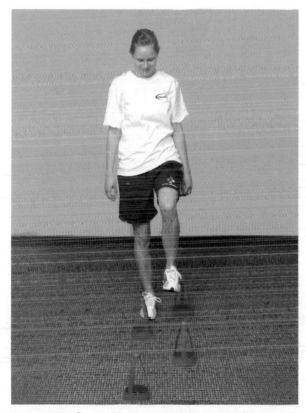

FIGURE 13–18. Cup walking to promote symmetry between the reconstructed and the uninvolved limbs.

controls hip and pelvic motion during midstance, gastrocnemius-soleus activity during push-off, and excessive hip hiking. These components of gait control are critical in the early phases of rehabilitation to decrease forces on the healing graft.

Double- and single-leg balance exercises in the stance position are beneficial early postoperatively. During the single-leg exercise, the foot is pointed straight ahead, the knee flexed 20° to 30°, the arms extended outward to horizontal, and the torso positioned upright with the shoulders above the hips and the hips above the ankles (Fig. 13–19A). The objective is to remain in this position until balance is disturbed. A minitrampoline or unstable platform may be used to make this exercise more challenging, because these devices promote greater dynamic limb control than that required to stand on a stable surface (see Fig. 13–19B). To provide a greater challenge, patients may assume the single-leg stance position and throw/catch a weighted ball against an inverted minitrampoline (Fig. 13–20) until fatigue occurs.

Perturbation-training techniques are initiated at approximately the 7th to 8th postoperative week during balance exercises. The therapist stands behind the patient and disrupts her or his body posture and position periodically to enhance dynamic knee stability. The techniques involve either direct contact with the patient (Fig. 13–21A) or disruption of the platform the patient is standing on (see Fig. 13–21B).

Half foam rolls are also used in this time period as part of the gait-retraining and balance program (Fig. 13–22). This exercise helps the patient develop balance and dynamic muscular control required to maintain an upright position and be able to walk from one end of the roll to the other. A center of balance, limb symmetry, quadriceps control in midstance, and postural positioning are benefits developed through this type of training. Use of the Biomechanical Ankle Platform System (Camp, Jackson, MI) in double-leg and single-leg stance is another effective balance and proprioceptive exercise (Fig. 13–23).

The use of more expensive devices adds another dimension to the proprioception program, because certain units objectively attempt to document balance and dynamic control. Two of the more common units include balance systems from Biodex (Fig. 13–24) (Biodex Medical Systems, Inc., Shirley, NY) and Neurocom (Neurocom, Clackamas, OR).

Conditioning

The primary consideration for a conditioning program throughout the rehabilitation period is to stress the cardiovascular system without compromising the knee joint. Depending on accessibility, a cardiovascular program is begun as soon as the patient can sufficiently tolerate the upright position with an upper extremity ergometer. The surgical limb should be elevated to minimize lower extremity

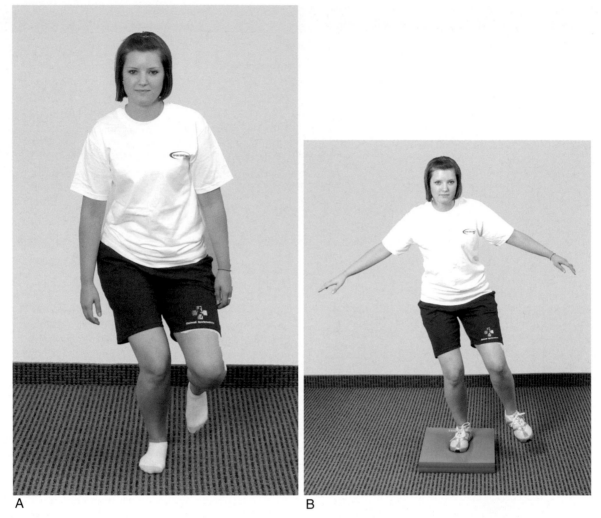

FIGURE 13–19. Single-leg balance exercise performed first on a stable surface (**A**) and then on an unstable surface (**B**).

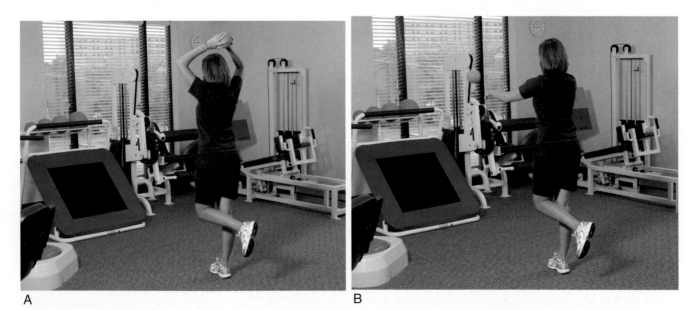

FIGURE 13–20. A and **B,** Single-leg balance exercise in which the patient throws and catches a weighted ball against an inverted minitrampoline.

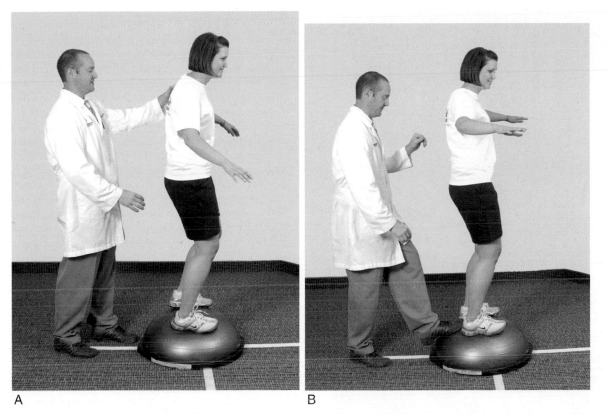

FIGURE 13–21. Perturbation training involving direct contact with the patient (**A**) and disruption of the platform the patient is standing on (**B**).

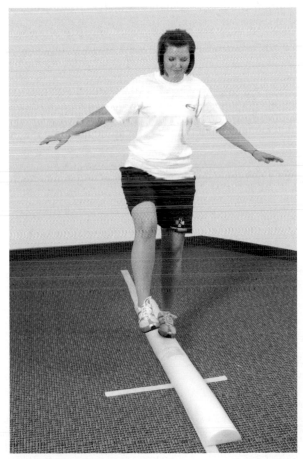

FIGURE 13–22. Gait and balance retraining using half foam rolls.

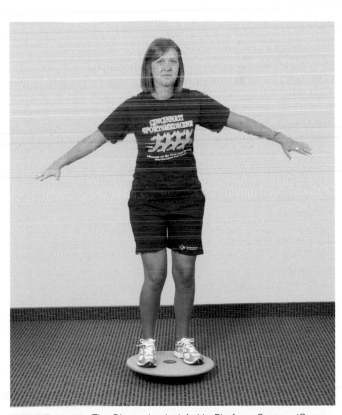

FIGURE 13–23. The Biomechanical Ankle Platform System (Camp, Jackson, MI) is used in double-leg and single-leg stance.

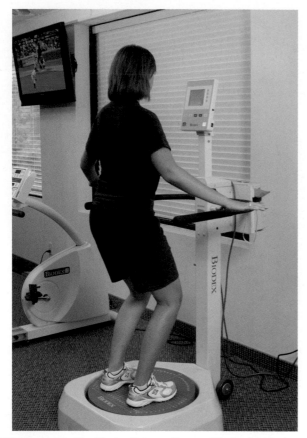

FIGURE 13–24. The Biodex Balance System (Biodex Medical Systems, Inc., Shirley, NY) may be used for balance training and to objectively measure balance and dynamic control.

swelling. This exercise is performed as tolerated. Stationary bicycling is begun in the 3rd postoperative week. Water walking may be initiated when the surgical wound has healed. Early goals of these programs include facilitation of full ROM, gait retraining, and cardiovascular reconditioning. In order to improve cardiovascular endurance, the program should be performed at least three times per week for 20 to 30 minutes, and the exercise should be performed to at least 60% to 85% of maximal heart rate. It is generally regarded that performing in the higher levels of percentage of maximal heart rate achieves greater cardiovascular efficiency and endurance.

Cross-country ski and stair-climbing machines are permitted during the 5th to 6th postoperative weeks. Protection against high stresses to the patellofemoral joint is strongly advocated. During bicycling, the seat height is adjusted to its highest level based on patient body size and a low resistance level is used initially. Stair-climbing machines are adjusted to produce a short step and low resistance.

An effective cardiovascular exercise program is an important component of the latter phases of rehabilitation. In addition to the previously described exercises, an aquatic program that includes lap work using freestyle or flutter kicking, water walking, water aerobics, and deep-water running is encouraged. Determining which cardiovascular exercises are appropriate is based on each patient's access to and preference for specific equipment.

Running and Agility Program

In order to initiate the running program, the patient must demonstrate no more than a 30% deficit in average torque for the quadriceps and hamstrings on isokinetic testing, have no more than 3 mm of increase in AP displacement on arthrometer testing, and be at least 9 weeks postoperative. It is important to note that the majority of patients initiate running at approximately 16 to 20 weeks postoperative. Only in exceptional cases does this program begin before this time period at which muscle strength has returned to normal, no pain or joint effusion is present, and no concurrent operative procedures were performed such as a complex meniscus repair or other ligament reconstruction.

The running program is designed based on the patient's athletic goals, particularly the position or physical requirements of the activity. For instance, an individual returning to short-duration, high-intensity activities should participate in a sprinting program rather than a long-distance endurance program. The running program is performed three times per week, on opposite days of the strength program. Because the running program may not reach aerobic levels initially, a cross-training program is used to facilitate cardiovascular fitness. The cross-training program is performed on the same day as the strength workout.

The first level consists of straight-ahead walk/run combinations. Running distances are 20, 40, 60, and 100 yards (18, 37, 55, 91 m) in both forward and backward directions. The initial running speed is approximately one quarter to one half of the patient's normal speed, which gradually progresses to three quarters to full speed. An interval-training–rest approach is applied in which the rest phase is two to three times the length of the training phase. After the patient is able to run straight ahead at full speed, lateral running and crossover maneuvers are begun. Short distances, such as 20 yards (18 m), are used to work on speed and agility. Side-to-side running over cups may be used to facilitate proprioception. At this time, sports-specific equipment is introduced to enhance skill development (e.g., a soccer ball for a soccer player to work on dribbling and passing activities). These variations are useful to motivate the patient and minimize training boredom.

The third level of the running program incorporates figure-eight running drills. Long and wide movement patterns over 20 yards (18 m) are initially used to encourage subtle cutting. As speed and confidence improve, the distance is decreased to approximately 10 yards (9 m). Progression through this phase is similar to that used in the lateral side-to-side program just described. Speed and agility are emphasized, and equipment is introduced to develop sports-specific skills.

The fourth phase in the running program introduces cutting patterns. These patterns include directional changes at 45° and 90° angles, which allow the patient to progress from subtle to sharp cuts.

Plyometric Training

Plyometric training is begun upon successful completion of the running program in order to minimize bilateral alterations in neuromuscular function and proprioception. Important parameters to consider when performing plyometric exercises include surface, footwear, and warm-up. The jump training should be done on a firm, yet forgiving surface such as a wooden gym floor. Very hard surfaces like concrete should be avoided. A cross-training or running shoe should be worn to provide adequate shock absorption as well as adequate stability to the foot. Checking wear patterns and outer sole wear will help avoid overuse injuries.

During the various jumps, the patient is instructed to keep the body weight on the balls of the feet and to jump and land with the knees flexed and shoulder-width apart to avoid knee hyperextension and an overall valgus lower limb position (Fig. 13–25). The patient should understand that the exercises are reaction and agility drills and, although speed is emphasized, correct body posture must be maintained throughout the drills.

The first exercise is level-surface box-hopping using both legs. A four-square grid of four equally sized boxes is created with tape on the floor. The patient is instructed to first hop from box 1 to box 3 (front-to-back; Fig. 13–26), and then from box 1 to box 2 (side-to-side; Fig. 13–27). The second level incorporates both of these directions into one sequence and also includes hopping in both right and left directions (e.g., box 1 to box 2 to box 4 to box 2 to box 1). Level three progresses to diagonal hops (Fig. 13–28), and level four includes pivot hops in 90° and 180° directions (Fig. 13–29). Once the patient can perform level four double-leg hops, the same exercises are done on a single leg. The next phase incorporates vertical box hops.

It is important to stress that plyometric exercise is intense and adequate rest must be included in the program. Individual sessions can be performed in a manner similar to that for interval training. Initially, the rest period lasts two to three times the length of the exercise period and is gradually decreased to one to two times the length of the exercise period. Plyometric training is performed two to three times weekly.

Improvement is measured by counting the number of hops in a defined time period. The initial exercise time period is 15

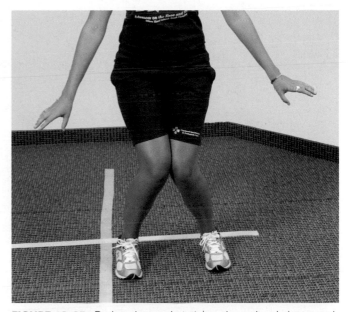

FIGURE 13–25. During plyometric training, the patient is instructed to keep the body weight on the balls of the feet, to jump and land with the knees flexed and shoulder-width apart to avoid knee hyperextension and an overall valgus lower limb position, as shown here.

seconds. The patient is asked to complete as many hops between the squares as possible in 15 seconds. Three sets are performed for both directions and the number of hops recorded. The program is progressed as the number of hops increases, as does patient confidence.

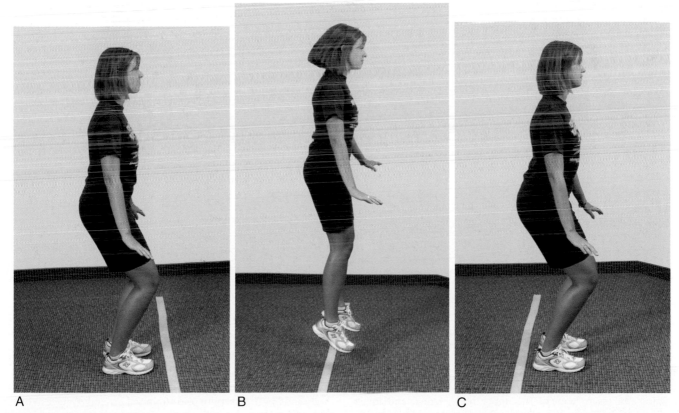

A   B   C

FIGURE 13–26. A–C, Initial plyometric training, jumping front-to-back on a level surface using both legs.

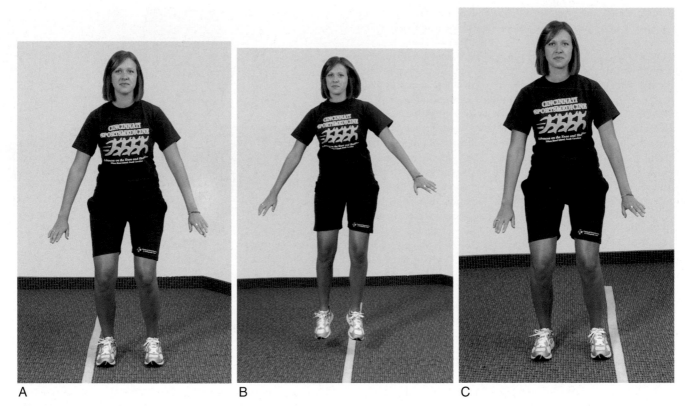

A   B   C

FIGURE 13–27. A–C, Initial plyometric training, jumping side-to-side on a level surface using both legs.

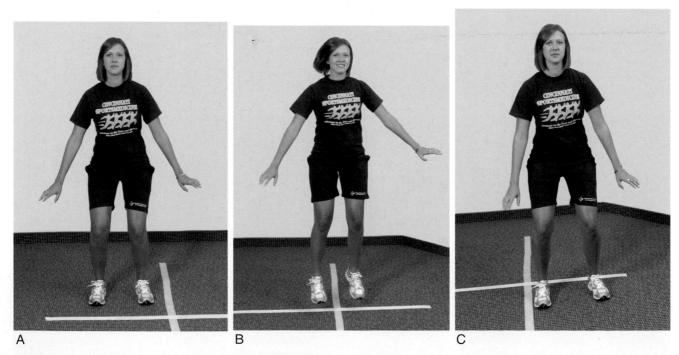

A   B   C

FIGURE 13–28. A–C, Plyometric training using diagonal hops, forward and backward.

The authors recommend that patients complete a course of Sportsmetrics training to reduce the risk of a noncontact reinjury before return to strenuous athletics. This training program teaches athletes to control the upper body, trunk, and lower body position; lower the center of gravity by increasing hip and knee flexion during activities; and develop muscular strength and techniques to land with decreased ground reaction forces. In addition, athletes are instructed to pre-position the body and lower extremity prior to initial ground contact in order to obtain the position of greatest knee joint stability and

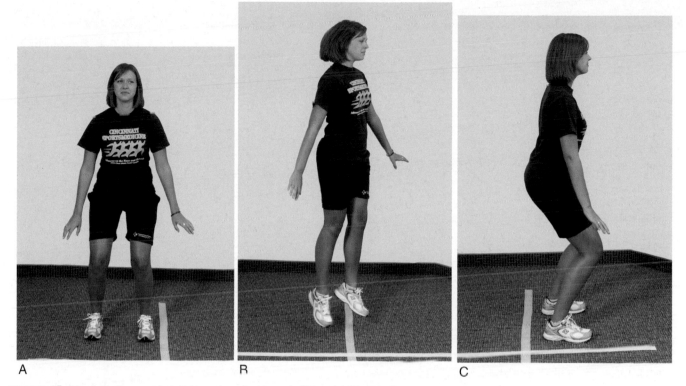

FIGURE 13–29. A–C, Plyometric training using pivot hops in 90° and 180° directions.

stiffness. The program consists of a dynamic warm-up, plyometric jump training, strengthening exercises, aerobic conditioning, agility, and risk-awareness training. The training is conducted three times a week on alternating days for 6 weeks and is described in detail in Chapter 19, Decreasing the Risk of ACL Injuries in Female Athletes.

Once the patient has completed the running and plyometric programs and strength and function testing reach normal values, return to sports is allowed. A trial of function is encouraged in which the patient is monitored for knee swelling, pain, overuse symptoms, and giving-way episodes. Some athletes will experience transient knee swelling upon return to strenuous activities and should be educated on how to recognize this problem and the importance of reducing activities until the swelling subsides. If swelling persists, the athlete is advised to reduce athletics for 2 to 6 weeks, consider use of nonsteroidal anti-inflammatories, and use ice and elevation. Upon successful return to activity, the patient is encouraged to continue with a maintenance program. During the in-season, a conditioning program of two workouts a week is recommended. In the off-season or preseason, this program should be performed three times a week to maximize gains in flexibility, strength, and cardiovascular endurance.

REHABILITATION PROTOCOL WITH DELAYED PARAMETERS FOR REVISION ACL RECONSTRUCTION, ALLOGRAFTS, AND COMPLEX KNEES

This protocol incorporates delays in return of full weight-bearing and knee flexion; initiation of certain strengthening, conditioning, running, and agility drills; and return to unrestricted activities (Table 13–7) for knees undergoing ACL revision,[13] allograft

reconstruction,[8] major concomitant operative procedures, or that have noteworthy articular cartilage damage.[10,11] Toe-touch-only weight-bearing is allowed for the first 2 postoperative weeks. The amount of weight patients are allowed after this time depends on the concomitant operative procedures performed as well as evaluation of postoperative pain and swelling, quadriceps muscle control, and ROM. The majority of patients are weaned from crutch support between the 6th and the 8th postoperative week.

Allowance of knee flexion of at least 135° is delayed according to the concomitant procedure performed. Knees that undergo a posterolateral reconstructive procedure are placed into a bivalved long-leg cast for the first 4 weeks[12] (see Chapter 23, Rehabilitation of PCL and Posterolateral Reconstructive Procedures). The patient removes the cast to perform ROM exercises several times a day and is instructed to reach 0° of extension but to avoid hyperextension. Patients who undergo a concomitant proximal patellar realignment are allowed 0° to 75° for the first 2 postoperative

---

Critical Points REHABILITATION PROTOCOL FOR REVISION ANTERIOR CRUCIATE LIGAMENT RECONSTRUCTION, ALLOGRAFTS, AND COMPLEX KNEES

- Toe-touch weight-bearing first 2 wk, full 6–8 wk.
- All knees 0° extension immediately.
- Knee flexion ≥ 135° delayed according to concomitant procedure performed.
- Long leg hinged knee brace first 8 wk in all except those who undergo a posterolateral procedure.
- Modifications in strengthening, conditioning, and strenuous training based on concomitant procedures performed.
- Return to activity delayed until at least the 6th postoperative mo; return to full activity usually 9–12 mo postoperative.

TABLE 13–7 Cincinnati Sportsmedicine and Orthopaedic Center Rehabilitation Protocol for Anterior Cruciate Ligament Reconstruction: Revision Knees, Allografts, and Complex Knees

	Postoperative Weeks					Postoperative Months			
	1–2	3–4	5–6	7–8	9–12	4	5	6	7–12
Brace: postoperative & functional	X	X	X	X	(X)			X	X
ROM minimum goals									
0°–90°	X	X							
0°–120°			X						
0°–135°				X					
Weight-bearing									
Toe touch	X								
25%–50% body weight		X							
75%–100% body weight			X						
Patella mobilization	X	X	X						
Modalities									
EMS	X	X	X	X					
Pain/edema management (cryotherapy)	X	X	X	X	X	X	X	X	X
Stretching									
Hamstring, gastrocnemius-soleus, iliotibial band, quadriceps	X	X	X	X	X	X	X	X	X
Strengthening									
Quadriceps isometrics, quadriceps-hamstring isometrics co-contraction, straight leg raises, active knee extension	X	X	X	X	X				
Closed-chain: gait retraining, toe-raises, wall-sits, mini-squats	X	X	X	X	X	X			
Knee flexion hamstring curls (90°)			X	X	X	X	X	X	X
Knee extension quads (90°-30°)			X	X	X	X	X	X	X
Hip abduction-adduction, multi-hip			X	X	X	X	X	X	X
Leg press (70°–10°)			X	X	X	X	X	X	X
Balance/proprioceptive training									
Weight-shifting, cup walking, BBS	X	X	X	X	X				
BBS, BAPS, perturbation training, balance board, minitrampoline						X	X	X	X
Conditioning									
UBC		X	X	X					
Bike (stationary)			X	X	X	X	X	X	X
Aquatic program				X	X	X	X	X	X
Elliptical machine				X	X	X	X	X	X
Swimming (kicking)						X	X	X	X
Walking						X	X	X	X
Stair-climbing machine						X	X	X	X
Ski machine						X	X	X	X
Running: straight								X	X
Cutting: lateral carioca, figure-eights									X
Plyometric training									X
Full sports									X

PHASE 1. WEEKS 1 TO 2

General Observation	Toe-touch weight-bearing to 25% body weight when
	• Pain controlled
	• Hemarthrosis controlled
	• Voluntary quadriceps contraction achieved
	• 0° extension

Evaluation		**Goals**
	Pain	Controlled
	Hemarthrosis	Mild
	Patellar mobility	Good
	ROM minimum	10°–80°
	Quadriceps contraction & patella migration	Good
	Soft tissue contracture	None

Frequency	**ROM**	**Duration**
3–4 x/day	ROM passive	
10 min	Meniscus repair (complex), MCL, revision, EA = 0°–90°	
	Patellar realignment = 0°–75°	
	Posterolateral procedure = 0°–90° (unless examination shows hyperelastic tissue type, then hold 15°–70° for 2 wk postoperative)	
	Patella mobilization	
	Ankle pumps (plantar flexion with resistance band)	
	Hamstring, gastrocnemius-soleus stretches	5 reps x 30 sec

3 x/day	**Strengthening**	
15 min	Straight leg raises (flexion)	3 sets x 10 reps
	Active quadriceps isometrics (based on ROM limits)	1 set x 10 reps
	Knee extension (active-assisted)	3 sets x 10 reps
As required	**Modalities**	
	EMS	20 min
	Cryotherapy	20 min
Goals	ROM (see above, depends on procedure)	
	Adequate quadriceps contraction	
	Control inflammation, effusion	

PHASE 2. WEEKS 3 TO 4

General Observation — 50% weight-bearing when
- Pain controlled
- Hemarthrosis controlled
- Voluntary quadriceps contraction achieved

Evaluation		**Goals**
	Pain	Controlled
	Effusion	Mild
	Patellar mobility	Good
	ROM minimum	0°–90°
	Quadriceps contraction & patella migration	Good
	Soft tissue contracture	None
	Joint arthrometer (3 wk, 20 lb)	<3 mm

Frequency	**ROM**	**Duration**
3–4 x/day	ROM passive, 0°–90°	
10 min	Patella mobilization	
	Ankle pumps (plantar flexion with resistance band)	
	Hamstring, gastrocnemius soleus stretches	5 reps x 30 secs
2–3 x/day	**Strengthening**	
20 min	Straight leg raises (flexion, extension, adduction)	3 sets x 10 reps
	Isometric training	1 set x 10 reps
	• Multiangle (0°, 60°)	
	• Active quadriceps (full extension)	
	• Quadriceps/hamstring co-contraction with electrical muscle stimulation	
	Toe-raise/heel-raise	3 sets x 10 reps
	Knee extension (90°-45°, no resistance)	3 sets x 10 reps
	Knee flexion (active, 0°- 90°)	3 sets x 10 reps
	Multi-hip machine (flexion, extension, abduction, adduction)	3 sets x 10 reps
	Leg press (70°-10°)	3 sets x 10 reps
	Closed-chain	3 sets x 20 reps to fatigue
	• Mini-squats (0°-45°, 50% weight-bearing)	
	• Wall-sits	
	• Wall-sits with EMS	
2 x/day	**Aerobic conditioning**	
10 min	UBC	
As required	**Modalities**	
	EMS	20 min
	Cryotherapy	20 min
Goals	ROM 0°–110°	
	Control inflammation, effusion	
	Adequate quadriceps contraction	
	50% weight-bearing	

PHASE 3. WEEKS 5 TO 6

General Observation — Full weight-bearing when
- Pain controlled without narcotics
- Effusion controlled
- ROM 0°–100°
- Muscle control throughout ROM
- Dynamic control varus/valgus

Evaluation		**Goals**
	Pain	Mild
	Effusion	Minimal
	Patellar mobility	Good
	ROM	0°–120°
	Muscle control	3/5
	Inflammatory response	None
	Joint arthrometer (6 wk, 30 lb)	<3 mm

Continued

PHASE 3. WEEKS 5 TO 6—Cont'd

Frequency	ROM	Duration
3 x/day	ROM passive, 0°–120°	
10 min	Patella mobilization	
	Ankle pumps (plantar flexion with resistance band)	
	Hamstring, gastrocnemius-soleus stretches	5 reps x 30 sec
2–3 x/day	**Strengthening**	
20 min	Straight leg raises (ankle weight, <10% of body weight)	3 sets x 10 reps
	Isometric training: multiangle (90°, 60°, 30°)	2 sets x 10 reps
	Heel-raise/toe-raise	3 sets x 10 reps
	Hamstring curls (active, 0°-90°)	3 sets x 10 reps
	Knee extension (90°-45°, with resistance)	3 sets x 10 reps
	Closed-chain	
	• Wall-sits	5 reps
	• Mini-squats	3 sets x 20 reps
	• Lunge (no resistance)	
	Multi-hip machine (flexion, extension, abduction, adduction)	3 sets x 10 reps
	Leg press (70°–10°)	3 sets x 10 reps
3 x/day	**Balance training**	
5 min	Weight shift side-to-side and forward-to-back	5 sets x 10 reps
	Balance board/two-legged	
1–2 x/day	Cup-walking	
5 min	Single-leg stance on stable platform	5 reps
2 x/day	**Aerobic conditioning**	
10 min	UBC	
	Water walking	
	Stationary bicycling (patellofemoral precautions)	
As required	**Modalities**	
	EMS	20 min
	Cryotherapy	20 min
Goals	ROM 0°–125°	
	Control inflammation, effusion	
	Muscle control	
	Full weight-bearing	
	Early recognition complications (motion loss, RSD, increased AP displacement, patellofemoral)	

PHASE 4. WEEKS 7 TO 8

General Observation	Independent ambulation when	
	• Pain controlled	
	• Effusion controlled	
	• ROM 0°–120°	
	• Muscle control throughout ROM	
	• Dynamic control varus/valgus	

Evaluation		**Goals**
	Pain	No RSD
	Effusion	Minimal
	Patellar mobility	Good
	ROM	0°–135°
	Muscle control	4/5
	Inflammatory response	None
	Gait	Symmetrical
	Joint arthrometer (8 wk)	<3 mm

Frequency	ROM	Duration
2 x/day	Hamstring, gastrocnemius-soleus stretches	5 reps x 30 sec
10 min		
2 x/day	**Strengthening**	
20 min	Straight leg raises (ankle weight, <10% body weight)	3 sets x 10 reps
	Straight leg raises, rubber tubing	3 sets x 30 reps
	Isometric training: multiangle (90°, 60°, 30°)	3 sets x 20 reps
	Heel-raise/toe-raise	3 sets x 10 reps
	Hamstring curls (active, 0°–90°)	3 sets x 10 reps
	Knee extension with resistance (90°-45°)	3 sets x 10 reps
	Leg press (70°–10°)	3 sets x 10 reps
	Closed-chain	3 sets x 20 reps to fatigue x 3
	• Wall-sits	
	• Mini-squats (rubber tubing, 0°-30°)	
	• Lunge	
	Multi-hip machine (flexion, extension, abduction, adduction)	3 sets x 10 reps
	Leg press (70°-10°)	3 sets x 10 reps

PHASE 4. WEEKS 7 TO 8—Cont'd

3 x/day
5 min
	Balance training
	   Balance board/two-legged
	   Lateral step-ups: 2"–4"	

2 x/day
10 min
	Aerobic conditioning (patellofemoral precautions)
	   UBC
	   Stationary bicycling
	   Water walking
	   Stair machine (low resistance, low stroke)
	   Ski machine (short stride, level, low resistance)
	   Elliptical machine (low resistance)	

As required	**Modalities** Cryotherapy	20 min
Goals	ROM 0°–135° Full weight-bearing, normal gait Control inflammation, effusion Muscle endurance Recognize complications (motion loss, RSD, increased AP displacement) Recognition of patellofemoral changes	

PHASE 5. WEEKS 9 TO 12

General Observation	Full weight-bearing ROM 0°–135° No effusion, painless ROM, joint stability Performs activities of daily living Can walk 20 min without pain	
Evaluation		**Goals**
	Manual muscle test: Hamstrings, quadriceps, hip abductors/adductors/ flexors/extensors	4/5
	Swelling	None
	Joint arthrometer (12 wk)	3 mm
	Patellar mobility	Good
	Crepitus	None/slight
Frequency	**ROM**	**Duration**
2 x/day 10 min	Hamstring, gastrocnemius-soleus, quadriceps, ITB stretches	5 reps x 30 sec

2 x/day
20 min
	Strengthening
	   Straight leg raises, rubber tubing
	   Hamstring curls (active, 0°–90°)
	   Knee extension with resistance (90°–45°)
	   Leg press (70°–10°)
	   Closed-chain
	     • Wall-sits
	     • Mini-squats (rubber tubing, 0°–40°)
	     • Lunge
	   Multi-hip machine (flexion, extension, abduction, adduction)
		3 sets x 30 reps
		3 sets x 10 reps
		3 sets x 10 reps
		3 sets x 10 reps
		3 sets x 20 reps to fatigue x 3
		
		3 sets x 10 reps
		3 sets x 10 reps

3 x/day
5 min
	Balance training
	   Balance board/two-legged
	   Single-leg stance on unstable platform
	   Perturbation training	

1–2 x/day
15–20 min
	Aerobic conditioning (patellofemoral precautions)
	   Stationary bicycling
	   Water walking
	   Swimming (straight leg kicking)
	   Walking
	   Stair machine (low resistance, low stroke)
	   Ski machine (short stride, level, low resistance)
	   Elliptical machine (low resistance)	

As required	**Modalities** Cryotherapy	20 min
Goals	Increase strength and endurance	

PHASE 6. WEEKS 13 TO 26

General Observation	No effusion, painless ROM, joint stability Performs activities of daily living Can walk 20 min without pain ROM 0°–135°

Continued

Evaluation		**Goals**
	Isometric test (% difference quadriceps & hamstrings)	30
	Swelling	None
	Joint arthrometer	<3 mm
	Patellar mobility	Good
	Crepitus	None/slight

Frequency	**ROM**	**Duration**
2 x/day 10 min	Hamstring, gastrocnemius-soleus, quadriceps, ITB stretches	5 reps x 30 sec
2 x/day 20 min	**Strengthening**	
	Straight leg raises, rubber tubing	3 sets x 30 reps
	Hamstring curls (active, 0°–90°)	3 sets x 10 reps
	Knee extension with resistance (90°–45°)	3 sets x 10 reps
	Leg press (70°–10°)	3 sets x 10 reps
	Multi-hip machine (flexion, extension, abduction, adduction)	3 sets x 10 reps
	Closed-chain	
	• Wall-sits	5 reps
	• Mini-squats	3 sets x 20 reps
	• Lateral step-ups (2"–4" block)	3 sets x 10 reps
3 x/day 5 min	**Balance training**	
	Balance board/two-legged	
	Single-leg stance on unstable platform	
	Plyoback with ball toss	
	Perturbation training	
3 x/wk 15–20 min	**Aerobic conditioning** (patellofemoral precautions)	
	Stationary bicycling	
	Water walking	
	Swimming (kicking)	
	Walking	
	Stair machine (low resistance, low stroke)	
	Ski machine (short stride, level, low resistance)	
3 x/week 10 min	**Running program** (6 mo, straight, 30% deficit isometric test)	
	Jog	¼ – 1 mile
	Walk	⅛ mile
	Backward run	20 yd
As required	**Modalities**	
	Cryotherapy	20 min
Goals	Increase strength and endurance	

General Observation	
	No effusion, painless ROM, joint stability
	Performs ADL
	Can walk 20 min without pain

Evaluation		**Goals**
	Isokinetic test (isometric + torque 300°/sec, % difference quadriceps & hamstrings)	10–15
	Swelling	None
	Joint arthrometer	3 mm
	Patellar mobility	Good
	Crepitus	None/slight
	Single-leg function tests (9 mo: hop distance, timed hop, % involved/uninvolved)	85

Frequency	**ROM**	**Duration**
2 x/day 10 min	Hamstring, gastrocnemius-soleus, quadriceps, ITB stretches	5 reps x 30 sec
1 x/day 20–30 min	**Strengthening**	
	Straight leg raises, rubber tubing (high speed)	3 sets x 30 reps
	Hamstring curls (active, 0°–90°)	3 sets x 10 reps
	Knee extension with resistance (90°–45°)	3 sets x 10 reps
	Leg press (70°-10°)	3 sets x 10 reps
	Multi-hip machine (flexion, extension, abduction, adduction)	3 sets x 10 reps
3 x/day 5 min	**Balance training**	
	Balance board/two-legged	
	Single-leg stance	
	Perturbation training	
3 x/wk 20–30 min	**Aerobic conditioning** (patellofemoral precautions)	
	Stationary bicycling	
	Water walking	
	Swimming (kicking)	
	Walking	
	Stair machine (low resistance, low stroke)	
	Ski machine (short stride, level, low resistance)	

PHASE 7. WEEKS 27 TO 52—Cont'd

3 x/wk 15–20 min	**Running program** (straight) Jog—interval training (20, 40, 60, 100 yd) Walk Backward run	¼ mile ⅛ mile 20 yd 20 yd
3 x/wk	**Cutting program**—lateral, carioca, figure-eights (20% deficit isokinetic test)	
3 x/wk	**Functional training** Plyometric training: box hops, level, double-leg Sports-specific drills (10%–15% deficit isokinetic test)	15 sec, 4–6 sets
As required	**Modalities** Cryotherapy	20 min
Goals	Increase function, strength, endurance Return to previous activity level	

AP, anteroposterior; BAPS, Biomechanical Ankle Platform System (Camp, Jackson, MI); BBS, Biodex Balance System (Biodex Medical Systems, Inc., Shirley, NY); EA, iliotibial band extra-articular procedure; EMS, electrical muscle stimulation; ITB, iliotibial band; MCL, medial collateral ligament; ROM, range of motion; RSD, reflex sympathetic dystrophy; UBC, upper body cycle (Biodex Medical Systems, Inc., Shirley, NY); X, when exercise is performed.

weeks. Flexion is slowly advanced to 135° by the 8th week. Knee flexion is also initially limited in knees that undergo a concomitant posterior cruciate ligament reconstruction[9] (see Chapter 23, Rehabilitation of PCL and Posterolateral Reconstructive Procedures) and/or complex meniscus repair[21] (see Chapter 30, Rehabilitation of Meniscus Repair and Transplantation Procedures).

Knee extension is limited in individuals who have abnormal hyperextension (≥10°) with physiologic laxity to 0° to 5° for approximately 3 weeks to allow for sufficient healing before stress is applied to push for 0°.

A postoperative long-leg hinged knee brace is used for approximately the first 8 weeks in patients placed in this protocol, except those who undergo a posterolateral procedure as described. The brace provides protection and support to the healing tissues and assists with patient comfort during this time period.

Modifications in strengthening, conditioning, and strenuous training are based on the concomitant procedures performed. Return to activity is delayed until at least the 6th postoperative month to allow for healing of all repaired and reconstructed tissues and return of joint and muscle function. It is the authors' opinion that allografts have a delay in maturation compared with autografts (see Chapter 5, Biology of Anterior Cruciate Ligament Graft Healing) and that the resultant time constraints postoperatively in terms of release to full activity are empirical at present. Evaluation is a key component to allow initiation of the functional program, which includes the assessment of symptoms and examination of knee motion, muscle strength, and ligament stability. The sum of the evaluation, not just one parameter, should determine return to function. In patients following this protocol, return to full activity is not usually expected to occur until the 9th to 12th month postoperative. It should also be noted that return to full activity does not guarantee return to pre-injury activity levels. Consideration of use of a derotation or functional brace includes patients who have undergone ACL revision or multiligament reconstruction or who demonstrate an increase in AP displacement of 3 mm or more postoperatively compared with the contralateral limb. In addition, patients who are apprehensive about returning to strenuous activities or who experience a subjective sensation of instability are candidates for functional bracing.

REFERENCES

1. American College of Sports Medicine: Position stand: progression models in resistance training for healthy adults. *Med Sci Sports Exerc* 34:364–380, 2002.
2. Barber-Westin, S. D.; Noyes, F. R.: The effect of rehabilitation and return to activity on anterior-posterior knee displacements after anterior cruciate ligament reconstruction. *Am J Sports Med* 21:264–270, 1993.
3. Barber-Westin, S. D.; Noyes, F. R.; Heckmann, T. P.; Shaffer, B. L.: The effect of exercise and rehabilitation on anterior-posterior knee displacements after anterior cruciate ligament autograft reconstruction. *Am J Sports Med* 27:84–93, 1999.
4. DeMaio, M.; Mangine, R. E.; Noyes, F. R.; Barber, S. D.: Advanced muscle training after ACL reconstruction: weeks 6 to 52. *Orthopedics* 15:757–767, 1992.
5. DeMaio, M.; Noyes, F. R.; Mangine, R. E.: Principles for aggressive rehabilitation after reconstruction of the anterior cruciate ligament. *Orthopedics* 15:385–392, 1992.
6. Kraemer, W. J.; Ratamess, N. A.: Fundamentals of resistance training: progression and exercise prescription. *Med Sci Sports Exerc* 36:674–688, 2004.
7. Mangine, R. E.; Noyes, F. R.; DeMaio, M.: Minimal protection program: advanced weight bearing and range of motion after ACL reconstruction—weeks 1 to 5. *Orthopedics* 15:504–515, 1992.
8. Noyes, F. R.; Barber, S. D.; Mangine, R. E.: Bone-patellar ligament-bone and fascia lata allografts for reconstruction of the anterior cruciate ligament. *J Bone Joint Surg Am* 72:1125–1136, 1990.
9. Noyes, F. R.; Barber-Westin, S.: Posterior cruciate ligament replacement with a two-strand quadriceps tendon–patellar bone autograft and a tibial inlay technique. *J Bone Joint Surg Am* 87:1241–1252, 2005.
10. Noyes, F. R.; Barber-Westin, S. D.: Anterior cruciate ligament reconstruction with autogenous patellar tendon graft in patients with articular cartilage damage. *Am J Sports Med* 25:626–634, 1997.
11. Noyes, F. R.; Barber-Westin, S. D.: Arthroscopic-assisted allograft anterior cruciate ligament reconstruction in patients with symptomatic arthrosis. *Arthroscopy* 13:24–32, 1997.
12. Noyes, F. R.; Barber-Westin, S. D.: Posterolateral knee reconstruction with an anatomical bone-patellar tendon–bone reconstruction of the fibular collateral ligament. *Am J Sports Med* 35:259–273, 2007.
13. Noyes, F. R.; Barber-Westin, S. D.: Revision anterior cruciate surgery with use of bone-patellar tendon–bone autogenous grafts. *J Bone Joint Surg Am* 83:1131–1143, 2001.
14. Noyes, F. R.; Berrios-Torres, S.; Barber-Westin, S. D.; Heckmann, T. P.: Prevention of permanent arthrofibrosis after anterior cruciate ligament reconstruction alone or combined with associated procedures: a prospective study in 443 knees. *Knee Surg Sports Traumatol Arthrosc* 8:196–206, 2000.
15. Noyes, F. R.; DeMaio, M.; Mangine, R. E.: Evaluation-based protocols: a new approach to rehabilitation. *Orthopedics* 14:1383–1385, 1991.
16. Noyes, F. R.; Mangine, R. E.; Barber, S.: Early knee motion after open and arthroscopic anterior cruciate ligament reconstruction. *Am J Sports Med* 15:149–160, 1987.

- Proprioception: The sense of awareness of the joint position. Achieved by a sensory pathway response that is first triggered by mechanoreceptors found in the synovial joints of the body. Components act together to transmit sensory information concerning joint position, movement, and strain via afferent pathways to the central nervous system (CNS). CNS sends electrical signals through efferent pathways to corresponding muscles surrounding the joint to alter muscle joint tone and function and provide stability.
- Kinesthesia: The sensation of joint movement
- Neuromuscular control: The afferent sensory recognition of joint position and the efferent response to that awareness. Provides the functional component referred to as *dynamic stabilization*.
- Motor responses depend on the level of processing of afferent inputs within the CNS. The processing may occur at the spinal cord, the brainstem, and the cerebral cortex. The site of processing affects the speed of motor responses. Sensory input processed at the CNS above the spinal cord level can be modified with training.
- After injury, interactions within the neuromuscular system are disrupted, which can result in diminished proprioception and kinesthesia, abnormal patterns of muscle activity, reduced joint stability. Problems may affect the contralateral limb.
- Open-loop control: A movement that is brief, predictable, produced in an unchanging environment, does not require sensory information for modification.
- Closed-loop control: Movements that rely on feedback from the sensory system.

quadriceps and a facilitation of the hamstrings. This protects against increasing strain on the ACL. The second mechanism is the joint receptors' indirect contribution to dynamic joint stability. In this mechanism, the joint receptors contribute to preparatory adjustments of muscles stiffness and dynamic joint stability. This is referred to as *presetting*.[31] The authors believe this concept of presetting is critical in providing joint stability during functional activities such as preparation for deceleration or cutting.

Motor responses depend on the level of processing of afferent inputs within the CNS. The processing may occur at three different levels: the spinal cord, the brainstem, and the cerebral cortex.[9] The site of processing affects the speed of motor responses. Spinal reflexes represent the shortest neuronal pathways and, consequently, the most rapid response to afferent stimuli.[11,48,58] Theoretically, these spinal reflexes are faster than ligamentous failure.[46,58] Conversely, sensory information mediated at the brainstem, cerebellum, and cortical levels include longer pathways and slower response times. Numerous studies[11,21,48] have documented that sensory input processed at the CNS above the spinal cord level can be modified with training. Thus, owing to the adaptability of the responses at the brainstem and the cerebellum, these pathways are believed to be important in providing dynamic knee stability.[18]

After injury, the complex interactions within the neuromuscular system are disrupted, which can result in diminished proprioception and kinesthesia, abnormal patterns of muscle activity,[15] and reduced joint dynamic stability.[4,7,34] Furthermore, injury to one knee can affect the proprioception on the contralateral (uninvolved) extremity.[28] Therefore, immediately after injury or surgery, the rehabilitation program must be directed toward creating an environment that promotes the restoration and development of motor responses and proprioception for both extremities.

Several other terms require classification. *Open-loop control* is defined as a movement that is brief, predictable, and produced in an unchanging environment that does not require sensory information for modification. Thus, these are movements that do not require feedback.[48] Conversely, movements that rely on feedback from the sensory system, such as reflexive movements, are considered *closed-loop control*.

Chmielewski and coworkers[12] defined motor skills in respect to the environment. Some motor skills, such as walking, stair-climbing, and extending the leg, although performed in a relatively stable environment, are referred to as *closed skills*. Conversely, *open skills* are performed in an environment that is changing and unpredictable. Examples of open skills include running in the woods, downhill skiing, or balancing on a wobble board. Other examples are playing sports such as basketball, soccer, or football.

EFFECTS OF INJURY ON PROPRIOCEPTION

Numerous authors[4-7,28] have shown a decrease in proprioception and kinesthesia after ACL injury. After ACL injury, deafferentization of peripheral sensory receptors occurs.[6,49] Changes in proprioception happen quickly. Lephart and associates[35] reported that these changes occur within 24 hours from the injury. Alterations in proprioception may persist for as long as 6 years.[17]

After an injury, changes occur within the joint that affect normal recruitment and timing patterns of the surrounding musculature.[20] Several theories regarding this deterioration of musculature activation have been proposed. One theory is that after an acute injury, an alteration occurs in the ratio of muscle spindle to GTO activity, leading to interference of the proprioception pathway. Another theory suggests that joint effusion after an acute injury alters the ability of the musculature to contract and, therefore, leads to decreased proprioception. A study by Palmieri-Smith and colleagues[44] showed that effusion of the knee of just 30 ml significantly decreased the activation of the

- A decrease in proprioception and kinesthesia occurs after anterior cruciate ligament (ACL) injury. Changes that occur within the joint affect normal recruitment and timing patterns of the surrounding musculature.
- There is a significant decrease in muscle activation timing and recruitment order in the lower extremity in response to anterior tibial translation in ACL-deficient knees compared with uninjured controls.
- After ACL rupture, patients walk with greater hamstring activity, a flexed knee, and minimal to no quadriceps electromyographic activity.
- Altered proprioception of the knee joint may last 1 to 3 yr after injury.

vastus medialis and lateralis muscles during a single-leg drop landing. Joint effusion of 30 ml is barely palpable by most clinicians.

Injury to the ACL can lead to significant problems for the athlete. One study by Wojtys and Hutson[59] showed there was a significant decrease in muscle activation timing and recruitment order in the medial and lateral quadriceps, medial and lateral hamstrings, and gastrocnemius in response to anterior tibial translation in individuals with ACL-deficient knees compared with an uninjured control group. This delay in muscle recruitment can lead to decreased stability of the joint because the musculature is the prime joint stabilizer owing to loss of ACL function. Beard and coworkers[7] examined the effects of applying 100 N of anterior shear force on ACL-deficient knees and noted a reflexive activation of the hamstring muscles. Paterno and associates[45] reported a significant difference in force production during a drop vertical jump in ACL-reconstructed knees compared with the contralateral limbs a mean of 27 months after ACL reconstruction. This study is one of many that show continued differences between ACL-reconstructed and uninvolved limbs for an extended period of time after surgery.[28,30,53,59]

Wilk and colleagues[28] reported that 24 to 48 hours after ACL injury, proprioception was altered bilaterally according to measurements on a stability system. The uninvolved lower extremity's ability to stabilize on a sway board (Biodex Stability System, Shirley, NY) was compromised for 6 to 8 weeks, with a gradual improvement in sway balance thereafter.

EFFECTS OF INJURY ON GAIT

After ACL injury, patients exhibit an alteration in gait patterns. Andriacchi and Birac[1] and Berchuck and coworkers[8] coined the term "quadriceps avoidance gait pattern" (see Chapter 6, Human Movement and Anterior Cruciate Ligament Function: Anterior Cruciate Ligament Deficiency and Gait Mechanics). Patients walk with greater hamstring activity, a flexed knee, and minimal to no quadriceps electromyographic activity. It has been clinically observed that these protective neuromuscular adaptations (quadriceps-avoidance gait) may persist for several months if not appropriately addressed in rehabilitation.

DURATION OF INJURY EFFECTS

Many theories exist regarding the length of time that a patient with an acute ACL injury experiences a decreased sense of proprioception and neuromuscular control; the exact duration remains unclear. Most sources cite anywhere from 1 to 3 years as the timeframe for altered proprioception of the knee joint. Harrison and associates[25] studied the differences between the reconstructed and the uninvolved legs during single-leg stance in patients after ACL reconstruction. These researchers found no significant differences in postural sway (with eyes both open and closed) between the involved and the uninvolved lower extremities during single-leg stance 10 to 18 months after surgery. This finding suggests that proprioception can be restored in a shorter timeframe than expected. Other studies propose that proprioception and joint position sense take much longer to be reestablished. Fremerey and colleagues[24] examined the differences of joint position sense at different time intervals and compared those data to information gathered preoperatively. This study showed that joint position sense of the knee was almost completely restored at the near-end range of knee flexion and knee extension 6 months postoperatively. However, the study also reported that proprioception at the midrange of knee motion was not fully restored at 6 months. In fact, some patients took over 3½ years to fully recover their joint position sense at midrange positions. This is critical to an athlete because a majority of activities that occur during competition do so at these midrange of motion positions. The lack of joint position sense at these levels may have a significant impact on the probability that the athlete will sustain a second injury.

Another theory also considered when studying the duration of decreased proprioception in patients with acute ACL injury is the preinjury level of activity of the individual. Roberts and coworkers[47] demonstrated that patients whose preinjury activity levels were high had a faster recovery of joint position sense after ACL reconstruction.

CLINICAL RELEVANCE

When designing a rehabilitation program for a patient who has sustained an ACL injury, the clinician must remember several critical components. One is the restoration of neuromuscular control almost immediately after ACL reconstruction to prevent deafferentation of the joint. The progression of the patient must be increased gradually, and therefore, it is the responsibility of the therapist to find a balance between a detrimentally slow progression and advanced techniques prematurely that could have dangerous results. The therapist must consider the additional stresses that neuromuscular training places on the joint and factor those stresses into the overall volume of work that the patient performs. One must find a delicate balance to maximize rehabilitation benefits but prevent fatigue without recovery that could lead to delays in rehabilitation and setbacks.

The therapist can use several techniques to progress the patient that do not involve the actual injured joint. One such technique is to incorporate neuromuscular training to the uninvolved side. Studies have shown that there can be a carry-over effect from training the uninvolved extremity; challenging the uninvolved side can lead to improvements in the involved side. Performing passive/active joint repositioning is valuable in restoring joint awareness in the patient. This technique can be performed immediately after surgery or injury. Another technique is to challenge the core, ideally, while the patient is in an athletic stance to produce the most relevance to the patient's sport. Core activities also help prepare the entire body for a return to activity when the patient is ready.

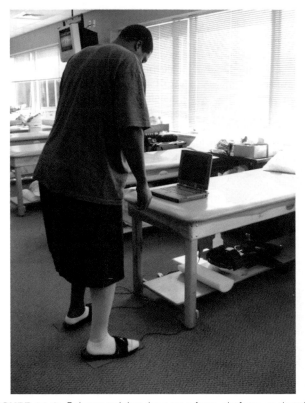

FIGURE 14–3. Balance training done on a force platform so that the patient obtains visual feedback regarding the amount of weight distribution between the lower extremities.

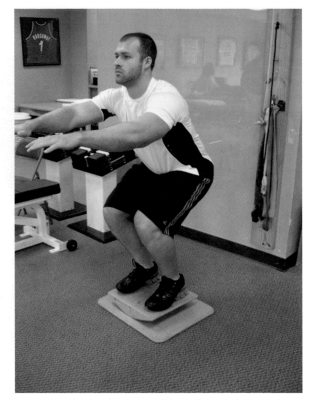

FIGURE 14–5. Rocker boards used for balance-training and perturbation-training drills.

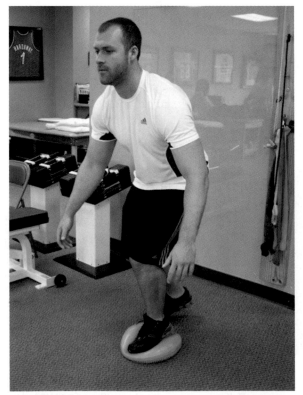

FIGURE 14–4. Wobble board used for balance-training drills.

Plyometric Exercises

Plyometric exercise is commonly referred to as jump training or stretch-shortening exercise drills. Wilk and coworkers[57] referred to plyometric training as "reactive neuromuscular training." Plyometrics are commonly used to increase performance in the advanced phase of rehabilitation and in injury prevention. Noyes and Barber-Westin designed and published on the beneficial effect of a 6-week neuromuscular-training program in female athletes (see Chapter 19, Decreasing the Risk of Anterior Cruciate Ligament Injuries in Female Athletes). An epidemiology study showed that this program may reduce the incidence of ACL injuries, and other knee injuries, in the female athlete.[26] The specially designed preventive program, referred to as "Sportmetrics,"[27] is discussed in Chapter 19, Decreasing the Risk of Anteror Cruciate Ligament Injuries in Female Athletes. This program and others have been used to reduce ACL injuries in athletes.

Plyometrics use the stretch-shortening cycle of muscle contraction. The stretch cycle elicits an eccentric contraction, whereas the shortening cycle creates a concentric contraction. Furthermore, plyometric training for the lower extremity must focus on proper technique and body position mechanics, with the goal of reducing the risk of serious injury. Proper technique, body position, and knee position are critical during the landing phase of the plyometric drills. Plyometric training for the lower extremity progresses from double-leg drills to single-leg drills, and from jumps from the ground to jumps off a box. Catching a ball or using resistance cords increases the challenge.

Technique Training

Technique training involves sports-specific or performance training with an emphasis on proper technique. Such drills include running and cutting, landing from a jump, and deceleration from running.

The clinician may offer both verbal and visual feedback to the patient. Phrases such as "land light as a feather," be a "shock absorber," and act as a "spring" can be used.[27] Technique training has been reported to reduce ACL injury.[39] Mandelbaum and associates[36] emphasized proper technique in their ACL preventive program, which was highly successful in reducing ACL injuries in soccer players. The Sportsmetrics program emphasizes proper landing from plyometric jumps.[27] If the exercise is not performed appropriately, the drill is stopped and the technique is corrected and practiced until the athlete exhibits correct landing technique.

REHABILITATION PROGRAM

Rehabilitation after ACL reconstruction has changed significantly since the mid 1990s. Today's programs emphasize immediate motion, immediate partial weight-bearing, immediate muscular training, closed kinetic chain exercises, and an earlier return to functional activities. The authors' rehabilitation program after ACL injury is shown in Table 14–1, and after reconstruction using a bone–patellar tendon–bone autograft appears in Table 14–2.

During the rehabilitation process, neuromuscular-training drills are integrated beginning the 1st day after ACL surgery or injury. The neuromuscular drills are progressed from simple to complex, isolated to combined, and blocked to random. *Blocked training* refers to a particular component of a skill in which each component is practiced before progressing to the next. Conversely, *random training* comprises different skills that are practiced interchangeably throughout a session. During the training, external feedback is given to the athlete in the form of instruction, technique guidance, examples, and other techniques. Occasionally, the athlete receives visual feedback from sources such as a mirror, a videotape, or a force pattern. These techniques may aid in technique modification and mastering a specific movement drill.

The program is based on 10 key components, listed in Table 14–3. The neuromuscular-training program is a four-phased program; examples of specific exercises and drills are found in Table 14–4. In this section, a brief discussion and examples of specific drills in each phase of the rehabilitation program are provided.

Phase I: Acute Phase Drills

Immediately after injury or surgery, numerous neuromuscular-training drills and activities may be initiated. In this phase, most of the drills are isolated in nature and a blocked-training technique is employed. Performing passive ROM is beneficial to joint position sense because it stimulates the mechanoreceptors. Furthermore, passive/active reposition sense techniques may be performed to improve proprioception. These activities are usually performed with the eyes closed. Performing weight-bearing exercises is also safe and beneficial. Mini-squats (0°–40°) can be done on a force platform, which provides visual feedback to the

patient regarding weight distribution, or on an unstable platform (Fig. 14–6). In addition, weight-shifting can be performed on the platform.

During the 2nd week after surgery, gait activities such as stepping over cones are initiated. This drill may be performed laterally or forward and backward (Figs. 14–7 and 14–8). Immediately after injury or surgery, the use of electrical stimulation to the quadriceps (Fig. 14–9) is strongly recommended to prevent "quadriceps shutdown" and assist in muscle reeducation, hypertrophy, and strength gains.[51]

Lateral lunges are performed on a stable floor surface without resistance. The goal of this exercise is to train patients to land from the lunge with a flexed knee; thus improving dynamic stability through co-contracture of the hamstrings and quadriceps (Fig. 14–10). Ambulation with a rubber band around the patient's hip is beneficial to improve hip muscular strength (Fig. 14–11). Another excellent exercise to improve stability through balance training is squats on a Biodex Stability System (see Fig. 14–2A). Lastly, patients are instructed to wear a compression sleeve when performing daily activities. Birmingham and colleagues[10] reported that wearing an elastic sleeve improved proprioception by 25%. A simple compression sleeve (see Fig. 14–2B) can significantly improve a patient's joint awareness.

Phase II: Dynamic Stability Drills

Phase II is referred to as the *dynamic stability phase*. Drills are gradually increased in degree of difficulty and complexity, with transition to more combined movement patterns. The training drills build from the previous phase and require that the patient has mastered specific techniques. One criterion, for instance, is the patient's ability to stabilize the knee with a single-leg stance at 30° of knee flexion.

Lateral lunge exercises are progressed from using a resistance cord in a straight plane (Fig. 14–12) to using a resistance cord in the diagonal plane (Fig. 14–13) and, finally, with rotation (Fig. 14–14). This drill can be progressed to landing on a unilateral surface such as foam (Fig. 14–15) or an air mattress (Fig. 14–16). The specific goal of this drill is the unilateral landing of the lunge. The patient is instructed to land with the knee flexed to 25° to 30° and the hip flexed approximately 30° to 45°, because this promotes a stable joint through quadriceps and hamstring co-activation.[56]

Other drills include front step-downs and lateral step-ups. The front step-down is an excellent functional training drill (Fig. 14–17). Chmielewski and coworkers[16] reported that the front step-down correlated to the patient's functional level and patient satisfaction. This drill may be performed with half-circle foam under the patient's foot or with a ball-catch (Fig. 14–18) to diminish the patient's conscious awareness of his or her knee joint. Squats on an unstable surface, such as on a BOSU ball (Fig. 14–19) or a Biodex Stability System, are excellent in this phase. In addition, hip rotation strengthening exercises are strongly emphasized through a variety of exercise drills (see Table 14–2, Early Rehabilitation Phase [Weeks 2–3]) along with foot and ankle exercise drills. Lastly, endurance exercises are gradually implemented. Numerous authors[33,43,60] have shown that once a joint is fatigued, proprioception is significantly decreased; in some cases, up to 75%. Wojtys and associates[60] reported a significantly slower response time in the quadriceps, hamstrings, and gastrocnemius after fatigue.

TABLE 14–2 Rehabilitation after Anterior Cruciate Ligament Bone–Patellar Tendon–Bone Reconstruction—Cont'd

Early Rehabilitation Phase (Weeks 2–3)

Criteria to Progress and Goals	Brace	Weight-Bearing	Exercises	Electrical Muscle Stimulation	Neuromuscular, Proprioception Training	Cryotherapy
Goals Maintain full passive knee extension (at least 0° to 5°–7° HE). Gradually increase knee flexion. Diminish swelling and pain. Muscle control and activation. Restore proprioception, neuromuscular control. Normalize patellar mobility.	Week 3: Discontinue locked brace. Some patients use ROM brace for ambulation. PROM, continue, should be 0° to 100°/105°.		Standing hamstring curls (active ROM). Bicycle if ROM allows. Overpressure into extension. PROM 0°–100° Patellar mobilization. Well-leg exercises. PRE program: start with 1 lb, progress 1 lb/wk. **Week 3: add** PROM 0°–105°. Pool-walking program if incision is closed. Eccentric quadriceps program 40°–100°, isotonic only. Lateral lunges, straight plane. Front step-downs. Lateral step-overs (cones). Stair-stepper machine.			

Progressive Strengthening/Neuromuscular Control Phase (Weeks 4–10)

Criteria to Progress and Goals	Brace	Exercises	Neuromuscular, Proprioception Training	Cryotherapy	Tests
Criteria AROM 0°–115°. Quadriceps strength > 60% contralateral side (isometric test, 60° flexion). KT < 3 mm Minimal to no joint effusion. No joint line, patellofemoral pain. **Goals** Restore full ROM (0°–125°). Improve lower extremity strength. Enhance proprioception, balance, neuromuscular control. Improve muscular endurance. Restore limb confidence and function.	No brace, may use knee sleeve to control swelling, support. ROM four to five times daily using the opposite leg. PROM: 0°–125° wk 4.	**Weeks 4–5:** Progress isometric strengthening. Leg press 0°–100°. Hamstring curls (isotonics). Hip abduction, adduction, flexion, extension. Lateral step-overs. Lateral lunges, straight plane, multiplane. Lateral step-ups. Front step-downs. Wall-squats. Vertical squats. Standing toe-calf-raises. Seated toe-calf-raises. Bicycle. Biodex Stability System (balance, squats). Stair-stepper machine. Pool program (backward running, hip and leg exercises)	**Weeks 4–5:** Tilt-board squats (perturbation). Passive/active reposition OKC. CKC repositioning on tilt-board with sports RAC **Week 6: add** Balance on tilt-board. Progress to balance and ball throws. **Week 8: add** plyometric leg press. Perturbation training.	Ice, compression, elevation.	**Week 4:** KT, 20 lb total AP **Weeks 6 and 8:** KT 30 lb, total AP

Week 6: add
Pool-running forward, agility drills.
Wall-slides/-squats

Week 8: add leg press sets, single leg;
0°–100°, 40°–100°
Isokinetic exercises 90°–40°
(120°/sec–240°/sec)
Walking program

Advanced Activity Phase (Weeks 10–16)

Criteria to Progress and Goals	Exercises	Neuromuscular, Proprioception Training	Tests

Criteria
AROM ≥ 0°–125°
Quadriceps strength 75% of contralateral side, knee extension flexor/extensor ratio 70%–75%.
No change in KT values, <3 mm over opposite side.
No pain, effusion.
Satisfactory clinical examination.
Isokinetic test:
  Quadriceps bilateral comparison 75% (180°/sec).
  Hamstrings equal bilateral.
  Quadriceps peak torque/BW 65% at 180°/sec (males), 55% at 180°/sec (females).
Hop test 80% of contralateral leg.
Subjective knee score (modified Cincinnati Knee Rating System) ≥ 80 points.
 	
Goals
Normalize lower extremity strength.
Enhance muscular power, endurance.
Improve neuromuscular control.
Perform selected sports-specific drills.
	Week 10:
	Running program (wk 10–12).
	Light sports program (golf).
	Continue strengthening drills
	  Leg press
	  Wall-squats
	  Hip abduction/adduction
	  Hip flexion/extension
	  Knee extension 90°–40°
	  Hamstring curls
	  Standing toe-calf
	  Seated toe-calf
	  Step-downs
	  Lateral step-ups
	  Lateral lunges
	
	Weeks 14–16:
	Initiate lateral agility drills, backward running.
		Week 10:
		Lateral step-overs (cones).
		Lateral lunges.
		Tilt-board drills.
		Sports RAC repositioning on tilt-board.
			Week 10:
			KT-2000 30 lb, manual maximum.
			Isokinetic test: Concentric knee extension, flexion 180°/sec, 300°/sec.

TABLE 14–2   Rehabilitation after Anterior Cruciate Ligament Bone–Patellar Tendon–Bone Reconstruction—Cont'd

Criteria to Progress and Goals	Return to Activity Phase (Weeks 16–22)		
	Exercises	Neuromuscular, Proprioception Training	Tests

Criteria
Full ROM
No change in KT values, <3 mm over opposite side.
Isokinetic test:
  Quadriceps bilateral comparison ≥ 80%.
  Hamstrings bilateral comparison ≥ 110%.
  Quadriceps torque/BW ratio ≥ 55%
  Hamstring/quadriceps ratio ≥ 70%.
Proprioceptive test: 100% contralateral side.
Function test: ≥85% contralateral side.
Satisfactory clinical examination.
Subjective knee score (modified Cincinnati Knee Rating System) ≥ 90 points.
 	
Goals
Gradual return to full, unrestricted sports.
Achieve maximal strength, endurance.
Normalize neuromuscular control.
Progress skill training.
	Continue strengthening exercises.
	Progress running, agility program.
	Progress sports-specific training:
	  Running/cutting/agility drills
	  Gradual return to sport drills
		Continue neuromuscular control drills.
		Continue plyometric drills.
			KT 30 lb, manual maximum.
			Isokinetic test.
			Functional tests.
			Repeat 6 mo, 12 mo.

AP, anteroposterior; AROM, active range of motion; BW, body weight; CKC, closed kinetic chain; CPM, continuous passive motion; EMS, electrical muscle stimulation; HE, hyperextension; KT, knee arthrometer; OKC, open kinetic chain; PRE, progressive resistive exercises; PROM, passive range of motion; ROM, range of motion; SLR, straight leg raise.

TABLE 14–3 Ten Key Components to the Neuromuscular-Training Program

1. Immediate stimulation of mechanoreceptors after injury and/or surgery.
2. Stimulation of mechanoreceptors of the contralateral extremity.
3. Facilitate co-contraction to enhance dynamic stability (immediately).
4. Control the knee from above and below (through the hip and foot/ankle).
5. Establish core stability early.
6. Perturbation training to enhance neuromuscular control.
7. Train to improve endurance.
8. Challenge the neuromuscular system.
9. Gradually increase challenges to the neuromuscular system.
10. Neuromuscular training never stops, enhancement continues for years.

Phase III: Neuromuscular Control Drills

The third phase of the neuromuscular-training program implements random designed drills performed in combined functional movement planes. The majority of these drills are designed to combine knee stabilization drills with sports-specific activities and other techniques to create higher levels of functional demands. Perturbation-training drills are initiated on a rocker board. These drills are progressed from bilateral squatting with perturbation (Fig. 14–20), to single-leg holds at 30° of flexion, to single-leg squats from 0° to 45° with holds, to single-leg holds at 30° flexion with a ball-throw/-catch (Fig. 14–21). During these drills, the clinician taps the rocker board or the patient to create a postural disturbance. The patient is instructed to maintain a horizontal platform position and to "right" the board after the perturbation force. The perturbation drills can also be

---

TABLE 14–4 Neuromuscular Control Drills Based on Phases of Recovery

Phase I	Phase II	Phase III	Phase IV
PROM knee flexion/ extension	Lateral lunges:	Single-leg squats with ball-catch and touch-cones	Plyometrics:
Passive/active joint positioning: 90°, 60°, 30°	Cord onto involved side	Lateral lunges:	Side-to-side floor over tape
Standing weight-bearing	Cord onto uninvolved side	Diagonal slight jump	Side-to-side floor four corners
Mini-squats on balance trainer	Cord 30° diagonal	Diagonal slight jump with ball-catch	Side-to-side one box
Weight-shifts on balance trainer	Cord 30° diagonal with rotation	Onto tilt-board (stabilize)	Side-to-side two boxes
Knee sleeve	Straight with ball catches	Onto tilt-board with ball-catch	Scissor jumps floor
EMS to quadriceps	Diagonal with ball catches	Tilt-board DSP with perturbation	Scissor jumps box
Quadriceps sets	Straight foam	Tilt-board DSP with perturbation and ball catch	Skip jumps
SLR flexion	Straight foam with rotation	Tilt board DSP with perturbation and rotational throws	Bounding drills
Hip abduction/ adduction	Straight foam with rotation with ball catch	Biodex squats with perturbation	Perturbation training
Multiangle isometrics 90°, 60°, 30°	Standing up and down with ball (stability position)	Biodex squat with ball-catch	Line-to-line lunges
Leg press 0°–100°	Standing balance position up and down with foam	Lateral lunge onto tremor	Running backward
Leg press 0°–45°	Standing DSP on foam	Lateral lunge onto tremor with ball catch	Running forward
Leg press with balance trainer	Standing single-leg one plyoball touching cones	Front jump lunge onto tremor	Lateral slides
Tilt-board squats	Front step-downs on foam	Front jump lunge onto tremor with ball-catch	Carioca
Cone-stepping	Front step-downs on foam	Front jump lunge onto tremor with taps	Running start/stop
Lateral lunges, no cord	½ circle foam	Side-to-side and up-and-down on tremor ball-catch	Running and cutting (gradual program cutting 30° to advanced 90°)
Biodex squats	Front step-downs on foam with TheraBand	Plyo leg press straight	Progress to sports-specific drills
Quadrant stepping:	Step-down lateral with sport cord around waist	Plyo leg press side-to-side	
Mini-squat on foam	Tilt board balance squats	Plyo leg press four corners	
Mini-squat on air mattress	Squats on rocker board	BOSU ball-squats with ball-catches	
Rubber band around hip walking	Front lunge onto box		
Wall-slides 0°–60° (5- to 7-sec hold)	Front lunge on foam		
	Wall-slides with physioball		
	Single-leg wall-slide		
	Single-leg wall-slides on box		
	Hip external/internal rotation tubing		
	Side-lying clams		
	Intrinsic foot exercise (towel gathering, marbles)		
	TheraBand inversion/eversion		

DSP, dynamic stabilization position; EMS, electrical muscle stimulation; PROM, passive range of motion; SLR, single-leg raise.

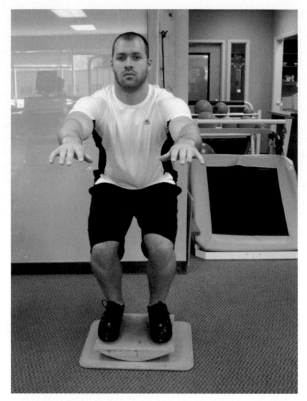

FIGURE 14–6. Mini-squats done from 0° to 40° on an unstable platform so that the patient may learn to distribute weight evenly during the exercise.

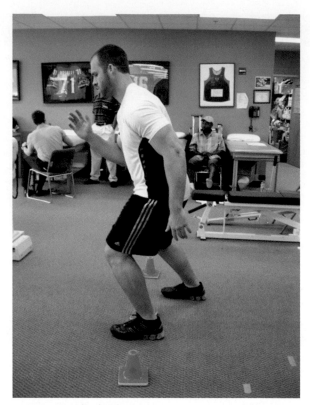

FIGURE 14–8. Lateral cone-walking done in the three-repetition sequence that is employed in the forward and backward cone-walking.

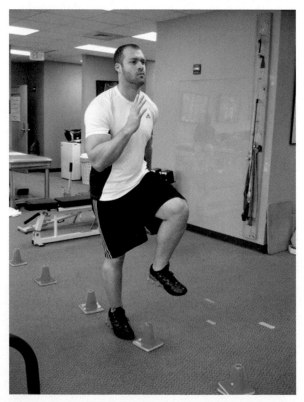

FIGURE 14–7. Forward and backward cone-walking. The patient is instructed to go through the cones three times each way; first, at normal speed; second, at a faster speed; and third, at a slower speed to emphasize knee and hip flexion.

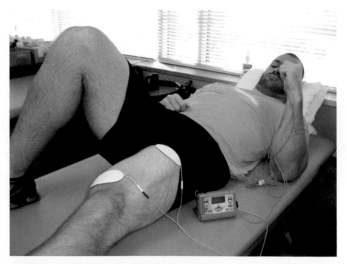

FIGURE 14–9. Neuromuscular stimulation applied to the quadriceps to facilitate a quadriceps muscular contraction (Empi Medical, St. Paul, MN).

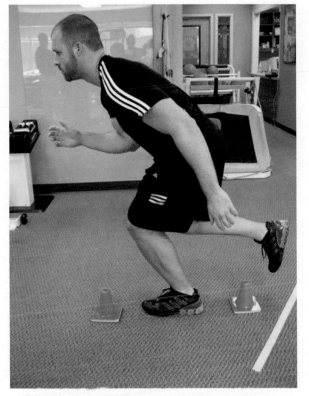

FIGURE 14–10. The desired flexed knee landing during the cone-walking drills. The flexed knee position is ideal for co-contraction of the hamstrings and the quadriceps musculature

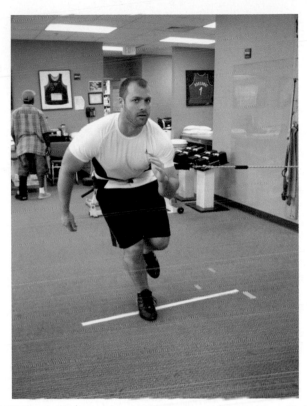

FIGURE 14–12. Lateral lunge performed in a straight plane with the resistance of a sportcord. The goal of this drill is to have the patient land unilaterally and pause in single-leg stance to promote balance and stability.

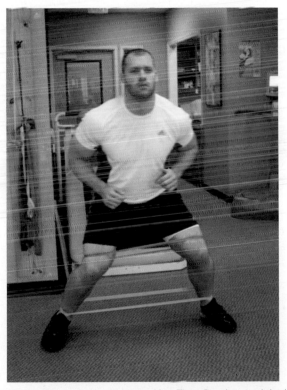

FIGURE 14–11. Ambulation done with a TheraBand around the hips. The TheraBand is used to create a greater contraction of the hip musculature and emphasize stability of the hip muscles to prepare for sports activities.

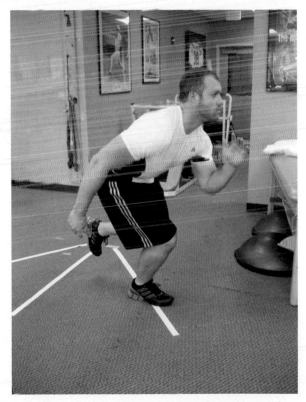

FIGURE 14–13. Sportcord lateral lunges performed in the diagonal plane.

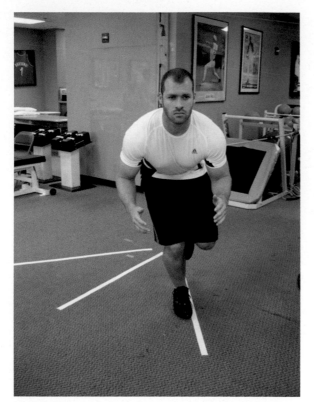

FIGURE 14–14. Sportcord lateral lunges performed with rotation.

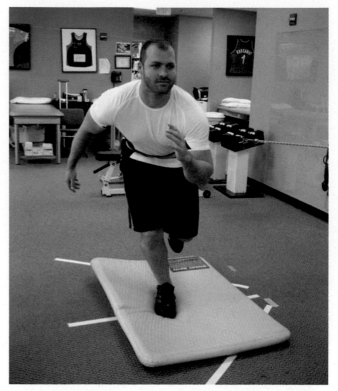

FIGURE 14–16. Sportcord lateral lunges performed onto an air mattress to create an unstable landing surface.

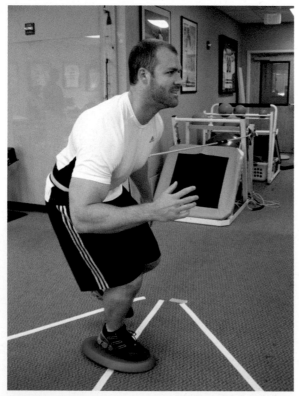

FIGURE 14–15. Sportcord lateral lunges performed onto an unstable surface such as a piece of foam. The air mattress is used to create an unstable surface for landing so that the patient's proprioception is challenged.

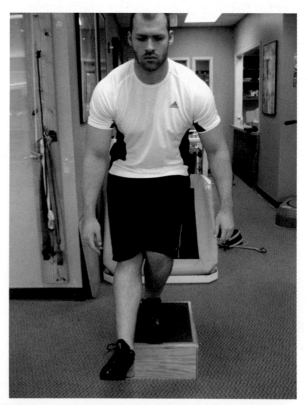

FIGURE 14–17. The front step-down performed on a box. The ability to perform this exercise correlates with the patient's functional level.

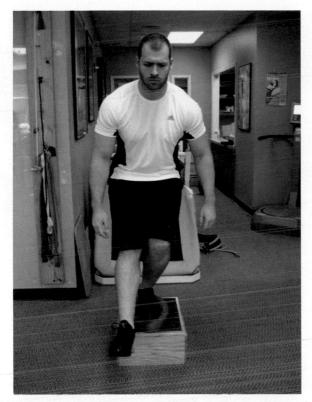

FIGURE 14–18. The front step-down performed with a foam pad underneath the patient's foot to challenge the proprioceptive system. The patient can be additionally challenged by adding a ball toss to the drill to decrease conscious awareness.

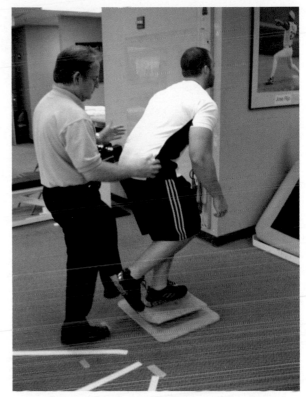

FIGURE 14–20. Mini-squats performed on a tilt board with perturbations. The patient is instructed to keep the board level as the clinician creates a disturbance either by tapping the board with a foot or by tapping the patient at the hips.

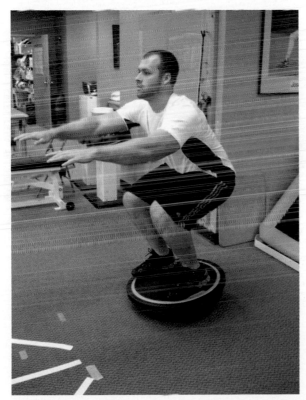

FIGURE 14–19. Mini-squats performed on a BOSU ball. The patient is instructed to perform a mini-squat and hold the position while catching a ball. The patient must hold this position until the ball is thrown back to the clinician.

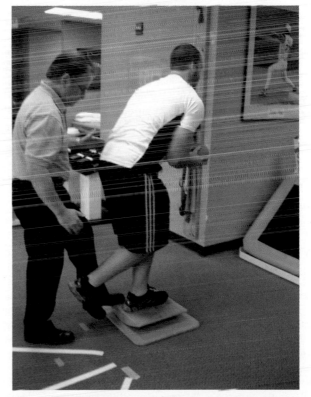

FIGURE 14–21. Single-leg balance holds on a tilt-board with ball toss and perturbations. The patient is instructed to maintain a single-leg stance while throwing a medicine ball into a toss-back trampoline while perturbations are given by the clinician.

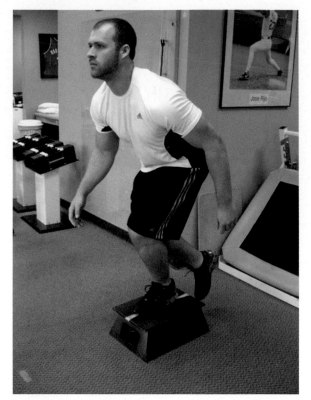

FIGURE 14–22. Lunges performed onto a tremor box device. The patient must lunge forward and land in the center of the platform. The patient is instructed to hold the position for a moment before returning to the starting position. This exercise can also have a ball toss added to increase the challenge.

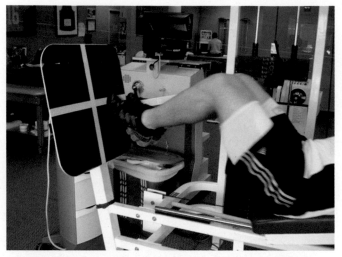

FIGURE 14–23. The four-corner plyometric leg press drill. The patient is told to explode off the platform and land in a different square as marked on the platform. The order of squares can begin with a blocked sequence and can then progress to a random sequence as determined by clinician.

Any problems with technique should result in the rehabilitation professional stopping the drill to both protect the motor skill and promote proper technique. In addition, during this phase, a functional assessment test may be performed to compare one extremity with the other.[2] Barber-Westin and colleagues[3] reported on ACL-reconstructed and normal patients performing the functional hop test.

performed on a Biodex Stability System. Other drills that challenge the neuromuscular system are step lunges onto the tremor device (Fig. 14–22) or a tilt-board. Plyometrics are also initiated in this phase and are performed bilaterally. Leg press plyometrics are initiated before floor-jumping drills, because it is easier to control the patient's body position. A preferred plyometric leg press drill is the four corners (Fig. 14–23), which combines proprioception and coordination.

Phase IV: Functional/Skills

The final phase is the skill and the return to activity phase. During this phase, four types of neuromuscular-training drills are employed: plyometrics, perturbation, technique, and sports-specific progression. The plyometric drills are progressed to jumping on the floor and/or over a cone or hurdle and then to box jumps. These drills include one-box jumps (Fig. 14–24), two-box jumps (Fig. 14–25), and four-box jumps. A running program is initiated with backward running to promote knee flexion and muscle co-activation. Running backward also results in higher electromyographic activity of the quadriceps and hamstrings than that of running forward.[23] From backward running, the patient progresses to side shuffles and cariocas, followed by forward running. Once forward running is achieved with a normal gait pattern, the patient is advanced to running and deceleration drills, and finally to running and cutting. After this progression is mastered, the patient may begin a sports-specific training program. Proper technique is critical during this phase.

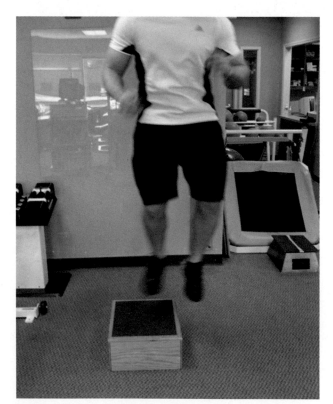

FIGURE 14–24. One-box-jump plyometrics. The patient jumps from the floor to the box and back down while being given cues to land with "quiet feet." This can be done front-to-back or side-to-side.

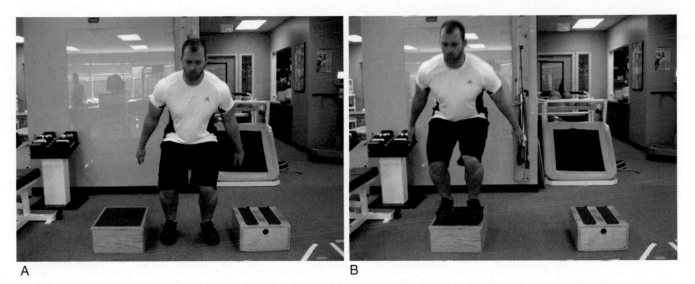

FIGURE 14–25. Two-box-jump plyometrics. **A,** The patient begins between two boxes on the floor. **B,** The patients jumps from the floor laterally to one box, back down to the floor, and then in the opposite direction to the second box. The patient is again instructed to land with "quiet feet."

CONCLUSIONS

After ACL injury, a significant compromise of the static and dynamic stabilization capabilities of the knee joint exists. ACL disruption can lead to changes in the muscular activation pattern of the muscles around the knee joint. After ACL injury or surgery, the rehabilitation program must restore motion, joint stability, and muscular strength and allow regeneration of the ACL graft. In addition, the therapy program must incorporate neuromuscular training to ensure a full functional return to activities without compromise. The neuromuscular system is a vital component to the rehabilitation program of a patient with an ACL injury to the knee.

REFERENCES

1. Andriacchi, T. P.; Birac, D.: Functional testing in the anterior cruciate ligament-deficient knee. *Clin Orthop Relat Res* 288:40–47, 1993.
2. Barber, S. D.; Noyes, F. R.; Mangine, R.; DeMaio, M.: Rehabilitation after ACL reconstruction: function testing. *Orthopedics* 15:969–974, 1992.
3. Barber-Westin, S. D.; Galloway, M.; Noyes, F. R.; et al.: Assessment of lower limb neuromuscular control in prepubescent athletes. *Am J Sports Med* 33:1853–1860, 2005.
4. Barrack, R. L.; Skinner, H. B.; Buckley, S. L.: Proprioception in the anterior cruciate deficient knee. *Am J Sports Med* 17:1–6, 1989.
5. Barrett, D. S.; Cobb, A. G.; Bentley, G.: Joint proprioception in normal, osteoarthritic and replaced knees. *J Bone Joint Surg Br* 73:53–56, 1991.
6. Beard, D. J.; Dodd, C. A. F.; Trundle, H. R.; Simpson, A. H. R. W.: Proprioception enhancement for anterior cruciate ligament deficiency. A prospective randomised trial of two physiotherapy regimes. *J Bone Joint Surg Br* 76:654–659, 1994.
7. Beard, D. J.; Kyberd, P. J.; Fergusson, C. M.; Dodd, C. A. F.: Proprioception after rupture of the anterior cruciate ligament. An objective indication of the need for surgery? *J Bone Joint Surg Br* 75:311–315, 1993.
8. Berchuck, M.; Andriacchi, T. P.; Bach, B. R.; Reider, B.: Gait adaptations by patients who have a deficient anterior cruciate ligament. *J Bone Joint Surg Am* 72:871–877, 1990.
9. Biedert, R. M.: Contribution of the three levels of nervous system motor control: spinal cord, lower brain, cerebral cortex. In Lephart, S., and Fu, F. (eds.): *Proprioception and Neuromuscular Control in Joint Stability*. Champaign, IL: Human Kinetics, 2000; pp. 23–29.
10. Birmingham, T. B.; Kramer, J. F.; Inglis, J. T.; et al.: Effect of a neoprene sleeve on knee joint position sense during sitting open kinetic chain and supine closed kinetic chain tests. *Am J Sports Med* 26:562–566, 1998.
11. Brooks, V. (ed.): *The Neural Basis of Motor Control*. New York: Oxford University Press, 1986.
12. Chmielewski, T.; Hewett, T. E.; Hurd, W. J.: Principles of neuromuscular control for injury prevention and rehabilitation. In Magee, D.; Zachazewski, J. F.; and Quillen, W. S. (eds.): *Scientific Foundations and Principles of Practice in Musculoskeletal Rehabilitation*. St. Louis: Saunders, 2007; pp. 375–387.
13. Chmielewski, T. L.; Hurd, W. J.; Rudolph, K. S.; et al.: Perturbation training improves knee kinematics and reduces muscle co-contraction after complete unilateral anterior cruciate ligament rupture. *Phys Ther* 85:740–749; discussion 750–754, 2005.
14. Chmielewski, T. L.; Rudolph, K. S.; Snyder-Mackler, L.: Development of dynamic knee stability after acute ACL injury. *J Electromyogr Kinesiol* 12:267–274, 2002.
15. Chmielewski, T. L.; Stackhouse, S.; Axe, M. J.; Snyder-Mackler, L.: A prospective analysis of incidence and severity of quadriceps inhibition in a consecutive sample of 100 patients with complete acute anterior cruciate ligament rupture. *J Orthop Res* 22:925–930, 2004.
16. Chmielewski, T. L.; Wilk, K. E.; Snyder-Mackler, L.: Changes in weight-bearing following injury or surgical reconstruction of the ACL: relationship to quadriceps strength and function. *Gait Posture* 16:87–95, 2002.
17. Denti, M.; Randelli, P.; Lo Vetere, D.; et al.: Motor control performance in the lower extremity: normals vs. anterior cruciate ligament reconstructed knees 5–8 years from the index surgery. *Knee Surg Sports Traumatol Arthrosc* 8:296–300, 2000.
18. Di Fabio, R. P.; Graf, B.; Badke, M. B.; et al.: Effect of knee joint laxity on long-loop postural reflexes: evidence for a human capsular-hamstring reflex. *Exp Brain Res* 90:189–200, 1992.
19. Diener, H. C.; Horak, F. B.; Nashner, L. M.: Influence of stimulus parameters on human postural responses. *J Neurophysiol* 59:1888–1905, 1988.
20. Dutton, M.: Neuromuscular control. In Dutton, M. (ed.): *Orthopaedic Examination, Evaluation and Intervention*. New York: McGraw-Hill, 2004; pp. 55–57.

21. Evarts, E. V.: Motor cortex reflexes associated with learned movement. *Science* 179(72):501–503, 1973.
22. Fitzgerald, G. K.; Axe, M. J.; Snyder-Mackler, L.: The efficacy of perturbation training in nonoperative anterior cruciate ligament rehabilitation programs for physical active individuals. *Phys Ther* 80:128–140, 2000.
23. Flynn, T. W.; Soutas-Little, R. W.: Mechanical power and muscle action during forward and backward running. *J Orthop Sports Phys Ther* 17:108–112, 1993.
24. Fremerey, R. W.; Lobenhoffer, P.; Zeichen, J.; et al.: Proprioception after rehabilitation and reconstruction in knees with deficiency of the anterior cruciate ligament. *J Bone Joint Surg Br* 82:801–806, 2000.
25. Harrison, E. L.; Duenkel, N.; Dunlop, R.; Russell, G.: Evaluation of single-leg standing following anterior cruciate ligament surgery and rehabilitation. *Phys Ther* 74:245–252, 1994.
26. Hewett, T. E.; Lindenfeld, T. N.; Riccobene, J. V.; Noyes, F. R.: The effect of neuromuscular training on the incidence of knee injury in female athletes. A prospective study. *Am J Sports Med* 27:699–706, 1999.
27. Hewett, T. E.; Stroupe, A. L.; Nance, T. A.; Noyes, F. R.: Plyometric training in female athletes. Decreased impact forces and increased hamstring torques. *Am J Sports Med* 24:765–773, 1996.
28. Hooks, T. R.; Wilk, K. E.; Reinold, M. M.: Comparison of proprioceptive deficits of the involved and noninvolved lower extremity following ACL injury and surgical reconstruction. *J Orthop Sports Phys Ther* 33:A59, 2003.
29. Houk, J.; Simon, W.: Responses of Golgi tendon organs to forces applied to muscle tendon. *J Neurophysiol* 30:1466–1481, 1967.
30. Hurd, W. J.; Axe, M. J.; Snyder-Mackler, L.: A 10-year prospective trial of a patient management algorithm and screening examination for highly active individuals with anterior cruciate ligament injury: part 2, determinants of dynamic knee stability. *Am J Sports Med* 36:48–56, 2008.
31. Johansson, H.: Role of knee ligaments in proprioception and regulation of muscle stiffness. *J Electromyogr Kinesiol* 1:158–179, 1991.
32. Johansson, H.; Sjolander, P.; Sojka, P.: Receptors in the knee joint ligaments and their role in the biomechanics of the joint. *Crit Rev Biomed Eng* 18:341–368, 1991.
33. Lattanzio, P. J.; Petrella, R. J.; Sproule, J. R.; Fowler, P. J.: Effects of fatigue on knee proprioception. *Clin J Sport Med* 7:22–27, 1997.
34. Lephart, S.; Kocher, M. S.; Fu, F.; et al.: Proprioception following anterior cruciate ligament reconstruction. *J Sport Rehabil* 1:188–196, 1992.
35. Lephart, S. M.; Pincivero, D. M.; Giraldo, J. L.; Fu, F. H.: The role of proprioception in the management and rehabilitation of athletic injuries. *Am J Sports Med* 25:130–137, 1997.
36. Mandelbaum, B. R.; Silvers, H. J.; Watanabe, D. S.; et al.: Effectiveness of a neuromuscular and proprioceptive training program in preventing anterior cruciate ligament injuries in female athletes: 2-year follow-up. *Am J Sports Med* 33:1003–1010, 2005.
37. Matthews, P. B.: Evolving views on the internal operation and functional role of the muscle spindle. *J Physiol* 320:1–30, 1981.
38. Matthews, P. B.: Recent advances in the understanding of the muscle spindle. *Sci Basis Med Annu Rev* 99–128, 1971.
39. Myklebust, G.; Engebretsen, L.; Braekken, I. H.; et al.: Prevention of anterior cruciate ligament injuries in female team handball players: a prospective intervention study over three seasons. *Clin J Sport Med* 13:71–78, 2003.
40. Nashner, L. M.; Shupert, C. L.; Horak, F. B.; Black, F. O.: Organization of posture controls: an analysis of sensory and mechanical constraints. *Prog Brain Res* 80:411–418, 1989.
41. Noyes, F. R.; Berrios-Torres, S.; Barber-Westin, S. D.; Heckmann, T. P.: Prevention of permanent arthrofibrosis after anterior cruciate ligament reconstruction alone or combined with associated procedures: a prospective study in 443 knees. *Knee Surg Sports Traumatol Arthrosc* 8:196–206, 2000.
42. Noyes, F. R.; Mangine, R. E.; Barber, S.: Early knee motion after open and arthroscopic anterior cruciate ligament reconstruction. *Am J Sports Med* 15:149–160, 1987.
43. Nyland, J. A.; Shapiro, R.; Stine, R. L.; et al.: Relationship of fatigued run and rapid stop to ground reaction forces, lower extremity kinematics, and muscle activation. *J Orthop Sports Phys Ther* 20:132–137, 1994.
44. Palmieri-Smith, R. M.; Kreinbrink, J.; Ashton-Miller, J. A.; Wojtys, E. M.: Quadriceps inhibition induced by an experimental knee joint effusion affects knee joint mechanics during a single-legged drop landing. *Am J Sports Med* 35:1269–1275, 2007.
45. Paterno, M. V.; Ford, K. R.; Myer, G. D.; et al.: Limb asymmetries in landing and jumping 2 years following anterior cruciate ligament reconstruction. *Clin J Sport Med* 17:258–262, 2007.
46. Pope, M. H.; Johnson, R. J.; Brown, D. W.: The role of musculature in injuries to the medial collateral ligament. *J Bone Joint Surg Am* 61:398–402, 1979.
47. Roberts, D.; Andersson, G.; Friden, T.: Knee joint proprioception in ACL-deficient knees is related to cartilage injury, laxity and age: a retrospective study of 54 patients. *Acta Orthop Scand* 75:78–83, 2004.
48. Schmidt, R.; Lee, T. (eds.): *Motor Control and Learning: A Behavioral Emphasis.* Champaign, IL: Human Kinetics, 1999.
49. Skinner, H. B.; Wyatt, M. P.; Hodgdon, J. A.; et al.: Effect of fatigue on joint position sense of the knee. *J Orthop Res* 4:112–118, 1986.
50. Snyder-Mackler, L.; Delitto, A.; Bailey, S. L.; Stralka, S. W.: Strength of the quadriceps femoris muscle and functional recovery after reconstruction of the anterior cruciate ligament. A prospective, randomized clinical trial of electrical stimulation. *J Bone Joint Surg Am* 77:1166–1173, 1995.
51. Snyder-Mackler, L.; Ladin, Z.; Schepsis, A. A.; et al.: Electrical stimulation of the thigh muscles after reconstruction of the anterior cruciate ligament. *J Bone Joint Surg Am* 73:1025–1036, 1991.
52. Sullivan, P. E.; Markos, P. D.; Minor, M. A. (eds.): An Integrated Approach to Therapeutic Exercise, Theory, and Clinical Application. Reston, Reston Publishing, 1982; pp. 25–160.
53. Swanik, C. B.; Lephart, S. M.; Giraldo, J. L.; et al.: Reactive muscle firing of anterior cruciate ligament–injured females during functional activities. *J Athl Train* 34:121–129, 1999.
54. Wilk, K. E.: Rehabilitation of isolated and combined posterior cruciate ligament injuries. *Clin Sports Med* 13:649–677, 1994.
55. Wilk, K. E.; Arrigo, C.; Andrews, J. R.; Clancy, W. G.: Rehabilitation after anterior cruciate ligament reconstruction in the female athlete. *J Athl Train* 34:177–193, 1999.
56. Wilk, K. E.; Escamilla, R. F.; Fleisig, G. S.; et al.: A comparison of tibiofemoral joint forces and electromyographic activity during open and closed kinetic chain exercises. *Am J Sports Med* 24:518–527, 1996.
57. Wilk, K. E.; Voight, M. L.; Keirns, M. A.; et al.: Stretch-shortening drills for the upper extremities: theory and clinical application. *J Orthop Sports Phys Ther* 17:225–239, 1993.
58. Williams, G. N.; Chmielewski, T.; Rudolph, K.; et al.: Dynamic knee stability: current theory and implications for clinicians and scientists. *J Orthop Sports Phys Ther* 31:546–566, 2001.
59. Wojtys, E. M.; Huston, L. J.: Neuromuscular performance in normal and anterior cruciate ligament–deficient lower extremities. *Am J Sports Med* 22:89–104, 1994.
60. Wojtys, E. M.; Wylie, B. B.; Huston, L. J.: The effects of muscle fatigue on neuromuscular function and anterior tibial translation in healthy knees. *Am J Sports Med* 24:615–621, 1996.

Gender Disparity in Anterior Cruciate Ligament Injuries

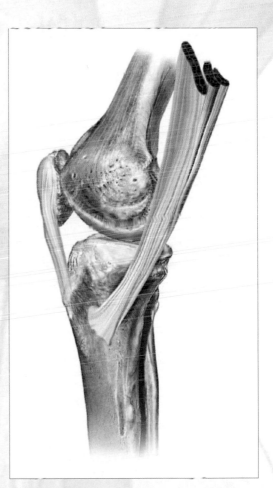

Chapter 15

Risk Factors for Anterior Cruciate Ligament Injuries in the Female Athlete

Sue D. Barber-Westin, BS ▪ *Frank R. Noyes*, MD

INTRODUCTION

The higher incidence of noncontact anterior cruciate ligament (ACL) injuries in female athletes than in male athletes participating in the same sport has received a significant amount of attention in the orthopaedic literature since the early 1990s. A study from the authors' institution published in 1994[63] was one of the first to report this problem, because female soccer players were found to have nearly six times the rate of serious knee ligament injuries than that of male players (0.87 and 0.29/100 player-hr, respectively; $P < .01$). The following year, Arendt and Dick[6] presented data from the National Collegiate Athletic Association (NCAA) of injuries sustained by soccer and basketball players over a 5-year period. The ACL injury rate in females was more than double that of males in soccer (0.31 and 0.13/1000 exposures, respectively; $P < .05$) and four times that of males in basketball (0.29 and 0.07/1000 exposures;

Critical Points INTRODUCTION

Higher incidence of noncontact ACL injuries in female athletes compared with male athletes participating in the same sport is well documented.

Definitive conclusions cannot currently be reached for either males or females regarding what factor(s) may predispose an athlete to an ACL rupture.

Reasons for the gender disparity in noncontact ACL injuries cannot be scientifically defined at present.

Majority of studies published to date have either examined a very small sample size of each gender, focused on only one possible risk category, or examined neuromuscular characteristics in a controlled laboratory environment instead of reactive or actual playing conditions.

ACL, anterior cruciate ligament.

respectively, $P < .05$). Messina and coworkers[70] reported that female high school basketball players had nearly four times the incidence of ACL injuries than male players (0.091 and 0.024/1000 player-hr, respectively; $P < .05$). Gwinn and associates[43] evaluated the incidence of ACL injuries in midshipmen at the U.S. Naval Academy over a 6-year period. These authors reported that women had a fourfold increase in this injury compared with men in intercollegiate soccer, basketball, and rugby collectively (0.511 and 0.129/1000 athlete-exposures, respectively; $P = .006$). During military training, women had nearly 11 times the incidence of ACL ruptures as men during obstacle course running (6.154 and 0.567/1000 athlete-exposures, respectively; $P = .004$). Agel and colleagues[1] reviewed 13 years of NCAA injury data and reported a continued gender disparity in ACL injury rates between collegiate female and male basketball and soccer players.

Despite the multitude of investigations that have been conducted on potential risk factors for noncontact ACL ruptures, definitive conclusions cannot currently be reached for either males or females regarding what factor(s) may predispose an athlete to this injury. In addition, the reasons for the increased incidence of this injury in female athletes over that in male athletes cannot be scientifically defined at present. The problems are that the majority of studies published to date have either examined a very small sample size of each gender (therefore containing insufficient power to avoid a type II statistical error[40]), focused on only one possible risk category, or examined neuromuscular characteristics in a controlled laboratory environment instead of actual playing conditions. The potential risk factors that have been proposed for this injury are shown in Table 15–1.

TABLE 15–1 Hypothesized Major Risk Factors for Anterior Cruciate Ligament Injury

Gender	Category	Risk Factor
Males and females	Familial	Genetics, possibly related to anatomic structures (size intercondylar notch)
Males and females	Environmental	Climate conditions Playing surface Footwear Interaction of footwear with playing surface Prophylactic knee braces
Females	Anatomic	Q-angle Size and shape of the intercondylar notch Size of the ACL Material properties of the ACL Foot pronation Body mass index Generalized ligament laxity
Females	Hormonal	Acute fluctuations of estrogen and progesterone during the menstrual cycle
Females	Neuromuscular/biomechanical	Movement and muscle activation patterns Ground reaction forces Knee adduction/abduction moments Knee and hip flexion angles during landing, jumping, cutting, pivoting Muscle strength Knee joint stiffness (see also Table 15–3)

ACL, anterior cruciate ligament.

This chapter reviews investigations related to these risk factors and emphasizes findings that may have a role in the gender disparity in noncontact ACL injury rates. Opinions expressed by scientists and researchers from the 2005 Hunt Valley II Meeting (sponsored by the American Orthopaedic Society for Sports Medicine [AOSSM])[41] regarding this problem are also provided in each major risk factor section as well as consensus statements generated from this meeting.

GENETIC PREDISPOSITION

Although the question has been raised for many years of a potential genetic predisposition for ACL rupture, only two studies have been published regarding this risk factor. Harner and coworkers[44] investigated familial and anatomic risk factors in a small series of 31 patients who had sustained noncontact bilateral ACL ruptures. Compared with a control group matched for age, sex, height, weight, and activity level, the patients demonstrated a significant difference in the incident rate of immediate family members who had sustained an ACL injury (35% and 4%, respectively; $P < .01$) and a significantly wider lateral femoral condyle (3.30 and 3.10 cm, respectively; $P < .05$). The authors concluded that there could have been a congenital predisposition to ACL injury that theoretically resulted from anatomic differences in the size of the femoral condyles.

Flynn and associates[34] conducted a questionnaire-based study of 171 patients who sustained either contact or noncontact ACL ruptures to determine whether a familial predisposition existed for this injury. The patients were matched with 171 uninjured control subjects according to age, gender, and primary sport. The data were not sorted according to mechanism of ACL rupture (contact vs. noncontact). The survey results revealed that patients who had sustained ACL ruptures were twice as likely to have a first-, second-, or third-degree relative who also had an ACL tear than the control subjects. Limitations of the study include those associated with recall of injury by the patients of their relatives' medical history and no medical documentation of the relatives' ACL ruptures.

AOSSM Consensus and Opinion

Owing to the paucity of published data, no conclusion or consensus was reached regarding genetic predisposition as a risk factor for noncontact ACL injuries by the Hunt Valley II Meeting participants.[41]

Critical Points GENETIC PREDISPOSITION

One study reported that, compared with a control group, patients with ACL ruptures demonstrated a significant difference in the incident rate of immediate family members who had sustained an ACL injury and a significantly wider lateral femoral condyle.

One study reported that patients who had sustained ACL ruptures were twice as likely to have a first-, second-, or third-degree relative who also had an ACL tear than control subjects.

AOSSM Consensus: No conclusion or consensus has been reached regarding genetic predisposition as a risk factor for noncontact ACL injuries owing to lack of data.

AOSSM, American Orthopaedic Society for Sports Medicine.

ENVIRONMENTAL

Climate Conditions

Few studies have been conducted to determine the effect of climate conditions, such as rainfall, heat, and humidity, on noncontact ACL injuries. In addition, no investigation to date has taken into account other risk factors (such as hormonal or neuromuscular) along with climate conditions that could confound possible conclusions. Orchard and colleagues[82] examined intrinsic (height, weight, age, body mass index (BMI), history of prior ACL injury) and environmental-related variables as risk factors for noncontact ACL injuries in male Australian football players. The incidence of noncontact ACL injuries in the 1643 players was 0.62 per 1000 athlete-exposures. The most significant risk factors were a history of a prior ACL injury and weather conditions (high evaporation and low rainfall) that resulted in a dry playing surface. The theories that high shoe-surface traction was a risk factor for noncontact ACL injury and that dry playing conditions increased friction and torsional resistance between shoes and natural grass were advanced by the authors. Of note was the higher incidence of all ACL injuries in this group (0.82/1000 athlete-exposures) compared with previously published data of American football players (0.25/100 athlete-exposures[93]) and American collegiate soccer male players (0.12/1000 athlete-exposures[7]). The authors attributed this difference to the prevailing climatic conditions in Australia, which commonly produced dry, hard ground conditions.

Playing Surface

Meyers and Barnhill[71] tracked male high school football injuries sustained in eight schools over 5 seasons. The rate of ACL injuries was nearly 50% higher on natural grass than on artificial turf (FieldTurf); however, a total of only 15 ACL ruptures were sustained in the 240 games surveyed. Olsen and coworkers[81] examined ACL injury rates in both men and women team handball players to determine whether an association existed between injury rates and two types of floor surfaces. Over a period of seven seasons (94,136 player-hr), the ACL injury rates were 0.24 per 1000 player-hours for men and 0.77 per 1000

player-hours for women ($P = .001$). The ACL injury rate for women was higher on artificial floors than that of women playing on wooden floors (0.96 and 0.41/1000 player-hr, respectively; $P = .03$). There was no difference in the ACL injury rate between floor surface types in the male players and there was no difference between genders in ACL injury rates on wooden floors. Unfortunately, the investigators had to eliminate two thirds of all ACL injuries that were incurred in the study group owing to unreliable floor-type exposure data.

Footwear

Lambson and associates[58] evaluated the effect of football cleat design on ACL injury rates (contact and noncontact) in 3119 high school football players who were followed for 3 seasons. A total of 42 ACL ruptures were recorded in this study. Shoes with long, irregular cleat designs produced significantly higher torsional resistance ($P < .05$) on both artificial and natural playing surfaces than the other cleat designs studied and were also associated with a significantly higher rate of ACL injuries ($P = .0062$). Whereas the authors recognized that many potential risk factors were not analyzed, they recommended that the long, irregular cleat design be discontinued in high school football players. The effect of footwear on ACL injuries in female athletes has not been investigated to date.

Prophylactic Knee Braces

No study to date has demonstrated that knee braces significantly reduce the incidence of ACL injuries in normal healthy athletes.[76] Only two epidemiologic investigations were published in the 1990s on this topic, both of which followed only male football players. Sitler and colleagues[102] conducted an investigation involving 1396 U.S. Military Academy cadets who played intramural tackle football and in whom the type of shoe, athlete exposure, brace compliance, playing surface, and knee injury history were controlled. The brace was a double-hinged, single, upright, off-the-shelf design (DonJoy, Inc., Carlsbad, CA) that was randomly assigned to players at the beginning of each of the 2 seasons surveyed. A statistically greater number of medial collateral ligament (MCL) injuries occurred in the control group than in the braced group ($P < .05$). Although a higher number of ACL injuries was found in the control group than in the braced group (12 vs. 4), the small number precluded statistical analysis. The second epidemiologic investigation published in this time period assessed only MCL injury patterns.[2]

AOSSM Consensus and Opinion

The Hunt Valley II Meeting participants concluded that data reported to date regarding environmental risk factors for ACL noncontact injuries has been "confusing and mixed."[41] The researchers did conclude that shoe-surface interaction may affect ACL injury risk both directly and indirectly.[41] The direct effect is through higher traction, which may transmit excessive load forces to the knee during cutting and pivoting. The indirect effect is through alterations in neuromuscular movement patterns in an attempt to adapt to variations in shoe and surface factors. Future studies examining the potential impact of these factors should include both intrinsic and extrinsic variables and use sound epidemiologic study design.

Critical Points ENVIRONMENTAL RISK FACTORS

Few studies have been conducted to determine the effect of environmental risk factors on noncontact ACL injuries.

High evaporation and low rainfall rates (which resulted in a dry playing surface) were found to be significant risk factors in one study. Authors hypothesized that
- High shoe-surface traction was a risk factor for noncontact ACL injury.
- Dry playing conditions increased friction and torsional resistance between shoes and natural grass.

ACL injury rate for women was higher on artificial floors than on wooden floors in one study.

Effect of footwear on ACL injury rates has not yet been studied in women.

No study to date has demonstrated that knee braces significantly reduce the incidence of ACL injuries in normal healthy athletes.

AOSSM Consensus: Shoe-surface interaction may affect ACL injury risk both directly and indirectly.

ANATOMIC

Many authors have proposed that inherent structural differences between genders are responsible or partially responsible for the disparity in noncontact ACL injury rates between genders. Although evidence exists to support differences between men and women in many of these factors including quadriceps femoris angle (Q-angle), femoral anteversion, tibial torsion, foot pronation, intercondylar notch size, and ACL size, no investigation has demonstrated that these differences alone are responsible for an increased risk of noncontact ACL injuries in female athletes.

Intercondylar Notch and ACL Size

An association between a small-sized intercondylar notch and an increased incidence of ACL ruptures has been reported or suggested by some authors,[5,36,50,59,67,97,105] but refuted by others.[47,65,92,108] The association, which remains debatable, has been reported by some investigators to be present in both genders.[41,54,97] A general speculation has been raised by some authors[41] that a small-sized notch will contain a small-sized ACL that is vulnerable to rupture owing to decreased strength properties. Variations in techniques used to determine notch size (plain non–weight-bearing and weight-bearing radiographs, magnetic resonance imaging [MRI], computed tomography [CT], photographic techniques), problems and lack of standardization with these techniques (such as uncontrolled knee flexion angles and rotation on radiographs), discrepancies in notch indices studied (lateral condylar width, total condylar width, notch width, notch width at two thirds notch height, notch width index, notch angle), and differences in statistical methods used to ascertain measurements account for the disagreement

---

Critical Points ANATOMIC RISK FACTORS

Hypothesis: Small-sized notch contains a small ACL that is vulnerable to rupture owing to decreased strength properties.

West Point study: Factors of narrow femoral notch, body mass index 1 SD or more above the mean, and generalized joint laxity correctly predicted 75% (6 of 8) of the noncontact ACL injuries in females.

Association between small-sized intercondylar notch and an increased incidence of ACL ruptures is not clear, published data are mixed owing to differences in study designs.

Size of the ACL cannot be reliably predicted from the size of the intercondylar notch.

Hypothesis: Excessive subtalar joint pronation leads to increased internal tibial rotation and resultant high forces on the ACL.

- Significantly higher navicular drop values bilaterally exist in patients with ACL ruptures compared with matched control subjects reported in two studies.
- Static measurements of pronation may not be representative of dynamic conditions.

No evidence exists to support that an excessive body mass index alone is a risk factor for noncontact ACL injuries.

No evidence exists that an increase in generalized ligament laxity in females is associated with the increased rate of noncontact ACL injuries.

AOSSM Consensus: No definite evidence exists that any anatomic factor is reliably associated across age groups and sexes with an increased rate of injury based on the amount of conflicting published data and variety of study designs.

---

among studies. The major problem is that no study to date has entered anatomic indices along with hormonal and neuromuscular factors into an appropriate statistical model to determine the effects of all of these potentially important risk factors.

Uhorchak and coworkers,[109] in the most comprehensive ACL risk factor study published to date, measured height, weight, BMI, condylar width, notch width, eminence width, tibial width, notch width index, generalized joint laxity, anteroposterior (AP) displacement on KT-2000 testing, isokinetic quadriceps and hamstrings concentric and eccentric strength, and hamstrings flexibility in a group of 895 West Point cadets (120 women, 739 men) upon their entrance into the academy. The cadets were followed for 4 years for ACL injuries, during which time 24 noncontact ACL ruptures occurred (16 in men, 8 in women). Using a hypothesis-driven logistic regression model, the factors of a narrow femoral notch, BMI 1 standard deviation (SD) or more above the mean, and generalized joint laxity explained 62.5% of the variability of the noncontact ACL tears in the female athletes. In addition, this model correctly predicted 75% (6 of 8) of the noncontact ACL injuries. The most predictive model in the men explained only 15% of the variability in the noncontact ACL injuries and was unable to predict any of the 16 injuries that occurred throughout the study period in the male athletes.

The shape of the intercondylar notch varies,[53] but this does not appear to be useful in predicting patients who may have an increased risk for ACL injury.[5,54,106] In addition, the size of the ACL cannot be reliably predicted from the size of the intercondylar notch.[4,75,106] A few investigators have attempted to determine whether a gender difference exists in the cross-sectional area, mass, and volume of the ACL in uninjured subjects using MRI[4,18,23,106] and in cadaveric specimens.[14,75] Charlton and associates[18] reported that, although a difference existed between uninjured men and women in the volume of the femoral notch and ACL, this difference was related to height and weight and not gender. Patients with smaller notches also had smaller ACLs. Anderson and colleagues[4] found no difference between male and female high school basketball players in the notch width index or in the size of the ACL when normalized for lean body weight (body weight x [100 – % body fat]). When adjusted for body weight, the mean ACL area was significantly greater in the male players ($P < .003$). There was a correlation of ACL area to height in the male players ($P = .03$) but not in the female players. Taller male players had large ACLs, but taller female players had ACLs of a size similar to that of shorter female players. The authors concluded from their data that the cause of ACL rupture in patients with narrow notches was not due to a smaller (more vulnerable) ligament, but to a normal-sized ACL in a stenotic notch. This finding supported that previously described by Muneta and coworkers[75] who, in a cadaveric study, found no correlation between the size of the intercondylar notch and that of the ACL.

Staeubli and associates[106] measured the widths of the cruciate ligaments and intercondylar notches in 51 uninjured subjects with MRI. The notch measurements were performed in three areas in the coronal plane: at the notch entrance, at the intersection of the cruciate ligaments, and at the notch outlet. The authors reported a significant difference between genders in the absolute width of the ACL at the cruciate intersection (men, 6.1 ± 1.1 mm, and women, 5.2 ± 1.0 mm; $P < .01$). The intercondylar notch widths were also significantly greater in males, as were height, weight, and bicondylar femoral width. The ACL and notch size measurements were not normalized for these variables. The ACL occupied only 31.9% of the notch in men and 31.1% of the notch in women, refuting the belief that the size and shape of the notch lead to an increased risk of ACL injury.

Chandrashekar and colleagues[14] studied the length, area, mass, and volume of the ACL in 20 cadaveric knees (10 males, 10 females, aged 17–50 yr) using a photographic three-dimensional scanning system. The male specimens had significantly larger values than the females for ACL length (29.82 mm ± 2.51 and 26.85 ± 2.82 mm, respectively; $P = .01$), mid-substance area (83.54 ± 24.89 mm^2 and 58.29 ± 15.32 mm^2, respectively; $P = .007$), mass (2.04 ± 0.26 g and 1.58 ± 0.42 g, respectively; $P = .009$), and volume (2967 ± 886 mm^3 and 1954 ± 516 mm^3, respectively; $P = .003$). There were no significant differences between genders in ACL mass density, notch width, or notch width index. ACL cross-sectional area and volume were not associated with body height or lean body mass in either gender. ACL mass strongly correlated with height in men ($R = 0.7$; $P < .02$), but not in women ($R = 0.43$; $P \geq .02$). The authors concluded that because the density of the ACL is similar between genders, the smaller ligament size in women may contribute to their increased rate of noncontact ACL rupture.

Foot Pronation

Excessive foot pronation has been suggested as a potential risk factor for ACL injuries.[3,9,66,115] Some authors have speculated that excessive subtalar joint pronation leads to increased internal tibial rotation and resultant high forces on the ACL. Two investigations involving small sample sizes reported significantly higher navicular drop values bilaterally in patients who sustained ACL ruptures compared with matched control subjects.[3,9] Allen and Glasoe[3] measured navicular drop in 18 subjects who had sustained ACL ruptures using a Metrecom three-dimensional digitizer. When compared with an age- and gender-matched control group, the mean values of the navicular drop of both the ACL-ruptured and the contralateral limbs of the patients were significantly larger than those in the control group ($P < .05$) by approximately 2 mm. No other risk factors were included in this investigation. Woodford-Rogers and coworkers[115] measured navicular drop, calcaneal alignment, and anterior tibial translation in the uninjured limb of 22 high school and collegiate athletes (14 males, 8 females) who had sustained noncontact ACL injuries. The data were compared with those of athletes matched by sport, team, position, and level of competition. The authors reported that the ACL-injured athletes had greater amounts of navicular drop of approximately 2.5 mm in the male subjects and 2 mm in the female subjects. Discriminant analysis of the data showed that navicular drop, calcaneal alignment, and anterior tibial translation (when combined) were predictors of classification of athletes into the ACL-injured and the ACL-noninjured groups, because 87.5% of the athletes were correctly classified (chi-square, 9.00; $P < .01$). Both of these studies suggested that excessive pronation may lead to an increased risk of ACL rupture.

A combination of postural "faults" was found to have a greater predictive value for ACL injury than a single problem (such as excessive pronation) by Loudon and associates.[66] In 20 female athletes with unilateral ACL ruptures, the combination of excessive knee hyperextension, navicular drop, and subtalar joint pronation was a strong discriminator between the patients and 20 control subjects. The authors concluded that

an association existed between noncontact ACL injuries in females who had a standing posture of genu recurvatum and subtalar joint overpronation.

Smith and colleagues[104] failed to find an association between excessive pronation and noncontact ACL injuries. The authors used a combination of navicular drop and calcaneal stance measures in 14 patients with ACL ruptures and compared the data with those of 14 control subjects matched for age, height, and weight. There was no significant difference in the navicular drop test between the patients and the controls. The authors cautioned that static measurements of pronation may not be representative of dynamic conditions and that future research should include not only dynamic analyses but other anatomic risk factors as well.

BMI

There is no evidence to support that an excessive BMI alone is a risk factor for noncontact ACL injuries. Ostenberg and Roos[83] found that BMI was not a risk factor for knee injuries in female soccer players, as did Knapik and coworkers[56] in military training–related injuries in female recruits. When combined with a narrow femoral notch and generalized joint laxity, a BMI greater than 1 SD above the mean did contribute to a high prediction of noncontact ACL injuries in Uhorchak and coworkers' series.[109]

Generalized Ligament Laxity

Some authors have reported that females appear to have greater inherent joint laxity than males.[12,60,88–90] Huston and Wojtys[52] reported that females had significantly greater anterior tibial translation than males (6.5 and 5.8 mm, respectively; $P < .05$), as did Rozzi and associates[90] (6.05 ± 1.46 mm and 4.80 ± 1.53 mm, respectively; $P = .02$). Seckin and colleagues[94] reported a significantly greater prevalence of generalized joint hypermobility in female high school students than in male students (16.2% and 7.2%, respectively; $P < .0001$). Remvig and coworkers[88] found considerable evidence in the literature of an increased prevalence of hypermobility among women. However, there is no evidence that an increase in generalized ligament laxity in females is associated with the increased rate of noncontact ACL injuries.

AOSSM Consensus and Opinion

The Hunt Valley II Meeting participants concluded that "there is no definite evidence that any anatomical factor is reliably associated across age groups and sexes with an increased rate of injury" based on the amount of conflicting published data and variety of study designs.[41]

HORMONAL

Sex Hormones in Human ACLs

Since the early 2000s, the hypothesis that fluctuations in sex hormones during certain periods of the menstrual cycle could be deleterious to the material and mechanical properties of the female ACL has been raised by several investigators. Some postulated that these harmful effects could explain the heightened risk of ACL ruptures in female athletes,[53] although a recent investigation on a synomolgus monkey model showed no direct effects of estrogen on ACL mechanical or material properties.[110] Estrogen and progesterone have been shown to significantly alter the structure and metabolism of collagen in human and animal models.[98] Other authors have raised the question of whether hormonal surges could have a deleterious effect on muscle and neuromuscular indices, thereby increasing the vulnerability of the ACL to rupture during certain phases of the menstrual cycle.[13]

In 1996, Liu and associates[64] conducted the first investigation to determine whether estrogen and progesterone target cells were located within the human ACL. Seventeen ACL specimens were obtained from patients undergoing a variety of surgical procedures, 13 from women and 4 from men. Both hormone receptors were found in the ACL fibroblasts, which led the authors to suggest that female sex hormones may have an effect on the ligament's structure and composition.

A few years later, Yu and colleagues[117] conducted an analysis of the effects of estrogen on human ACL fibroblast proliferation and procollagen synthesis. An ACL sample was obtained from a 32-year-old female patient undergoing a total knee replacement. A dose-dependent effect of estrogen was demonstrated, because the proliferation of ACL fibroblasts decreased as estrogen concentration was increased. This effect was most striking in the early periods of hormone exposure (days 1 and 3 after administration) and became less pronounced with time. In addition, a dose-dependent effect was found with type I procollagen synthesis, which decreased with increased estrogen concentration. Type I collagen is associated with mechanical strength of connective tissues.

In a second investigation, Yu and coworkers[118] studied the effects of varying levels of estrogen and progesterone on human ACL fibroblast proliferation and procollagen synthesis. Cell lines were obtained from ligaments in two young female patients. The authors reported that estrogen had a dominant

inhibitory effect on human ACL fibroblast proliferation and type I procollagen synthesis and that progesterone reduced this effect. A dose-dependent increase in ACL fibroblast proliferation and type I procollagen synthesis occurred when progesterone concentration was increased and estrogen concentration held constant. The dose-dependent effects of progesterone were more pronounced at lower levels of estrogen concentration than at higher levels. The authors concluded from these investigations that the acute hormonal fluctuations that occur during the menstrual cycle may induce changes in the metabolism of the ACL, weakening the ligament's strength and increasing its vulnerability to injury.

Faryniarz and associates[31] measured estrogen and relaxin receptors from resected ACL specimens in eight women and seven men an average of approximately 5 weeks after their injury. Whereas there was no significant difference between genders in the concentration of estrogen receptors in ACL cells, women had higher levels of relaxin-binding sites. The authors concluded that estrogen alone may not play a role in the gender disparity in noncontact ACL injury rates. However, their data were considered preliminary and the authors remarked that subtle differences between genders in estrogen concentration in human ACLs may be detected in a study with a larger sample size.

Influence of Sex Hormones on AP Tibial Translation

Several investigators have measured fluctuations in AP tibial displacement measured with a KT-2000 throughout the menstrual cycle.[12,27,45,98,99] Heitz and colleagues[45] followed seven active women aged 21 to 32 years with serial radioimmunoassay procedures to determine levels of estrogen and progesterone throughout a 28- to 30-day menstrual cycle. The subjects' hormone levels and AP tibial displacement were measured on days 1, 10, 11, 12, 13, 20, 21, 22, and 23 of the menstrual cycle. Day 1 corresponded to the ovulatory phase; days 10 to 13, to the follicular phase (peak estrogen surge); and days 20 to 23, to the luteal phase (peak progesterone surge). Statistically significant increases in AP displacement (at 134 N) were reported between day 1 and the follicular phase (5.6 ± 1.34 mm and 6.4 ± 1.64 mm, respectively; $P < .05$) and between day 1 and the luteal phase (5.6 ± 1.34 mm and 7.0 ± 1.66 mm, respectively; $P = .006$).

Deie and coworkers[27] followed 16 women aged 21 to 23 years with serial measurements of AP displacement, basal body temperature, and serum levels of estrogen and progesterone obtained two to three times per week over 4 consecutive weeks. The authors reported statistically significant increases in AP displacement between the follicular and the ovulatory phases (4.7 ± 0.8 mm and 5.3 ± 0.7 mm, respectively; $P < .05$) and between the follicular and the luteal phases (4.7 ± 0.8 mm and 5.2 ± 0.7 mm, respectively; $P < .05$). However, the differences in AP displacement are relatively small and of questionable clinical significance.

Shultz and associates[98] conducted a rigorous investigation on 22 women aged 18 to 30 years in which daily tests were conducted to determine levels of estrogen, progesterone, and testosterone, as well as anterior tibial displacement, over one complete menstrual cycle. The authors reported that interaction of all three hormones explained 63% of the variance in anterior tibial translation. However, considerable variability was reported between subjects regarding the contribution of each hormone separately and all three collectively and in the associated time delay in which the change in anterior tibial displacement was detected after a hormonal surge. In addition, not all subjects demonstrated an increase in anterior tibial displacement; whereas some women had 4- to 5-mm differences across the cycle, others had little to no change.

In a second study, Shultz and colleagues[99] compared the anterior tibial translation values of 22 female subjects collected daily over the course of one complete menstrual cycle with those of 20 males who were tested once per week for 4 weeks. The women underwent daily tests to determine the levels of estrogen, progesterone, and testosterone. The female subjects had significantly greater anterior tibial translation than the male subjects ($P < .05$) over the study period. However, these measurements varied daily and appeared to occur on days in which estrogen and progesterone levels were significantly elevated (early luteal phase). The authors stressed that it remains unknown whether the differences in knee joint laxity between genders accounts for the increased risk of ACL injury in females.

Beynnon and coworkers[12] compared AP tibial translation values between 17 healthy women aged 17 to 29 years collected at five time periods (early follicular, late follicular, midluteal, late luteal during one menstrual cycle, and early follicular of the next cycle) with measurements obtained from 17 male control subjects aged 18 to 31 years. The females had significantly greater AP values ($P = .01$) at each time period. There was no significant difference within the female subjects in AP translation over time.

Association between Phases of the Menstrual Cycle and ACL Ruptures

In three investigations, hormone levels were measured after ACL ruptures in a total of 144 female athletes to determine whether an association existed between the incidence of this injury and a phase of the cycle.[13,103,112] Wojtys and associates[112] measured estrogen, progesterone, and luteinizing hormone metabolites in the urine of 65 female athletes within 24 hours of their ACL injury and at the start of their next menstrual cycle. The luteinizing hormone, identifiable by serum or urine specimens, determines when ovulation occurs and allows accurate identification of the follicular and luteal phases. Fifty-one of the women did not use oral contraceptives; in these subjects, significantly more ACL ruptures occurred during the ovulatory phase than expected (>2.5 times), and fewer injuries occurred during the luteal phase than expected (Table 15-2). Fourteen women were taking oral contraceptives; in this subgroup, there was no significant association found between the phase of the cycle and the incidence of ACL rupture. However, the number of subjects taking oral contraceptives was too low to draw statistically relevant conclusions.

Slauterbeck and colleagues[103] used questionnaires and saliva samples obtained within 72 hours of ACL ruptures in 38 female athletes to document cycle phase. Thirty-one of the women did not use oral contraceptives. There were a significantly greater number of ACL injuries during the follicular phase of the cycle than expected. Only 1 subject suffered an ACL rupture during the ovulatory phase.

TABLE 15-2 Phase of the Menstrual Cycle in Which Anterior Cruciate Ligament Ruptures Occurred According to Oral Contraceptive Use

Phase	Expected rate % (N)	No Oral Contraception Use Subgroup (N = 51)* % (N)	Oral Contraception Use Subgroup (N = 14)† % (N)
Follicular	32 (9/28)	25 (13/51)	14 (2/14)
Ovulatory	18 (5/28)	47 (24/51)	29 (4/14)
Luteal	50 (14/28)	27 (14/51)	57 (8/14)

*Significant association (chi-square = 29.8; $P < .001$).
†No significant association (chi-square = 2.38; $P = .07$).

Beynnon and coworkers[13] measured serum concentrations of estrogen and progesterone in 42 female recreational alpine skiers within 2 hours of the ACL rupture. The subjects were matched with 46 controls. The investigators segregated the menstrual cycle into two phases, preovulatory and postovulatory, according to levels of progesterone measured. The data revealed that significantly more ACL ruptures occurred during the preovulatory phase than expected. After considering skier experience and ability, the female subjects were estimated to be three times more likely to tear their ACL during the preovulatory phase. The authors concluded that their data were similar to those reported by others,[103,113] with an apparent association toward a greater proportion of female athletes suffering ACL ruptures in the preovulatory (follicular) phase than in later phases of the cycle. Whether this observation is due to deleterious effects of hormonal fluctuations on collagen metabolism or to changes in muscle contraction and neuromuscular control remains to be determined.

Influence of Hormone Fluctuations and Oral Contraceptives on Knee Kinematics

As of the time of writing, a study conducted at the authors' laboratory[19] was the only one published to date that assessed whether hormonal cycling in women affected loading on the knee during high-risk tasks. Twenty-five women, 12 of whom were not taking oral contraceptives and 13 of whom were on oral contraceptives, and 12 males underwent neuromuscular testing. The female subjects completed the same tests six times over an 8-week period during which time serum concentrations of estrogen and progesterone were measured. Each subject was tested twice during the follicular, luteal, and ovulatory phases. The tests included a horizontal jump, a vertical jump, and a drop-jump from a 30-cm box onto a single leg. Hip and knee kinematics and peak externally applied moments were calculated. The male subjects underwent the same tests on one occasion. The results showed no significant difference between genders or between the two female subgroups in moments or knee flexion angles. The authors concluded that fluctuations in hormones throughout the menstrual cycle are not solely responsible for the gender disparity in noncontact ACL injury rates; rather, that the problem most likely is a result of a "complex interaction between ligament structural properties, fatigue, and neuromuscular control."[19]

AOSSM Consensus and Opinion

Participants of the Hunt Valley II Meeting agreed that further well-controlled investigations are required to understand the implications of fluctuating or surging female hormones on ACL injury risk and knee function.[41] Although there appears to be an uneven distribution of ACL injuries in the follicular phase of the menstrual cycle, more data are required before definitive conclusions may be reached. There was no consensus among panel members regarding the role of oral contraceptives on knee injury risk or function.

NEUROMUSCULAR/BIOMECHANICS

Several neuromuscular and biomechanical factors have been hypothesized by various investigators to be responsible for the disparity between genders in noncontact ACL injury rates (Table 15–3). Differences between female and male athletes in movement patterns; muscle strength, activation, and recruitment patterns; and knee joint stiffness have been demonstrated under controlled preplanned and reactive conditions in the laboratory. As well, videotape analyses of noncontact ACL injuries demonstrate certain lower extremity positions and characteristics that lend support to the theory that these differences may likely play a role in this problem.[57,80]

Biomechanical Function of the Hamstring Musculature

Many noncontact ACL ruptures occur when an athlete lands from a jump.[33,35,39,55] Ground reaction forces measured during various jumping models have been reported to be 3 to 14 times body weight.[29,72,73,79,100,101] When analyzed on videotape, noncontact ACL injuries frequently occur with a forceful valgus and tibial rotation motion with the knee close to full extension.[80] The hamstring musculature is important in stabilizing the knee

joint because it functions as a joint compressor and restrains anterior tibial translation.[68,74] The biomechanical function of the pes anserinus (sartorius, gracilis, and semitendinosus muscles) was assessed many years ago in a study involving 15 fresh cadaver knees.[77] The anatomic courses and insertions of the three muscles relative to the knee joint and tibia were recorded at standard positions of knee flexion. On 5 of these specimens, biplane radiographs were collected to determine the orientation and load lines of the muscles at 0°, 30°, 60°, and 90° of flexion. A gentle pull on the muscle belly was done to simulate muscle

Critical Points NEUROMUSCULAR/BIOMECHANICAL RISK FACTORS

Differences between female and male athletes in movement patterns; muscle strength, activation, and recruitment patterns; and knee joint stiffness have been demonstrated under controlled preplanned and reactive conditions in multiple studies.

Hamstring musculature is important in stabilizing the knee joint, because it functions as a joint compressor and restrains anterior tibial translation.

High quadriceps activity can serve as a major intrinsic force in noncontact ACL injuries.

Gender differences in movement patterns on landing, take-off, cutting, stop-jump tasks, squatting are documented, but results of studies vary. Overall, females tend to assume posture positions of small knee and hip flexion angles, greater tibial rotation, and an overall lower limb valgus alignment during these activities.

Muscle activation patterns differ according to study design: reactive (unplanned) versus preplanned tasks.

Marked differences between adolescent and adult male and female athletes in quadriceps and hamstrings peak torques are well documented. Females appear to reach peak hamstrings strength at age 11.

AOSSM Consensus: Only that the role of "knee valgus" needs to be "better understood," the positions of the hip and the knee are likely associated with a higher risk of injury.

TABLE 15–3 Hypothesized Neuromuscular and Biomechanical Risk Factors for Noncontact Anterior Cruciate Ligament Injury in the Female Athlete

Category	Risk Factor	Hypothesized Gender Difference
Movement patterns	Knee flexion Hip flexion Hip internal rotation Hip abduction External tibial rotation Abduction moment Adduction moment	Compared with males, females have • Smaller knee and hip flexion angles during high-risk activity. • Greater internal hip rotation, hip abduction, external tibial rotation, and knee abduction-adduction moments during high-risk activity.
Muscle strength, activation, recruitment patterns	Lower extremity muscle strength and activity Hip muscle strength Lower extremity muscle recruitment patterns Fatigue Core stability	Compared with males, females have • Smaller quadriceps and hamstrings muscle torques. • Slower times to reach lower extremity muscle peak torques. • Higher quadriceps activity and reduced hamstrings activity during athletic maneuvers. • Weaker hip muscles. • Poorer core stability. • Different muscle activation patterns during preplanned and unplanned athletic tasks. • Faster time to fatigue. Females recruit quadriceps first in response to anterior tibial translation force whereas males recruit hamstrings.
Knee stiffness		Compared with males, females have • Decreased inherent passive and active knee joint stiffness.

contractions. The spatial relations of the muscles and tendons that form the pes anserinus were recorded by placing fine wire markers under direct visualization into the superficial aspect of the midportion of each muscle belly and tendon. The wires extended from a proximal point on the thigh to the insertion in the tibia. The dissection was limited to a subcutaneous exposure in order not to disturb the structures under study.

Mechanical tests of the forces produced on the knee joint under known loading conditions of the pes anserinus were performed on 8 unembalmed extremities. The three muscles were loaded individually and then collectively with weights up to 7.72 kg, which provided easily measurable forces on the leg (Fig. 15–1). The flexion force produced was measured by a circular bearing attached to the distal aspect of the leg, which allowed the tibia to be rotated without significantly changing the knee joint's axial center of rotation. Rotation was measured by two Steinmann pins that were inserted through the tibial tubercle in a transverse plane. A cord to measure rotation force ($F_{rotation}$) was attached at right angles to one pin. This cord was loaded prior to testing, which allowed the limbs to be positioned in external tibial rotation up to 15°.

The flexion force of the pes anserinus was greatest at 90° of knee flexion (Fig. 15–2). As the knee was extended, the tendon insertion angle became more acute relative to the tibia, resulting in a decrease in the mechanical advantage of the muscle and a subsequent decrease in the flexion moment about the knee joint despite equal muscle loading conditions. The difference in the mean values of the flexion force at the four knee positions was statistically significant ($P < .05$).

The rotation force of the pes anserinus was greatest at 90° of knee flexion (Fig. 15–3). The decrease in the angle of tendon insertion relative to the tibial with knee extension explains the decrease in rotation force in a manner similar to that noted for the flexion force. There was a statistically significant difference in the mean values of the rotation force at the four knee flexion positions ($P < .05$).

The rotation force of the pes anserinus under the same muscle load increased with increasing external tibial rotation at the four knee flexion positions (Fig. 15–4). The rotation force produced at 15° of external tibial rotation was approximately double that measured at 0° of external tibial rotation. The wind-up effect, although present at 90° of knee flexion, was smaller in magnitude than that measured at 30° of knee flexion. The difference in the mean rotation force values was significant at the four knee flexion positions ($P < .05$).

There was no significant change in the flexion force of the pes anserinus at the different positions of external tibial rotation. The wind-up effect is due in part to a change with external tibial rotation in the angle of muscle tendon insertion of the pes anserinus relative to the tibia (Fig. 15–5). The tibia may be viewed as a cylinder undergoing external rotation whereby the tendon insertion course angle increases from α_1 to α_2. The component of the force that produces the rotation effect (F_T) is equal to ($F \sin \alpha$) and thus increases as the angle α increases.

These data indicate that the sartorius, gracilis, and semitendinosus muscles have a marked functional dependence on the angle of knee flexion and degrees of external tibial rotation. They actively oppose extension by stabilizing the knee posteriorly and preventing knee hyperextension and anterior subluxation of the tibia. In addition, these muscles actively oppose external tibial rotation. The mechanical advantage of the pes anserinus increases as the knee goes into further flexion. At 0° of extension, the flexion force is reduced to 49% of that measured at 90° of flexion. Other investigators have reported that a quadriceps-hamstrings co-contraction cannot reduce ACL strain from full extension to approximately 20° of flexion.[78,85]

Consequences of High Quadriceps Forces on the ACL

Grood and associates[42] examined the knee extension exercise in cadavers to determine the conditions in which the ACL was

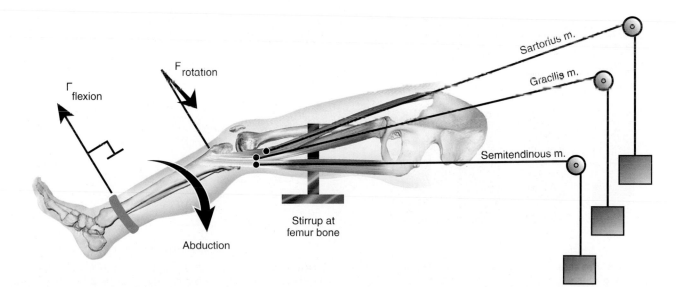

FIGURE 15–1. Mechanical test apparatus. Fixture enables loading of the three muscles at present knee flexion-external tibial rotation leg positions and measurement of corresponding flexion, rotation, and adduction forces. *(Redrawn from Noyes, F. R.; Sonstegard, D. A.: Biomechanical function of the pes anserinus at the knee and the effect of its transplantation. J Bone Joint Surg Am 55:1225–1241, 1973. Reprinted with permission from The Bone and Joint Surgery, Inc.)*

KNEE FLEXION

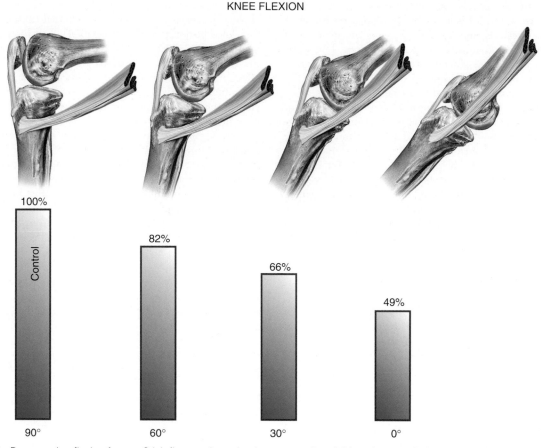

FIGURE 15–2. Pes anserine flexion forces. Stick figures show that knee extension yields a decrease in insertion course angles with respect to the tibia. Resulting loss in mechanical advantage is indicated by reduced flexion forces with extension ($P < .05$). *(Redrawn from Noyes, F. R.; Sonstegard, D. A.: Biomechanical function of the pes anserinus at the knee and the effect of its transplantation. J Bone Joint Surg Am 55:1225–1241, 1973. Reprinted with permission from The Bone and Joint Surgery, Inc.)*

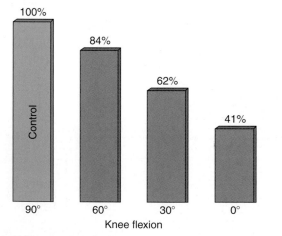

FIGURE 15–3. Pes anserine rotation forces. Reduction in mechanical advantage with knee extension is accompanied by corresponding decreases in rotation forces ($P < .05$). *(Redrawn from Noyes, F. R.; Sonstegard, D. A.: Biomechanical function of the pes anserinus at the knee and the effect of its transplantation. J Bone Joint Surg Am 55:1225–1241, 1973. Reprinted with permission from The Bone and Joint Surgery, Inc.)*

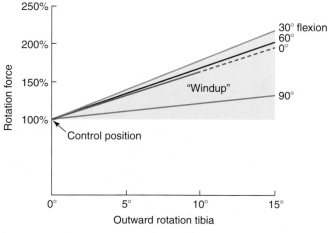

FIGURE 15–4. Rotation wind-up forces. The rotation forces under the same muscle loadings increase significantly with external tibial rotation at each knee flexion position tested ($P < .05$). *(Redrawn from Noyes, F. R.; Sonstegard, D. A.: Biomechanical function of the pes anserinus at the knee and the effect of its transplantation. J Bone Joint Surg Am 55:1225–1241, 1973. Reprinted with permission from The Bone and Joint Surgery, Inc.)*

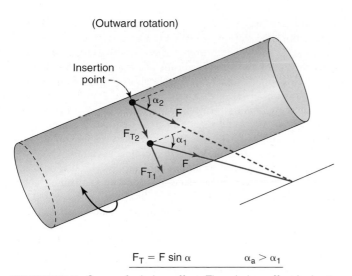

(Outward rotation)

$$F_T = F \sin \alpha \qquad \alpha_a > \alpha_1$$

FIGURE 15–5. Cause of wind-up effect. The wind up effect is due to an increase in the angle of tendon insertion ($\alpha_1 - \alpha_2$) with external tibial rotation. Muscle mechanical advantages are thereby increased and produce greater rotation forces under the same loadings. *(Redrawn from Noyes, F. R.; Sonstegard, D. A.: Biomechanical function of the pes anserinus at the knee and the effect of its transplantation. J Bone Joint Surg Am 55:1225–1241, 1973. Reprinted with permission from The Bone and Joint Surgery, Inc.)*

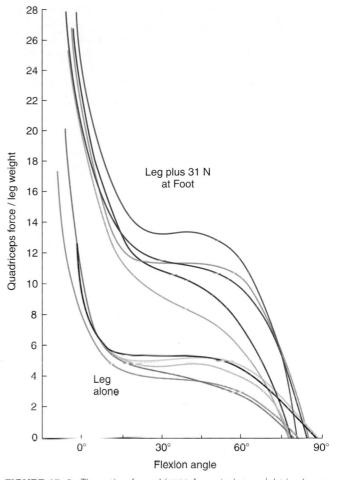

FIGURE 15–6. The ratio of quadriceps force to leg weight is shown for five specimens as a function of flexion angle. The *lower group of curves* demonstrate the force measured when extending the leg against its own weight. The *upper group of curves* show the forces measured when 31 N was placed at the foot. *(Redrawn from Grood, E. S.; Suntay, W. J.; Noyes, F. R.; Butler, D. L.: Biomechanics of the knee-extension exercise. Effect of cutting the anterior cruciate ligament. J Bone Joint Surg Am 66:725–734, 1984. Reprinted with permission from The Bone and Joint Surgery, Inc.)*

loaded, the quadriceps force that developed during knee flexion-extension, and the forces that were incurred on the extensor mechanism as the knee was extended. An open kinetic chain knee extension exercise was simulated both without resistance and with 31 N (7 lb) of resistance provided by an ankle weight placed at the foot. The quadriceps force required to extend the knee remained at a constant value of 177 N between 50° and 15°, but then rose rapidly to reach 350 N at 0° (Fig. 15–6). The addition of resistance doubled the quadriceps force that was required to extend the knee, resulting in large muscle forces on the ACL and patellofemoral joint.

DeMorat and colleagues[28] reported that a high quadriceps load (4500 N) simulated in cadaveric knees at 20° of flexion produced significant anterior tibial translation (mean, 19.5 mm). Whereas all 11 knees sustained damage to the ACL, not all suffered complete failure. The authors concluded that the quadriceps can serve as a major intrinsic force in noncontact ACL injuries.

Colby and coworkers[21] measured hamstring and quadriceps muscle activation and knee flexion angles during eccentric motion of sidestep cutting, cross-cutting, stopping, and landing in 15 collegiate athletes. A high-level quadriceps muscle activation occurred just before foot-strike and peaked in mideccentric motion. The peak quadriceps muscle activation occurred between 39° (stopping) and 53° (cross-cutting) of knee flexion and averaged between 126% (landing) and 161% (stopping) of that measured in a maximum isometric contraction. Hamstring muscle activation was submaximal at and after foot-strike. The minimal hamstring muscle activation occurred between 21° (stopping) and 34° (cutting) of knee flexion and averaged between 14% (landing) and 40% (cross-cutting) that of a maximum isometric contraction. The knee flexion position at which foot-strike occurred during all four activities averaged 22° (range, 14° on stopping to 29° on cross-cutting). The authors concluded that the combination of the high level of quadriceps activity, low level of hamstrings activity, and low angle of knee flexion during eccentric contractions in these maneuvers could

produce significant anterior translation of the tibia. The subjects included 9 men and 6 women; a gender comparison was not conducted.

Gender Differences in Movement Patterns on Landing and Take-Off

A study conducted at the authors' laboratory[48] using a two-camera, video-based optoelectronic digitizer and a multicomponent force plate was one of the first to demonstrate gender differences in movement patterns. Eleven high school female volleyball players were matched with 9 male athletes according to age, height, and weight and taken through jumping tasks and isokinetic lower extremity muscle strength testing. The males demonstrated greater knee extension moments on landing and take-off, which were interpreted to be likely due to their high use of the hamstrings musculature. Males also had a greater mean hamstring-to-quadriceps ratio on isokinetic testing at 360°/sec. Interestingly, males had significantly greater peak landing forces than females (6.1 and 4.2 times body weight, respectively; $P < .01$). The hypothesis was advanced that male athletes most likely use different mechanisms than those used by female athletes to compensate for these high landing forces. The investigation did not find significant gender differences with respect to knee abduction-adduction moments, knee flexion angles on landing and take-off, flexion moments, and ankle and hip flexion-extension and abduction-adduction moments.

Huston and associates[51] found significant differences between genders on the knee flexion angle measured at impact from a drop-jump. Ten males and 10 females, matched for height, performed three drop-jumps from heights of 20, 40, and 60 cm. The men consistently demonstrated greater knee flexion angles than the women at 20 cm (8° and 5.4°, respectively; $P < .05$), 40 cm (10° and 5.4° respectively; $P < .05$), and 60 cm (16° and 7°, respectively; $P < .05$). The authors hypothesized that ground reaction forces are likely to be greater in women per unit body weight than in men because women land with a straighter knee.

Lephart and colleagues[62] evaluated kinematic and ground reaction forces in 30 collegiate athletes on single-leg landing and single-leg forward hopping. In both tasks, the females had significantly less knee flexion and lower leg internal rotation

after impact than males and also took less time to reach their maximum knee flexion subsequent to impact (Figs. 15–7 and 15–8). The authors interpreted these findings to indicate that women experience a more abrupt absorption of impact forces on landing. The women also demonstrated greater hip internal rotation with lower leg external rotation from the point of impact to the maximum rotation position. There was no difference in vertical ground reaction forces between genders.

Decker and coworkers[26] examined kinetic, kinematic, and energetic indices of 9 female and 12 male recreational athletes during a two-legged drop-jump task. The females demonstrated significantly greater knee extension and ankle plantar flexion angles at initial ground contact ($P < .05$). The female group also had greater energy absorption from the knee and ankle than from the hip ($P < .05$), whereas the male group had equal amounts of energy absorption from all lower extremity joints. The female group performed 34% less negative hip work, 30% more negative knee work, and 52% more negative ankle work than the male group ($P < .05$). There were no differences between the groups in vertical ground reaction forces. The findings indicated that females were in a more erect posture on initial impact than the males; however, the general external loading conditions were

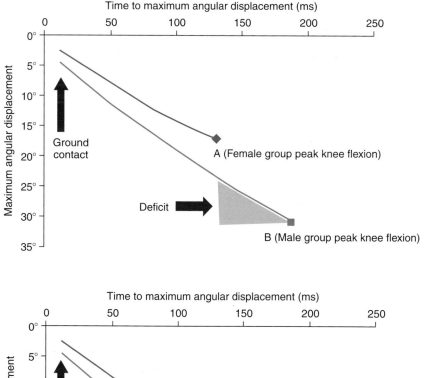

FIGURE 15–7. In the single-leg hop-landing task, points A and B represent the maximum angular displacement of knee flexion and the time to achieve this position after ground contact. The deficit represents a significant ($P < .05$) difference in knee position between females and males after ground contact. *(Redrawn from Lephart, S. M.; Ferris, C. M.; Riemann, B. L.; et al.: Gender differences in strength and lower extremity kinematics during landing. Clin Orthop 401:162–169, 2002.)*

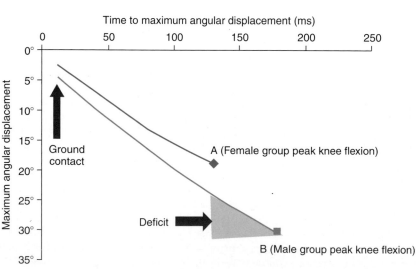

FIGURE 15–8. In the forward hop-landing task, points A and B represent the maximum angular displacement of knee flexion and the time to achieve this position after ground contact. The deficit represents a significant ($P < 0.05$) difference in knee position between females and males after ground contact. *(Redrawn from Lephart, S. M.; Ferris, C. M.; Riemann, B. L.; et al.: Gender differences in strength and lower extremity kinematics during landing. Clin Orthop 401:162–169, 2002.)*

similar between genders. The women preferred to use the ankle musculature to absorb impact forces, which was accompanied with greater knee extension and ankle plantar flexion angles. Conversely, the males demonstrated greater knee flexion and less plantar flexion angles on impact, allowing a transfer of the forces to the larger muscles such as the hip extensors.

Salci and associates[91] reported that female collegiate volleyball players landed with lower knee and hip flexion angles and higher ground reaction forces than male players during simulated spike and block maneuvers. Sell and colleagues[96] conducted an investigation involving high school basketball players in which both planned and reactive (to a visual cue) stop-jump tasks were performed vertically, horizontally to the left, and horizontally to the right. During the reactive tasks, females had lower maximum knee flexion angles than males (68.4° and 74.9°, respectively; $P = .001$), greater maximum knee valgus angles (–7.5° and –4.2°, respectively; $P < .05$), greater anterior shear force at peak posterior ground reaction force ($P < .05$), and greater knee flexion moment at peak posterior ground reaction force ($P < .05$). During the horizontal jump to the left, females had significantly lower maximum knee flexion angles ($P = .007$), lower knee flexion at posterior ground reaction force ($P = .006$), and greater knee valgus at posterior ground reaction force ($P < .05$). The authors hypothesized that these differences could place greater strain on the female ACL. For all subjects, the horizontal jump to the left (to the medial aspect of the right knee) produced greater vertical and posterior ground reaction forces, proximal anterior tibial shear force, valgus and flexion moments, and lowest knee flexion angles than the other jumps. In addition, measured knee kinematics and kinetics were significantly altered during the reactive (unplanned) jumps. The authors recommended that future study designs take into account jump direction and simulate as closely as possible actual playing conditions to more accurately study ACL risk factors.

In contrast to many other studies, Fagenbaum and Darling[30] reported that female athletes had significantly greater knee flexion angles (from 10°–14°) on landing than male athletes ($P < .05$), all of whom were collegiate basketball players attending the same university. The females demonstrated greater knee flexion both before and upon contact. Women also landed with greater knee flexion acceleration than men ($P < .05$). Cowling and Steele[22] measured knee, hip, and trunk flexion angles in 11 females and 9 males matched for sport during a dynamic and abrupt deceleration single-leg task. No significant differences were found between genders in flexion angles on landing.

Gender Differences in Movement Patterns on Cutting

Malinzak and coworkers[69] reported that female athletes had smaller knee flexion angles, greater valgus angles, increased quadriceps muscle activation, and decreased hamstring muscle activation during the stance cycle of straight running and two preplanned cutting maneuvers. The authors believed that these differences in lower extremity motion patterns could have been due to differences in anatomic structures, motor controls, or physiologic characteristics, although none of these factors was measured. Another investigation reported that during running, females had significantly greater hip internal rotation, peak hip adduction, and peak knee abduction and were in a greater abducted knee position throughout stance than males.[32]

Pollard and associates[86] studied three-dimensional hip and knee joint kinematics and moments during a randomly cued cutting maneuver in 24 experienced collegiate soccer players. The authors reported no differences between genders in peak knee joint abduction or internal rotation angles during the first 0° to 40° of knee flexion across the stance phase. There were also no differences with respect to peak hip internal rotation angles. Females did demonstrate significantly less hip abduction than the males ($P = .03$). No gender differences were found for peak knee adduction, knee external rotation, hip abduction, or hip external rotation joint moments. The authors speculated that the failure to find differences in mechanics could have been a result of years of training and exposure to the same sport.

Besier and colleagues[10,11] studied external knee moments and knee flexion angles during straight running, sidestepping, and crossover cutting in male subjects in two investigations. The data revealed that large increases occurred during cutting and sidestepping in varus-valgus and internal-external rotation moments compared with straight running ($P < .05$). The authors concluded that these movements placed the ACL at higher risk of injury, particularly at low knee flexion angles. During sidestepping, combined external loads of flexion, valgus, and internal rotation were observed, potentially increasing the load on both the ACL and the MCL. During cutting, combined flexion and varus loads could place large loads on the fibular collateral ligament. Female athletes were not included in these investigations.

Chaudhari and coworkers[20] observed a correlation between frontal plane lower limb alignment and knee moments, because subjects who assumed a valgus lower limb position during a 90° lateral run-to-cut maneuver had significantly higher knee abduction moments than those who had a neutral or varus lower limb position (Fig. 15–9; $P < .01$). Of the 21 subjects tested, 67% of females assumed a lower limb valgus alignment compared with 22% of males.

Gender Differences in Movement Patterns on Stop-Jump Tasks

A gender comparison of knee kinetics in three stop-jump tasks (Fig. 15–10) found that women had significantly greater proximal anterior shear forces, extension moments and valgus moments on landing than men (Fig. 15–11).[17] The investigators believed that the increased proximal shear force was due to a high quadriceps muscle force, a low hamstrings muscle force, a straight knee on landing, or a combination of all of these factors. There was no difference between male and female athletes in knee valgus-varus moments, thereby refuting that this moment is responsible for the gender disparity in noncontact ACL injury rates. Chappell and associates[16] also assessed the effect of fatigue on knee kinetics in these same stop-jump tasks. Female subjects had significantly greater peak proximal tibial anterior shear forces than males, greater knee extension moments at peak proximal tibial anterior shear force, and smaller knee flexion angles ($P = .001$, all comparisons) in both unfatigued and fatigued states. The mean valgus moment at the peak proximal tibial anterior shear force of female subjects increased 96% from the unfatigued to the fatigued condition (from 0.026–0.051 times body height x weight). Male subjects decreased mean valgus moment by 43% between test conditions. The authors concluded that fatigue increased the risk of ACL injury more in females than in males.

FIGURE 15–9. Top, Peak external knee abduction moment. **Bottom,** Peak external knee adduction moment. The valgus group was significantly more positive than the neutral + varus and neutral groups for all values (P < .01). *Error bars* denote the 95% confidence intervals of the group means. *(From Chaudhari, A. M.; Hearn, B. K.; Leveille, L. A.; et al.: The effects of dynamic limb alignment on knee moments during single limb landing: implications for the analysis of the non-contact injury to the anterior cruciate ligament. Proceedings of the 2003 Summer Bioengineering Conference, June 25–29, Key Biscayne, FL, 2003.)*

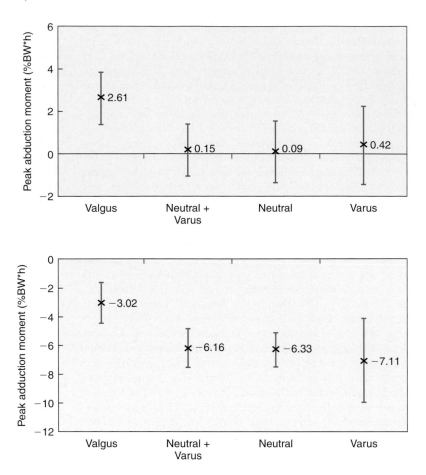

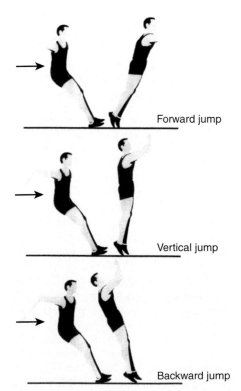

FIGURE 15–10. Three stop-jump tasks. *(From Chappell, J. D.; Yu, B.; Kirkendall, D. T.; Garrett, W. E.: A comparison of knee kinetics between male and female recreational athletes in stop-jump tasks. Am J Sports Med 30:261–267, 2002.)*

A third investigation from Chappell and colleagues[15] was conducted to determine whether gender differences existed during the preparation for landing in the vertical stop-jump task. Female recreational athletes displayed less knee and hip flexion, less hip external rotation, and increased hip abduction than male athletes upon preparation for landing. The authors hypothesized that the athletes "preprogrammed" these lower extremity motions during the flight phase of the last step of the approach run in this task.

Yu and coworkers[116] studied lower extremity kinematics during a stop-jump task in soccer players aged 11 to 16 years. The athletes were divided into six age groups, with each group composed of five female and five male subjects. Female players older than 12 years had decreased knee and hip flexion angles (Figs. 15–12 and 15–13) than the male athletes on landing. All players younger than 12 years had valgus knee angles at initial foot contact with the ground. Female players increased the amount of knee valgus motion as age increased. However, male players older than 12 years demonstrated a varus knee angle at initial contact. The authors acknowledged the small sample size as a limitation of the study.

Gender Differences in Movement Patterns on Squatting

During a dynamic single-leg squat in 18 healthy intercollegiate athletes (9 men, 9 women), Zeller and associates[119] reported that female athletes had significantly greater ankle dorsiflexion, ankle pronation, hip adduction, and hip flexion than males. The

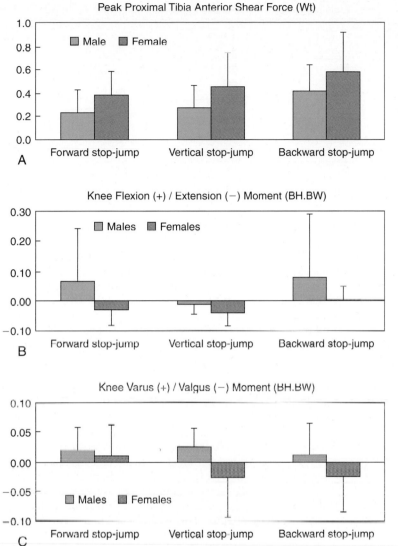

FIGURE 15–11. Comparisons of peak proximal tibia anterior shear force (**A**), knee flexion-extension moment (**B**), and knee varus-valgus moment (**C**) during the landing phase of three stop-jump tasks. Results are normalized by body weight (Wt) (peak shear force) or by body weight x height (BH.BW) (knee flexion-extension moment and varus-valgus moment). (*A–C, Redrawn from Chappell, J. D.; Yu, B.; Kirkendall, D. T.; Garrett, W. E.: A comparison of knee kinetics between male and female recreational athletes in stop-jump tasks. Am J Sports Med 30:261–267, 2002.)*

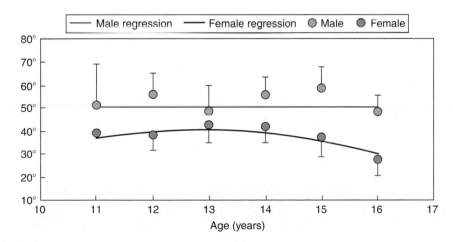

FIGURE 15–12. Age and gender effects on hip flexion angles at initial contact. Age and gender significantly affected the hip flexion angle of youth soccer players at initial foot contact with the ground. *(Redrawn from Yu, B.; McClure, S. B.; Onate, J. A.; et al.: Age and gender effects on lower extremity kinematics of youth soccer players in a stop-jump task. Am J Sports Med 33:1356–1364, 2005.)*

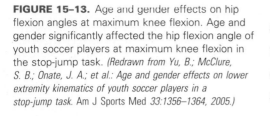

FIGURE 15-13. Age and gender effects on hip flexion angles at maximum knee flexion. Age and gender significantly affected the hip flexion angle of youth soccer players at maximum knee flexion in the stop-jump task. *(Redrawn from Yu, B.; McClure, S. B.; Onate, J. A.; et al.: Age and gender effects on lower extremity kinematics of youth soccer players in a stop-jump task. Am J Sports Med 33:1356–1364, 2005.)*

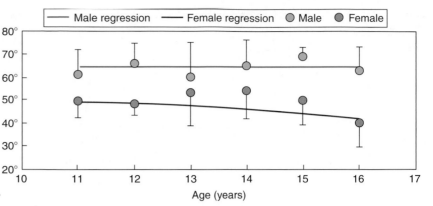

women began the movement in greater valgus alignment and remained in this alignment throughout the squat. In addition, the women had less trunk lateral flexion than the men. The investigation revealed that women had poor hip control, which resulted in an adducted position that in turn allowed the femur to internally rotate, which placed the knee into a valgus position.

Gender Differences in Muscle Strength, Activation, and Recruitment Patterns

Marked differences between adolescent and adult male and female athletes in quadriceps and hamstrings peak torques, even when normalized for body weight, have been documented by numerous investigations.[8,48,52,62,91] One of the largest studies conducted to date on 853 females and 177 males aged 9 to 17 demonstrated that significant gender differences in lower extremity strength become evident at age 14 (see Chapter 16, Lower Limb Neuromuscular Control and Strength in Prepubescent and Adolescent Male and Female Athletes).[8] This investigation revealed that females appear to reach peak hamstrings strength at age 11, with no significant difference found in this factor between girls 11 years of age and those up to 17 years of age. No difference in isokinetic muscle strength values between boys and girls younger than 14 years has been reported by many laboratories.[24,25,46,49,87,95,107]

Huston and Wojtys[52] studied lower extremity muscle strength, endurance, reaction time, and recruitment order in response to an anterior tibial translation force in 100 elite collegiate athletes and 40 matched nonathletic controls. The female athletes had significantly weaker knee flexor and extensor peak torques (normalized for body weight, 60°/sec and 240°/sec) and endurance values than the male athletes and were only marginally stronger than the female controls. The female athletes had slower time-to-peak torque values for knee flexors than the male athletes (430 and 328 msec, respectively; P < .001). Only 28% of the female athletes recruited their hamstrings first in response to an anterior tibial translation force compared with 45% of the other three subgroups. The preferred order of muscle recruitment in the female athletes was quadriceps, hamstrings, and gastrocnemius. In contrast, the preferred order of muscle recruitment in the male athletes, male controls, and female controls was hamstrings, quadriceps, and gastrocnemius.

Rozzi and associates[90] failed to find a gender difference in time-to-peak torque in 34 healthy collegiate athletes tested at 180°/sec. On a single-leg drop jump test, no differences were detected between genders in mean onset times for the quadriceps or hamstrings musculatures. The female athletes demonstrated greater electromyographic (EMG) peak amplitude and area of the lateral hamstring on landing. In addition, the female athletes had greater anterior tibial displacements and reduced knee joint proprioception (time to detect the knee moving into extension) than the male athletes. These investigators postulated that the female athletes adopted compensatory mechanisms of increased hamstring activity to achieve knee stability in the presence of increased inherent joint instability.

Cowling and Steele[22] measured muscle activation patterns in 11 females and 7 males during a dynamic and abrupt deceleration single-leg task. There were no significant differences between genders in quadriceps muscle activation patterns on landing. However, males had a significant delay in the onset of semimembranosus muscle burst peak time relative to initial contact compared with females (113 ± 46 msec and 173 ± 54 msec, respectively; P < .05). The authors postulated that this delay allowed peak hamstring muscle activity to coincide with the anterior tibiofemoral joint forces generated just after initial contact and enable the hamstrings to act as a synergist to the ACL.

Zeller and associates[119] measured muscle activity during a single-leg dynamic squat in nine female and nine male collegiate athletes. The women had greater quadriceps femoris activation than the men in both the area under the linear envelope (78.8% ± 26.1% and 34.4% ± 16.4% of maximal voluntary isometric contraction, respectively; P < .05) and muscle activation (83.4% ± 14.5% and 36.2% ± 14.5% of maximal voluntary isometric contraction, respectively; P < .05). Chappell and colleagues[15] measured muscle activation during the preparation for landing in the vertical stop-jump in recreational athletes. The females had greater quadriceps and hamstrings muscle activation than the males during landing preparation, but had lower hamstring activation after landing (foot-strike).

Leetun and associates[61] measured hip abduction and external rotation isometric strength, abdominal muscle function, and back extensor and quadratus lumborum endurance in 79 female and 60 male intercollegiate athletes. The athletes were tested prior to the onset of their sport season and then followed for that season for injuries. The male athletes had greater hip isometric abduction (P < .05) and external rotation (P < .001) strength than the females. Only 1 athlete in the series sustained an ACL injury.

Gender Differences in Knee Stiffness

Wojtys and colleagues[111] measured passive and active anterior shear stiffness of the knee joint in 10 men and 13 women. The subjects were placed in a knee testing apparatus that recorded anterior tibial translation and muscle activity with surface electromyography. Tests were conducted in a passive state and then in an active state in response to an anterior tibial translation force that was 20% of the subject's body weight. Knee shear stiffness values were obtained by dividing the load of the anteriorly directed force by the anterior displacement of the knee joint. All subjects had uninjured, physiologically lax knees ($\geq$6 mm anterior tibial translation on KT-1000 testing). There was no difference between the men and women in passive anterior tibial translation. Whereas there was no significant difference between genders in passive shear stiffness, men produced significantly higher active stiffness values during a maximum co-contraction (70.9 and 40.7 N/mm, respectively; $P = .005$). Men increased knee joint stiffness by 379% compared with the passive state, and women increased this value by 212%. There was no association between muscle strength, time-to-peak torque, or body height and the ability to increase shear stiffness. No difference was found between genders in EMG activity levels of the lower extremity.

In a separate investigation, Wojtys and coworkers[114] reported that female athletes involved in pivoting sports had significantly smaller increases in torsional stiffness of the knee under internal rotation loading conditions than male athletes (159% $\pm$ 13% and 275% $\pm$ 39%; $P = .001$). The 24 athletes were matched for age, height, weight, BMI, shoe size, and activity level.

A reduction in active muscle stiffness in females compared with males was reported by Granata and associates[37,38] during isometric knee flexion and extension and hopping tasks. These authors noted that effective stiffness increased linearly with the applied torque load. The gender difference was amplified at higher loads, leading the investigators to conclude that this finding had implications for potential injury during functional loading tasks.

Padua and colleagues[84] found no differences between genders in leg stiffness during two-legged hopping tasks when the data were normalized for body mass. Significant differences were detected in stiffness prior to normalization, leading the authors

to conclude that this finding was due to the lighter mass of the female subjects. No gender associations were found for joint angles at initial ground contact or joint excursions of the knees and ankles. Females recruited 46% greater quadriceps activity than the males and 37% greater soleus activity; however, no difference was found between genders in hamstrings activity during the hopping tasks.

AOSSM Consensus and Opinion

Even though numerous well-controlled investigations have been conducted regarding potential neuromuscular risk factors, the participants of the Hunt Valley II Meeting could agree only that the role of "knee valgus" needs to be "better understood" and that the positions of the hip and knee are likely associated with a higher risk of injury.

CONCLUSIONS

In order to determine which risk factors for noncontact ACL ruptures are significant and which may play a more negligible role, future investigations must include greater sample sizes, analyze factors from all of the major categories (anatomic, environmental, hormonal, and neuromuscular), and follow athletes for at least 1 entire athletic season for injury. Epidemiologically sound study methodology must be followed, including tracking injury exposures and conducting power analyses to avoid a type II statistical error. Athletes from multiple sports should be included in order to determine whether certain factors are sports-specific in terms of injury risk. Future studies need to incorporate reactive tasks, because there appear to be significant differences in movement and muscle activation patterns under these conditions versus those of controlled preplanned maneuvers. As technology improves, these studies may hopefully be able to move out of the laboratory and measure neuromuscular indices under actual playing conditions.

REFERENCES

1. Agel, J.; Arendt, E. A.; Bershadsky, B.: Anterior cruciate ligament injury in National Collegiate Athletic Association basketball and soccer: a 13-year review. *Am J Sports Med* 33:524–530, 2005.
2. Albright, J. P., et al.: Medial collateral ligament knee sprains in college football. Effectiveness of preventive braces. *Am J Sports Med* 22:12–18, 1994.
3. Allen, M. K.; Glasoe, W. M.: Metrecom measurement of navicular drop in subjects with anterior cruciate ligament injury. *J Athl Train* 35:403–406, 2000.
4. Anderson, A. F.; Dome, D. C.; Gautam, S.; et al.: Correlation of anthropometric measurements, strength, anterior cruciate ligament size, and intercondylar notch characteristics to sex differences in anterior cruciate ligament tear rates. *Am J Sports Med* 29:58–66, 2001.
5. Anderson, A. F.; Lipscomb, A. B.; Liudahl, K. J.; Addlestone, R. B.: Analysis of the intercondylar notch by computed tomography. *Am J Sports Med* 15:547–552, 1987.
6. Arendt, E.; Dick, R.: Knee injury patterns among men and women in collegiate basketball and soccer. NCAA data and review of literature. *Am J Sports Med* 23:694–701, 1995.
7. Arendt, E. A.; Agel, J.; Dick, R.: Anterior cruciate ligament injury patterns among collegiate men and women. *J Athl Train* 34:86–92, 1999.
8. Barber-Westin, S. D.; Noyes, F. R.; Galloway, M.: Jump-land characteristics and muscle strength development in young athletes: a gender comparison of 1140 athletes 9 to 17 years of age. *Am J Sports Med* 34:375–384, 2006.

9. Beckett, M. E.; Massie, D. L.; Bowers, K. D.; Stoll, D. A.: Incidence of hyperpronation in the ACL injured knee: a clinical perspective. *J Athl Train* 27:58–62, 1992.
10. Besier, T. F.; Lloyd, D. G.; Ackland, T. R.; Cochrane, J. L.: Anticipatory effects on knee joint loading during running and cutting maneuvers. *Med Sci Sports Exerc* 33:1176–1181, 2001.
11. Besier, T. F.; Lloyd, D. G.; Cochrane, J. L.; Ackland, T. R.: External loading of the knee joint during running and cutting maneuvers. *Med Sci Sports Exerc* 33:1168–1175, 2001.
12. Beynnon, B. D.; Bernstein, I. M.; Belisle, A.; et al.: The effect of estradiol and progesterone on knee and ankle joint laxity. *Am J Sports Med* 33:1298–1304, 2005.
13. Beynnon, B. D.; Johnson, R. J.; Braun, S.; et al.: The relationship between menstrual cycle phase and anterior cruciate ligament injury: a case-control study of recreational alpine skiers. *Am J Sports Med* 34:757–764, 2006.
14. Chandrashekar, N.; Slauterbeck, J.; Hashemi, J.: Sex-based differences in the anthropometric characteristics of the anterior cruciate ligament and its relation to intercondylar notch geometry: a cadaveric study. *Am J Sports Med* 33:1492–1498, 2005.
15. Chappell, J. D.; Creighton, R. A.; Giuliani, C.; et al.: Kinematics and electromyography of landing preparation in vertical stop-jump: risks for noncontact anterior cruciate ligament injury. *Am J Sports Med* 35:235–241, 2007.

16. Chappell, J. D.; Herman, D. C.; Knight, B. S.; et al.: Effect of fatigue on knee kinetics and kinematics in stop-jump tasks. *Am J Sports Med* 33:1022–1029, 2005.

17. Chappell, J. D.; Yu, B.; Kirkendall, D. T.; Garrett, W. E.: A comparison of knee kinetics between male and female recreational athletes in stop-jump tasks. *Am J Sports Med* 30:261–267, 2002.

18. Charlton, W. P.; St. John, T. A.; Ciccotti, M. G.; et al.: Differences in femoral notch anatomy between men and women: a magnetic resonance imaging study. *Am J Sports Med* 30:329–333, 2002.

19. Chaudhari, A. M.; Lindenfeld, T. N.; Andriacchi, T. P.; et al.: Knee and hip loading patterns at different phases in the menstrual cycle: implications for the gender difference in anterior cruciate ligament injury rates. *Am J Sports Med* 35:793–800, 2007.

20. Chaudhari, A. M.; Hearn, B. K.; Leveille, L. A.; et al.: The effects of dynamic limb alignment on knee moments during single limb landing: implications for the analysis of the non-contact injury to the anterior cruciate ligament. Proceedings of the 2003 Summer Bioengineering Conference, June 25–29, Key Biscayne, FL, 2003.

21. Colby, S.; Francisco, A.; Yu, B.; Kirkendall, D.; et al.: Electromyographic and kinematic analysis of cutting maneuvers. Implications for anterior cruciate ligament injury. *Am J Sports Med* 28:234–240, 2000.

22. Cowling, E. J.; Steele, J. R.: Is lower limb muscle synchrony during landing affected by gender? Implications for variations in ACL injury rates. *J Electromyogr Kinesiol* 11:263–268, 2001.

23. Davis, T. J.; Shelbourne, K. D.; Klootwyk, T. E.: Correlation of the intercondylar notch width of the femur to the width of the anterior and posterior cruciate ligaments. *Knee Surg Sports Traumatol Arthrosc* 7:209–214, 1999.

24. De Ste Croix, M. B.; Armstrong, N.; Welsman, J. R.; Sharpe, P.: Longitudinal changes in isokinetic leg strength in 10- to 14-year-olds. *Ann Hum Biol* 29:50–62, 2002.

25. De Ste Croix, M. B. A.; Armstrong, N.; Welsman, J. R.: Concentric isokinetic leg strength in pre-teen, teenage and adult males and females. *Biol Sport* 16:75–86, 1999.

26. Decker, M. J.; Torry, M. R.; Wyland, D. J.; et al.: Gender differences in lower extremity kinematics, kinetics and energy absorption during landing. *Clin Biomech (Bristol, Avon)* 18:662–669, 2003.

27. Deie, M.; Sakamaki, Y.; Sumen, Y.; et al.: Anterior knee laxity in young women varies with their menstrual cycle. *Int Orthop* 26:154–156, 2002.

28. DeMorat, G.; Weinhold, P.; Blackburn, T.; et al.: Aggressive quadriceps loading can induce noncontact anterior cruciate ligament injury. *Am J Sports Med* 32:477–483, 2004.

29. Dufek, J. S.; Bates, B. T.: The evaluation and prediction of impact forces during landings. *Med Sci Sports Exerc* 22:370–377, 1990.

30. Fagenbaum, R.; Darling, W. G.: Jump landing strategies in male and female college athletes and the implications of such strategies for anterior cruciate ligament injury. *Am J Sports Med* 31:233–240, 2003.

31. Faryniarz, D. A.; Bhargava, M.; Lajam, C.; et al.: Quantitation of estrogen receptors and relaxin binding in human anterior cruciate ligament fibroblasts. *In Vitro Cell Dev Biol Anim* 42:176–181, 2006.

32. Ferber, R.; Davis, I. M.; Williams, D. S., 3rd: Gender differences in lower extremity mechanics during running. *Clin Biomech (Bristol, Avon)* 18:350–357, 2003.

33. Ferretti, A.; Papandrea, P.; Conteduca, F.; Mariani, P. P.: Knee ligament injuries in volleyball players. *Am J Sports Med* 20:203–207, 1992.

34. Flynn, R. K.; Pedersen, C. L.; Birmingham, T. B.; et al.: The familial predisposition toward tearing the anterior cruciate ligament: a case control study. *Am J Sports Med* 33:23–28, 2005.

35. Gerberich, S. G.; Luhmann, S.; Finke, C.; et al.: Analysis of severe injuries associated with volleyball activities. *Physician Sportsmed* 15:75–79, 1987.

36. Good, L.; Odensten, M.; Gillquist, J.: Intercondylar notch measurements with special reference to anterior cruciate ligament surgery. *Clin Orthop Relat Res* 263:185–189, 1991.

37. Granata, K. P.; Padua, D. A.; Wilson, S. E.: Gender differences in active musculoskeletal stiffness. Part II. Quantification of leg stiffness during functional hopping tasks. *J Electromyogr Kinesiol* 12:127–135, 2002.

38. Granata, K. P.; Wilson, S. E.; Padua, D. A.: Gender differences in active musculoskeletal stiffness. Part I. Quantification in controlled

39. measurements of knee joint dynamics. *J Electromyogr Kinesiol* 12:119–126, 2002.

39. Gray, J.; Taunton, J. E.; McKenzie, D. C.; et al.: A survey of injuries to the anterior cruciate ligament of the knee in female basketball players. *Int J Sports Med* 6:314–316, 1985.

40. Greenfield, M. L.; Kuhn, J. E.; Wojtys, E. M.: A statistics primer. Power analysis and sample size determination. *Am J Sports Med* 25:138–140, 1997.

41. Griffin, L. Y.; Albohm, M. J.; Arendt, E. A.; et al.: Understanding and preventing noncontact anterior cruciate ligament injuries: a review of the Hunt Valley II meeting, January 2005. *Am J Sports Med* 34:1512–1532, 2006.

42. Grood, E. S.; Suntay, W. J.; Noyes, F. R.; Butler, D. L.: Biomechanics of the knee-extension exercise. Effect of cutting the anterior cruciate ligament. *J Bone Joint Surg Am* 66:725–734, 1984.

43. Gwinn, D. E.; Wilckens, J. H.; McDevitt, E. R.; et al.: The relative incidence of anterior cruciate ligament injury in men and women at the United States Naval Academy. *Am J Sports Med* 28:98–102, 2000.

44. Harner, C. D.; Paulos, L. E.; Greenwald, A. E.; et al.: Detailed analysis of patients with bilateral anterior cruciate ligament injuries. *Am J Sports Med* 22:37–43, 1994.

45. Heitz, N. A.; Eisenman, P. A.; Beck, C. L.; Walker, J. A.: Hormonal changes throughout the menstrual cycle and increased anterior cruciate ligament laxity in females. *J Athl Train* 34:144–149, 1999.

46. Henderson, R. C.; Howes, C. L.; Erickson, K. L.; et al.: Knee flexor-extensor strength in children. *J Orthop Sports Phys Ther* 18:559–563, 1993.

47. Herzog, R. J.; Silliman, J. F.; Hutton, K.; et al.: Measurements of the intercondylar notch by plain film radiography and magnetic resonance imaging. *Am J Sports Med* 22:204–210, 1994.

48. Hewett, T. E.; Stroupe, A. L.; Nance, T. A.; Noyes, F. R.: Plyometric training in female athletes. Decreased impact forces and increased hamstring torques. *Am J Sports Med* 24:765–773, 1996.

49. Holm, I.; Steen, H.; Olstad, M.: Isokinetic muscle performance in growing boys from pre-teen to maturity. An eleven-year longitudinal study. *Isok Exer Sci* 13:153–158, 2005.

50. Houseworth, S. W.; Mauro, V. J.; Mellon, B. A.; Kieffer, D. A.: The intercondylar notch in acute tears of the anterior cruciate ligament: a computer graphics study. *Am J Sports Med* 15:221–224, 1987.

51. Huston, L. J.; Vibert, B.; Ashton-Miller, J. A.; Wojtys, E. M.: Gender differences in knee angle when landing from a drop-jump. *Am J Knee Surg* 14:215–219, 2001.

52. Huston, L. J.; Wojtys, E. M.: Neuromuscular performance characteristics in elite female athletes. *Am J Sports Med* 24:427–436, 1996.

53. Hutchinson, M. R.; Ireland, M. L.: Knee injuries in female athletes. *Sports Med* 19:288–302, 1995.

54. Ireland, M. L.; Ballantyne, B. T.; Little, K.; McClay, I. S.: A radiographic analysis of the relationship between the size and shape of the intercondylar notch and anterior cruciate ligament injury. *Knee Surg Sports Traumatol Arthrosc* 9:200–205, 2001.

55. Kirkendall, D. T.; Garrett, W. E., Jr.: The anterior cruciate ligament enigma. Injury mechanisms and prevention. *Clin Orthop* 372:64–68, 2000.

56. Knapik, J. J.; Wright, J. E.; Mawdsley, R. H.; Braun, J.: Isometric, isotonic, and isokinetic torque variations in four muscle groups through a range of joint motion. *Phys Ther* 63:938–947, 1983.

57. Krosshaug, T.; Nakamae, A.; Boden, B. P.; et al.: Mechanisms of anterior cruciate ligament injury in basketball: video analysis of 39 cases. *Am J Sports Med* 35:359–367, 2007.

58. Lambson, R. B.; Barnhill, B. S.; Higgins, R. W.: Football cleat design and its effect on anterior cruciate ligament injuries. A three-year prospective study. *Am J Sports Med* 24:155–159, 1996.

59. LaPrade, R. F.; Burnett, Q. M.: Femoral intercondylar notch stenosis and correlation to anterior cruciate ligament injuries. A prospective study. *Am J Sports Med* 22:198–203, 1994.

60. Larsson, L. G.; Baum, J.; Mudholkar, G. S.: Hypermobility: features and differential incidence between the sexes. *Arthritis Rheum* 30:1426–1430, 1987.

61. Leetun, D. T.; Ireland, M. L.; Willson, J. D.; et al.: Core stability measures as risk factors for lower extremity injury in athletes. *Med Sci Sports Exerc* 36:926–934, 2004.

62. Lephart, S. M.; Ferris, C. M.; Riemann, B. L.; et al.: Gender differences in strength and lower extremity kinematics during landing. *Clin Orthop* 401:162–169, 2002.

63. Lindenfeld, T. N.; Schmitt, D. J.; Hendy, M. P.; et al.: Incidence of injury in indoor soccer. *Am J Sports Med* 22:364–371, 1994.

64. Liu, S. H.; al-Shaikh, R.; Panossian, V.; et al.: Primary immunolocalization of estrogen and progesterone target cells in the human anterior cruciate ligament. *J Orthop Res* 14:526–533, 1996.

65. Lombardo, S.; Sethi, P. M.; Starkey, C.: Intercondylar notch stenosis is not a risk factor for anterior cruciate ligament tears in professional male basketball players: an 11-year prospective study. *Am J Sports Med* 33:29–34, 2005.

66. Loudon, J. K.; Jenkins, W.; Loudon, K. L.: The relationship between static posture and ACL injury in female athletes. *J Orthop Sports Phys Ther* 24:91–97, 1996.

67. Lund-Hanssen, H.; Gannon, J.; Engebretsen, L.; et al.: Intercondylar notch width and the risk for anterior cruciate ligament rupture. A case-control study in 46 female handball players. *Acta Orthop Scand* 65:529–532, 1994.

68. MacWilliams, B. A.; Wilson, D. R.; DesJardins, J. D.; et al.: Hamstrings cocontraction reduces internal rotation, anterior translation, and anterior cruciate ligament load in weight-bearing flexion. *J Orthop Res* 17:817–822, 1999.

69. Malinzak, R. A.; Colby, S. M.; Kirkendall, D. T.; et al.: A comparison of knee joint motion patterns between men and women in selected athletic tasks. *Clin Biomech (Bristol, Avon)* 16:438–445, 2001.

70. Messina, D. F.; Farney, W. C.; DeLee, J. C.: The incidence of injury in Texas high school basketball. A prospective study among male and female athletes. *Am J Sports Med* 27:294–299, 1999.

71. Meyers, M. C.; Barnhill, B. S.: Incidence, causes, and severity of high school football injuries on FieldTurf versus natural grass: a 5-year prospective study. *Am J Sports Med* 32:1626–1638, 2004.

72. Mizrahi, J.; Susak, Z.: Analysis of parameters affecting impact force attenuation during landing in human vertical free fall. *Eng Med* 11:141–147, 1982.

73. Mizrahi, J.; Susak, Z.: In-vivo elastic and damping response of the human leg to impact forces. *J Biomech Eng* 104:63–66, 1982.

74. More, R. C.; Karras, B. T.; Neiman, F.; et al.: Hamstrings—an anterior cruciate ligament protagonist: an in vitro study. *Am J Sports Med* 21:231–237, 1993.

75. Muneta, T.; Takakuda, K.; Yamamoto, H.: Intercondylar notch width and its relation to the configuration and cross-sectional area of the anterior cruciate ligament. A cadaveric knee study. *Am J Sports Med* 25:69–72, 1997.

76. Najibi, S.; Albright, J. P.: The use of knee braces, part 1: prophylactic knee braces in contact sports. *Am J Sports Med* 33:602–611, 2005.

77. Noyes, F. R.; Sonstegard, D. A.: Biomechanical function of the pes anserinus at the knee and the effect of its transplantation. *J Bone Joint Surg Am* 55:1225–1241, 1973.

78. O'Connor, J. J.: Can muscle co-contraction protect knee ligaments after injury or repair? *J Bone Joint Surg Br* 75:41–48, 1993.

79. Oggero, E.; Pagnacco, G.; Morr, D. R.; et al.: The mechanics of drop landing on a flat surface—a preliminary study. *Biomed Sci Instrum* 33:53–58, 1997.

80. Olsen, O. E.; Myklebust, G.; Engebretsen, L.; Bahr, R.: Injury mechanisms for anterior cruciate ligament injuries in team handball: a systematic video analysis. *Am J Sports Med* 32:1002–1012, 2004.

81. Olsen, O. E.; Myklebust, G.; Engebretsen, L.; et al.: Relationship between floor type and risk of ACL injury in team handball. *Scand J Med Sci Sports* 13:299–304, 2003.

82. Orchard, J.; Seward, H.; McGivern, J.; Hood, S.: Intrinsic and extrinsic risk factors for anterior cruciate ligament injury in Australian footballers. *Am J Sports Med* 29:196–200, 2001.

83. Ostenberg, A.; Roos, H.: Injury risk factors in female European football. A prospective study of 123 players during one season. *Scand J Med Sci Sports* 10:279–285, 2000.

84. Padua, D. A.; Carcia, C. R.; Arnold, B. L.; Granata, K. P.: Gender differences in leg stiffness and stiffness recruitment strategy during two-legged hopping. *J Mot Behav* 37:111–125, 2005.

85. Pandy, M. G.; Shelburne, K. B.: Dependence of cruciate-ligament loading on muscle forces and external load. *J Biomech* 30:1015–1024, 1997.

86. Pollard, C. D.; Davis, I. M.; Hamill, J.: Influence of gender on hip and knee mechanics during a randomly cued cutting maneuver. *Clin Biomech (Bristol, Avon)* 19:1022–1031, 2004.

87. Ramos, E.; Frontera, W. R.; Llopart, A.; Feliciano, D.: Muscle strength and hormonal levels in adolescents: gender related differences. *Int J Sports Med* 19:526–531, 1998.

88. Remvig, L.; Jensen, D. V.; Ward, R. C.: Epidemiology of general joint hypermobility and basis for the proposed criteria for benign joint hypermobility syndrome: review of the literature. *J Rheumatol* 34:804–809, 2007.

89. Rosene, J. M.; Fogarty, T. D.: Anterior tibial translation in collegiate athletes with normal anterior cruciate ligament integrity. *J Athl Train* 34:93–98, 1999.

90. Rozzi, S. L.; Lephart, S. M.; Gear, W. S.; Fu, F. H.: Knee joint laxity and neuromuscular characteristics of male and female soccer and basketball players. *Am J Sports Med* 27:312–319, 1999.

91. Salci, Y.; Kentel, B. B.; Heycan, C.; et al.: Comparison of landing maneuvers between male and female college volleyball players. *Clin Biomech (Bristol, Avon)* 19:622–628, 2004.

92. Schickendantz, M. S.; Weiker, G. G.: The predictive value of radiographs in the evaluation of unilateral and bilateral anterior cruciate ligament injuries. *Am J Sports Med* 21:110–113, 1993.

93. Scranton, P. E., Jr.; Whitesel, J. P.; Powell, J. W.; et al.: A review of selected noncontact anterior cruciate ligament injuries in the National Football League. *Foot Ankle Int* 18:772–776, 1997.

94. Seckin, U.; Tur, B. S.; Yilmaz, O.; et al.: The prevalence of joint hypermobility among high school students. *Rheumatol Int* 25:260–263, 2005.

95. Seger, J. Y.; Thorstensson, A.: Muscle strength and electromyogram in boys and girls followed through puberty. *Eur J Appl Physiol* 81:54–61, 2000.

96. Sell, T. C.; Ferris, C. M.; Abt, J. P.; et al.: The effect of direction and reaction on the neuromuscular and biomechanical characteristics of the knee during tasks that simulate the noncontact anterior cruciate ligament injury mechanism. *Am J Sports Med* 34:43–54, 2006.

97. Shelbourne, K. D.; Davis, T. J.; Klootwyk, T. E.: The relationship between intercondylar notch width of the femur and the incidence of anterior cruciate ligament tears. A prospective study. *Am J Sports Med* 26:402–408, 1998.

98. Shultz, S. J.; Kirk, S. E.; Johnson, M. L.; et al.: Relationship between sex hormones and anterior knee laxity across the menstrual cycle. *Med Sci Sports Exerc* 36:1165–1174, 2004.

99. Shultz, S. J.; Sander, T. C.; Kirk, S. E.; Perrin, D. H.: Sex differences in knee joint laxity change across the female menstrual cycle. *J Sports Med Phys Fitness* 45:594–603, 2005.

100. Simpson, K. J.; Kanter, L.: Jump distance of dance landings influencing internal joint forces: I. Axial forces. *Med Sci Sports Exerc* 29:916–927, 1997.

101. Simpson, K. J.; Pettit, M.: Jump distance of dance landings influencing internal joint forces: II. Shear forces. *Med Sci Sports Exerc* 29:928–936, 1997.

102. Sitler, M.; Ryan, J.; Hopkinson, W.; et al.: The efficacy of a prophylactic knee brace to reduce knee injuries in football. A prospective, randomized study at West Point. *Am J Sports Med* 18:310–315, 1990.

103. Slauterbeck, J. R.; Fuzie, S. F.; Smith, M. P.; et al.: The menstrual cycle, sex hormones, and anterior cruciate ligament injury. *J Athl Train* 37:275–278, 2002.

104. Smith, J.; Szczerba, J. E.; Arnold, B. L.; et al.: Role of hyperpronation as a possible risk factor for anterior cruciate ligament injuries. *J Athl Train* 32:25–28, 1997.

105. Souryal, T. O.; Freeman, T. R.: Intercondylar notch size and anterior cruciate ligament injuries in athletes. A prospective study. *Am J Sports Med* 21:535–539, 1993.

106. Staeubli, H. U.; Adam, O.; Becker, W.; Burgkart, R.: Anterior cruciate ligament and intercondylar notch in the coronal oblique plane: anatomy complemented by magnetic resonance imaging in cruciate ligament-intact knees. *Arthroscopy* 15:349–359, 1999.

107. Sunnegardh, J.; Bratteby, L. E.; Nordesjo, L. O.; Nordgren, B.: Isometric and isokinetic muscle strength, anthropometry and physical activity in 8 and 13 year old Swedish children. *Eur J Appl Physiol Occup Physiol* 58:291–297, 1988.

108. Teitz, C. C.; Lind, B. K.; Sacks, B. M.: Symmetry of the femoral notch width index. *Am J Sports Med* 25:687–690, 1997.

109. Uhorchak, J. M.; Scoville, C. R.; Williams, G. N.; et al.: Risk factors associated with noncontact injury of the anterior cruciate ligament: a prospective four-year evaluation of 859 West Point cadets. *Am J Sports Med* 31:831–842, 2003.

110. Wentorf, F. A.; Sudoh, K.; Moses, C.; et al.: The effects of estrogen on material and mechanical properties of the intra- and extra-articular knee structures. *Am J Sports Med* 34:1948–1952, 2006.

111. Wojtys, E. M.; Ashton-Miller, J. A.; Huston, L. J.: A gender-related difference in the contribution of the knee musculature to sagittal-plane shear stiffness in subjects with similar knee laxity. *J Bone Joint Surg Am* 84:10–16, 2002.

112. Wojtys, E. M.; Huston, L.; Boynton, M. D.; et al.: The effect of the menstrual cycle on anterior cruciate ligament injuries in women as determined by hormone levels. *Am J Sports Med* 30:182–188, 2002.

113. Wojtys, E. M.; Huston, L. J.; Lindenfeld, T. N.; et al.: Association between the menstrual cycle and anterior cruciate ligament injuries in female athletes. *Am J Sports Med* 26:614–619, 1998.

114. Wojtys, E. M.; Huston, L. J.; Schock, H. J.; et al.: Gender differences in muscular protection of the knee in torsion in size-matched athletes. *J Bone Joint Surg Am* 85:782–789, 2003.

115. Woodford-Rogers, B.; Cyphert, L.; Denegar, C. R.: Risk factors for anterior cruciate ligament injury in high school and college athletes. *J Athl Train* 29:343–346, 1994.

116. Yu, B.; McClure, S. B.; Onate, J. A.; et al.: Age and gender effects on lower extremity kinematics of youth soccer players in a stop-jump task. *Am J Sports Med* 33:1356–1364, 2005.

117. Yu, W. D.; Liu, S. H.; Hatch, J. D.; et al.: Effect of estrogen on cellular metabolism of the human anterior cruciate ligament. *Clin Orthop Relat Res* 366:229–238, 1999.

118. Yu, W. D.; Panossian, V.; Hatch, J. D.; et al.: Combined effects of estrogen and progesterone on the anterior cruciate ligament. *Clin Orthop Relat Res* 383:268–281, 2001.

119. Zeller, B. L.; McCrory, J. L.; Kibler, W. B.; Uhl, T. L.: Differences in kinematics and electromyographic activity between men and women during the single-legged squat. *Am J Sports Med* 31:449–456, 2003.

Chapter 16

Lower Limb Neuromuscular Control and Strength in Prepubescent and Adolescent Male and Female Athletes

Sue D. Barber-Westin, BS ■ Frank R. Noyes, MD

INTRODUCTION

An estimated 30 million children aged 5 to 18 years participate in organized sports programs each year in the United States.[1] Unfortunately, approximately one third of these athletes sustain injuries frequently in the ankle or knee that require medical treatment.[1,47,62,78] Several studies have reported that female athletes have a four- to eightfold higher incidence of serious knee ligament injury than males participating in the same sport.[4,15,36,51] The mechanisms responsible for the disparity between genders in knee ligament injury rates, especially in regard to the anterior cruciate ligament (ACL), are controversial and not scientifically

FIGURE 16–1. A, Knee joint stability is influenced by the muscles, ligaments, and bony geometry, which act together to resist external adduction moments that are incurred during weight-bearing activities. **B**, An abnormally high adduction moment may result in laxity of the lateral soft tissues and loss of normal lateral tibiofemoral joint contact. Termed *lateral condylar lift-off*, this phenomenon increases the potential for an anterior cruciate ligament (ACL) rupture, especially if the knee is in 30° or less of flexion.

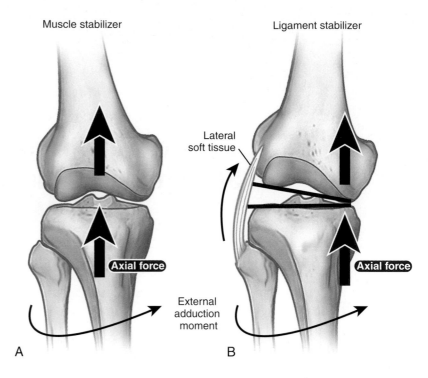

defined at present. Theories have included anatomic variations, environmental influences, hormonal fluctuations, and genetic factors.[34] Investigators have described gender differences in neuromuscular indices including muscle strength, running, cutting, sidestepping, and landing characteristics in adolescent and adult populations that are believed to be at least partially responsible for the differences in knee ligament injury rates.*

A valgus lower limb alignment commonly occurs during non-contact ACL injuries, when an athlete either lands from a jump or attempts to accelerate into a jump.[11,28,30] Scientists have reported significant differences between genders in knee and hip flexion angles[44] and ground reaction forces placed on the lower extremity upon landing.[42,57,68,69,76] Experimental studies show that, in a cadaver model, a valgus torque combined with an anterior tibial force results in statistically significant larger strain in the ACL than that produced from an anterior tibial force alone ($P < .0001$).[10] Markolf and coworkers[54] measured in vitro forces in the ACL during isolated and combined loading states in cadaver knees. Increases in ACL forces occurred when a valgus or varus moment was applied with an anterior tibial load compared with those measured when an anterior tibial load only was applied. In addition, high valgus or varus moments increase the risk for medial or lateral tibiofemoral joint lift-off and the potential for a knee ligament rupture (Fig. 16–1).[54] It is unknown whether one can extrapolate these laboratory findings to an increased risk of ACL injury when an athlete lands or collapses into a valgus position, with little distance separating the right and the left knee.

This chapter summarizes a series of four studies conducted by the authors that measured the effects of chronological age and gender in athletes 9 to 17 years of age on isokinetic lower extremity strength, lower limb alignment during a drop-jump test, and lower limb symmetry during single-leg-hop tests. The ages for the hypotheses developed for the studies were based

on the mean time to achieve peak height velocity (mean, 11.5 yr for girls and 13.5 yr for boys[88]) and skeletal maturity (mean, 13.3 yr for girls and 14.3 yr for boys[3]). All studies were approved by a local hospital's institutional review board.

NEUROMUSCULAR TESTING METHODS

A total of 1140 athletes (916 female and 224 male athletes) 9 to 17 years of age were recruited from area schools and youth athletic leagues to participate in the authors' investigational sports injury test (SIT). The students participated in a variety of organized sports, including soccer, basketball, volleyball, baseball, football, and track and field. Before the SIT, the athletes were screened to ensure that no participant had sustained an injury that required medical treatment. All testing was done on a voluntary basis.

The goal of the SIT was to collect data on a large number of young athletes that included

- Demographics (height, weight, body mass index [BMI], age).
- History of athletic participation.
- Lower limb dominance.
- Lower limb isokinetic muscle strength.
- Lower limb alignment on a videographic drop-jump test.
- Lower limb symmetry on single-leg-hop tests.

Videographic Drop-Jump Screening Test

A drop-jump videographic screening test was developed as described in detail previously.[65] Minimal equipment is required and the software is available from the authors' nonprofit foundation. A camcorder equipped with a memory stick is placed on a stand 102.24 cm (40.25 inches) in height. The stand is positioned approximately 365.76 cm (12 ft) in front of a box 30.48 cm (12 inches) in

---

*See references 18, 27, 41, 42, 44, 45, 50, 55, 56, 91–94.

Critical Points NEUROMUSCULAR TESTING METHODS

Sports injury test done on 1140 athletes (916 female, 224 male) 9–17 yr of age.

Videographic Drop Jump Screening Test

- Equipment: camcorder, memory stick, software, stand 102.24 cm in height, Velcro circles, reflective markers.
- No verbal instructions other than "land straight in front of the box to be in the correct angle for the camera to record properly."
- Athlete jumps off box, lands, jumps up into a maximum vertical jump. Repeats three times.
- Three sequences: pre-land, land, take-off.
- Sequences captured; images imported into software. Calculates absolute centimeters of distance between right and left hips, knees, ankles.
- Knee separation distance normalized according to hip separation distance.

Reliability

- Test-retest intraclass correlation coefficient (ICC) > .90 hip separation distance all three phases.
- Within-test ICC > .90 all sequences.

Isokinetic Evaluation of Knee Extensor and Flexor Strength

- Knee extensor, flexor isokinetic testing 300°/sec athletes > 11 yr of age, 180°/sec athletes 9–10 yr of age.
- Ten repetitions; highest peak torque used for analyses. Peak torques normalized for body weight.

Isokinetic Evaluation of Internal and External Tibial Rotation Strength

- Internal rotation, external rotation peak torques obtained 120°/sec, 180°/sec.
- Partial supine position, hip flexed 60°, knee flexed 90°.
- Foot and ankle secured to a footplate.
- Eight repetitions completed for each speed; highest peak torque used for analysis.
- Peak torques normalized for body weight.

Single-Leg Functional Hop Testing

Timed Side-Hop Test

- Course created on floor using masking tape to mark three boxes 46 × 46 cm.
- Athletes were encouraged to hop as fast as possible, but to maintain balance.
- Two tests completed for each limb; mean times calculated with stopwatch to the nearest .01 sec.

Crossover Hop Test

- Strip made with masking tape on floor, extends approximately 6 m.
- Athletes hop three consecutive times on one foot, crossing diagonally over the tape on each hop.
- Total distance hopped measured and each leg tested twice; average distance calculated.

Limb symmetry calculated for each test by dividing the mean of the right limb by the mean of the left limb and multiplying the result by 100. Limb symmetry < 85% abnormal.

---

height and 38.1 cm (15 inches) in width. One-inch Velcro circles are placed on each of the four corners of the box that faces the camera. Athletes wear fitted, dark shorts and low-cut gym shoes. Reflective markers are placed at the greater trochanter and the lateral malleolus of both the right and the left legs, and Velcro circles are placed on the center of each patella. A research assistant demonstrates the jump-land sequence, and one practice trial is done to ensure the athlete understands the test. No verbal instruction regarding how to land or jump is provided. Athletes are told only to land straight in front of the box to be in the correct angle for the camera to record properly. The athletes perform a jump-land sequence by first jumping off the box, landing, and immediately performing a maximum vertical jump. This sequence is repeated three times.

After completion of the test, a research assistant views all three trials, and the one that best represents the athlete's jumping ability is selected for measurement. Advancing the videographic frame-by-frame, the following images are captured as still photographs: (1) pre-land, the frame in which the athlete's toes just touch the ground after the jump off of the box; (2) land, the frame in which the athlete is at the deepest point; and (3) take-off, the frame that demonstrates the initial forward and upward movement of the arms and the body as the athlete prepares to go into the maximum vertical jump.

The captured images are imported into a hard drive of a desktop computer and digitized on the computer screen. A calibration procedure is done by placing the cursor and clicking in the center of each Velcro marker on each of the four corners of the drop-jump box. The anatomic reference points represented by the reflective markers are selected by clicking in a designated sequence the cursor for each image.

The absolute centimeters of separation distance between the right and the left hip and normalized separation distances for the knees and ankles, standardized according to the hip separation distance, are analyzed. Normalized knee separation distance is calculated as knee separation distance divided by hip separation distance and normalized ankle separation distance is calculated as ankle separation distance divided by hip separation distance (Fig. 16–2).

The reliability of the drop-jump videographic test was determined in 17 female athletes who underwent the test twice, 7 weeks apart.[61] The reliability of the absolute centimeters of hip separation distances was evaluated. Hip separation distance was expected to be highly reliable, thus providing the basis for normalization of knee and ankle separation distances. Then, in 10 other subjects, reliability within the videographic test was assessed by capturing two of the three jump-land sequence trials and comparing the absolute centimeters of hip, knee, and ankle separation distances between the two sequences on the same day of testing. For the test-retest trial, the intraclass correlation coefficients (ICC) for the hip separation distance demonstrated high reliability (pre-land, .96; land, .94; take-off, .94). For the within-test trial, the ICC for the hip, knee, and ankle separation distance were all .90 or higher, demonstrating excellent reliability of the videographic test and software capturing procedures.

Isokinetic Evaluation of Knee Extensor and Flexor Strength

Isokinetic knee extensor and flexor testing was conducted (concentric mode) at 300°/sec (Fig. 16–3) in athletes over the age of 11 years. For the children who were 9 to 10 years of age, this test was performed at 180°/sec. Other investigators have reported acceptable reliability of isokinetic measurements in children and adults

FIGURE 16–2. The videographic test produced photographs of three phases of the drop-jump test. The centimeters of distance between the hips, the knees, and the ankles was calculated along with normalized knee and ankle separation distance (according to the hip separation distance). Shown is the test result of a 14-year-old female. *(From Noyes, F. B.; Barber-Westin, S. D.; Fleckenstein, C.; et al.: The drop-jump screening test: difference in lower limb control by gender and effect of neuromuscular training in female athletes. Am J Sports Med 33:197–207, 2005.)*

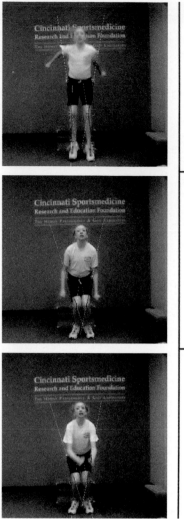

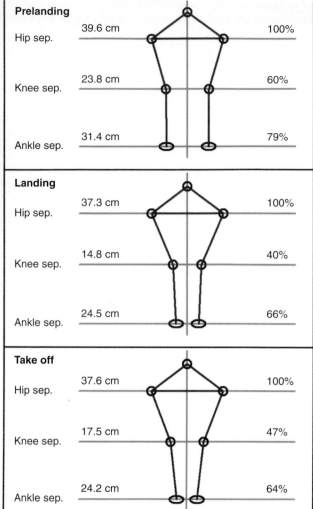

Prelanding

Hip sep.	39.6 cm	100%
Knee sep.	23.8 cm	60%
Ankle sep.	31.4 cm	79%

Landing

Hip sep.	37.3 cm	100%
Knee sep.	14.8 cm	40%
Ankle sep.	24.5 cm	66%

Take off

Hip sep.	37.6 cm	100%
Knee sep.	17.5 cm	47%
Ankle sep.	24.2 cm	64%

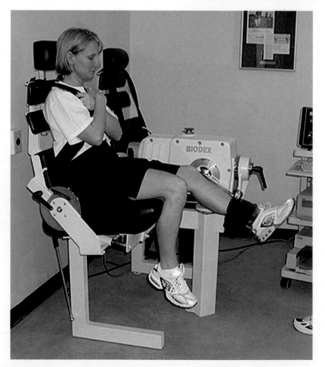

FIGURE 16–3. Isokinetic knee extensor and flexor testing.

at these test velocities.[48,58,60] The athletes first completed a dynamic warm-up session that lasted 5 minutes. They were then positioned in the chair of the device with appropriate torso, pelvis, and thigh straps placed according to the manufacturer's protocol. The lever arm of the dynamometer was aligned with the lateral epicondyle of the knee, with the knee flexed to 90°. The chair was adjusted for each athlete as required to ensure proper positioning. The range of motion during the test was fixed from 90° to 0°. Gravitational factors were calculated by the dynamometer and automatically compensated for during the tests. The athletes performed three to four submaximal trials to become familiar with the machine and test velocity. A total of 10 repetitions were completed and the highest peak torque value used for analyses. Mean peak torque values (in Newton-meters [Nm]) were normalized for body weight (BW) in kilograms. Verbal encouragement was given throughout the tests, because the athletes were told to kick as hard and as fast as possible, but no visual feedback was available.

Isokinetic Evaluation of Internal and External Tibial Rotation Strength

An isokinetic assessment of knee internal tibial rotation (IR) and external tibial rotation (ER) strength was conducted on a calibrated Biodex System 3 (Biodex Medical Systems, Inc., Shirley, NY).

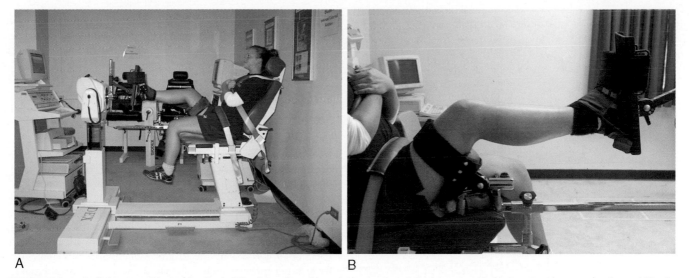

A   B

FIGURE 16–4. A, Subject positioning for the isokinetic testing of internal and external tibial rotation. **B**, Foot and ankle strapping for stabilization. (**A** and **B**, Reprinted from Noyes, F. R.; Barber-Westin, S. D.: Isokinetic profile and differences in tibial rotation strength between male and female athletes 11 to 17 years of age. Isok Exer Sci 13:251–259, 2005; with permission from IOS Press.)

The IR and ER peak torques of each limb were obtained at 120°/sec and 180°/sec. Testing was preceded by a dynamic warm-up that lasted approximately 5 minutes. The patients were positioned in the device in a partial supine position with the hip flexed 60° and the knee flexed 90° as described by Hester and Falkel (Fig. 16-4).[39] Appropriate torso, pelvis, and thigh straps were placed according to the manufacturer's protocol. In addition, the foot and ankle were tightly secured to a footplate using Velcro (VELCRO USA, Manchester, NH) straps.[39] The athletes were instructed to relax so that the neutral position with regard to tibial rotation and the range of internal and external tibial motion could be obtained.[72,89] Five submaximal repetitions were done before each test to promote familiarization with the dynamometer velocity speeds and to set the range of motion limits for both IR and ER.

There were 2-minute rest periods between the two velocity speed tests. The testing sequence of the dominant and nondominant limbs was randomized among the subjects. Verbal encouragement was given throughout the tests, because the athletes were told to rotate their lower leg through full range with maximal effort, but no visual feedback was available. A total of eight repetitions were completed at each speed and the single highest peak torque value used for analyses. Peak torque values were normalized for BW in kilograms and were expressed as (Nm/BW). Time-to-peak torque was measured in milliseconds (msec). The ratio of the mean peak torque of IR was calculated relative to that of ER (ratio IE = IR/ER × 100) in a manner described by Segawa and associates.[82] The ratio of the mean peak torque of both IR and ER were also calculated relative to that of knee flexion. The ratio IR-F was calculated as IR/flexion × 100, and the ratio ER-F was calculated as ER/flexion × 100. The ratio of the mean peak torque of IR (IR-E) and ER (ER-E) were also calculated relative to that of knee extension in a manner similar to that described for knee flexion.

Single-Leg Functional Hop Testing

Two single-leg functional hop tests were conducted: a timed side-hop and a crossover hop for distance. The athletes were provided with instructions and one practice trial was conducted for each test. In the timed side-hop test, a course was created on the floor using masking tape to mark three boxes that were 46 × 46 cm (Fig. 16–5).[7] The athletes were encouraged to hop as fast as possible, but to maintain balance to be able to complete the test. If the athlete did not clear the lines, double bounced between hops, or could not hold balance on landing, a zero was recorded. Two tests were completed for each limb, with mean times calculated with a standard stopwatch to the nearest .01 sec.

In the crossover hop for distance test, a marking strip made of masking tape was placed on the floor that extended approximately 6 m (Fig. 16–6).[63] The athletes hopped three consecutive times on one foot, crossing diagonally over the tape on each hop. They were encouraged to go as far as possible while maintaining balance and control. The total distance hopped was measured and each leg tested twice, with the average distance calculated. The reliability of this test has been reported by other investigators to be excellent.[5,12,29]

Limb symmetry was calculated for each test by dividing the mean of the right limb by the mean of the left limb and

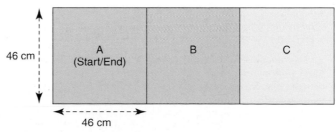

FIGURE 16–5. Single-leg timed side-hop function test. Subject begins in box A. Standing on one leg, the subject hops to box B, box C, then back to box B and box A to complete one course repetition. One trial consists of three repetitions. The subject must successfully cross the lines, maintain single-legged balance, and hold each landing without placing the opposite foot down on the floor. (From Barber-Westin, S. D.; Noyes, F. R.; Galloway, M.: Jump-land characteristics and muscle strength development in young athletes: a gender comparison of 1140 athletes 9 to 17 years of age. Am J Sports Med 34:375–384, 2006.)

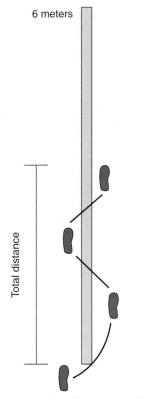

6 meters

Total distance

FIGURE 16–6. Crossover hop for distance test. The athlete hops three consecutive times on one foot, crossing diagonally over the tape on each hop. Subjects are encouraged to hop as far as possible while maintaining balance and control. *(From Noyes, F. R.; Barber, S. D.; Mangine, R. E.: Abnormal lower limb symmetry determined by function hop tests after anterior cruciate ligament rupture. Am J Sports Med 19:513–518, 1991.)*

multiplying the result by 100. Prior studies on populations aged 17 to 34 reported that less than 85% limb symmetry on single-leg-hop tests was abnormal and representative of a general lower limb functional limitation.[6,63]

STUDY #1: VIDEOGRAPHIC DROP-JUMP SCREENING TEST

In this investigation, 325 female and 130 male athletes aged 11 to 19 underwent the videographic drop-jump screening test.[65] A neuromuscular-training program[40,42] (Sportsmetrics) was completed by 62 of the females; their jump-landing characteristics were reexamined within 1 week of the final training session. This subgroup also underwent an isokinetic evaluation of knee extensor and flexor strength before and after the neuromuscular-training program. The training sessions, described in detail in Chapter 19, Decreasing the Risk of ACL Injuries in Female Athletes, lasted approximately 1 hr/day, 3 days a week on alternating days and consisted of stretching, plyometric jump-training, and weight training under the supervision of a certified instructor. Participation in the training program was strictly voluntary and no attempt was made to influence certain individuals over others to complete the training with respect to the results of the initial videographic tests. Power and sample-size calculations were done to evaluate the primary study findings, the effect of training on absolute knee separation distance and normalized knee separation distance. With 62 trained females, it was found that this investigation had sufficient power (90%) to detect significant differences at a level of 0.05.

There was no statistically significant effect of age or lower limb dominance in either the female or the male athletes for the normalized mean knee and ankle separation distances for each phase (pre-land, landing, and take-off) of the jump-land sequence.

Critical Points STUDY #1: VIDEOGRAPHIC DROP-JUMP SCREENING TEST

$N = 325$ female and 130 male athletes aged 11–19 yr. Neuromuscular-training program completed by 62 females; jump-landing characteristics reexamined within 1 wk of the final training session.

Hypothesis #1: Female athletes have an overall lower limb valgus alignment, indicated by abnormally decreased knee separation distances, on landing and acceleration into a vertical jump on a videographic drop-jump test.

- Hypothesis supported: marked overall lower limb valgus alignment found in 63% of the female athletes on landing, 80% on take-off.

Hypothesis #2: Male athletes have a more neutrally aligned lower limb position, with a greater amount of separation distance between the knees, on landing and acceleration into a vertical jump compared with females on a drop-jump test.

- Hypothesis not supported: marked overall lower limb valgus alignment in 75% of male athletes on landing, 72% on take-off.

Hypothesis #3: A neuromuscular-training program will produce significantly greater knee separation distance in female athletes, thereby producing a more neutrally aligned lower limb alignment on a drop-jump test.

- Hypothesis supported: statistically significant increases found after training in the subgroup of 62 females in the absolute and the normalized knee and ankle separation distances for all phases of the jump-land sequence.

- Significant improvement after training knee flexor peak torque values in dominant and nondominant legs.

Implication of Findings

- Study goal was to provide a general indicator of an athletes' lower limb axial alignment in the coronal plane in a straightforward drop-jump and vertical take-off task. The authors do not propose that this videographic analysis can be used as a risk indicator for a knee ligament injury.

- Excessive valgus moments about the knee joint with subsequent high anterior tibial shear forces may be one of the anterior cruciate ligament injury mechanisms in females.

- Excessive valgus loading may decrease tibiofemoral contact, or condylar lift-off, and reduce normal joint contact geometry that contributes to knee joint stability.

- 75% of males had valgus-aligned lower limb position on landing. The significance of this finding is unknown and may represent an aberration requiring further study.

- It is unknown whether the improvement in knee separation distance after training will transfer to reduce the risk of a serious knee ligament injury in female athletes.

- Some female athletes may require further training to improve overall alignment and land in a more neutrally aligned position.

Hypothesis #1: Female Athletes Have an Overall Lower Limb Valgus Alignment, Indicated by Abnormally Decreased Knee Separation Distances, on Landing and Acceleration into a Vertical Jump on a Videographic Drop-Jump Test

The hypothesis was supported, because a marked overall lower limb valgus alignment (indicated by a knee separation distance of ≤ 60%) was found in 63% of the female athletes on landing (Fig. 16–7) and in 80% on take-off.

Hypothesis #2: Male Athletes Have a More Neutrally Aligned Lower Limb Position, with a Greater Amount of Separation Distance between the Knees, on Landing and Acceleration into a Vertical Jump Compared with Females on a Drop-Jump Test

The hypothesis was not supported, as a marked overall lower limb valgus alignment was found in 75% of the male athletes on landing (see Fig. 16–7) and in 72% on take-off. There was no statistically significant difference between male and female athletes in the mean normalized knee and ankle separation distance during the landing and take-off phases. The female athletes had significantly higher mean normalized knee and ankle separation distances during the pre-land phase only.

The normalized knee separation distances for both genders are shown in Figure 16–8, the normalized ankle separation distances are shown in Figure 16–9, and the absolute values for the hip, knee, and ankle separation distances are shown in Table 16–1. There were no correlations between knee and ankle separation distances for each phase of the jump-land sequence in either the female or the male athletes.

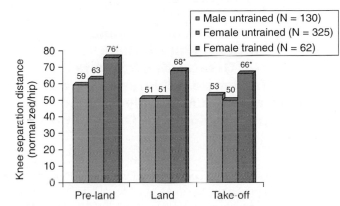

FIGURE 16–8. The mean normalized knee separation distances for the three phases of the drop-jump test are shown for the male athletes, untrained female athletes, and trained female athletes. After training, female athletes had statistically significant increases in the mean normalized knee separation distance in all three phases (P < .001) and had statistically greater mean normalized knee separation distances than males for all phases (P < .0001). (From Noyes, F. R.; Barber-Westin, S. D., Fleckenstein, C.; et al.: The drop-jump screening test: difference in lower limb control by gender and effect of neuromuscular training in female athletes. Am J Sports Med 33:197–207, 2005.)

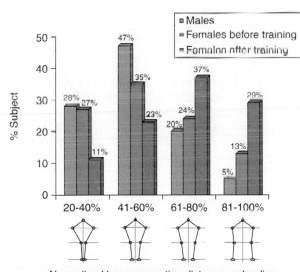

FIGURE 16–7. The distribution of male athletes and the 62 female athletes before and after training according to normalized knee separation distance on landing. Whereas there was no difference in the distribution of male and untrained female athletes among the categories shown, a significant difference was present between male and trained females (P < .0001). The stick figures are representative of the knee separation distance but not of the ankle separation distance. (From Noyes, F. R.; Barber-Westin, S. D.; Fleckenstein, C.; et al.: The drop-jump screening test: difference in lower limb control by gender and effect of neuromuscular training in female athletes. Am J Sports Med 33:197–207, 2005.)

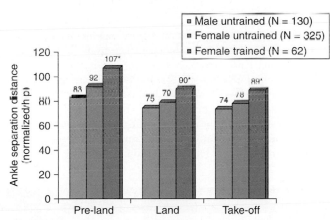

FIGURE 16–9. The mean normalized ankle separation distances for the three phases of the drop-jump test are shown for the male athletes, untrained female athletes, and trained female athletes. After training, female athletes had statistically significant increases in the mean normalized ankle separation distance in all three phases (P < .001) and had statistically greater mean normalized ankle separation distances than males for all phases (P < .0001). (From Noyes, F. R.; Barber-Westin, S. D.; Fleckenstein, C.; et al.: The drop-jump screening test: difference in lower limb control by gender and effect of neuromuscular training in female athletes. Am J Sports Med 33:197–207, 2005.)

TABLE 16–1   Absolute Hip, Knee, and Ankle Separation Distances in 455 Athletes during a Videographic Drop-Jump Screening Test*

Gender	Pre-Land			Land			Take-off		
	Hip	Knee	Ankle	Hip	Knee	Ankle	Hip	Knee	Ankle
Untrained females ($N = 325$)	41 ± 3	28 ± 6	40 ± 8	41 ± 3	23 ± 9	35 ± 8	41 ± 3	23 ± 9	34 ± 8
Trained females ($N = 62$)	41 ± 3	$31 \pm 5^{\dagger}$	$44 \pm 7^{\dagger}$	42 ± 3	$29 \pm 8^{\dagger}$	$38 \pm 7^{\dagger}$	42 ± 3	$28 \pm 8^{\dagger}$	$38 \pm 7^{\dagger}$
Males ($N = 130$)	44 ± 5	26 ± 5	36 ± 6	42 ± 5	22 ± 8	31 ± 6	42 ± 5	23 ± 8	31 ± 6

*Data shown are mean ± standard deviation in centimeters.
†Significantly greater than pretrained females ($P < .001$) and males ($P < .0001$).

Hypothesis #3: A Neuromuscular-Training Program Will Produce Significantly Greater Knee Separation Distance in Female Athletes, thereby Producing a More Neutrally Aligned Lower Limb Position on a Drop-Jump Test

The neuromuscular-training program was effective, supporting the hypothesis, because statistically significant increases were found after training in the subgroup of 62 females in the absolute (see Table 16–1) and the normalized knee (see Fig. 16–8) and ankle (see Fig. 16–9) separation distances for all phases of the jump-land sequence ($P < .001$). After training, the female athletes had statistically greater mean normalized knee and ankle separation distances than the male athletes for all phases of the jump-land sequence ($P < .0001$). In addition, after training, a statistically significant difference was found in the distribution of female athletes who had less than 60%, 61% to 80%, or greater than 80% knee separation distance on landing ($P = .003$) and take-off ($P = .006$). The distribution in the percentage change in knee and ankle separation distances after training is shown for all three phases of the jump-land sequence in Table 16–2.

Another important finding of this investigation was the significant improvement after training in knee flexor peak torque values in both the dominant and the nondominant legs ($P < .0001$). In the dominant leg, knee flexor peak torque increased from 40 ± 8 Nm (mean ± standard deviation) before training to 44 ± 7 Nm after training; and in the nondominant leg, from 38 ± 8 Nm to 42 ± 8 Nm. Knee extensor peak torque improved slightly (but not significantly) in both legs. In the dominant leg, extensor peak torque improved from 54 ± 9 Nm to 56 ± 13 Nm, and in the nondominant leg, from 54 ± 10 Nm to 57 ± 15 Nm.

Statistically significant improvements were found in the hamstrings-to-quadriceps ratio for the nondominant leg, which increased from $71 \pm 15\%$ before training to $77 \pm 16\%$ after

training ($P = .01$). There was no significant increase in this ratio in the dominant leg. No correlations were found between knee extensor and flexor strength and normalized knee and ankle separation distances for any phase of the jump-land sequence before or after training.

Implication of Findings

The authors developed and studied a videographic drop-jump screening test to record lower limb axial alignment in the coronal plane using a single standard videographic camera. The testing procedure was designed to be relatively easy to perform by researchers, coaches, trainers, or therapists in any facility. The goal was to provide a general indicator of an athlete's lower limb axial alignment in the coronal plane in a straightforward drop-jump and vertical take-off task. The authors do not propose that this videographic analysis can be used as a risk indicator for a knee ligament injury. The test depicts only hip, knee, and ankle positions in a single plane during one maneuver, and it is recognized that noncontact ACL injuries may occur in side-to-side or cutting motions. A more sophisticated multicamera system would be required to measure these types of motions. The use of even just a second camera to measure the degrees of knee flexion on landing would provide additional information[44]; however, the goal was to use one camera to make the measurements easier to perform from a screening standpoint. Because of these limitations, it may be that the single-plane videographic drop-jump test was not sensitive enough to depict relevant differences in landing patterns between the sexes.

Authors have reported that 58% to 61% of noncontact injuries occur on landing from a jump.[28,30] The final position of the knee joint on landing is influenced by the center of gravity of the upper body and the trunk over the lower extremity. Equally important are the positions of trunk-hip adduction or abduction, foot-ankle pronation-supination, and foot separation distance. These effects combine together to produce either a varus or a valgus moment about the knee joint that must be balanced by the lower

TABLE 16–2   Change in Normalized Knee and Ankle Separation Distances after Neuromuscular Training in 62 Female Athletes

% Change	Pre-Land*		Land*		Take-Off*	
	Knee	Ankle	Knee	Ankle	Knee	Ankle
None	24 (38)	27 (44)	21 (33)	33 (53)	22 (35)	35 (56)
5–10	12 (19)	9 (15)	11 (18)	3 (4)	8 (13)	1 (2)
11–15	9 (15)	8 (13)	5 (8)	5 (8)	7 (11)	8 (13)
16–20	9 (15)	3 (4)	6 (10)	9 (15)	4 (6)	6 (10)
>20	8 (13)	15 (24)	19 (31)	12 (19)	21 (34)	12 (19)

*Values represent number (%) of athletes.

limb musculature (see Fig. 16–1).[42] If the athlete is off-balance, or has contact with another player, a loss of trunk and lower limb control and position may occur and the knee joint may go into a hyperextended or severe valgus position. The knee position measured in the coronal plane in the authors' single-plane videographic analysis is a reflection of rotations in both the coronal and the transverse planes (internal-external femoral and tibial rotation). This test does not distinguish between these individual motions, which requires more sophisticated instrumentation.[42]

Although there are many potential mechanisms for ACL injury, it has been postulated that excessive valgus moments about the knee joint with subsequent high anterior tibial shear forces may be one of the ACL injury mechanisms in females.[33,46,53] Excessive valgus loading may result in decreased tibiofemoral contact or condylar lift-off[54] and a reduction in the normal joint contact geometry that contributes to knee joint stability. This position, coupled with a highly activated quadriceps muscle that produces maximum anterior shear forces with the knee joint at low flexion angles ($\leq 30°$),[23,35,67] can lead to ACL rupture.

Hamstrings muscle activation with the knee joint at or near full knee extension ($\leq 30°$) produces insufficient posterior tibia shear forces to protect the ACL owing to the small angle of inclination of the hamstring tendons.[73] Noyes and Sonstegard[66] described a decreased mechanical advantage of the inner hamstrings when the knee is extended, because the hamstring flexion force at 0° is approximately half that at 90°. Similarly, the rotation force of the inner hamstrings declines with knee extension, because the rotation force at 0° is 41% that of the rotation force that occurs at 90°. A rotation "wind-up" effect exists, in which the IR forces increase significantly with ER owing to an increase in muscle mechanical advantage.

The authors hypothesized that the majority of untrained female athletes would demonstrate an abnormal lower limb position on landing from a drop-jump and on acceleration into a vertical jump. A normalized knee separation distance of less than 60% occurred in 63% of the untrained females on landing and in 80% on take-off. It was also hypothesized that the majority of young male athletes would demonstrate a neutrally aligned lower limb position on landing and acceleration into a vertical jump. This hypothesis was not supported, because 75% of the males had marked knee separation distances on landing and 72% on take-off, indicating a valgus-aligned lower limb position. The significance of this finding is unknown and may represent an aberration requiring further study (Fig. 16–10). It may be that this single-plane videographic test was not sensitive enough to depict relevant differences in landing patterns between the sexes. Other studies that used multicamera systems or force plates to investigate the drop-jump test found significant differences between females and males regarding knee flexion angles,[44] knee extension moments,[16,42] knee valgus moments,[16] and ground reaction forces.[42] A prior investigation determined that untrained female athletes had lower knee extension moments than males and postulated that this was explained by the male subjects' high use of the hamstrings as a knee flexor at landing.[44]

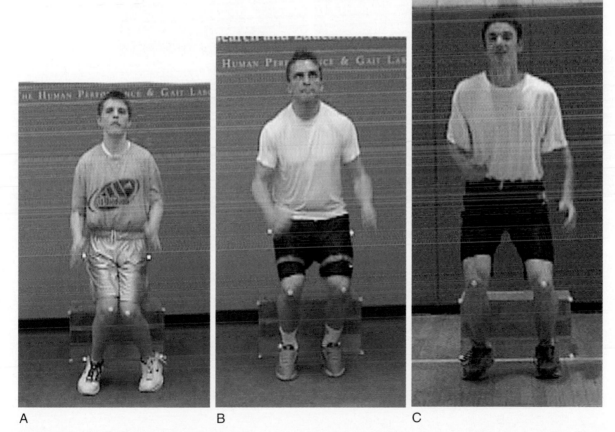

FIGURE 16–10. The drop-jump take-off sequences from three male athletes. **A,** Athlete 1: A 12-year-old soccer player demonstrates poor knee separation distance of 10.6 cm (28% normalized). **B,** Athlete 2: A 17-year-old basketball player demonstrated 29.3 cm (65% normalized) knee separation distance. **C,** Athlete 3: A neutral alignment is evident in this 16-year-old football player, who demonstrated 38.4 cm (82% normalized) knee separation distance. (**A–C,** From Noyes, F. R.; Barber-Westin, S. D.; Fleckenstein, C.; et al.: The drop-jump screening test: difference in lower limb control by gender and effect of neuromuscular training in female athletes. Am J Sports Med 33:197–207, 2005.)

The authors believed that a neuromuscular-training program would increase knee separation distance in female athletes, thereby leading to a more neutral overall lower limb position during the drop-jump test (Fig. 16–11). The goals of the training program were to teach athletes to control the upper body, trunk, and lower body position; lower the center of gravity by

increasing hip and knee flexion on landing; and develop muscular strength and techniques to land with decreased ground reaction forces. In addition, athletes were taught to pre-position the body and lower extremity before landing in order to land in the position of greatest knee joint stability and stiffness, with the goal of obtaining ankle and knee separation distances within approximately

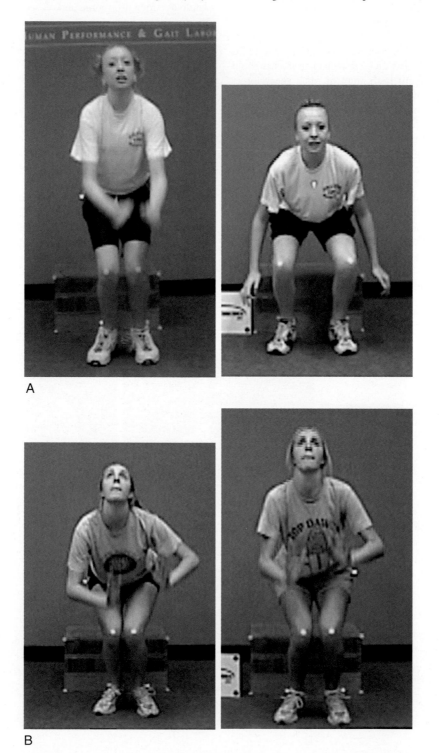

FIGURE 16–11. The drop-jump take-off sequences from three female athletes before and after neuromuscular training. **Athlete A**, A 14-year-old basketball player demonstrated marked improvement in knee separation distance (from 17 cm to 37 cm) and in ankle separation distance (from 24 cm to 36 cm) after training (*right*). The normalized knee separation distance improved from 47% to 92%, and the normalized ankle separation distance improved from 64% to 92%. **Athlete B**, A 14-year-old volleyball player demonstrated poor upper body position and no improvement in knee or ankle separation distance after training (*right*). She was encouraged to pursue additional training.

Continued

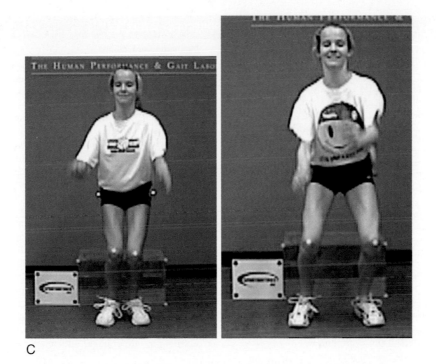

C

FIGURE 16–11 cont'd. Athlete C, A 12-year-old basketball player showed slight overcorrection from a valgus position (knee separation distance, 14 cm) before training (*left*) to a varus position (knee separation distance, 37 cm) after training (*right*). The normalized knee separation distance improved from 38% to 98%. The normalized ankle separation distance improved dramatically from 65% to 111%. (*A–C, from Nuyes, F. R.; Barber Westin, S. D., Fleckenstein, C.; et al.: The drop-jump screening test: difference in lower limb control by gender and effect of neuromuscular training in female athletes. Am J Sports Med 33:197–217, 2005.*)

80% that of the hip separation distance. The neuromuscular training program was previously shown to be effective in inducing changes in neuromuscular indices (see Chapter 19, Decreasing the Risk of ACL Injuries in Female Athletes),[42] including decreasing peak landing forces and peak adduction and abduction moments and improving hamstrings-to-quadriceps ratios. A correlation was found between the ability of the athlete to control knee adduction and abduction moments and the peak landing forces (*P* = .006). Decreased abduction or abduction moments may lessen the risk of lift-off of the medial or lateral femoral condyle, improve tibiofemoral contact stabilizing forces,[54] and decrease the risk of ligament injury. Other training techniques that use verbal and visual feedback have also been successful in reducing ground reaction forces.[25,49,57,69,76]

In the female athletes, significant increases were found after training in the absolute and normalized knee and ankle separation distances for all phases of the jump-land sequence (*P* < .001). As a result, the female athletes had significantly greater normalized knee and ankle separation distances than the males for each phase. The neuromuscular-training program was reported to be effective in another study in decreasing the incidence of noncontact serious knee ligament injuries in female athletes.[40] In that report, 8 of 463 untrained females sustained a serious noncontact knee ligament injury compared with 0 of 366 trained females and 1 of 434 untrained male athletes. Untrained females had a 3.6 times higher incidence of knee injury than trained females (*P* = .05) and 4.8 times higher than males (*P* = .03).

It is unknown whether the improvement in knee separation distance after training will transfer to reduce the risk of a serious knee ligament injury in female athletes. The increased incidence of knee ligament injuries in female athletes is multifactorial and it

is currently unknown which factors are dominant and which play a smaller role. A number of intrinsic factors inherent in women have been suggested, including a narrow intercondylar notch, smaller-sized ACL, pelvic-hip-knee-foot alignment, generalized knee laxity, foot pronation, and hormonal fluctuations.[33] Extrinsic factors related to athletic conditioning, skill, training, and equipment have also been discussed. Although issues related to differences in neuromuscular control, muscle reaction patterns,[45,93] and coordination and control of body and lower extremity positions during athletics are usually related to extrinsic factors, it may be that these factors are both intrinsic and extrinsic in their development.

It is important to note that some female athletes may require further training to demonstrate improvements in knee and ankle separation distance and land in a more neutrally aligned position. The pictorial sequence of the filmed drop-jump provides important information to athletes, parents, and coaches and can be useful in detecting athletes who require further neuromuscular training (see Fig. 16–11).

STUDY #2: NEUROMUSCULAR INDICES IN PREPUBESCENT ATHLETES

In this study, 27 girls and 25 boys who were participating in organized athletics were recruited from area schools and youth soccer leagues to participate.[7] There was no difference between the girls and the boys for mean age (9.7 ± 0.5 yr and 9.6 ± 0.5 yr, respectively), height (136 ± 7 cm and 133 ± 5 cm, respectively), weight (39 ± 11 kg and 36 ± 5 kg, respectively), or BMI (18 ± 4 and 18 ± 2, respectively). There was no difference between the girls and the boys in the mean years of sports

Critical Points STUDY #2: NEUROMUSCULAR INDICES IN PREPUBESCENT ATHLETES

$N = 27$ girls and 25 boys participating in organized athletics. Matched age, height, weight, body mass index, years of sports participation.

Hypothesis #1: No significant difference exists between prepubescent boys and prepubescent girls in overall lower limb alignment during a drop-jump test.
- Hypothesis supported: marked decrease in normalized knee separation distance in 19 males (76%) and 25 females (93%) on landing.

Hypothesis #2: No significant difference exists between prepubescent boys and prepubescent girls in knee extensor and flexor strength.
- Hypothesis supported: no difference between genders in knee extensor and flexor peak torques.
- No correlations between extensor and flexor peak torque values and overall lower limb alignment in drop-jump test.

Hypothesis #3: No significant difference exists between prepubescent boys and prepubescent girls in lower limb symmetry on single-leg function testing.
- Hypothesis supported: lower limb asymmetry found in 77% of females and 84% of males in the timed side-hop test, and 55% of females and 56% of males in the triple-hop test.

Implication of Findings
- Valgus lower limb alignment occurred in boys and girls even though the boys had greater ankle and knee separation distances throughout the drop-jump sequence, presumably owing to hip adduction and internal rotation.
- Predominance of valgus posture would be expected to lead these children to a higher injury risk. However, this risk may be offset by their smaller stature and body mass and the relatively slower velocities involved in their sporting activities.
- Whether neuromuscular training would be effective in improving overall lower limb alignment to a more neutral position in children on a drop-jump test is unknown.
- Finding of a lack of a difference in all of the isokinetic muscle strength values between the boys and the girls agrees with other recent studies in children of similar ages. Gender-related strength differences are not expected to become apparent until the mid-teens.
- Results of the functional tests could be due to motor development skills and neuromuscular indices such as balance, proprioception, and hip muscle strength not analyzed in this study.
- Consideration should be given to incorporate neuromuscular-training techniques that educate proper landing mechanisms and body positioning, and train to improve balance and muscle strength, into younger athletes.

participation before testing (4.8 ± 1.4 yr and 4.6 ± 0.7 yr, respectively) or the mean age in which they had begun organized sports participation (4.8 ± 1.3 yr and 4.9 ± 0.9 yr, respectively).

In order to evaluate the primary study outcome (knee separation distance on landing and take-off), sample-size calculations and the power to detect a difference between genders were determined by an independent statistician. With 27 female and 25 male subjects in this study, it was found that the investigation had sufficient power (>90%) to detect differences of at least 15% between gender in knee separation distance at a significance level of 0.05.

Hypothesis #1: No Significant Difference Exists between Prepubescent Boys and Prepubescent Girls in Overall Lower Limb Alignment during a Drop-Jump Test

The hypothesis was supported, because a marked decrease in normalized knee separation distance of less than 60% was found in 19 males (76%) and 25 females (93%) on landing (Fig. 16–12).

There was no difference between the female and the male athletes in the mean centimeters of hip separation for each phase of the jump-land sequence. The mean hip separation distance was 36 ± 3 cm on pre-land and 35 ± 3 cm on landing and take-off for both genders. There was no association between normalized knee and normalized ankle separation distances for either gender on pre-land, landing, or take-off.

The male athletes had greater absolute ankle separation distances than the females (pre-land, 35 ± 5 cm and 28 ± 5 cm, respectively; landing, 32 ± 6 cm and 24 ± 6 cm, respectively; take-off, 32 ± 6 cm and 24 ± 5, respectively; $P < .001$), and greater normalized ankle separation distances as shown in Table 16–3. A wider 95% confidence interval (CI) range was noted for the male athletes than for the female values for all three phases of the test.

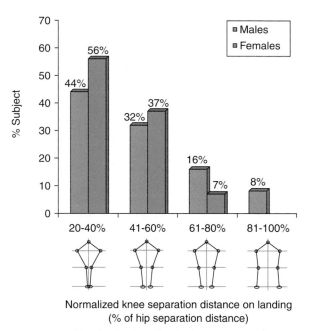

FIGURE 16–12. The distribution of male and female athletes according to normalized knee separation distance on landing. These percentile groups were chosen arbitrarily. There was no difference in the distribution of athletes among the categories shown. The *stick figures* are representative of the knee separation distance but not of the ankle separation distance. *(From Barber-Westin, S. D.; Galloway, M.; Noyes, F. R.; et al.: Assessment of lower limb neuromuscular control in prepubescent athletes. Am J Sports Med 33:1853–1860, 2005.)*

Male athletes also had greater absolute knee separation distances on pre-land and landing than females (pre-land, 22 ± 4 cm and 17 ± 4 cm, respectively; landing, 18 ± 7 cm and 14 ± 5 cm, respectively; $P < .05$), and greater normalized knee separation distances in these phases, as shown in Table 16–4.

TABLE 16–3 Videographic Drop-Jump Test: Normalized Ankle Separation Distances

Phase	Males				Females			
	Mean	SD	SE	95% CI	Mean	SD	SE	95% CI
Pre-land	96	12	2.4	91–101	79*	11	2.1	75–83
Land	92	20	4.0	84–100	71*	13	2.5	66–76
Take-off	91	20	3.9	83–99	70*	11	2.2	66–74

*$P < .001$ compared with male mean value.
95% CI, 95% confidence interval; SD, standard deviation; SE, standard error.

TABLE 16–4 Videographic Drop-Jump Test: Normalized Knee Separation Distances

Phase	Males				Females			
	Mean	SD	SE	95% CI	Mean	SD	SE	95% CI
Pre-land	60	10	1.9	56–64	48*	10	1.9	44–52
Land	49	18	3.6	42–56	41†	12	2.4	36–46
Take-off	49	18	3.5	42–56	44	10	2.0	40–48

*$P < .001$ compared with male mean value.
†$P < .05$ compared with male mean value.
95% CI, 95% confidence interval; SD, standard deviation; SE, standard error.

A wider 95% CI range was found for the male athletes on landing and take-off than for the females.

Hypothesis #2: No Significant Difference Exists between Prepubescent Boys and Prepubescent Girls in Knee Extensor and Flexor Strength

The hypothesis was supported, because there was no difference between genders in knee extensor and flexor peak torques (Table 16–5). No correlations were found between extensor and flexor peak torque values and overall lower limb alignment in the three phases of the drop-jump test. There was also no correlation between the isokinetic indices and BW or BMI for either gender.

Hypothesis #3: No Significant Difference Exists between Prepubescent Boys and Prepubescent Girls in Lower Limb Symmetry on Single-Leg Function Testing

The hypothesis was supported, because lower limb asymmetry (<85%) was found in 77% of the females and 84% of the males in the timed side-hop test, and in 55% of the females and 56% of the males in the triple-hop test. There was no difference between genders in the mean limb symmetry values for the timed side-hop test (68% ± 22% and 74% ± 22%, respectively) or the crossover hop for distance test (78% ± 21% and 76% ± 21%, respectively). There were no correlations between limb symmetry and knee isokinetic extension and flexion peak torques for either gender.

TABLE 16–5 Isokinetic Knee Extensor and Flexor Strength (180°/sec)

Variable	Extensor/Flexor	Leg	Females*	Males*
Peak torque (Nm/BW)	Extensor	Dominant	93 ± 23	94 ± 14
		Nondominant	101 ± 21	99 ± 14
	Flexor	Dominant	80 ± 17	82 ± 20
		Nondominant	78 ± 15	82 ± 20
Ham/quad ratio (%)		Dominant	77 ± 12	81 ± 15
		Nondominant	73 ± 10	75 ± 19
Total work (Nm)	Extensor	Dominant	57 ± 13	55 ± 11
		Nondominant	62 ± 13	59 ± 12†
	Flexor	Dominant	49 ± 11	51 ± 12
		Nondominant	53 ± 12†	50 ± 14
Time-to-peak torque (msec)	Extensor	Dominant	162 ± 60	195 ± 93
		Nondominant	172 ± 58	186 ± 58
	Flexor	Dominant	183 ± 63	214 ± 74
		Nondominant	211 ± 94	225 ± 82

*All values are mean ± standard deviation.
†$P < .05$ compared with dominant leg.
BW, body weight; ham/quad, hamstrings/quadriceps.

Implication of Findings

The authors hypothesized that no difference exists between genders in overall lower limb alignment during a drop-jump test. A valgus lower limb alignment assumed during athletic maneuvers has been hypothesized to increase the risk for a serious knee ligament injury, based on studies involving adolescent and adult athletes.[33,46] It was believed that prepubescent children would not demonstrate these gender differences because their muscle strength and motor skills had not yet fully developed.

The data indicated that 76% of boys and 93% of girls had a marked valgus alignment (<60% knee separation distance) during the videographic drop-jump test. This valgus lower limb alignment occurred even though the boys had greater ankle and knee separation distances throughout the drop-jump sequence. For example, the boys had a mean knee separation distance on landing of 49% ± 18% (95% CI, 42%–56%) compared with the girls who had a mean knee separation distance of 41% ± 12% (95% CI, 36%–46%). The mean normalized ankle separation distance of the males of 92% on landing has a theoretical advantage in providing a broader base (Fig. 16–13). However, the majority of boys still showed an overall lower extremity valgus alignment on landing and take-off, presumably owing to hip adduction and internal rotation. The predominance of this posture in the subjects would be expected to lead them to a higher injury risk. However, this risk may be offset in children by their smaller stature and body mass and the relatively slower velocities involved in their sporting activities.

Whether neuromuscular training would be effective in improving overall lower limb alignment to a more neutral position in children on a drop-jump test is unknown. Few controlled studies have been conducted to investigate injury-prevention strategies in children.[14,52,59] There are no formal national education or certification requirements for coaches in the United States, and it is unknown how many coaches have had formal training in conditioning and training, growth and development, or injury prevention.[59] The continued analysis of knee ligament injury mechanisms is strongly advised, because newer coaching techniques and strategies may become effective in addressing the ACL injury problem.

The finding of a lack of a difference in all of the isokinetic muscle strength values between the boys and the girls agrees with other studies in children of similar ages.[21,22,86] Gender-related strength differences are not expected to become apparent until the mid-teens.[21,22,38,43,79,83] One purpose of conducting isokinetic testing in the study was to assess whether a correlation existed between knee extensor and flexor strength and knee or ankle separation distances, of which none was found.

The authors hypothesized that there would be no difference between boys and girls in lower limb symmetry as determined by single-leg-hop tests. One previous study assessed the reliability of two sports-related functional tests that involved speed and

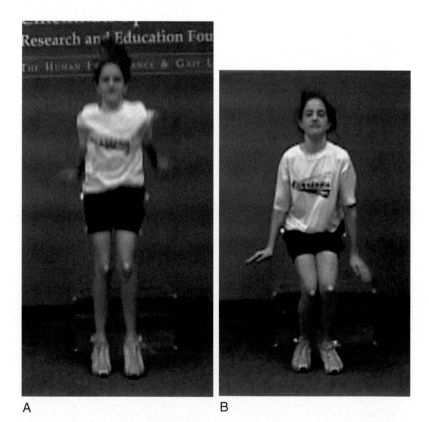

A   B

FIGURE 16–13. The videographic drop-jump test photographs for the toe-touch and take-off phases are shown for two subjects. **A** and **B**, A 10-year-old female subject demonstrated poor knee separation distance in both pre-land (11 cm, 31% normalized) and take-off (12 cm, 33% normalized) phases.

Continued

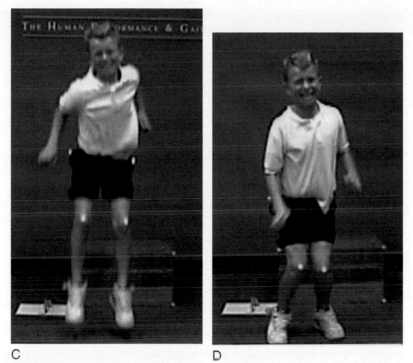

C   D

FIGURE 16–13—cont'd. C and **D**, A 9-year-old male subject demonstrated good knee separation distance on pre-land (24 cm, 68% normalized); however, on take-off, the valgus position is apparent with a large decrease in knee separation distance (13 cm, 38% normalized). (**A–D**, From Barber-Westin, S. D.; Galloway, M.; Noyes, F. R.; et al.: *Assessment of lower limb neuromuscular control in prepubescent athletes.* Am J Sports Med 33:1853–1860, 2005.)

agility during double-legged activities (slalom and hurdle tests) in 11 athletes (8 boys and 3 girls) who were all 11 years of age.[2] The intraclass correlation coefficients (ICCs) demonstrated adequate reliability of these tests. The standing balance of children 10 years of age and younger has been shown to be poorer than that of adults owing to their developing vestibular system.[17] Postural sway has been shown to be greater in children 9 to 10 years of age than in those 15 to 18 years of age.[95] In our study, abnormal limb symmetry was found in 77% of the females and 84% of the males in the timed side-hop test and in 55% of the females and 56% of the males in the triple-hop test. The timed side-hop test induced medial and lateral forces, and the children had a difficult time maintaining balance on one leg while hopping in these directions.

There was no correlation between knee extensor and flexor strength and lower limb symmetry on the single-leg-hop tests. Prior studies have shown a relationship between extensor strength and single-leg-hop testing in older populations 16 to 48 years of age.[6,63] The results of the functional tests could be due to motor development skills and neuromuscular indices such as balance, proprioception, and hip muscle strength not analyzed in this study. Cross-sectional investigations using single-leg-hop tests on children and adolescents up to 18 years of age are necessary to determine whether an age effect exists similar to those that exist for isokinetic muscle strength[19] and standing balance.[17]

The overall results of this investigation showed that a high percentage of male and female athletes 9 to 10 years of age had a noteworthy valgus lower limb alignment during a drop-jump screening test and a lack of symmetry between lower limbs in single-leg-hop tests. These same indices have been hypothesized to increase the risk for serious knee ligament injuries in adolescent and adult athletes. Consideration should be given to incorporate neuromuscular training techniques that educate proper landing mechanisms and body positioning, and train to improve balance and muscle strength, into younger athletes.

STUDY #3: NEUROMUSCULAR INDICES IN ATHLETES 9 TO 17 YEARS OF AGE

The number of athletes that participated in the tests for this investigation are shown in Table 16–6.[8] In order to be able to compare data collected in this investigation with those previously reported,[20–22,79,86] each subject was assigned to a category according to chronological age. This allowed establishment of age-related reference values, with age groups being as small as possible.[9] The height and weight of the subjects fell within the 50th to 75th percentile according to Tanner-Whitehouse clinical growth charts.[87,88]

There was no statistically significant effect of lower limb dominance on any of the tests. The mean values provided for the isokinetic and videographic drop-jump tests are representative of the dominant limb. There was no difference in the results of the videographic drop-jump data when the knee and ankle separation distances were normalized to body height or BMI. Therefore, normalized data according to the hip separation distance are provided for consistency with other published data.[7,65]

Significant increases were noted with age in BMI, height, and weight between each of the age categories in both the female and the male athletes ($P < .05$). There was no significant difference in height, weight, or BMI between male and female athletes aged 9 to 14. Males 15, 16, and 17 years of age had significantly greater values for these indices ($P < .05$).

TABLE 16–6   Subject Data

Age Group (yr)	Total N*	Number of Athletes Tested		
		Videographic Drop-Jump Test	Isokinetic Test	Function Test
Female Athletes				
9–12	170	94	156	56
13	115	64	107	34
14	219	92	206	57
15	188	62	175	41
16–17	224	84	209	59
Total	916	396	853	247
Male Athletes				
9–12	52	49	51	39
13	25	17	17	9
14	25	13	16	4
15	47	21	37	9
16–17	75	40	56	16
Total	224	140	177	77

*Number of athletes who completed at least one test.

Critical Points STUDY #3: NEUROMUSCULAR INDICES IN ATHLETES 9–17 YEARS OF AGE

$N = 1140$ athletes tested; each subject was assigned to a category according to chronological age.

Hypothesis #1: A significant increase in isokinetic knee extensor and flexor strength occurs with age in both male and female athletes.

- Hypothesis supported for knee extensor strength in both female and male athletes.
- Hypothesis supported for isokinetic knee flexion strength in the male athletes, not in the female athletes. Normalized mean flexor peak torque was only slightly greater in female athletes 11 yr of age compared with those 9–10 yr of age, with no improvement thereafter. In the male athletes, normalized mean flexor peak torque significantly increased from ages 9–14.

Hypothesis #2: Males aged 14 and older have significantly greater lower limb muscle strength than age-matched females.

- Hypothesis supported: from ages 14–17, male athletes had significantly greater mean extensor and flexor peak torques than age-matched female athletes.

Hypothesis #3: Age and gender do not influence lower limb symmetry on single-leg-hop functional testing.

- Hypothesis supported: no significant difference in mean lower limb symmetry between any age groups for either gender.

Hypothesis #4: Age and gender do not influence overall lower limb alignment on a drop-jump test.

- Hypothesis supported: no effect of age in either female or male athletes on mean normalized ankle and knee separation distances on landing or take-off.
- No significant difference in percent of athletes with <60%, 61%–80%, or >80% normalized knee separation distance.
- Few significant differences were found between genders within the age categories in the mean normalized knee separation distances.

Implications of Findings

- Females: increase extensor peak torque of 20% observed between ages 9 and 13. However, only 16% increase in flexor peak torque measured between ages 9 and 11. Emphasis on hamstring strengthening programs needs to be pursued in young female athletes to enable them to continue to achieve strength gains past the age of 11.
- Male subjects: increase in mean extensor peak torque of 38% found between ages 9 and 14, increase in mean flexor peak torque of 23% from ages 9 and 14.
- No difference between genders in lower extremity muscle strength until the age of 14.
- No difference in limb symmetry between the age categories in either the male or the female athletes.
- Although males aged 9–12 had greater mean ankle separation distances than age-matched females, and males aged 14 had greater knee separation distances on take-off than females, the majority of all athletes had a distinct valgus lower limb alignment on landing.

Hypothesis #1: A Significant Increase in Isokinetic Knee Extensor and Flexor Strength Occurs with Age in Both Male and Female Athletes

This hypothesis was supported for knee extensor strength in both female and male athletes. In the female athletes, a significant increase in the normalized mean extensor peak torque was noted from the ages of 9 to 13 ($P < .001$; Fig. 16–14). The average extensor peak torque in the 13-year-olds was 20% greater than that of the 9-year-old subjects. There were no significant increases in this factor after the age of 13. In the male athletes, significant increases in mean extensor peak torque were found from ages 9 to 14 ($P < .001$). The average extensor peak torque in the 14-year-olds was 38% greater than that of the 9-year-old subjects. There were no significant differences in this factor after the age of 14.

Whereas this hypothesis was supported for isokinetic knee flexion strength in male athletes, it was not supported in the female athletes. The normalized mean flexor peak torque

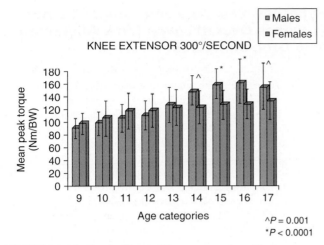

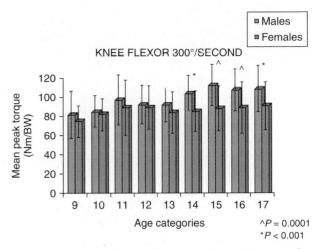

FIGURE 16–14. No significant difference was found in the mean extensor peak torque ratio values between females and males in the 9- to 13-year-old age groups. However, from the ages of 14 to 17, males had significantly greater mean extensor peak torque ratio values than females. *(From Barber-Westin, S. D.; Noyes, F. R.; Galloway, M.: Jump-land characteristics and muscle strength development in young athletes: a gender comparison of 1140 athletes 9 to 17 years of age. Am J Sports Med 34:375–384, 2006.)*

FIGURE 16–15. No significant difference was found in the mean flexor peak torque ratio values between females and males in the 9- to 13-year-old age groups. However, from the ages of 14 to 17, males had significantly greater mean flexor peak torque ratio values than females. *(From Barber-Westin, S. D.; Noyes, F. R.; Galloway, M.: Jump-land characteristics and muscle strength development in young athletes: a gender comparison of 1140 athletes 9 to 17 years of age. Am J Sports Med 34:375–384, 2006.)*

was only slightly greater in female athletes 11 years of age than in those 9 to 10 years of age (Fig. 16–15). There was no significant difference in flexor peak torques in athletes older than the age of 11. Hamstrings-to-quadriceps ratios slightly declined with age (from 82% at age 10 to 70% at age 17). In the male athletes, normalized mean flexor peak torque significantly increased from 80 ± 26 Nm/BW at age 9 to 104 ± 16 Nm/BW at age 14 ($P < .001$). Hamstrings-to-quadriceps ratios declined significantly from ages 9 (mean, 87%) to 14 (mean, 72%; $P < .001$), after which this value remained constant. There was no correlation between age and extensor or flexor peak torque absolute values, peak torque normalized values, or the hamstrings-to-quadriceps ratio for either gender.

Hypothesis #2: Males Aged 14 and Older Have Significantly Greater Lower Limb Muscle Strength than Age-matched Females

This hypothesis was supported, because from ages 14 to 17, male athletes had significantly greater mean extensor and flexor peak torques than age-matched female athletes (Table 16–7). There was no significant difference between genders in the hamstrings-to-quadriceps ratio in any age group.

Hypothesis #3: Age and Gender Do not Influence Lower Limb Symmetry on Single-Leg-Hop Functional Testing

The hypothesis was supported, because no statistically significant difference was found in the mean lower limb symmetry

---

TABLE 16–7   Statistically Significant Differences between Male and Female Athletes in Knee Extensor and Flexor Strength

Age Group (yr)	Extensor*					Flexor*				
	Male (Nm)	Female (Nm)	Male (Nm/BW) (range)	Female (Nm/BW) (range)	P Value[†]	Male (Nm)	Female (Nm)	Male (Nm/BW) (range)	Female (Nm/BW) (range)	P Value[†]
14	92 ± 24	71 ± 15	147 ± 23 (135–159)	122 ± 25 (119–125)	.0002	64 ± 15	49 ± 13	104 ± 16 (96–112)	85 ± 20 (82–88)	.0002
15	116 ± 34	77 ± 15	157 ± 25 (149–165)	126 ± 24 (123–129)	<.0001	81 ± 23	53 ± 12	112 ± 26 (104–120)	88 ± 19 (85–91)	<.0001
16	120 ± 26	81 ± 16	160 ± 33 (148–172)	126 ± 25 (122–130)	<.0001	80 ± 16	57 ± 12	107 ± 20 (100–114)	89 ± 21 (86–92)	<.0001
17	128 ± 34	85 ± 19	153 ± 33 (141–165)	131 ± 27 (125–137)	.001	90 ± 19	59 ± 13	108 ± 22 (100–116)	91 ± 18 (87–95)	.0002

*Values shown are mean ± standard deviation (95% confidence intervals)
[†]Comparison of normalized data.
BW, body weight.

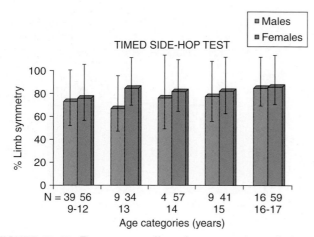

FIGURE 16–16. There was no effect of age or gender on limb symmetry in the timed side-hop test. *(From Barber-Westin, S. D.; Noyes, F. R.; Galloway, M.: Jump-land characteristics and muscle strength development in young athletes: a gender comparison of 1140 athletes 9 to 17 years of age. Am J Sports Med 34:375–384, 2006.)*

Hypothesis #4: Age and Gender Do not Influence Overall Lower Limb Alignment on a Drop-Jump Test

The hypothesis was supported, because there was no effect of age found in either the female or the male athletes on the mean normalized ankle and knee separation distances on landing (Fig. 16–18) or take-off. There was no significant difference in the percentage of athletes within the categories of less than 60%, 61% to 80%, or greater than 80% normalized knee separation distance (Fig. 16–19). A distinct overall lower limb valgus alignment (<60% knee separation distance) was measured in 78% of female athletes aged 9 to 12, 81% of athletes aged 13, 83% of athletes aged 14, 71% of athletes aged 15, and 74% of athletes aged 16 to 17. In the male athletes, a distinct valgus alignment was found in 79% of those aged 9 to 12, 70% of athletes aged 13, 62% of athletes aged 14, 67% of athletes aged 15, and 80% of athletes aged 16 to 17.

Significant differences were found in the male athletes between the age groups in mean ankle separation distances for all three phases of the drop-jump test ($P < .005$). The ankle separation distances were greatest in the 9- to 12-year-olds and smallest in the 15-year-olds. Significant differences were found between genders in the mean ankle separation distances in the pre-land phase (Table 16–8). Although male athletes had greater mean ankle separation distances in the 9- to 12-year-old group, female athletes had greater mean values in the 13-, 15-, and 16- to 17-year old groups. Few significant differences were found between genders within the age categories in the mean normalized knee separation distances.

values between any of the age groups for either the female or the male athletes in the single-leg-hop tests (Figs. 16–16 and 16–17). There was no correlation between extensor and flexor peak torques and limb symmetry.

There were no significant differences between male and female athletes in the single-leg-hop tests, except in the cross-over hop for distance test in which the 15-year-old males had a greater mean limb symmetry value than the females ($P < .05$).

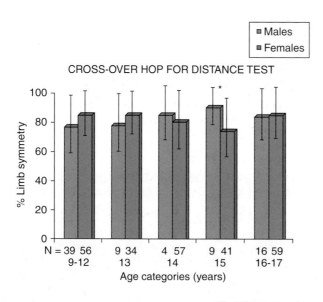

*$P < 0.05$ compared to females aged 15

FIGURE 16–17. There was no effect of age on limb symmetry for either gender in the crossover hop for distance test. Males 15 years of age had greater mean limb symmetry values than age-matched females. *(From Barber-Westin, S. D.; Noyes, F. R.; Galloway, M.: Jump-land characteristics and muscle strength development in young athletes: a gender comparison of 1140 athletes 9 to 17 years of age. Am J Sports Med 34:375–384, 2006.)*

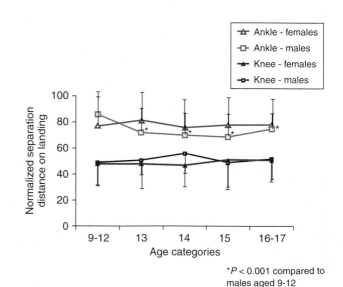

*$P < 0.001$ compared to males aged 9-12

FIGURE 16–18. Normalized ankle and knee separation distances on landing during a videographic drop-jump test in 396 female and 140 male athletes. There was no effect of age on these data in the female athletes. An age effect was found in the male athletes in the mean ankle separation distance, but not in the mean knee separation distance. *(From Barber-Westin, S. D.; Noyes, F. R.; Galloway, M.: Jump-land characteristics and muscle strength development in young athletes: a gender comparison of 1140 athletes 9 to 17 years of age. Am J Sports Med 34:375–384, 2006.)*

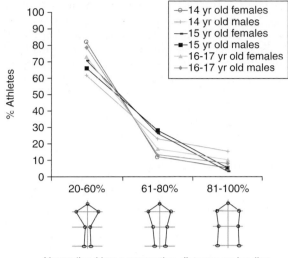

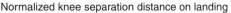

FIGURE 16–19. There was no significant difference between either the male or the female athletes aged 14 to 17 in the percentage of subjects with <60%, 61%–80%, or >80% normalized knee separation distance. The *stick figures* are representative of the knee separation distance but not of the ankle separation distance. *(From Barber-Westin, S. D.; Noyes, F. R.; Galloway, M.: Jump-land characteristics and muscle strength development in young athletes: a gender comparison of 1140 athletes 9 to 17 years of age. Am J Sports Med 34:375–384, 2006.)*

Study Implications

The first hypothesis was that a significant increase in lower limb muscle strength occurs with age in both male and female athletes. There is disparity in the literature regarding age effects on knee extensor and flexor strength within gender owing to the few comprehensive cross-sectional or longitudinal studies that have been published. No age effects were found in females or males when tested at a low-velocity speed (30°/sec) after stature and mass were accounted for in two investigations.[21,22] Other authors reported that an age effect existed in both genders for extensor and flexor torques at velocity speeds ranging from 120°/sec to 130°/sec.[80] Another report claimed that an age effect existed for males, but not for females, in knee extensor and flexor peak torques at 300°/sec.[41] De Ste Croix and colleagues[22] tested 46 subjects aged 8 to 9 years, 47 subjects aged 13 to 14 years, and 48 subjects aged 18 to 27 years. Knee extensor and flexor strength increased with age, regardless of how the data were analyzed (absolute, body mass–related, or body

mass–adjusted). Ramos and coworkers[79] tested 18 subjects aged 11 to 12 years, 21 subjects aged 13 to 14 years, and 18 subjects aged 17 to 18 years, and reported increases in absolute and BW-corrected peak torque with age in both males and females.

In the authors' study, an increase in knee extensor peak torque of 20% was observed in the female subjects between the ages of 9 and 13. However, only a small (nonsignificant) mean increase of 16% in knee flexor peak torque was measured between the ages of 9 to 11, with no significant improvement noted in athletes older than 11 years. In the male subjects, an increase in mean knee extensor peak torque of 38% was found between the ages of 9 and 14 and an increase in mean knee flexor peak torque of 23% from the ages of 9 and 14.

The second hypothesis was that males aged 14 and older have significantly greater lower limb muscle strength than age-matched females. Three investigations on isokinetic testing in children reported no differences between boys and girls in knee extensor or flexor strength up to the age of 14, even after controlling for body mass and stature.[21,22,79] Our data was in agreement, because there was no difference between genders in lower extremity muscle strength until the age of 14. One of the most important findings from this investigation was the difference between the male and the female athletes in strength increases in knee flexor peak torque according to the age categories. Whereas flexor peak torques in males gradually increased from ages 9 to 14, such increases were noted in females only from ages 9 to 11. In addition, the increases noted in extensor and flexor peak torques with age in males was approximately double those of females, even after controlling for BW. One theory of the increased incidence of ACL injury in female athletes compared with males relates to the quadriceps-dominance effect, or greater quadriceps activation measured during functional activities.[16,53] An increased quadriceps muscle force combined with a decreased hamstring muscle force and decreased knee flexion angle produce an increased proximal tibial anterior shear force that may result in excessive strain on the ACL.[16,45,53,80] It would appear from this study that an emphasis on hamstring-strengthening programs needs to be further pursued in young female athletes to enable them to continue to achieve strength gains past the age of 11.

The third hypothesis was that age and gender do not influence lower limb symmetry on single-leg-hop functional testing. There was no difference in limb symmetry between the age categories in either the male or the female athletes. Although the mean values of the two hop tests indicated adequate limb symmetry was present within most age categories, the large standard deviations prevent definitive conclusions. In a previous study from the authors'

TABLE 16–8 Statistically Significant Differences between Male and Female Athletes in Normalized Knee and Ankle Separation Distances (%) in the Drop-Jump Test

Age Group (yr)	Knee/Ankle	Test Phase	Males*	Females*	P Value[†]
9–12	Ankle	Pre-land	93 ± 13 (89–97)	87 ± 18 (83–91)	.04
	Ankle	Land	86 ± 20 (80–92)	77 ± 19 (73–81)	.009
	Ankle	Take-off	85 ± 19 (80–90)	75 ± 18 (71–79)	.003
13	Ankle	Pre-land	81 ± 12 (75–87)	94 ± 21 (89–99)	.02
14	Knee	Take-off	58 ± 13 (51–65)	48 ± 16 (45–51)	.04
15	Ankle	Pre-land	78 ± 14 (72–84)	91 ± 20 (86–96)	.005
	Ankle	Land	69 ± 15 (62–76)	78 ± 19 (73–83)	.05
16–17	Knee	Pre-land	60 ± 9 (57–63)	66 ± 14 (63–69)	.03
	Ankle	Pre-land	82 ± 14 (78–86)	91 ± 18 (87–95)	.004

*Values shown are mean ± standard deviation (95% confidence intervals).
[†]P values adjusted (Bonferroni/Dunn).

institution that involved 93 subjects aged 17 to 34 years, 90% had limb symmetry of at least 85%. A relationship between extensor strength and single-leg-hop testing was reported in one study[6]; however, a second investigation failed to find a significant correlation.[63] No association was found in the current investigation between extensor or flexor strength and limb symmetry values. Studies conducted elsewhere have presented wide variability in regard to a correlation between extensor strength and limb symmetry on single-leg-hop testing; moderate correlation coefficients ($R = 0.60$–0.78) were reported by Greenberger and Paterno,[31] Sachs and associates,[81] Wilk and colleagues,[90] and Barber and coworkers.[6] However, low correlation coefficients were described by other investigators,[71,74,75,84] and no definitive conclusion may be reached regarding this association.

The fourth hypothesis was that age and gender do not influence overall lower limb alignment on a drop-jump test. Some authors have postulated that female athletes tend to land from a jump in a noteworthy valgus lower limb alignment, in contrast to male athletes who land in a more neutrally aligned position, and that a valgus alignment position increases the risk for a knee ligament injury.[33,46] However, based on data from prior investigations, we believed no difference in lower limb alignment on a drop-jump task would be detected between genders.[7,65] The results showed that, although males aged 9 to 12 had greater mean ankle separation distances than age-matched females, and males aged 14 had greater knee separation distances on take-off than females, the majority of all athletes had a distinct valgus lower limb alignment on landing. Valgus knee alignment on take-off and landing has been hypothesized to predispose an athlete to ACL rupture and indeed is commonly seen during noncontact ACL injuries.[11,28,30]

Hass and associates[37] recently reported an age-dependent effect on knee biomechanics during landing between 16 prepubescent (aged 8–11 yr) and 16 postpubescent (aged 18–25 yr) females. The postpubescent group had reduced knee flexion upon initial contact (4.5°) and increased medial knee forces, but decreased landing forces and knee extensor moments than

the younger group. Although the study's results suggested the presence of a developmental effect on landing mechanisms, the authors concluded that further work is required on the effects of age, developmental level, and motor control during landing.

Chappell and colleagues[16] reported no difference between genders aged 19 to 25 years in the magnitude of knee varus-valgus moments during three stop-jump tasks. Those authors concluded that the female knee varus-valgus moment may not be responsible for the gender differences in ACL strain during those tasks. The increased incidence of knee injuries in female athletes is most likely due to many factors. Whereas a valgus alignment position assumed on landing may increase the risk for a knee ligament injury, the fact that there was no difference detected in alignment between genders in the authors' study in such a large number of athletes indicates that other factors most likely have a role in the increased ACL injury rate in females. In addition, injury mechanisms other than a valgus knee position have been noted during ACL ruptures,[11] including a sudden deceleration, acceleration, or change of direction in response to avoiding contact with another player or in reaction to a ball or play. Differences between genders in muscle reaction and firing patterns,[45,93] coordination, control of body and lower extremity positions during athletics, lower extremity and hip strength, and external-internal knee flexion moments all most likely contribute to this problem. Neuromuscular training (see Chapter 19, Decreasing the Risk of ACL Injuries in Female Athletes) is effective in improving lower limb alignment on the drop-jump test,[65] increasing hamstrings strength, increasing knee flexion angles on landing,[42,44,76] and reducing deleterious moments and ground reaction forces.

STUDY #4: TIBIAL ROTATION STRENGTH IN MALE AND FEMALE ATHLETES 11 TO 17 YEARS OF AGE

The study population comprised 94 athletes (47 females and 47 males), aged 11 to 17 years, who participated in a variety of organized sports including soccer, basketball, volleyball,

---

Critical Points STUDY #4: TIBIAL ROTATION STRENGTH IN MALE AND FEMALE ATHLETES 11–17 YEARS OF AGE

$N = 94$ athletes (47 female, 47 male), aged 11–17 yr.

Hypothesis #1: A significant increase in internal tibial rotation (IR) and external tibial rotation (ER) strength occurs with age in both male and female athletes.

- Hypothesis true for male athletes, but not for female athletes. Male athletes aged 14–17 yr had significantly greater mean IR and ER peak torques than males aged 11–13 yr.

Hypothesis #2: No difference exists between male and female athletes aged 11–13 in IR and ER strength.

- Hypothesis supported: no significant difference between male and female athletes 11–13 yr of age regarding IR and ER strength.

Hypothesis #3: Male athletes aged 14–17 have significantly greater IR and ER strength than age-matched female athletes.

- Hypothesis supported for IR only: males aged 14–17 yr had a significantly greater mean IR peak torque and faster mean time-to-reach IR peak torque, than age-matched females.

Implications of Findings

- First study to conduct lower extremity tibial rotational strength testing in athletes 11–17 yr of age to assess age- and gender-related effects.

- Joint angular positions based on biomechanical studies that demonstrated the rotational force of the pes anserinus musculature (sartorius, gracilis, semitendinosus) is greatest at 90° of knee flexion.

- Significant decrease in rotational force exists as the knee is extended, declining as much as 41% when the knee is fully extended (0°) compared with the strength measured at 90° of flexion.

- Further rotational strength testing is required in cross-sectional or longitudinal studies before a conclusion can be reached on the effects of aging on IR and ER peak torques.

- No difference between genders aged 11–13 yr in mean ER and IR peak torque values, time-to-peak torque, or IE ratios.

- IR peak torques for males were 17% greater than those of the females at 180°/sec.

- Appears to be no difference in ER strength between genders.

- First study to report that male athletes have faster times-to-reach peak torque for IR than age-matched female athletes.

baseball, football, and track and field.[64] In order to evaluate the primary study outcomes (mean peak torque and time-to-peak torque), sample-size calculations and the power to detect a difference of 10% between gender and age group mean scores were determined by an independent statistician. With 94 patients in this study, it was found that the investigation had sufficient power (>80%) to detect differences in mean peak IR and ER torque and time-to-peak torque of at least 10% between genders and age group categories.

There were no significant effects of lower limb dominance in all of the athletes aged 11 to 13 years. In the female athletes aged 14 to 17 years, the mean value of the dominant lower limb was significantly stronger than that of the nondominant limb in IR at 120°/sec (31 ± 7 and 27 ± 8, respectively; $P < .05$). No other effects of lower limb dominance were found in the isokinetic indices in all of the athletes 14 to 17 years of age.

Hypothesis #1: A Significant Increase in IR and ER Strength Occurs with Age in Both Male and Female Athletes

The hypothesis was proved true for the male athletes, but not for the female athletes. Male athletes aged 14 to 17 years had significantly greater mean IR and ER peak torques (Table 16–9), and significantly greater extensor and flexor peak torques (Table 16–10), than males aged 11 to 13 years. There was no significant difference in all of the lower limb muscle strength indices in female athletes between the ages of 11 to 13 years and 14 to 17 years.

There were no age effects for either gender on the IE ratio. Only one age effect was found for the rotation-flexion and rotation-extension ratios: females aged 11 to 13 years had a significantly greater mean IR-E ratio than females aged 14 to 17 years.

TABLE 16–9   Tibial External and Internal Rotation Peak Torque Indices

Rotation	Velocity	Age Group (yr)	Peak Torque (Nm/BW)* Males	Peak Torque (Nm/BW)* Females	Time-to-Peak Torque (msec)* Males	Time-to-Peak Torque (msec)* Females	IE Ratio (%)* Males	IE Ratio (%)* Females
External	120°/sec	11–13	32 ± 8	33 ± 11	274 ± 100	312 ± 216		
		14–17	39 ± 9†	35 ± 12	284 ± 113	329 ± 126		
	180°/sec	11–13	31 ± 8	31 ± 13	257 ± 133	243 ± 153		
		14–17	36 ± 9†	33 ± 13	209 ± 54	238 ± 130		
Internal	120°/sec	11–13	29 ± 7	33 ± 8	270 ± 126	284 + 157		
		14–17	35 ± 12‡	31 ± 7	234 ± 84	323 ± 168‖		
	180°/sec	11–13	25 ± 7	28 ± 6	242 ± 177	233 ± 130		
		14–17	30 ± 9‡	25 ± 7§	191 ± 155	266 ± 134		
IE ratio¶	120°/sec	11–13					92 ± 24	101 ± 21
		14–17					93 ± 20	95 ± 25
	180°/sec	11–13					84 ± 25	99 ± 27
		14–17					83 ± 17	86 ± 31

*Data shown are mean ± SD for the dominant limb.
†$P < .01$ compared with 11- to 13-year-old males.
‡$P < .05$ compared with 11- to 13-year-old males.
§$P = .05$ compared with 14- to 17-year-old males.
‖$P = .02$ compared with 14- to 17-year-old males.
¶Data are shown as percentages.
BW, body weight; IE, internal rotation–to–external rotation.

TABLE 16–10   Knee Flexor and Extensor Peak Torques and Their Relation to Tibial Rotation Strength (180°/sec)

	11–13 Yr Males	11–13 Yr Females	14–17 Yr Males	14–17 Yr Females
Flexor peak torque (Nm/BW)	104 ± 22	100 ± 22	127 ± 20†	101 ± 14‡
Internal rotation-flexion ratio*	24 ± 8	29 ± 6§	23 ± 6	26 ± 9
External rotation-flexion ratio*	30 ± 7	32 ± 11	29 ± 6	33 ± 13
Extensor peak torque (Nm/BW)	139 ± 27	131 ± 23	167 ± 23†	138 ± 14‡
Internal rotation-extension ratio*	18 ± 5	22 ± 5‖¶	18 ± 6	18 ± 4
External rotation-extension ratio*	22 ± 6	24 ± 7	22 ± 6	24 ± 9

*Data are shown as percentages.
†$P < .001$ compared with 11- to 13-year-old males.
‡$P < .0001$ compared with 14- to 17-year-old males.
§$P < .05$ compared with 11- to 13-year-old males.
‖$P = .01$ compared with 11- to 13-year-old males.
¶$P = .01$ compared with 14- to 17-year-old females.

Hypothesis #2: No Difference Exists between Male and Female Athletes Aged 11 to 13 in IR and ER Strength

The hypothesis was supported, because there was no significant difference between male and female athletes 11 to 13 years of age regarding IR and ER strength (Fig. 16–20). Females aged 11 to 13 years had significantly greater mean IR-F and IR-E ratios than age-matched males.

Hypothesis #3: Male Athletes Aged 14 to 17 Have Significantly Greater IR and ER Strength than Age-matched Female Athletes

The hypothesis was supported for IR only, because males aged 14 to 17 years had a significantly greater mean IR peak torque (at 180°/sec) and a significantly faster mean time-to-reach IR peak torque than age-matched females (see Table 16–9). There was no significant difference between the male and the female athletes for mean ER peak torque.

In a subgroup of 14- to 17-year-old athletes matched for BMI, males had significantly greater IR peak torques at 120°/sec than females ($P < .05$). Males in this subgroup also had significantly greater knee extensor ($P < .01$) and flexor peak torques ($P = .0001$) than females.

Study Implications

This is the first study to conduct lower extremity tibial rotational strength testing in athletes 11 to 17 years of age with the specific purposes of assessing age- and gender-related effects. During a potential injury situation, dynamic muscular stabilization of the knee joint, particularly the hamstring muscles, may potentially reduce ACL strain.[24,45,61,77,80] Several investigators have demonstrated that female athletes have weaker knee flexor peak torques, and take longer to develop flexor peak torque, than males even after normalizing for BW.[18,32,42,45] The impetus for this study was the paucity of

published data regarding the IR and ER isokinetic strength of the hamstring musculature.

The isokinetic test design and protocol was performed in a manner similar to that of other investigations.[39,82,89] The joint angular positions were based on biomechanical studies that demonstrated that the rotational force of the pes anserinus musculature (sartorius, gracilis, semitendinosus) is greatest at 90° of knee flexion.[66,85] A significant decrease in rotational force exists as the knee is extended, declining as much as 41% when the knee is fully extended (0°) compared with the strength measured at 90° of flexion. Hip flexion angle also affects the generation of internal rotational torque, with greater torque generated at higher hip flexion angles (when the knee is flexed 90°).[70,85] The test protocol was similar to that described by other investigators with respect to hip and knee flexion angles, stabilization of the foot, and the resting position used to determine the neutral position before the onset of testing.[39,82,89]

A limitation of this study is the fact that it is not possible to isolate and measure the specific muscles that act as the primary internal rotators (semitendinosus, gracilis, popliteus, semimembranosus, and sartorius) and external rotators (biceps muscle, long and short head)[13] with dynamometer systems. However, the testing procedure does provide a functional assessment of lower limb isokinetic capabilities. The data showed few effects of lower limb dominance on rotational strength, which agreed with the results of Osternig and coworkers[72] and Hester and Falkel.[39] The results of the IE ratios were also similar with those reported previously, because the mean ER peak torque slightly exceeded that of IR peak torque at both velocities.[39,72]

The first hypothesis, that a significant increase in IR and ER strength occurs with age in both genders, was proved for males but not for females. Male athletes aged 14 to 17 years had significantly greater mean IR (17% for both test velocities) and ER (14%–18%) peak torques than males aged 11 to 13 years. In contrast, females aged 14 to 17 years had only 6% greater ER strength than that measured in 11- to 13-year-old females. Further rotational strength testing is required in cross-sectional or longitudinal studies before a conclusion can be reached on the effects of aging on IR and ER peak torques. Our study did demonstrate a hierarchy of isokinetic peak torques in the musculature about the knee, which was similar in both genders and age groups (see Fig. 16–20).

Our second hypothesis, that no difference exists between genders aged 11 to 13 years in IR and ER strength, was supported. Other investigators have successfully used a variety of isokinetic velocity speeds to measure knee extension and flexion peak torque in children, ranging from 12°/sec[86] to 300°/sec.[26] No significant gender-related knee flexion and extension strength differences have been reported by authors in children between the ages of 8 and 14 years.[21,22,86] Our investigation showed no difference between genders aged 11 to 13 years in mean ER and IR peak torque values, time-to-peak torque, or IE ratios.

Our third hypothesis, that male athletes aged 14 to 17 years have significantly greater tibial rotation isokinetic muscle strength than age-matched female athletes, was supported. The IR peak torques for the males were 17% greater than those of the females at 180°/sec. Viola and associates[89] reported that the noninjured limb IR of males was approximately 25% stronger than the uninjured limb IR of females at 120°/sec; and approximately 11% stronger at 180°/sec. These data were not normalized for BW. Segawa and associates[82] reported that (after normalization for BW) the male noninjured limb IR was approximately 16%

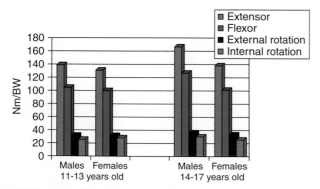

FIGURE 16–20. Overall isokinetic peak torque averages for knee extensor, flexor, external rotation, and internal rotation for the dominant limb at 180°/sec. A hierarchy of isokinetic muscle strength about the knee can be seen, which is similar between genders and age groups. *(Reprinted from Noyes, F. R.; Barber-Westin, S. D.: Isokinetic profile and differences in tibial rotation strength between male and female athletes 11 to 17 years of age. Isok Exer Sci 13:251–259, 2005; with permission from IOS Press.)*

stronger than the female uninjured limb IR at 120°/sec. There appears to be no difference in ER strength between genders, according to the data from our study and those of other investigators.[89,93]

Our study is the first we are aware of to report that male athletes have faster times-to-reach peak torque for IR than age-matched female athletes. Gender differences in muscular protection of the knee joint during weight-bearing and non–weight bearing activities have been reported by many authors, but only a few have included IR data. Wojtys and colleagues[93] compared the amount of IR and rotational stiffness in collegiate athletes participating in high-risk sports with those participating in low-risk endurance sports. Gender comparisons were performed regarding the amount of passive and active IR in response to a medially directed 80-N force (with the subjects seated) and the resultant amount of apparent knee joint stiffness. Male athletes participating in high-risk sports had significantly less IR (mean, 3°) during muscle activation, and significantly greater (42%) apparent joint stiffness than the female athletes. However, Lephart and coworkers[50] found that collegiate women who participated in high-risk sports had less knee flexion and IR maximum angular displacements during single-leg landing and forward hop landing tasks than age- and activity-matched males. McLean and associates[55] reported that women had an average of 5° less IR during a sidestep maneuver, along with less hip flexion, hip abduction, hip internal rotation, and knee flexion than age-matched males. The protection provided by the dynamic neuromuscular control of the lower extremity is multifactorial and beyond the scope of the authors' study.

CONCLUSIONS

The important findings from the four studies are

1. There is no influence of age or gender on overall lower limb alignment as calculated from a single coronal plane videographic drop-jump test. A marked overall lower limb valgus alignment is present in 62% of female athletes and in 75% of male athletes on landing from a drop-jump.

2. A neuromuscular-training program significantly improves overall lower limb alignment in a drop-jump test in the majority of female athletes.

3. There is no influence of age or gender on limb symmetry on single-leg-hop tests between male and female athletes 9 to 17 years of age.

4. In female athletes, a significant increase (mean, 20%) in normalized knee extensor strength occurs from the ages of 9 to 13. There is no statistically significant increase in extensor strength after the age of 13.

5. In male athletes, a significant increase (mean, 38%) in normalized knee extensor strength occurs from ages 9 to 14. There is no statistically significant increase in extensor strength after the age of 14.

6. In female athletes, only slight increases occur in normalized knee flexor strength from ages 9 to 11, with no further increases expected thereafter.

7. In male athletes, a significant increase (mean, 23%) occurs in normalized knee flexor strength from ages 9 to 14. There is no statistically significant increase in flexor strength after the age of 14.

8. Whereas there are no differences between genders in normalized knee extensor and flexor strength from ages 9 to 13, male athletes aged 14 and older have significantly greater normalized extensor and flexor strength than those of age-matched female athletes.

9. Male athletes aged 14 to 17 years have significantly greater normalized IR strength (17%) than age matched female athletes. Male athletes also have a significantly faster mean time-to-reach IR peak torque than female athletes.

10. There is no difference between genders in normalized ER muscle strength.

11. A hierarchy of isokinetic peak torques exists in the musculature about the knee, which was similar in both genders and age groups. In males, the peak torque measured during ER was approximately 28% of that measured in the flexors and 20% of that measured in the extensors. In females, the peak torque measured during ER was approximately 35% of that measured in the flexors and 25% of that measured in the extensors.

REFERENCES

1. Adirim, T. A.; Cheng, T. L.: Overview of injuries in the young athlete. *Sports Med* 33:75–81, 2003.
2. Alricsson, M.; Harms-Ringdahl, K.; Werner, S.: Reliability of sports-related functional tests with emphasis on speed and agility in young athletes. *Scand J Med Sci Sports* 11:229–232, 2001.
3. Anderson, M.; Messner, M. B.; Green, W. T.: Distribution of lengths of the normal femur and tibia in children from one to eighteen years of age. *J Bone Joint Surg Am* 46:1197–1202, 1964.
4. Arendt, E.; Dick, R.: Knee injury patterns among men and women in collegiate basketball and soccer. NCAA data and review of literature. *Am J Sports Med* 23:694–701, 1995.
5. Bandy, W.; Rusche, K.; Tekulve, F. X.: Reliability and limb symmetry for five unilateral functional tests of the lower extremities. *Isok Exer Sci* 4:108–111, 1994.
6. Barber, S. D.; Noyes, F. R.; Mangine, R. E.; et al.: Quantitative assessment of functional limitations in normal and anterior cruciate ligament–deficient knees. *Clin Orthop* 255:204–214, 1990.
7. Barber-Westin, S. D.; Galloway, M.; Noyes, F. R.; et al.: Assessment of lower limb neuromuscular control in prepubescent athletes. *Am J Sports Med* 33:1853–1860, 2005.
8. Barber-Westin, S. D.; Noyes, F. R.; Galloway, M.: Jump-land characteristics and muscle strength development in young athletes: a gender comparison of 1140 athletes 9 to 17 years of age. *Am J Sports Med* 34:375–384, 2006.
9. Beenakker, E. A.; van der Hoeven, J. H.; Fock, J. M.; Maurits, N. M.: Reference values of maximum isometric muscle force obtained in 270 children aged 4–16 years by hand-held dynamometry. *Neuromuscul Disord* 11:441–446, 2001.
10. Berns, G. S.; Hull, M. L.; Patterson, H. A.: Strain in the anteromedial bundle of the anterior cruciate ligament under combination loading. *J Orthop Res* 10:167–176, 1992.
11. Boden, B. P.; Dean, G. S.; Feagin, J. A., Jr.; Garrett, W. E., Jr.: Mechanisms of anterior cruciate ligament injury. *Orthopedics* 23:573–578, 2000.
12. Bolgla, L. A.; Keskula, D. R.: Reliability of lower extremity functional performance tests. *J Orthop Sports Phys Ther* 26:138–142, 1997.
13. Buford, W. L., Jr.; Ivey, F. M., Jr.; Nakamura, T.; et al.: Internal/external rotation moment arms of muscles at the knee: moment arms for the normal knee and the ACL-deficient knee. *Knee* 8:293–303, 2001.
14. Chalmers, D. J.: Injury prevention in sport: not yet part of the game? *Inj Prev* 8(suppl 4):IV22–IV25, 2002.
15. Chandy, T. A.; Grana, W. A.: Secondary school athletic injury in boys and girls: A three-year comparison. *Physician Sportsmed* 13:106–111, 1985.

16. Chappell, J. D.; Yu, B.; Kirkendall, D. T.; Garrett, W. E.: A comparison of knee kinetics between male and female recreational athletes in stop-jump tasks. *Am J Sports Med* 30:261–267, 2002.

17. Cherng, R. J.; Chen, J. J.; Su, F. C.: Vestibular system in performance of standing balance of children and young adults under altered sensory conditions. *Percept Mot Skills* 92(3 pt 2):1167–1179, 2001.

18. Cowling, E. J.; Steele, J. R.: Is lower limb muscle synchrony during landing affected by gender? Implications for variations in ACL injury rates. *J Electromyogr Kinesiol* 11:263–268, 2001.

19. De Ste Croix, M.; Deighan, M.; Armstrong, N.: Assessment and interpretation of isokinetic muscle strength during growth and maturation. *Sports Med* 33:727–743, 2003.

20. De Ste Croix, M. B.; Armstrong, N.; Chia, M. Y.; et al.: Changes in short-term power output in 10- to 12-year-olds. *J Sports Sci* 19:141–148, 2001.

21. De Ste Croix, M. B.; Armstrong, N.; Welsman, J. R.; Sharpe, P.: Longitudinal changes in isokinetic leg strength in 10- to 14-year-olds. *Ann Hum Biol* 29:50–62, 2002.

22. De Ste Croix, M. B. A.; Armstrong, N.; Welsman, J. R.: Concentric isokinetic leg strength in pre-teen, teenage and adult males and females. *Biol Sport* 16:75–86, 1999.

23. DeMorat, G.; Weinhold, P.; Blackburn, T.; et al.: Aggressive quadriceps loading can induce noncontact anterior cruciate ligament injury. *Am J Sports Med* 32:477–483, 2004.

24. Draganich, L. F.; Vahey, J. W.: An in vitro study of anterior cruciate ligament strain induced by quadriceps and hamstrings forces. *J Orthop Res* 8:57–63, 1990.

25. Dufek, J. S.; Bates, B. T.: The evaluation and prediction of impact forces during landings. *Med Sci Sports Exerc* 22:370–377, 1990.

26. Ellenbecker, T. S.; Roetert, E. P.: Concentric isokinetic quadriceps and hamstrings strength in elite junior tennis players. *Isok Exer Sci* 5:3–6, 1995.

27. Ferber, R.; Davis, I. M.; Williams, D. S., 3rd: Gender differences in lower extremity mechanics during running. *Clin Biomech (Bristol, Avon)* 18:350–357, 2003.

28. Gerberich, S. G.; Luhmann, S.; Finke, C.; et al.: Analysis of severe injuries associated with volleyball activities. *Physician Sportsmed* 15:75–79, 1987.

29. Goh, S.; Boyle, J.: Self-evaluation and functional testing two to four years post ACL reconstruction. *Aust J Physiother* 43:255–262, 1997.

30. Gray, J.; Taunton, J. E.; McKenzie, D. C.; et al.: A survey of injuries to the anterior cruciate ligament of the knee in female basketball players. *Int J Sports Med* 6:314–316, 1985.

31. Greenberger, H. B.; Paterno, M. V.: Relationship of knee extensor strength and hopping test performance in the assessment of lower extremity function. *J Orthop Sports Phys Ther* 22:202–206, 1995.

32. Griffin, J. W.; Tooms, R. E.; vander Zwaag, R.; et al.: Eccentric muscle performance of elbow and knee muscle groups in untrained men and women. *Med Sci Sports Exerc* 25:936–944, 1993.

33. Griffin, L. Y.; Agel, J.; Albohm, M. J.; et al.: Noncontact anterior cruciate ligament injuries: risk factors and prevention strategies. *J Am Acad Orthop Surg* 8:141–150, 2000.

34. Griffin, L. Y.; Albohm, M. J.; Arendt, E. A.; et al.: Understanding and preventing noncontact anterior cruciate ligament injuries: a review of the Hunt Valley II Meeting, January 2005. *Am J Sports Med* 34:1512–1532, 2006.

35. Grood, E. S.; Suntay, W. J.; Noyes, F. R.; Butler, D. L.: Biomechanics of the knee-extension exercise. Effect of cutting the anterior cruciate ligament. *J Bone Joint Surg Am* 66:725–734, 1984.

36. Gwinn, D. E.; Wilckens, J. H.; McDevitt, E. R.; et al.: The relative incidence of anterior cruciate ligament injury in men and women at the United States Naval Academy. *Am J Sports Med* 28:98–102, 2000.

37. Hass, C. J.; Schick, E. A.; Tillman, M. D.; et al.: Knee biomechanics during landings: comparison of pre- and postpubescent females. *Med Sci Sports Exerc* 37:100–107, 2005.

38. Henderson, R. C.; Howes, C. L.; Erickson, K. L.; et al.: Knee flexor-extensor strength in children. *J Orthop Sports Phys Ther* 18:559–563, 1993.

39. Hester, J. T.; Falkel, J.: Isokinetic evaluation of tibial rotation: assessment of a stabilization technique. *J Orthop Sports Phys Ther* 6:46–51, 1984.

40. Hewett, T. E.; Lindenfeld, T. N.; Riccobene, J. V.; Noyes, F. R.: The effect of neuromuscular training on the incidence of knee injury in female athletes. A prospective study. *Am J Sports Med* 27:699–706, 1999.

41. Hewett, T. E.; Myer, G. D.; Ford, K. R.: Decrease in neuromuscular control about the knee with maturation in female athletes. *J Bone Joint Surg Am* 86:1601–1608, 2004.

42. Hewett, T. E.; Stroupe, A. L.; Nance, T. A.; Noyes, F. R.: Plyometric training in female athletes. Decreased impact forces and increased hamstring torques. *Am J Sports Med* 24:765–773, 1996.

43. Holm, I.; Steen, H.; Olstad, M.: Isokinetic muscle performance in growing boys from pre-teen to maturity. An eleven-year longitudinal study. *Isok Exer Sci* 13:153–158, 2005.

44. Huston, L. J.; Vibert, B.; Ashton-Miller, J. A.; Wojtys, E. M.: Gender differences in knee angle when landing from a drop-jump. *Am J Knee Surg* 14:215–219, 2001.

45. Huston, L. J.; Wojtys, E. M.: Neuromuscular performance characteristics in elite female athletes. *Am J Sports Med* 24:427–436, 1996.

46. Hutchinson, M. R.; Ireland, M. L.: Knee injuries in female athletes. *Sports Med* 19:288–302, 1995.

47. Jones, S. J.; Lyons, R. A.; Sibert, J.; et al.: Changes in sports injuries to children between 1983 and 1998: comparison of case series. *J Public Health Med* 23:268–271, 2001.

48. Kellis, E.; Kellis, S.; Gerodimos, V.: Reliability of isokinetic concentric and eccentric strength in circumpubertal soccer players. *Pediatr Exerc Sci* 11:218–228, 1999.

49. Lees, A.: Methods of impact absorption when landing from a jump. *Eng Med* 10:207–211, 1981.

50. Lephart, S. M.; Ferris, C. M.; Riemann, B. L.; et al.: Gender differences in strength and lower extremity kinematics during landing. *Clin Orthop* 401:162–169, 2002.

51. Lindenfeld, T. N.; Schmitt, D. J.; Hendy, M. P.; et al.: Incidence of injury in indoor soccer. *Am J Sports Med* 22:364–371, 1994.

52. MacKay, M.; Scanlan, A.; Olsen, L.; et al.: Looking for the evidence: a systematic review of prevention strategies addressing sport and recreational injury among children and youth. *J Sci Med Sport* 7:58–73, 2004.

53. Malinzak, R. A.; Colby, S. M.; Kirkendall, D. T.; et al.: A comparison of knee joint motion patterns between men and women in selected athletic tasks. *Clin Biomech (Bristol, Avon)* 16:438–445, 2001.

54. Markolf, K. L.; Burchfield, D. M.; Shapiro, M. M.; et al.: Combined knee loading states that generate high anterior cruciate ligament forces. *J Orthop Res* 13:930–935, 1995.

55. McLean, S. G.; Lipfert, S. W.; van den Bogert, A. J.: Effect of gender and defensive opponent on the biomechanics of sidestep cutting. *Med Sci Sports Exerc* 36:1008–1016, 2004.

56. McLean, S. G.; Neal, R. J.; Myers, P. T.; Walters, M. R.: Knee joint kinematics during the sidestep cutting maneuver: potential for injury in women. *Med Sci Sports Exerc* 31:959–968, 1999.

57. McNair, P. J.; Prapavessis, H.; Callender, K.: Decreasing landing forces: effect of instruction. *Br J Sports Med* 34:293–296, 2000.

58. Merlini, L.; Dell'Accio, D.; Granata, C.: Reliability of dynamic strength knee muscle testing in children. *J Orthop Sports Phys Ther* 22:73–76, 1995.

59. Micheli, L. J.; Glassman, R.; Klein, M.: The prevention of sports injuries in children. *Clin Sports Med* 19:821–834, 2000.

60. Molnar, G. E.; Alexander, J.; Gutfeld, N.: Reliability of quantitative strength measurements in children. *Arch Phys Med Rehabil* 60:218–221, 1979.

61. More, R. C.; Karras, B. T.; Neiman, F.; et al.: Hamstrings—an anterior cruciate ligament protagonist: an in vitro study. *Am J Sports Med* 21:231–237, 1993.

62. Moti, A. W.; Micheli, L. J.: Meniscal and articular cartilage injury in the skeletally immature knee. *Instr Course Lect* 52:683–690, 2003.

63. Noyes, F. R.; Barber, S. D.; Mangine, R. E.: Abnormal lower limb symmetry determined by function hop tests after anterior cruciate ligament rupture. *Am J Sports Med* 19:513–518, 1991.

64. Noyes, F. R.; Barber-Westin, S. D.: Isokinetic profile and differences in tibial rotation strength between male and female athletes 11 to 17 years of age. *Isok Exer Sci* 13:251–259, 2005.

65. Noyes, F. R.; Barber-Westin, S. D.; Fleckenstein, C.; et al.: The drop-jump screening test: difference in lower limb control by gender

and effect of neuromuscular training in female athletes. *Am J Sports Med* 33:197–207, 2005.

66. Noyes, F. R.; Sonstegard, D. A.: Biomechanical function of the pes anserinus at the knee and the effect of its transplantation. *J Bone Joint Surg Am* 55:1225–1241, 1973.

67. O'Connor, J. J.: Can muscle co-contraction protect knee ligaments after injury or repair? *J Bone Joint Surg Br* 75:41–48, 1993.

68. Olsen, O. E.; Myklebust, G.; Engebretsen, L.; et al.: Relationship between floor type and risk of ACL injury in team handball. *Scand J Med Sci Sports* 13:299–304, 2003.

69. Onate, J. A.; Guskiewicz, K. M.; Sullivan, R. J.: Augmented feedback reduces jump landing forces. *J Orthop Sports Phys Ther* 31:511–517, 2001.

70. Oshimo, T. A.; Greene, T. A.; Jensen, G. M.; Lopopolo, R. B.: The effect of varied hip angles on the generation of internal tibial rotary torque. *Med Sci Sports Exerc* 15:529–534, 1983.

71. Ostenberg, A.; Roos, E.; Ekdahl, C.; Roos, H.: Isokinetic knee extensor strength and functional performance in healthy female soccer players. *Scand J Med Sci Sports* 8(5 pt 1):257–264, 1998.

72. Osternig, L. R.; Bates, B. T.; James, S. L.: Patterns of tibial rotary torque in knees of healthy subjects. *Med Sci Sports Exerc* 12:195–199, 1980.

73. Pandy, M. G.; Shelburne, K. B.: Dependence of cruciate-ligament loading on muscle forces and external load. *J Biomech* 30:1015–1024, 1997.

74. Petschnig, R.; Baron, R.; Albrecht, M.: The relationship between isokinetic quadriceps strength test and hop tests for distance and one-legged vertical jump test following anterior cruciate ligament reconstruction. *J Orthop Sports Phys Ther* 28:23–31, 1998.

75. Pincivero, D. M.; Lephart, S. M.; Karunakara, R. G.: Relation between open and closed kinematic chain assessment of knee strength and functional performance. *Clin J Sport Med* 7(1):11–16, 1997.

76. Prapavessis, H.; McNair, P. J.: Effects of instruction in jumping technique and experience jumping on ground reaction forces. *J Orthop Sports Phys Ther* 29:352–356, 1999.

77. Prietto, C. A.; Caiozzo, V. J.: The in vivo force-velocity relationship of the knee flexors and extensors. *Am J Sports Med* 17:607–611, 1989.

78. Radelet, M. A.; Lephart, S. M.; Rubinstein, E. N.; Myers, J. B.: Survey of the injury rate for children in community sports. *Pediatrics* 110:e28, 2002.

79. Ramos, E.; Frontera, W. R.; Llopart, A.; Feliciano, D.: Muscle strength and hormonal levels in adolescents: gender-related differences. *Int J Sports Med* 19:526–531, 1998.

80. Renstrom, P.; Arms, S. W.; Stanwyck, T. S.; et al.: Strain within the anterior cruciate ligament during hamstring and quadriceps activity. *Am J Sports Med* 14:83–87, 1986.

81. Sachs, R. A.; Daniel, D. M.; Stone, M. L.; Garfein, R. F.: Patellofemoral problems after anterior cruciate ligament reconstruction. *Am J Sports Med* 17:760–765, 1989.

82. Segawa, H.; Omori, G.; Koga, Y.; et al.: Rotational muscle strength of the limb after anterior cruciate ligament reconstruction using semitendinosus and gracilis tendon. *Arthroscopy* 18:177–182, 2002.

83. Seger, J. Y.; Thorstensson, A.: Muscle strength and electromyogram in boys and girls followed through puberty. *Eur J Appl Physiol* 81:54–61, 2000.

84. Sekiya, I.; Muneta, T.; Ogiuchi, T.; et al.: Significance of the single-legged hop test to the anterior cruciate ligament-reconstructed knee in relation to muscle strength and anterior laxity. *Am J Sports Med* 26:384–388, 1998.

85. Shoemaker, S. C.; Markolf, K. L.: In vivo rotatory knee stability. Ligamentous and muscular contributions. *J Bone Joint Surg Am* 64:208–216, 1982.

86. Sunnegardh, J.; Bratteby, L. E.; Nordesjo, L. O.; Nordgren, B.: Isometric and isokinetic muscle strength, anthropometry and physical activity in 8- and 13-year-old Swedish children. *Eur J Appl Physiol Occup Physiol* 58:291–297, 1988.

87. Tanner, J. M.; Buckler, J. M.: Revision and update of Tanner-Whitehouse clinical longitudinal charts for height and weight. *Eur J Pediatr* 156:248–249, 1997.

88. Tanner, J. M.; Davies, P. S.: Clinical longitudinal standards for height and height velocity for North American children. *J Pediatr* 107:317–329, 1985.

89. Viola, R. W.; Sterett, W. I.; Newfield, D.; et al.: Internal and external tibial rotation strength after anterior cruciate ligament reconstruction using ipsilateral semitendinosus and gracilis tendon autografts. *Am J Sports Med* 28:552–555, 2000.

90. Wilk, K. E.; Romaniello, W. T.; Soscia, S. M.; et al.: The relationship between subjective knee scores, isokinetic testing, and functional testing in the ACL-reconstructed knee. *J Orthop Sports Phys Ther* 20:60–73, 1994.

91. Wojtys, E. M.; Ashton-Miller, J. A.; Huston, L. J.: A gender-related difference in the contribution of the knee musculature to sagittal-plane shear stiffness in subjects with similar knee laxity. *J Bone Joint Surg Am* 84:10–16, 2002.

92. Wojtys, E. M.; Huston, L. J.: Neuromuscular performance in normal and anterior cruciate ligament–deficient lower extremities. *Am J Sports Med* 22:89–104, 1994.

93. Wojtys, E. M.; Huston, L. J.; Schock, H. J.; et al.: Gender differences in muscular protection of the knee in torsion in size-matched athletes. *J Bone Joint Surg Am* 85:782–789, 2003.

94. Wojtys, E. M.; Huston, L. J.; Taylor, P. D.; Bastian, S. D.: Neuromuscular adaptations in isokinetic, isotonic, and agility training programs. *Am J Sports Med* 24:187–192, 1996.

95. Wolff, D. R.; Rose, J.; Jones, V. K.; et al.: Postural balance measurements for children and adolescents. *J Orthop Res* 16:271–275, 1998.

Chapter 17

Differences in Neuromuscular Characteristics between Male and Female Athletes

Timothy Sell, PhD, PT ■ *Scott Lephart*, PhD, ATC

INTRODUCTION

Joint stability may be defined as the state of a joint remaining or promptly returning to proper alignment through an equalization of forces.[71] This requires a synergy between bones, joint capsules, ligaments, muscles, tendons, and sensory receptors.[83] The static components of joint stability include the ligaments, joint capsule, cartilage, friction, and the bony geometry of the articulation.[35,48] These components are typically assessed through joint stress testing and have commonly defined clinical joint stability.[71] These static components provide the foundation for joint stability during functional activities by guiding joint arthrokinematics. However, during physically demanding tasks such as running, jumping, and cutting, these components may not provide the restraint necessary to prevent joint injury. During these tasks, stability is provided by dynamic components that include the neuromuscular control of the skeletal muscles crossing the joint.[71] The functional joint stability accomplished through the integration and complementary relationship between the static and the dynamic components of joint stability is referred to as *dynamic joint stability*.

Dynamic joint stability is influenced by the neuromuscular control of the muscles crossing the joint. Relative to joint stability, neuromuscular control is the unconscious activation of the dynamic restraints occurring in preparation for and in response to joint motion and loading for the purpose of maintaining and restoring functional joint stability.[71] Neuromuscular control of joint stability is a complex interaction between components of the nervous system and those of the musculoskeletal system and typically is accomplished through two different control systems, *feedback* and *feed-forward control*.[23] In a system that uses feedback control, sensors continually measure the parameter of interest based on an optimal value. A deviation from this optimal value will initiate an error signal. In response to this error signal, the system will trigger a compensatory response. Feed-forward systems also require measurement of a parameter, but measurement occurs only intermittently. The sensory components of this system are designed to measure a potential disturbance or change in the parameter of interest. Once a potential disturbance has been detected, the system initiates an error signal. In response to this error signal, the system institutes commands to counteract the anticipated effects of the disturbance. The commands instituted by this system are largely shaped by previous experience with similar disturbances. Feed-forward control systems are considered to be anticipatory in nature compared with feedback control systems, which are characterized by responses only to current stimulus. Both are essential for optimal maintenance of dynamic knee stability.

NONCONTACT ANTERIOR CRUCIATE LIGAMENT INJURIES AND FEMALE ATHLETES

The role of dynamic joint stability in the prevention of knee injuries has been a focus of research at the University of Pittsburgh and the Neuromuscular Research Laboratory since 1995 in response to the demonstrated differences in noncontact anterior cruciate ligament (ACL) injury rates between male and female athletes. Female athletes suffer ACL injuries at a significantly higher rate than male athletes in matched sports.[1–3,9,15,17,26–28,59,63] The majority of these injuries occur through a noncontact mechanism of injury in which no external forces are applied directly to the knee joint.[10,57,64] The forces that cause the injury are applied to the knee joint through ground reaction forces and internal soft tissue and muscle forces. An examination of gender-specific characteristics is an important first step in determining potential risk factors and prevention of these injuries. Researchers have investigated numerous potential risk factors for noncontact ACL injuries including anatomic, hormonal, environmental, neuromuscular, and biomechanical characteristics. The primary and current focus in female noncontact ACL injury prevention (risk factor identification and training) is on the neuromuscular and biomechanical factors of joint stability owing to their potential for modification through intervention programs.[12,29,31,50,52,62,70,87]

The authors' initial studies included the examination of the proprioceptive, electromyographic (EMG), balance, and strength characteristics of female athletes. The gender differences observed in these neuromuscular characteristics may result in altered neuromuscular control, which has been observed in the laboratory. This chapter provides an overview of the authors' studies examining gender differences in neuromuscular and biomechanical characteristics of athletes who are susceptible to noncontact ACL injury. Studies are also presented that examine the effects of fatigue on neuromuscular characteristics.

PROPRIOCEPTION

Proprioception is the afferent information arising from the internal peripheral areas of the body that contribute to postural control, joint stability, and conscious sensations. These include the conscious submodalities of proprioception: joint position sense, active and passive kinesthesia, the sense of heaviness or resistance, and appreciation of movement velocity. Proprioception is an important component to establish and maintain functional joint stability.[15,67] Alterations in the acquisition, processing, and integration of proprioceptive information can affect functional joint stability. The presence of knee joint proprioception deficits in females may contribute to their increased rate of ACL injury,

because the lack of proprioception inhibits recruitment of the dynamic stabilizers that prevent anterior tibial translation.

The proprioceptive characteristics of male and female athletes were examined in 34 collegiate-level athletes.[75] Knee joint proprioception was measured by assessing the threshold to detect passive motion with a custom-built testing device (Department of Engineering, University of Pittsburgh). The device was capable of rotating the knee joint at 0.5°/sec, which is necessary to reduce the input of musculotendinous mechanoreceptors. Subjects were tested in a seated position while wearing a pneumatic sleeve on their tested lower leg, a blindfold over their eyes, and headphones with white noise in order to reduce cutaneous input, visual input, and auditory input, respectively (Fig. 17–1). Participants were instructed to signal (with a button signal) when joint motion was sensed. Direction of movement was randomized across six trials (three in each direction), with data averaged for each direction. The amount of rotation before the participants' signal was recorded as the threshold to detect passive motion. Testing was performed at a knee flexion angle of 15° with movement into both flexion and extension. This position was chosen because most noncontact ACL injuries occur with the knee close to full extension.[10,57,65] Reliability of the device was demonstrated to be high.[47]

No differences were observed between male and female athletes when the knee was rotated into flexion, but a significant difference was found when the knee was rotated toward full extension (Fig. 17–2). The ACL becomes tauter as the knee extends, and although the female subjects in this study had greater knee joint laxity, this may provide evidence for the increased risk of ACL injury (noncontact) in female athletes. The decreased ability to detect motion toward a dangerous position[10,57,65] of full extension could prevent preactivation of protective muscle forces such as the hamstrings.

Critical Points PROPRIOCEPTION

- Proprioception is the afferent information arising from the internal peripheral areas of the body that contribute to postural control, joint stability, and conscious sensations including the conscious submodalities of proprioception.
- Female athletes demonstrate decreased proprioception as measured with threshold to detect passive motion. The inability to detect motion toward a position of potential injury may indicate an increased risk for injury.
- Female gymnasts have superior proprioception compared with female nongymnasts. The superior proprioception may be due to development of advanced neurosensory pathways owing to enhanced central and peripheral mechanisms as a result of long-term athletic training or genetically predetermined increased kinesthetic awareness or those individuals with superior kinesthetic awareness participate and remain participants in gymnastics owing to the physical requirements of faster reaction times.

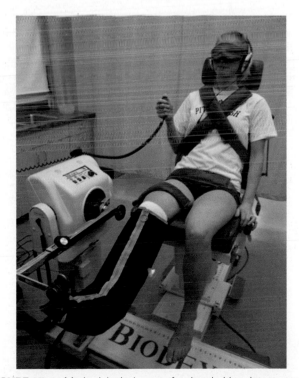

FIGURE 17–1. Methodological set-up for threshold to detect passive motion (TTDPM).

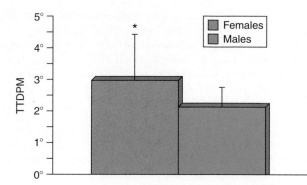

FIGURE 17–2. Gender differences in TTDPM (*P = .039). *(From Rozzi, S. L.; Lephart, S. M.; Gear, W. S.; Fu, F. H.: Knee joint laxity and neuromuscular characteristics of male and female soccer and basketball players. Am J Sports Med 27:312–319, 1999.)*

Although proprioception differences exist between genders, differences also exist in proprioception abilities within the female athletic population.[44] A comparison of the threshold to detect passive motion was conducted between female gymnasts and a group of healthy, age-matched participants. The instrumentation and methodology of testing were similar to that of the gender comparison study described previously. Gymnasts recognized movement significantly faster than the nongymnasts (Fig. 17–3). It is recognized that the superior kinesthetic awareness observed in the gymnasts may be due to one or multiple factors:

1. Development of advanced neurosensory pathways owing to enhanced central and peripheral mechanisms as a result of long-term athletic training.
2. Genetically predetermined increased kinesthetic awareness.
3. Individuals with superior kinesthetic awareness participate and remain active in gymnastics owing to the physical requirements of faster reaction times.

The results of this study do not provide definitive support for any of these explanations, but it may be asserted that training can improve proprioceptive capabilities.

The authors' proprioception research has been expanded to include multiple modalities of proprioception testing and multiple planes of movement. Recently, a reliability study was completed that examined force sense reproduction, velocity sense reproduction, active/passive position sense, and threshold to detect passive motion of knee flexion and extension and internal

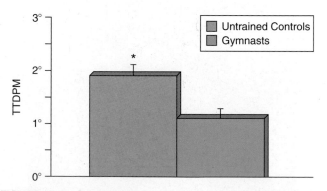

FIGURE 17–3. Gymnasts demonstrate superior TTDPM compared with untrained controls (*P = .011). *(From Lephart, S. M.; Giraldo, J. L.; Borsa, P. A.; Fu, F. H.: Knee joint proprioception: a comparison between female intercollegiate gymnasts and controls. Knee Surg Sports Traumatol Arthrosc 4:121–124, 1996.)*

and external rotation. This study also compared these characteristics between genders. The preliminary results indicated adequate reliability for force sense and threshold to detect passive motion for both planes of movement. The data further revealed proprioception deficits in female athletes in the direction of internal tibial rotation.

BALANCE AND POSTURAL STABILITY

Postural stability is the ability to maintain the body in equilibrium by maintaining the projected center of mass within the limits of the base of support.[81] Similar to joint stability, maintenance of postural stability is a dynamic process that involves establishing an equilibrium between destabilizing and stabilizing forces.[56] Sensory information for this stability is derived from vision, the vestibular system, and somatosensory feedback.[38] Somatosensory feedback is also necessary for dynamic knee stability and is incorporated into the sensorimotor system in order to maintain stability both in dynamic tasks and in static posture.[38,71] Although researchers have cautioned against extrapolating data from static conditions to dynamic athletic situations, postural stability testing can provide valuable information regarding sensory integration, processing, and motor planning.[85]

The sensorimotor system provides the sensory information and action components that influence the perception, cognition, and action processes that are paramount to dynamic knee stability.[71] Sensorimotor processes involved in dynamic knee stability include the neurosensory and neuromuscular mechanisms involved in the acquisition of a sensory stimulus, the conversion of the stimulus to a neural signal, transmission of the signal to the central nervous system (CNS), processing and integration of the signal within the CNS, and the motor responses resulting in muscle activation for joint stability during locomotion and functional tasks.[46] Accurate sensory information is critical to this system.[71] Without accurate sensory information, the proper corrective actions cannot be planned and executed.

Overall, the authors' research demonstrates that female athletes have superior balance than male athletes. A study was conducted that measured and compared the balance of male college-aged athletes and female National Collegiate Athletic Association (NCAA) Division I athletes using the Biodex Stability System (Biodex, Inc., Shirley, NY).[75] The Biodex software generates a stability index value that is based on the amount of time the platform is off-level. Female athletes had a significantly greater stability index than their male counterparts (Fig. 17–4). In another study, single-leg balance was measured on a traditional force plate (Kistler Corporation, Worthington, OH; Model #4060-1011000).[80] Testing methodology and data processing were based on that described by Goldie and coworkers[24,25]

Critical Points BALANCE AND POSTURAL STABILITY

- Postural stability is the ability to maintain the body in equilibrium; it is a dynamic process that involves establishing an equilibrium between destabilizing and stabilizing forces.
- Female athletes demonstrate superior single-leg balance ability when measured during static tasks.
- Static measurements of balance and postural stability may not be the most appropriate test to assess athletes. Future research should utilize more dynamic measures of postural stability.

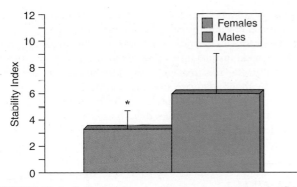

FIGURE 17–4. Collegiate female athletes demonstrate significantly greater single-leg balance than male athletes (*P = .002). (From Rozzi, S. L.; Lephart, S. M.; Gear, W. S.; Fu, F. H.: Knee joint laxity and neuromuscular characteristics of male and female soccer and basketball players. Am J Sports Med 27:312–319, 1999.)

and included both an eyes-closed and an eyes-open condition. Comparisons were made between male and female high school basketball players. Females demonstrated significantly better single-leg balance scores for both the eyes-closed and the eyes-opened conditions (Fig. 17–5).

It is interesting to note that many noncontact ACL injury prevention training programs include activities designed to improve balance[12,29,31,42,51,62] despite the fact that females have significantly better single-leg balance and that single-leg balance deficits have not been identified as a risk factor for ACL injury. The lack of balance deficits seems to contradict the research demonstrating that females have proprioceptive deficits. The authors proposed that the measurement of static single-leg balance might not adequately challenge the underlying motor control and peripheral somatosensory system. A more dynamic test of postural control would be more appropriate and likely to reveal potential deficits related to the acquisition, processing, and integration of somatosensory information and functional joint stability. Currently, the authors are conducting a study examining single-leg balance (static) and dynamic postural control. The goals of this study are to establish the reliability of a test of dynamic postural control, determine the relationships between static balance tests and dynamic balance tests, and determine whether gender differences are present in dynamic postural control.

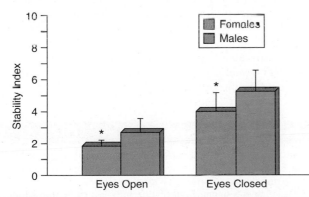

FIGURE 17–5. Female high school basketball players demonstrate better single-leg balance than male basketball players under both conditions of eyes open (*P < .001) and eyes closed (*P < .001). (From Sell, T. C.; Myers, J. B.; Youk, A. O.; et al.: Neuromechanical Predictors of Dynamic Stability. Dissertation. Pittsburgh: Department of Sports Medicine and Nutrition, University of Pittsburgh, 2004.)

EMG ACTIVITY

The electromyogram measures the electrical manifestation of the contracting muscle.[4] It is the electrical signal that propagates from the neuromuscular junction along the muscle fiber and is termed the *muscle action potential*.[33] Measurement of EMG activity provides information regarding the amount of electrical activity in the contracting muscle, which provides insight into the magnitude of tension developed.[86] Many variables can influence this signal and thus create difficulty in interpreting these data. These variables include velocity of muscle shortening or lengthening, rate of tension buildup, fatigue, and reflex activity.[89] Muscle activation patterns, amplitude, and quantity provide important insight into the neuromuscular control of joint stability.

Dynamic knee stability is dependent on the neuromuscular control over the musculature of the knee in order to reduce strain in the ACL. For this control to be effective, the CNS must be able to anticipate destabilizing forces and act appropriately.[8] Benvenuti and associates[6] examined EMG activity of upper arm musculature during reaction-time arm movements and demonstrated that when destabilizing forces are anticipated, the CNS is capable of adjusting muscle activation patterns to oppose these forces, supporting the notion that anticipatory postural adjustments are planned in detail. EMG activity of the knee musculature has been investigated and compared between genders during athletic tasks in an attempt to quantify the role of the knee extensors and flexors in dynamic knee stability.[7,14,19]

The authors measured the EMG activity of the vastus medialis, vastus lateralis, medial hamstrings, lateral hamstrings, and gastrocnemius with surface electrodes while athletes performed a drop-land task.[75] Comparisons between genders were performed for the activity onset time after initial contact and peak amplitude after initial contact. In addition, the area of activity (integrated) for the first 1 second of the contraction after landing was calculated for each muscle. No significant differences were observed for onset time for any of the muscles. Analysis of the peak amplitude and integrated electromyographic (IEMG) activity revealed a significant difference between genders for the lateral hamstrings; females had a greater peak amplitude and IEMG activity (Fig. 17–6) than males. Activation of the lateral hamstrings in response to the landing is an attempt by female athletes to prevent the anterior tibial translation that occurs as the knee flexes. It may also be an attempt to counteract potential anterolateral subluxations due to its insertion on the fibular head.

Gender differences have also been observed in EMG activation during reactive stop-jump tasks and stop-jump tasks designed to simulate tasks during which noncontact ACL injuries occur.[78] The IEMG activity of the vastus lateralis and

---

Critical Points ELECTROMYOGRAPHIC ACTIVITY

- Measurement of electromyographic (EMG) activity provides information regarding the amount of electrical activity in the contracting muscle, which supplies insight into the magnitude of tension developed.
- Female athletes demonstrate compensatory EMG activation of the hamstrings musculature, possibly in an attempt to prevent anterior tibial translation.

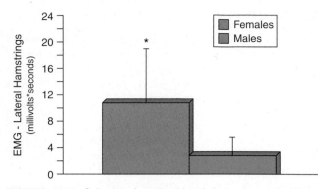

FIGURE 17–6. Collegiate female athletes demonstrate significantly higher integrated electromyographic activity of the lateral hamstrings than male athletes (*P = .001). *(From Rozzi, S. L.; Lephart, S. M.; Gear, W. S.; Fu, F. H.: Knee joint laxity and neuromuscular characteristics of male and female soccer and basketball players. Am J Sports Med 27:312–319, 1999.)*

semitendinosus was measured during the 150 msec prior to peak posterior ground reaction force (maximum deceleration) while male and female high school basketball players performed reactive jumps. This particular time point was chosen because deceleration is the most common characteristic among those tasks during which noncontact ACL injuries occur.[10,65] In addition, a co-contraction value (vastus lateralis and semitendinosus) was calculated during this same time period. Female athletes performed these reactive jumps with a greater IEMG activity of the semitendinosus (Fig. 17–7) and a higher co-contraction value.

Similar gender differences were observed during an examination of stop-jump tasks to the medial aspect of the knee. The authors' biomechanical analyses of jump direction demonstrated that stop-jump tasks directed to the medial aspect of the knee (such as an inside cut) are more dangerous than vertical jumps and stop-jump tasks to the lateral aspect of the knee.[78] Athletes perform these jumps with the greatest vertical and posterior ground reaction forces, greatest proximal anterior tibia shear force, highest valgus and flexion moments, and lowest knee flexion angles. Female athletes use the same IEMG activation patterns during these jumps as during the reactive jumps. The gender differences observed in semitendinosus activity during these stop-jump tasks are consistent with a previous study[75] and reinforce the concept that females use compensatory

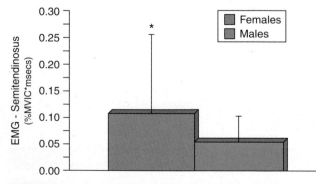

FIGURE 17–7. Female high school basketball players demonstrate significantly higher integrated electromyographic activity of the semitendinosus than male basketball players (*P < .05). *(From Sell, T. C.; Ferris, C. M.; Abt, J. P.; et al.: The effect of direction and reaction on the neuromuscular and biomechanical characteristics of the knee during tasks that simulate the noncontact anterior cruciate ligament injury mechanism. Am J Sports Med 34:43–54, 2006.)*

strategies to counter the decreased knee joint proprioception in order to achieve functional joint stabilization.

Analyses of EMG activation patterns, timing, amplitude, and quantity provide insight into the attempt to achieve functional joint stability in the presence of destabilizing forces and moments. Without adequate strength, even efficient and timely activation of the stabilizing muscles of the knee may not provide the necessary force to counteract these potentially injurious joint forces and moments. Therefore, strength and the ability to generate high torque are also important to functional joint stability.

STRENGTH

Muscular strength can assist dynamic knee stability by producing force that aids to counteract the destabilizing forces occurring during dynamic activities. For the knee joint, these forces are primarily provided by knee flexors and knee extensors. Knee strength testing provides information regarding the potential force production capabilities of those muscles crossing the knee joint. The authors' research has consistently demonstrated gender differences in athletes for both the knee extensors and the knee flexors. The isokinetic knee extensor and flexor strength of 15 female NCAA Division I volleyball, basketball, and soccer athletes was tested (60°/sec) and compared with those of males of similar age and activity level who had previously participated in soccer and basketball.[43] A Biodex System III Dynamometer (Biodex Medical Inc., Shirley, NY) provided scores of peak torque that were normalized to each participant's body weight. Females produced significantly less peak torque for both the knee extensors and the knee flexors compared with males (Figs. 17–8 and 17–9). Similar observations of isokinetic strength (60°/sec) have been made in high school athletes for knee extensors and knee flexors.[80] Male high school basketball players demonstrated significantly stronger knee extensors and flexors than female basketball players when normalized to body weight (see Figs. 17–8 and 17–9).

The authors recognize the significant contributions, including strength, of the joints proximal and distal (to the knee) to functional joint stability of the knee. An analysis and gender comparison was conducted of hip strength of high school basketball players.[18] Hip external rotation and abductor strength was assessed with a hand-held dynamometer. Measurements of strength were normalized to each participant's segment length and body weight. No significant gender differences were observed in hip abductor strength, although females had less strength than males. Females demonstrated significantly less hip external rotation strength than males. These differences in hip strength reinforce the need to include proximal strengthening exercises for the knee joint.

Critical Points STRENGTH

- Muscular strength can assist dynamic knee stability by producing force that can help to counteract the destabilizing forces occurring during dynamic activities.
- Female athletes demonstrate significantly less strength for both the knee extensors and the knee flexors than male athletes.
- Female athletes demonstrate significantly less hip external rotation strength than male athletes.
- The differences in strength at the knee and hip demonstrate the importance of training for both joints.

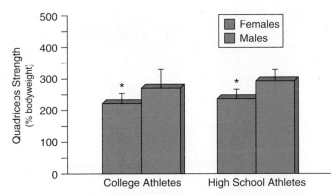

FIGURE 17–8. Female athletes demonstrate significantly less isokinetic quadriceps strength (60°/sec, normalized to body weight) than male athletes at both the collegiate (*$P < .05$) and the high school (*$P < .05$) level. *(From Lephart, S. M.; Ferris, C. M.; Riemann, B. L.; et al.: Gender differences in strength and lower extremity kinematics during landing. Clin Orthop Relat Res 401:162–169, 2002; and Sell, T. C.; Myers, J. B.; Youk, A. O.; et al.: Neuromechanical Predictors of Dynamic Stability. Dissertation. Pittsburgh: Department of Sports Medicine and Nutrition, University of Pittsburgh, 2004.)*

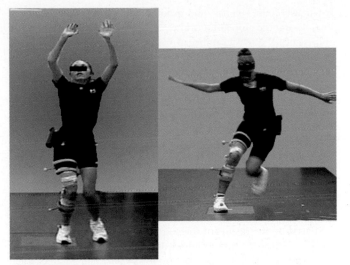

FIGURE 17–10. Participants performing jump landing and cutting tasks.

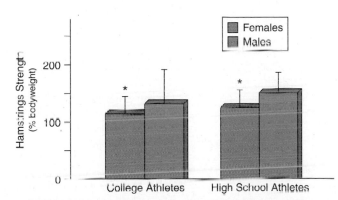

FIGURE 17–9. Female athletes demonstrate significantly less isokinetic hamstrings strength (60°/sec, normalized to body weight) than male athletes at both the collegiate (*$P < .05$) and the high school (*$P < .05$) level. *(From Lephart, S. M.; Ferris, C. M.; Riemann, B. L.; et al.: Gender differences in strength and lower extremity kinematics during landing. Clin Orthop Relat Res 401:162–169, 2002; and Sell, T. C.; Myers, J. B.; Youk, A. O.; et al.: Neuromechanical Predictors of Dynamic Stability. Dissertation. Pittsburgh: Department of Sports Medicine and Nutrition, University of Pittsburgh, 2004.)*

BIOMECHANICS

The differences observed in proprioception, EMG activity, and strength can lead to differences in neuromuscular control of the knee during dynamic tasks. The result of this difference in neuromuscular control is evident in biomechanical differences observed in dynamic tasks. The authors have examined the

biomechanics of males and females performing several different tasks (Fig. 17–10) to determine how neuromuscular control (deficits) affects landing kinematics and kinetics.

The landing kinematics and ground reaction forces of 15 female NCAA Division I collegiate basketball, volleyball, and soccer athletes were measured.[43] These data were compared with those of male recreational athletes matched for age and activity level. Landing kinematics and vertical ground reaction forces were examined while the participants performed single-leg landings and forward hops. During the single-leg hops, the female athletes demonstrated greater internal rotation of the hip, less knee flexion (Fig. 17–11), less lower leg maximum angular displacement, and decreased time to maximum angular displacement (flexion) than their male counterparts. Females also demonstrated less knee flexion, lower leg internal rotation, and decreased time to maximum angular displacement (flexion) than males during the forward hop. Ground reaction forces were not significantly different between genders during the two tasks studied.

A series of jump tasks were developed to better replicate those tasks during which noncontact ACL injuries occur.[10,57,65] Two of the most common components include a sharp deceleration, such as a cutting maneuver or stop-jump, and a quick change in direction. Olsen and colleagues[65] also described that many of these injuries occur with a valgus collapse of the knee. The joint

Critical Points BIOMECHANICS

- The gender differences observed in proprioception, EMG activity, and strength can lead to differences in neuromuscular control of the knee during dynamic tasks.
- Female athletes demonstrate decreased knee flexion, an increased knee valgus angle, greater ground reaction forces, increased knee flexion moment, increased knee valgus moment, and greater proximal tibia anterior shear force during tasks implicated in noncontact ACL injuries.
- These differences can lead to increased risk for ACL injury and/or increased ACL strain.

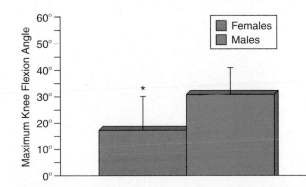

FIGURE 17–11. Female collegiate athletes demonstrate significantly less maximum knee flexion angle during a single-leg landing than male athletes (*$P < .05$). *(From Lephart, S. M.; Ferris, C. M.; Riemann, B. L.; et al.: Gender differences in strength and lower extremity kinematics during landing. Clin Orthop Relat Res 401:162–169, 2002.)*

kinematic, joint kinetics, and ground reaction forces were examined during the stop-jump in three different directions (left, right, and vertical). Each jump began with a two-legged broad jump to two force plates, followed by an immediate (as fast as possible) jump in the designated direction. The results of this study indicated that direction had a significant effect on biomechanics during these stop-jump tasks. Jumps to the medial aspect of the studied knee (e.g., jumps to the left during an examination of the right knee) resulted in the highest vertical ground reaction forces, greatest deceleration forces (posterior ground reaction forces), highest proximal anterior tibia shear force, highest valgus and flexion moments, and lowest knee flexion angles. They concluded that this particular jump was the most dangerous owing to the potential risk of injury[30] and increased ACL strain.[19,53,76] This type of jump also mirrors the observations of Olsen and colleagues.[65]

Based on the results of the comparison of jump direction, the authors examined the potential differences in joint kinematics, joint kinetics, and ground reaction forces between genders when performing the most dangerous of the three jumps, jumps to the medial aspect of the knee. Females performed jumps to the left with significantly less flexion at the time of peak posterior ground reaction force (PPGRF) and had less total flexion. Females also performed these tasks with a significantly greater knee valgus angle at PPGRF (Fig. 17–12). PPGRF was chosen as a time point because it is a common characteristic across the multitude of tasks that have been identified as those during which noncontact ACL injuries occur.[10,57,65] Tasks such as landing, stopping, stop-jump, and cutting all have one common component—a sharp deceleration. Deceleration during a dynamic task can be measured by posterior ground reaction forces. They concluded that female athletes perform the most dangerous of landing tasks differently than males and in a manner that increases their susceptibility to ligament injury.

The majority of biomechanical analyses of dynamic tasks have been performed during controlled laboratory experiments.[13,20,31,43,49,68,77] Whereas these studies have been valuable, they may not represent the best simulation of actual athletic competition. Actual athletic competition requires the participant to react on a millisecond-by-millisecond basis to unanticipated events.

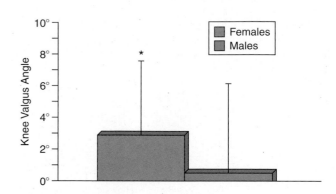

FIGURE 17–12. Female high school athletes perform jumps to the medial aspect of the knee with a significantly greater valgus angle than that of male athletes (*$P < .05$). *(From Sell, T. C.; Ferris, C. M.; Abt, J. P.; et al.: The effect of direction and reaction on the neuromuscular and biomechanical characteristics of the knee during tasks that simulate the noncontact anterior cruciate ligament injury mechanism. Am J Sports Med 34:43–54, 2006.)*

Knowledge of the task to be performed allows individuals to preplan movement patterns. To better replicate these unanticipated events, the authors designed and implemented a novel testing model.[78] Eighteen male and 17 female high school basketball players performed a series of 30 jumps in three different directions under two different conditions (planned and reactive). The task was a stop-jump maneuver that began with a two-legged broad jump to two force plates, followed by an immediate jump in one of three directions (left, right, or vertical). For half of the jumps (randomized order), the participants had to react to a visual cue for jump direction. The visual cue was triggered by a laser coupled with a photocell that was instrumented with a videographic monitor via a Matlab program (Release 12, The MathWorks, Natick, MA). Comparisons between the planned and the reactive tasks revealed significant differences for most of the biomechanical variables. During the reactive jumps, female participants landed with less knee flexion at PPGRF and a greater maximum knee flexion angle and experienced greater deceleration forces, knee flexion moments, and knee valgus moments (Table 17–1). These differences indicate that these laboratory experiments may be different from actual game situations.

TABLE 17–1 Comparison between Jump Tasks (Planned vs. Reactive)		
	Planned*	**Reactive***
Knee flexion angle at PPGRF (°)[†]	29.5 ± 11.8	24.4 ± 10.4
Maximum knee flexion angle (°)[†]	68.6 ± 12.8	71.7 ± 11.0
Knee valgus angle at PPGRF (°)	0.4 ± 6.4	0.5 ± 5.6
Maximum knee valgus angle (°)	−4.7 ± 8.7	−5.8 ± 9.3
Maximum vertical ground reaction force (body weight)	2.23 ± 0.90	2.18 ± 0.88
Maximum posterior ground reaction force (body weight)[†]	−0.70 ± 0.24	−0.81 ± 0.29
Proximal anterior tibia shear force at PPGRF (body weight)	0.318 ± 0.198	0.283 ± 0.171
Maximum proximal anterior shear force (body weight)	0.97 ± 0.23	0.93 ± 0.23
Knee flexion moment at PPGRF (body weight x height)[†]	−0.040 ± 0.045	−0.054 ± 0.039
Maximum knee flexion moment (body weight x height)	−0.152 ± 0.037	−0.161 ± 0.047
Knee valgus moment at PPGRF (body weight x height)	−0.017 ± 0.025	−0.013 ± 0.025
Maximum knee valgus moment (body weight x height)[†]	−0.044 ± 0.019	−0.050 ± 0.020
Vastus lateralis IEMG	0.122 ± 0.338	0.076 ± 0.054
Semitendinosus IEMG	0.077 ± 0.099	0.068 ± 0.097
Co-contraction value	0.088 ± 0.089	0.073 ± 0.063

*Data shown are mean ± standard deviation.
[†]Significant difference observed between tasks (P < .05).
IEMG, integrated electromyogram; PPGRF, peak posterior ground reaction force.
From Sell, T. C.; Ferris, C. M.; Abt, J. P.; et al.: The effect of direction and reaction on the neuromuscular and biomechanical characteristics of the knee during tasks that simulate the noncontact anterior cruciate ligament injury mechanism. *Am J Sports Med* 34:43–54, 2006.

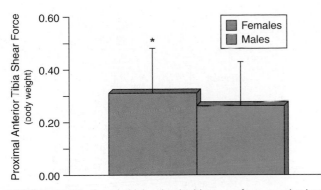

FIGURE 17–13. Female high school athletes perform reactive jumps with significantly greater proximal tibia anterior shear force than male athletes (*$P < .05$). *(From Sell, T. C.; Ferris, C. M.; Abt, J. P.; et al.: The effect of direction and reaction on the neuromuscular and biomechanical characteristics of the knee during tasks that simulate the noncontact anterior cruciate ligament injury mechanism. Am J Sports Med 34:43–54, 2006.)*

A secondary analysis was performed to compare biomechanical characteristics of males and females during reactive tasks. Females performed the reactive tasks with less flexion, greater valgus angle, greater proximal anterior tibia shear force (Fig. 17–13), and a greater knee flexion moment. The differences observed between genders are consistent with what is observed under planned conditions, but the differences between planned and reactive tasks demonstrate the need to develop testing models that better replicate actual game conditions.

Dynamic knee stability is essential in reducing the destabilizing forces during dynamic activities. Athletes must be able to perform the activities required in their sport while reducing those forces that can lead to joint injury. At the knee, one of those forces is proximal tibia anterior shear force. Proximal tibia anterior shear force is the most direct loading mechanism of the ACL[11,53-55] and may be estimated through inverse dynamics. Yu and coworkers[89] described how proximal tibia anterior shear force (estimated through inverse dynamics) may be an indicator of ACL loading. Females have been shown to perform dynamic tasks with greater proximal tibia anterior shear force. A regression analysis was conducted to determine the biomechanical and neuromuscular predictors of proximal tibia anterior shear force.[79] The analysis included knee flexion angle, knee valgus angle, knee flexion moment, knee valgus moment, PPGRF, IEMG activity of the vastus lateralis and semitendinosus, and gender. These variables were chosen because of their previously identified relationships with ACL strain and/or ACL injury.[11,53-55]

The analysis revealed that an equation based on PPGRF, knee flexion-extension moment, knee flexion angle, IEMG activity of the vastus lateralis, and gender (female) significantly predicts proximal tibia anterior shear force during stop-jump tasks. The equation indicates that a sharper deceleration, greater quadriceps activity, and landing with increased flexion will increase the proximal tibia anterior shear forces. Females perform these tasks with a greater flexion moment, IEMG activity of the vastus lateralis, and greater deceleration than males, further demonstrating their increased propensity for ACL injury, because each of these differences would predict landing in a greater proximal tibia anterior shear force.

Biomechanical analyses of tasks implicated in knee injuries are a continued focus of the authors' laboratory. Research has been expanded to incorporate emerging technology, including the use of wireless three-dimensional accelerometers that have the potential to be used during actual competition. Current work involves studying the relationships among knee joint forces as measured through inverse dynamics, tibial accelerations as measured with a wireless three-dimensional accelerometer, and tibial translation as measured with dual radiography.

FATIGUE

The effects of fatigue (both central and peripheral) have been studied on neuromuscular and biomechanical characteristics.[5,74] Muscular fatigue may disrupt or degrade the compensatory stabilizing mechanisms necessary to maintain joint stability in the presence of destabilizing forces and moments.[74] Numerous studies indicate that athletic injuries are more common in the later stages of activity and competition.[16,21,23,61,66,73,84] The reasons for this are unclear, but may be due to the effects of fatigue on decreased motor control,[36,88] increased knee joint laxity,[34,74,82] decreased balance skill,[36] and decreased proprioception.[32,40,41,60] The authors conducted two studies examining the effects of fatigue on neuromuscular and biomechanical characteristics.

The first study examined knee joint laxity, kinesthesia (via threshold to detect passive motion), lower extremity balance, and surface EMG activity during a landing maneuver of male and female athletes before and after a peripheral muscular fatigue protocol.[74] The fatigue protocol was designed to induce peripheral fatigue of the knee flexors and extensors and was implemented using a Biodex Isokinetic Dynamometer. Seventeen male and 17 female collegiate athletes performed three sets of maximum contraction at 180°/sec, or until their torque production fell below 25% of their initial peak torque production. The fatigue protocol had a significant effect on the neuromuscular characteristics of both males and females. The ability to detect joint motion, measured through threshold to detect passive motion, was decreased during knee joint motion toward full extension (Fig. 17–14). In addition, both males and females demonstrated an increase in the contraction onset time for the medial hamstrings and gastrocnemius and increased IEMG activity of the vastus lateralis and vastus medialis. The results of this series of neuromuscular testing indicate that both males and females are at an increased risk for ligamentous injury under fatigued conditions.

The second study examined the kinematic characteristics of the hip and knee during a single-leg stop-jump task before and after an exhaustive run. The exhaustive run was designed to induce general/central fatigue and was performed on a treadmill using a modified Astrand protocol.[39,69] Lower extremity kinematic measurements were taken of male and female college-aged

---

Critical Points FATIGUE

- Muscular fatigue may disrupt compensatory stabilizing mechanisms necessary to maintain joint stability. Athletic injuries are more common in the later stages of activity and competition.
- Fatigue decreases the ability of athletes to detect knee joint motion.
- Fatigue decreases the amount of knee flexion during dynamic tasks.
- Fatigue affects both genders equally and may be a risk factor for injury during the latter stages of athletic events.

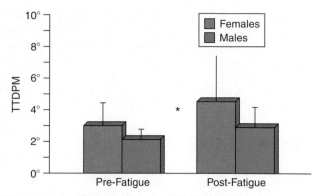

FIGURE 17–14. Fatigue effects on TTDPM. A significant treatment effect (decreased kinesthesia) was present in both male and female athletes after fatigue (*$P < .05$). *(From Rozzi, S. L.; Lephart, S. M.; Fu, F. H.: Effects of muscular fatigue on knee joint laxity and neuromuscular characteristics of male and female athletes. J Athl Train 34:106–114, 1999.)*

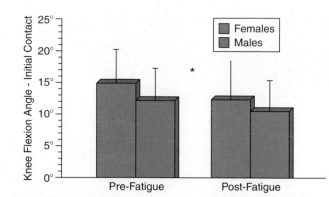

FIGURE 17–15. Fatigue effects on knee flexion angle at initial contact during a single-leg stop-jump task. A significant treatment effect (decreased flexion angle) was present after fatigue in both male and female athletes (*$P < .05$). *(From Benjaminse, A.; Habu, A.; Sell, T. C.; et al.: Fatigue alters lower extremity kinematics during a single-leg stop-jump task. Knee Surg Sports Traumatol Arthrosc 16:400–407, 2008.)*

recreational athletes. All subjects demonstrated a decreased knee flexion angle at initial contact and decreased maximum valgus angle (Fig. 17–15).[5] Landing with less knee flexion may be an attempt to improve knee stability by decreasing the available knee valgus-varus and internal-external rotation. Unfortunately, this landing may also increase ACL strain[19,53–55,76] and place individuals at greater risk for ACL rupture at the latter stages of games/competition. Overall, it appears as though fatigue affects both genders equally.

CURRENT RESEARCH

The authors continue to conduct research on injury prevention and control in female athletes, but have expanded and applied subject models to Army soldiers and Naval Special Warfare operators. These models use the public health approach to the injury control process.[37,58,72] This model integrates a five-step process designed to determine injury patterns and ultimately evaluate the effectiveness of intervention programs to reduce the incidence of injuries. Human performance testing has been incorporated in order to enhance training techniques. The ultimate goals of these projects are to reduce the incidence and severity of injuries, minimize the necessity for surgery, promote longevity, enhance performance, and optimize military readiness.

SUMMARY

The authors' studies have demonstrated that female athletes have decreased proprioception, compensatory EMG patterns, enhanced static balance, and decreased lower extremity strength than male athletes. These differences result in altered neuromuscular control as observed in the kinematic and kinetic characteristics of the knee during dynamic tasks. Future research should incorporate these characteristics in prospective studies to determine the risk factors for noncontact ACL injury and the development of intervention programs to reduce the incidence of these debilitating injuries.

REFERENCES

1. Agel, J.; Arendt, E. A.; Bershadsky, B.: Anterior cruciate ligament injury in National Collegiate Athletic Association basketball and soccer: a 13-year review. *Am J Sports Med* 33:524–531, 2005.
2. Arendt, E.; Agel, J.; Dick, R.: Anterior cruciate ligament injury patterns among collegiate men and women. *J Athl Train* 34:86–92, 1999.
3. Arendt, E.; Dick, R.: Knee injury patterns among men and women in collegiate basketball and soccer. NCAA data and review of literature. *Am J Sports Med* 23:694–701, 1995.
4. Basmajian, J. V.: *Muscles Alive, Their Functions Revealed by Electromyography*, 4th ed. Baltimore: Williams & Wilkins, 1978.
5. Benjaminse, A.; Habu, A.; Sell, T. C.; et al.: Fatigue alters lower extremity kinematics during a single-leg stop-jump task. *Knee Surg Sports Traumatol Arthrosc* 16:400–407, 2008.
6. Benvenuti, F.; Stanhope, S. J.; Thomas, S. L.; et al.: Flexibility of anticipatory postural adjustments revealed by self-paced and reaction-time arm movements. *Brain Res* 761:59–70, 1997.
7. Besier, T. F.; Lloyd, D. G.; Ackland, T. R.: Muscle activation strategies at the knee during running and cutting maneuvers. *Med Sci Sports Exerc* 35:119–127, 2003.
8. Besier, T. F.; Lloyd, D. G.; Ackland, T. R.; Cochrane, J. L.: Anticipatory effects on knee joint loading during running and cutting maneuvers. *Med Sci Sports Exerc* 33:1176–1181, 2001.
9. Bjordal, J. M.; Arnly, F.; Hannestad, B.; Strand, T.: Epidemiology of anterior cruciate ligament injuries in soccer. *Am J Sports Med* 25:341–345, 1997.
10. Boden, B. P.; Dean, G. S.; Feagin, J. A., Jr.; Garrett, W. E., Jr.: Mechanisms of anterior cruciate ligament injury. *Orthopedics* 23:573–578, 2000.
11. Butler, D. L.; Noyes, F. R.; Grood, E. S.: Ligamentous restraints to anterior-posterior drawer in the human knee. A biomechanical study. *J Bone Joint Surg Am* 62:259–270, 1980.
12. Caraffa, A.; Cerulli, G.; Projetti, M.; et al.: Prevention of anterior cruciate ligament injuries in soccer. A prospective controlled study of proprioceptive training. *Knee Surg Sports Traumatol Arthrosc* 4:19–21, 1996.
13. Chappell, J. D.; Yu, B.; Kirkendall, D. T.; Garrett, W. E.: A comparison of knee kinetics between male and female recreational athletes in stop-jump tasks. *Am J Sports Med* 30:261–267, 2002.
14. Cowling, E. J.; Steele, J. R.: Is lower limb muscle synchrony during landing affected by gender? Implications for variations in ACL injury rates. *J Electromyogr Kinesiol* 11:263–268, 2001.
15. Cox, J. S.; Lenz, H. W.: Women midshipmen in sports. *Am J Sports Med* 12:241–243, 1984.
16. Feagin, J. A., Jr.; Lambert, K. L.; Cunningham, R. R.; et al.: Consideration of the anterior cruciate ligament injury in skiing. *Clin Orthop Rel Res* 216:13–18, 1987.

17. Ferretti, A.; Papandrea, P.; Conteduca, F.; Mariani, P. P.: Knee ligament injuries in volleyball players. *Am J Sports Med* 20:203–207, 1992.
18. Ferris, C. M.: *Relationship of pelvis and hip neuromechanical characteristics to the knee during a stop-jump task.* Dissertation. Pittsburgh: Department of Sports Medicine and Nutrition, University of Pittsburgh, 2003.
19. Fleming, B. C.; Renstrom, P. A.; Beynnon, B. D.; et al.: The effect of weightbearing and external loading on anterior cruciate ligament strain. *J Biomech* 34:163–170, 2001.
20. Ford, K. R.; Myer, G. D.; Toms, H. E.; Hewett, T. E.: Gender differences in the kinematics of unanticipated cutting in young athletes. *Med Sci Sports Exerc* 37:124–129, 2005.
21. Gabbett, T. J.: Incidence, site, and nature of injuries in amateur rugby league over three consecutive seasons. *Br J Sports Med* 34:98–103, 2000.
22. Gabbett, T. J.: Incidence of injury in junior and senior rugby league players. *Sports Med* 34:849–859, 2004.
23. Ghez, C.; Krakauer, J.: The organization of movement. In Kandel, E. R.; Schwartz, J. H.; Jessell, T. M. (eds.): *Principles of Neural Science.* New York: McGraw-Hill, Health Professions Division; 2000; pp. 653–673.
24. Goldie, P. A.; Bach, T. M.; Evans, O. M.: Force platform measures for evaluating postural control: reliability and validity. *Arch Phys Med Rehabil* 70:510–517, 1989.
25. Goldie, P. A.; Evans, O. M.; Bach, T. M.: Steadiness in one-legged stance: development of a reliable force-platform testing procedure. *Arch Phys Med Rehabil* 73:348–354, 1992.
26. Gomez, E.; DeLee, J. C.; Farney, W. C.: Incidence of injury in Texas girls' high school basketball. *Am J Sports Med* 24:684–687, 1996.
27. Gwinn, D. E.; Wilckens, J. H.; McDevitt, E. R.; et al.: The relative incidence of anterior cruciate ligament injury in men and women at the United States Naval Academy. *Am J Sports Med* 28:98–102, 2000.
28. Harrer, M. F.; Berson, L.; Hosea, T. M.; Leddy, T. P.: Lower extremity injuries: females vs. males in the sport of basketball. Paper presented at American Orthopaedic Society for Sports Medicine 22nd Annual Meeting. June 16–20, 1996, Lake Buena Vista, FL.
29. Hewett, T. E.; Lindenfeld, T. N.; Riccobene, J. V.; Noyes, F. R.: The effect of neuromuscular training on the incidence of knee injury in female athletes. A prospective study. *Am J Sports Med* 27:699–706, 1999.
30. Hewett, T. E.; Myer, G. D.; Ford, K. R.; et al.: Biomechanical measures of neuromuscular control and valgus loading of the knee predict anterior cruciate ligament injury risk in female athletes: a prospective study. *Am J Sports Med* 33:492–501, 2005.
31. Hewett, T. E.; Stroupe, A. L.; Nance, T. A.; Noyes, F. R.: Plyometric training in female athletes. Decreased impact forces and increased hamstring torques. *Am J Sports Med* 24:765–773, 1996.
32. Hiemstra, L. A.; Lo, I. K.; Fowler, P. J.: Effect of fatigue on knee proprioception: implications for dynamic stabilization. *J Orthop Sports Phys Ther* 31:598–605, 2001.
33. Hillstrom, H. J.; Triolo, R. J.: EMG theory. In Craik, R. L.; Oatis, C. A. (eds.): *Gait Analysis: Theory and Application*, 1st ed. St. Louis: Mosby, 1995; pp. 271–292.
34. Huston, L. J.; Wojtys, E. M.: Neuromuscular performance characteristics in elite female athletes. *Am J Sports Med* 24:427–436, 1996.
35. Johansson, H.; Sjolander, P.: The neurophysiology of joints. In Wright, V.; Radin, E. L. (eds.): *Mechanics of Joints: Physiology, Pathophysiology, and Treatment.* New York: Marcel Dekker, 1993; pp. 243–290.
36. Johnston, R. B., 3rd; Howard, M. E.; Cawley, P. W., Losse, G. M.: Effect of lower extremity muscular fatigue on motor control performance. *Med Sci Sports Exerc* 30:1703–1707, 1998.
37. Jones, B. H.; Knapik, J. J.: Physical training and exercise-related injuries. Surveillance, research and injury prevention in military populations. *Sports Med* 27:111–125, 1999.
38. Kandel, E. R.; Schwartz, J. H.; Jessell, T. M.: Posture. *Principles of Neural Science*, 3rd ed. Norwalk, CT: Appleton & Lange; 1991; pp. 816–831.
39. Kang, J.; Chaloupka, E. C.; Mastrangelo, M. A.; et al.: Physiological comparisons among three maximal treadmill exercise protocols in trained and untrained individuals. *Eur J Appl Physiol* 84:291–295, 2001.
40. Lattanzio, P. J.; Petrella, R. J.: Knee proprioception: a review of mechanisms, measurements, and implications of muscular fatigue. *Orthopedics* 21:463–470, 1998.
41. Lattanzio, P. J.; Petrella, R. J.; Sproule, J. R.; Fowler, P. J.: Effects of fatigue on knee proprioception. *Clin J Sport Med* 7:22–27, 1997.
42. Lephart, S. M.; Abt, J. P.; Ferris, C. M.; et al.: Neuromuscular and biomechanical characteristic changes in high school athletes: a plyometric versus basic resistance program. *Br J Sports Med* 39:932–938, 2005.
43. Lephart, S. M.; Ferris, C. M.; Riemann, B. L.; et al.: Gender differences in strength and lower extremity kinematics during landing. *Clin Orthop Relat Res* 401:162–169, 2002.
44. Lephart, S. M.; Giraldo, J. L.; Borsa, P. A.; Fu, F. H.: Knee joint proprioception: a comparison between female intercollegiate gymnasts and controls. *Knee Surg Sports Traumatol Arthrosc* 4:121–124, 1996.
45. Lephart, S. M.; Pincivero, D. M.; Rozzi, S. L.: Proprioception of the ankle and knee. *Sports Med* 25:149–155, 1998.
46. Lephart, S. M.; Riemann, B. L.; Fu, F. H.: Introduction to the sensorimotor system. In Lephart, S.; Fu, F. H. (eds.): *Proprioception and Neuromuscular Control in Joint Stability.* Champaign, IL: Human Kinetics, 2000; pp. xxiv–xxv.
47. Lephart, S. M.; Warner, J. J. P.; Borsa, P. A.; Fu, F. H.: Proprioception of the shoulder joint in healthy, unstable, and surgically repaired shoulders. *J Shoulder Elbow Surg* 3:371–380, 1994.
48. Lew, W. D.; Lewis, J. L.; Craig, E. V.: Stabilization by capsule, ligaments, and labrum: stability at the extremes of motion. In Matsen, F. A.; Fu, F. H.; Hawkins, R. J. (eds.) *The Shoulder: A Balance of Mobility and Stability.* Rosemont, IL: American Academy of Orthopaedic Surgeons, 1993; pp. 69–89.
49. Malinzak, R. A.; Colby, S. M.; Kirkendall, D. T.; et al.: A comparison of knee joint motion patterns between men and women in selected athletic tasks. *Clin Biomech (Bristol, Avon)* 16:438–445, 2001.
50. Mandelbaum, B. R.; Silvers, H. J.; Watanabe, D. S.; et al.: ACL prevention strategies in the female athlete and soccer. Implementation of a neuromuscular training program to determine its efficacy on the incidence of ACL injury. Paper presented at American Academy of Orthopaedic Surgeons—Specialty Society Day, February 16, 2000, San Francisco.
51. Mandelbaum, B. R.; Silvers, H. J.; Watanabe, D. S.; et al.: Effectiveness of a neuromuscular and proprioceptive training program in preventing anterior cruciate ligament injuries in female athletes. 2-year follow-up. *Am J Sports Med* 33:1003–1010, 2005.
52. Mandelbaum, B. R.; Silvers, H. J.; Watanabe, D. T.; et al.: Effectiveness of a neuromuscular and proprioceptive training program in preventing the incidence of ACL injuries in female athletes: year two. Paper presented at American Orthopaedic Society of Sports Medicine, February 8, 2003, New Orleans.
53. Markolf, K. L.; Burchfield, D. M.; Shapiro, M. M.; et al.: Combined knee loading states that generate high anterior cruciate ligament forces. *J Orthop Res* 13:930–935, 1995.
54. Markolf, K. L.; Gorek, J. F.; Kabo, J. M.; Shapiro, M. S.: Direct measurement of resultant forces in the anterior cruciate ligament. An in vitro study performed with a new experimental technique. *J Bone Joint Surg Am* 72:557–567, 1990.
55. Markolf, K. L.; Mensch, J. S.; Amstutz, H. C.: Stiffness and laxity of the knee—the contributions of the supporting structures. A quantitative in vitro study. *J Bone Joint Surg Am* 58:583–594, 1976.
56. McCollum, G.; Leen, T.: The form and exploration of mechanical stability limits in erect stance. *J Mot Behav* 21:225–238, 1989.
57. McNair, P. J.; Marshall, R. N.; Matheson, J. A.: Important features associated with acute anterior cruciate ligament injury. *N Z Med J* 103:537–539, 1990.
58. Mercy, J. A.; Rosenberg, M. L.; Powell, K. E.; et al.: Public health policy for preventing violence. *Health Aff (Millwood)* 12:7–29, 1993.
59. Messina, D. F.; Farney, W. C.; DeLee, J. C.: The incidence of injury in Texas high school basketball. A prospective study among male and female athletes. *Am J Sports Med* 27:294–299, 1999.
60. Miura, K.; Ishibashi, Y.; Tsuda, E.; et al.: The effect of local and general fatigue on knee proprioception. *Arthroscopy* 20:414–418, 2004.
61. Molsa, J.; Airaksinen, O.; Nasman, O.; Torstila, I.: Ice hockey injuries in Finland. A prospective epidemiologic study. *Am J Sports Med* 25:495–499, 1997.
62. Myklebust, G.; Engebretsen, L.; Braekken, I. H.; et al.: Prevention of anterior cruciate ligament injuries in female team handball players: a prospective intervention study over three seasons. *Clin J Sport Med* 13:71–78, 2003.

63. Myklebust, G.; Maehlum, S.; Holm, I.; Bahr, R.: A prospective cohort study of anterior cruciate ligament injuries in elite Norwegian team handball. *Scand J Med Sci Sports* 8:149–153, 1998.
64. Noyes, F. R.; Matthews, D. S.; Mooar, P. A.; Grood, E. S.: The symptomatic anterior cruciate–deficient knee. Part II: the results of rehabilitation, activity modification, and counseling on functional disability. *J Bone Joint Surg Am* 65:163–174, 1983.
65. Olsen, O. E.; Myklebust, G.; Engebretsen, L.; Bahr, R.: Injury mechanisms for anterior cruciate ligament injuries in team handball: a systematic video analysis. *Am J Sports Med* 32:1002–1012, 2004.
66. Pettrone, F. A.; Ricciardelli, E.: Gymnastic injuries: the Virginia experience 1982–1983. *Am J Sports Med* 15:59–62, 1987.
67. Pincivero, D. M.; Lephart, S. M.; Karunakara, R. A.: Reliability and precision of isokinetic strength and muscular endurance for the quadriceps and hamstrings. *Int J Sports Med* 18:113–117, 1997.
68. Pollard, C. D.; Davis, I. M.; Hamill, J.: Influence of gender on hip and knee mechanics during a randomly cued cutting maneuver. *Clin Biomech* 19:1022–1031, 2004.
69. Pollock, L. M.; Wilmore, J. H.; Fox, S. M.: *Health and Fitness through Physical Activity*. New York: Wiley, 1978.
70. Prapavessis, H.; McNair, P. J.: Effects of instruction in jumping technique and experience jumping on ground reaction forces. *J Orthop Sports Phys Ther* 29:352–356, 1999.
71. Riemann, B. L.; Lephart, S. M.: The sensorimotor system. Part I. The physiologic basis of functional joint stability. *J Athl Train* 37:71–79, 2002.
72. Robertson, L. S.: *Injury Epidemiology*. New York: Oxford University Press, 1992.
73. Rodacki, A. L.; Fowler, N. E.; Bennett, S. J.: Vertical jump coordination: fatigue effects. *Med Sci Sports Exerc* 34:105–116, 2002.
74. Rozzi, S. L.; Lephart, S. M.; Fu, F. H.: Effects of muscular fatigue on knee joint laxity and neuromuscular characteristics of male and female athletes. *J Athl Train* 34:106–114, 1999.
75. Rozzi, S. L.; Lephart, S. M.; Gear, W. S.; Fu, F. H.: Knee joint laxity and neuromuscular characteristics of male and female soccer and basketball players. *Am J Sports Med* 27:312–319, 1999.
76. Sakane, M.; Fox, R. J.; Woo, S. L.; et al.: In situ forces in the anterior cruciate ligament and its bundles in response to anterior tibial loads. *J Orthop Res* 15:285–293, 1997.
77. Salci, Y.; Kentel, B. B.; Heycan, C.; et al.: Comparison of landing maneuvers between male and female college volleyball players. *Clin Biomech (Bristol, Avon)* 19:622–628, 2004.
78. Sell, T. C.; Ferris, C. M.; Abt, J. P.; et al.: The effect of direction and reaction on the neuromuscular and biomechanical characteristics of the knee during tasks that simulate the noncontact anterior cruciate ligament injury mechanism. *Am J Sports Med* 34:43–54, 2006.
79. Sell, T. C.; Ferris, C. M.; Abt, J. P.; et al.: Predictors of proximal tibia anterior shear force during a vertical stop-jump. *J Orthop Res* 25:1589–1597, 2007.
80. Sell, T. C.; Myers, J. B.; Youk, A. O.; et al.: *Neuromechanical Predictors of Dynamic Stability*. Dissertation. Pittsburgh: Department of Sports Medicine and Nutrition, University of Pittsburgh, 2004.
81. Shumway-Cook, A.; Woollacott, M. H.: *Motor Control: Theory and Practical Applications*, 2nd ed. Philadelphia: Lippincott Williams & Wilkins, 2001.
82. Skinner, H. B.; Wyatt, M. P.; Stone, M. L.; et al.: Exercise-related knee joint laxity. *Am J Sports Med* 14:30–34, 1986.
83. Solomonow, M.; Krogsgaard, M.: Sensorimotor control of knee stability. A review. *Scand J Med Sci Sports* 11:64–80, 2001.
84. Stuart, M. J.; Smith, A.: Injuries in Junior A ice hockey. A three-year prospective study. *Am J Sports Med* 23:458–461, 1995.
85. Williams, G. N.; Chmielewski, T.; Rudolph, K.; et al.: Dynamic knee stability: current theory and implications for clinicians and scientists. *J Orthop Sports Phys Ther* 31:546–566, 2001.
86. Winter, D. A.: *Biomechanics and Motor Control of Human Movement*, 2nd ed. New York: Wiley, 1990.
87. Wojtys, E. M.; Huston, L. J.; Taylor, P. D.; Bastian, S. D.: Neuromuscular adaptations in isokinetic, isotonic, and agility training programs. *Am J Sports Med* 24:187–192, 1996.
88. Wojtys, E. M.; Wylie, B. B.; Huston, L. J.: The effects of muscle fatigue on neuromuscular function and anterior tibial translation in healthy knees. *Am J Sports Med* 24:615–621, 1996.
89. Yu, B.; Chappell, J. D.; Garrett, W. E.: Letters to the editor: author's response. *Am J Sports Med* 34:313–315, 2006.

Chapter 18

Gender Differences in Muscular Protection of the Knee

Jennifer Kreinbrink, BS ▪ *Edward M. Wojtys*, MD

INTRODUCTION: PROTECTION SYSTEM

The protection system of the knee joint relies on the body's ability to sense the surrounding environment (proprioception) and to generate a timely motor response (muscle activation) while coordinating neuromuscular patterns that correctly position the torso and lower extremity to minimize soft tissue strain and impact load.

The proprioceptive pathways through which humans detect the musculoskeletal challenges that are presented daily derive information from multiple afferent systems, including vision, hearing, and sensation. These systems provide the signals and warnings to which a response is generated at various levels of consciousness (motor programs) during walking, jumping, running, turning, sitting, and other activities. As the complexity of movement increases, so does the need for detailed information about the environment in which function occurs.

Suboptimal responses by the neuroprotection system can lead to injuries and accidents. These shortcomings may be the result of inadequate input from the environment (proprioception), slow neuroprocessing, or an inadequate motor response. A goal of functional testing is to identify these neuromuscular factors before injuries occur. Therefore, when examining the results of functional testing, these three factors must be kept in mind. Unfortunately, the elements that contribute to injury are usually not readily apparent and are often difficult to trace and identify. Separating afferent from efferent problems can be difficult. Failure to correctly recognize these elements may result in ineffectual training and/or repeated injury.

The gender predisposition to some musculoskeletal injuries, such as anterior cruciate ligament (ACL) ruptures, has led many investigators to the conclusion that there must be gender differences in the muscle protection system of the knee. Whereas gender differences in the protective system have been detected, the role they play in ACL and other injuries remains unclear.

PROPRIOCEPTION

Proprioception refers to an individual's awareness of joint and body movement and their position in space. Motor control feedback via the gamma motor system can modify muscle stiffness or transjoint resistance of muscles to control joint movement and positioning during planned and unexpected events. Therefore, skeletal muscle plays an important role in knee joint proprioception. An individual's ability to detect knee joint position and motion is a major component required for reflex response, allowing joint stabilization and protection to develop. When

Critical Points PROTECTION SYSTEM

Gender differences have been detected in the knee protective system; however, the role these systems play in anterior cruciate ligament (ACL) and other injuries continues to be defined.

Critical Points PROPRIOCEPTION

- Knee joint proprioception is influenced by muscles in the torso and lower limb as well as joint laxity and muscle fatigue.
- Some injured female athletes have demonstrated a lower level of lower extremity proprioception than their male counterparts; however, uninjured female athletes tend to have higher levels of stability than healthy male athletes.

errors in these systems occur, or when these systems function at suboptimal levels, increased ligament strain, articular cartilage shear, and/or bone impact may result. High risk positioning of the lower extremity may also occur.[13,20]

Several authors have reported gender differences in proprioception.[21,39,40,53] Rozzi and coworkers[40] investigated joint proprioception in 34 (17 male, 17 female) collegiate soccer and basketball athletes by measuring the threshold to detection of passive motion using a device that moved the knee joint at a constant 0.5°/sec velocity through flexion and extension. A rotational transducer provided angular displacement values. Compared with male athletes, females took significantly longer to detect the threshold of knee joint motion in extension (2.11° ± 0.63° and 2.95° ± 1.47°, respectively; $P = .039$). However, no significant gender difference was observed during flexion. The clinical significance of a mean difference of 0.84° of angular motion between genders is unknown.

Hewett and associates[21] assessed proprioception using single-leg postural balance at the knee on a dynamic platform in ACL-deficient subjects. Uninjured females demonstrated greater knee joint stability than males, which the authors attributed to a lower center of gravity. In contrast, males had significantly greater single-leg stability after an ACL rupture, and females took longer to regain adequate levels of single-leg balance postoperatively.[21] A clear gender difference cannot be extracted from these results.

Although injury research often focuses on the lower limbs, the core of the torso may be the key to understanding body positioning. Therefore, the core muscle of the torso should not be overlooked in the investigation of proprioception. Zazulak and colleagues[53] evaluated core proprioception and knee joint control. Two-hundred seventy-seven collegiate athletes (137 male, 140 female) underwent core proprioceptive measurements by passive trunk rotation in the seated position through 20° in the transverse plane. With auditory and visual stimuli diminished, the athletes were instructed to reproduce the initial position after displacement. The difference between the perceived and the actual angle was calculated as the active proprioceptive repositioning error. After testing, the athletes were followed for 3 years, during which 25 (14 male, 11 female) sustained knee injuries. Analysis of the active proprioceptive repositioning error revealed that females who sustained knee ligament or meniscal injuries demonstrated significantly greater error in active repositioning than uninjured females. Male athletes did not demonstrate this problem. In addition, uninjured female athletes had significantly better core proprioception than uninjured male athletes, which supports previous studies.[20,40] Zazulak and coworkers[52] also reported that after an unexpected perturbation, the maximal trunk displacement in females who suffered knee ligament injuries was significantly greater than that of females who did not experience injury. No significant difference in maximal trunk displacement between injured and uninjured males was found. Therefore, the core stability of female athletes may be a greater factor in lower extremity injury susceptibility than that in males.[52] In fact, lateral trunk displacement was the lone significant predictor of ligament injury in female athletes ($P = .001$) in this investigation, with 100% sensitivity and 72% specificity rates reported. This was not true for male athletes, because their sole predictor of injury was a history of low back pain.[52]

Other factors that may influence proprioceptive function include joint laxity and muscle fatigue, both of which also affect muscle function. Rozzi and associates[39] reported that female athletes had greater knee laxity that resulted in a decreased sensitivity to knee position change. Many clinicians have suspected that joint laxity is a risk factor for knee injury, but the evidence is not overwhelming. The best evidence may be that provided by Uhorchak and colleagues[43] in their risk factor analysis for ACL injury in military cadets.

Regarding muscle fatigue, Rozzi and associates[39] showed in male and female collegiate basketball and soccer athletes that induced fatigue altered proprioception, especially in knee extension. Wojtys and coworkers[51] evaluated the effects of muscle fatigue on anterior tibial translation, muscle reaction time, and recruitment order in 10 athletes (6 male, 4 female) whose physical activity included jumping, pivoting, and twisting. Each athlete completed baseline measurements and then underwent a vigorous isokinetic workout until quadriceps and hamstrings torques decreased by 50% or greater. Eight of the 10 fatigued athletes demonstrated greater anterior tibial translation during dynamic testing (average percentage increase, 32.5%), indicating that fatigue did increase joint laxity. Fatigued athletes did not alter their muscle recruitment order in response to an anterior tibial translation. However, after fatigue, muscle reaction time slowed significantly in the three response phases (spinal reflex, intermediate, and voluntary). Although the investigation found a change in muscle reaction time and laxity of the knee, no gender difference was reported for these factors, nor was a correlation established between fatigue and a decrease in proprioception.

Earlier studies have evaluated the effect of ACL-deficiency on proprioception, although gender was not specifically examined.[6,11,48] More recent studies have focused on gender differences. In general, these studies show that injured female athletes have poorer lower extremity proprioception than their male athlete counterparts.[21,40,52] However, uninjured female athletes tend to have higher levels of stability than healthy male athletes.

Considering the consequences of serious knee injury, proprioceptive prescreening of female athletes, especially in high-risk sports, prior to athletic participation may help focus training and conditioning programs.[20,52,53]

MUSCLE RESPONSE

Time to Peak Torque

Neuromuscular activation patterns influence dynamic knee joint stability potential, which may contribute to knee injury susceptibility.[10,19,23,25] Gender-related differences in these activation patterns have been reported by numerous investigators.[8,10,27,33,40,41,44,47]

Using isokinetic peak torque strength testing of 100 Division I athletes (60 male, 40 female), Huston and Wojtys[27] detected significant gender differences. Female athletes and controls generated similar time to peak knee flexion torques, which were slower than male athletes. Male athletes were able to generate peak knee extension and flexion torques faster than male or

---

Critical Points MUSCLE RESPONSE

- Females' initial quadriceps activation and a slowed hamstring response may lead to ineffective knee stabilization.
- Mature male athletes have stronger quadriceps and hamstring muscles than mature females when corrected for body weight.

TABLE 18–1	Time to Peak Torque during Isokinetic Testing					
			Subjects*			
			Males		Females	
Reference	Subject Age and Athletic Involvement	Testing Condition	Athletes	Nonathletes	Athletes	Nonathletes
Huston et al., 1996[27]	Divsion I collegiate athletes and recreationally active college students	Quadriceps, 60°/sec	408[‡§]	463	420[‡]	448
		Hamstrings, 60°/sec	328[‖]	443	430	426
		Quadriceps, 240°/sec	153[§]	150	158	170
		Hamstrings, 240°/sec	150[‖]	170	169	164
Bowerman et al., 2006[8]	18- to 25-yr-old collegiate athletes and college students	Quadriceps, 60°/sec	475.93 (±133.83)	476.40 (±134.19)	522.96 (±102.46)	503.57 (±123.63)
		Hamstrings, 60°/sec	519.26 (±183.78)	539.60 (±176.36)	556.30 (±139.65)	540.71 (±177.76)
Rozzi et al., 1999[40]	Collegiate soccer and basketball athletes	Quadriceps, 180°/sec	338.23 (±124.16)		371.88 (±154.67)	
		Hamstrings, 180°/sec	214.71 (±46.38)		220.63 (±51.83)	
Barber-Westin et al., 2005[4†]	9- to 10-yr-old soccer, football, basketball, baseball, and hockey athletes	Quadriceps, 180°/sec	195 (±93)		162 (±60)	
		Hamstrings, 180°/sec	214 (±74)		183 (±63)	
Noyes & Barber-Westin, 2005[33]	11- to 13-yr-old basketball, soccer, volleyball, baseball, and track & field athletes	Ex rotation, 120°/sec	274 (±100)		312 (±216)	
		Ex rotation, 180°/sec	257 (±133)		243 (±153)	
		Int rotation, 120°/sec	270 (±126)		284 (±157)	
		Int rotation, 180°/sec	242 (±177)		233 (±130)	
	14- to 17-yr-old basketball, soccer, volleyball, baseball, and track & field athletes	Ex rotation, 120°/sec	284 (±113)		329 (±126)	
		Ex rotation, 180°/sec	209 (±54)		238 (±130)	
		Int rotation, 120°/sec	234 (±84)		323 (±168)[¶]	
		Int rotation, 180°/sec	191 (±155)		266 (±134)	

*Data shown are mean in milliseconds ± standard deviation.
†Only dominant limb reported.
‡Significantly faster than the male controls.
§Significantly faster than the female controls.
‖Significantly faster than all other groups.
¶Significantly slower than 14- to 17-yr-old males.
Ex, external; Int, internal.

female controls (Table 18–1). The slowed response of the hamstring in females was most striking.

Considering the young age at which many ACL injuries occur, muscle function maturation should be considered in the evaluation of injury susceptibility. Noyes and Barber-Westin[33] examined the gender- and age-related differences in time to peak torque for internal and external tibial rotation with isokinetic strength testing. They separated 94 athletes into two age groups: 11 to 13 years of age (20 male, 20 female) and 14 to 17 years of age (27 male, 27 female). Older male athletes were faster (28%) in internal rotation peak torque of the hamstrings than age-matched female athletes (see Table 18–1). In contrast, multiple investigators have reported no gender differences in isokinetic peak torques for quadriceps and/or hamstrings in collegiate athletes,[8,40] nonathlete controls,[8] and athletes 13 years of age or younger[4,33] (see Table 18–1).

Muscle Reaction Time

In an attempt to identify more relevant functional gender differences, several investigators have assessed peak muscle torque during weight-bearing perturbations and athletic tasks. Shultz and associates[41] examined muscle response times in 64 collegiate lacrosse and soccer athletes (32 male, 32 female) after applying an unexpected rotational perturbation force to the lower extremity. Female athletes' muscle response times for the quadriceps muscles were faster than male athletes with comparable recruitment patterns (Table 18–2). The Division I collegiate athletes

TABLE 18–2 Time to Peak Torque during Functional Testing

Reference	Subject Age and Athletic Involvement	Testing Condition	Muscle	Subjects*	
				Males	Females
Shultz et al., 2001[41]	Division I collegiate soccer and lacrosse athletes	Perturbation: External rotation	Lateral quadriceps	100.0 (±24.0)	90.8 (±16.3)[‡]
			Medial quadriceps	99.0 (±22.8)	87.1 (±18.0)[‡]
		Perturbation: Internal rotation	Lateral quadriceps	98.8 (±22.4)	89.8 (±12.6)[‡]
			Medial quadriceps	95.7 (±20.4)	86.3 (±13.6)[‡]
Carcia et al., 2005[10]	Recreationally active college students	Rotary perturbation in single-leg stance	Medial gastrocnemius	61.2 (±6.7)	62.8 (±8.4)
			Lateral gastrocnemius	63.9 (±10.2)	66.3 (±11.5)
			Medial hamstring	73.3 (±21.1)	73.9 (±17.3)
			Lateral hamstring	86.9 (±24.4)	93.1 (±30.8)
			Medial quadriceps	112.1 (±28.6)	98.2 (±21.1)[‡]
			Lateral quadriceps	118.0 (±28.4)	98.6 (±18.3)[‡]
Wojtys et al., 2002[47]	19- to 31-year-old sedentary to elite-level athletes	Anterior tibial translation	Hamstrings	383 (±157)	488 (±167)
			Quadriceps	412 (±143)	419 (±123)
Cowling & Steele, 2001[12]	20- to 24-year-old activity-matched subjects	Muscle burst peak time to peak F_s[†] after single-leg drop landing	Rectus femoris	39 (±24)	43 (±31)
			Semimembranosus	54 (±27)[§]	77 (±15)
			Gastrocnemius	47 (±45)	49 (±37)

*Data shown are mean in milliseconds ± standard deviation.
[†]Denotes tibiofemoral joint shear force.
[‡]Significantly faster than male athletes.
[§]Significant delay in timing compared with females.

displayed faster muscle response times than the recreational athletes.

Carcia and colleagues[10] measured the response times of the quadriceps, hamstrings, and gastrocnemius muscles after a weight-bearing rotary perturbation in 20 recreationally active adults (10 male, 10 female). Males and females responded with similar muscle recruitment order patterns at various angles of flexion (10°, 20°, 30°), and females generated faster quadriceps muscle response times than males at all angles (see Table 18–2).

Using a posterior force to the calf muscle to simulate anterior tibial translation, Huston and Wojtys[27] reported that female athletes activated their quadriceps first and faster than their male counterparts, raising concerns about what role the quadriceps could directly play in ACL injuries. In contrast, Cowling and Steele[12] reported a delay in the semimembranosus (hamstring) muscle of male athletes during abrupt single-leg landing compared with athletic level–matched female athletes.

In summary, preferential quadriceps activation and a slowed hamstring response may lead to a neuromuscular imbalance producing ineffective knee stabilization.[10,27,41,49] Powerful or unopposed quadriceps contractions, especially close to knee extension, have the potential to cause ACL injury.[46] Further research is necessary to better understand these relationships, especially in terms of muscle activity mode injury rates.

Strength

The timely ability to generate high levels of muscle force across the knee joint may decrease functional joint laxity and result in less stress and strain on the passive structures that constrain knee motion.[7,8,15,16,27,47,49] A poor muscle strength–to–body weight ratio may be a risk factor for lower extremity injury.[30,43]

Besides the peak torque–to–body weight ratio, the balance of forces expressed as the hamstring-to-quadriceps (H:Q) ratio is

an additional performance measurement that may provide insight into the gender differences in injury susceptibility. Evidence suggests that the hamstring muscles have the potential to unload the ACL,[46] whereas the quadriceps appear to function as the ACL antagonist.[46] The suspected relationship between the H:Q peak torque ratio and ACL injury susceptibility has been investigated by several authors.[2,8,9,22,38] This factor may be critical in ACL protection.[2,4,5,8,9,22,38,49]

Bowerman and coworkers[8] tested the peak isokinetic muscle torque (60°/sec) of 54 healthy collegiate athletes and 53 age-matched nonathletes. Males were stronger than females for both quadriceps and hamstring muscles (Table 18–3). Unfortunately, measurements were not normalized to body weight in this study. Not surprisingly, athletes generated higher quadriceps and hamstring peak torques. Similar findings were reported by Wojtys and associates[47] in 23 healthy volunteers (10 male, 13 female) whose activity level ranged from sedentary to elite-level athletes. Lephart and colleagues[30] also reported similar results, as did Bowerman and coworkers[8] in 15 Division I collegiate athletes and 15 age-matched male controls under the same testing conditions after normalizing for body weight (see Table 18–3). Male recreational athletes generated greater quadriceps and hamstring peak isokinetic torques (180°/sec) than their female counterparts with body weight normalization.[35] In addition, Hewett and coworkers[22] and Anderson and associates[2] reported that female high school athletes had lower H:Q ratios than male athletes. Conversely, Bowerman and coworkers[8] and Rosene and colleagues[38] found no gender difference in H:Q ratios among collegiate soccer, volleyball, softball, basketball, football, tennis, and track athletes. However, their strength levels were not corrected for body weight (Table 18–4).

Related studies have focused on the progression of muscle strength through adolescence to maturity. Barber-Westin and coworkers[5] reported isokinetic muscle strength data (300°/sec normalized to body weight) on 1140 athletes (177 male, 853

TABLE 18–3 Peak Torque Strength during Isokinetic Testing

Reference	Subject Age and Athletic Involvement	Testing Condition	Males Athletes	Males Nonathletes	Females Athletes	Females Nonathletes
Bowerman et al., 2006[8]	18- to 25-yr-old collegiate athletes and college students	Quadriceps, 60°/sec	253.14 (±64.97) Nm[‡][‖]	232.57 (±47.99) Nm	167.55 (±28.75) Nm[§]	137.22 (±30.84) Nm
		Hamstrings, 60°/sec	131.81 (±39.70) Nm[†][‖]	113.24 (±28.86) Nm	86.90 (±14.09) Nm[§]	63.74 (±14.67) Nm
Wojtys et al., 2002[47][†]	19- to 31-yr-old sedentary subjects to elite-level athletes	Quadriceps, 60°/sec	89 (±10) ft-lb/lb body weight[‖]		69 (±14) ft-lb/lb body weight	
		Hamstrings, 60°/sec	45 (±7) ft-lb/lb body weight		37 (±8) ft-lb/lb body weight	
Lephart et al., 2002[30][†]	Division I collegiate basketball, volleyball, and soccer athletes	Quadriceps, 60°/sec	271.68 (±59.27) Nm[‖]		222.93 (±30.86) Nm	
		Hamstrings, 60°/sec	131.72 (±21.89) Nm[‖]		113.74 (±23.66) Nm	
Piniverco et al., 2003[35][†]	20- to 28-yr-old recreationally active subjects	Quadriceps, 180°/sec	2.11 (±0.22) Nm/kg[‖]		1.53 (±0.21) Nm/kg	
		Hamstrings, 180°/sec	1.23 (±0.15) Nm/kg[‖]		0.93 (±0.14) Nm/kg	

*Data shown are mean ± standard deviation.
†Denotes measurements normalized to body weight.
‡Significantly greater than all other groups.
§Significantly greater than controls.
‖Significantly greater than female athletes.

TABLE 18-4 Hamstring-to-Quadriceps Ratio for Mean Peak Torque during Isokinetic Testing

Reference	Subject Age and Athletic Involvement	Testing Condition	Males Athletes	Males Nonathletes	Females Athletes	Females Nonathletes
Bowerman et al., 2006[8][†]	18- to 25-yr-old collegiate athletes and college students	60°/sec	52.01% (±8.51%)[§]	48.86% (±6.39%)	52.40% (±7.30%)[§]	46.79% (±6.00%)
Hewett et al., 1996[22][†]	High school volleyball athletes	Dominant leg; 60°/sec	62 (±8)[‖]		41 (±7)	
		Nondominant leg; 60°/sec	67 (±7)[‖]		47 (±8)	
Anderson et al., 2001[2][†]	High school varsity basketball athletes	60°/sec	61.8[‖]		56.8	
		240°/sec	73.5[‖]		62.9	
Rosene et al., 2001[38][†][‡]	Collegiate volleyball, soccer, basketball, and softball athletes	60°/sec	50.86 (±11.24)		50.14 (±7.74)	
		120°/sec	54.50 (±12.12)		56.44 (±20.76)	
		180°/sec	59.71 (±13.82)		59.40 (±10.86)	
Barber-Westin et al., 2005[4][†]	9- to 10-yr-old soccer, football, basketball, baseball, and hockey athletes	Dominant leg; 180°/sec	81% (±15%)		77% (±22%)	
		Nondominant leg; 180°/sec	75% (±19%)		73% (±10%)	
Buchanan et al., 2003[9][†]	11- to 13-yr-old basketball athletes	60°/sec	0.47 (±0.03)		0.41 (±0.04)	
	15- to 17-yr-old basketball athletes	60°/sec	0.43 (±0.03)		0.51 (±0.04)	
			Mature	**Immature**	**Mature**	**Immature**
Ahmad et al., 2006[1]	10- to 13-yr-old (immature) & 14- to 18-yr-old (mature) soccer athletes	Hand-held dynamometer	1.48 (±0.33)	1.58 (±0.46)	2.06 (±0.55)[¶]	1.73 (±0.32)

*Data shown are mean ± standard deviation.
†Denotes measurements normalized to body weight.
‡Only measurements for right leg reported.
§Significantly greater than male and female controls.
‖Significantly greater than females.
¶Significantly greater than all other groups.

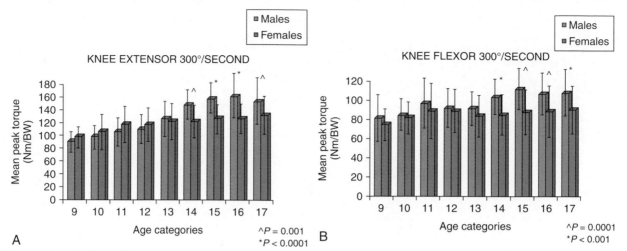

FIGURE 18–1. No significant difference was found in the main extension (**A**) or flexion (**B**) peak torque ratio values between girls and boys in the 9- to 13-yr-old age groups. However, from the ages of 14–17 yr, boys had significantly greater mean extension and flexion peak torque ratio values than did girls ($P < .001$ to $< .0001$). (**A** and **B**, Redrawn from Barber-Westin, S. D.; Noyes, F. R.; Galloway, M.: Jump-land characteristics and muscle strength development in young athletes: a gender comparison of 1140 athletes 9 to 17 years of age. Am J Sports Med 34:375–384, 2006. Reprinted with permission of SAGE Publications, Inc.)

female), ranging in age from 9 to 17 years. An increase in the mean knee extension peak torque was seen for both male and female subjects with maturation (Fig. 18–1A). At age 13 years, females produced 20% more extension peak torque than at age 9, but failed to produce a difference after age 13. Similarly, males at age 14 years produced 38% more extension peak torque than at age 9 with no difference found after age 14. There was no gender difference in the peak extension torque mean until the age of 14, when male athletes surpassed the females.

Male athletes demonstrated an increase in mean knee flexion peak torque (23%) from age 9 to 14 years, whereas female athletes produced a much smaller increase (16%), with no difference between ages 9 to 11 years (see Fig. 18–1B). There was no increase in hamstring peak torque after the age of 11 in females, despite an increase in quadriceps strength (see earlier). Similar to the peak extension torque, a gender difference in mean flexion peak torques became evident after the age of 14 years. This hamstring strength deficit in females, along with the increased quadriceps strength that occurs with maturation, may contribute to a muscle force imbalance across the knee and ACL strain patterns during activities. Therefore, hamstring strengthening programs, in particular, for young female athletes appear to be an essential component of knee injury prevention programs.

Ramos and associates[37] examined the isokinetic strength (60°/sec) of knee extensor muscles in young athletes. Dominant knees in 57 males and females ages 11 to 18 years were tested and strength levels were corrected for body weight. The female athletes aged 11 to 12 years displayed 95% of the strength of age-matched male athletes. At ages 13 to 14, females generated 90% of male strength. By age 17, male athletes were much stronger in extension than females of the same age. Female athletes displayed only 74% of the strength of age-matched male athletes. Similar to the data reported by Barber-Westin and co-workers,[4,5] the strength changes in females in the prepubescent years were similar to that of age-matched males, but the increases in female strength slowed and then essentially stopped after puberty while the strength of male athletes continued to increase. Ahmad and colleagues[1] reported similar results for H:Q co-activation ratios in 123 immature and mature soccer

players (70 male, 53 female). In contrast, several investigators have found no significant gender or age difference in H:Q ratio in young athletes[4,5,9] (see Table 18–4).

In conclusion, H:Q strength ratios across various age and athletic groups have mixed results. Most show that mature male athletes have significantly stronger quadriceps and hamstring muscles than mature female athletes when corrected for body weight. When determining the relevance of these studies, it is important to consider the relationship between the testing mode (often shortening contractions) and the muscle function needed most in vivo (lengthening contractions). Unfortunately, these commonly used testing procedures may not reflect the features of athletic activities.

FUNCTIONAL BIOMECHANICS

Knee

Excessive joint laxity and the decreased ability to generate muscle resistance across the knee are believed to contribute to injury susceptibility. Several authors[1,8,15,16,27,40,47] have demonstrated joint knee laxity differences between male and female athletes that may, in part, reflect passive muscle properties.

The ability to increase active muscular resistance to motion (stiffness) across the knee joint has the potential to dissipate

---

Critical Points FUNCTIONAL BIOMECHANICS

Knee

- Male athletes have greater active resistance to knee joint perturbations than female athletes.

Lower Extremity

- Females usually land in greater knee extension and produce higher ground reaction forces than male athletes after drop-landing tasks.

Core

- Females appear to have decreased levels of core stability and hip muscle strength compared with their male counterparts.

damaging loads across knees that can injure ligaments and other passive structures.[7,15,16,47,49] Males are capable of producing greater active stiffness across the knee than females.[15,16,47,49]

Granata and coworkers[16] tested active muscle stiffness at the ankle by applying a perturbation at three different weight load conditions (0 kg, 6 kg, and 20% maximum voluntary exertion). These loads created a knee flexion or extension moment. The 23 healthy subjects (12 male, 11 female) were positioned with their knees at 45° prior to perturbation. Males exhibited a mean stiffness of 25 to 164 Nm/rad greater than the mean values of female subjects. Females produced 56% to 73% of male subjects' muscles stiffness at each load. Male subjects maintained a higher stiffness in the hamstrings and quadriceps at all weight load conditions tested (Table 18–5).

Wojtys and associates[47] measured the active and passive sagittal-plane knee stiffness of 23 healthy volunteers (10 male, 13 female) and also concluded that male subjects produced higher levels of knee joint stiffness than female subjects. Most importantly, the dynamic capacity in males was much greater than that measured in females (379% and 212%, respectively; see Table 18–5).

Granata and associates[15] studied a two-legged-hopping task at frequencies of 2.5 Hz and 3.0 Hz while testing 30 subjects (15 male, 15 female) whose ages ranged from 21 to 62 years. Males maintained greater knee joint stiffness than females. A subgroup of younger and more physically active subjects (ages 21–31 yr) demonstrated results similar to that of the group at large: males produced greater knee joint stiffness (see Table 18–5). The lower extremity stiffness of athletic female subjects was 77% and 81% of that observed in male athletic and nonathletic subjects, respectively. Blackburn and colleagues[7] reported similar results in physically active males and females (see Table 18–5).

Because there is a rotational component to many knee injuries in sports, Wojtys and coworkers[49] tested the dynamic rotational stiffness of 24 Division I athletes (12 male, 12 female) who competed in high-risk ACL injury pivoting sports. The data were compared with those of 28 collegiate athletes (14 male, 14 female) participating in low injury–risk nonpivoting sports such as running, bicycling, and crew. Males generated a larger percentage increase in dynamic knee joint resistance to rotation at both 30° and 60° of knee flexion. Male athletes who participated in pivoting sports had a greater percentage increase (275% at 30° knee flexion) in dynamic knee joint resistance than the other three groups (159% females in pivoting sports, 191% control females, and 170% males in nonpivoting sports). Female athletes participating in pivoting sports had the lowest percentage increase in active knee joint resistance to rotation (see Table 18–5). These findings raised concerns about the current training and conditioning of female athletes in these high-risk sports. Because it was unlikely that these sports at the Division I level attracted a group of weaker female athletes, the current training routines may not be effective in producing muscle use patterns that resist undesirable rotational movements at the knee. Differences in muscle tendon unit stiffness can be attributed to muscle, tendon, or both. Most recent studies have focused on muscle. Interestingly, investigations using ultrasound have documented impressive gender differences in the gastrocnemius muscle[28] and patellar tendon.[31] More importantly, tendon viscoelastic performance has been linked to postural balance and may be the mechanism by which muscle-tendon stiffness plays a role in injury risk.[34]

In summary, multiple investigators have reported that male athletes have significantly greater active resistance to knee joint perturbations. Several physiologic explanations exist for these differences, including structural and mechanical factors in the tendon along with response and performance factors in muscle. Because these gender differences have been detected in several different studies using a variety of models for investigation, systemic factors such as hormones should be considered in the search for explanations of these differences.

Lower Extremity

Biomechanical factors and neuromuscular responses in the lower extremity both above and below the knee may influence knee injury susceptibility. Muscle use patterns while performing

---

TABLE 18–5   Gender and Athletic Differences in Muscle Stiffness at the Knee

Reference	Subject Age and Athletic Involvement	Testing Condition	Subjects* Males[†]	Females
Blackburn et al., 2004[7]	18- to 28-yr-old recreationally active	Knee flexion at 30°	221.7 (±40.7) Nm/rad	160.7 (±23.2) Nm/rad
Granata et al., 2002[15]	21- to 62-yr-old recreationally active	Hopping at 2.5 Hz Hopping at 3.0 Hz	31 (±8) kN/m 43 (±8) kN/m	24 (±5) kN/m 35 (±7) kN/m
Granata et al., 2002[16]	21- to 33-yr-old recreationally active	Quadriceps: 0-kg perturbation	97.6 (±31.1) Nm/rad	72.2 (±30.3)
		Quadriceps: 6-kg perturbation	262.2 (±78.3)	170.1 (±29.0)
		Quadriceps: 20% MVE perturbation	326.9 (±105.9)	182.5 (±43.2)
		Hamstrings: 0-kg perturbation	73.3 (±25.1)	53.6 (±16.2)
		Hamstrings: 6-kg perturbation	196.8 (±36.9)	130.5 (±22.2)
		Hamstrings: 20% MVE perturbation	159.1 (±51.0)	94.0 (±22.0)
Wojtys et al., 2002[47]	19- to 31-yr-old sedentary subjects to elite-level athletes	Knee flexion at 30° tibial translation	70.9 N/mm	40.7 N/mm
Wojtys et al., 2003[49]	Division I collegiate athletes	Knee flexion at 30° tibial rotation Knee flexion at 60° tibial rotation	218% (±22%) 231% (±21%)	178% (±9%) 185% (±12%)

*Data shown are mean ± standard deviation.
[†]Significantly greater than females.
MVE, maximum voluntary exertion.

dynamic athletic tasks, such as drop-landings, cutting, and, pivoting have been studied with mixed results in terms of gender.[22,25,26,36,42]

One viewpoint is that muscle strength often predicts activity characteristics and joint positioning in vivo. For example, landing from a jump with the knee joint near full extension may be the result of weak quadriceps muscles. Unfortunately, the increased percentage of ground reaction force transferred through the knee because of a more extended knee position may increase the likelihood of knee injury. Because noncontact jump-landings are one of the most frequent mechanisms of ACL injury in females, Huston and associates[26] assessed knee flexion angle in 20 healthy activity level–matched individuals (10 male, 10 female) during drop landings. Even though it is not a very challenging task, when starting from heights of 40 cm and 60 cm, females landed in more knee extension than their age- and size-matched male counterparts (Table 18–6).

Quatman and colleagues[36] examined landing forces of 33 adolescent basketball athletes (17 male, 16 female) during a drop-landing followed by a vertical jump looking for gender and maturation differences. At baseline testing, all athletes were Tanner stage 2 or 3. In the following year, all athletes were Tanner stage 4 or 5. Male athletes were more efficient at reducing ground reaction forces during landing as they matured (9.5% on the dominant side and 18.2% on the nondominant side). Unfortunately, female athletes did not demonstrate this favorable trend, producing higher ground reaction forces and higher loading rates than the mature male athletes (see Table 18–6). This lack of adaptation suggests a generalized phenomenon: males improve their neuromuscular efficiency more than females as they mature. Therefore, targeting these age groups of athletes in the high-risk sports for focused training and conditioning appears to be a worthwhile approach as the athlete approaches puberty.

In a more specific athletic task–related muscle strength test, 30 Division I or II soccer athletes (15 male, 15 female) were tested at a 35° and 55° cutting maneuver after a 5-m run.[42] After adjusting for body weight, male athletes produced a greater peak knee flexor moment during early deceleration than their female counterparts who demonstrated a greater average quadriceps activation than male athletes (191% and 151% maximum voluntary isometric contraction, respectively; see Table 18–6).

In summary, these studies demonstrate discrete gender differences in neuromuscular and activation response during simulated athletic tasks. Therefore, until better explanations are available, targeting these muscle activity patterns and performance deficits in athletic performance may be the most effective method of injury prevention.

Core

Core stability can be defined as the capacity of the lumbar-pelvic-hip muscle complex to control lower trunk movement and maintain stability of the vertebral column after skeletal perturbation.[45] Therefore, the core musculature may influence the kinematics and load-bearing capacity of the knee by determining what loads are transmitted from the torso.[17,19,29] Core stabilization potential and muscle endurance should not be overlooked in investigations of lower extremity injury potential.[17,19,29,52] Several clinical tests of core stability (e.g., isometric side-bridge) have been conducted to test these relationships.[14,31]

Leetun and coworkers[29] explored the relationship between core strength and the injury rate of 139 collegiate basketball and cross-country athletes (60 male, 79 female) during a competitive athletic season. During the season, 28 female and 13 male (41 of 139) athletes experienced back or lower extremity injuries. Injured athletes were weaker in hip abduction and hip external rotation strength (Table 18–7). Gender differences were seen in hip abduction, hip external rotation strength, and side-bridge

TABLE 18–6	Gender Differences during Athletic Tasks			
			Subjects*	
Reference	Subject Age and Athletic Involvement	Testing Condition	Males	Females
	Knee Angle at Impact			
Huston et al., 2001[26]	23- to 33-year-old recreational to competitive team sport athletes	Drop landing from 20 cm	8°	5.4°
		Drop landing from 40 cm	10°‡	5.4°
		Drop landing from 60 cm	16°‡	7°
	Maximum Ground Reaction Forces			
Quatman et al., 2006[36]†	Prepubescent (Tanner 2–3) basketball athletes	Two-footed drop landing from a 31-cm box	2.1 BW (±0.4 BW)	2.2 BW (±0.6 BW)
	Pubescent (Tanner 4–5) basketball athletes		1.9 BW (±0.5 BW)§	2.2 BW (±0.4 BW)
	Peak Knee Flexor Moments			
Sigward et al., 2006[42]	Division I and II collegiate soccer athletes	Side-step cutting at 35° and 55°	2.1 (±0.8) Nm/kg-BW‖	1.4 (±0.7) Nm/kg-BW

*Data shown are mean ± standard deviation.
†Only dominant limb reported.
‡Significantly greater knee angle than females at impact.
§Significantly reduced force from prepubescent age.
‖Significantly greater than female controls.
BW, body weight.

TABLE 18–7   Gender Differences in Core Strength

Reference	Subject Age and Athletic Involvement	Testing Condition	Subjects*	
			Males	**Females**
Leetun et al., 2004[29]	Collegiate cross-country and basketball athletes	Hip abduction	32.6 (±7.3) BW	29.2 (±6.1) BW
		Hip external rotation	21.6 (±4.3) BW[†]	18.4 (±4.1) BW
		Side bridge	84.3 (±32.5) sec[†]	58.9 (±26.0) sec
		Back extension	130.4 (±40.0) sec	123.4 (±48.4) sec
McGill et al., 1999[31]	20- to 26-yr-old recreationally active	Trunk extensor	146 (±51) sec	189 (±60) sec[‡]
		Trunk flexor	144 (±76) sec	149 (±99) sec
		Side bridge; left side	94 (±34) sec[†]	72 (±31) sec
		Side bridge; right side	97 (±35) sec[†]	77 (±35) sec
Evans et al., 2007[14]	19- to 23-yr-old elite-level athletes	Trunk extensor	157.4 (±42.9) sec	167.4 (±55.0) sec
		Trunk flexor	224.4 (±128.0) sec	222.0 (±86.1) sec
		Side bridge; left side	121.2 (±44.4) sec[†]	91.4 (±35.0) sec
		Side bridge; right side	126.6 (±44.9) sec[†]	91.1 (±38.0) sec

*Data shown are mean ± standard deviation.
[†]Significantly greater than female athletes.
[‡]Significantly greater than male athletes.
BW, body weight.

endurance (quadratus lumborum strength). Male athletes displayed greater core stability strength (see Table 18–7) similar to results for side-bridge endurance testing.[14,31] It is noteworthy that, of the 139 athletes in Leetun and coworkers' study,[29] only 1 athlete (a female) experienced a season ending ACL injury. This individual's core strength was significantly lower than the average female athlete.

Core muscle fatigue can affect lower extremity muscle performance. McGill and associates[31] compared isometric endurance values for low back stabilization in male and female athletes participating in soccer, rowing, and golf. Lateral endurance (side-bridge) was not sports-specific, but it was gender-related. Women produced better endurance times in the trunk extensor exercise than males (189 ± 60 sec and 146 ± 51 sec, respectively).[31] However, gender differences in trunk extensor exercises were not observed by Evans and colleagues[14] and Leetun and coworkers[29] (see Table 18–7).

Essential to core stability, the gluteus medius helps stabilize the hip and in turn supports the lumbopelvic complex. A weakness in the hip musculature can result in suboptimal positioning and loading of the lower extremity during athletic activity.[19,32] Gender differences in hip muscle activity were reported in 16 Division I soccer athletes (8 male, 8 female) during a single-legged forward take-off and landing task.[17] The gluteus medius muscle activity was almost three times higher in males than in females (electromyography root mean square: 7.16 ± 3.16 and 2.62 ± 0.95, respectively).

Understandably, hip positioning can affect lower limb alignment and limb muscle function, because femoral adduction and internal rotation can produce a misaligned lower extremity. Unfortunately, the full implications of these apparent muscle deficiencies and the associated limb positions during athletic tasks such as jump landing are not understood at present. However, the hypothesis is that limb malalignment is hazardous while landing from a jump or decelerating in a pivot-cut maneuver.

In summary, females appear to have decreased levels of core stability and hip muscle strength than their male counterparts. Core strengthening (rectus abdominis, quadratus lumborum, and lumbar extensors) can be achieved with curl-ups, side planks, and birddog exercises[45] (Figs. 18–2 to 18–4). Particular

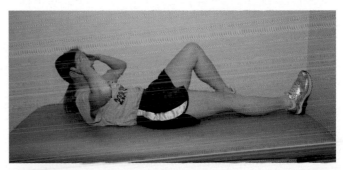

FIGURE 18–2. Demonstration of a curl-up, a core-strengthening exercise. Lying on the back, the shoulders are lifted off the ground, with this position held for 2 sec. To prevent undo strain to the neck, the hands are kept at the level of the forehead.

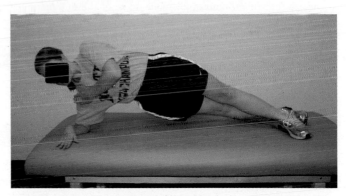

FIGURE 18–3. Demonstration of the side plank, a core-strengthening exercise. While the athlete lies on one side, the elbow, bent to 90°, is used for support. The free hand of the opposite shoulder is placed for additional support. The torso is kept straight as the buttocks are lifted off the ground.

attention to femoral abduction and external rotation strength appears to be justified because of their potential role in maintaining favorable lower extremity alignment during high-risk athletic tasks.

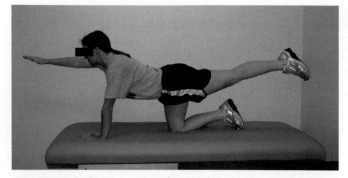

FIGURE 18–4. Demonstration of the birddog, a core-strengthening exercise. The athlete is positioned on all fours, with knees under hips and hands under the shoulders. The buttocks and abdominals are squeezed. Then, the athlete reaches forward with one arm and reaches back with the opposite leg. This position is held for 5 sec, then the alternate side is exercised.

TRAINING PROGRAMS

Neuromuscular training may be the most efficient route to knee injury prevention.[3,18,23,50] Intrinsic factors including neuromuscular balance and dynamic joint laxity appear to be modifiable with appropriate training.[19,23,27]

Hewett and coworkers[22] developed a jump-training neuromuscular program for female athletes to address perceived deficits in lower extremity strength and poor body positioning during landing (see Chapter 19, Decreasing the Risk of Anterior Cruciate Ligament Injuries in Female Athletes). Eleven female high school volleyball athletes underwent 2-hour training sessions 3 days a week for 6 weeks. Upon completion of training, 10 of the 11 female athletes decreased their peak landing forces by 22%. The peak landing forces before and after training were lower than those of the untrained male athletes (Table 18–8). With training, peak hamstring torque increased 13% in the dominant leg and 26% in the nondominant leg in female athletes (see Table 18–8). Consequently, the H:Q ratio improved to nearly that of the untrained male: 13% in the dominant leg and 26% in the nondominant leg.

Knee muscle resistance to translational movements that generate tibial femoral shear can be examined by determining tibial control characteristics. An analysis of muscle activation patterns in response to an anterior tibial translation in the elite female athletes with excellent quadriceps and hamstring peak torques[27]

Critical Points TRAINING PROGRAMS

- Intrinsic factors (neuromuscular balance and dynamic joint laxity) appear to be modifiable with appropriate training.
- Progress in the development of injury prevention programs has been hindered by our limited understanding of the mechanisms of injury, especially with the ACL.

showed that the females favored the initial activation of their hamstrings. Interestingly, the 5 weakest female athletes activated their quadriceps initially in response to the same stimulus. This quadriceps dominance may be a risk factor for ACL injury because the quadriceps is an ACL antagonist. These worrisome findings appear to justify balanced lower extremity muscle conditioning, especially in injured athletes.

A perturbation-enhanced training program that incorporated strength training and agility drills was able to normalize quadriceps-hamstring balance in female collegiate athletes who presented with the "quadriceps dominant" activation pattern.[24] After training, both medial and lateral hamstrings were activated earlier (Fig. 18–5). Most importantly, after 10 1-hour sessions in the perturbation-enhanced training program, female athletes increased their active knee muscle stiffness across the knee (see Fig. 18–5). Theoretically, these results may explain the positive trends seen in some injury prevention programs and they help reduce the risk of injury to the knee.[24] Unfortunately, males did not display significant changes with training.

In an effort to determine which type of training might be most beneficial to athletes at risk, Wojtys and associates[50] tested the effects of isotonic, isokinetic, and agility exercise regimens on the ability to resist anterior tibial translation, muscle reaction time, and time to peak muscle torque. Thirty-two healthy active volunteers trained for 30 minutes, 3 times a week for 6 weeks. After normalizing strength values with respect to body weight, the isokinetic group was stronger in knee extension and ankle plantar flexion peak torques after training. The isokinetic protocol was the only training regimen that decreased the time to peak torque in the quadriceps, hamstrings, and gastrocnemius muscles (Fig. 18–6). Surprisingly, the muscle reaction times for the isokinetic-training groups were significantly slower in the medial hamstrings (39.1 msec) and medial quadriceps (32.4 msec) muscles (Table 18–9). The isotonic and agility groups predictably showed no increase in isokinetic strength after completing the training regimen (see Table 18–9). The

TABLE 18–8	**Effects of a Jump-Training Neuromuscular Program**			
		Subjects*		
Quantitative Measurement	**Testing Condition**	**Untrained Females**	**Trained Females**	**Untrained Males**
Peak landing forces		2538 (±525) N[†]	2082 (±333) N[†]	3702 (±800)
Peak hamstring torque	Dominant leg	41 (±7) Nm	46 (±7) Nm	61 (±13) Nm
	Nondominant leg	37 (±7) Nm	46 (±8) Nm[‡]	66 (±16) Nm
H:Q ratio	Dominant leg	55 (±9)	62 (±7)[‡]	62 (±8)
	Nondominant leg	47 (±8)	59 (±9)[‡]	67 (±7)

*Data shown are mean ± standard deviation.
[†]Significantly lower than untrained male athletes.
[‡]Significantly greater than untrained females.
H:Q ratio, hamstrings-to-quadriceps peak torque ratio.
Adapted from Hewett, T. E.; Stroupe, A. L.; Nance, T. A.; et al.: Plyometric training in female athletes. Decreased impact forces and increased hamstring torques. *Am J Sports Med* 24:765–773, 1996.

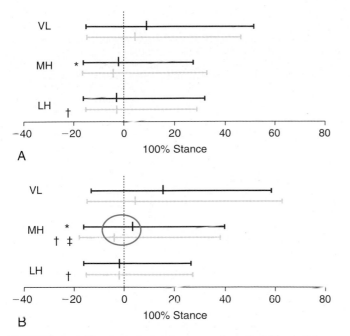

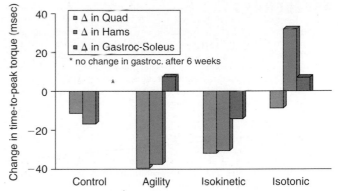

FIGURE 18-6. The average change in time to peak muscle torque in the quadriceps, hamstrings, and gastrocnemius muscles between 0 and 6 wk. *(Redrawn from Wojtys, E. M.; Huston, L. J.; Taylor, P. D.; et al.: Neuromuscular adaptations in isokinetic, isotonic, and agility training programs. Am J Sports Med 24:187–192, 1996. Reprinted with permission of SAGE Publications, Inc.)*

FIGURE 18-5. Muscle timing of the vastus lateralis (VL), medial hamstrings (MH), and lateral hamstrings (LH) for males (**A**) and females (**B**). *Red lines* represent values before training; *orange bars* represent values after training. The *left side of the bar* is onset of muscle activity, the *right side of the bar* indicates when the muscle turned off. The *vertical dashed line* represents heel-strike; the *small vertical lines* represent the time of the peak muscle activity. Significant difference between groups at *P* < .1 before training is denoted with an *asterisk*, after training between groups with a *dagger*, and within groups after training with a *double dagger*. (**A** and **B**, *Reprinted with permission from Springer Science + Business Media: Hurd, W. J.; Chmielewski, T. L.; Snyder-Mackler, L.: Perturbation-enhanced neuromuscular training alters muscle activity in female athletes. Knee Surg Sports Traumatol Arthrosc 14:60–69, 2006.)*

agility-training group generated the greatest decrease (38 msec) in time to peak hamstring torque among the groups. The muscle reaction time of the agility-trained group displayed significant improvements at all levels of function: spinal cord, intermediate, and voluntary response.

To summarize, gender differences exist in neuromuscular factors such as proprioception, muscle activation, and coordination. Also apparent are differences in athletic task performance and techniques. Whereas a relationship between these neuromuscular factors and performance characteristics is expected, their effect on injury risk remains unclear, in part because the mechanism of injury is still not understood, especially for the ACL. This lack of mechanistic understanding hinders attempts at risk factor surveillance and injury prevention program development.

ACKNOWLEDGMENTS

The authors would like to thank Kristi Overgaard of the University of Michigan, Department of Orthopaedics, for her advice, editing expertise, and dedication to this chapter.

TABLE 18-9   Effects on Muscle Strength and Response Times after 6 Weeks of Training

Quantitative Measurement	Testing Condition	Training Groups			
		Controls	Agility	Isokinetic	Isotonic
Peak torques*	Knee Extension	−2.20%	−0.70%	7.2%‡	−0.30%
	Knee Flexion	−0.60%	0.90%	−0.30%	1.50%
	Ankle Plantar Flexion	−1.90%	2.30%	18.9%‡	3.80%
Voluntary response†	Gastrocnemius	11.8	−15.7‡	15.1	5.1
	Lateral Hamstring	−4.1	−20	21.7	0.5
	Medial Hamstring	−4.5	−34.4‡	39.1§	2.5
	Lateral Quadriceps	0.8	−27.9‡	0.4	8.3
	Medial Quadriceps	5.7	−9.7	32.4§	10.9

*Data equals percentage of strength: peak torque (ft-lb) divided by body weight (lb).
†Average change in muscle reaction time (milliseconds).
‡Significantly greater than control group.
§Significantly less than control group.
Adapted from Wojtys, E. M.; Huston, L. J.; Taylor, P. D.; et al.: Neuromuscular adaptations in isokinetic, isotonic, and agility training programs. *Am J Sports Med* 24:187–192, 1996.

REFERENCES

1. Ahmad, C. S.; Clark, A. M.; Heilmann, N.; et al.: Effect of gender and maturity on quadriceps-to-hamstring strength ratio and anterior cruciate ligament laxity. *Am J Sports Med* 34:370–374, 2006.
2. Anderson, A. F.; Dome, D. C.; Gautam, S.; et al.: Correlation of anthropometric measurements, strength, anterior cruciate ligament size, and intercondylar notch characteristics to sex differences in anterior cruciate ligament tear rates. *Am J Sports Med* 29:58–66, 2001.
3. Baratta, R.; Solomonow, M.; Zhou, B. H.; et al.: Muscular coactivation. The role of the antagonist musculature in maintaining knee stability. *Am J Sports Med* 16:113–122, 1988.
4. Barber-Westin, S. D.; Galloway, M.; Noyes, F. R.; et al.: Assessment of lower limb neuromuscular control in prepubescent athletes. *Am J Sports Med* 33:1853–1860, 2005.
5. Barber-Westin, S. D.; Noyes, F. R.; Galloway, M.: Jump-land characteristics and muscle strength development in young athletes: a gender comparison of 1140 athletes 9 to 17 years of age. *Am J Sports Med* 34:375–384, 2006.
6. Barrett, D. S.: Proprioception and function after anterior cruciate reconstruction. *J Bone Joint Surg Br* 73:833–837, 1991.
7. Blackburn, J. T.; Riemann, B. L.; Padua, D. A.; et al.: Sex comparison of extensibility, passive, and active stiffness of the knee flexors. *Clin Biomech (Bristol, Avon)* 19:36–43, 2004.
8. Bowerman, S. J.; Smith, D. R.; Carlson, M.; King, G. A.: A comparison of factors influencing ACL injury in male and female athletes and non-athletes. *Phys Ther Sport* 7:144–152, 2006.
9. Buchanan, P. A.; Vardaxis, V. G.: Sex-related and age-related differences in knee strength of basketball players ages 11–17 years. *J Athl Train* 38:231–237, 2003.
10. Carcia, C. R.; Shultz, S. J.; Granata, K. P.; et al.: Females recruit quadriceps faster than males at multiple knee flexion angles following a weight-bearing rotary perturbation. *Clin J Sport Med* 15:167–171, 2005.
11. Corrigan, J. P.; Cashman, W. F.; Brady, M. P.: Proprioception in the cruciate deficient knee. *J Bone Joint Surg Br* 74:247–250, 1992.
12. Cowling, E. J.; Steele, J. R.: Is lower limb muscle synchrony during landing affected by gender? Implications for variations in ACL injury rates. *J Electromyogr Kinesiol* 11:263–268, 2001.
13. Dugan, S. A.: Sports-related knee injuries in female athletes: what gives? *Am J Phys Med Rehabil* 84:122–130, 2005.
14. Evans, K.; Refshauge, K. M.; Adams, R.: Trunk muscle endurance tests: reliability and gender differences in athletes. *J Sci Med Sport* 10:447–455, 2007.
15. Granata, K. P.; Padua, D. A.; Wilson, S. E.: Gender differences in active musculoskeletal stiffness. Part II. Quantification of leg stiffness during functional hopping tasks. *J Electromyogr Kinesiol* 12:127–135, 2002.
16. Granata, K. P.; Wilson, S. E.; Padua, D. A.: Gender differences in active musculoskeletal stiffness. Part I. Quantification in controlled measurements of knee joint dynamics. *J Electromyogr Kinesiol* 12:119–126, 2002.
17. Hart, J. M.; Garrison, J. C.; Kerrigan, D. C.; et al.: Gender differences in gluteus medius muscle activity exist in soccer players performing a forward jump. *Res Sports Med* 15:147–155, 2007.
18. Hewett, T. E.; Lindenfeld, T. N.; Riccobene, J. V.; et al.: The effect of neuromuscular training on the incidence of knee injury in female athletes. A prospective study. *Am J Sports Med* 27:699–706, 1999.
19. Hewett, T. E.; Myer, G. D.; Ford, K. R.: Anterior cruciate ligament injuries in female athletes: part 1, mechanisms and risk factors. *Am J Sports Med* 34:299–311, 2006.
20. Hewett, T. E.; Paterno, M. V.; Myer, G. D.: Strategies for enhancing proprioception and neuromuscular control of the knee. *Clin Orthop Relat Res* 402:76–94, 2002.
21. Hewett, T. E.; Paterno, M. V.; Noyes, F. R.: Differences in single leg balance on an unstable platform between female and male normal, ACL-deficient and ACL-reconstructed knees. Paper presented at the 25th Annual Meeting of the American Orthopaedic Society for Sports Medicine, June 19–22, 1999, Traverse City, MI.
22. Hewett, T. E.; Stroupe, A. L.; Nance, T. A.; et al.: Plyometric training in female athletes. Decreased impact forces and increased hamstring torques. *Am J Sports Med* 24:765–773, 1996.
23. Hewett, T. E.; Zazulak, B. T.; Myer, G. D.; et al.: A review of electromyographic activation levels, timing differences, and increased anterior cruciate ligament injury incidence in female athletes. *Br J Sports Med* 39:347–350, 2005.
24. Hurd, W. J.; Chmielewski, T. L.; Snyder-Mackler, L.: Perturbation-enhanced neuromuscular training alters muscle activity in female athletes. *Knee Surg Sports Traumatol Arthrosc* 14:60–69, 2006.
25. Huston, L. J.; Greenfield, M. L.; Wojtys, E. M.: Anterior cruciate ligament injuries in the female athlete. Potential risk factors. *Clin Orthop Relat Res* 372:50–63, 2000.
26. Huston, L. J.; Vibert, B.; Ashton-Miller, J. A.; et al.: Gender differences in knee angle when landing from a drop-jump. *Am J Knee Surg* 14:215–219; discussion 219–220, 2001.
27. Huston, L. J.; Wojtys, E. M.: Neuromuscular performance characteristics in elite female athletes. *Am J Sports Med* 24:427–436, 1996.
28. Kubo, K.; Kanehisa, H.; Azuma, K.; et al.: Muscle architectural characteristics in young and elderly men and women. *Int J Sports Med* 24:125–130, 2003.
29. Leetun, D. T.; Ireland, M. L.; Willson, J. D.; et al.: Core stability measures as risk factors for lower extremity injury in athletes. *Med Sci Sports Exerc* 36:926–934, 2004.
30. Lephart, S. M.; Ferris, C. M.; Riemann, B. L.; et al.: Gender differences in strength and lower extremity kinematics during landing. *Clin Orthop Relat Res* 401:162–169, 2002.
31. McGill, S. M.; Childs, A.; Liebenson, C.: Endurance times for low back stabilization exercises: clinical targets for testing and training from a normal database. *Arch Phys Med Rehabil* 80:941–944, 1999.
32. Nadler, S. F.; Malanga, G. A.; DePrince, M.; et al.: The relationship between lower extremity injury, low back pain, and hip muscle strength in male and female collegiate athletes. *Clin J Sport Med* 10:89–97, 2000.
33. Noyes, F. R.; Barber-Westin, S. D.: Isokinetic profile and differences in tibial rotation strength between male and female athletes 11 to 17 years of age. *Isok Exer Sci* 13:251–259, 2005.
34. Onambele, G. N.; Burgess, K.; Pearson, S. J.: Gender-specific in vivo measurement of the structural and mechanical properties of the human patellar tendon. *J Orthop Res* 25:1635–1642, 2007.
35. Pincivero, D. M.; Gandaio, C. M.; Ito, Y.: Gender-specific knee extensor torque, flexor torque, and muscle fatigue responses during maximal effort contractions. *Eur J Appl Physiol* 89:134–141, 2003.
36. Quatman, C. E.; Ford, K. R.; Myer, G. D.; et al.: Maturation leads to gender differences in landing force and vertical jump performance: a longitudinal study. *Am J Sports Med* 34:806–813, 2006.
37. Ramos, E.; Frontera, W. R.; Llopart, A.; et al.: Muscle strength and hormonal levels in adolescents: gender-related differences. *Int J Sports Med* 19:526–531, 1998.
38. Rosene, J. M.; Fogarty, T. D.; Mahaffey, B. L.: Isokinetic hamstrings:quadriceps ratios in intercollegiate athletes. *J Athl Train* 36:378–383, 2001.
39. Rozzi, S. L.; Lephart, S. M.; Fu, F. H.: Effects of muscular fatigue on knee joint laxity and neuromuscular characteristics of male and female athletes. *J Athl Train* 34:106–114, 1999.
40. Rozzi, S. L.; Lephart, S. M.; Gear, W. S.; et al.: Knee joint laxity and neuromuscular characteristics of male and female soccer and basketball players. *Am J Sports Med* 27:312–319, 1999.
41. Shultz, S. J.; Perrin, D. H.; Adams, M. J.; et al.: Neuromuscular response characteristics in men and women after knee perturbation in a single-leg, weight-bearing stance. *J Athl Train* 36:37–43, 2001.
42. Sigward, S. M.; Powers, C. M.: The influence of gender on knee kinematics, kinetics and muscle activation patterns during side-step cutting. *Clin Biomech (Bristol, Avon)* 21:41–48, 2006.
43. Uhorchak, J. M.; Scoville, C. R.; Williams, G. N.; et al.: Risk factors associated with noncontact injury of the anterior cruciate ligament: a prospective four-year evaluation of 859 West Point cadets. *Am J Sports Med* 31:831–842, 2003.
44. White, K. K.; Lee, S. S.; Cutuk, A.; et al.: EMG power spectra of intercollegiate athletes and anterior cruciate ligament injury risk in females. *Med Sci Sports Exerc* 35:371–376, 2003.
45. Willson, J. D.; Dougherty, C. P.; Ireland, M. L.; et al.: Core stability and its relationship to lower extremity function and injury. *J Am Acad Orthop Surg* 13:316–325, 2005.
46. Withrow, T. J.; Huston, L. J.; Wojtys, E. M.; et al.: The relationship between quadriceps muscle force, knee flexion, and anterior cruciate ligament strain in an in vitro simulated jump landing. *Am J Sports Med* 34:269–274, 2006.

47. Wojtys, E. M.; Ashton-Miller, J. A.; Huston, L. J.: A gender-related difference in the contribution of the knee musculature to sagittal-plane shear stiffness in subjects with similar knee laxity. *J Bone Joint Surg Am* 84:10–16, 2002.
48. Wojtys, E. M.; Huston, L. J.: Neuromuscular performance in normal and anterior cruciate ligament–deficient lower extremities. *Am J Sports Med* 22:89–104, 1994.
49. Wojtys, E. M.; Huston, L. J.; Schock, H. J.; et al.: Gender differences in muscular protection of the knee in torsion in size-matched athletes. *J Bone Joint Surg Am* 85:782–789, 2003.
50. Wojtys, E. M.; Huston, L. J.; Taylor, P. D.; et al.: Neuromuscular adaptations in isokinetic, isotonic, and agility training programs. *Am J Sports Med* 24:187–192, 1996.
51. Wojtys, E. M.; Wylie, B. B.; Huston, L. J.: The effects of muscle fatigue on neuromuscular function and anterior tibial translation in healthy knees. *Am J Sports Med* 24:615–621, 1996.
52. Zazulak, B. T.; Hewett, T. E.; Reeves, N. P.; et al.: Deficits in neuromuscular control of the trunk predict knee injury risk: a prospective biomechanical-epidemiologic study. *Am J Sports Med* 35:1123–1130, 2007.
53. Zazulak, B. T.; Hewett, T. E.; Reeves, N. P.; et al. The effects of core proprioception on knee injury: a prospective biomechanical-epidemiological study. *Am J Sports Med* 35:368–373, 2007.

Chapter 19

Decreasing the Risk of Anterior Cruciate Ligament Injuries in Female Athletes

Sue D. Barber-Westin, BS ∎ *Frank R. Noyes*, MD

SCIENTIFIC RATIONALE AND SUPPORTING INVESTIGATIONS FOR SPORTSMETRICS NEUROMUSCULAR RETRAINING PROGRAM

The purpose of this chapter is to present the scientific rationale, supporting data, and specific strategies for the implementation of a neuromuscular knee ligament injury prevention–training program, Sportsmetrics. Although many knee ligament injury prevention–training programs have been published,* few have presented scientific justification that the training effectively improved neuromuscular deficiencies and reduced the incidence of noncontact anterior cruciate ligament (ACL) injuries in female athletes (Table 19–1). Some programs had small sample sizes and were thus underpowered to avoid the potential for a type II statistical error.[7,11,28,29,33,35] Most studies were not randomized, and several did not contain a control group studied concurrently with a trained group. Although some investigations cited a reduction in noncontact ACL injury rates, others failed to find a statistically significant effect.[11,28,29,33–35] Some programs have been published even though the investigators did not follow athletes over a season or a period of time to determine whether a reduction in ACL injuries occurred as a result of preventive training.[14,16,21]

The Sportsmetrics program is effective in inducing changes in neuromuscular indices in female athletes, because studies have shown improved overall lower limb alignment on a drop-jump test,[24] increased hamstrings strength,[13,24,36] increased knee flexion angles on landing,[13,31] and reduced deleterious abduction/adduction moments and ground reaction forces.[13] Sportsmetrics also significantly reduces the risk of noncontact ACL injuries in female athletes participating in basketball, soccer, and volleyball.[12]

A pilot laboratory study was conducted at the authors' institution using 11 high school female volleyball players to determine the effect of Sportsmetrics training on landing mechanics and lower extremity strength.[13] The mean age of the female subjects was 15 ± 0.6 years, and they had participated in organized volleyball for an average of 2 ± 1 years before the study was initiated. A control group of 9 male subjects was selected and matched to the females according to height, weight, and age. The Sportsmetrics training program, described in detail later in this chapter, was performed 3 times a week (2-hr sessions) for 6 weeks. The athletes were taken through a series of tests before and after the training program. These tests included isokinetic muscle testing at 360°/sec and force analysis testing with a two-camera, video-based, optoelectronic digitizer for

---

*See references 2, 6, 11, 14, 16, 19, 22, 27–29, 33, 35.

TABLE 19-1 Anterior Cruciate Ligament Injury Prevention Training Programs

Reference	Number of Athletes, Type of Sports, Number of Seasons in Study	Duration of Training	Plyometrics	Strength	Agility	Balance	Flexibility	Total Number of Exposures	Number of ACL Injuries	Study Limitations
Ettlinger et al., 1995[6]	4000 trained patrollers and instructors, gender unknown 22 "ski areas" control, number not given, gender unknown Alpine skiers 3 ski seasons	1 hr reviewing video clips of injuries, awareness-training sessions, small group discussions; prevention strategies	No	No	No	No	No	Not given	179, 62% decline in serious knee ligament injuries among trained patrollers and instructors No decline in control group.	Not randomized, no exposure data, no medical documentation of ACL injuries "Any mention of a grade II or III ACL sprain or grade III knee sprain included," unknown which knee ligaments torn, unknown number of contact vs. noncontact
Caraffa et al., 1996[2]	300 trained males 300 control males Soccer players 3 seasons	20 min every day x 30 consecutive day preseason	No	No	No	Yes	Yes	Not given	10 in trained group, 70 in control group	Not randomized, no exposure data, unknown number of training sessions completed
Heidt et al., 2000[11]	42 trained females 258 control females Soccer players, high school 1 season	3 sessions/wk for 7 wk	Yes	Yes	Yes	No	Yes	Not given	1 in trained group, 8 in control group	Not randomized, no exposure data, no statistically significant difference ACL injury rates trained vs. control group
Soderman et al., 2000[33]	62 trained females 78 control females Soccer players, mean age 20 yr 1 season	10–15 min every day x 30 consecutive day preseason, then 3 x/wk in season	No	No	No	Yes	No	Not given for ACL injuries	4 in trained group, 1 in control group	No exposure data for ACL injuries, trained at home not controlled, variability in amount of training completed, no statistically significant difference ACL injury rates trained vs. control group

Continued

TABLE 19–1 Anterior Cruciate Ligament Injury Prevention Training Programs—Cont'd

Reference	Number of Athletes, Type of Sports, Number of Seasons in Study	Duration of Training	Plyometrics	Strength	Agility	Balance	Flexibility	Total Number of Exposures	Number of ACL Injuries	Study Limitations
Myklebust, 2003[22]	263 trained females 1587 control females Team handball, 3 top divisions Norwegian Handball Federation 3 seasons (1 control, 2 intervention)	15 min, 3 x/wk for 5–7 wk	Landing technique	No	Planting, cutting, jumping control, awareness	Yes, on mats and boards	Yes	568,433 hr	All divisions: 29 control season (1.48), 23 first intervention season (1.14), 17 second intervention season (1.09) No difference. Significant reduction ACL injury elite division only.	Not randomized, poor team compliance with training, combined contact and noncontact ACL injuries in elite division statistics, elite division bias — better compliance training
Olsen et al., 2005[27]	808 trained females 778 control females 150 trained males 101 control males Team handball, high school 1 season	15–20 min, average 27 sessions	Landing technique	Yes	Planting, cutting, jumping control, awareness	Yes, on mats and boards	Yes	93,812 trained 87,483 control	Not given	ACL ruptures not sorted per group, all knee ligament injuries combined
Petersen et al., 2005[28]	134 trained females 142 control females Team handball, several divisions, adult players 1 season	10 min, 3 x/wk for 8 wk	Yes	No	Planting, cutting, jumping control, awareness	Yes	No	Not given	1 in trained group (0.04), 5 in control group (0.21)	Not randomized, no statistically significant difference ACL injury rates trained vs. control group
Mandelbaum et al., 2005[19]	1885 trained females 3818 control females Soccer, 14–18 yr of age 2 yr	20 min, replaced traditional warm-up	Yes	Yes	Yes	No	Yes	67,860 trained 137,447 control	6 in trained group (0.09), 67 in untrained group (0.49), $P < .0001$	Not randomized, voluntary enrollment training, unknown number of training sessions completed
Pfeiffer et al., 2006[29]	577 trained females 862 control females Soccer, basketball, volleyball High school athletes 1 season	20 min, 2 x/wk throughout season	Yes	No	Landing technique control and awareness	No	No	17,954 trained 38,662 control	3 in trained group (0.167) 3 in control group (0.078)	Not randomized, no statistically significant difference ACL injury rates trained vs. control group

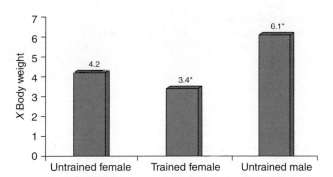

FIGURE 19–1. Bar graph shows decrease in peak landing forces with training in female subjects before and after training and relative to age- and weight-matched athletic male subjects. *P < .01. *(From Hewett, T. E.; Stroupe, A. L.; Nance, T. A.; Noyes, F. R.: Plyometric training in female athletes. Decreased impact forces and increased hamstring torques. Am J Sports Med 24:765–773, 1996.)*

measuring motion and a multicomponent force plate for measuring ground reaction force. The subjects performed 10 jumps on the force plate that simulated volleyball jumping and landing maneuvers.

After 6 weeks of training, peak landing forces from a volleyball block jump decreased 22% (P = .006), or an average of 456N (103lb); all but 1 of the female subjects demonstrated a decrease in these forces (Fig. 19–1). Knee adduction and abduction moments, which induce a lateral or medial torque to the knee joint, decreased approximately 50% (Fig. 19–2). These moments were significant predictors of peak landing forces. The importance of this finding is that decreased abduction or abduction moments may lessen the risk of lift-off of the medial or lateral femoral condyle, improve tibiofemoral contact stabilizing forces,[20] and reduce the risk of knee ligament injury.

Female athletes demonstrated lower landing forces than male athletes, and lower adduction and abduction moments after training compared with pretraining values. External knee extension moments (which are balanced by an internal flexion,

hamstring muscle) of male athletes were three times higher than those of female athletes. The training did not significantly alter these extension moments.

After training, hamstring-to-quadriceps muscle peak torque ratios increased 26% on the nondominant side and 13% on the dominant side, correcting side-to-side imbalances in the female athletes. In addition, hamstring muscle power increased 44% on the dominant side and 21% on the nondominant side. Whereas peak torque ratios of male athletes were significantly greater than those of the female athletes before training, the ratios were similar between genders after training.

A second study was conducted in a group of 62 high school female athletes to determine whether Sportsmetrics training altered lower limb alignment on a drop-jump task and isokinetic lower limb muscle strength.[24] This investigation is described in detail in Chapter 16, Lower Limb Neuromuscular Control and Strength in Prepubescent and Adolescent Male and Female Athletes. Before training, 80% of the female athletes had a valgus overall lower limb alignment on landing from a drop-jump. After training, 34% of the females demonstrated this alignment (P < .0001). Significant increases were also noted after training in knee flexion peak torque in both the dominant and the nondominant limbs (P < .0001).

In order to determine whether Sportsmetrics training reduced the incidence of noncontact ACL injuries in female athletes, a controlled, prospective investigation was conducted in 1263 high school athletes.[12] One group of 366 females underwent 6 weeks of Sportsmetrics training and a second group of 463 females was not trained. Included in the study was a group of 434 untrained male athletes. All athletes were followed throughout a single soccer, volleyball, or basketball season. Weekly reports submitted by athletic trainers included the number of practice and competition exposures and mechanism of injury. All ACL injuries were confirmed by arthroscopy, and medial collateral ligament (MCL) injuries were confirmed by manual valgus testing.

The total number of athlete-exposures were 23,138 for the untrained group, 17,222 for the trained group, and 21,390 for the male control group. There were 14 serious knee ligament injuries, which were sustained in 10 of 463 untrained female athletes (8 noncontact), 2 of 366 trained female athletes (0 noncontact), and 2 of 434 male athletes (1 noncontact). The knee injury incidence per 1000 athlete-exposures was 0.43 in untrained female athletes, 0.12 in trained female athletes, and 0.09 in male athletes (P = .02, chi-square analysis). Untrained female athletes had a 3.6 times higher incidence of knee injury than trained female athletes (P = .05) and 4.8 times higher than male athletes (P = .03). The incidence of knee injury in trained female athletes was not significantly different from that in untrained male athletes (Fig. 19–3; P = .86).

The risk factors that have been hypothesized to increase the potential for an ACL injury are discussed in Chapter 15, Risk Factors for Anterior Cruciate Ligament Injuries in the Female Athlete. The final position of the knee joint on landing, pivoting, and cutting is influenced by the center of gravity of the upper body and the trunk over the lower extremity. Equally important are trunk-hip adduction or abduction, foot-ankle pronation-supination, and foot separation distance. These effects add together to produce either a varus or a valgus moment about the knee joint that must be balanced by the lower limb musculature. If the athlete is off-balance, or contacts another player, a loss of trunk and lower limb control and position may occur

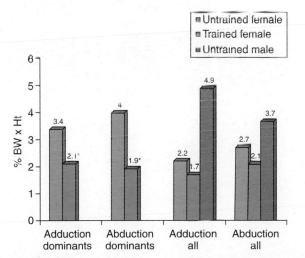

FIGURE 19–2. Bar graph shows peak knee adduction and abduction moment data at landing before and after training. The female subjects were grouped according to the dominant moment (adduction or abduction) and all the female subjects grouped together (all). *P < .05 compared with untrained females. *(From Hewett, T. E.; Stroupe, A. L.; Nance, T. A.; Noyes, F. R.: Plyometric training in female athletes. Decreased impact forces and increased hamstring torques. Am J Sports Med 24:765–773, 1996.)*

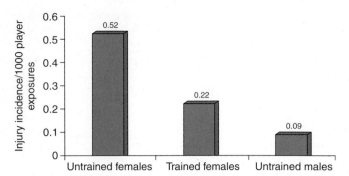

FIGURE 19–3. Serious knee injuries per 1000 player-exposures in soccer and basketball players. *(From Hewett, T. E.; Stroupe, A. L.; Nance, T. A.; Noyes, F. R.: Plyometric training in female athletes. Decreased impact forces and increased hamstring torques. Am J Sports Med 24:765–773, 1996.)*

and the knee joint may go into a hyperextended or valgus position. Although there are many potential mechanisms for ACL injury, it has been postulated that excessive valgus moments about the knee joint with subsequent high anterior tibial shear forces may be one of the most common to occur in females.[8,15,18] Excessive valgus loading may result in decreased tibiofemoral contact, or condylar lift-off,[20] and a reduction in the normal joint contact geometry that contributes to knee joint stability. This position, coupled with a highly activated quadriceps muscle that produces maximum anterior shear forces with the knee joint at low flexion angles (0°–30°),[5,10,26] and a relatively inactive hamstrings musculature, could potentially lead to ACL rupture. The function of the hamstrings is dependent on the angle of knee flexion and degrees of external tibial rotation.[25] The mechanical advantage of these muscles increases as the knee is flexed. At 0° of extension, the flexion force is only 49% of that generated at 90° of flexion. Withrow and coworkers[37] measured the relative strain in the anteromedial region of the ACL in cadaver knees during a simulated jump landing

maneuver. Increased hamstring muscle forces during the knee flexion phase significantly reduced the peak relative strain in the ACL by greater than 70% compared with the baseline condition ($P = .005$). The authors concluded that it may be possible to limit ACL strain by accentuating hip flexion during knee flexion phase of jump landings because this increases the tension in the active hamstring muscles.

The time in which an ACL rupture occurs was recently estimated to range from 17 to 50 msec after initial ground contact.[17] It is evident that there is not enough time for an athlete, upon sensing a knee injury about to occur, to alter the body or lower extremity position to prevent the injury. In order to have a significant impact on reducing the incident rate of this injury, a training program must teach athletes to control the upper body, trunk, and lower body position; lower the center of gravity by increasing hip and knee flexion during activities; and develop muscular strength and techniques to land with decreased ground reaction forces. In addition, athletes should be taught to pre-position the body and lower extremity prior to initial ground contact in order to obtain the position of greatest knee joint stability and stiffness. The program should consist of a dynamic warm-up, plyometric jump training, strengthening exercises, aerobic conditioning, agility, and risk awareness training.[9]

SPORTS INJURY TEST

The authors developed a sports injury test (SIT) in order to obtain a profile of each athlete before and after Sportsmetrics training. The SIT measures (1) knee and ankle position on landing and take-off from a drop-jump during a video test (described in detail in Chapter 16, Lower Limb Neuromuscular Control and Strength in Prepubescent and Adolescent Male and Female Athletes), (2) lower limb symmetry[1,23] and a general assessment of lower limb control on single-leg hop tasks (Fig. 19–4), (3) isokinetic lower extremity muscle strength, (4) hamstring flexibility, and (5) vertical jump height. Athletes participating in sports-specific Sportsmetrics training

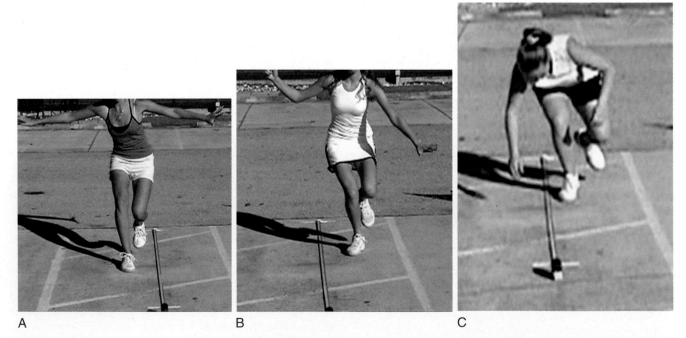

FIGURE 19–4. Single hop for distance video screening allows a qualitative assessment of an athlete's ability to control the upper and lower extremities upon landing, which may be rated as either good (**A**), fair (**B**), or complete failure, fall to ground (**C**).

programs, discussed later in this chapter, also undergo a 10-yard dash, a 20-yard dash, a T-drill run, and a 1-mile run. A history is collected for each athlete regarding prior injuries to the knees and ankles. The SIT is completed just prior to the initiation of training and within 1 week of completion of training.

SPORTSMETRICS NEUROMUSCULAR TRAINING PROGRAM COMPONENTS

The essential elements of the Sportsmetrics neuromuscular training program are a dynamic warm-up, plyometric jump training, strengthening, and flexibility. It is recommended that this training program be conducted either during the off-season or just prior to the beginning of the athlete's sport season. The training is conducted 3 times a week on alternating days for 6 weeks.

As is described later, sports-specific speed and agility components may be incorporated into the training program if desired by an athlete or team. Sports-specific programs have been developed for soccer (Sportsmetrics Soccer), basketball (Sportsmetrics Basketball), and tennis (Sportsmetrics Tennis) players. A maintenance-training program (Sportsmetrics Warm-up for Injury Prevention and Performance [WIPP]) may be performed upon completion of the 6 weeks of formal Sportsmetrics to continue to instill the skills and techniques learned during the athlete's sports season. For athletes who have already suffered an injury or had ACL reconstruction, Sportsmetrics Return to Play is recommended as end-stage rehabilitation training.

Training may be accomplished either in classes led by an instructor who has completed certification training from the authors' foundation or from an instructional step-by-step videotape series. Athletes who do not train with a certified instructor are encouraged to perform the training either in front of a mirror or with a partner so that mistakes in technique, form, and body alignment may be detected and corrected. A list of certified instructors and sites is available at http://www.sportsmetrics.net.

Dynamic Warm-up

The purpose of the dynamic warm-up is to prepare the body for activity with functional-based activities that incorporate sports-specific motions. The goals are to raise core body temperature; increase heart rate; increase blood flow to the muscles; and improve flexibility, balance, and coordination. Upon completion of this warm-up, the athlete will be physically prepared for training. All of the exercises should be performed across the width of a court or field or for approximately 20 to 30 seconds.

1. **Toe walk**. The athlete walks up on the toes with the legs straight. The heel of the foot should not touch the ground and the hips should remain neutral throughout.
2. **Heel walk**. The athlete walks on the heels with the legs straight. The toes should not touch the ground, the knees should not lock, and the hips should remain neutral.
3. **Straight leg march**. The athlete walks with both legs straight, alternating lifting up each leg as high as possible without compromising form. The knees are kept straight and posture is erect; the body should not lean backward. The arms are swung in opposition.
4. **Leg cradle** (Fig. 19–5). The athlete walks forward, keeping the entire body straight and neutrally aligned. One leg is lifted in front of the body, bending at the knee. The knee is rotated outward and the foot inward. The foot is held with both hands, standing on one leg, and held in this position for 3 seconds. The foot is placed back down and the exercise is repeated with the opposite leg.

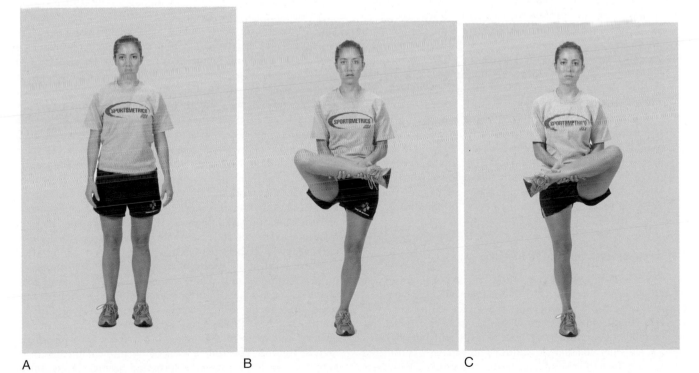

A   B   C

FIGURE 19–5. A–C, Leg cradle.

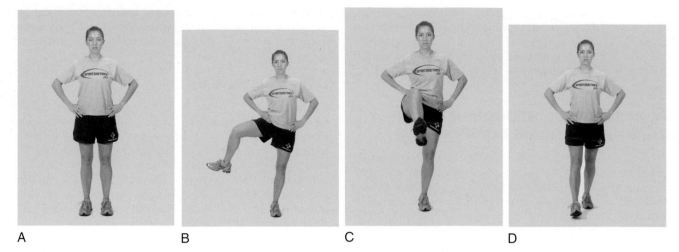

FIGURE 19–6. A–D, Dog and bush walk.

5. **Dog and bush (hip rotator) walk** (Fig. 19–6). The athlete is instructed to pretend that there is an obstacle directly in front of her or him. The athlete faces forward and keeps the shoulders and hips square. One leg is extended at the hip and the knee kept softly bent. The leg is externally rotated out at the hip and the knee is bent to approximately 90°. The leg is rotated and brought up and over the obstacle and then placed back on the ground. The exercise is repeated with the opposite leg.

6. **High knee skip**. The athlete begins to skip. One knee is driven up in the air as high as possible, while the other leg hops off the ground. As the athlete lands, the exercise is immediately repeated on the opposite side. The opposite arm of the high knee is swung up in the air to help gain height.

7. **High knees**. The athlete begins to jog forward. With each step, the knees are driven up as high as possible using short, choppy steps. The athlete remains facing forward, keeping the shoulders and hips square throughout the exercise.

8. **Glut kicks**. The athlete begins to jog forward. Each step, the athlete kicks the feet back as if trying to reach the gluts with the heel, using short, choppy steps. The athlete remains facing forward, keeping the shoulder and hips square throughout the exercise.

9. **Stride out**. The athlete begins jogging forward with an exaggerated running form. The knees are driven as high as possible and the feet are kicked back, as if trying to make a large complete circle with the legs. The athlete should stay up on the balls of his or her feet throughout the exercise.

10. **All-out sprint**. The athlete sprints forward as fast as possible while keeping proper technique and running form.

Plyometrics/Jump Training

In reference to ACL injury prevention–training programs, Griffin and associates[9] stated, "The rationale to include plyometric exercises is based on evidence that the stretch-shortening cycle activates neural, muscular, and elastic components and, therefore, should enhance joint stability (dynamic stiffening)." Plyometrics help develop muscle control and strength considered critical to reduce the risk of knee ligament injuries. These exercises are well known to increase muscular power, vertical jump height, acceleration speed, and running speed.[3,4,32] However, if done improperly, these exercises would not be expected to have a beneficial effect in reducing the risk of a noncontact ACL injury. Therefore, the philosophy of the plyometric and jump-training component in the Sportsmetrics program is to place a major emphasis on correct jumping and techniques throughout the 6 weeks of training. Specific drills and instruction are used to teach the athlete to pre-position the entire body safely when accelerating or decelerating on landing. The selection and progression of the exercises entail neuromuscular retraining and proceed from simple jumping drills (to instill correct form) to multidirectional, single-foot hops and plyometrics with an emphasis on quick turnover (to add movements that mimic sports-specific motions). The jump training is divided into three 2-week phases. Each 2-week phase has a different training focus and the exercises change correspondingly (Table 19–2).

Phase 1, termed the *technique development phase*, aims to teach the athlete proper form and technique for eight different jumps. Four basic techniques are stressed: correct posture and body alignment throughout the jump (spine erect, shoulders back, chest over knees), jumping straight up with no excessive side-to-side or forward-backward movement, soft landings including toe-to-midfoot rocking and bent knees, and instant recoil preparation for the next jump. The athletes are taught these techniques through verbal queues from instructors such as "on your toes," "straight as an arrow," "light as a feather," "shock absorber," and "recoil like a spring." Constant feedback is offered by instructors, and mirrors are used in the training sessions to provide direct visual feedback as frequently as possible. Throughout each session, exercises are increased by duration or repetition. If the athlete becomes fatigued and cannot perform the jumps with the proper technique, she or he is encouraged to stop and rest. Approximately 30 seconds of recovery time is allowed between each exercise.

Phase 2, called the *fundamentals phase*, continues to emphasize proper technique and quality jumping form. Six jumps from phase 1 are continued, but these are performed for longer periods of time. In addition, three new jumps of increased difficulty are incorporated. Phase 3, the *performance phase*, increases the quantity and speed of the jumps to develop a truly plyometric exercise routine. The athlete is encouraged to complete as many jumps as possible with proper form and to concentrate on the height achieved in each jump.

TABLE 19–2   Sportsmetrics Neuromuscular Training Program: Jump-Training Component

Phase	Jumps	Duration		Emphasis, Goals
1: Technique development		**Week 1**	**Week 2**	Proper form and technique for each jump.
	Wall jump	20 sec	25 sec	Correct posture, body alignment throughout each jump.
Weeks 1–2	Tuck jump	20 sec	25 sec	Jump straight up with no excessive side-to-side or
	Squat jump	10 sec	15 sec	forward-backward movement.
	Barrier jump (side-to-side)	20 sec	25 sec	Soft landings that include toe-to-midfoot rocking and
	Barrier jump (forward-back)	20 sec	25 sec	bent knees.
	180° jump	20 sec	25 sec	Deep knee flexion.
	Broad jump (stick 5 sec)	5 reps	10 reps	Instant recoil preparation for the next jump, no double
	Bounding in place	20 sec	25 sec	bouncing.
2: Fundamentals		**Week 3**	**Week 4**	Proper technique to build a base of strength, power, agility.
Weeks 3–4	Wall jump	25 sec	30 sec	Focus on well-performed, quality jumps.
	Tuck jump	25 sec	30 sec	Same jumps from phase 1 done for longer duration.
	Jump, jump, jump, vertical jump	5 total	8 total	New, more difficult jumps introduced to build on skills
	Squat jump	15 sec	20 sec	mastered from phase 1.
	Barrier hop side-to-side*	25 sec	30 sec	
	Barrier hop forward-back*	25 sec	30 sec	
	Scissors jump	25 sec	30 sec	
	Single-leg hop* (stick)	5 reps	5 reps	
	Bounding for distance	1 run	2 runs	
3: Performance		**Week 5**	**Week 6**	Enhance basic skill and muscle control learned in first 2 phases.
Weeks 5–6	Wall-jump	20 sec	20 sec	Increase quantity, speed of jumps with well-performed,
	Jump up, down, 180°, vertical	5 total	10 total	quality jumping technique.
	Squat jump	25 sec	25 sec	
	Mattress jump side-to-side	30 sec	30 sec	
	Mattress jump forward-back	30 sec	30 sec	
	Hop, hop, hop, stick*	5 reps	5 reps	
	Jump into bounding	3 runs	4 runs	

*Repeat on both sides for duration or repetitions listed.

1. **Wall jump** (wk 1–6). Also known as ankle bounces, this jump is performed with the knees slightly bent and both arms raised overhead (Fig. 19–7A). From this position, the athlete bounces up and down off his or her toes (see Fig. 19–7B). The knees should be soft and the hips, knees, and ankles in neutral alignment. This jump is performed first to prepare the athlete mentally and physically for plyometric training. This also provides the trainer an opportunity to observe and begin positive feedback and instruction.

Mistakes to correct include slouched posture, too much knee flexion, and eyes watching the feet with the head down. The athlete should be told to keep the eyes and head focused up, bend the knees slightly, and maintain neutral alignment.

2. **Tuck jump** (wk 1–6). The athlete begins in an upright neutral stance with the feet shoulder-width apart (Fig. 19–8A). The athlete jumps up, bending the knees together to bring the thighs up toward the chest as high as possible (see Fig. 19–8B).

Mistakes to correct include lowering the chest to the knees rather than lifting the knees to the chest, bringing the knees together during take-off or landing, double-bouncing between jumps, and producing a loud landing with a lack of muscle control. The athlete should be told to lift the knees up to the chest, control and keep the landing quiet, land on the balls of the feet, keep the knees bent when landing in order to go immediately into the next jump, keep the knees and ankles at shoulder/hip width at all times, keep the back straight, shoulders back, and keep the head/eyes up with each jump.

3. **Squat jump** (wk 1–6). The athlete begins in a fully crouched position as deep as comfortable (Fig. 19–9A). The knees and feet are directed forward and are in alignment with the hips. The upper body is upright with the chest open. The hands touch or reach toward the ground on the outside of the heels. The athlete jumps up, reaching as high as possible (see Fig. 19–9B), and then returns to the crouched position with hands reaching back toward the heels (see Fig. 19–9C).

Mistakes to correct include landing with body/knees forward and/or off-balance, bringing the knees together during take-off or landing, and producing a loud landing with a lack of muscle control. The athlete should be told to keep the hands reaching back toward the heels (not forward), keep the knees tracking under the hips on take-off and landing, maintain the knees and ankles at shoulder/hip width at all times, keep the back straight and the shoulders back, and keep the head/eyes up with each jump.

4. **Barrier jump side-to-side** (wk 1–2). A cone or barrier approximately 6 to 8 inches in height is used. The athlete stands in a modified squat position (Fig. 19–10A). The athlete then jumps from one side of the barrier to the other side with the feet kept together (see Fig. 19–10B), and lands in the same amount of knee flexion as the starting position (see Fig. 19–10C).

Mistakes to correct include landing or taking off with stiff, straight, or wobbly knees; jumping side-to-side quickly

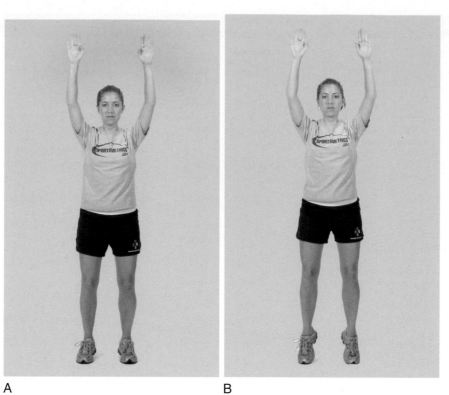

A   B

FIGURE 19–7. A and **B,** Wall jump.

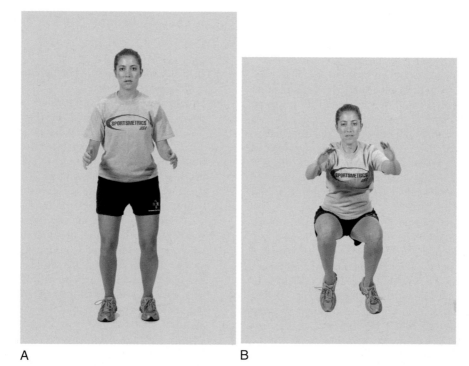

A   B

FIGURE 19–8. A and **B,** Tuck jump.

without bringing the entire body over the barrier; double-bouncing on landing and take-off; and not landing with the feet together. The athlete should be told to bend the knees up to clear the barrier, land quietly on the balls of the feet and rock back to the heels, control the landing to be able to immediately take off again, keep the back straight with the shoulders back, keep head/eyes up with each jump, keep the knees tracking under the hips and toes pointed forward on take-off and landing, and keep the feet parallel to each other.

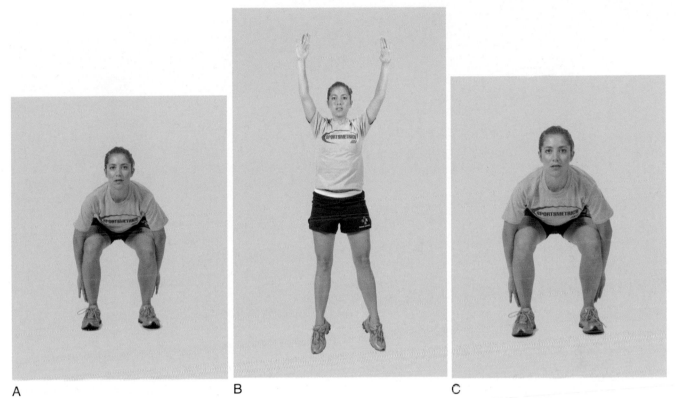

FIGURE 19–9. A–C, Squat jump.

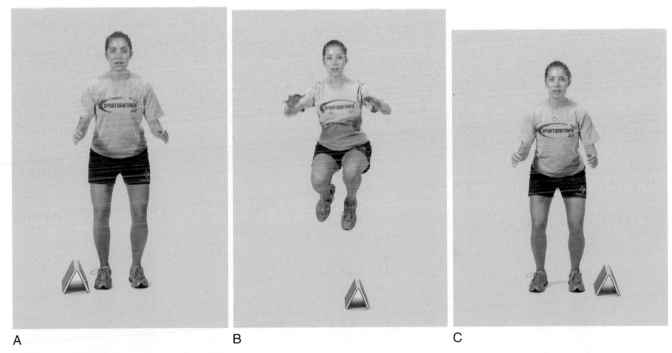

FIGURE 19–10. A–C, Barrier jump side-to-side.

5. **Barrier jump forward-backward** (wk 1–2). A cone or barrier approximately 6 to 8 inches in height is used. The athlete stands facing the barrier in a modified squat position (Fig. 19–11A). The athlete jumps forward and backward with the feet kept together (see Fig. 19–11B), and lands in the same amount of knee flexion as the starting position (see Fig. 19–11C).

Mistakes to correct include landing or taking off with stiff, straight, or wobbly knees; jumping forward-backward quickly without bringing the entire body over the barrier;

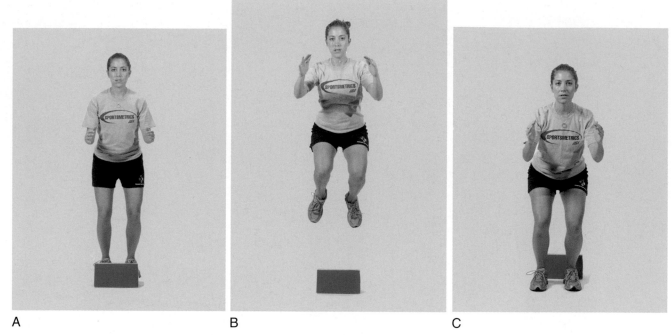

A   B   C

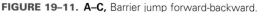
FIGURE 19–11. A–C, Barrier jump forward-backward.

double-bouncing on landing and take-off; and separating the feet to clear the barrier. The athlete should be told to lift the knees up to the chest to clear the barrier, land quietly on the balls of the feet and rock back to the heels, control the landing to be able to immediately take off again, keep the back straight with the shoulders back, keep the head/ eyes up with each jump, and keep the knees tracking under the hips and the toes pointed forward on take-off and landing.

6. **180° jump** (wk 1–2). The athlete begins from an upright neutral stance with the feet shoulder-width apart (Fig. 19–12A). The athlete jumps with both feet straight up into the air and makes a 180° turn in midair (see Fig. 19–21B) before landing (see Fig. 19–12C). The landing is held for two seconds, and then the direction is reversed and the jump repeated.

Mistakes to correct include over- or underrotating; not turning the body 180°; not rotating the body as a unit; landing loud, straight, stiff-legged, with staggered feet or one

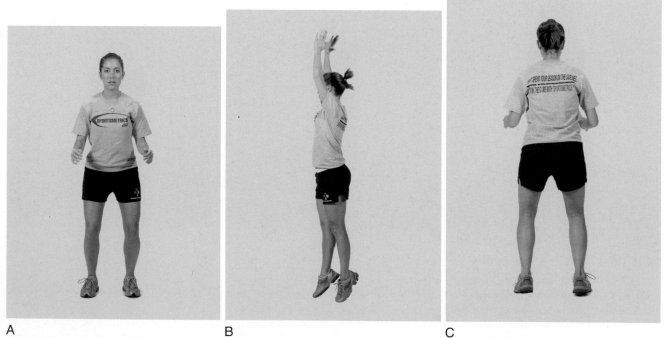

A   B   C

FIGURE 19–12. A–C, 180° jump.

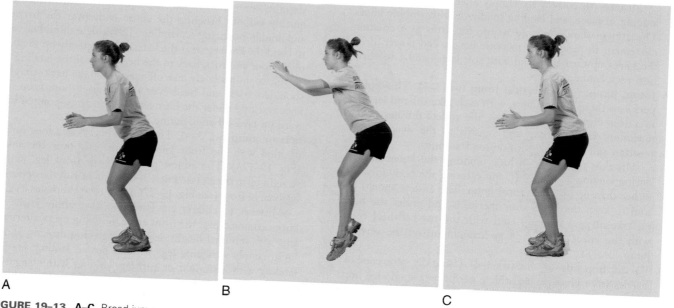

FIGURE 19–13. A–C, Broad jump.

foot landing before the other; always jumping in the same direction (in a circle); rotating back and forth with minimal height during jump; and separating the feet beyond the desired "feet shoulder-/hip-width" distance.

The athlete should be told to jump straight up and rotate the body as a unit from the head to the toes; land with soft, slightly flexed knees; always jump in opposing directions (one jump over the right shoulder, the next over the left); keep the knees tracking under the hips on take-off and landing; maintain knees and ankles at shoulder/hip width at all times; keep the back straight with the shoulders back, and keep the head/eyes up with each jump.

7. **Broad jump** (wk 1–2). The athlete starts from an upright neutral stance (Fig. 19–13A) and jumps forward as far as

possible (see Fig. 19–13B), taking off with both feet. The athlete lands on both feet, remains in a deep crouch position (see Fig. 19–13C) for 5 seconds, and then repeats the jump.

Mistakes to correct include not holding or sticking the landing, pointing the knees inward during landing and take-off, and landing in a straight-legged or upright position. The athlete should be told to track the knees over the heels and under the hips on take-off and landing, land with a soft toe ball heel rock with the knees flexed, and hold the landing for 5 seconds.

8. **Bounding in place** (wk 1–2). The athlete begins this jump on a single leg, with the opposite leg bent behind. Staying in one place, the leg positions are alternated by driving the back leg forward and upward. The rhythm and height are progressively increased throughout the exercise (Fig. 19–14).

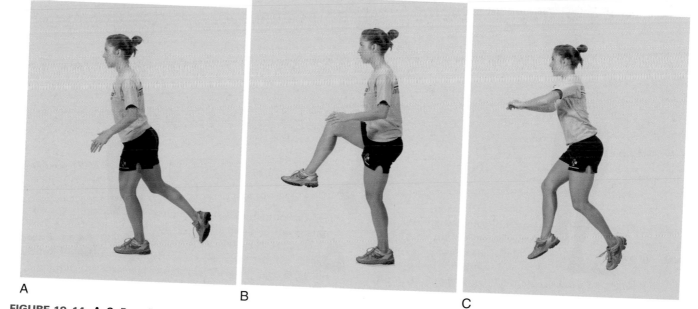

FIGURE 19–14. A–C, Bounding in place.

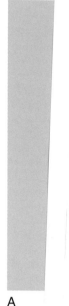

A

FIGURE

The
diate
right
deep

N
strai
The
crou
land

16. Ma
is p

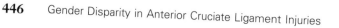

8. **Superman (alternating arms/legs)**. The athlete lies face down and places the forehead on top of the back of one hand. The other arm is extended out on the ground. The abdominal muscles are tightened and the upper body is raised to lift the extended arm. At the same time, from the hip and gluteals, the leg opposite from the extended arm is raised. The toes and fingers on the lifted leg and arm are extended. The abdominals remained tightened. This exercise is done for 30 seconds during weeks 1 to 3 and for 60 seconds during weeks 4 to 6.

Mistakes to correct are lifting the head up, overly arching the back, and lifting the leg to the side. The athlete should be told to keep the spine as neutral as possible, focusing the eyes on the mat/ground directly below; lift from the trunk; lift the leg and arm only to the point of tension in the lower back; and keep the abdominals tight.

9. **Abdominals (Russian twists)**. The athlete lies on the ground, bends the knees, and places the heels on the floor. The athlete bends at the hips, not the waist, to bring the upper body to a 45° angle and holds this position. Moving the trunk as a unit, the athlete rotates the upper body side-to-side allowing the hands to touch the ground next to the hip with each rotation (Fig. 19–24). This exercise is done 1 day each week for 30 seconds in phase I, 60 seconds in phase II, and 90 seconds in phase III.

Mistakes to correct are slouched posture, rounded shoulders, and twisting only the shoulders and not the torso. The athlete should be told to keep the back straight and shoulders relaxed, keep the upper body at a 45° angle, and to move the trunk as a unit, making sure that both hands are touching the ground with each rotation.

10. **Abdominals (plank)**. The athlete lies face down and places the elbows under the shoulders with the forearms on the floor (Fig. 19–25A). The legs are placed a hip-distance apart and the toes curled under. The athlete lifts the body up onto the elbows and toes (see Fig. 19–25B). A neutral posture is maintained. The position is held with tight abdominals. This exercise is done 1 day each week for 30 seconds in phase I, 60 seconds in phase II, and 90 seconds in phase III.

Mistakes to correct include maintaining a slouched or arched midsection, placing the head down with chin resting on chest, and keeping the elbows and/or toes too close together. The athlete should be told to make sure to maintain a neutral posture, keep the neck and shoulders relaxed, keep the body in a straight line parallel to the ground, maintain head in a neutral position, and keep the abdominals tight at all times.

11. **Abdominals (bicycle kicks)**. The athlete lies on the back with the knees bent into the chest, placing the fingertips on the back of the head. The upper body is raised off the ground until the shoulders no longer touch the ground and holds this

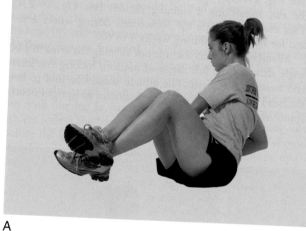

A

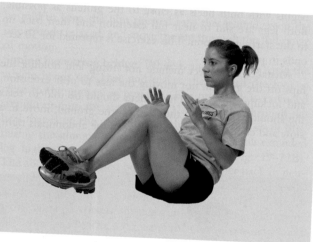

B

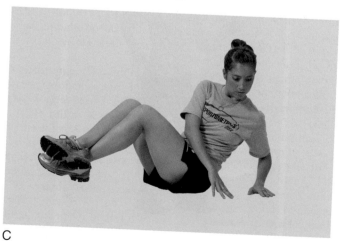

C

FIGURE 19–24. **A–C,** Abdominals (Russian twists).

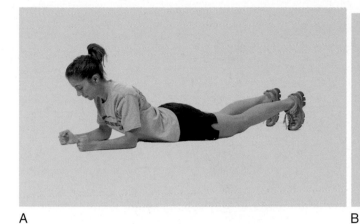
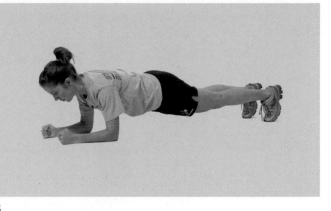

A   B

FIGURE 19–25. A and **B,** Abdominals (plank).

position. The legs are moved in a cyclic motion, bringing the heels into the gluteus and extending the legs out as close to the floor as possible (Fig. 19–26). This exercise is performed 1 day each week for 30 seconds in phase I, 60 seconds in phase II, and 90 seconds in phase III.

Mistakes to correct include not keeping the upper body off the ground, rotating the upper body, and cycling the legs close to body. The athlete should be told to keep the chest open and lift from the waist, keep the elbows open and upper body stationary, and fully bend and straighten the legs close to the ground.

12. **Hip flexor TheraBand kicking.** The athlete places one end of a piece of TheraBand around the ankle, with the other end around the ankle of a partner or anchored to a stationary object. With the athlete's back to the partner or stationary object, the athlete steps forward to produce moderate tension in the band while the leg with the TheraBand around it is in approximately 15° of hip extension (Fig. 19–27A). Then, the athlete drives the knee that is back up and forward with maximal effort against the resistance of the band until the thigh is parallel with the ground (see Fig. 19–27B). The leg is returned to a slightly extended position after each exertion. This exercise consists of two sets of 10 repetitions, with 30 seconds rest between each set. A third set is performed of 20 repetitions in phase I, 30 repetitions in phase II, and 40 repetitions in phase III.

Mistakes to correct include swinging the leg up and back, hiking the hip, and moving the torso. The athlete should be told to keep head and neck straight, look straight down, keep shoulders and hips square, keep the upper body

stationary, and always return the working leg to a slightly extended position before kicking forward again.

13. **Steamboats (hip flexion).** The athlete places a resistance band around the thighs, halfway between the hips and the knees. The exercise is begun with the feet shoulder width apart and one knee is bent slightly so that the foot is off the ground. The athlete balances on the one leg and begins kicking forward and backward on the bent leg at the hip. The upper body is kept still and does not sway. This exercise is done for 30 seconds on each leg during weeks 1 to 3 and for 60 seconds during weeks 4 to 6. It may replace hip flexor TheraBand kicking.

Mistakes to correct include flexing or extending at the knee, simply bending and straightening the knee and not moving at the hip, swaying the upper body back and forth with kicking movements, and not kicking forward or backward enough to feel resistance of the band. The athlete should be told to keep the back straight, the shoulders back, and the head/eyes up, maintain slight bend in both knees at all times, keep the upper body stationary, kick the leg back and forth through full range of motion, keep the hips level at all times, and do not hike the hip with motion.

14. **Hip abductor TheraBand kicking.** The athlete places one end of a piece of TheraBand around the ankle with the other end around the ankle of a partner or anchored to a stationary object. The athlete stands in line with the partner or stationary object so that the leg with the resistance is farthest away from the partner or object (Fig. 19–28A). The athlete steps sideways to produce moderate tension in the band, kicks the outside leg out sideways against the

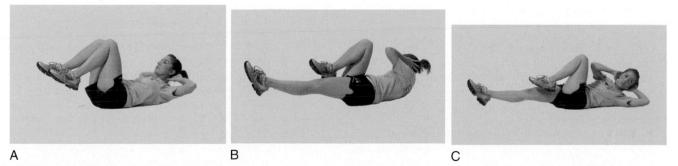

A   B   C

FIGURE 19–26. A–C, Abdominals (bicycle kicks).

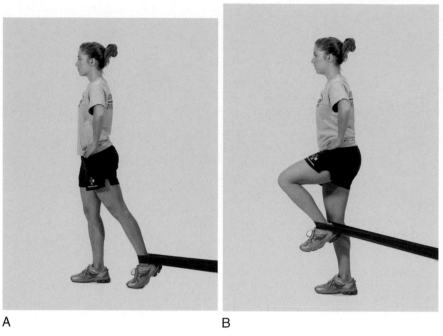

FIGURE 19–27. A and **B,** Hip flexor TheraBand kicking.

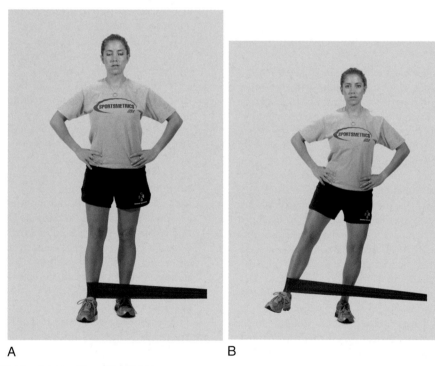

FIGURE 19–28. A and **B,** Hip abductor TheraBand kicking.

resistance of the band (see Fig. 19–28), and returns to the starting position. This exercise consists of two sets of 10 repetitions, with 30 seconds rest between sets. A third set is performed of 20 repetitions in phase I, 30 repetitions in phase II, and 40 repetitions in phase III. This activity is performed 2 days a week.

Mistakes to correct are swinging the leg out and back without control, and leaning the upper body to the side while kicking. The athlete should be told to keep the head and neck straight, look straight ahead, keep shoulders and hips square, keep upper body stationary, and keep movements slow and controlled.

15. **Lateral walking with TheraBand.** The athlete places a resistance band around the thighs, halfway between the hips and the knees. The exercise is begun with the feet shoulder-width apart. The athlete steps out to the side approximately 2 to 3 feet. Slowly and under control, the athlete follows with the other foot to regain the "feet shoulder-width apart" position. Once finished, the athlete reverses directions so that the opposite foot leads the exercise. This exercise is

done for 30 seconds during weeks 1 to 3 and for 60 seconds during weeks 4 to 6. It may replace hip abduction Thera-Band kicking.

Mistakes to correct include allowing the feet to come together between steps, allowing the leg that follows to "snap" back to the starting position, walking with the knees locked in the straight position, bending forward at the waist, rounding the shoulders, and looking down at the feet/ground. The athlete should be told to keep the back straight, the shoulders back, and the head/eyes up, keep the steps to a distance that allows for leg control throughout the activity, keep motion slow and under control at all times, and make sure that all motion is coming from the hips and legs.

Flexibility

Passive stretching is done at the conclusion of training, with each stretch held for 20 to 30 seconds and repeated twice on each side. Stretching is considered essential to achieve maximum muscle length to allow muscles to work with power through a complete range of motion. The major muscle groups targeted are the hamstrings, iliotibial band, quadriceps, hip flexor, gastrocnemius, soleus, deltoid, triceps, biceps, pectoralis, and latissimus dorsi.

1. **Hamstrings.** While seated, the athlete extends the right leg fully and bends the left leg, placing the inside of the foot along the left calf (Fig. 19–29A). The back is kept straight and the chest is brought toward the knee. The athlete reaches with both hands toward the toes (see Fig. 19–29B). The hands are placed on the floor alongside the legs or hold on to the toes. Switch the side and repeat.

   Mistakes to correct are rounding the shoulders when leaning into stretch, bringing the chin into the chest when stretching, allowing the knee of the leg on the ground to bend, and bouncing into the stretch. The athlete should be told to keep the back straight when leaning forward into the stretch, bend forward at the waist, and keep the shoulders back and head up for the duration of the stretch.

2. **Iliotibial band.** While seated, the athlete bends the right knee and places the right foot flat on the floor. The left foot and ankle are placed on the right thigh just above the knee. Both hands are placed on the floor behind the hips and the chest is pressed toward the knee and foot. The upper torso, neck, and shoulders remain neutral and open and the upper back is not rounded (Fig. 19–30). This stretch may be performed while lying on the back to support the spine and neck.

3. **Quadriceps.** While standing, the athlete grabs the foot or ankle and lifts it up behind the body. The lower leg and foot are gently pulled up, directly behind the upper leg, with no twisting inward or outward (Fig. 19–31). The stretch is held for 20 seconds, released, and repeated on the same side. Then, the opposite side is stretched with the same sequence.

   Mistakes to correct include allowing the foot to rest on the buttocks, pulling the leg and/or foot inward or outward, and locking the knee of the leg being used for balance. The athlete should be told to pull straight up on the foot and leg, and to keep the back straight, shoulders back, and head/eyes up.

4. **Hip flexor.** The athlete stands with the feet in a lunge position and the front knee slightly bent. The athlete pushes up on the rear toe. The hips are pressed forward while the buttocks are tightened until a stretch is felt in the front of the hip. The upper torso remains upright and centered directly over the hips (Fig. 19–32).

   Mistakes to correct include leaning the upper body forward, not pressing the hips forward, and bouncing into the stretch. The athlete should be told to keep the upper body upright and centered directly over the hips, press or rock the hips forward to initiate stretch, and keep the back straight, shoulders back, and head/eyes up.

5. **Gastrocnemius.** The athlete stands in a long lunge position with the front knee slightly bent, but not extended past the ankle. The hands are placed on the front of the thigh and the body is leaned forward while keeping the back leg straight. The rear heel is pressed down (Fig. 19–33). This stretch may also be done by placing both hands against a wall and leaning forward. The stretch is held for 20 seconds, released, and repeated.

   Mistakes to correct are allowing the back heel to rise off the ground, bouncing into the stretch, allowing the knee of the back leg to bend, and not maintaining upper body posture. The athlete should be told to keep the back straight, the shoulders back, and head/eyes up; keep the back leg straight; and keep the heel on the ground at all times.

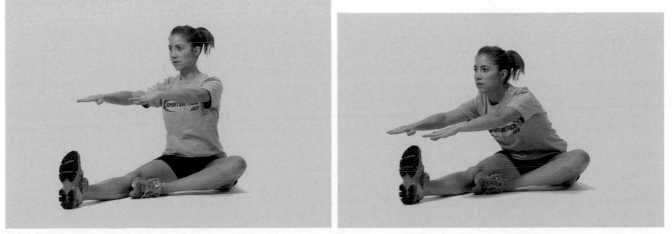

A   B

FIGURE 19–29. A and **B,** Hamstrings stretch.

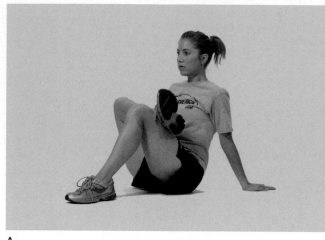
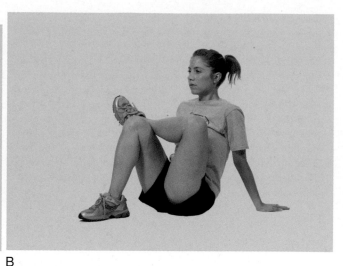

A   B

FIGURE 19–30. **A** and **B,** Iliotibial band stretch.

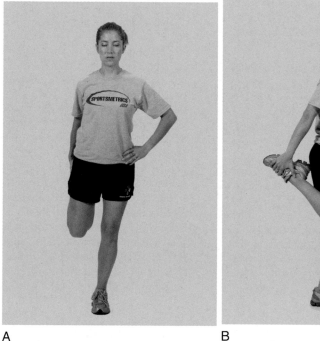
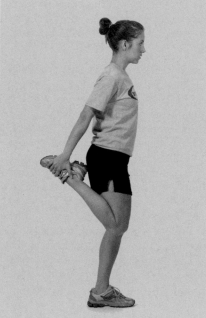

A   B

FIGURE 19–31. **A** and **B,** Quadriceps stretch.

6. **Soleus**. The athlete stands with one foot forward and one foot back, in a short lunge position. Both knees are bent and the athlete is instructed to sit the hips down into the back heel, with the majority of body weight on the back leg (Fig. 19–34). The heel is kept on the floor. This stretch may be performed by placing both hands against a wall for balance.

7. **Deltoid**. While either standing or sitting, the athlete brings the left arm across the body, placing the elbow in close to the chest. The palm of the hand faces the rear. The arm is clasped at the elbow and gently pressed into and across the body (Fig. 19–35). Both shoulders stay relaxed and low. The head, neck, and spine all remain neutral.

8. **Triceps, latissimus dorsi**. While either standing or sitting, the athlete extends the right arm above the head. The elbow is bent behind the head while the palm of the hand is brought toward the center of the upper back. The elbow is grasped with the left hand and gently pressed down and back (Fig. 19–36).

9. **Pectoralis, biceps**. While standing, the athlete clasps the hands behind the back. With the shoulders and neck relaxed, the elbows are extended, the chest opened, and the hands lifted up. The posture should remain upright and neutral and the knees slightly flexed (Fig. 19–37).

10. **Low back**. The athlete kneels on the floor with the hands close to the buttocks. The athlete bends forward with the arms fully extended reaching out onto the floor. The head is lowered between the arms with the forehead close to or resting on the floor. The hands are gradually moved out farther from the body without rising up from the heels (Fig. 19–38).

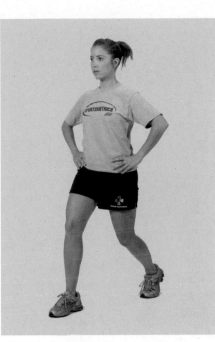

FIGURE 19–32. Hip flexor stretch.

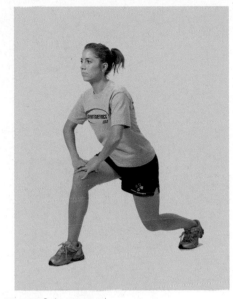

FIGURE 19–34. Soleus stretch.

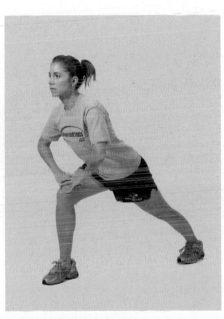

FIGURE 19–33. Gastrocnemius stretch.

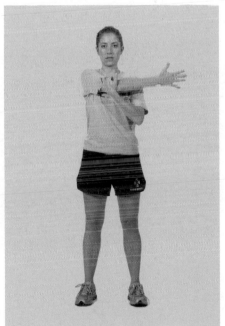

FIGURE 19–35. Deltoid stretch.

SPORTSMETRICS TRAINING PROGRAM OPTIONS

Sportsmetrics Warm-up for Injury Prevention and Performance

Designed as a maintenance program, WIPP is recommended upon completion of the 6 weeks of formal Sportsmetrics training to continue to instill the skills and techniques learned during Sportsmetrics for the athlete's entire sports season. WIPP training is conducted in place of the normal warm-up before a practice or a game and lasts approximately 20 minutes. The program integrates select elements from the four basic components of Sportsmetrics and focuses on the essential training concepts of control of the upper body, trunk, and lower body position on landing, increased hip and knee flexion angles on landing, and techniques to land softly to decrease ground reaction forces (Table 19–3).

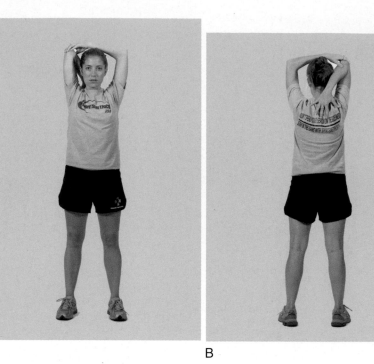

A   B

FIGURE 19–36. A and **B,** Triceps, latissimus dorsi stretch.

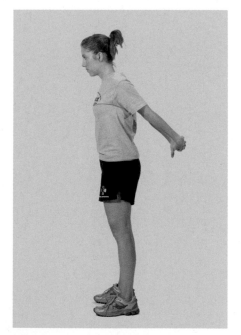

FIGURE 19–37. Pectoralis, biceps stretch.

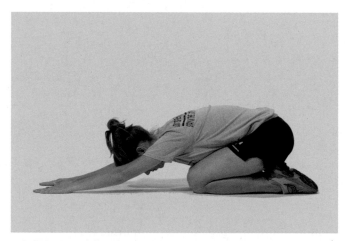

FIGURE 19–38. Low back stretch.

Sports-Specific Training

Sportsmetrics Soccer and Basketball

Soccer and basketball represent two of the highest-risk sports for noncontact ACL injuries in female athletes. Sports-specific training programs were designed for these activities that allow all training to be conducted on the field or court. These programs incorporate strength training, cardiovascular conditioning, and agility drills that mirror the typical demands of the sports. Seventeen of the jumps from Sportsmetrics are included in the training.

These programs should be performed in the athlete's off or preparatory season at least 3 days/week. No equipment other than a basketball or soccer ball for each athlete is required. As in Sportsmetrics training, emphasis is placed on the athlete performing every exercise or drill with proper technique, body alignment, and form. If an athlete exhibits compromised form, the exercise should be stopped by the instructor. The athlete should then perform one more repetition of the task, focusing on correcting obvious deficiencies.

Sportsmetrics Soccer includes the components of Sportsmetrics in addition to agility drills and three different cardiovascular workouts that are both aerobic and anaerobic (Table 19–4). Each cardiovascular workout has a slightly different combination of short bursts of hard running and longer-distance/lower-intensity movements. The intensity of each running maneuver is monitored using a Rating of Perceived Exertion (RPE) scale from 1 to 10, with a

TABLE 19–3   Sportsmetrics Warm-up for Injury Prevention and Performance Training Program

Component	Exercise	Duration (sec)	Comments	Transition between Exercises (sec)
Dynamic warm-up	Straight leg march	20		5
Dynamic warm-up	Hand walk	20		10
Dynamic warm-up	Cradle walk	20		5
Dynamic warm-up	Hip rotator walk	20		20
Jump training	Tuck jump	30		10
Jump training	Squat jumps	30		10
Jump training	180° jump	30		10
Jump training	Scissor jump	30		10
Jump training	Barrier hop side-to-side	30	15 sec each leg	75
Strength training	Steamboats	60	30 sec each leg	10
Strength training	Lateral step	60	30 sec each direction	40
Strength training	Supine hamstring	60	30 sec each leg	15
Strength training	Abdominal crunch	60		10
Strength training	Modified plank	60		15
Flexibility	Hamstring stretch	40	20 sec each leg	15
Flexibility	Hip flexor stretch	40	20 sec each leg	15
Flexibility	Quadriceps stretch	40	20 sec each leg	25
Flexibility	Calf stretch	40	20 sec each leg	20
Agility	Quick feet	60	30 sec each direction	20
Agility	Nebraska drill	60	30 sec each run	—

TABLE 19–4   Sportsmetrics Soccer Training Program

Component	Day(s)	Exercise	Duration (sec/reps/runs/laps)	Rating of Perceived Exertion
Dynamic warm-up	1–18 (all)	Heel-toe walk Straight leg march Hand walk Forward lunge Backward lunge Leg cradle walk Dog and bush walk	Across width of soccer field or 20 sec (all)	
Agility drills	1–18 1–18 1–18	Quick feet Tire drill high knees Diagonal run	Based on individual athlete	
Jump training	1–12 1–12 1–18 1–6 1–6 1–6 1–6 1–6 7–12 7–12 7–12 7–12 7–12 7–12 13–18 13–18 13–18 13–18 13–18	Wall jump Tuck jump Squat jump Barrier jump side-to-side Barrier jump forward-backward 180° jump Broad jump Bounding in place Jump, jump, jump, vertical Barrier hop side-to-side Barrier hop forward-backward Scissors jump Single-leg hop Bounding for distance Tuck jump holding ball—knees to ball Combo hop (forward, side-to-side over ball, backward-forward, side-to-side over ball, backward) Single leg hop diagonal Scissor jump holding ball Jump into bounding	20–30 sec 20–30 sec 10–20 sec 20–25 sec 20–25 sec 20–25 sec 5–10 reps 20–25 sec 5–8 reps 25–30 sec 25–30 sec 25–30 sec 5 reps 1–2 runs 30 sec 25–30 sec 25–30 sec 30 sec 5 reps	
Strength training	1–18 (all)	Standing squat Calf raise Long stride lunge Standing abductor ball roll Backward lunge	45 sec–2 min (all)	

Continued

TABLE 19–4	Sportsmetrics Soccer Training Program—Cont'd			
Component	**Day(s)**	**Exercise**	**Duration (sec/reps/runs/laps)**	**Rating of Perceived Exertion**
		Tricep dips		
		Push-ups		
		Supine throw-in with partner		
		Abdominals (ball side-to-side)		
		Bridge with ball roll		
		Plank with leg raise		
Cardiovascular training	1, 4, 7, 10, 13, 16	Exaggerate stride hard	1–2 laps	8
	1, 4, 7, 10, 13, 16	Recovery lap dribbling ball	1 lap	6
	2, 5, 8, 11, 14, 17	Maximum effort sprint	1–2 laps	10
	2, 5, 8, 11, 14, 17	Recovery—skip	½–1 lap	6
	2, 5, 8, 11, 14, 17	Recovery—shuffle right	½–1 lap	6
	2, 5, 8, 11, 14, 17	Maximum effort sprint	1–2 laps	10
	2, 5, 8, 11, 14, 17	Recovery—jog backward	½–1 lap	6
	2, 5, 8, 11, 14, 17	Recovery—shuffle left	½–1 lap	6
	3, 6, 9, 12, 15, 18	Run hard	1 lap	8
	3, 6, 9, 12, 15, 18	Recover—backward jog	½–1 lap	6
	3, 6, 9, 12, 15, 18	Run hard	1 lap	8
	3, 6, 9, 12, 15, 18	Recover—caricoa right	½–1 lap	6
	3, 6, 9, 12, 15, 18	Run hard	½–1 lap	8
	3, 6, 9, 12, 15, 18	Recover—caricoa left	½–1 lap	6
	3, 6, 9, 12, 15, 18	Run hard	1 lap	8
	3, 6, 9, 12, 15, 18	Recover—skip	½–1 lap	6
	3, 6, 9, 12, 15, 18	Run hard	1 lap	8
	3, 6, 9, 12, 15, 18	Recover—forward jog	½–1 lap	6
Flexibility	1–18 (all)	Hamstrings	20–30 sec repeat 2 times each side	
		Quadriceps		
		Iliotibial band		
		Hip flexor		
		Gastrocnemius/soleus		
		Deltoid		
		Triceps		
		Pectorals/biceps		
		Low back		

rating of 1 indicating the lightest intensity and a rating of 10 designating an all-out maximum effort.

Sportsmetrics Basketball was designed to address fundamental strength, coordination, agility, and aerobic fitness (Table 19–5). The dynamic warm-up, jump/plyometric drills, and stretches are essentially the same as the original Sportsmetrics program with the addition of a basketball whenever possible to enhance balance, postural/body control, and trunk strength. The strength exercises are functional body weight exercises emphasizing total body conditioning. Agility drills and cardiovascular workouts, based upon basketball movement patterns and drills, round out the training.

Sportsmetrics Tennis

Although not considered a high-risk sport for noncontact ACL injuries, tennis carries the risk of other lower extremity injuries

TABLE 19–5	Sportsmetrics Basketball Training Program		
Component	**Day(s)**	**Exercise**	**Duration (sec/reps/runs/laps)**
Dynamic warm-up	1–18 (all)	Heel-toe walk	From sideline to sideline (all)
		Straight leg march	
		Hand walk	
		Forward lunge	
		Backward lunge	
		Leg cradle walk	
		Dog and bush walk	
Agility drills	1–18	Quick feet	Based on individual athlete
	1–18	Defensive slides	
	1–18	Diagonal run	
Jump training	1–12	Wall jump	20–30 sec
	1–12	Tuck jump	20–30 sec
	1–18	Squat jump	10–20 sec
	1–6	Barrier jump side-to-side	20–25 sec
	1–6	Barrier jump forward-backward	20–25 sec

	1–6	180° jump	20–25 sec
	1–6	Broad jump	5–10 reps
	1–6	Bounding in place	20–25 sec
	7–12	Jump, jump, jump, vertical	5–8 reps
	7–12	Barrier hop side-to-side	25–30 sec
	7–12	Barrier hop forward-backward	25–30 sec
	7–12	Scissors jump	25–30 sec
	7–12	Single-leg hop	5 reps
	7–12	Bounding for distance	1–2 runs
	13–18	Tuck jump holding ball-knees to ball	30 sec
	13–18	Combo hop (forward, side-to-side over ball, backward-forward, side-to-side over ball, B)	25–30 sec
	13–18	Single leg hop diagonal	25–30 sec
	13–18	Scissor jump holding ball	30 sec
	13–18	Jump into bounding	5 reps
Strength training	1–18	Baseline–to–foul line chest pass	45 sec–1 min
	1–18	Long stride lunge with knee lift	45 sec–2 min
	1–6	Lateral lunge—moving	45 sec–1 min
	1–18	Backward lunge	45 sec–2 min
	1–18	Calf raise	45 sec–2 min
	1–18	Tricep dips	45 sec–2 min
	1–6	Bridging with leg raised	45 sec–1 min
	1–18	Push-ups	45 sec–2 min
	1–18	Abdominals with partner, rotation pass	45 sec–2 min
	1–18	Abdominals with partner, overhead pass	45 sec–2 min
	1–18	Modified plank, alternate leg raise	45 sec–2 min
	7–18	Baseline–to–half court overhead pass	40 sec–1 min
	7–12	Diagonal lunge—stationary	1'15"–1'30"
	7–12	Bridging with foot on ball	1'15"–1'30"
	13–18	Diagonal lunge—moving	1'45"–2'
	13–18	Bridging with ball roll	1'45"–2'
Cardiovascular training	1, 4, 7, 10, 13, 15	Sprint drills	
	2, 5, 8, 11, 14, 17	Sixer sprints	
	3, 6, 9, 12, 15, 18	Suicides	
Flexibility training	1–18 (all)	Hamstrings	20–30 sec repeat 2 times each side
		Quadriceps	
		Iliotibial band	
		Hip flexor	
		Gastrocnemius/soleus	
		Deltoid	
		Triceps	
		Pectorals/biceps	
		Low back	

and overuse syndromes. A recent review of the literature regarding tennis injuries found that the lower extremity was the most common area injured.[30] The concepts developed in traditional Sportsmetrics of decreased landing forces, increased knee and hip flexion angles during activity, improvement in balance and posture, and increased strength and agility may be effective in reducing the risk of other lower extremity injuries during tennis. Emphasis is placed on the athlete performing every exercise or drill with proper technique, body alignment, and form. The program incorporates strength training, cardiovascular conditioning, and skill/agility drills that match the demands of the sport (Table 19–6). Performed three times a week for 6 weeks, the training may be conducted during season or off-season. All training is performed on the court, and the authors recommend the use of clay courts if possible.

The foundation of the program duplicates traditional Sportsmetrics, because the athletes begin with dynamic warm-up exercises and jump training. The program strives to teach athletes to control the upper body, trunk, and lower body position; lower their center of gravity by increasing hip and knee flexion; and develop muscular strength and techniques to land with decreased ground reaction forces. In addition, athletes are taught to pre-position the body and lower extremity prior to initial ground contact in order to obtain the position of greatest knee joint stability and stiffness.

In addition to the jumps from the traditional Sportsmetrics program, the athletes perform level surface box (four-square) hops over barriers in a variety of patterns of increasing difficulty each week (Fig. 19–39). The patterns involve right-left, forward-backward, and diagonal directions to simulate the constant change of direction required during competitive tennis. While maintaining proper body position and knee flexion angles, the athletes are encouraged to perform as many hops as possible in 20 to 25 seconds.

After jump training, the players are taken through a series of rigorous speed, agility, footwork, and skill drills. The drills emphasize body posture, knee and hip flexion position, and

TABLE 19–6   Sportsmetrics Tennis Training Program

Component	Day(s)	Exercise	Duration (sec/reps/runs/sets/laps)
Dynamic warm-up	1–18 (all)	1 lap around two courts/side-step/arm circles	Two courts
		1 lap around two courts carioca	Two courts
		Straight leg march	Baseline-net-baseline
		Forward lunge	Baseline-net-baseline
		Lateral lunge	Baseline-net-baseline
Jump training	1–18	Wall jump	20–25 sec
	1–18	Tuck jump	20–25 sec
	1–18	Squat jump	10–20 sec
	1–3	Barrier jump side-to-side	20 sec
	1–3	Barrier jump forward-backward	20 sec
	1–6	180° jump	20–25 sec
	1–6	Broad jump	5–10 reps
	7–12	Jump, jump, jump, vertical	5–8 reps
	7–12	Single-leg hop	5–8 reps
	13–18	Scissors jump	20 sec
	4–6	Barrier four-square, patterns 1 and 2	25 sec
	7–9	Barrier four-square, patterns 3 and 4	25 sec
	10–12	Barrier four-square, patterns 5 and 6	25 sec
	13–15	Barrier four-square, patterns 7 and 8	25 sec
	16–18	Barrier four-square, patterns 9 and 10	25 sec
Strength training	1–18 (all)	Medicine ball forehand	2 sets 6–16 reps
		Medicine ball backhand	2 sets 6–16 reps
		Medicine ball overhead	2 sets 6–16 reps
		Medicine ball backward, between legs	2 sets 6–16 reps
		Backward lunge, add hand weight day 7	1–2 reps, baseline-net-baseline
		Single-leg toe raise, add hand weight day 7	3 sets, 10–20 reps
		Seated press-ups	10–20 reps
		Wall push-ups	3 sets, 10–20 reps
		Biceps curls, free weights	3 sets, 10 reps
		Mini–arm circles, tennis ball against wall	2 sets, 60 sec
		Wall-sits	3 sets, 45–60 sec
		Wall-sits, ball pressed between legs	3 sets, 45–60 sec
		Abdominals: crunches	30–60 sec
		Abdominals: bicycle	30–60 sec
		Abdominals: crunches, twisting	30 sec
		Abdominals: plank, alternate leg raise	60–90 sec
		Abdominals: Superman, alternating	2 sets, 10 reps
Agility/skill/cardiovascular training	1–18	Cross-shadow, singles sideline-sideline	2 sets, 8 reps
		Net zigzag, baseline-net-baseline	2 sets, 9 cones
		Shadow swing baseline	2 sets, 10 sec
		Forehand with resistance belt	2 sets, 20 sec
		Backhand with resistance belt	2 sets, 20 sec
		Forehand/backhand baseline reaction	1 set, 30 sec/30 sec rest/2 min
		Short/deep ball reaction: forehand	2 sets, 8 reps
		Short/deep ball reaction: backhand	2 sets, 8 reps
		Forehand/backhand alternating reaction	2 sets, 8 reps
		Sprints: baseline-net	10 reps
		Ladder: various patterns	2 reps
Flexibility training	1–18 (all)	Hamstrings	20–30 sec repeat 2 times each side
		Quadriceps	
		Iliotibial band	
		Hip flexor	
		Gastrocnemius/soleus	
		Deltoid	
		Triceps	
		Pectorals/biceps	
		Low back	

balance techniques taught in the jump-training element of the program. Some of the tasks include use of a resistance belt during groundstroke and approach shot training, net zigzag that includes nine sharp cuts around cones placed between the baseline and the net, short sprints, and a cross-shadow drill which stresses balance and appropriate footwork along the baseline. In addition, muscle strengthening exercises include backward lunges, medicine ball tossing, single-leg toe-raises, wall-sits, seated press-ups, and wall push-ups. Athletes perform a variety of upper body free weight strength exercises. Free weights are added to the lunges and single-leg toe raises during the 3rd week of training to increase the difficulty of these tasks. A variety of abdominal exercises round

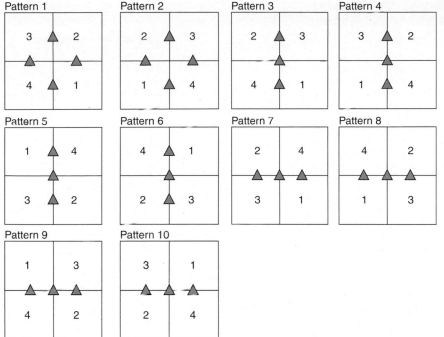

FIGURE 19–39. Barrier four-square hop patterns. The *red triangles* designate barriers.

out the program, starting with 100 repetitions the 1st week and working up to 250 repetitions the last week of training.

Sportsmetrics Speed and Conditioning Program

The Sportsmetrics Speed and Conditioning Program incorporates complex conditioning in addition to the other components of Sportsmetrics. The conditioning program encompasses a series of vigorous speed and agility drills comprising quick feet, sharp cuts, straight sprints, backward running, and unpredicted agility patterns (Table 19-7). With each drill, athletes concentrate on correct running form, body posture, and proper

technique associated with cutting, pivoting, and decelerating. The entire program may be performed on a court or field with minimal equipment. It should be conducted in the athlete's off or preparatory season, 3 days a week for 6 weeks. A few examples of the speed and agility training drills are listed later. The four-square hops shown in Figure 19-39 are included in the training (termed dot drill). This program is under prospective investigation to determine its effectiveness on both improving performance and reducing the rate of ACL noncontact injuries.

1. **Quick feet.** The athlete begins this drill at the end of a straight line, lined up parallel to the line. Moving down the line, to the left, the athlete steps the left foot forward and

TABLE 19-7 Sportsmetrics Speed and Conditioning Training Program			
Component	**Day(s)**	**Exercise**	**Duration (sec/reps/runs/laps)**
Dynamic warm-up	1–18 (all)	Heel-toe walk	Half court
		Straight leg march	Half court
		Leg cradle walk	Half court
		Dog and bush walk	Half court
		High knee skip	Half court
		High knee/butt kicks	Half court
		Stride out	Half court
		All-out sprint	Baseline-to-baseline
Jump training	1–18	Wall jump	20–25 sec
	1–12	Tuck jump	20–25 sec
	1–18	Squat jump	10–20 sec
	1–6	Barrier jump side-to-side	20 sec
	1–6	Barrier jump forward-backward	20 sec
	1–6	180° jump	20–25 sec
	1–6	Broad jump	5–10 reps
	1–6	Bounding in place	20–25 sec
	7–12	Jump, jump, jump, vertical	5–8 reps

Continued

TABLE 19–7 Sportsmetrics Speed and Conditioning Training Program—Cont'd

Component	Day(s)	Exercise	Duration (sec/reps/runs/laps)
	7–12	Barrier hop side-to-side	25–30 sec
	7–12	Barrier hop forward-backward	25–30 sec
	7–12	Single-leg hop	5–8 reps
	7–12	Scissors jump	25–30 sec
	7–12	Single-leg hop	5 reps
	7–12	Bounding for distance	1–2 runs
	13–18	Step, jump up, down, vertical	30 sec
	13–18	Mattress jumps side-to-side	30 sec
	13–18	Mattress jumps forward-backward	30 sec
	13–18	Hop, hop, hop, stick	5 reps each leg
	13–18	Jump into bounding	3–4 reps
Speed and agility training	1–18	Dot drill: various jump patterns	5 reps x 3
	1–3	Serpentine run	3 reps
	1–3,	Partner push-off	5 reps x 5 sec
	7–9,	Partner push-off	10 reps x 10 sec
	13–15	Partner push-off	10 reps x 15 sec
	1–6	Sprint/backpedal	6 reps
	1–9	Quick feet	2 reps x 45 sec
	1–9	Sprint-stop listen reaction drills	2 reps x 30 sec
	1–3	Four laps around field	1 rep
	4–6	Shuttle run	2 reps
	4–6	Resisted sprint with band	To baseline x 2
	10–12	Resisted sprint with band 25 yd	3 x 15 sec
	16–18	Resisted sprint with band 12 yd	4 x 15 sec
	4–6	100-yd shuttle run, 3 x 100 yd	4 reps
	7–9	Square drill	3 reps
	7–9	Half eagles into sprint, jog back	6 reps
	7–9	50-yd shuttle, up and back x 3	4 reps
	10–12	Nebraska drill	3 reps
	10–12	Box drill, 90° turns	3 reps
	10–18	Ladder drills	2 reps
	10–12	Mirror, reaction to partner	4 reps x 45 sec
	10–12	50-yd cone drill	4 reps
	13–15	Illinois drill	4 reps
	13–15	Sprint, 180°, backpedal	7 reps
Speed and agility training	13–18	Wheel reaction drill	6 reps x 60 sec
	13–18	Jingle jangle, 20 yd x 5	5 reps
	16–18	T-drill	4 reps
	16–18	Sprint, 260°, sprint	7 reps
Strength training	1–18	Explosion squats, band	30 sec
	1–18	Power lunges	30 sec
	1–18	Single-leg heel-raise	30 sec
	1–3	Supine hamstring bridge	30 sec
	4–18	Single-leg hamstring bridge	30 sec
	1–18	Seated scapular retraction	30 sec
	1–18	Seated latissimus pull	30 sec
	1–18	Seated scapular protraction	30 sec
	1–18	Seated external rotation	30 sec
	1–18	Partner internal rotation	30 sec
	1–18	Abdominals (variety)	30 sec
	1–18	Hip flexion strengthening (variety)	time, reps vary
	1–18	Hip abduction/adduction strengthening (variety)	time, reps vary
Flexibility training	1–18 (all)	Hamstrings Quadriceps Iliotibial band Hip flexor Gastrocnemius/soleus Deltoid Triceps Pectorals/biceps Low back	20–30 sec repeat 2 times each side

diagonally over the line followed quickly by the right foot. As soon as the right foot crosses the line, the athlete steps the left foot backward and diagonally (back over the line), again followed quickly by the right foot. This pattern is continued along the length of the line for 30 seconds. At the end of the first 30 seconds, the athlete proceeds back to the starting position, moving to the right, leading with the right foot and following with the left for 30 seconds.

Mistakes to correct include overlapping the feet while traveling along the line, rotating the upper body, leading with the wrong foot, taking very wide steps, bending forward at the waist, rounding the shoulders, and looking down at the feet/ground. The athlete should be told to keep the toes and knees pointed forward; keep the back straight, shoulders back, and head/eyes up; make the steps short and choppy, with feet not going wider than shoulder width; and keep speed under control until proper pattern is achieved.

2. **Ladder drill 1**. A 15-foot ladder is placed along a sideline. The athlete begins at the left end of the ladder and steps the right foot forward and diagonally over the ladder into the first square followed quickly by the left foot (Fig. 19–40). As soon as the left foot crosses the ladder, the right foot steps backward and diagonally (back over the ladder), again followed quickly by the left foot. This pattern is continued along the 15-foot distance until the right end of the ladder is reached. Then, the same pattern is repeated leading with the left foot back to the starting point. The athlete should travel back and forth along the distance of the ladder for 30 seconds. The athlete should be told to keep the feet shoulder-width apart at all times; make all steps quick, short, and choppy; keep the knees slightly bent and relaxed; keep the back straight and the head up with eyes forward; and try not to land on any portion of the ladder.

3. **Ladder drill 2**. A 15-foot agility ladder is placed flat on the floor. The athlete begins the drill at the bottom of the ladder, with the feet outside of the first ladder "square" (Fig. 19–41). The right foot steps forward into the first ladder "square" followed quickly by the left foot. As soon as the left foot touches down in the ladder "square," the right foot steps forward and laterally (to the outside right of the ladder) so that it is parallel to the ladder and in line with the ladder's rung. Once the right foot touches down outside of the ladder, the left foot steps

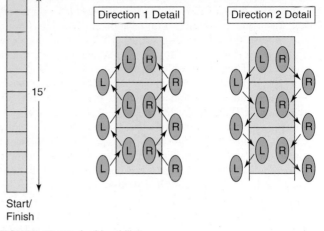

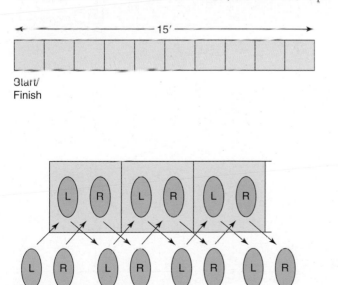

FIGURE 19–40. Ladder drill 1.

forward and laterally (to the outside left of the ladder) so that it is parallel to the ladder and in line with the rung. Once the left foot is down, the right foot steps forward and laterally into the next ladder "square," followed immediately by the left foot. This pattern is continued along the length of the ladder in order to move in and out of each of the ladder "squares." Upon reaching the end of the ladder, the same pattern described previously is followed, but the footwork moves backward in order to return to the starting position.

The athlete should be told to make all steps quick, short, and choppy; keep the knees slightly bent and relaxed; keep the back straight and head up with eyes forward; and try not to land on any portion of the ladder.

4. **T-drill**. A T-shaped course is created with three cones and a start/finish marker as shown in Figure 19–42. The first cone is placed 30 feet in front of the start/finish marker. The other two cones are placed so that each is exactly 15 feet from (and in line with) the first cone. This forms a 30-foot line that is perpendicular to the line formed by the start/finish marker

FIGURE 19–41. Ladder drill 2.

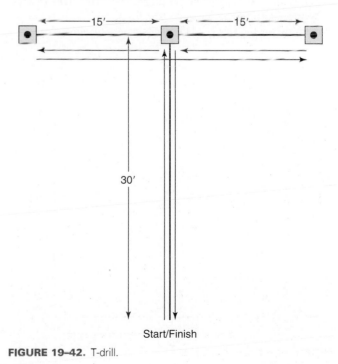

FIGURE 19–42. T-drill.

and the first cone. The athlete begins at the base of the "T" and sprints forward to the cone straight ahead. Upon reaching the cone, the athlete immediately shuffles left toward the cone to the left making sure that the feet do not cross at any point during the shuffle. The athlete taps the top of the cone. Then, the athlete shuffles right, making sure that the feet do not cross at any time. The athlete moves past the middle cone and shuffles to the cone located on the far right. The athlete taps the top of that cone and then shuffles left back toward the center cone. Once the center cone is reached, the athlete taps the top of the middle cone and immediately runs backward to the start/finish marker. Two repetitions of the course are completed, with at least 15 seconds rest between each repetition. A stopwatch is used to record the time of each repetition.

The athlete should be told to keep the head and neck straight, look straight ahead, keep the shoulders and hips square, do not round shoulders forward, make sure the back is straight, lean slightly forward for the duration of the activity, and make sure that the feet do not cross at any point during shuffle activities.

5. **Beanbag game.** A square course is created with flat markers placed on each corner of a 40- x 40-foot area on a gym floor (Fig. 19–43). Eight beanbags are placed in the center of the square. The athletes are divided into four groups (each group should contain the same number of athletes, if possible). Each group lines up behind one of the flat markers that will be their "home-base," and faces the beanbags. On the command "GO," one athlete from each team sprints to the center of the square and retrieves one of the beanbags for their team. Each athlete then sprints back to their home-base and places the beanbag on the flat marker so that the entire beanbag is on the marker. As soon as the beanbag is completely on the marker, the next team member leaves home-base and sprints to retrieve another beanbag. This teammate has the choice of going to the center of the square for a beanbag or running to the home-base of an opposing team to retrieve their bean-bag. After retrieving each beanbag, the team member must return the beanbag to their home-base so that it is resting entirely on the marker before their next teammate can take

off. The object of the game is for one team to get three bean-bags resting on their home base, and yell "BEANBAG," before anyone else. The first team to do this wins and receives a point. The game is played for 5 minutes in phase I, 7 minutes in phase II, and 9 minutes in phase III.

6. **Forward/backward sprints.** Starting on the baseline of a standard basketball court, the athlete sprints forward until the opposite baseline is reached (approximately 94 ft) and then immediately runs backward at ¾ speed to the starting baseline. The athlete completes 5 repetitions in phase I, 6 repetitions in phase II, and 7 repetitions in phase III, with 15 seconds rest between each repetition.

The athlete should be told to keep the head and neck straight, look straight ahead, keep the shoulders and hips square, do not round the shoulders forward, keep the back straight, lean slightly forward for the duration of the activity, and decelerate each sprint with a bent knee.

7. **Shuttle sprints.** Five cones are placed in a zigzag pattern within an 18- × 48-foot area (Fig. 19–44). Beginning to the left of the first cone, the athlete sprints across to the next cone in the pattern. Upon approaching the second cone, the athlete decelerates the sprint with choppy steps in order to allow for tapping the top of the cone once it is reached. As soon as the second cone is tapped, the athlete immediately accelerates across to the next cone and repeats the deceler-ate/tap/accelerate sequence until the last cone in the pattern is reached. Once the last cone is reached, the athlete rounds the cone and runs through the pattern again back to the start/finish line. One repetition involves running up and back the course. The athlete completes 2 repetitions with at least 15 seconds rest between each repetition. A stopwatch is used to time each repetition.

The athlete should be told to keep the head and neck straight, look straight ahead, keep the shoulders and hips

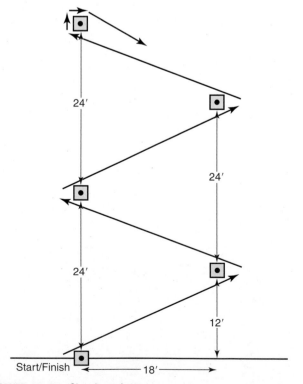

FIGURE 19–44. Shuttle sprints.

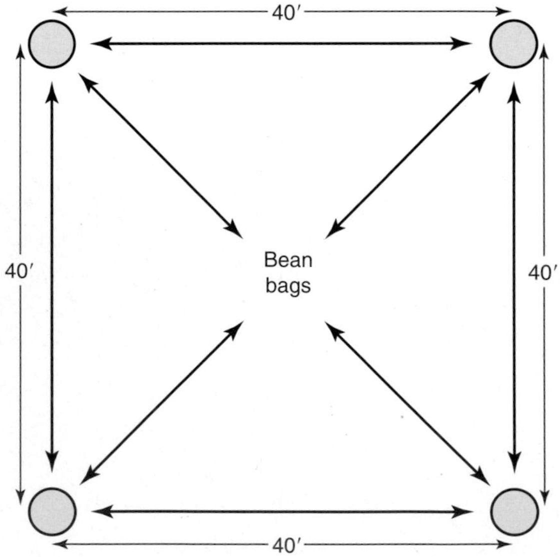

FIGURE 19–43. Beanbag game.

square, do not round the shoulders forward, keep the back straight, lean slightly forward for the duration of the activity, decelerate each sprint with a bent knee, and stay tight to the cones throughout the activity.

8. **Reaction agility drill 1.** During this drill, the athlete reacts to verbal cues given by an instructor who stands on the base-line. The athlete starts in the center of the court with the back facing the instructor (Fig. 19–45) and runs backward toward the instructor. The instructor commands the athlete to turn left or right, upon which time the athlete shuffles left or right. The instructor then commands the athlete to run backward diagonally toward the closest sideline, then sprint straight forward. The final command instructs the athlete to go to the left, center, or right of the cones. The length of each command is based on the instructor and space available. The drill is performed twice with 30 seconds rest.

9. **Reaction agility drill 2.** The athlete stands in the center of the court facing the instructor who is standing on the baseline. The instructor uses hand motions to indicate the direction the athlete should move toward. For example, if the instructor points straight forward, the athlete will backpedal away from the instructor. If the instructor points to the right, the athlete will side shuffle to the left. If the instructor points diagonally to the right, the athlete will backpedal diagonally to the left. The length of each command is based on the instructor and space available. The drill is performed twice for 30 seconds, with 30 seconds rest between repetitions. As athletes progress, the time for this drill is increased to 45 seconds.

Sportsmetrics Return to Play

The Sportsmetrics Return to Play program was developed for athletes who have suffered an injury or undergone ACL recon-struction as an end-stage component to rehabilitation. Part of the problem in today's managed care environment is that few physical therapy visits are allowed after surgery. By the time an athlete is nearing completion of rehabilitation, her or his visits are typically no longer covered. In the Return to Play program, the athlete trains at home using instructional videotapes, but

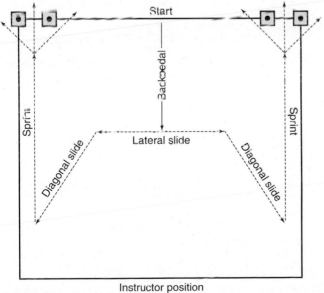

FIGURE 19–45. Reaction agility drill.

must see the physical therapist three times during training: before training begins, 2 weeks later prior to the start of the sec-ond phase of Sportsmetrics, and then 2 weeks later before the start of the third phase of training. In this manner, the therapist can watch and educate the athlete regarding proper form and positioning for each jump.

The indications to initiate this training program are isoki-netic lower extremity muscle strength of at least 80% of that of the contralateral side, successful completion of a running pro-gram, and no symptoms of pain, swelling, or instability with any activity.

STRATEGIES FOR IMPLEMENTATION OF NEUROMUSCULAR TRAINING

Educate Health Care Professionals to Conduct Formal Neuromuscular Training

In order to implement Sportsmetrics on a national basis, a for-mal course was devised to educate and certify health care profes-sionals and coaches who wished to conduct training in their communities. The 13-hour formal course teaches (1) the the-ories of why female athletes have an increased incidence of seri-ous knee ligament injuries compared with males, (2) the scientific basis of Sportsmetrics, (3) the necessity for neuromus-cular training versus plyometric performance-enhancement training, (4) the verbal cues and methods required to teach the program to produce a change in landing mechanics and body positioning, (5) the differences between Sportsmetrics and other neuromuscular-training programs, (6) marketing strategies and ways to implement training in the community, (7) the necessity to conduct sports injury testing (see Chapter 16, Lower Limb Neuromuscular Control and Strength in Prepubescent and Ado-lescent Male and Female Athletes) and produce research data, and (8) for those involved in rehabilitation clinics, the imple-mentation of Sportsmetrics as a component of rehabilitation after ACL reconstruction.

Participants are given a detailed demonstration of every jump and spend a few hours practicing the jumps themselves and con-ducting mock instructions for the teaching staff. Each partici-pant is taken through the sports injury test and given step by-step instruction on the video drop-jump test (see Chapter 16, Lower Limb Neuromuscular Control and Strength in Prepubescent and Adolescent Male and Female Athletes). A for-mal written examination is conducted to ascertain that the par-ticipant has adequate knowledge of knee anatomy and strength training and plyometric concepts. A practical examination is done in which the participant trains a local athlete to demon-strate to our staff that he or she understands the correct verbal cues and training methodology to produce the desired result of proper body positioning and landing mechanics.

Step-by-Step Instructional Videotapes of Training

Because not all athletes have access to a certified instructor, a two-volume instructional videotape set and detailed manual are available. The first volume focuses on technique and teaching the proper form for body positioning and landing position.

The second volume provides a step-by-step analysis of the training program and includes the dynamic warm-up, jumps, and flexibility exercises.

Problems Encountered and Suggested Solutions

In the authors' experience, young athletes are easily convinced to participate in performance enhancement training. However, unless they or someone they know has gone through a serious knee ligament injury, they simply do not comprehend the consequences of such an injury. It takes considerable effort on the part of the health care professional to educate and motivate athletes to undergo 6 weeks of training (3 times/wk) to prevent an injury. In a similar manner, coaches are difficult to convince unless they have lost a number of athletes to ACL injuries. It appears that this problem is going to require further education of health care professionals; mission statements from national organizations such as the American Academy of Orthopaedic Surgeons, the National Institutes of Health, and the American Orthopaedic Society for Sports Medicine; and continued media attention before widespread training and the benefits of an injury prevention program are realized.

Many high school athletes either participate in multiple sports or play their one particular sport yearround. This is especially true with soccer players, who in some communities never have an off-season. The integration of neuromuscular training into the schedules of these athletes is challenging. Solutions include incorporating Sportsmetrics training into an existing sports-specific training and conditioning program or to make the neuromuscular training itself sports-specific.

REFERENCES

1. Barber, S. D.; Noyes, F. R.; Mangine, R. E.; et al.: Quantitative assessment of functional limitations in normal and anterior cruciate ligament–deficient knees. *Clin Orthop* 255:204–214, 1990.
2. Caraffa, A.; Cerulli, G.; Projetti, M.; et al.: Prevention of anterior cruciate ligament injuries in soccer. A prospective controlled study of proprioceptive training. *Knee Surg Sports Traumatol Arthrosc* 4: 19–21, 1996.
3. Chu, D. A.: Explosive power. In Foran, B. (ed.): *High-Performance Sports Conditioning*. Champaign, IL: Human Kinetics, 2001; pp. 83–98.
4. Delecluse, C.; Van Coppenolle, H.; Willems, E.; et al.: Influence of high-resistance and high-velocity training on sprint performance. *Med Sci Sports Exerc* 27:1203–1209, 1995.
5. DeMorat, G.; Weinhold, P.; Blackburn, T.; et al.: Aggressive quadriceps loading can induce noncontact anterior cruciate ligament injury. *Am J Sports Med* 32:477–483, 2004.
6. Ettlinger, C. F.; Johnson, R. J.; Shealy, J. E.: A method to help reduce the risk of serious knee sprains incurred in alpine skiing. *Am J Sports Med* 23:531–537, 1995.
7. Greenfield, M. L.; Kuhn, J. E.; Wojtys, E. M.: A statistics primer. Power analysis and sample size determination. *Am J Sports Med* 25:138–140, 1997.
8. Griffin, L. Y.; Agel, J.; Albohm, M. J.; et al.: Noncontact anterior cruciate ligament injuries: risk factors and prevention strategies. *J Am Acad Orthop Surg* 8:141–150, 2000.
9. Griffin, L. Y.; Albohm, M. J.; Arendt, E. A.; et al.: Understanding and preventing noncontact anterior cruciate ligament injuries: a review of the Hunt Valley II meeting, January 2005. *Am J Sports Med* 34:1512–1532, 2006.
10. Grood, E. S.; Suntay, W. J.; Noyes, F. R.; Butler, D. L.: Biomechanics of the knee-extension exercise. Effect of cutting the anterior cruciate ligament. *J Bone Joint Surg Am* 66:725–734, 1984.
11. Heidt, R. S., Jr.; Sweeterman, L. M.; Carlonas, R. L.; et al.: Avoidance of soccer injuries with preseason conditioning. *Am J Sports Med* 28:659–662, 2000.
12. Hewett, T. E.; Lindenfeld, T. N.; Riccobene, J. V.; Noyes, F. R.: The effect of neuromuscular training on the incidence of knee injury in female athletes. A prospective study. *Am J Sports Med* 27:699–706, 1999.
13. Hewett, T. E.; Stroupe, A. L.; Nance, T. A.; Noyes, F. R.: Plyometric training in female athletes. Decreased impact forces and increased hamstring torques. *Am J Sports Med* 24:765–773, 1996.
14. Holm, I.; Fosdahl, M. A.; Friis, A.; et al.: Effect of neuromuscular training on proprioception, balance, muscle strength, and lower limb function in female team handball players. *Clin J Sport Med* 14:88–94, 2004.
15. Hutchinson, M. R.; Ireland, M. L.: Knee injuries in female athletes. *Sports Med* 19:288–302, 1995.
16. Irmischer, B. S.; Harris, C.; Pfeiffer, R. P.; et al.: Effects of a knee ligament injury prevention exercise program on impact forces in women. *J Strength Cond Res* 18:703–707, 2004.
17. Krosshaug, T.; Nakamae, A.; Boden, B. P.; et al.: Mechanisms of anterior cruciate ligament injury in basketball: video analysis of 39 cases. *Am J Sports Med* 35:359–367, 2007.
18. Malinzak, R. A.; Colby, S. M.; Kirkendall, D. T.; et al.: A comparison of knee joint motion patterns between men and women in selected athletic tasks. *Clin Biomech (Bristol, Avon)* 16:438–445, 2001.
19. Mandelbaum, B. R.; Silvers, H. J.; Watanabe, D. S.; et al.: Effectiveness of a neuromuscular and proprioceptive training program in preventing anterior cruciate ligament injuries in female athletes: 2-year follow-up. *Am J Sports Med* 33:1003–1010, 2005.
20. Markolf, K. L.; Burchfield, D. M.; Shapiro, M. M.; et al.: Combined knee loading states that generate high anterior cruciate ligament forces. *J Orthop Res* 13:930–935, 1995.
21. Myer, G. D.; Ford, K. R.; McLean, S. G.; Hewett, T. E.: The effects of plyometric versus dynamic stabilization and balance training on lower extremity biomechanics. *Am J Sports Med* 34:445–455, 2006.
22. Myklebust, G.; Engebretsen, L.; Braekken, I. H.; et al.: Prevention of anterior cruciate ligament injuries in female team handball players: a prospective intervention study over three seasons. *Clin J Sport Med* 13:71–78, 2003.
23. Noyes, F. R.; Barber, S. D.; Mangine, R. E.: Abnormal lower limb symmetry determined by function hop tests after anterior cruciate ligament rupture. *Am J Sports Med* 19:513–518, 1991.
24. Noyes, F. R.; Barber-Westin, S. D.; Fleckenstein, C.; et al.: The drop-jump screening test: difference in lower limb control by gender and effect of neuromuscular training in female athletes. *Am J Sports Med* 33:197–207, 2005.
25. Noyes, F. R.; Sonstegard, D. A.: Biomechanical function of the pes anserinus at the knee and the effect of its transplantation. *J Bone Joint Surg Am* 55:1225–1241, 1973.
26. O'Connor, J. J.: Can muscle co-contraction protect knee ligaments after injury or repair? *J Bone Joint Surg Br* 75:41–48, 1993.
27. Olsen, O. E.; Myklebust, G.; Engebretsen, L.; et al.: Exercises to prevent lower limb injuries in youth sports: cluster randomised controlled trial. *BMJ* 330(7489):449, 2005.
28. Petersen, W.; Braun, C.; Bock, W.; et al.: A controlled prospective case control study of a prevention training program in female team handball players: the German experience. *Arch Orthop Trauma Surg* 125:614–621, 2005.
29. Pfeiffer, R. P.; Shea, K. G.; Roberts, D.; et al.: Lack of effect of a knee ligament injury prevention program on the incidence of noncontact anterior cruciate ligament injury. *J Bone Joint Surg Am* 88:1769–1774, 2006.
30. Pluim, B. M.; Staal, J. B.; Windler, G. E.; Jayanthi, N.: Tennis injuries: occurrence, aetiology, and prevention. *Br J Sports Med* 40:415–423, 2006.
31. Prapavessis, H.; McNair, P. J.: Effects of instruction in jumping technique and experience jumping on ground reaction forces. *J Orthop Sports Phys Ther* 29:352–356, 1999.
32. Rimmer, E.; Sleivert, G.: Effects of a plyometric intervention program on sprint performance. *J Strength Cond Res* 14:295–301, 2000.

33. Soderman, K.; Werner, S.; Pietila, T.; et al.: Balance board training: prevention of traumatic injuries of the lower extremities in female soccer players? A prospective randomized intervention study. *Knee Surg Sports Traumatol Arthrosc* 8:356–363, 2000.
34. Wedderkopp, N.; Kaltoft, M.; Holm, R.; Froberg, K.: Comparison of two intervention programmes in young female players in European handball—with and without ankle disc. *Scand J Med Sci Sports* 13:371–375, 2003.
35. Wedderkopp, N.; Kaltoft, M.; Lundgaard, B.; et al.: Prevention of injuries in young female players in European team handball.

A prospective intervention study. *Scand J Med Sci Sports* 9:41–47, 1999.
36. Wilkerson, G. B.; Colston, M. A.; Short, N. I.; et al.: Neuromuscular changes in female collegiate athletes resulting from a plyometric jump-training program. *J Athl Train* 39:17–23, 2004.
37. Withrow, T. J.; Huston, L. J.; Wojtys, E. M.; Ashton-Miller, J. A.: Effect of varying hamstring tension on anterior cruciate ligament strain during in vitro impulsive knee flexion and compression loading. *J Bone Joint Surg Am* 90:815–823, 2008.

Posterior Cruciate Ligament and Posterolateral Ligament Structures

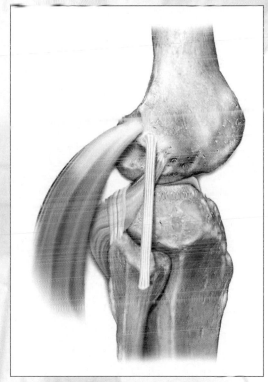

Chapter 20

Function of the Posterior Cruciate Ligament and Posterolateral Ligament Structures

Frank R. Noyes, MD ■ *Sue D. Barber-Westin*, BS

INTRODUCTION

The purpose of this chapter is to provide a summary of the important biomechanical principles gained from studies from the authors' laboratory and other investigations regarding the posterior cruciate ligament (PCL) and posterolateral structures (PLS). The primary posterolateral structures of the knee joint are the fibular collateral ligament (FCL) and popliteus muscle-tendon-ligament unit (PMTL), including the popliteofibular ligament (PFL) and posterolateral capsule (PLC). Additional PLS that may be injured and require repair are the iliotibial band femoral and tibial attachments, meniscal tibial and femoral attachments (including fascicles), the fabellofibular ligament, and the lateral and anterior capsule. All of these structures are illustrated in Chapter 2, Lateral, Posterior, and Cruciate Knee Anatomy. Data from these investigations provide the basis for the diagnosis of abnormal knee motion limits in single and combined ligament injuries and allow the surgeon to plan the appropriate ligament reconstructive procedure.

EFFECT OF SECTIONING THE PCL AND PLS ON THE LIMITS OF KNEE MOTION

A series of studies were conducted in cadaveric knees to measure the limits of anteroposterior (AP) translation, internal-external tibial rotation, and varus-valgus rotation (using a six-degrees-of-freedom electrogoniometer) under specific forces and moments with a verified testing apparatus previously described.[8,24,25,31,64,97]

The PCL and PLS were sectioned in 15 knees first separately and then in combination to measure the resultant abnormal knee motion limits to simulate isolated and combined ligament ruptures.[25] The PLS in this investigation included the FCL, PMTL, and PLC. A 100-N force was applied to determine the AP limits, 5 Nm was used for internal-external rotation limits, and 20 Nm was used for adduction-abduction (varus-valgus) limits from 0° to 100° of knee flexion.

In these ligament-cutting experiments, the popliteus tendon was sectioned from the femoral attachment, which effectively removed the entire popliteus muscle tendon and PFL static

Cadaveric studies measured limits of anteroposterior (AP) translation, internal-external tibial rotation, varus-valgus rotation under specific forces and moments.

100 N force applied to determine the AP limits, 5 Nm for internal-external rotation limits, 20 Nm for adduction-abduction (varus-valgus) limits from 0° to 100° of knee flexion.

Effect on Limits of Knee Extension

- No primary restraint to hyperextension, structures work together: entire posterior knee capsule, oblique popliteal ligament, fabellofibular ligament, posterior fibers posterior cruciate ligament (PCL), and anterior cruciate ligament (ACL).

Effect on AP Translation Limits0

- PCL primary restraint to posterior tibial translation throughout knee flexion.
- Increased posterior translation at 30°–45° flexion associated injury to posterolateral structures (PLS), medial ligament structures.

Effect on Internal-External Tibial Rotation Limits

- No increase external tibial rotation PCL cut alone.
- PLS primary restraint external tibial rotation low knee flexion positions; test 20°–40° flexion.
- Increases in external tibial rotation at 90° indicate injury to PLS and PCL

Effect on Adduction-Abduction Rotation Limits

- PLS primary restraint adduction-abduction rotation limits.
- Loss PLS converts both cruciate ligaments into primary restraints for varus loading.
- Combined rupture PCL/PLS requires surgical restoration of all structures.
- Abnormal medial or lateral joint opening (gap test) at arthroscopy: concurrent medial or lateral ligament reconstruction.

function. In other experiments to be described,[67] the PFL was sectioned independently of the popliteus tendon attachment to investigate the individual function of this ligament. The PLC was removed, including all soft tissue structures posterior to the FCL, to ensure that the individual soft tissue components were removed. This included, in addition to the PLC, additional tissue components comprising the fabellofibular ligament and capsular arm of the biceps femoris short head.

Effect on Limits of Extension

The normal fully hyperextended knee position averaged 5.6° ± 3.8°. After sectioning the PCL or PLS alone, only slight and clinically insignificant increases in hyperextension were noted (such as 2.6° ± 0.09° when the PLS was cut). When both the PCL and the PLS were sectioned, the increase in hyperextension was 4.0° ± 1.4°.

The data indicate that there is no primary restraint in the knee that resists hyperextension. Many structures work in synergy to resist hyperextension, and it is therefore not surprising that sectioning only the PLS or PCL results in a small increase. Other structures anatomically positioned to resist hyperextension include the entire posterior knee capsule (femoral-meniscal tibial attachments), oblique popliteal ligament, fabellofibular ligament, and the posterior fibers of the PCL and anterior cruciate ligament (ACL).

Effect on AP Translation Limits

The normal anterior and posterior translation knee limits are shown in Figure 20–1A. The increase in these limits when the PCL is cut are shown in Figure 20–1B, and the further increase

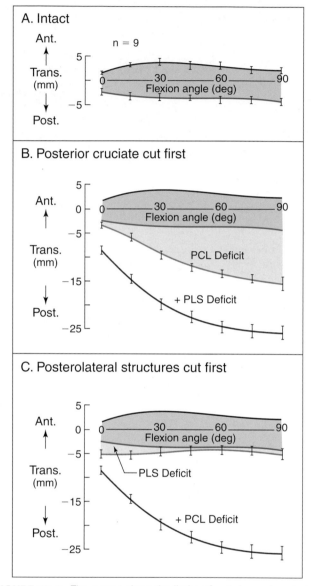

FIGURE 20–1. The curves show the limits of anterior and posterior translation (vertical axis) when a 100-N anteroposterior (AP) force was applied. **A,** Intact knees. The curves show the average limits of motion and the standard deviation for nine knees. The range of total AP translation of the intact knee is shown in *shaded green* in **A, B,** and **C. B,** Posterior cruciate ligament (PCL) is cut first. The increase in posterior translation after cutting the PCL is shown in the *orange-shaded* area (PCL deficit). The limit of posterior translation, and therefore the amount of increase, is controlled by the remaining intact structures. The *unshaded portion* (+ PLS deficit) shows the added increase when the posterolateral structures (fibular collateral ligament [FCL], capsule, popliteus muscle-tendon-ligament [PMTL]) were cut after the PCL had first been removed. A concurrent external rotation took place with this cut. **C,** Posterolateral structures are cut first. There was only a small increase (PLS deficit) in the posterior limit near full extension when the posterolateral structural elements were cut first. A concurrent external rotation was also present. *(A–C, From Grood, E. S.; Stowers, S. F.; Noyes, F. R.: Limits of movement in the human knee. Effect of sectioning the posterior cruciate ligament and posterolateral structures. J Bone Joint Surg Am 70:88–97, 1988.)*

TABLE 20–1   Increased Motion Compared With Normal Motion that Occurred when the Indicated Structures Were Sectioned*

	Angle of Flexion				
	0°	15°	30°	60°	90°
Anterior limit (mm)					
All cut	0.5 ± 0.8	0.6 ± 0.6	0.7 ± 0.7	0.4 ± 1.3	0.8 ± 1.0
Posterior limit (mm)					
PCL cut	1.0 ± 1.6	3.6 ± 1.6	6.4 ± 1.5	9.6 ± 1.3	11.4 ± 1.9
PLS cut	3.1 ± 0.7	1.9 ± 0.8	1.4 ± 1.1	0.7 ± 0.8	0.5 ± 0.7
All cut	6.6 ± 2.7	11.3 ± 3.1	15.8 ± 3.0	20.7 ± 3.4	21.5 ± 3.4
External rotation limit (°)					
PCL cut	0.4 ± 0.5	0.2 ± 0.5	0.2 ± 0.6	0.4 ± 0.9	0.6 ± 1.2
PLS cut	8.5 ± 2.6	11.8 ± 3.0	13.0 ± 2.3	5.2 ± 9.0	5.3 ± 2.6
All cut	10.5 ± 4.0	14.2 ± 3.7	18.0 ± 3.8	21.0 ± 3.1	20.9 ± 2.8
Varus angulation limit (°)					
FCL cut	2.5 ± 0.4	4.5 ± 0.4	5.7 ± 0.2	5.5 ± 0.6	4.3 ± 0.9
PCL cut	0.4 ± 0.6	0.4 ± 0.6	0.4 ± 0.6	0.8 ± 0.6	1.4 ± 0.6
PLS cut	6.4 ± 2.3	7.9 ± 2.0	9.0 ± 2.0	8.3 ± 3.7	6.8 ± 4.5
All cut	8.1 ± 2.5	11.3 ± 3.0	14.2 ± 3.3	18.9 ± 3.4	21.2 ± 3.0
Valgus angulation limit (°)					
PCL cut	0.3 ± 0.6	0.3 ± 1.0	0.5 ± 1.7	0.7 ± 1.9	0.5 ± 1.0

*All values are given as mean ± standard deviation (SD).
FCL, fibular collateral ligament; PCL, posterior cruciate ligament; PLS, posterolateral structures (FCL, capsule, popliteus muscle-tendon-ligament [PMTL]).

in these limits when the PLS are also sectioned are shown in Figure 20-1C. The values for the increase in motion limits are given in Table 20–1.

The data show that the PCL is a primary restraint to posterior tibial translation throughout knee flexion, with the exception of a small increase in posterior translation at full extension when the PLS are cut. The clinical finding of a knee with increased posterior translation at 30° to 45° of knee flexion, similar to the posterior translation limit at 90° (Fig. 20–2), indicates associated injury to the PLS and the medial structures.

It should be noted that a complete description of the translation limits requires an anatomic measurable point on the tibia, which is selected at the midcoronal point of the tibia. The limits of posterior translation to the medial and lateral tibiofemoral joints are described in a subsequent study.[64]

In a knee with a combined deficiency of the PCL and the PLS, the abnormal posterior tibial translation is at least four to five times the normal limit throughout knee flexion.

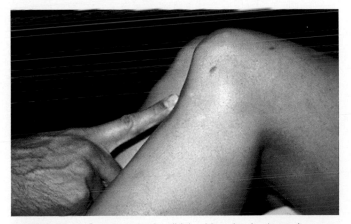

FIGURE 20–2. Severe posterior tibial subluxation is shown in a chronic PCL-deficient knee, which is either due to physiologic laxity of the remaining secondary restraints or the result of a traumatic injury.

Effect on Internal-External Tibial Rotation Limits

The normal knee motion limits to internal and external tibial rotation are shown in Figure 20–3A. There is no increase in external tibial rotation when the PCL is cut alone (see Fig. 20–3B). This finding demonstrates that the PLS are the primary restraint for external tibial rotation throughout knee flexion. When the PLS only are sectioned, an increase in external tibial rotation occurs (see Fig. 20–3C), which is greatest at 30° of knee flexion. The amount of external tibial rotation decreases as the knee is flexed, showing the influence of the PCL in limiting external tibial rotation after the PLS are sectioned.

These data indicate that the PLS provide the primary restraint to external tibial rotation at low knee flexion positions and, therefore, should be tested in this range (20°–40° flexion). Increases in external tibial rotation at 90° indicate injury to both the PLS and the PCL, consistent with the dial test (see Chapter 22, Posterolateral Ligament Injuries: Diagnosis, Operative Techniques, and Clinical Outcomes). The data are in disagreement with the classic interpretation of the posterolateral drawer test at 90° flexion, indicating injury to only the PLS. The resisting function of the FCL, popliteus tendon, and PFL is described in separate studies later in this chapter.

Gollehon and coworkers[22] reported an increase in external tibial rotation of 20° flexion after sectioning the PLS at 30° of flexion. Sectioning of the PCL along with the PLS did not produce further significant increases in external tibial rotation (Fig. 20–4).

Effect on Adduction-Abduction Rotation Limits

The normal limits of adduction and abduction rotation are shown in Figure 20–5A. Sectioning the PCL produces very small changes in these limits (see Fig. 20–5B). When the PLS are sectioned alone, large increases in adduction occur (see

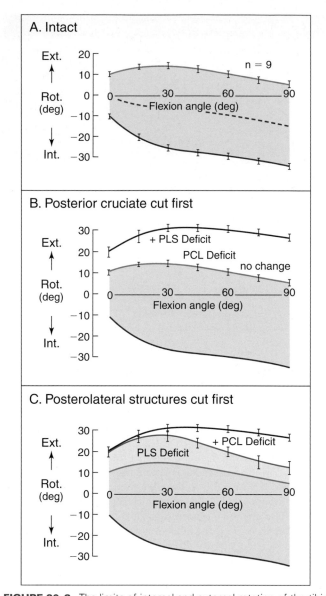

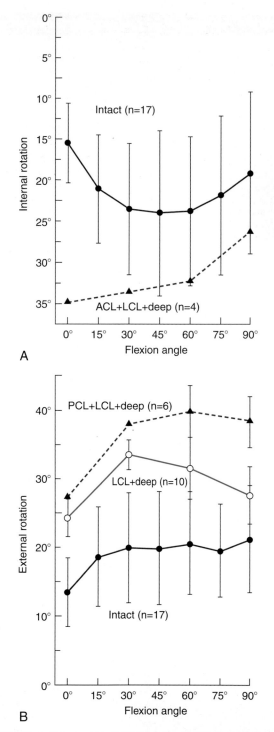

FIGURE 20–3. The limits of internal and external rotation of the tibia when a 5-N torque was applied. The fully extended position, measured in the intact knee, was used as the zero-rotation reference. **A,** Intact knees. The *upper curve* shows the limit of external rotation. The *broken line* shows the average position of the knee during passive flexion with the tibia hanging freely. The range of tibial rotation in the intact knee is shaded in **A, B,** and **C. B,** PCL is cut first. No change was found in external tibial rotation. **C,** Posterolateral structures (FCL, capsule, PMTL) are cut first. Increases in external tibial rotation occurred at low flexion angles. With added PCL sectioning, the increase in external tibial rotation occurred at high flexion angles. (*A–C, From Grood, E. S.; Stowers, S. F.; Noyes, F. R.: Limits of movement in the human knee. Effect of sectioning the posterior cruciate ligament and posterolateral structures. J Bone Joint Surg Am 70:88–97, 1988.*)

FIGURE 20–4. Primary internal and external tibial rotations resulting from 4.5 Nm of internal and external tibial torque in intact knees and after ligament sectioning. **A,** Increased internal rotation occurred only with combined section of the lateral collateral ligament (LCL [FCL]), deep structures (PMTL and capsule), and anterior cruciate ligament (ACL). **B,** Increased external rotation occurred at all angles of flexion with combined section of the LCL and deep structures, with additional increases at 60° and 90° when the PCL was sectioned. The *broken lines* indicate a lack of statistical difference from the adjacent curve unless otherwise stated. (*A and B, From Gollehon, D. L.; Torzilli, P. A.; Warren, R. F.: The role of the posterolateral and cruciate ligaments in the stability of the human knee. A biomechanical study. J Bone Joint Surg Am 69:233–242, 1987.*)

Fig. 20–5C), indicating that these structures are the primary restraint to this knee motion. Once the PLS are removed, the PCL becomes a primary restraint and large increases in the adduction limit occur with knee flexion.

The limits to adduction (varus angulation) are graphed in Figure 20–6[25] after sectioning the FCL, the PLS (PMTL and PLC), and all structures (PCL, FCL, PMTL, and PLC). The

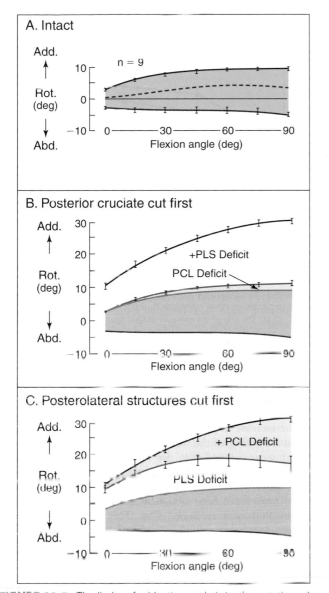

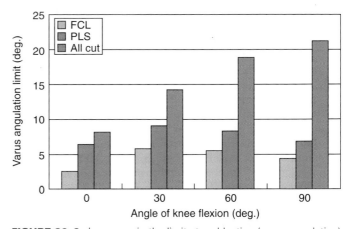

FIGURE 20–6. Increases in the limits to adduction (varus angulation) are shown after sectioning the FCL, the posterolateral capsule (PLC; PMTL and PLC), and all structures (PCL, FCL, PMTL, and PLC). The data demonstrate that the FCL is the primary restraint for lateral joint opening, with further increases after the remaining posterolateral structures are sectioned. *(From Grood, E. S.; Stowers, S. F.; Noyes, F. R.: Limits of movement in the human knee. Effect of sectioning the posterior cruciate ligament and posterolateral structures. J Bone Joint Surg Am 70:88 .97, 1988.)*

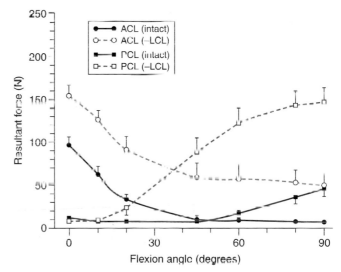

FIGURE 20–5. The limits of adduction and abduction rotation when a 20 Nm moment was applied. The fully extended position, measured in the intact knee, was used as the zero-rotation reference. **A,** Intact knees. The *upper curve* shows the limit of adduction rotation, and the *lower curve,* the limit of abduction rotation. The *broken line* shows the amount of adduction when the knee is passively flexed, with the tibia upside down to ensure tibiofemoral contact in both the medial and the lateral compartment. **B,** PCL is cut first. **C,** Posterolateral structures (FCL, capsule, PMTL) are cut first. *(A–C, From Grood, E. S.; Stowers, S. F., Noyes, F. R.: Limits of movement in the human knee. Effect of sectioning the posterior cruciate ligament and posterolateral structures. J Bone Joint Surg Am 70:88–97, 1988.)*

FIGURE 20–7. Graph shows the forces generated in the ACL and the PCL by 10.0 Nm of applied varus bending moment before (INTACT) and after section of the LCL (FCL) and the posterolateral structures (LCL). The increases in the mean force in the ACL after ligamentous section were significant at all angles of flexion; the increases in the mean force in the PCL were significant from 45° to 90° of flexion. The mean values for eight specimens are shown; the *error bars* indicate the standard error of the mean (SEM). *(From Markolf, K. L.; Wascher, D. C.; Finerman, G. A.: Direct in vitro measurement of forces in the cruciate ligaments. Part II: the effect of section of the posterolateral structures. J Bone Joint Surg Am 75:387–394, 1993.)*

data demonstrate that the FCL is the primary restraint for lateral joint opening, with further increases after the remaining PLS are sectioned.

Markolf and associates[52] developed an in vitro system in cadaveric knees in which load transducers were used to measure ACL and PCL forces under different loading situations. After sectioning the FCL and the other PLS, large increases were noted in resisting tensile forces in both cruciate ligaments under varus loading (Fig. 20–7) and in the PCL under posterior tibial loads and external tibial torques (Fig. 20–8). These findings

are in agreement with prior studies, because the loss of the PLS converts both cruciate ligaments into primary restraints for varus loading, in which the ligaments are poorly positioned with small lever arms to resist this motion.

The importance of load-sharing of the PLS with the PCL is demonstrated in many studies, which reinforces the need in knees with combined PCL-PLS ruptures to also perform

increase in posterior translation of the lateral tibial plateau compared with the intact state averaged 17.8 mm and 23.5 mm at 30° and 90° of flexion, respectively. The increase in posterior translation of the medial tibial plateau over the intact state averaged 7.6 mm and 12.3 mm at 30° and 90° of flexion, respectively.

External Tibial Rotation

The mean values of the external tibial rotation limits for the intact knees and after sectioning the PLS and PLS/PCL are shown in Table 20–2. Cutting the PLS caused a significant increase (P < .01) in external tibial rotation at both 30° (mean increase, 13.0°) and 90° (mean increase, 5.4°) of flexion. Sectioning the PCL along with the PLS caused a further increase in external tibial rotation at 30° (mean increase, 5.0°; not significant) and at 90° of flexion (mean increase 15.1°, P < .01). Considerable variability was present between specimens in the amount of measured external tibial rotation at 30° (see Fig. 20–13) and 90° (see Fig. 20–14) of flexion.

From these data, a classification system of rotatory subluxations was devised based on two concepts: the final position of the medial and lateral tibial plateaus under defined loading conditions (such as with either internal or external tibial rotation at a

defined knee flexion angle) and the position of each plateau. There are three possible positions for each plateau: anterior subluxation, normal position, or posterior subluxation. For each of these positions of the lateral tibial plateau, there exist three corresponding positions for the medial tibial plateau (Fig. 20–18).

This study showed that in normal knees under the conditions of external tibial rotation (5 Nm) and a posterior force (100 N) at 30° of flexion, the lateral tibial plateau displaced a mean of 7.5 ± 2.9 mm. After sectioning the PLS, a further increase to 15.5 ± 3.5 mm was noted, representing an increase of 8 mm of posterior tibial subluxation of the lateral tibia plateau from normal. This is the amount that the clinician may palpate on the lateral tibiofemoral step-off with external tibial rotation in knees with ruptures to the PLS (compared with the opposite knee). After sectioning the PCL (in addition to the PLS), a mean posterior translation of 25.3 ± 5.2 mm was demonstrated, representing a 17.8-mm increase from normal.

Under the same loading conditions at 90° of flexion, sectioning only the PLS resulted in a small (2.7-mm) increase in posterior translation of the lateral tibial plateau. These data agree with the external tibial knee motion limits previously reported,[25] in which small and insignificant increases in external tibial rotation occurred at 90° after PLS sectioning. When the PCL was also sectioned, the lateral tibial plateau demonstrated a gross posterior subluxation, with a mean posterior translation of 34.2 ± 3.5 mm (23.5 mm from normal).

TABLE 20–2 External Rotation Limits (100 N Posterior Force, 5 Nm External Moment)	
Flexion	**External Rotation (°; Mean ± SD)**
30°	
Intact	18.2 ± 3.9
PLS* cut	31.2 ± 5.0
PLS, PCL cut[†]	36.2 ± 4.7
90°	
Intact	17.4 ± 3.5
PLS cut	22.8 ± 5.0
PLS, PCL cut[†]	37.9 ± 3.0

*PLS, posterolateral structures including fibular collateral ligament (FCL).
[†]PCL, posterior cruciate ligament and ligaments of Humphry and Wrisberg cut in addition to the PLS and FCL.
SD, standard deviation.

Effect of Physiologic Laxity

Normal knees that had greater physiologic laxity (greater posterior tibial translation and degrees of external rotation) had larger amounts of posterior subluxation of the lateral tibial plateau when the PLS were sectioned. It is important to note that the posterior subluxation of the lateral tibial plateau varied from 10 mm to 18 mm at 30° of flexion and from 9 mm to 18 mm at 90° of flexion. This represents the displacement required to tense the PCL to resist further posterior subluxation of the lateral tibial plateau. In intact knees that had low values for posterior tibial displacements, ligament cutting resulted in a small increase in posterior

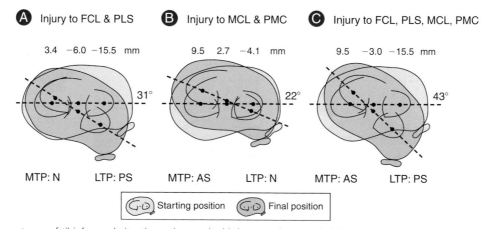

A Injury to FCL & PLS   **B** Injury to MCL & PMC   **C** Injury to FCL, PLS, MCL, PMC

3.4 −6.0 −15.5 mm   9.5 2.7 −4.1 mm   9.5 −3.0 −15.5 mm

31°   22°   43°

MTP: N   LTP: PS   MTP: AS   LTP: N   MTP: AS   LTP: PS

Starting position   Final position

FIGURE 20–18. Three types of tibiofemoral situations observed with increased external tibial rotation. **A,** Abnormal posterior translation of the lateral tibial plateau (at 30° of knee flexion under the loading conditions described in the study). **B,** Abnormal anterior translation of the medial tibial plateau under loading conditions of 5 Nm (at 30° of knee flexion). **C,** Abnormal posterior translation of the lateral tibial plateau plus abnormal anterior translation of the medial tibial plateau after sectioning both the medial and the lateral ligament structures. AS, anterior subluxation; FCL, fibular collateral ligament; LTP, lateral tibial plateau; MCL, medial collateral ligament; MTP, medial tibial plateau; N, normal position; PLS, posterolateral structures (FCL, PMTL); PMC, posterior medial capsule; PS, posterior subluxation. *(A–C, From Noyes, F. R.; Stowers, S. F.; Grood, E. S.; et al.: Posterior subluxations of the medial and lateral tibiofemoral compartments. An in vitro ligament sectioning study in cadaveric knees. Am J Sports Med 21:407–414, 1993.)*

subluxation, which was often lower than that measured in the normal "physiologically loose" knees.

From a clinical standpoint, knees that normally have low values for posterior subluxation that have substantial damage to the PLS may demonstrate only minimal increases in posterior tibial subluxation on external tibial rotation due to the secondary resistance provided by the PCL. Conversely, in knees with physiologic laxity, large increases in posterior tibial plateau subluxation may be detected after isolated PLS rupture because there is little resistance provided by the PCL. This finding explains the importance of individualizing the examination to each patient and determining his or her laxity profile. The surgeon should expect substantial differences in ligament stress tests in "tight" versus "loose" jointed knees, which determine the amount of displacement before other secondary ligament restraints block further joint displacements.

The data in this experiment confirm the significant increase in posterior subluxation of the lateral tibial plateau at 30° knee flexion after sectioning the PLS, but not at 90° flexion. In addition, the data show that there is no significant increase in external tibial rotation after the PCL is sectioned. The data also confirm that the diagnosis of injury to the PLS is based on the final posterior position of the lateral tibial plateau and not on the degrees of external tibial rotation. This is because an increase in external tibial rotation may occur with anterior subluxation of the medial tibial plateau when damage to the medial ligamentous structures is present.

In a prior study, the authors[62] reported that the clinician may frequently diagnose a posterolateral injury when, in fact, the increase in external tibial rotation is due to a medial collateral ligament (MCL) injury. For this reason, during clinical testing for tibial rotatory subluxation, the examiner must palpate the position of the medial and lateral tibial plateaus to qualitatively determine whether an anterior position of the medial plateau and a posterior position of lateral tibial plateau occur with external tibial rotation. This is why the rotation tests should be done in the supine position (and not the prone position) to enable the examiner to observe and palpate the relative step-off of both the medial and the lateral tibial plateaus at 30° and 90° of flexion. Still, it may be difficult to quantify the amount of posterior subluxation of the lateral tibial plateau with PLS injuries, and additional tests such as lateral joint opening under varus loading and varus recurvatum help to confirm the diagnosis.

In Figure 20–19, the external rotation dial test is shown for a cadaveric knee measured with a three-dimensional goniometer with 5 Nm load under conditions already described.[62] The increase in the external rotation limit and anterior translation of the medial tibial plateau is shown in the normal knee and then after sectioning the ACL and SMCL. The tibial rotation increased from 7° to 16° and was associated with a lateral shift in the axis of tibial rotation. This resulted in an increase in anterior translation of the medial tibial plateau from 3.2 mm to 8.5 mm (anteromedial subluxation). In this study, an examination of cadaveric knees was performed by 11 experienced knee surgeons who were blinded as to the sectioned ligaments and asked to determine a diagnosis. More than half of the surgeons misinterpreted the increase in external tibial rotation as an injury to the PLS. This indicates that tests for rotatory subluxations of the knee joint are limited by the ability to quantitatively determine the millimeters of AP translation of the medial or lateral tibiofemoral joint under external rotation loads and variability between examiners should be expected.

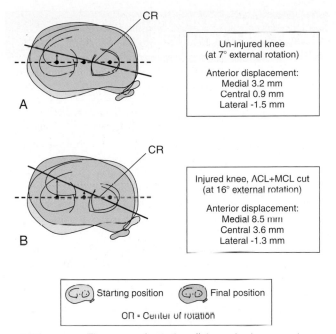

Un-injured knee
(at 7° external rotation)

Anterior displacement:
Medial 3.2 mm
Central 0.9 mm
Lateral -1.5 mm

Injured knee, ACL+MCL cut
(at 16° external rotation)

Anterior displacement:
Medial 8.5 mm
Central 3.6 mm
Lateral -1.3 mm

Starting position   Final position
CR = Center of rotation

FIGURE 20–19. The external rotation dial test in the normal uninjured knee (**A**) and after sectioning the ACL and MCL (**B**). The increase in external tibial rotation from 7° to 16° is shown, along with an increase in anterior translation of the MTP and shift in the axis of tibial rotation. (A and B, From Noyes, F. R.; Cummings, J. F.; Grood, E. S.; et al.: The diagnosis of knee motion limits, subluxations, and ligament injury. Am J Sports Med 19.163–171, 1991.)

EFFECT OF PCL AND POSTEROLATERAL RECONSTRUCTION ON RESTORING NORMAL KNEE MOTION LIMITS

Sekiya and coworkers[77] conducted an in vitro cadaveric study using a robotic testing system in which the PCL was reconstructed with a two-strand construct (Achilles and semitendinosus tendons), the PFL was reconstructed with a gracilis tendon, and the popliteus tendon was reattached to its femoral origin. The specimens were subjected to a 134-N posterior tibial load and a 5-Nm external tibial torque at multiple flexion angles. The authors reported that the forces in the posterolateral grafts were significantly higher than those in the native PLS. A possible explanation for the increased loads on the posterolateral reconstruction is the fact that the two-strand PCL reconstruction did not restore normal posterior tibial translation, because significant increases in posterior tibial translation were detected from 0° to 90° of flexion compared with intact knees. The PCL grafts were tensioned to a defined load, but not to the load required to reduce posterior tibial translation to normal; therefore, the PCL reconstruction forces were low after the reconstruction. For this reason, additional loads were placed upon the posterolateral grafts.

The data from the investigation by Sekiya and coworkers[77] and a subsequent study[32] show the dependence of posterolateral reconstructions on a functional PCL reconstruction. Harner and associates[32] studied the effect of deficiency of the posterolateral structures on PCL Achilles tendon graft reconstructions in 10 cadaver knees. The authors reported that a functional PCL reconstruction (posterior tibial translation restored to within 2.4 ± 1.4 mm of the intact knee, 90° flexion) subjected to sectioning of the PLS resulted in a significant increase in posterior

tibial translation (6.0 ± 2.7 mm at 30°, 4.6 ± 1.5 mm at 90° of
flexion; $P < .05$). In addition, the forces in the PCL graft significantly increased for posterior tibial load, external tibial torque,
combined posterior and external torque, and varus torque.
These data support other studies that conclude that a PCL
reconstruction may stretch out or fail if a concurrent injury to
the PLS is not diagnosed and concurrently surgically
addressed.[52,59]

LaPrade and colleagues[40] conducted a biomechanical analysis
of an anatomic posterolateral reconstruction in which a two-
graft technique was used to replace the FCL, popliteus tendon,
and PFL. The reconstructions were performed using Achilles
tendon–bone constructs in 10 cadaver knees aged 62 to 74 years
(Fig. 20–20). It should be noted that in the LaPrade and colleagues[40] reconstruction, the PFL does not attach to the popliteus
tendon at its normal anatomic attachment, and therefore, this
represents an anatomic reconstruction of the popliteus tendon
and FCL. The knees were tested under a 5-Nm varus moment
and 5 Nm external rotation torque first with the posterolateral
structures intact; second, with the FCL, popliteus tendon,
and PFL sectioned; and third, after the posterolateral

reconstruction. There was no significant difference between
the intact and the reconstructed knees for varus translation at
0°, 60°, and 90° or for external tibial rotation at 0°, 30°, 60°,
and 90° of flexion. The authors concluded that this technique
restored static stability and provides the scientific basis for
patient outcome studies. The authors of this chapter agree with
this conclusion, because both the popliteus tendon (static attachments) and the FCL were reconstructed.

Apsingi and coworkers[2] reported on the kinematics of cadaveric knees with a combined PCL and posterolateral ligament
deficiency. The authors used both a single-bundle and a double-bundle PCL reconstruction that was combined with a femoral-fibular graft reconstruction for the posterolateral structures.
The combined PCL and posterolateral reconstruction restored
all the laxity limits to normal, and the double-bundle PCL
reconstruction was not reported to have an advantage over the
single-bundle reconstruction. Of importance, the nonanatomic
femoral-fibular reconstruction involved two femoral tunnels
with the graft passed in an anterior-to-posterior direction
through the fibula. The location of the two femoral tunnels
was determined by selecting isometric points on the lateral femoral condyle and not by attaching the two graft arms to any specific anatomic location. The two graft ends passed through the
two femoral tunnels were tensioned independently to restore
the adduction and external rotation limits to normal. The anterior limb was tensioned at 20° of flexion to match the laxity of
the intact knee to varus loading. The posterior limb was tensioned at 90° of flexion to match the intact knee motion limit
to external rotation torque. Each graft arm was only 5 mm in
diameter. The data from this study and others on femoral-fibular reconstructions, if interpreted incorrectly, may suggest that
the more simplified femoral-fibular reconstruction is all that is

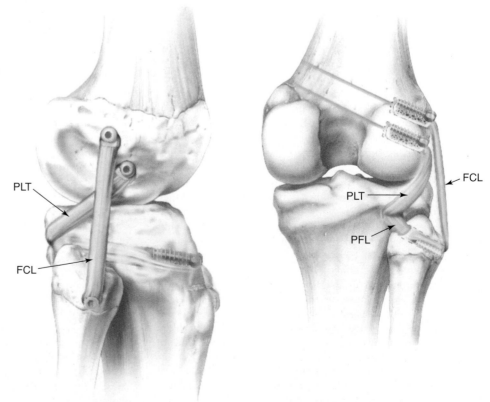

FIGURE 20–20. The posterolater knee
reconstruction described by LaPrade.
Left, Lateral view, right knee. **Right,**
Posterior view, right knee. FCL, fibular
collateral ligament; PFL, popliteofibular
ligament; PLT, popliteus tendon. *(From
LaPrade, R. F.; Johansen, S.; Wentorf, F. A.; et al.:
An analysis of an anatomical posterolateral knee
reconstruction: an in vitro biomechanical study
and development of a surgical technique. Am J
Sports Med 32:1405–1414, 2004.)*

required for posterolateral insufficiency instead of the more complex anatomic reconstruction recommended by the senior author and LaPrade.[40] It is true that in a time-zero cadaveric study, a single graft appropriately tensioned will restore varus and external rotation motion limits to normal.

Two points are worthy of emphasis. Apsingi and coworkers[2] did not measure the effects of the femoral-fibular reconstruction on decreasing or unloading the PCL graft. Markolf and associates[50] showed that an FCL reconstruction alone was insufficient to decrease or unload PCL graft forces. The Markolf and associates data[50] provide added support to the concept of restoring all of the functional components of the PLS at the time of surgery. Second, a small-diameter graft passed through the fibula and secured to the femoral condyle may be insufficient to resist the large adduction and external rotation loads that occur postoperatively. The anatomic reconstruction advocated by Noyes[60] and LaPrade[40] places two larger-diameter grafts at both the femoral, the fibular, and the tibial attachment sites of respective PLS. The graft function, therefore, does not depend upon only a fibular attachment site, and the popliteus tendon graft is passed through a distal tibial tunnel. A third point on the application of biomechanical studies to clinical cases involves whether to select an isometric point on the femur for the FCL and popliteus tendon[50,82] or, as described by some authors, to select the anatomic attachment site to restore native anatomy.[40,60] Sigward and associates[82] reported, in a cadaveric knee study, the femoral fixation sites for isometry of posterolateral reconstructions. A coordinate grid system was located across the lateral femoral condyle, permitting the placement of 21 holes in the femur, 5 mm apart, for the measurement of suture length changes with knee flexion. The authors did compute a mean location for the FCL and popliteus tendon attachment; however, the femoral isometric points showed major differences between knees. This wide variability between specimens indicates that one mean value for the ideal isometric point for a graft placement would most likely be incorrect for knees undergoing surgery. Future clinical studies are necessary to determine the ideal success rates from knees in which either an isometric point is selected at surgery or an anatomic attachment site is selected. Until these studies are available, the senior author recommends anatomic attachment points and an anatomic reconstruction for posterolateral instability as described in Chapter 22, Posterolateral Ligament Injuries: Diagnosis, Operative Techniques, and Clinical Outcomes.

CLINICAL EFFECTS OF POSTERIOR TIBIAL SUBLUXATION OF THE PCL-DEFICIENT KNEE

Morrison[58] and Denham and Bishop[16] estimated that PCL forces up to 50% body weight occur during level walking. Even higher PCL forces have been calculated during stair-climbing, ascending stairs, and descending stairs[4] (see Chapter 23, Rehabilitation of Posterior Cruciate Ligament and Posterolateral Reconstructive Procedures, for other studies on estimated PCL forces during activity). In a study at the authors' laboratory[10] involving 10 patients with complete PCL ruptures, the amount of posterior tibial translation that occurred during a double-stance static squat test was measured. A lateral radiograph was obtained of both lower limbs, which was used to compute the amount of posterior tibial translation and sagittal plane forces

---

Critical Points CLINICAL EFFECTS OF POSTERIOR TIBIAL SUBLUXATION OF THE POSTERIOR CRUCIATE LIGAMENT– DEFICIENT KNEE

- Posterior cruciate ligament (PCL) forces up to 50% body weight occur during level walking.
- Higher PCL forces occur during stair-climbing, ascending stairs, descending stairs.
- Posterior tibial subluxation occurs in PCL-deficient knees during activities of daily living in high knee flexion positions, but not at low flexion positions in which smaller posterior shear forces are present.
- Quadriceps neutral angle may vary from 60° to 90° between knees, not objective measurement diagnosis of posterior tibial subluxation.
- PCL-deficient patients frequently note an anterior shifting of the tibia, as the tibia moves forward from its subluxated position, when they attempt to stand from a seated position.
- Significantly increased contact pressures in medial tibiofemoral and patellofemoral compartments occur in PCL-deficient knees.

---

on the PCL-deficient knee and the normal knee. A stress radiograph was taken with an 11-kg posterior force (108 N) to provide an objective measurement of the amount of posterior translation in the PCL-deficient knee compared with the opposite normal knee.

In low knee flexion angles, only 3 of the 10 knees had a posterior subluxation (from 5–9 mm) during the squat test. However, in high knee flexion positions, 9 knees had an abnormal posterior tibial subluxation (mean, 5.9 ± 2.8 mm; range, 3–12 mm). These data support the concept that posterior tibial subluxation occurs in PCL-deficient knees during activities of daily living in high knee flexion positions, but not necessarily at low flexion positions in which smaller posterior shear forces are present. In strenuous activities such as sudden stopping, deceleration, or walking down a ramp, a posterior subluxation of the tibia is expected to occur. If the subluxation reaches 8 to 10 mm, minimal function of the menisci occurs (particularly the medial meniscus) and increased tibiofemoral stresses (as in postmedial meniscectomized knees) may be expected. As the tibia becomes more vertical with knee flexion, an increase in tibiofemoral compressive forces occurs from increased quadriceps and patellar tendon forces. However, the increased tibiofemoral compressive forces are not sufficient to overcome the posterior tibial shear forces and a resultant abnormal posterior tibial translation occurs.

As noted by Daniel and colleagues,[14] the quadriceps neutral angle is the angle of knee flexion at which the course of the patellar tendon is perpendicular to the articular surface of the tibia. The neutral knee flexion angle may vary from 60° to 90°, with a mean of 71°. Below this angle, the patellar tendon lies anterior to the tibial tubercle and produces a posterior tibial shear force. Conversely, at a greater flexion angle, the patellar tendon has a line of action coursing posterior to the attachment to the tibial tubercle, producing an anterior tibial shear force. The quadriceps neutral angle varies sufficiently between knees and is not an objective measurement in terms of the diagnosis of posterior tibial subluxation. However, patients with PCL-deficient knees frequently note an anterior shifting of the tibia from its posterior subluxated position when they attempt to stand from a seated position, which can be easily demonstrated in the clinic.

Experimental studies have documented significantly increased contact pressures in the medial tibiofemoral and patellofemoral compartments after PCL sectioning.[21,43,84] Skyhar and coworkers[84] reported that PCL sectioning caused significant increases in contact pressure on the medial tibiofemoral compartment (29.1 ± 11.6 Pa) at all knee flexion angles compared with intact specimens (19 ± 3.4 Pa; $P < .05$). A significant elevation in contact pressure in the patellofemoral compartment was found only at 60° of flexion. Gill and associates[21] analyzed patellofemoral contact pressures under simulated muscle loads in both PCL-sectioned and PCL-reconstructed cadaver knees (Achilles tendon single-bundle allograft). Significantly greater peak contract pressures were measured in the PCL-deficient knees than in the intact knees under both an isolated quadriceps (400 N) and a combined quadriceps and hamstrings (400 N/200 N) load. The PCL-reconstructed knees also had elevated pressures, which were not significantly different from those measured in the PCL-deficient specimens. There was no effect of knee flexion angle on these findings. The residual posterior tibial translation after the PCL reconstruction was not determined.

MENISCOFEMORAL LIGAMENTS

Gupte and colleagues[27] conducted an analysis of 16 anatomic studies involving 1022 cadaveric knees and reported that 91% had at least one meniscofemoral ligament (MFL). The anterior meniscofemoral ligament (aMFL) was identified in 390 knees (48%), the posterior meniscofemoral ligament (pMFL) was identified in 569 knees (70%), and both the aMFL and the pMFL were found in 257 knees (32%). It is important to identify the aMFL and pMFL (when present) to determine the true PCL anatomic footprint for graft placement, particularly when a two-strand graft construct is used.[30] The anatomic attachment of the aMFL is distal to the PCL attachment (Fig. 20–21), which gives the appearance that the PCL footprint is adjacent to the articular cartilage when, in fact, the true PCL attachment is a few more millimeters proximal.

The cross-sectional area of the aMFL ranges from 6.8 to 7.8 mm^2, and the cross-sectional area of the pMFL ranges from 6.7 to 12.7 mm^2.[27] For the surgeon, this indicates that these structures will be encountered at the time of PCL surgery. The mean ultimate loads of the aMFL and pMFL have been reported to be 265 ± 152 N and 443 ± 287 N, respectively.[38] A comparison of the ultimate strength of the MFLs and the

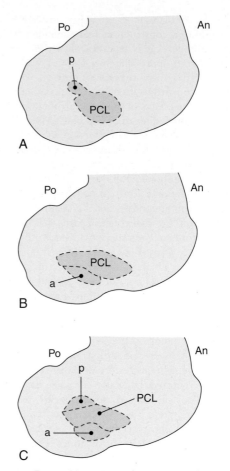

FIGURE 20–21. Femoral insertions of the meniscofemoral ligaments in relation to the insertion of the PCL. Diagrammatic views of the left lateral femoral condyle in sagittal section demonstrate its anterior (An) and posterior (Po) aspects. **A,** Specimen with posterior meniscofemoral ligament (p) and PCL. **B,** Specimen with anterior meniscofemoral ligament and PCL. **C,** Specimen with PCL and coexisting anterior and posterior meniscofemoral ligaments. *(A–C, From Gupte, C. M.; Bull, A. M.; Thomas, R. D.; Amis, A. A.: A review of the function and biomechanics of the meniscofemoral ligaments. Arthroscopy 19:161–171, 2003.)*

PCL is not possible because published cadaveric data are from older specimens tested at reduced failure loads than would be expected.

Gupte and colleagues[27] reviewed the numerous theories and evolutionary perspectives on the function of the MFL and concluded that there are insufficient data to support a functional role of these structures in humans. In animals such as sheep, horses, and dogs, the lateral meniscus posterior horn is attached by virtue of the pMFL without a separate posterior tibial attachment. In humans, the posterior horn of the lateral meniscus has two separate attachments into the tibia and, when the pMFL is present, an additional attachment into the femur. In rare cases, the posterolateral meniscus tibial attachment is absent and attaches only by the femoral pMFL, which must be preserved with any surgical procedure such as PCL reconstruction. The Wrisberg-type discoid lateral meniscus may have the pMFL as the only attachment, with an absent posterior tibial attachment. Gupte and colleagues[27] noted that the pMFL is tight in both knee extension and deep knee flexion. It has been theorized that the pMFL may pull the lateral meniscus into the joint during

---

Critical Points MENISCOFEMORAL LIGAMENTS

- Most knees have at least one meniscofemoral ligament (MFL).
- One third of knees have both MFLs.
- Insufficient data to support a functional role of these structures.
- Identify anterior meniscofemoral ligament (aMFL) and posterior meniscofemoral ligament (pMFL) (when present) to determine true posterior cruciate ligament (PCL) anatomic footprint for graft placement.
- In some knees with isolated PCL ruptures, secondary ligament restraints including the MFL structures resist posterior tibial subluxation, particularly at low knee flexion angles.
- 90° knee flexion, neutral tibial rotation is the best position to test for maximum posterior translation.
- Amount of posterior translation determined by secondary restraints will vary depending on physiologic laxity.

flexion, causing clicking and snapping symptoms leading to meniscus deteroriation.[17] It is possible that the pMFL provides additional resistance to posterior displacement of the lateral meniscus posterior horn during maximum tibial external rotation; however, this has not been experimentally proved.

The effect of the MFLs acting as a secondary restraint to posterior tibial translation was investigated by Gupte and co-workers[28] in cadaveric knees. These authors postulated that the MFLs provide to the PCL a "synergistic reinforcement" in resisting posterior tibial translation. In this study, the PCL was first divided and the increase in posterior tibial translation measured, then the MFLs were divided (Figs. 20–22 and 20–23). The data showed that the MFLs contributed 28% of the restraining force at 90° of knee flexion without any restraint for rotatory subluxations. The data show that partial or isolated tears of the PCL may be supported in part by intact MFL structures, resulting in less overall posterior tibial translation. This suggests the potential benefit of preserving when possible at surgery the function of the MFLs, which is often difficult in double-bundle PCL reconstructions. This also provides the rationale for protecting knees with isolated PCL ruptures, using a postoperative brace at full extension with a calf pad for 4 weeks to allow initial healing. The secondary ligament restraints maintain a normal tibiofemoral joint position at full extension, maintaining a normal PCL tibiofemoral attachment distance.

Bergfeld and associates[5] conducted a cadaveric study on 20 knees in which total AP translation was measured in four different flexion angles after cutting the PCL and MFLs. Testing was performed with the tibia in neutral, internal, and external rotation (5 Nm torque). Statistically significant decreases in posterior tibial translation occurred with internal and external tibial rotation (Fig. 20–24 and Table 20–3). The authors concluded that 90° knee flexion and neutral tibial rotation was the best position to test for maximum posterior translation and that the medial and lateral secondary restraints were tensioned to reduce the posterior limit with internal-external tibial rotation. Because the MFLs were cut, other structures limited posterior translation in internal tibial rotation and not the MFLs, as had been reported previously.[11] Note in Chapter 3, The Scientific Basis for Examination and Classification of Knee Ligament Injuries, after sectioning the PCL, the posterior tibial translation increased 12.1 ± 0.6 mm and 15 of 22 specimens had increases greater than 10 mm. This indicates that the amount of posterior translation determined by secondary restraints will vary depending on their physiologic laxity. Therefore, the frequently reported value of greater than 10 mm posterior translation indicating injury to the secondary restraints cannot be used. The secondary restraints may be lax owing to either physiologic laxity or injury.

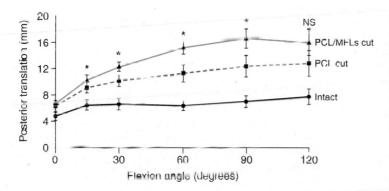

FIGURE 20–22. Graph shows the effect of division of the PCL on posterior laxity in the intact knee, and the effect of division of the meniscofemoral ligaments (MFLs) in the PCL-deficient knee. Division of the PCL resulted in an increase in posterior translation at all angles of flexion in the intact knee (paired T-test and analysis of variance [ANOVA], $P < .005$). Division of the MFLs resulted in an increase in posterior translation in the PCL-deficient knee between 15° and 90° of flexion (*, $P < .005$; NS, not significant, SEM bars are shown). (From Gupte, C. M.; Bull, A. M.; Thomas, R. D.; Amis, A. A.: The meniscofemoral ligaments: secondary restraints to the posterior drawer. Analysis of anteroposterior and rotary laxity in the intact and posterior-cruciate-deficient knee. J Bone Joint Surg Br 85:765–773, 2003.)

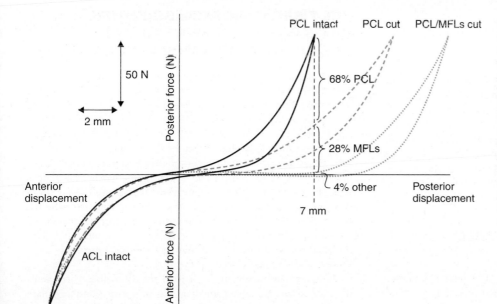

FIGURE 20–23. Graph shows mean load-displacement curves for intact, PCL-deficient, and PCL-MFL–deficient knees tested at 90° flexion. Note the hysteresis effect of the AP drawer cycle. Note also the relative percentage contributions of the PCL and MFLs to resisting posterior drawer at displacement of 7 mm. The crossed hairlines mark the assumed AP neutral and zero load. (From Gupte, C. M.; Bull, A. M.; Thomas, R. D.; Amis, A. A.: The meniscofemoral ligaments: secondary restraints to the posterior drawer. Analysis of anteroposterior and rotary laxity in the intact and posterior-cruciate-deficient knee. J Bone Joint Surg Br 85:765–773, 2003.)

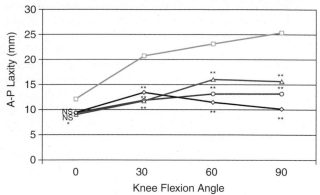

Anterior-Posterior Laxity vs. Knee Flexion Angle

FIGURE 20–24. Graph illustrates anterior-posterior (A-P) laxity with the knee in 0°, 30°, 60°, and 90° of flexion. The test was performed under four conditions: with the posterior cruciate and MFLs intact (*diamonds*), with the ligaments transected and the tibia in neutral rotation (*squares*), with the ligaments transected and the tibia in internal rotation (*circles*), and with the ligaments transected and the tibia in external rotation (*triangles*). A *double asterisk* indicates a significant difference at $P \leq .001$, a *single asterisk* indicates a significant difference at $P \leq .05$, and NS indicates no significant difference ($P > .05$) compared with the laxity measured with the ligaments transected and the tibia in neutral rotation. *(From Bergfeld, J. A.; McAllister, D. R.; Parker, R. D.; et al.: The effects of tibial rotation on posterior translation in knees in which the posterior cruciate ligament has been cut. J Bone Joint Surg Am 83:1339–1343, 2001.)*

TABLE 20–3 Anterior-Posterior Laxity for Each Condition at Each Knee Flexion Angle

Condition	Anterior-Posterior Laxity* (mm)			
	0° Flexion	30° Flexion	60° Flexion	90° Flexion
PCL and MFL intact	9.4	13.5	11.5	10.2
PCL and MFL transected				
Neutral tibial rotation	12.1[c]	20.8[a]	23.3[a]	25.5[a]
Internal tibial rotation	9.3[c,e]	11.8[c,e]	13.2[c,d]	13.2[b,d]
External tibial rotation	9.0[c]	11.7[c]	16.1[a]	15.7[a]

*a, b, and c indicate $P \leq .001$, $P \leq .05$, and $P < .05$, respectively, compared with the intact condition; d and e indicate $P \leq .05$ and $P > .05$, respectively, compared with the test performed with the ligaments transected and the tibia in external rotation.

MFL, meniscofemoral ligament; PCL, posterior cruciate ligament.

Gupte and colleagues[26] introduced the concept of a "meniscal tug test" at arthroscopy, which involves placing tension on the aMFL with a nerve hook and observing movement in the posterior horn of the lateral meniscus. The aMFL was confirmed in 88% of 68 knees, whereas the pMFL was identified in only 9%. The authors concluded that this test could be used to distinguish between fibers of the PCL and the MFLs, which is helpful in avoiding a misdiagnosis of a partial versus a complete PCL tear.

POPLITEOMENISCAL FASCICLE ATTACHMENTS

Staubli and Birrer[85] conducted anatomic dissections of the popliteus tendon and its fascicles and described their relationship to the lateral meniscus attachments in cadaveric knees. These authors

Critical Points POPLITEOMENISCAL FASCICLE ATTACHMENTS

- Structural lesions of the popliteus system observed in approximately 19% of control knees compared with 86% to 95% of anterior cruciate ligament (ACL)–deficient knees in one study.[85]
- Popliteomeniscal fasciculi contribute to lateral meniscus stability, difficult to objectively determine abnormal meniscus displacements at arthroscopy.
- Surgeon determines whether an anterior subluxation of the posterior horn lateral meniscus is present with partial disruption of meniscus attachments, requiring operative repair. This is common with ACL ruptures.

also compared arthroscopic examinations of the popliteus-lateral meniscus attachments in a normal control group of 107 patients with those of 68 patients with acute and chronic ACL disruptions. Structural lesions of the popliteus meniscus attachments were observed in approximately 19% of control knees compared with 86% to 95% of ACL-deficient knees. The authors concluded that the surgeon should determine whether an anterior subluxation and disruption of lateral meniscus attachments is present, requiring operative repair at the time of ACL reconstruction.

Simonian and coworkers,[83] in a cadaveric study, transected the anteroinferior fascicle and then the posterosuperior fasciculi to determine the contribution of these structures to lateral meniscus stability. The mean lateral meniscal motion under a 10-N load was 3.6 mm. After the anteroinferior fascicle was cut, an increase in anterior displacement of the posterior horn of the lateral meniscus of 1.8 mm (50%) occurred, and when both fasciculi were cut, an increase of 2.8 mm (78%) was reported. The authors concluded that the popliteomeniscal fasciculi contributed to lateral meniscus stability and acknowledged the difficulty in objectively determining abnormal meniscus displacements at the time of arthroscopic surgery. Tests for abnormal lateral meniscus displacement at the time of arthroscopic surgery and the repair of the popliteomeniscal fascicles are discussed in Chapter 28, Meniscus Tears: Diagnosis, Repair Techniques, and Clinical Outcomes.

PCL FIBER FUNCTION: SCIENTIFIC BASIS FOR PLACEMENT OF PCL GRAFTS AT TIBIOFEMORAL LOCATIONS

The anatomy of the cruciate ligaments has been described for over a century in qualitative terms as having two major bundles or bands. The Weber brothers in 1836[94] and Fick in 1911[20] published some of the first anatomic descriptions of the ACL and PCL; however, these authors did not conduct biomechanical studies to support their descriptions. The PCL has been classically described as a structure composed of an anterolateral bundle that is tense in flexion and a posteromedial bundle that is tense in extension. This nomenclature is still used today, even though it is incorrect because it does not precisely describe the function of the PCL fibers and gives the surgeon inadequate data for determining placement of PCL graft strands (see Chapter 21, Posterior Cruciate Ligament: Diagnosis, Operative Techniques, and Clinical Outcomes).

Inderster and associates[37] divided the PCL into three bundles: anterolateral, posteromedial, and posterior oblique. These authors reported that the femoral-to-tibial distances of the

Critical Points POSTERIOR CRUCIATE LIGAMENT FIBER FUNCTION: SCIENTIFIC BASIS FOR PLACEMENT OF POSTERIOR CRUCIATE LIGAMENT GRAFTS AT TIBIOFEMORAL LOCATIONS

- Posterior cruciate ligament (PCL) classical description: antero-lateral bundle tense in flexion, posteromedial bundle tense in extension. Does not describe function of PCL fibers, gives surgeon inadequate data for determining placement and tensioning PCL grafts.
- PCL ligament length pattern is highly dependent on a proximal-to-distal direction of the femoral attachment.
- Transitional zone in proximal one third of PCL femoral attachment, approximately 11 mm from the articular cartilage distally, extending approximately 10 mm from the roof in a posterior direction.
- The bulk of the PCL lengthens with knee flexion, approximately one third of the posterior fibers lengthen with knee extension.
- Graft placed within PCL attachment will have portions that undergo different elongations along every 2–3 mm in graft diameter, progressing proximal-to-distal.
- One- and two-strand reconstructions attached in three different locations within PCL femoral footprint in a cadaveric investigation.[45] Central tibial tunnel used.
  - One strand (distal and middle position) restored posterior translation limits to normal.
  - One strand (deep and proximal) gave abnormal increase in posterior translation.
  - Two strands (distal locations, tensioned at 90°) shared applied load.
  - Two strands (one strand anterior, one proximal): reciprocal loading relationship.
  - Tension in single-strand PCL graft nearly doubles with knee flexion.
  - Placement of second graft strand in either distal or middle position is most ideal.
- All graft constructs capable of restoring posterior translation limit to normal. However, the constructs do so by inducing high tensile forces in the graft that may be deleterious, producing eventual graft elongation.

anterolateral and posteromedial bundles increased with knee flexion from 0° to 90°, whereas the length of the posterior oblique bundle remained the same. Accordingly, they recommended a more posterior position of a PCL reconstruction at the femoral attachment of the posterior oblique bundle. The authors did not induce posterior loads on the tibia to determine femoral-tibial length changes under loading conditions, nor did they measure tibial displacements after PCL reconstruction.

Covey and colleagues[12,13] described a fiber continuum of the PCL consisting of four regions: anterior, central, posterior longitudinal, and posterior oblique. This four-fiber region classification was confirmed by Makris and coworkers[44] according to fiber orientation and osseous sites of attachment visualized in 24 cadaver knees. The anterior fiber region attachment was located at the most anterior portion of the femoral attachment and inserted into the anterior portion of the tibial attachment. The central fiber region was the widest portion, representing the middle part of the femoral attachment, and inserted into the middle and slightly lateral aspect of the tibial attachment. The anterior and central fiber regions represented nearly 80% of the PCL, with the posterior fiber regions accounting for the remaining 15% to 20%. The posterior fiber region consisted of a posterior longitudinal attachment to the tibia medially and a posterior oblique region attachment to the tibia laterally.

These investigations reported that under operative conditions, most of the PCL's attachment sites exhibit nonisometric behavior. Only the small posterior fiber attachment sites (which account for 15% of the PCL[44]) demonstrate near isometry. In addition, Covey and colleagues[12] reported marked loosening of most PCL fibers by an applied quadriceps force at knee flexion angles less than 75° when compared with an unloaded state. Internal tibial rotation slackened certain fibers (anterior, central) near extension, but significantly tightened others (central, posterior) with flexion. The authors concluded that the joint angle and type of load applied to the knee joint produce different functional roles to the four fiber regions of the PCL.

Quantitative data from many investigators have been reported using a variety of techniques to determine the length-tension behavior of the PCL fibers under loaded conditions. These measurement conditions include the use of force measurement sensors,[3,46,52] wire cables,[18] mercury strain gauges,[19,39] and photogrammetric techniques.[15,88,90,91] Ahmad and associates[1] performed an analysis of PCL bundle length change and angle of orientation with knee flexion and extension. The anterolateral bundle was observed to become more vertical with increased knee flexion and the posteromedial bundle became more horizontal. Therefore, the posteromedial bundle has a better orientation to resist posterior tibial translation owing to its horizontal position. The study data are in agreement with other studies showing the marked changes in the length of PCL fibers with knee flexion and extension based on their femoral attachment.

The use of an instrumented spatial linkage during application of joint loads (followed by digitization of the tibia and femoral surfaces and ligament attachment locations) allows the length of discrete fiber strands or regions within a ligament to be measured based on tibiofemoral attachment sites and the change in distance (fiber length) with knee motion.[23,33,76] This information is required to determine locations of graft attachments whose tibiofemoral length changes the least with knee flexion or, alternatively, graft attachment locations at which the fiber length changes the most. The surgeon should select graft attachment locations that have the least amount of change in tibiofemoral length, and tension the graft at the knee flexion position where the graft length is the longest (and therefore functional). For example, if a graft is tensioned at a knee flexion angle where the tibiofemoral fiber length is at its shortest, the graft will initially constrain knee flexion or extension and fail as the graft construct (tibiofemoral distance) lengthens with further knee flexion or extension.

The PCL ligament length pattern is highly dependent on a proximal-to-distal direction of the femoral attachment, and not an anterior-to-posterior direction, as proposed by the anterolateral-posteromedial bundle concept previously discussed. In Figure 20–25, the tibiofemoral separation distances are shown for a number of proximal-to-distal locations that pass through the PCL femoral attachment. A transitional zone (<2 mm length change) adjacent to the center of rotation is shown. All attachment locations distal to line A-A lengthen with knee flexion, and all fibers proximal to this line shorten with knee flexion. In Figure 20–26, the average tibiofemoral separation length is shown along three femoral attachment site locations. Two sites are within the PCL femoral attachment and one is outside the PCL attachment. These data demonstrate that the fiber length change is minimal in an anterior-to-posterior direction within the PCL attachment. These experimental findings were

FIGURE 20–25. Contour map for one typical knee. The *number* on each contour line indicates the magnitude of the maximum length change. *Line A-A* represents the most isometric line and runs almost in the AP direction. *Point CR* indicates the intersection of the best-fit flexion axis with the lateral surface of the medial femoral condyle. Note that line A-A passes near point CR. The *curves at the right* show the changes in the tibiofemoral separation distances that occurred for selected femoral attachments. Attachments proximal to the isometric line were shorter at 90° than at full extension. Attachments distal to the line were longer at 90°. Attachments along line A-A had a length at 90° that was nearly identical to its length at 0°. *(From Grood, E. S.; Hefzy, M. S.; Lindenfeld, T. N.: Factors affecting the region of most isometric femoral attachments. Part I: the posterior cruciate ligament. Am J Sports Med 17:197–207, 1989.)*

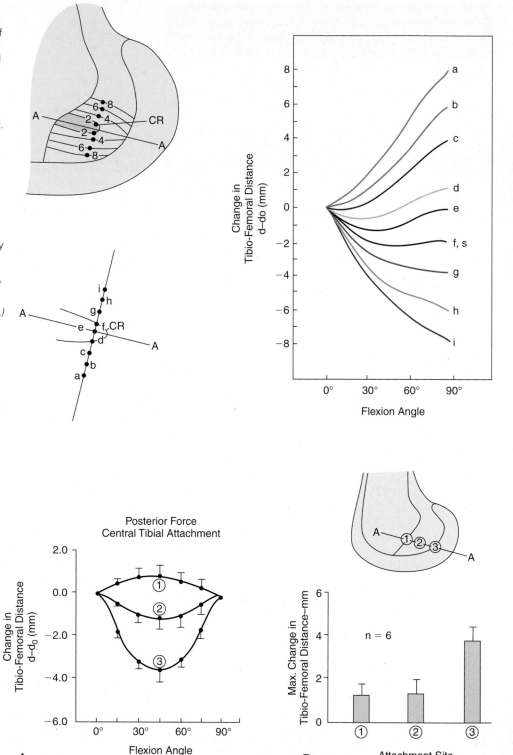

FIGURE 20–26. A, The curves show the average tibiofemoral separation distance versus knee flexion for three femoral attachment sites located along the most isometric line. **B,** The bar chart shows the average and the SD of the difference between the maximum and the minimum tibiofemoral separation distance for each of the three femoral attachment sites. *(A and B, From Grood, E. S.; Hefzy, M. S.; Lindenfeld, T. N.: Factors affecting the region of most isometric femoral attachments. Part I: the posterior cruciate ligament. Am J Sports Med 17:197–207, 1989.)*

corroborated by Sidles and colleagues,[81] Ogata and McCarthy,[65] and Trus and coworkers.[89]

The changes in tibial attachment location show only a small effect on the tibiofemoral separation distance, as demonstrated in Figure 20–27. These experimental conditions are valid assuming a PCL fiber follows a straight path between attachment sites. Native PCL fibers do not follow straight paths, but may have curvatures induced from other fibers. As yet, there is no description of fiber anatomy suggesting major PCL fiber curvature from one attachment site to another.

A simplified planar model may be used to explain the larger effect of the femoral attachment on PCL fiber length change in comparison with the tibial attachment. The model is shown in Figure 20–28, where the tibia is stationary and the femur

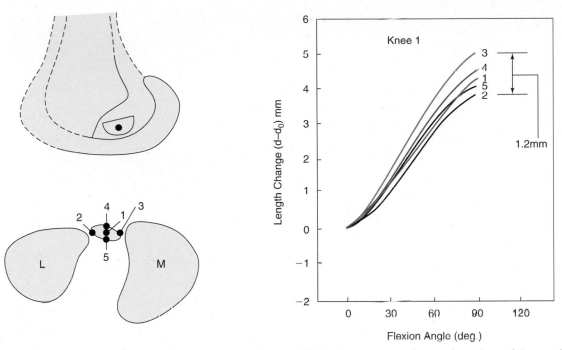

FIGURE 20–27. The curves show the relation between the change in the tibiofemoral separation distance from that at full extension and the flexion angle for five tibial attachment sites in one typical knee. *(From Grood, E. S.; Hefzy, M. S.; Lindenfeld, T. N.: Factors affecting the region of most isometric femoral attachments. Part I: the posterior cruciate ligament. Am J Sports Med 17:197–207, 1989.)*

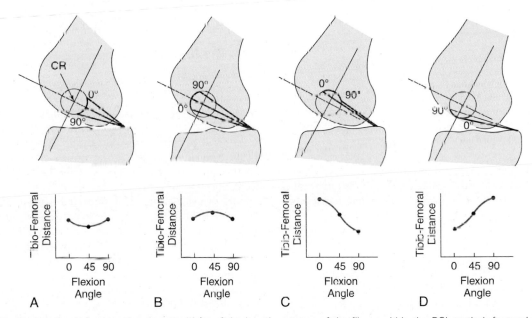

FIGURE 20–28. The mechanism governing the sensitivity of the length patterns of the fibers within the PCL to their femoral attachments. **A,** Fiber is attached posterior to the center of rotation (CR) and has a concave length pattern. **B,** Fiber is attached anterior to the CR and has a convex length pattern. **C** and **D,** Length patterns of fibers with femoral attachments located proximal and distal to the CR. The fiber with proximal attachment (**C**) becomes longer with flexion, whereas the fiber with distal attachment (**D**) becomes shorter with flexion. *(A–D, From Grood, E. S.; Hefzy, M. S.; Lindenfeld, T. N.: Factors affecting the region of most isometric femoral attachments. Part I: the posterior cruciate ligament. Am J Sports Med 17:197–207, 1989.)*

rotates about a fixed center. The femur is positioned at 45°, and the change in tibiofemoral distance is shown relative to the center of rotation with knee extension and flexion to 90°. The planar model does not describe the true three-dimensional behavior of the PCL fibers, which is more complex. However, the model does show how the fiber length change is dependent on its femoral attachment relative to the center of femoral rotation, which

is simplified to a fixed point. The reader is referred to Chapter 3, The Scientific Basis for Examination and Classification of Knee Ligament Injuries, for further information on ACL and PCL fiber function.

In Figure 20–29, the center transitional zone (<2 mm change in tibiofemoral length) is shown. The zone is located in the proximal one third of the PCL femoral attachment toward the

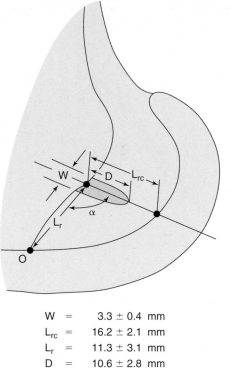

W	=	3.3 ± 0.4 mm
L_{rc}	=	16.2 ± 2.1 mm
L_r	=	11.3 ± 3.1 mm
D	=	10.6 ± 2.8 mm
α	=	105.8 ± 10.0 deg

FIGURE 20–29. The geometric variables that describe the location and orientation of the most isometric line. *(From Grood, E. S.; Hefzy, M. S.; Lindenfeld, T. N.: Factors affecting the region of most isometric femoral attachments. Part I: the posterior cruciate ligament. Am J Sports Med 17:197–207, 1989.)*

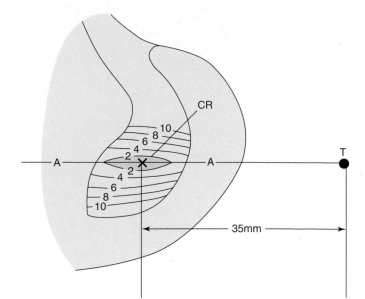

FIGURE 20–30. Contour map obtained from the single-hinge model in which the knee rotates around a single axis of rotation. A tibial attachment site (T) 35 mm away from this axis was used in the analysis. The *number* on each contour line indicates the magnitude of the maximum length change found as the knee was rotated from 0° to 90°. *Line A-A* represents the "most isometric" line. This line, besides being an axis of symmetry for the contour map, passes through the center of rotation and the tibial attachment site when the knee is positioned midway between the limits of flexion. The *shaded region* indicates the region within which a maximum length change of less than 2 mm was found. *(From Grood, E. S.; Hefzy, M. S.; Lindenfeld, T. N.: Factors affecting the region of most isometric femoral attachments. Part I: the posterior cruciate ligament. Am J Sports Med 17:197–207, 1989.)*

roof of the intercondylar region, 11 mm from the articular cartilage distally, extending approximately 10 mm from the roof in a posterior direction. The data show that the majority of the PCL lengthens with knee flexion. The contour map showing the length change from 0° to 90° is shown in a planar manner in Figure 20–30. A previous study showed that a graft placed into a nonisometric location, just distal to the transitional zone, demonstrated a few millimeters increase in tibiofemoral distance with knee flexion, providing greater control of posterior tibial displacement than a graft placed in a so-called isometric zone.[23] These data show that any graft placed within the PCL attachment will have portions that undergo different elongations along every 2 to 3 mm in graft cross-sectional area, progressing in a proximal-to-distal direction.

In a second investigation at the authors' laboratory,[76] several attachment sites at the proximal and distal origins located around the circumference of the PCL femoral attachment were studied. The peripheral attachment sites originated on the proximal border of the PCL (anterior, middle, posterior, and posterior oblique) and on the distal border (anterior, middle, and posterior). The limbs were loaded to 100 N and the knees flexed from 0° to 120°. This was one of the first studies to examine PCL fiber length changes at knee flexion angles greater than 90°. The changes in tibiofemoral length for the seven selected peripheral attachment points are shown in Figure 20–31. These data confirm that proximal PCL fibers lengthen with knee extension, whereas distal fibers lengthen with knee flexion. In Figure 20–32, the flexion angles in which the fiber length elongations were the least (within 5% of the maximum length and,

therefore, the functional zone) are graphed for each attachment point. The data as a whole show a progressive loading of fibers from distal to proximal within the PCL attachment with progressive knee flexion. There is a smaller effect proceeding from anterior to posterior. These data contradict the description of PCL fiber function that divides the PCL into an anterolateral bundle (which is tight in flexion) and a posteromedial bundle (which is tight in flexion).

The surgeon has the option of placing a PCL graft strand into different regions of the PCL femoral attachment site that determines the functional range of the graft with knee flexion and the knee flexion position to tension the graft. This was investigated in a third cadaveric study in the authors' laboratory in 12 cadaver knees (Fig. 20–33).[45] The one-strand and two-strand reconstructions were attached in three different locations within the PCL femoral footprint (Figs. 20–34 to 20–36). A bone–patellar tendon–bone (B-PT-B) graft was used to provide secure fixation and prevent slippage in the fixture apparatus. The shallow edge of the graft was placed 2 mm from the articular cartilage margin. The center of the deep proximal strand was within 1 to 2 mm of the proximal edge of the PCL attachment. Within the femoral tunnels, the graft orientation was chosen to place the fibers on either the shallow or the distal side of the tunnel, with the bone placed along the deep side. A central tibial tunnel was chosen. A 50-N posterior force was applied to the tibia for the single-strand construct, and a 100-N force was applied to the two-strand PCL reconstructions. The tension in the graft strand was adjusted to restore posterior

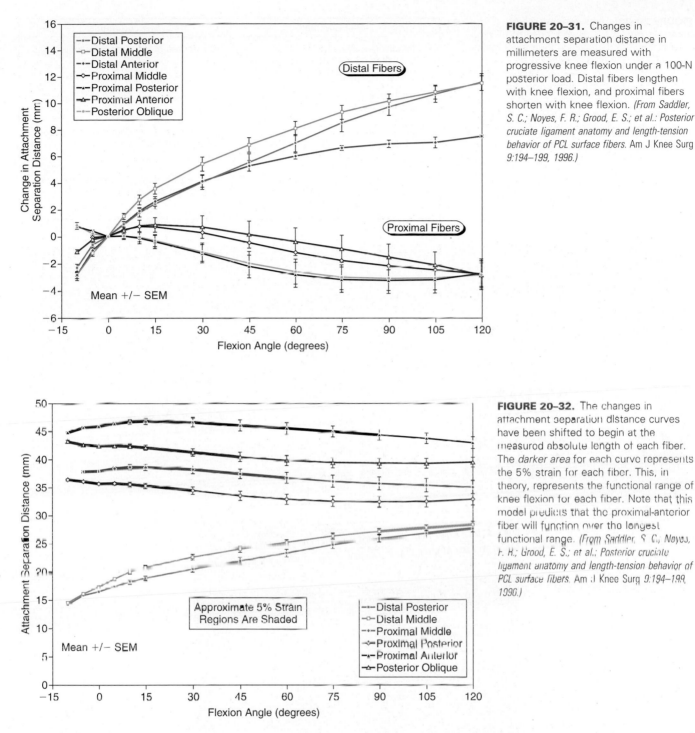

FIGURE 20–31. Changes in attachment separation distance in millimeters are measured with progressive knee flexion under a 100-N posterior load. Distal fibers lengthen with knee flexion, and proximal fibers shorten with knee flexion. *(From Saddler, S. C.; Noyes, F. R.; Grood, E. S.; et al.: Posterior cruciate ligament anatomy and length-tension behavior of PCL surface fibers. Am J Knee Surg 9:194–199, 1996.)*

FIGURE 20–32. The changes in attachment separation distance curves have been shifted to begin at the measured absolute length of each fiber. The *darker area* for each curve represents the 5% strain for each fiber. This, in theory, represents the functional range of knee flexion for each fiber. Note that this model predicts that the proximal-anterior fiber will function over the longest functional range. *(From Saddler, S. C.; Noyes, F. R.; Grood, E. S.; et al.: Posterior cruciate ligament anatomy and length-tension behavior of PCL surface fibers. Am J Knee Surg 9:194–199, 1996.)*

translation to within ± 1 mm of the intact knee. The graft tensioning was performed at 90° flexion for all grafts except the proximal (deep) graft, which was tensioned at 30° knee flexion. This was done to remain consistent with prior data on the increased tibiofemoral separation distance of a graft placed at this location.

In Figure 20–37, the increase in graft tension with knee flexion is shown along with the posterior translation limit. The one-strand graft restored the knee joint to a normal posterior translation limit, with a more than doubling of graft tension with knee flexion (maximum, 118 ± 15 N; $P < .001$). In Figure 20–38, the one-strand reconstruction placed at the distal and middle (S_2) position shows a similar tension relationship with knee flexion

and also restored knee posterior translation limits to normal. In contrast, the single-graft strand placed into a deep and more proximal position (Fig. 20–39) showed less overall graft tensile loading and an abnormal increase in posterior translation with knee flexion. The difference in the behavior from the two shallow grafts was significant ($P < .001$). The more proximal graft position and graft tensioning did not restore normal posterior translation limits and, therefore, is not a position recommended for PCL reconstruction.

The more complex behavior of a two-strand PCL reconstruction is shown in Figure 20–40 where the two strands were both placed into the more distal locations and tensioned at 90°.

FIGURE 20–33. Tests performed and measurements made using six-degree-of-freedom knee kinematics that include the three rotations (flexion/extension, adduction/abduction, and external/internal) and three translations (anterior/posterior, medial/lateral, and proximal/distal). *(From Mannor, D. A.; Shearn, J. T.; Grood, E. S.; et al.: Two-bundle posterior cruciate ligament reconstruction. An in vitro analysis of graft placement and tension. Am J Sports Med 28:833–845, 2000.)*

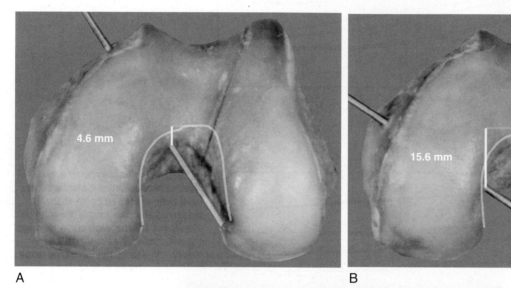

Test Performed	Measurements

I. Intact Knee (N = 12)
  a. 50 N posterior force
  b. 100 N posterior force
	Six degree of freedom knee kinematics

II. PCL and MFL sectioned (N = 12) Same as in I	Same as in I

III. One-strand PCL reconstructions
  S_1 (N = 12), S_2 (N = 7), D (N = 5)
  50 N posterior force
	Six degree of freedom knee kinematics
	Strand tension

IV. Two-strand PCL reconstructions
  S_1-S_2 (N = 7), S_1-D (N = 5)
  100 N posterior force
	Six degree of freedom knee kinematics
	Tension in both strands

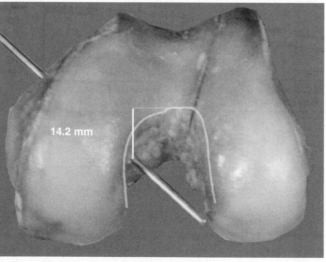

A

4.6 mm

B

15.6 mm

C

14.2 mm

FIGURE 20–34. A–C, The transverse view of the three femoral tunnel positions. The measurements are taken posteriorly from the point at which the trochlear groove meets the intercondylar notch. *(From Mannor, D. A.; Shearn, J. T.; Grood, E. S.; et al.: Two-bundle posterior cruciate ligament reconstruction. An in vitro analysis of graft placement and tension. Am J Sports Med 28:833–845, 2000.)*

Both strands shared the applied load, as shown. In contrast, a two-strand construct in which one strand was placed anterior and a second was placed more proximal resulted in a marked difference in load-sharing, with a reciprocal loading relationship found between strands (Fig. 20–41). In both situations, posterior

translation limits were restored to normal. Similar results were reported by Carson and associates[9] who conducted an in vitro study of cadaveric knees using a two-bundle (two femoral tunnels) and tibial inlay graft and measured forces in the anterolateral and posteromedial bundles. A reciprocal loading pattern

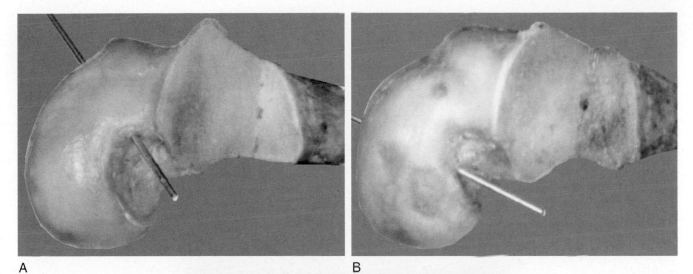

A   B

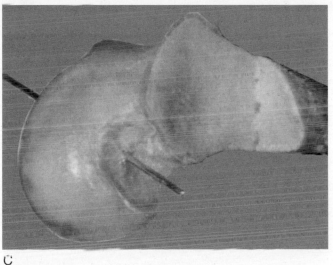

C

FIGURE 20–35. A–C, The oblique view of the three femoral tunnel positions. *(From Mannor, D. A.; Shearn, J. T.; Grood, E. S.; et al.: Two-bundle posterior cruciate ligament reconstruction. An in vitro analysis of graft placement and tension. Am J Sports Med 28:833–845, 2000.)*

was reported when the anterolateral bundle was placed anterior and the posteromedial bundle was placed posterior to the center of femoral rotation. These authors recommended that tensioning and fixation of the anterolateral and posteromedial bundles be performed at 90° and 0°, respectively.

To further investigate these findings, a fourth cadaveric study was conducted on 19 lower limbs to determine the tension that develops in various two-strand PCL graft constructs.[80] The test conditions are shown in Figure 20–42 for the graft strand configurations. A one-strand PCL reconstruction was performed and the measured graft tension compared with three different two-strand reconstructions. The location of the single- and two-strand graft configurations are shown in Figure 20–43. The one-strand graft was placed in the anterior one third and middle of the PCL femoral attachment. The two-strand PCL graft reconstructions placed one strand in the anterior femoral region (AD$_2$) and the second graft strand in either the distal, the middle, or the proximal third of the PCL attachment. The reconstructions were tensioned (with a custom-designed instrumented spatial linkage) to restore posterior translation to ± 1 mm of the intact knee (90° flexion, 100 N posterior load). The two-strand graft configurations were all tensioned to share load,

with the exception that the proximal strand (MP) was tensioned to carry 20% of the load and the anterior strand was tensioned to carry 80%. The tension in each graft strand was directly measured during knee motion using strain-gauge load-cells following a methodology previously described.[80]

The relationship between graft strand placement within the PCL femoral attachment and the tension and function of the graft strand are shown in Table 20–4. In Figure 20–44, the tension in the single-strand PCL graft is shown to nearly double with knee flexion. Under a 100-N posterior load, the graft tension reached over 200 N. This doubling of the tensile load as a multiple of the applied posterior load has been shown in numerous experiments conducted in laboratory studies. With the knee at 90° of flexion, the PCL is elevated approximately 60° from the sagittal AP plane. At this flexion position, the PCL resists nearly all (95%) of the applied posterior force. In this study, the graft tensions required to restore normal posterior translation limits ranged from 230 to 300 N.

The graft strand tensions for the two-strand PCL reconstructions are shown in Figures 20–45 to 20–47. The average tension and the peak tension decreased for the two-strand reconstructions in which the second graft strand was placed in

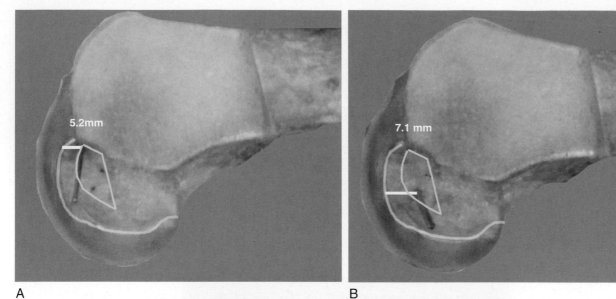

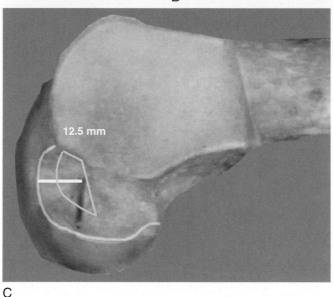

FIGURE 20–36. A–C, The sagittal view of the three femoral tunnel positions. *(From Mannor, D. A.; Shearn, J. T.; Grood, E. S.; et al.: Two-bundle posterior cruciate ligament reconstruction. An in vitro analysis of graft placement and tension. Am J Sports Med 28:833–845, 2000.)*

either a distal or a middle position and able to share the posterior resisting load (Table 20–5). This represented the most ideal arrangement for the two graft strands, particularly when the second graft strand was placed in the middle third of the PCL attachment. In contrast, placement of the second graft strand in a more proximal location resulted in a reciprocal loading behavior between both graft strands, with higher loads placed on the anterior graft strand in comparison with those in the other two-strand configurations.

The data in this experiment support the conclusions of prior studies previously described that small changes in graft position in a proximal-to-distal direction within the PCL attachment have a pronounced effect on graft tension behavior. The hypothesis of this study is that load-sharing between two-strand PCL reconstructions is more ideal in terms of graft function in the long term in preventing posterior tibial subluxation with increasing knee flexion. In addition, the lower graft strand loads in a load-sharing configuration would be more protective against deleterious graft elongation that would be expected to occur under higher loads. It

should be noted that under the conditions of the experiment, all of the two-strand reconstructions restored the posterior translation limit to within ± 1 mm of the intact knee, whereas the single-strand reconstruction resulted in a slight overconstraint of 2 mm (which occurred at the 30° flexion position; Fig. 20–48).

Petersen and associates,[68] in a cadaveric study, examined the effect of the femoral tunnel position of a two-bundle PCL reconstruction using a robotic testing system. These authors reported a significant effect of the femoral tunnel position in fiber tension behaviors. An anterior position of the two tunnels (anterolateral 7 mm, posteromedial 4 mm from femoral articular cartilage) was recommended. A more posterior (deep) placement of the tunnels was not recommended. One problem should be noted in that the PCL reconstructions (80 N tension at 90° knee flexion) resulted in a residual posterior tibial translation (7–10 mm at 90° knee flexion). It is preferred that biomechanical experiments tension grafts until the abnormal posterior translation is eliminated and not to an arbitrary graft tension, as in this study.

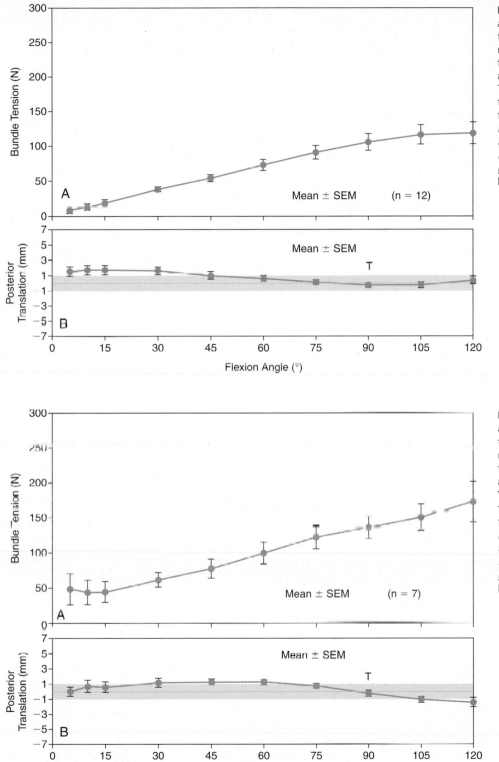

FIGURE 20–37. Strand tension (**A**) and change in posterior translation from intact (**B**) for the S$_1$ one-strand reconstruction with a 50-N posterior force. The T indicates the flexion angle at which the strand was tensioned. The *shaded area* for posterior translation represents the translation for the intact knee ± 1 mm. *(A and B, From Mannor, D. A.; Shearn, J. T.; Grood, E. S.; et al.: Two-bundle posterior cruciate ligament reconstruction. An in vitro analysis of graft placement and tension. Am J Sports Med 28:833–845, 2000.)*

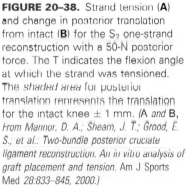

FIGURE 20–38. Strand tension (**A**) and change in posterior translation from intact (**B**) for the S$_2$ one-strand reconstruction with a 50-N posterior force. The T indicates the flexion angle at which the strand was tensioned. The *shaded area* for posterior translation represents the translation for the intact knee ± 1 mm. *(A and B, From Mannor, D. A.; Shearn, J. T.; Grood, E. S.; et al.: Two-bundle posterior cruciate ligament reconstruction. An in vitro analysis of graft placement and tension. Am J Sports Med 28:833–845, 2000.)*

Markolf and colleagues[47] conducted a cadaveric study in which one- and two-strand PCL reconstructions were performed to determine whether the second graft strand placed in a posterior position (two placements, center and proximal PCL footprint) provided an advantage in terms of tensile load-sharing between graft fibers. The posteriorly placed grafts provided a resistance to posterior tibial translation, developed tension in the low knee flexion range, and developed greater than the normal PCL forces measured prior to PCL reconstructions. One problem not explained in the study is that under 100 N posterior tibial load, the PCL would be expected (as the primary restraint in an oblique position) to develop close to or greater than the 100-N applied posterior forces. In the experimental results, the PCL only developed forces of approximately 30 to 50 N in

FIGURE 20–39. Strand tension (**A**) and change in posterior translation from intact (**B**) for the D one-bundle reconstruction with a 50-N posterior force. The T indicates the flexion angle at which the strand was tensioned. The *shaded area* for posterior translation represents the translation for the intact knee ± 1 mm. (*A and B, From Mannor, D. A.; Shearn, J. T.; Grood, E. S.; et al.: Two-bundle posterior cruciate ligament reconstruction. An in vitro analysis of graft placement and tension. Am J Sports Med 28:833–845, 2000.*)

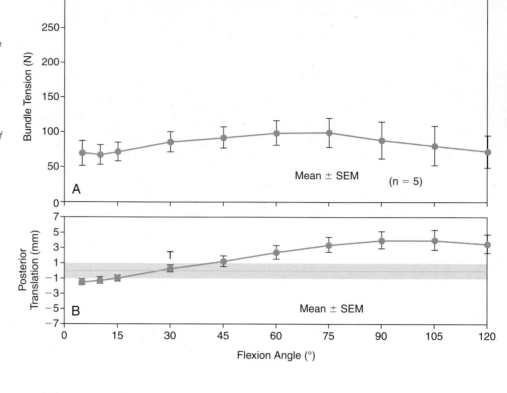

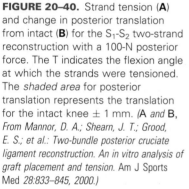

FIGURE 20–40. Strand tension (**A**) and change in posterior translation from intact (**B**) for the S_1-S_2 two-strand reconstruction with a 100-N posterior force. The T indicates the flexion angle at which the strands were tensioned. The *shaded area* for posterior translation represents the translation for the intact knee ± 1 mm. (*A and B, From Mannor, D. A.; Shearn, J. T.; Grood, E. S.; et al.: Two-bundle posterior cruciate ligament reconstruction. An in vitro analysis of graft placement and tension. Am J Sports Med 28:833–845, 2000.*)

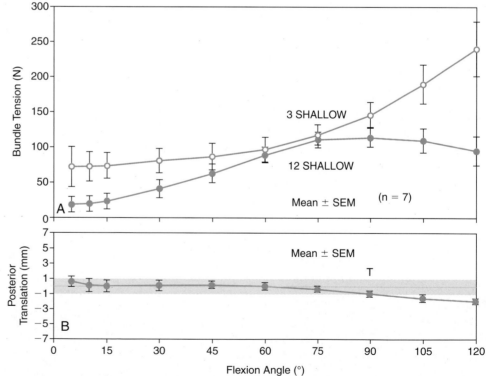

the 20° to 40° flexion range, which is considerably lower than would be expected. Therefore, it is difficult to interpret the data because the PCL and graft forces were less than expected.

Race and Amis[70] examined the separate functions of the anterolateral (aPCL) and posteromedial (pPCL) PCL bundles under loaded conditions in cadaveric knees. The results showed that approaching knee extension, ligamentous restraints other than the PCL provide a significant contribution to resisting posterior tibial translation (Fig. 20–49). With increasing knee flexion, the aPCL and the pPCL provide a posterior resisting force. These results question the traditional concept that the pPCL provides a posterior resistance close to knee extensions because the pPCL

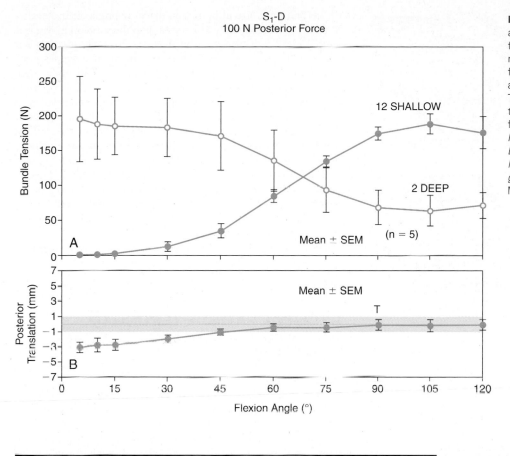

S₁-D
100 N Posterior Force

FIGURE 20–41. Strand tension (**A**) and change in posterior translation from intact (**B**) for the S₁-D two-strand reconstruction with a 100-N posterior force. The T indicates the flexion angle at which the strands were tensioned. The *shaded area* for posterior translation represents the translation for the intact knee + 1 mm. *(A and B, From Mannor, D. A.; Shearn, J. T.; Grood, E. S.; et al.: Two-bundle posterior cruciate ligament reconstruction. An in vitro analysis of graft placement and tension. Am J Sports Med 28:833–845, 2000.)*

Configurations Tested	Measurements
I. Intact Knee (N = 14)	Flexion angle, A/P Translation
II. PCL and MFL sectioned (N = 14)	Same as I
III. One-strand PCL reconstruction AD₁ (N = 5)	Flexion Angle, A/P Translation, Strand Tension
IV. Two-strand PCL reconstruction AD₂-MD (N = 5) AD₂-MM (N = 5) AD₂-MP (N = 4)	Same as III

FIGURE 20–42. Knee configurations tested and measurements made. AD₁, one-strand anterior-distal reconstruction; AD₂-MD, two-strand anterior-distal, middle-distal reconstruction; AD₂-MM, two-strand anterior-distal, middle-middle reconstruction; AD₂-MP, two-strand anterior-distal, middle-proximal reconstruction; A/P, anterior/posterior; MFL, meniscofemoral ligaments; PCL, posterior cruciate ligament. *(From Shearn, J. T.; Grood, E. S.; Noyes, F. R.; Levy, M. S.: Two-bundle posterior cruciate ligament reconstruction: how bundle tension depends on femoral placement. J Bone Joint Surg Am 86:1262–1270, 2004.)*

is aligned nearly perpendicular to a posterior loading direction. Further, with knee flexion, the pPCL is oriented in a more advantageous position because it is less vertical in terms of resisting posterior tibial displacement. These data support those from the senior author,[45] as already discussed. In addition, surgical reconstruction of the knee with significant posterior instability at low flexion angles implies damaged medial and posterolateral structures described in the bumper model analogy in Chapter 3, The Scientific Basis for Examination and Classification of Knee Ligament Injuries.

Race and Amis[72] demonstrated in a cadaveric study that a single anterolateral bundle reconstruction alone would not prevent abnormal posterior tibial translation at high flexion angles. Markolf and coworkers[48] studied in cadavers the effect of a single PCL graft placed in three tunnels (anterior, central, and posterior) within the PCL femoral footprint. The authors reported that if a single graft is used, a central location provided the best match for the PCL. The anterolateral and

posteromedial tunnel positions did not control posterior tibial translation and underwent potentially deleterious high forces. A problem in the experimental design was that the posteromedial graft was tensioned at 90° knee flexion (its shortest position) and, therefore, underwent very high tensile loads as the knee approached full extension. It is important at surgery to determine the length change of the graft construct (tibiofemoral separation distance during knee flexion-extension), as is discussed later.

Wiley and associates[96] studied in cadavers the effect of single- and double-bundle PCL grafts and reported that the double-bundle reconstruction had statistically lower posterior tibial translation. Both graft constructs were placed into the distal two thirds, or more shallow, PCL femoral attachment (avoiding a posterior or deep graft placement) and both grafts were tensioned at 90° knee flexion. The single-bundle PCL reconstruction was placed more proximally in the PCL attachment.

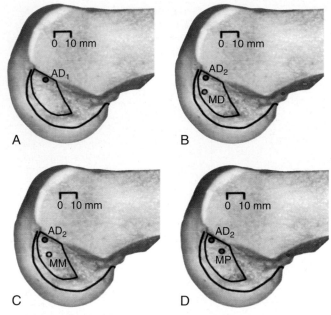

FIGURE 20–43. Sagittal views of the femur in 90° of flexion. **A,** One-strand anterior-distal reconstruction. The anterior-distal attachment (AD_1) is 6.7 mm from the trochlear groove and 10.6 mm from the cartilage edge. **B,** Two-strand anterior-distal, middle-distal reconstruction. The anterior-distal attachment (AD_2) is 5.2 mm from the trochlear groove and 6.3 mm from the cartilage edge. **C,** Two-strand anterior-distal, middle-middle reconstruction. The middle-middle attachment (MM) is 14.8 mm from the trochlear groove and 9.5 mm from the cartilage edge. **D,** Two-strand anterior-distal, middle-proximal reconstruction. The middle-proximal attachment (MP) is 12.1 mm from the trochlear groove and 13.3 mm from the cartilage edge. *(A–D, From Shearn, J. T.; Grood, E. S.; Noyes, F. R.; Levy, M. S.: Two-bundle posterior cruciate ligament reconstruction: how bundle tension depends on femoral placement. J Bone Joint Surg Am 86:1262–1270, 2004.)*

The primary conclusion of these studies is that most of the graft constructs are capable of restoring the posterior translation limit to normal after PCL sectioning. However, the constructs do so by inducing high tensile forces in the graft that may be deleterious and result in graft elongation and failure. To the extent that the in vitro data apply to in vivo graft function, the surgeon may select a position of the second graft strand that induces either load-sharing or reciprocal loading. Placement of the two graft strands in the middle region avoids the large tibio-femoral separations and resultant graft tensions that affect grafts placed closer to the periphery of the PCL attachment. These findings contradict those of other studies that recommend that

the second graft strand be placed distal or proximal in relation to the PCL attachment.[70,71] Even though the surgeon may select a more ideal graft placement in regard to load-sharing between graft strands, or the more ideal placement of a single graft strand, the data show that due to the diameter of the graft, there will be asymmetrical graft loading with portions of the graft at the outside diameter undergoing different elongation and tension than other portions. This makes it difficult for any graft strand to reproduce the complex microgeometry of the PCL in which different length collagen fibers are brought into the loading sequence as knee flexion occurs.

Data are not currently available from clinical studies to determine whether two-strand PCL grafts are more successful in restoring posterior tibial translation than single-strand PCL grafts. There are no clinical data that compare two-strand PCL grafts implanted in an equal load-sharing configuration versus a reciprocal load-sharing (proximal-distal grafts) configuration. These are important areas for future study to improve the success rate of PCL reconstructions.

CYCLICAL FATIGUE TESTING OF ONE- AND TWO-STRAND PCL GRAFT CONSTRUCTS

Several potential mechanisms exist for failure of a PCL graft after implantation, and it is important to design operative techniques and a postoperative rehabilitation program that diminish high tensile forces when possible. Because the PCL is the primary restraint to posterior tibial subluxation, any activities that involve high knee flexion or hamstring activation (descending stairs, walking down a ramp, squatting) may induce deleterious graft tensile forces.[4,10,51,66] In the early postoperative period, before graft maturation occurs and an adequate quadriceps muscle force production is able to counteract these forces, graft elongation or failure might occur. All of the muscles that cross the knee joint are involved in increasing joint contact forces by allowing normal knee joint geometry to decrease high tibial shear forces (see Chapter 23, Rehabilitation of Posterior Cruciate Ligament and Posterolateral Reconstructive Procedures).[10,49,57] Improper graft tensioning (at the knee position of the shortest length) will produce high tensile forces as the graft elongates with knee flexion or extension. Abrasion of collagen strands against bone tunnels is a known cause of graft thinning and rupture.[6,53,79]

The cyclical fatigue of a PCL graft after implantation has been reported in only a few studies.[6,53,79] The failure mechanism of cyclical fatigue involves the nonuniform distribution of loads. For example, a single graft strand placed into the PCL femoral

TABLE 20–4	Posterior Translation with Graft Tensioning*					
Reconstruction	**Knees (N)**	**Change in Posterior Translation (mm)†**	**Anterior-Distal Strand Tension (N)**	**Second Strand Tension (N)**	**Total Strand Tension (N)**
One-strand (anterior-distal)	5	−0.7 ± 0.3	230.3 ± 23	NA	230.3 ± 23
Two-strand (anterior-distal, middle-distal)	5	−0.1 ± 0.3	123.3 ± 6	152.3 ± 14	275.6 ± 19
Two-strand (anterior-distal, middle-middle)	5	−0.1 ± 0.4	148.0 ± 12	155.1 ± 15	303.1 ± 22
Two-strand (anterior-distal, middle-proximal)	4	0.6 ± 0.5	246.9 ± 20	40.8 ± 16	287.7 ± 25

*The data are for 90° of flexion with a 100-N posterior force applied to the proximal part of the tibia. The values are given as the mean ± the standard error of the mean.
†Compared with the intact knee.
NA, not available.

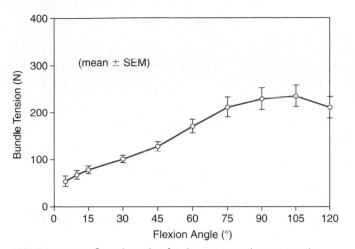

FIGURE 20–44. Strand tension for the one-strand reconstruction. SEM, standard error of the mean. *(From Shearn, J. T.; Grood, E. S.; Noyes, F. R.; Levy, M. S.: Two-bundle posterior cruciate ligament reconstruction: how bundle tension depends on femoral placement. J Bone Joint Surg Am 86:1262–1270, 2004.)*

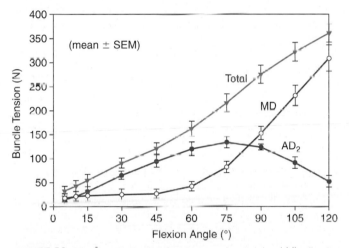

FIGURE 20–45. Strand tension for the anterior-distal, middle-distal reconstruction. AD$_2$, anterior strand; MD, middle-distal strand; SEM, standard error of the mean. *(From Shearn, J. T.; Grood, E. S.; Noyes, F. R.; Levy, M. S.: Two-bundle posterior cruciate ligament reconstruction: how bundle tension depends on femoral placement. J Bone Joint Surg Am 86:1262–1270, 2004.)*

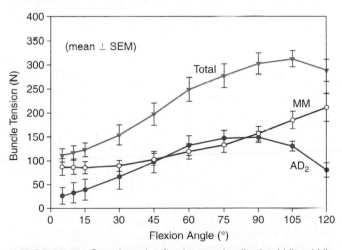

FIGURE 20–46. Strand tension for the anterior-distal, middle-middle reconstruction. AD$_2$, anterior strand; MM, middle-middle strand; SEM, standard error of the mean. *(From Shearn, J. T.; Grood, E. S.; Noyes, F. R.; Levy, M. S.: Two-bundle posterior cruciate ligament reconstruction: how bundle tension depends on femoral placement. J Bone Joint Surg Am 86:1262–1270, 2004.)*

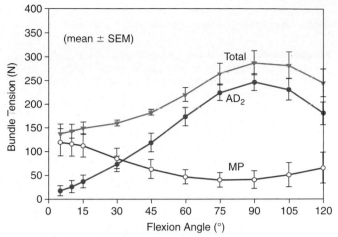

FIGURE 20–47. Strand tension for the anterior-distal, middle-proximal reconstruction. AD$_2$, anterior strand; MP, middle-proximal strand; SEM, standard error of the mean. *(From Shearn, J. T.; Grood, E. S.; Noyes, F. R.; Levy, M. S.: Two-bundle posterior cruciate ligament reconstruction: how bundle tension depends on femoral placement. J Bone Joint Surg Am 86:1262–1270, 2004.)*

TABLE 20–5 Anterior Strand Tension

Reconstruction	Average Tension* (N)	Peak Tension* (N)	Angle at Peak Tension	Slope* (N/30° flexion)
One strand (AD)	149.3 ± 11	236.2 ± 23	105°	49.9 ± 4
Two-strand (AD MD)	74.7 ± 7	133.9 ± 12	75°	18.9 ± 4
Two-strand (AD-MM)	88.6 ± 9	148.0 ± 12	90°	25.7 ± 5
Two-strand (AD-MP)	133.2 ± 14	246.9 ± 20	90°	60.0 ± 6

*The values are given as the mean ± the standard error of the mean.
AD, anterior-distal; AD-MD, anterior-distal, middle-distal; AD-MM, anterior-distal, middle-middle; AD-MP, anterior-distal, middle-proximal.

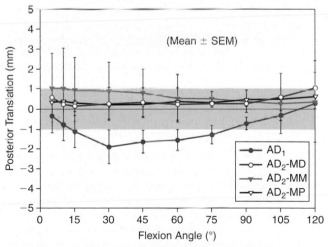

FIGURE 20–48. Change in posterior translation compared with the intact knee. The *gray-shaded area* represents translation within ± 1 mm of that in the intact knee. AD$_1$, single-strand anterior-distal reconstruction; AD$_2$-MD, two-strand anterior-distal, middle-distal reconstruction; AD$_2$-MM, two-strand anterior-distal, middle-middle reconstruction; AD$_2$-MP, two-strand anterior-distal, middle-proximal reconstruction. *(From Shearn, J. T.; Grood, E. S.; Noyes, F. R.; Levy, M. S.: Two-bundle posterior cruciate ligament reconstruction: how bundle tension depends on femoral placement. J Bone Joint Surg Am 86:1262–1270, 2004.)*

FIGURE 20–49. Graph of average percentage contribution to resisting posterior displacement against flexion angles for the anterolateral posterior cruciate ligament (aPCL), the posteromedial posterior cruciate ligament (pPCL), and combined other structures (N = 9). (From Race, A.; Amis, A. A.: Loading of the two bundles of the posterior cruciate ligament: an analysis of bundle function in a-P drawer. J Biomech 29:873–879, 1996.)

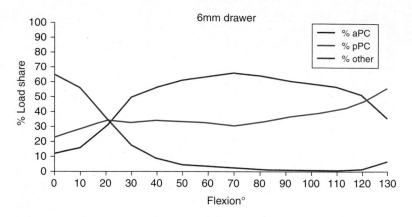

Critical Points CYCLICAL FATIGUE TESTING OF ONE- AND TWO-STRAND POSTERIOR CRUCIATE LIGAMENT GRAFT CONSTRUCTS

- Design operative techniques and postoperative rehabilitation program that diminish high tensile forces.
- High knee flexion activities, hamstring activation (descending stairs, walking down a ramp, squatting), produce deleterious graft tensile forces.
- Early postoperative period, before adequate quadriceps muscle force able to counteract forces, graft elongation or failure may occur.
- A single diameter graft of a fixed length does not function as a native posterior cruciate ligament (PCL).
- A proximal-to-distal change in graft position of only a few millimeters results in significant changes in graft tension-length relationships.
- Cyclical fatigue testing of PCL grafts show marked effect, produce premature graft failure after few hundred knee flexion cycles.
- All graft configurations show marked sensitivity to cyclical loading.
- Only the two-strand construct (one anterior strand, one central strand) showed two- to threefold increase in number of cycles to graft failure.
- Number of cycles to failure would be reached in the first 2 weeks of rehabilitation unless appropriate measures were taken to limit posterior translation loads and number of flexion-extension cycles.
- In vitro data indicate need to build into protocols measures to protect PCL grafts early postoperatively.

attachment with knee flexion-extension would subject the individual graft fibers to different tensions and lengths. The native PCL has different fiber lengths that are brought into the loading profile; however, a single-diameter graft of a fixed length does not function as a native PCL fiber. This means that individual fibers would, at certain periods, be carrying the majority of the applied load, potentially resulting in an overload situation and graft fiber elongation. The biomechanical studies already presented show that a proximal-to-distal change in graft position of 2 to 3 mm results in significant changes in graft tension-length relationships. As well, a PCL graft strand may be subjected to angulation (bending) or torsional forces at the bone insertion site. A native ligament has two fibrocartilagenous zones[63] owing to diffuse insertional forces over a wide area and decreased stiffness that prevents stress concentration effects.

It is theorized that collagen graft fibers placed into a bone tunnel do not undergo remodeling to restore a normal attachment site,[7,95] and therefore, stress concentration effects are always present, particularly at higher in vivo loads when activity is resumed.

The transfer of a B-PT-B construct may be highly beneficial in this regard because there is evidence that the bone-tendon junction does remodel to a normal attachment site.[75]

Studies of cyclical fatigue testing of PCL grafts after implantation have reported a marked effect of this loading that produced premature graft failure. In three studies, the flexion angle of the graft construct was fixed and a load applied in a cyclical manner to test a one-strand B-PT-B graft.[6,53,55] This type of loading is less ideal in terms of understanding graft cyclical fatigue properties because single tensile loading does not reproduce the loading profile that a graft would be subjected to with knee flexion-extension motion. Mehalik[56] studied the cyclical behavior of one-strand Achilles tendon grafts in knees cycled to 90° of flexion and reported an increase in posterior translation of approximately 1.7 mm after 1000 cycles (posterior load, 50 N; flexion limit, 105°).

Markolf and colleagues[53] performed a cyclical loading study of a B-PT-B allograft using a tibial tunnel and a tibial inlay technique. After 2000 cycles, the graft length of the inlay and tunnel methods increased 5.9 mm and 9.8 mm, respectively (load level, 50–300 N). The authors concluded that grafts undergo thinning and increase in length with both fixation techniques. There was greater thinning and degradative effects of the angulated grafts in tibial tunnels than with the tibial inlay grafts. For example, 10 of 31 grafts (32%) failed at the acute angle of tibial attachment prior to 2000 cycles, whereas all of the 31 tibial inlay graft constructs survived the testing procedure. The data suggest that a 10-mm wide B-PT-B graft replacement for PCL reconstruction, with either a tunnel or an inlay technique, might result in unacceptable graft elongation under the loading profile. However, the relationship of the cyclical loading behavior to the other mechanical properties of the graft was not studied, and it is possible that significant disuse and age effects resulted in increased elongation or premature failure.

Bergfeld and coworkers[6] compared a tibial tunnel graft technique with a tibial inlay technique using a 10-mm central third B-PT-B graft in cadavers. Both reconstructions restored posterior translation limits to within 2 mm (150 N loading). A tensile load on the PCL graft at the femoral site of 89 N was used. After 72 cycles (from 0°–90°), the "laxity" of both reconstructions increased as a result of graft stretching, with thinning of the graft found at the tibial tunnel exit but not in the tibial inlay group. The authors acknowledged that the conditions of tensioning may have overconstrained knees in the inlay group.

In a study from the authors' laboratory,[79] the cyclical behavior of a PCL B-PT-B graft was reported using cadaveric knee joints cycled from 5° to 120° under 100 N posterior loading. The conditions of the experiment were already described and four graft constructs used are shown in Figure 20–42. The behavior of a normal PCL under cyclical loading is shown in Figure 20–50, where at 2048 cycles, the increase in posterior translation under loading was less than 1 mm. The return of 2.5 mm of posterior translation for the four PCL reconstruction techniques is shown in Table 20–6. All of the graft configurations showed a marked sensitivity to cyclical loading. The return of 7.5 mm of posterior translation was also low in terms of the numbers of cycles. Only the two-strand construct with one anterior graft strand and a second strand placed in the middle configuration showed a two- to threefold increase in the number of cycles to graft failure (Fig. 20–51). Even so, this number of cycles to failure would be reached in the first 2 weeks of rehabilitation unless appropriate measures were taken to limit

flexion-extension cycles or the maximum of 120°. The results further showed that 76% of the grafts failed at or adjacent to the femoral attachment region (19 of 25 grafts), with 20% (5 of 25 grafts) in the mid-substance, and 4% (1 of 25 grafts) at the tibial attachment ($P < .001$).

Hiraga and colleagues[35] reported the results of cyclical loading tests on four types of PCL reconstruction in cadaveric knees. The knee joints were cycled between 0 and 100 N for 1000 cycles. Increases in posterior tibial translation were attributed to slippage of the graft and/or permanent elongation of the graft construct. The knees were positioned at 90° of flexion, and the cyclical loading involved repetitive AP displacements. This is in contrast to the study by Shearn and coworkers[79] in which the knees were cycled between 0° and 120° of knee flexion. It is important that differences in cyclical loading techniques be understood, because the cyclical loading under both posterior load and knee flexion-extension is more detrimental in terms of inducing graft elongation or failure than unidirectional loading. Hiraga and colleagues[35] reported that no grafts failed under the reduced loading of 100 N; however, there were increases in posterior tibial translation after only 100 cycles in all reconstruction groups. The greatest increase was found in semitendinosus-gracilis (STG) grafts that were fixated with an EndoButton (Smith & Nephew, Naples, FL), which was then an STG graft fixed with an interference screw and an Endopearl device (Linvatec, Largo, FL). There was no difference between B-PT-B tibial tunnel and B-PT-B

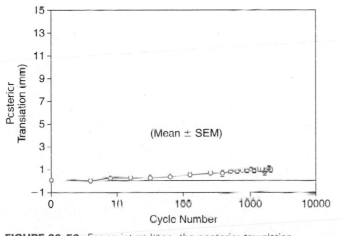

FIGURE 20–50. For an intact knee, the posterior translation increased during a cyclical fatigue test at 90° flexion ($N = 8$ for cycle numbers 384, 640, 896, 1152, 1408, 1664, 1920; $N = 12$ for the other cycle numbers). *(From Shearn, J. T.; Grood, E. S.; Noyes, F. R.; Levy, M. S. One- and two-strand posterior cruciate ligament reconstructions: cyclic fatigue testing. J Orthop Res 23:958–963, 2005.)*

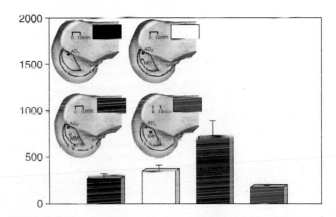

FIGURE 20–51. Cycle number corresponding to a 7.5-mm posterior translation increase. *(From Shearn, J. T.; Grood, E. S.; Noyes, F. R.; Levy, M. S. One- and two-strand posterior cruciate ligament reconstructions: cyclic fatigue testing. J Orthop Res 23:958–963, 2005.)*

TABLE 20–6	Cyclical Data for the Reconstructed Knees				
Reconstruction	**N**	**Cycle Number to 2.5 mm**	**Rate of Posterior Translation Return for 2.5 mm***	**Cycle Number to 7.5 mm**	**Rate of Posterior Translation Return for 7.5 mm***
AD₁	4†	137 ± 44	2.3 ± 0.7	267 ± 52	2.5 ± 0.4
AD₂-MD	4	171 ± 15	1.5 ± 0.2	347 ± 63	2.1 ± 0.5
AD₂-MM	4†	158 ± 21	1.5 ± 0.1	694 ± 188	1.2 ± 0.3
AD₂-MP	4†	80 ± 10	3.1 ± 0.5	176 ± 14	4.0 ± 0.4

*Mean ± standard error of the mean in mm/100 cycles.

†Specimen excluded from 7.5-mm group.

‡Specimen excluded from 2.5-mm group.

AD₁, one-strand anterior-distal; AD₂-MD, two-strand anterior-distal, middle-distal; AD₂-MM, two-strand anterior-distal, middle-middle; AD₂-MP, two-strand anterior-distal, middle-proximal.

tibial inlay reconstructions, with increases in residual posterior translation of approximately 3 mm reported for both tunnel and inlay grafts.

To the extent that these in vitro results apply to in vivo PCL graft constructs, the data indicate the potential need to protect PCL grafts in the initial postoperative period. The in vitro data represent the worst-case scenario for a PCL graft, in that the PCL construct was loaded to 100 N and up to 120° of knee flexion, which would be expected to induce graft tensile loads already reported of 200 to 300 N. In addition, a 5-mm B-PT-B graft was used in contrast to larger-diameter grafts used in vivo, which would undoubtedly require greater number of cycles to ultimate failure. There are insufficient in vitro and in vivo biomechanical and clinical data on the effects of these variables to scientifically construct a rational treatment program. The authors stress that the surgeon will need to select empirical rules in terms of the postoperative treatment rehabilitation protocol.

REFERENCES

1. Ahmad, C. S.; Cohen, Z. A.; Levine, W. N.; et al.: Codominance of the individual posterior cruciate ligament bundles. An analysis of bundle lengths and orientation. *Am J Sports Med* 31:221–225, 2003.
2. Apsingi, S.; Nguyen, T.; Bull, A. M.; et al.: Control of laxity in knees with combined posterior cruciate ligament and posterolateral corner deficiency: comparison of single-bundle versus double-bundle posterior cruciate ligament reconstruction combined with modified Larson posterolateral corner reconstruction. *Am J Sports Med* 36:487–494, 2008.
3. Arms, S. W.; Pope, M. H.; Johnson, R. J.; et al.: The biomechanics of anterior cruciate ligament rehabilitation and reconstruction. *Am J Sports Med* 12:8–18, 1984.
4. Berchuck, M.; Andriacchi, T. P.; Bach, B. R.; Reider, B.: Gait adaptations by patients who have a deficient anterior cruciate ligament. *J Bone Joint Surg Am* 72:871–877, 1990.
5. Bergfeld, J. A.; McAllister, D. R.; Parker, R. D.; et al.: The effects of tibial rotation on posterior translation in knees in which the posterior cruciate ligament has been cut. *J Bone Joint Surg Am* 83:1339–1343, 2001.
6. Bergfeld, J. A.; McAllister, D. R.; Parker, R. D.; et al.: A biomechanical comparison of posterior cruciate ligament reconstruction techniques. *Am J Sports Med* 29:129–136, 2001.
7. Blickenstaff, K. R.; Grana, W. A.; Egle, D.: Analysis of a semitendinosus autograft in a rabbit model. *Am J Sports Med* 25:554–559, 1997.
8. Butler, D. L.; Noyes, F. R.; Grood, E. S.: Ligamentous restraints to anterior-posterior drawer in the human knee. A biomechanical study. *J Bone Joint Surg Am* 62:259–270, 1980.
9. Carson, E. W.; Deng, X. H.; Allen, A.; et al.: Evaluation of in situ graft forces of a 2-bundle tibial inlay posterior cruciate ligament reconstruction at various flexion angles. *Arthroscopy* 23:488–495, 2007.
10. Castle, T. H., Jr.; Noyes, F. R.; Grood, E. S.: Posterior tibial subluxation of the posterior cruciate–deficient knee. *Clin Orthop* 284:193–202, 1992.
11. Clancy, W. G., Jr.; Shelbourne, K. D.; Zoellner, G. B.; et al.: Treatment of knee joint instability secondary to rupture of the posterior cruciate ligament. Report of a new procedure. *J Bone Joint Surg Am* 65:310–322, 1983.
12. Covey, D. C.; Sapega, A. A.; Marshall, R. C.: The effects of varied joint motion and loading conditions on posterior cruciate ligament fiber length behavior. *Am J Sports Med* 32:1866–1872, 2004.
13. Covey, D. C.; Sapega, A. A.; Sherman, G. M.: Testing for isometry during reconstruction of the posterior cruciate ligament. Anatomic and biomechanical considerations. *Am J Sports Med* 24:740–746, 1996.
14. Daniel, D. M.; Stone, M. L.; Barnett, P.; Sachs, R.: Use of the quadriceps active test to diagnose posterior cruciate ligament disruption and measure posterior laxity of the knee. *J Bone Joint Surg Am* 70:386–391, 1988.
15. de Lange, A.; Van Dijk, R.; Huiskes, R.: Three-dimensional experimental assessment of knee ligament length patterns: in vitro. *Trans Orthop Res Soc* 8:10, 1983.
16. Denham, R. A.; Bishop, R. E.: Mechanics of the knee and problems in reconstructive surgery. *J Bone Joint Surg Br* 60:345–352, 1978.
17. Dickhaut, S. C.; DeLee, J. C.: The discoid lateral-meniscus syndrome. *J Bone Joint Surg Am* 64:1068–1073, 1982.
18. Dorlot, J. M.; Christel, P.; Meunier, A.: The displacement of the bony insertion sites of the anterior cruciate ligament during the flexion of the knee. *Trans Orthop Res Soc* 8:328, 1983.
19. Edwards, R. G.; Lafferty, J. F.; Lange, K. O.: Ligament strain in the human knee. *J Basic Eng* 92:131–136, 1970.
20. Fick, R.; von Bardeleben, K. (eds.): Anatomie und Mechanik der Gelenke. Part I: Anatomie der Gelenke; Part II: Allgemeine Gelenk- und Muskelmechanik; Part III: Spezielle Gelenk- und Muskelmechanik. Jena, Germany; Gustav Fischer, 1911.
21. Gill, T. J.; DeFrate, L. E.; Wang, C.; et al.: The effect of posterior cruciate ligament reconstruction on patellofemoral contact pressures in the knee joint under simulated muscle loads. *Am J Sports Med* 32:109–115, 2004.
22. Gollehon, D. L.; Torzilli, P. A.; Warren, R. F.: The role of the posterolateral and cruciate ligaments in the stability of the human knee. A biomechanical study. *J Bone Joint Surg Am* 69:233–242, 1987.
23. Grood, E. S.; Hefzy, M. S.; Lindenfeld, T. N.: Factors affecting the region of most isometric femoral attachments. Part I: the posterior cruciate ligament. *Am J Sports Med* 17:197–207, 1989.
24. Grood, E. S.; Noyes, F. R.; Butler, D. L.; Suntay, W. J.: Ligamentous and capsular restraints preventing straight medial and lateral laxity in intact human cadaver knees. *J Bone Joint Surg Am* 63:1257–1269, 1981.
25. Grood, E. S.; Stowers, S. F.; Noyes, F. R.: Limits of movement in the human knee. Effect of sectioning the posterior cruciate ligament and posterolateral structures. *J Bone Joint Surg Am* 70:88–97, 1988.
26. Gupte, C. M.; Bull, A. M.; Atkinson, H. D.; et al.: Arthroscopic appearances of the meniscofemoral ligaments: introducing the "meniscal tug test." *Knee Surg Sports Traumatol Arthrosc* 14:1259–1265, 2006.
27. Gupte, C. M.; Bull, A. M.; Thomas, R. D.; Amis, A. A.: A review of the function and biomechanics of the meniscofemoral ligaments. *Arthroscopy* 19:161–171, 2003.
28. Gupte, C. M.; Bull, A. M.; Thomas, R. D.; Amis, A. A.: The meniscofemoral ligaments: secondary restraints to the posterior drawer. Analysis of anteroposterior and rotary laxity in the intact and posterior-cruciate-deficient knee. *J Bone Joint Surg Br* 85:765–773, 2003.
29. Gupte, C. M.; Smith, A.; Jamieson, N.; et al.: Meniscofemoral ligaments—structural and material properties. *J Biomech* 35:1623–1629, 2002.
30. Gupte, C. M.; Smith, A.; McDermott, I. D.; et al.: Meniscofemoral ligaments revisited. Anatomical study, age correlation and clinical implications. *J Bone Joint Surg Br* 84:846–851, 2002.
31. Haimes, J. L.; Wroble, R. R.; Grood, E. S.; Noyes, F. R.: Role of the medial structures in the intact and anterior cruciate ligament–deficient knee. Limits of motion in the human knee. *Am J Sports Med* 22:402–409, 1994.
32. Harner, C. D.; Vogrin, T. M.; Hoher, J.; et al.: Biomechanical analysis of a posterior cruciate ligament reconstruction. Deficiency of the posterolateral structures as a cause of graft failure. *Am J Sports Med* 28:32–39, 2000.
33. Hefzy, M. S.; Grood, E. S.: Sensitivity of insertion locations on length patterns of anterior cruciate ligament fibers. *J Biomech Eng* 108:73–82, 1986.
34. Heller, L.; Langman, J.: The menisco-femoral ligaments of the human knee. *J Bone Joint Surg Br* 46:307–313, 1964.

35. Hiraga, Y.; Ishibashi, Y.; Tsuda, E.; Toh, H. T.: Biomechanical comparison of posterior cruciate ligament reconstruction techniques using cyclic loading tests. *Knee Surg Sports Traumatol Arthrosc* 14:13–19, 2006.

36. Hughston, J. C.; Eilers, A. F.: The role of the posterior oblique ligament in repairs of acute medial (collateral) ligament tears of the knee. *J Bone Joint Surg Am* 55:923–940, 1973.

37. Inderster, A.; Benedetto, K. P.; Klestil, T.; et al.: Fiber orientation of posterior cruciate ligament: an experimental morphological and functional study, part 2. *Clin Anat* 8:315–322, 1995.

38. Jamieson, N.; Bull, A. M.; Amis, A. A.: Meniscofemoral ligaments—incidence, anatomy and strength. *J Bone Joint Surg Br* 82(suppl II):139, 2000.

39. Kennedy, J. C.; Hawkins, R. J.; Willis, R. B.: Strain gauge analysis of knee ligaments. *Clin Orthop Relat Res* 129:225–229, 1977.

40. LaPrade, R. F.; Johansen, S.; Wentorf, F. A.; et al.: An analysis of an anatomical posterolateral knee reconstruction: an in vitro biomechanical study and development of a surgical technique. *Am J Sports Med* 32:1405–1414, 2004.

41. LaPrade, R. F.; Tso, A.; Wentorf, F. A.: Force measurements on the fibular collateral ligament, popliteofibular ligament, and popliteus tendon to applied loads. *Am J Sports Med* 32:1695–1701, 2004.

42. Last, R. J.: Some anatomical details of the knee joint. *J Bone Joint Surg Br* 30:683–688, 1948.

43. MacDonald, P.; Miniaci, A.; Fowler, P.; et al.: A biomechanical analysis of joint contact forces in the posterior cruciate deficient knee. *Knee Surg Sports Traumatol Arthrosc* 3:252–255, 1996.

44. Makris, C. A.; Georgoulis, A. D.; Papageorgiou, C. D.; et al.: Posterior cruciate ligament architecture: evaluation under microsurgical dissection. *Arthroscopy* 16:627–632, 2000.

45. Mannor, D. A.; Shearn, J. T.; Grood, E. S.; et al.: Two-bundle posterior cruciate ligament reconstruction. An in vitro analysis of graft placement and tension. *Am J Sports Med* 28:833–845, 2000.

46. Markolf, K. L.; Gorek, J. F.; Kabo, J. M.; et al.: Direct measurement of resultant forces in the anterior cruciate ligament. An in vitro study performed with a new experimental technique. *J Bone Joint Surg Am* 72:557–567, 1990.

47. Markolf, K. L.; Feeley, B. T.; Jackson, S. R.; McAllister, D. R.: Biomechanical studies of double-bundle posterior cruciate ligament reconstructions. *J Bone Joint Surg Am* 88:1788–1794, 2006.

48. Markolf, K. L.; Feeley, B. T.; Jackson, S. R.; McAllister, D. R.: Where should the femoral tunnel of a posterior cruciate ligament reconstruction be placed to best restore anteroposterior laxity and ligament forces? *Am J Sports Med* 34:604–611, 2006.

49. Markolf, K. L.; Graff-Radford, A.; Amstutz, H. C.: In vivo knee stability. A quantitative assessment using an instrumented clinical testing apparatus. *J Bone Joint Surg Am* 60:664–674, 1978.

50. Markolf, K. L.; Graves, B. R.; Sigward, S. M.; et al.: Effects of posterolateral reconstructions on external tibial rotation and forces in a posterior cruciate ligament graft. *J Bone Joint Surg Am* 89:2351–2358, 2007.

51. Markolf, K. L.; O'Neill, G.; Jackson, S. R.; McAllister, D. R.: Effects of applied quadriceps and hamstrings muscle loads on forces in the anterior and posterior cruciate ligaments. *Am J Sports Med* 32:1144–1149, 2004.

52. Markolf, K. L.; Wascher, D. C.; Finerman, G. A.: Direct in vitro measurement of forces in the cruciate ligaments. Part II: the effect of section of the posterolateral structures. *J Bone Joint Surg Am* 75:387–394, 1993.

53. Markolf, K. L.; Zemanovic, J. R.; McAllister, D. R.: Cyclic loading of posterior cruciate ligament replacements fixed with tibial tunnel and tibial inlay methods. *J Bone Joint Surg Am* 84:518–524, 2002.

54. Maynard, M. J.; Deng, X.; Wickiewicz, T. L.; Warren, R. F.: The popliteofibular ligament. Rediscovery of a key element in posterolateral stability. *Am J Sports Med* 24:311–316, 1996.

55. McAllister, D. R.; Markolf, K. L.; Oakes, D. A.; et al.: A biomechanical comparison of tibial inlay and tibial tunnel posterior cruciate ligament reconstruction techniques. Graft pretension and knee laxity. *Am J Sports Med* 30:312–317, 2002.

56. Mehalik, J. N.: Posterior cruciate ligament reconstruction: an investigation of surgical variables: graft attachment location, knee flexion angle at graft fixation, and postoperative knee mobilization. In

Department of Aerospace Engineering and Engineering Mechanics. Cincinnati, OH: University of Cincinnati, 1992.

57. Morrison, J. B.: Function of the knee joint in various activities. *Biomed Eng* 4:573–580, 1969.

58. Morrison, J. B.: The mechanics of the knee joint in relation to normal walking. *J Biomech* 3:51–61, 1970.

59. Noyes, F. R.; Barber-Westin, S. D.: Posterior cruciate ligament revision reconstruction, part 1: causes of surgical failure in 52 consecutive operations. *Am J Sports Med* 33:646–654, 2005.

60. Noyes, F. R.; Barber-Westin, S. D.: Posterolateral knee reconstruction with an anatomical bone–patellar tendon–bone reconstruction of the fibular collateral ligament. *Am J Sports Med* 35:259–273, 2007.

61. Noyes, F. R.; Barber-Westin, S. D.: Surgical reconstruction of severe chronic posterolateral complex injuries of the knee using allograft tissues. *Am J Sports Med* 23:2–12, 1995.

62. Noyes, F. R.; Cummings, J. F.; Grood, E. S.; et al.: The diagnosis of knee motion limits, subluxations, and ligament injury. *Am J Sports Med* 19:163–171, 1991.

63. Noyes, F. R.; DeLucas, J. L.; Torvik, P. J.: Biomechanics of anterior cruciate ligament failure: an analysis of strain-rate sensitivity and mechanisms of failure in primates. *J Bone Joint Surg Am* 56:236–253, 1974.

64. Noyes, F. R.; Stowers, S. F.; Grood, E. S.; et al.: Posterior subluxations of the medial and lateral tibiofemoral compartments. An in vitro ligament sectioning study in cadaveric knees. *Am J Sports Med* 21:407–414, 1993.

65. Ogata, K.; McCarthy, J. A.: Measurements of length and tension patterns during reconstruction of the posterior cruciate ligament. *Am J Sports Med* 20:351–355, 1992.

66. Ohkoshi, Y.; Yasuda, K.; Kaneda, K.; et al.: Biomechanical analysis of rehabilitation in the standing position. *Am J Sports Med* 19:605–611, 1991.

67. Pasque, C.; Noyes, F. R.; Gibbons, M.; et al.: The role of the popliteofibular ligament and the tendon of popliteus in providing stability in the human knee. *J Bone Joint Surg Br* 85:292–298, 2003.

68. Petersen, W.; Lenschow, S.; Weimann, A.; et al.: Importance of femoral tunnel placement in double-bundle posterior cruciate ligament reconstruction: biomechanical analysis using a robotic/universal force-moment sensor testing system. *Am J Sports Med* 34:456–463, 2006.

69. Petersen, W. J.; Loerch, S.; Schanz, S.; et al.: The role of the posterior oblique ligament in controlling posterior tibial translation in the posterior cruciate ligament–deficient knee. *Am J Sports Med* 36:495–501, 2008.

70. Race, A.; Amis, A. A.: Loading of the two bundles of the posterior cruciate ligament: an analysis of bundle function in a-P drawer. *J Biomech* 29:873–879, 1996.

71. Race, A.; Amis, A. A.: PCL reconstruction. In vitro biomechanical comparison of "isometric" versus single- and double-bundled "anatomic" grafts. *J Bone Joint Surg Br* 80:173–179, 1998.

72. Race, A.; Amis, A. A.: The mechanical properties of the two bundles of the human posterior cruciate ligament. *J Biomech* 27:13–24, 1994.

73. Robinson, J. R.; Bull, A. M.; Thomas, R. R.; Amis, A. A.: The role of the medial collateral ligament and posteromedial capsule in controlling knee laxity. *Am J Sports Med* 34:1815–1823, 2006.

74. Robinson, J. R.; Sanchez-Ballester, J.; Bull, A. M.; et al.: The posteromedial corner revisited. An anatomical description of the passive restraining structures of the medial aspect of the human knee. *J Bone Joint Surg Br* 86:674–681, 2004.

75. Rodeo, S. A.; Arnoczky, S. P.; Torzilli, P. A.; et al.: Tendon-healing in a bone tunnel. A biomechanical and histological study in the dog. *J Bone Joint Surg Am* 75:1795–1803, 1993.

76. Saddler, S. C.; Noyes, F. R.; Grood, E. S.; et al.: Posterior cruciate ligament anatomy and length-tension behavior of PCL surface fibers. *Am J Knee Surg* 9:194–199, 1996.

77. Sekiya, J. K.; Haemmerle, M. J.; Stabile, K. J.; et al.: Biomechanical analysis of a combined double-bundle posterior cruciate ligament and posterolateral corner reconstruction. *Am J Sports Med* 33:360–369, 2005.

78. Shahane, S. A.; Ibbotson, C.; Strachan, R.; Bickerstaff, D. R.: The popliteofibular ligament. An anatomical study of the posterolateral corner of the knee. *J Bone Joint Surg Br* 81:636–642, 1999.

79. Shearn, J. T.; Grood, E. S.; Noyes, F. R.; Levy, M. S.: One- and two-strand posterior cruciate ligament reconstructions: cyclic fatigue testing. *J Orthop Res* 23:958–963, 2005.

80. Shearn, J. T.; Grood, E. S.; Noyes, F. R.; Levy, M. S.: Two-bundle posterior cruciate ligament reconstruction: how bundle tension depends on femoral placement. *J Bone Joint Surg Am* 86:1262–1270, 2004.

81. Sidles, J. A.; Larson, R. V.; Garbini, J. L.; et al.: Ligament length relationship in the moving knee. *J Orthop Res* 6:593–610, 1988.

82. Sigward, S. M.; Markolf, K. L.; Graves, B. R.; et al.: Femoral fixation sites for optimum isometry of posterolateral reconstruction. *J Bone Joint Surg Am* 89:2359–2368, 2007.

83. Simonian, P. T.; Sussmann, P. S.; van Trommel, M.; et al.: Popliteomeniscal fasciculi and lateral meniscal stability. *Am J Sports Med* 25:849–853, 1997.

84. Skyhar, M. J.; Warren, R. F.; Ortiz, G. J.; et al.: The effects of sectioning of the posterior cruciate ligament and the posterolateral complex on the articular contact pressures within the knee. *J Bone Joint Surg Am* 75:694–699, 1993.

85. Staubli, H.-U.; Birrer, S.: The popliteus tendon and its fascicles at the popliteal hiatus: gross anatomy and functional arthroscopic evaluation with and without anterior cruciate ligament deficiency. *Arthroscopy* 6:209–220, 1990.

86. Sudasna, S.; Harnsiriwattanagit, K.: The ligamentous structures of the posterolateral aspect of the knee. *Bull Hosp Jt Dis Orthop Inst* 50:35–40, 1990.

87. Sugita, T.; Amis, A. A.: Anatomic and biomechanical study of the lateral collateral and popliteofibular ligaments. *Am J Sports Med* 29:466–472, 2001.

88. Trent, P. S.; Walker, P. S.; Wolf, B.: Ligament length patterns, strength, and rotational axes of the knee joint. *Clin Orthop Relat Res* 117:263–270, 1976.

89. Trus, P.; Petermann, J.; Gotzen, L.: Posterior cruciate ligament (PCL) reconstruction—an in vitro study of isometry. Part I: tests using a string linkage model. *Knee Surg Sports Traumatol Arthrosc* 2:100–103, 1994.

90. Van Dijk, R.: Length measurements on the cruciate ligaments: measuring technique and results. In *The Behavior of the Cruciate Ligaments in the Human Knee.* Dissertation, University of Nijmegen, Netherlands; 1983; pp. 89–126.

91. van Dijk, R.; Huiskes, R.; Selvik, G.: Roentgen stereophotogrammetric methods for the evaluation of the three dimensional kinematic behaviour and cruciate ligament length patterns of the human knee joint. *J Biomech* 12:727–731, 1979.

92. Veltri, D. M.; Deng, X.-H.; Torzilli, P. A.; et al.: The role of the popliteofibular ligament in stability of the human knee. A biomechanical study. *Am J Sports Med* 24:19–27, 1996.

93. Veltri, D. M.; Deng, X. H.; Torzilli, P. A.; et al.: The role of the cruciate and posterolateral ligaments in stability of the knee. A biomechanical study. *Am J Sports Med* 23:436–443, 1995.

94. Weber, W.; Weber, E.: Mechanik der menschlichen. Part II. Ueber das kniegelenk. In Gehwerkzeuge. Gottingen, Germany; 1836; pp. 161–202.

95. Weiler, A.; Peine, R.; Pashmineh-Azar, A.; et al.: Tendon healing in a bone tunnel. Part I: biomechanical results after biodegradable interference fit fixation in a model of anterior cruciate ligament reconstruction in sheep. *Arthroscopy* 18:113–123, 2002.

96. Wiley, W. B.; Askew, M. J.; Melby, A., 3rd; Noe, D. A.: Kinematics of the posterior cruciate ligament/posterolateral corner–injured knee after reconstruction by single- and double-bundle intra-articular grafts. *Am J Sports Med* 34:741–748, 2006.

97. Wroble, R. R.; Grood, E. S.; Cummings, J. S.; et al.: The role of the lateral extra-articular restraints in the anterior cruciate ligament–deficient knee. *Am J Sports Med* 21:257–262; discussion 263, 1993.

Chapter 21

Posterior Cruciate Ligament: Diagnosis, Operative Techniques, and Clinical Outcomes

Frank R. Noyes, MD ■ *Sue D. Barber-Westin*, BS

INDICATIONS

Complete ruptures to the posterior cruciate ligament (PCL) account for approximately 3% of all knee ligament injuries in the general population.[160] However, in the trauma setting, the reported incidence of complete PCL ruptures has been as high as 37% of serious knee-related cases.[40] These injuries are classified as either low-velocity in nature, such as those that occur from contact with another player in sports, or high-velocity, such as a dashboard injury in a motor vehicle accident.[44] The mechanism of PCL rupture in athletes is usually a fall on the flexed knee with a plantar-flexed foot or hyperflexion of the knee.[36] High-velocity injuries frequently involve dislocations with multiple ligament ruptures that require immediate medical attention. In this chapter, the different types of PCL reconstructive techniques are described in detail to allow the

surgeon to select the procedure most suited for the specific knee injury. In addition, the initial diagnosis and management of acute PCL ruptures is addressed in the "Preoperative Planning" section.

The proper management of complete ruptures to the PCL requires thorough knowledge of anatomy, diagnosis, surgical reconstruction, and rehabilitation concepts. Some aspects of the treatment of complete isolated PCL ruptures are controversial owing to the unknown natural history in regard to long-term symptoms, functional limitations, and risk of joint arthritis. Whereas some studies (that included patients with partial PCL deficiency) report that patients do well when treated conservatively,[29,44,116,136–138,148,149] other investigations describe noteworthy symptoms and functional limitations years after the injury that can be disabling[13,30,34,66] (Table 21–1). A high percentage of knees with complete PCL

TABLE 21–1 Investigations on PCL Natural History

Reference	Enrolled (*N*)/Followed (*N*) Acute/Chronic Initial Visit	Partial (*N*)/ Complete (*N*) PCL Rupture	Time of Follow-up from Injury	Symptoms	Limitations	Investigators' Comments
Shelbourne & Muthukaruppan, 2005[137]	*N* = 271 215 completed questionnaires All acute	129 partial 86 complete All isolated PCL	Mean 7.8 yr (range, 1–18 yr)	30% pain (complete PCL ruptures) 47% subjective ratings consistently excellent or good	62% abnormal Cincinnati knee scores (complete PCL ruptures)	No correlation Cincinnati knee scores and PCL laxity.
Shelbourne et al., 1999[136]	*N* = 133 68 clinic visit 65 completed questionnaire All acute	87 partial 46 complete All isolated PCL	Mean 5.4 yr (range, 2.3–11.4 yr)	Instability: 53% none 25% during strenuous activity 13% during recreational activity 8% during ADL	50% returned same sports level 48% decreased sports level 1% no sports 1% problems ADL	No increase in arthritis. No correlation Cincinnati knee scores, symptoms, limitations with PCL laxity grade.
Boynton & Tietjens, 1996[13]	*N* = 43 38 clinic visit All chronic	20 partial 10 complete All isolated PCL	Mean 13.4 yr (range, 5–38 yr)	81% occasional pain 56% occasional swelling	74% limited in activities	Positive correlation Cincinnati overall knee score, symptom score, function score with PCL laxity grade. 53% x-ray deterioration medial TF. Results varied, no clear prognostic factors.
Shino et al., 1995[138]	*N* = 22 Excluded 7 (4 significant damage MFC, 3 early PCL reconstruction) *N* = 15 9 clinic visit 4 completed questionnaire Acute/chronic initial visit	Unknown All isolated PCL	Mean 51 mo (range, 24–96 mo)	IKDC subjective: 3 normal 5 nearly normal 5 abnormal	11 (73%) returned same sport level	Recommend early PCL reconstruction in patients with medial tibiofemoral damage, repairable meniscus tears. Patients 2+ or 3+ posterior drawer, no joint damage tolerated athletics.
Keller et al., 1993[66]	*N* = 54 40 office visit Acute/chronic unknown	37 partial 3 complete All isolated PCL	Mean 6 yr (range, 1–28 yr)	90% pain 35% pain ADL	65% limited in activities 43% problems with walking	Correlation decreased Cincinnati score with time from injury, PCL laxity grade. No correlation quadriceps strength and knee score. Knee deterioration began < 5 yr after injury.
Torg et al., 1989[149]	*N* = 43 Acute/chronic unknown	Unknown 14 isolated PCL 29 combined ligament injury	Mean 5.6 yr (range, 1–35 yr)		Functional results isolated: 5 excellent 7 good 2 fair/poor (problems ADL) Results combined: 4 excellent 10 good 15 fair/poor	Combined injuries poorer results, more likely to develop arthrosis. Predictive indicators: meniscectomy, presence of arthrosis, quadriceps weakness.
Tibone et al., 1988[148]	*N* = 10 Acute/chronic unknown	Unknown All isolated PCL	Mean 6 yr (range, 1–30 yr)	4 pain with sports 3 occasional pain	6/8 patients who played sports returned, activity levels unknown	All but 1 decreased quadriceps strength.

TABLE 21–1 Investigations on PCL Natural History—Cont'd

Reference	Enrolled (*N*)/Followed (*N*) Acute/Chronic Initial Visit	Partial (*N*)/Complete (*N*) PCL Rupture	Time of Follow-up from Injury	Symptoms	Limitations	Investigators' Comments
Parolie & Bergfeld, 1986[116]	*N* = 25 11 acute 14 chronic	5 partial 20 complete All isolated PCL	Mean 6.2 yr (range, 2.2–16 yr)	48% stiffness 24% occasional pain 28% pain after exercise 12% instability with exercise 8% instability with ADL	68% returned prior sports activities 32% returned lower levels	No relationship between isolated posterior instability and ability to return to sports.
Cross & Powell, 1984[29]	*N* = 116 86 no PCL surgery 30 reconstructed 3 acute 113 chronic	37 partial 76 complete 96 isolated 20 combined 19 meniscectomy	3 mo–20 yr	NA for patients no PCL surgery	48% excellent 33% good 19% fair/poor (problems with ADL)	No relationship degree posterior instability and functional result.
Dandy & Pusey, 1982[30]	*N* = 20 All chronic	Unknown All isolated PCL	Mean 7.2 yr (range, 1–38 yr)	70% pain walking long distances 55% pain stairs or squatting 45% giving-way walking uneven ground	18% returned to sports without problems	No relationship degree posterior instability and severity patient symptoms.

ADL, activities of daily living; IKDG, International Knee Documentation Committee; MFC, medial femoral condyle; NA, not available; PCL, posterior cruciate ligament; TF, tibiofemoral.

Critical Points INDICATIONS

- Mechanism of injury, low versus high velocity.
- Complete PCL rupture usually associated with other ligament injuries.
- Isolated PCL rupture treated conservatively; however, represents serious injury, high chance of functional deterioration, arthritis over time.
- Indications for chronic isolated complete PCL rupture: pain and instability with athletics or other activities, swelling, ≥10 mm increased posterior tibial translation at 90° flexion.
- Results of PCL reconstruction in chronic knees less favorable as arthritic symptoms persist.

PCL, posterior cruciate ligament.

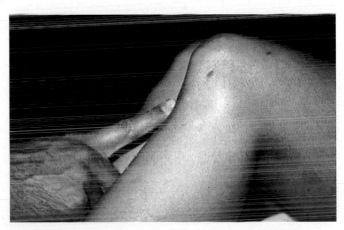

FIGURE 21–1. Severe posterior tibial subluxation is shown in a chronic posterior cruciate ligament (PCL)–deficient knee. There is loss of the normal anterior tibiofemoral step-off.

ruptures develop articular cartilage deterioration over time that usually occurs on the medial femoral condyle and patellofemoral surfaces owing to increased joint pressures.[13,49,50,147] Posterior tibial subluxation after PCL rupture has a deleterious effect to the knee similar to that of a medial meniscectomy, because there is loss of medial meniscus function and increased joint contact stress. There is less of an effect to the lateral meniscus, which retains load-bearing function. Posterior tibial subluxation results in a loss of normal joint kinematics and in coupled external tibial rotation with joint loading. Accordingly, a PCL rupture would be expected to have a more deleterious effect in a varus-angulated knee with associated loss of the medial meniscus and, in particular, larger athletes desiring a return to strenuous athletics. All of these factors alone or together result in substantial medial tibiofemoral loads and risk of joint deterioration.

The indications for surgical reconstruction in knees with a chronic isolated complete PCL rupture are pain and instability with athletics or other activities, swelling, and 10 mm or more of increased posterior tibial translation at 90° flexion (Fig. 21–1). PCL reconstruction is most frequently performed in dislocated knees with gross instability due to other ligament injuries to the anterior cruciate ligament (ACL), medial collateral ligament (MCL; see Chapter 24, Medial and Posteromedial Ligament Injuries: Diagnosis, Operative Techniques, and Clinical Outcomes), or posterolateral structures (see Chapter 22, Posterolateral Ligament Injuries: Diagnosis, Operative Techniques, and Clinical Outcomes). Indications for surgery in acute isolated PCL ruptures are discussed later in this chapter.

If symptomatic meniscal tears or early patellofemoral or tibiofemoral articular cartilage damage is present, early PCL reconstruction is recommended with the goal of decreasing joint deterioration over time. The results of PCL reconstruction in knees with chronic ruptures are not as favorable as those that undergo reconstruction for acute injuries. This is because patients present with pain and swelling due to joint deterioration that often persists even though some benefit may be gained from improved knee stability obtained from the operative procedure.[95]

CONTRAINDICATIONS

Contraindications to PCL reconstruction include acute partial and complete isolated tears that will heal and provide partial function with conservative treatment. Advanced symptomatic patellofemoral or tibiofemoral arthritis is a frequent contraindication. Unfortunately, many patients present with chronic PCL deficiency and severe associated joint arthritis. It is important to distinguish joint instability symptoms from symptomatic arthritis, in which a ligament reconstruction would provide little to no benefit.

Chronic PCL ruptures with varus angulation and early medial tibiofemoral arthritis or with increased lateral joint opening and associated posterolateral insufficiency, require high tibial osteotomy (HTO) before PCL reconstruction.

Dislocated knees require initial observation, vascular evaluation (ankle/brachial index), possible arteriography, early protected range of motion, and rehabilitation to restore muscle function before PCL reconstruction. The authors discourage the use of external fixators to initially stabilize the knee joint, because the use of these devices frequently results in arthrofibrosis and pin track infection and limits the ability to perform a ligament reconstruction. It is important to document with lateral radiographs that tibiofemoral reduction has been maintained and a residual posterior subluxation is not present.

In addition, patients with chronic PCL deficiency who have severe muscle atrophy, loss of knee motion, or hyperextension gait abnormalities require extensive rehabilitation and gait retraining (see Chapter 34, Correction of Hyperextension Gait Abnormalities: Preoperative and Postoperative Techniques) before reconstruction.[107]

A select group of morbidly obese patients sustain serious knee dislocations with minimal trauma. The lack of protective muscle function and the extreme body weight place abnormal tensile loads on ligament reconstructions, and a high rate of failure of a PCL reconstruction is expected. The preferred treatment for these patients is short-term plaster immobilization (and occasionally external fixation) to allow healing of soft tissues, followed by rehabilitation to return muscle function and knee motion. In only exceptional circumstances would operative repair (acute or chronic) be warranted in these patients, although consideration for surgical reconstruction is warranted after appropriate weight reduction.

PCL ANATOMY

The PCL arises from a depression posterior to the intra-articular upper surface of the tibia and courses anteromedially behind the ACL to the lateral surface of the medial femoral condyle and is described in detail in Chapter 2, Lateral, Posterior, and

Critical Points CONTRAINDICATIONS

- Partial isolated PCL tears.
- Advanced symptomatic patellofemoral or tibiofemoral arthrosis.
- Varus-angulated knees with early medial tibiofemoral arthrosis; osteotomy required before PCL reconstruction.
- Dislocated knee: vascular evaluation, protected range of knee motion, return of muscle function before PCL reconstruction.
- Loss of knee motion, quadriceps weakness, hyperextension gait abnormalities: requires extensive rehabilitation and gait retraining before PCL reconstruction.

PCL, posterior cruciate ligament.

Critical Points POSTERIOR CRUCIATE LIGAMENT ANATOMY

- PCL arises from a depression posterior to the intra-articular upper surface of the tibia, courses anteromedially behind ACL to lateral surface of medial femoral condyle.
- Contains type I, type II, type IV mechanoreceptors.
- 91% of knees have at least one meniscofemoral ligament.
- PCL complex anatomic structure comprised of a continuum of fibers of different lengths and attachment characteristics.
- PCL attachment extends from high in the notch (11:30–5:00, right knee).
- Anterior portion of PCL attachment follows articular cartilage within 2–3 mm of its edge.
- Posterior third of PCL is 5 mm from the articular margin.
- Proximal edge of PCL is straight or oval, with the attachment tapered in width along its posterior portion.
- PCL femoral attachment described using rule of thirds to define the proximal-middle-distal thirds (deep to shallow in the femoral notch), and anterior-middle-posterior thirds.
- PCL fibers function from proximal-to-distal in length changes with knee flexion.
- PCL graft femoral attachment location strongly influences graft tension, ability of reconstruction to restore posterior stability.

ACL, anterior cruciate ligament; PCL, posterior cruciate ligament.

Cruciate Knee Anatomy (Fig. 21–2). The PCL has an average length of 38 mm and an average width of 13 mm.[51,155] The cross-sectional area of the PCL is variable and increases from tibial to femoral insertions.[58] It is approximately 50% larger than the ACL at its femoral origin and 20% larger than the ACL at its tibial insertion.

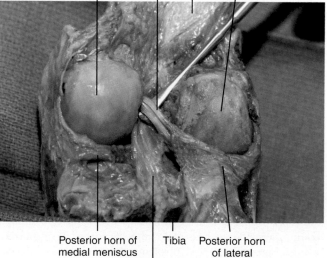

FIGURE 21–2. PCL femoral and tibial attachments. Note the prominent posterior meniscofemoral ligament and broad posterior tibial attachment.

Free nerve endings and mechanoreceptors have been identified in the femoral and tibial attachment sites and on the surface of the PCL.[65,131] The mechanoreceptors resemble Golgi tendon organs and are believed to have a proprioceptive function in the knee.[67]

In a histologic study of the PCL in cadaveric knees, Katonis and coworkers[65] reported a neural innervation similar to that of the ACL. Specifically, the PCL contains type I or Ruffini's corpuscles, which have a slow threshold to pressure changes; type II (Vater-Pacini corpuscles), which are more rapid acting, and type IV (free nerve endings) for pain reception. The mechanoreceptors are located at each ligament bony attachment and on the surface of the PCL.

The meniscofemoral ligaments are in close proximity to the PCL. They arise from the posterior horn of the lateral meniscus and insert near the PCL insertion site on the lateral aspect of the medial femoral condyle.[58] The anterior meniscofemoral ligament (ligament of Humphry) courses anterior to the PCL, and the posterior meniscofemoral ligament (ligament of Wrisberg) runs obliquely behind the PCL. Frequently, the anterior meniscofemoral ligament interdigitates with the PCL fiber attachments on the medial femoral condyle (Fig. 21–3).[87] At least one of the meniscofemoral ligaments is present in 91% of knees, and both ligaments may be found in 50% of knees in young individuals.[55,58,87] The biomechanical function of the meniscofemoral ligaments is discussed in detail in Chapter 28, Meniscus Tears: Diagnosis, Repair Techniques, and Clinical Outcomes.

The traditional division of the PCL into separate anterolateral and posteromedial bundles oversimplifies PCL fiber function. The PCL is a complex anatomic structure composed of a continuum of fibers of different lengths and attachment characteristics. The length-tension behaviors of the fibers that resist posterior tibial translation (with knee flexion) are controlled primarily by femoral attachment regions.[28,46,54,76,77,129,135,140] The distal fibers lengthen with increasing knee flexion and the proximal fibers shorten with knee flexion.[87,129] A detailed description of the length-tension behavior of the PCL appears in Chapter 20, Function of the Posterior Cruciate Ligament and Posterolateral Ligament Structures.

The anatomy of the PCL femoral attachment site has been studied extensively.[87,129] Variation exists between knees in the shape of this attachment, from the common elliptical shape to a more rounded and thicker shape (Fig. 21–4).[87] Differing measurement systems have been proposed to describe the femoral

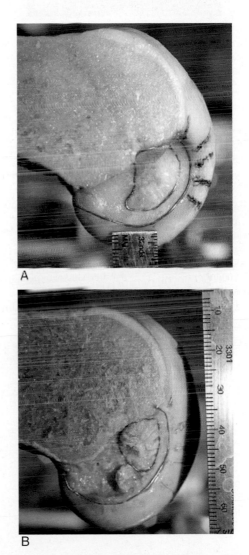

A

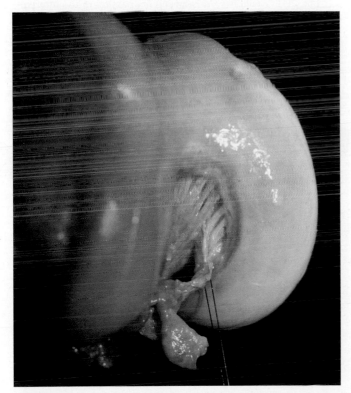

FIGURE 21–3. Anterior meniscofemoral ligament (ligament of Humphry) attachment on the femur interdigitates with the PCL distal fibers. *(From Mejia, E. A.; Noyes, F. R.; Grood, E. S.: Posterior cruciate ligament femoral insertion site characteristics. Importance for reconstructive procedures. Am J Sports Med 30:643–651, 2002.)*

FIGURE 21–4. Composite of the shapes of different PCL insertion sites as seen on lateral views. Variability is noted between specimens from an oval to an elliptical PCL footprint configuration. Note the differences in anterior-to-posterior and proximal-to-distal dimensions in the PCL footprint. The most common shape of the PCL footprint is elliptical. **A,** Note that the fibers insert proximally to the intercondylar roof. The PCL footprint is smaller in its anteroposterior dimension. **B,** Note the prominent posterior meniscofemoral ligaments.

(Continued)

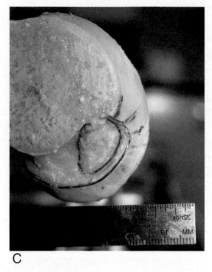

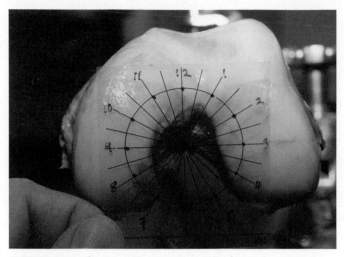

FIGURE 21–4—cont'd.   C, A more oval PCL attachment with greater proximal-to-distal width. *(A–C, From Mejia, E. A.; Noyes, F. R.; Grood, E. S.: Posterior cruciate ligament femoral insertion site characteristics. Importance for reconstructive procedures.* Am J Sports Med *30:643–651, 2002.)*

FIGURE 21–5. Clock markings on the medial femoral condyle as projected from a transparent sheet of acetate onto the notch viewed axially from a knee at 90° of flexion. *(From Mejia, E. A.; Noyes, F. R.; Grood, E. S.: Posterior cruciate ligament femoral insertion site characteristics. Importance for reconstructive procedures.* Am J Sports Med *30:643–651, 2002.)*

attachment site. The most accurate of these methods uses a clock reference position (Fig. 21–5), with measurement lines perpendicular to the articular cartilage edge and measurement lines parallel to the femoral shaft (Fig. 21–6).

In general, the PCL attachment extends from high in the notch (11:30 to 5 o'clock position on a right knee) along the medial femoral condyle notch. The anterior portion of the PCL attachment follows the articular cartilage within 2 to 3 mm of its edge and gradually recedes deeper with the notch until, at the 5 o'clock position, the posterior third is 5 mm from the articular margin. Therefore, the distal boundary of the PCL femoral attachment does not parallel the articular margin as reported by others[51,154] but is farthest away from the cartilage margin posteriorly.

The distance of the distal edge of the attachment to the articular cartilage margin is 3.2 ± 0.8 mm at the roof, 5.8 ± 2.2 mm at its midportion, and 7.9 ± 2.2 mm at its "lowest" extent.[129] The distal and proximal measurements for the PCL femoral attachment are shown in Table 21–2. The proximal edge of the PCL is usually straight or partially oval, with the attachment tapered in width along its posterior portion.

The PCL attachment measurements parallel to the intercondylar roof are shown in Table 21–3. The length of the radial measurement lines extending from the intercondylar roof is shown in Table 21–4. This method provides a means to measure the middle and lower portions of the PCL and provides information on the distance from the lowest cartilage margin to the most posterior portion of the PCL attachment.

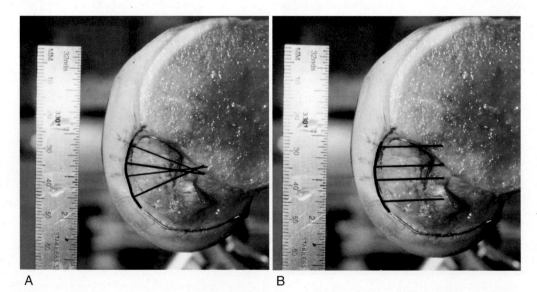

FIGURE 21–6. A, Measurement lines referenced from clock positions perpendicular to the cartilage edge. These reference lines represent the shortest distance to the distal margin of the PCL attachment. **B,** Measurement lines referenced from a clock position parallel to the femoral shaft.

(Continued)

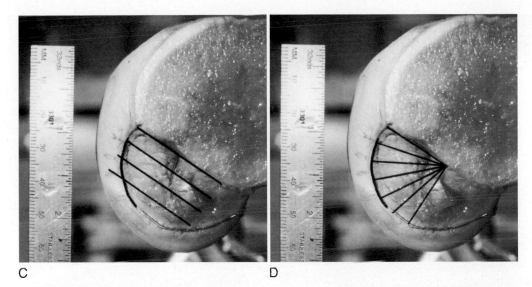

C   D

FIGURE 21–6—cont'd. **C,** Measurement lines referenced from a clock position parallel to the intercondylar roof (5-mm increments). **D,** Measurement lines referenced radially from the intercondylar roof. These lines are directed from a center located at the most proximal extent of the PCL attachment onto the roof of the intercondylar notch. This point is, on average, located at approximately 60% of the roof depth. The line progresses from the 12 o'clock position (*top line*) to the 6 o'clock position (*bottom line*). (A–D, From Mejia, E. A.; Noyes, F. R.; Grood, E. S.: *Posterior cruciate ligament femoral insertion site characteristics. Importance for reconstructive procedures.* Am J Sports Med 30:643–651, 2002.)

TABLE 21–2   PCL Femoral Attachment Measurements Made with the Femoral Condyle Articular Cartilage Clock System

Measurement	Distal (mm)	Proximal (mm)	Thickness (mm)
Perpendicular to the cartilage			
12 o'clock	2.54 ± 1.0	12.92 ± 2.8	10.38 ± 2.8
1 o'clock	2.38 ± 0.7	14.33 ± 2.2	11.96 ± 2.0
2 o'clock	2.38 ± 0.5	14.79 ± 1.8	12.42 ± 1.7
3 o'clock	2.54 ± 0.5	14.83 ± 2.0	12.50 ± 1.7
4 o'clock	2.71 ± 0.7	13.92 ± 2.4	11.71 ± 2.2
Parallel to the femoral shaft			
12 o'clock	2.54 ± 1.0	12.75 ± 2.8	10.25 ± 2.8
1 o'clock	2.38 ± 0.7	13.75 ± 2.8	11.38 ± 2.8
2 o'clock	2.46 ± 0.7	14.63 ± 2.0	12.17 ± 1.9
3 o'clock	2.63 ± 0.8	13.42 ± 2.2	10.83 ± 2.2
4 o'clock	3.78 ± 1.0	11.06 ± 2.6	7.39 ± 2.9

From Mejia, E. A.; Noyes, F. R.; Grood, E. S.: Posterior cruciate ligament femoral insertion site characteristics. Importance for reconstructive procedures. *Am J Sports Med* 30:643–651, 2002.

TABLE 21–3   Length of Measurement Lines Parallel to the Intercondylar Roof

Line location (mm)	Distal (mm)	Proximal (mm)	Thickness (mm)
0	3.50 ± 1.7	13.82 ± 2.8	10.36 ± 3.3
5	2.50 ± 0.7	16.96 ± 2.5	14.54 ± 2.0
10	3.67 ± 1.3	15.21 ± 3.7	11.46 ± 3.7
15	4.25 ± 1.1	13.25 ± 3.9	9.00 ± 4.9

From Mejia, E. A.; Noyes, F. R.; Grood, E. S.: Posterior cruciate ligament femoral insertion site characteristics. Importance for reconstructive procedures. *Am J Sports Med* 30:643–651, 2002.

TABLE 21–4   Length of Measurement Lines Radial to the Intercondylar Roof

Number	Distal (mm)	Proximal (mm)	Thickness (mm)
0	3.17 ± 1.9	12.92 ± 4.7	9.75 ± 4.2
1	2.33 ± 0.7	15.00 ± 2.5	12.67 ± 2.0
2	2.63 ± 0.7	14.96 ± 2.0	12.33 ± 1.8
3	2.54 ± 0.5	14.04 ± 1.7	11.50 ± 1.9
4	2.75 ± 0.9	12.88 ± 1.8	10.13 ± 1.9
5	3.08 ± 0.9	1.46 ± 2.1	8.38 ± 2.1
6	3.21 ± 1.1		

From Mejia, E. A.; Noyes, F. R.; Grood, E. S.: Posterior cruciate ligament femoral insertion site characteristics. Importance for reconstructive procedures. *Am J Sports Med* 30:643–651, 2002.

The use of measurement lines perpendicular to the cartilage edge is preferred for describing the distal attachments of the PCL (see Fig. 21–6A). The disadvantage of this system is that the 12 o'clock and usually the 1 o'clock measurements cannot be made parallel to the femoral shaft, but must be made perpendicular to the cartilage (Fig. 21–7).

Therefore, more than one measurement system is required to describe the anterior, middle, and posterior portions of the PCL femoral origin. Location of the center of the clock face midway in the notch is difficult but critical for identification of the landmarks required to map the PCL femoral attachment. This location should be identified with the knee at 90° of flexion. Ideally, sagittal, anteroposterior, and notch descriptions are required to anatomically represent the entire PCL attachment.

A clear understanding of the anatomy of the native PCL is critical to determining what portion of the ligament will be reconstructed. The terms "high," "low," "shallow," and "deep" are only general descriptors. Because there may be considerable confusion regarding femoral graft tunnel placement during PCL reconstruction, the PCL femoral attachment is described using

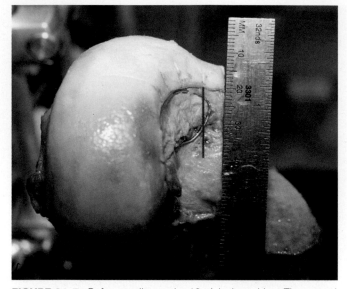

FIGURE 21–7. Reference line at the 12 o'clock position. The curved PCL attachment is shown extending to the intercondylar roof. *(From Mejia, E. A.; Noyes, F. R.; Grood, E. S.: Posterior cruciate ligament femoral insertion site characteristics. Importance for reconstructive procedures. Am J Sports Med 30:643–651, 2002.)*

the rule of thirds (Fig. 21–8A and B) to define the proximal-middle-distal thirds (deep to shallow in the femoral notch) and anterior-middle-posterior thirds (high to low), with a small posterior oblique portion in the sagittal plane.[87,91] This provides a grid for the identification of the tunnel locations for the graft strands and is preferred over the historical division of an anterolateral or a posteromedial bundle (see Fig. 21–8C).

It is well appreciated the PCL graft femoral attachment location strongly influences graft tension and the ability of the reconstruction to restore posterior stability.[5,47,129,135] Investigations by Grood and associates[53] and Sidles and colleagues[140] demonstrate that the femoral attachment location determines the graft tibiofemoral separation distance with knee flexion-extension, much more so than the tibial attachment location. The proximal-distal femoral location of a graft has a greater effect on the attachment separation distance than the anterior-posterior (AP) femoral location, which is the basis for the rule of thirds (see Fig. 21–8B). A graft placed in the distal and middle thirds elongates with knee flexion, whereas a graft placed in the proximal third elongates with knee extension. These concepts are used to select PCL graft attachment locations and tensioning described in the "Operative Techniques" section.

VASCULAR ANATOMY AND VARIATIONS

The vascular supply to the cruciate ligaments is provided mostly by the middle genicular artery, which is a branch of the popliteal artery that penetrates the posterior capsule of the knee.[4,130] The PCL is covered with a well-vascularized synovial sleeve that contributes to its blood supply. The distal portion of the PCL also receives some vascular supply from capsular vessels originating from the inferior genicular arteries and the popliteal artery.

Detailed knowledge of posteromedial knee anatomy, especially the vascular structures, is required to avoid complications

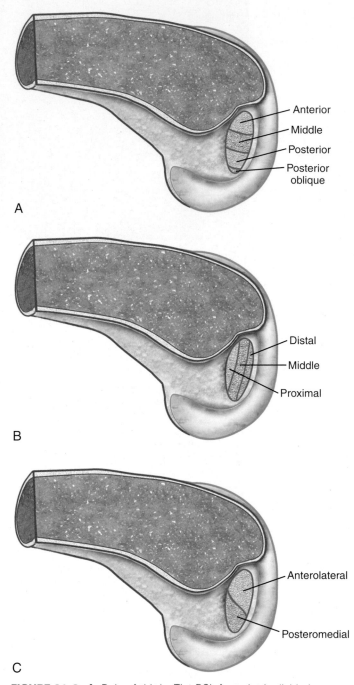

FIGURE 21–8. A, Rule of thirds: The PCL footprint is divided into anterior, middle, and posterior thirds. The anterior third extends past the midline (12:30, left knee) and the posterior region extends to 5 o'clock. The smaller posterior oblique portion of the PCL footprint is also represented. The PCL footprint is elliptical in most knees, but variations exist. **B,** Rule of thirds: The PCL footprint is further divided into the distal, middle, and proximal thirds. This allows for more exact referencing of graft strand placement during PCL reconstruction. The PCL fibers in the distal two thirds lengthen with knee flexion while the proximal fibers shorten. The reverse occurs with knee extension. **C,** Classical division of anterolateral and posteromedial bundles provides an incorrect description of PCL fiber length change, because it describes anterior PCL fibers that lengthen and posterior fibers that shorten with knee flexion.

the level of the supracondylar ridge, superomedial and superolateral genicular arteries are given off.

At the level of the knee joint, four major arteries are distributed: the medial and lateral sural arteries, a cutaneous branch that travels with the small saphenous vein to supply superficial tissues, and the middle genicular artery. Finally, the medial and lateral inferior genicular arteries are given off just distal to the knee joint.

Two branches deserve particular attention. The medial inferior genicular artery arises from the medial aspect of the distal portion of the popliteal artery and runs medially, deep to the medial head of the gastrocnemius, and approximately 2 to 3 mm from the superior surface of the popliteus muscle. It continues around the medial aspect of the proximal tibia, deep to the superficial medial collateral ligament (SMCL). The middle genicular artery arises at the level of the femoral condyles proximal to the joint line and passes anteriorly to pierce the oblique popliteal ligament and posterior joint capsule and supply the cruciate ligaments.

This "normal" vascular pattern has been reported to occur in approximately 88% of cases.[31,84] In approximately 5% to 7% of cases, the popliteal artery will divide at least an inch or more proximal to the distal border of the popliteus muscle.[26,31,84] In slightly less than half of these cases, with a high division of the popliteal artery, the anterior tibial artery passes anterior, not posterior, to the popliteus muscle belly.[153] The number of variations of the anterior tibial artery according to Mauro and coworkers[84] is illustrated in Figure 21–9. Therefore, with a tibial inlay approach,

when using a posteromedial approach to a tibial inlay PCL reconstruction (see Chapter 2, Lateral, Posterior, and Cruciate Knee Anatomy). The popliteal artery originates at the adductor hiatus and passes through the popliteal fossa. Before passing deep to the fibrous arch over the soleus muscle, it divides into the anterior and posterior tibial arteries at the distal aspect of the popliteus muscle.

Proximal to the knee joint, several muscular branches arise and supply the adductor magnus and hamstring muscles. At

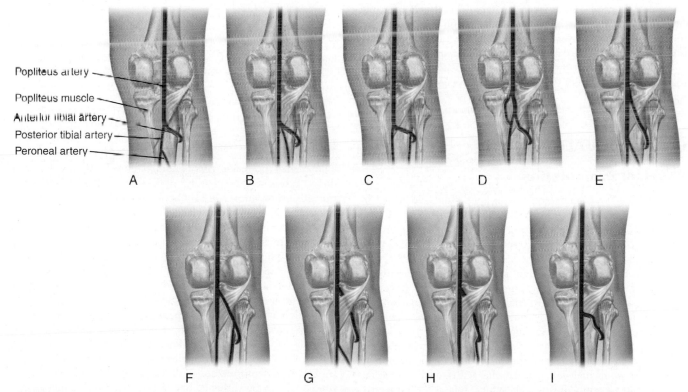

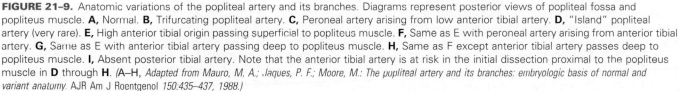

FIGURE 21–9. Anatomic variations of the popliteal artery and its branches. Diagrams represent posterior views of popliteal fossa and popliteus muscle. **A,** Normal. **B,** Trifurcating popliteal artery. **C,** Peroneal artery arising from low anterior tibial artery. **D,** "Island" popliteal artery (very rare). **E,** High anterior tibial origin passing superficial to popliteus muscle. **F,** Same as E with peroneal artery arising from anterior tibial artery. **G,** Same as E with anterior tibial artery passing deep to popliteus muscle. **H,** Same as F except anterior tibial artery passes deep to popliteus muscle. **I,** Absent posterior tibial artery. Note that the anterior tibial artery is at risk in the initial dissection proximal to the popliteus muscle in **D** through **H**. *(A–H, Adapted from Mauro, M. A.; Jaques, P. F.; Moore, M.: The popliteal artery and its branches: embryologic basis of normal and variant anatomy. AJR Am J Roentgenol 150:435–437, 1988.)*

the dissection is always proximal to the popliteus muscle with a meticulous technique, because the anterior tibial artery is at risk for transection in approximately 3% to 4% of knees.

An unusual variation in the vascular pattern involves the popliteal artery passing medial and then beneath the medial head of the gastrocnemius. Various subtypes of this abnormal pattern have been described. An abnormal vascular pattern may manifest clinically as the popliteal artery entrapment syndrome, which is characterized by vascular claudication symptoms.[70,125,143] Arterial insufficiency occurs most commonly with entrapment of the artery deep to the medial gastrocnemius muscle, but can also occur when the artery is entrapped deep to the popliteus muscle (persistence of ventral component of artery) or deep to an abnormal accessory head of the gastrocnemius. A history of pain in the lower extremity with activity and disappearance with rest, particularly in a young patient, should alert the surgeon to the possibility that an abnormal vascular pattern may exist. Further evaluation with magnetic resonance imaging (MRI) or angiography may be warranted.[45,74]

Embryologic development helps to explain these abnormal vascular patterns. In the embryo, the lower extremity blood supply is derived from the sciatic or axial artery (a branch of the internal iliac artery) as well as the femoral artery (a branch of the external iliac artery). The proximal sciatic artery regresses, whereas the middle and distal sciatic artery persists to form the definitive popliteal and peroneal arteries.

The anterior tibial artery arises as a branch of the popliteal artery and initially courses anterior to the popliteus muscle. In humans, the early anterior tibial artery is replaced with the superficial popliteal artery and passes posterior to the popliteus muscle, which then gives rise to the anterior tibial artery. Furthermore, during embryonic life, the medial head of the gastrocnemius migrates medially and cranially. It is with this migration that the popliteal artery can be caught and swept medially with the muscle.[84,125]

CLINICAL EVALUATION

Physical Examination

A comprehensive examination of the knee joint is required to detect all abnormalities. This includes assessment of (1) the patellofemoral joint and extensor mechanism malalignment, which may occur if increased external tibial rotation exists owing to posterolateral ligament injury that accompanies the PCL rupture; (2) patellofemoral and tibiofemoral crepitus, indicative of articular cartilage damage; (3) gait abnormalities (excessive hyperextension or varus thrust) during walking and jogging[107]; and (4) abnormal knee motion limits and subluxations compared with those of the contralateral knee.[109]

Experienced clinicians are aware that patients with chronic deficiency of the PCL and posterolateral structures may develop an abnormal gait pattern characterized by excessive knee hyperextension during the stance phase.[107] Subjective complaints of knee instability and giving-way during routine daily activities, along with severe quadriceps atrophy, often accompany this gait abnormality. Gait analysis and retraining are required in patients who demonstrate abnormal knee hyperextension patterns before proceeding with any ligament reconstruction (see Chapter 34, Correction of Hyperextension

---

Gait Abnormalities: Preoperative and Postoperative Techniques).[107] The failure to do so may lead to failure of reconstructed ligaments if the abnormal gait pattern is resumed postoperatively.

Diagnostic Clinical Tests

The medial posterior tibiofemoral step-off on the posterior drawer test is performed at 90° of flexion. The amount of posterior tibial translation will vary between knees with isolated PCL ruptures due to physiologic laxity or injury to the secondary posterolateral or medial soft tissue restraints. Posterior tibial translation progressively increases with injury to the secondary restraints. The importance of determining abnormal medial or lateral joint opening and increases in external-internal tibial rotation cannot be overemphasized, because the failure to correct these associated subluxations places PCL graft reconstructions under high in vivo forces postoperatively and risk of graft failure. The diagnostic tests and their interpretation are discussed in Chapter 20, Function of the Posterior Cruciate Ligament and Posterolateral Ligament Structures, and are shown in Table 22–1.

The exact determination of the extent of a PCL tear (partial vs. complete) can be difficult, but is essential from a therapeutic standpoint. The clinical posterior drawer test can be highly subjective, with the forces applied too variable to allow accurate determination of the status of the PCL. MRI is not always accurate in diagnosing partial PCL tears (Fig. 21–10). Frequently, this test may indicate that the ligament is completely ruptured; however, ligament continuity may still exist with some portions

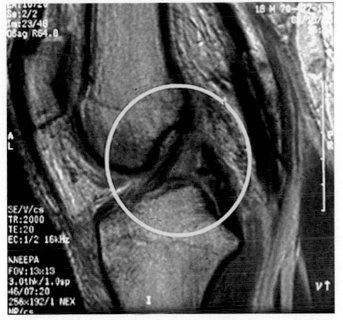

FIGURE 21–10. A partial PCL rupture is shown. Even though the magnetic resonance imaging (MRI) scan suggests a complete rupture, there were remaining PCL fibers resisting posterior tibial subluxation.

functioning to limit posterior tibial subluxation to only a few millimeters. Patten and associates[117] reported only a 67% sensitivity rate of the ability of MRI to distinguish complete from partial PCL tears by identifying focal areas of ligamentous discontinuity.

The quantitative measurement of posterior tibial subluxation in knees with PCL ruptures or reconstruction is therefore important.[60] The knee arthrometer is the most frequently used device to measure posterior tibial translation after PCL injury and reconstruction. However, the knee arthrometer underestimates the true amount of posterior translation in PCL-deficient and reconstructed knees, often by several millimeters.[60,78,146] Stress radiography is the most accurate and reproducible technique currently available,[37,43,60,78,119,132] yet only a few studies to date have used this method to document posterior tibial translation after PCL reconstruction. The authors recommend that PCL clinical investigations incorporate stress radiography to provide a more valid measure of posterior tibial translation (Fig. 21–11). To correct for tibial rotation, which can produce errors in measurement, the radiograph should be as close to a pure lateral as possible, with the two femoral condyles superimposed upon themselves. A horizontal line is placed across the medial tibial plateau and a perpendicular line determines the posterior position of each femoral condyle. A similar measurement is made for the most posterior position of the medial and lateral tibial plateau. The amount of tibial translation is the average of both of these measurements.

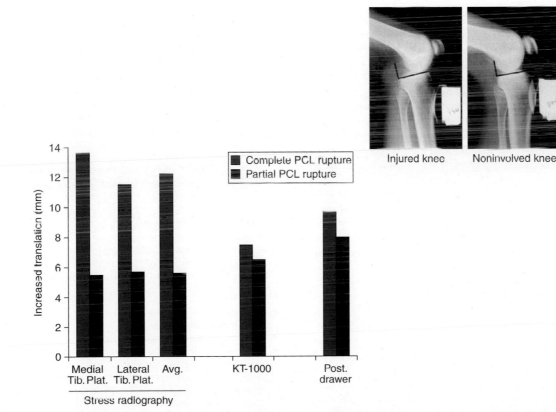

Injured knee   Noninvolved knee

FIGURE 21–11. The results of lateral stress radiography on 20 patients with PCL deficiency (9 complete ruptures and 11 partial ruptures). The differences in the measurements between complete and partial PCL ruptures for the medial tibial plateau, the lateral tibial plateau, and the average of both plateaus were statistically significant ($P < .01$). Differences in the KT-1000 and posterior drawer measurements between complete and partial PCL ruptures were not significant. The KT measurements at 70° flexion underestimated the magnitude of posterior tibial subluxation for complete PCL ruptures. *(From Hewett, T. E.; Noyes, F. R.; Lee, M. D.: Diagnosis of complete and partial posterior cruciate ligament ruptures. Stress radiography compared with KT-1000 arthrometer and posterior drawer testing. Am J Sports Med 25:648–655, 1997.)*

The integrity of the ACL is determined by Lachman and pivot shift testing. The result of the pivot shift test is recorded on a scale of 0 to 3, with a grade of 0 indicating no pivot shift; grade I, a slip or glide; grade II, a jerk with gross subluxation or clunk; and grade III, gross subluxation with impingement of the posterior aspect of the lateral side of the tibial plateau against the femoral condyle. A KT-2000 arthrometer test may be done at 20° of flexion (134 N force) to quantify total AP displacement.

Medial and lateral ligament insufficiency are determined by varus and valgus stress testing at 0° and 30° of knee flexion. The surgeon estimates the amount of joint opening (in millimeters) between the initial closed contact position of each tibiofemoral compartment, performed in a constrained manner avoiding internal or external tibial rotation, and the maximal opened position. The result is recorded according to the increase in the tibiofemoral compartment of the affected knee compared with that of the opposite normal knee.

The tibiofemoral rotation dial test at 30° and 90° is done to determine whether increases in external tibial rotation exist with posterior subluxation of the lateral tibial plateau (see Fig. 22–3).[109] This test is described in further detail in Table 22–1.

The presence of a varus recurvatum in both the supine and the standing positions is carefully assessed. The difference in results of these tests must be done between the injured and the contralateral normal knee owing to inherent physiologic looseness present in some individuals.

Radiographic Assessment

Radiographs taken during the initial examination include AP, lateral at 30° of knee flexion, weight-bearing posteroanterior (PA) at 45° of knee flexion, and patellofemoral axial views.

Posterior stress radiographs are done with an 89-N force applied to the proximal tibia.[60] A lateral radiograph is taken of each knee at 90° of flexion. The limb is placed in neutral rotation with the tibia unconstrained and the quadriceps relaxed. The difference in posterior tibial displacement between the reconstructed knee and the contralateral knee is recorded. More than 8 mm of increase in posterior tibial translation on stress testing indicates a complete PCL rupture.[132]

Medial or lateral stress radiographs may be required of both knees. The patient is seated (0° knee extension) in neutral tibial rotation with the tibia unconstrained. Approximately 89 N of varus or valgus force is applied and comparison made of the millimeters of medial or lateral tibiofemoral compartment opening between knees.

Full standing radiographs of both lower extremities, from the femoral heads to the ankle joints, are done in knees in which varus lower extremity alignment is detected on clinical examination. The mechanical axis and weight-bearing line are measured to determine whether HTO is indicated before PCL reconstruction (see Chapter 31, Primary, Double, and Triple Varus Knee Syndromes: Diagnosis, Osteotomy Techniques, and Clinical Outcomes).[35,105] If the varus malalignment is not corrected, there is a risk that either a PCL or an ACL graft may fail owing to the varus thrusting forces and concurrent increased lateral joint opening producing high graft tension loads.[96]

Patients complete questionnaires and are interviewed for the assessment of symptoms, functional limitations, sports and occupational activity levels, and patient perception of the overall knee condition according to the Cincinnati Knee Rating System (CKRS).[6]

PREOPERATIVE PLANNING

Acute Ruptures of the PCL

Controversy exists in the treatment of midsubstance complete PCL ruptures, primarily owing to the lack of a scientifically-proven operative procedure that can predictably restore posterior stability and PCL function. In comparison, surgical procedures to reattach the native PCL in cases of bony avulsion injuries or peel-off injuries directly at the PCL attachment site have more predictable healing rates.[12,73,151,152] Even in cases of PCL rupture directly at the attachment site, usually sufficient ligament substance remains for a direct repair. In select situations, an augmentation using the semitendinosus tendon may facilitate PCL repair.

Augmentation of partial PCL tears is controversial.[3,63,156] Graft reconstruction of the so-called posteromedial portion of the PCL has been described in which the "anterolateral bundle" is still intact and functional. The authors have no experience with this technique and have not performed augmentation procedures in the acute setting. Stress radiography plays an

---

Critical Points PREOPERATIVE PLANNING

Acute Ruptures
- Reattach native PCL bony avulsion injuries, peel-off injuries directly at PCL attachment, predictable healing rates.
- Select knees, augmentation with semitendinosus tendon may facilitate PCL repair, add postoperative protection.
- Partial or acute isolated PCL tears
  - Immobilize 4 wk in full knee extension brace or bivalved cylinder cast.
  - Lateral radiograph verifies no posterior tibial subluxation.
  - 2 wk: 0°–90° of motion maintaining anterior tibial translation load. Patient sleeps in brace, no unsupervised knee motion.
  - 4 wk: active quadriceps extension out of brace, 50% weight-bearing, crutch support, maintain brace protection.
  - 5–6 wk: wean from the brace and crutch support, rehabilitation (see Chapter 23, Rehabilitation of Posterior Cruciate Ligament and Posterolateral Reconstructive Procedures).
- Acute PCL injuries with associated rupture to medial or posterolateral structures: delay reconstruction until neurovascular status and other injuries are resolved and major knee ligament surgery can be safely performed.
- Associated posterolateral ruptures: acute anatomic repair required within 14 days before scarring occurs.
- PCL graft reconstruction in select athletes before secondary restraints stretch out with subsequent reinjury, arthritis.

Chronic Injuries
- Assess patient symptoms, goals, athletic desires: may indicate PCL reconstruction required.
- Varus malalignment: osteotomy before PCL reconstruction.
- PCL plus medial or posterolateral ligament injury, complex instability pattern, usually surgical candidate.
- Severe arthrosis: not expected to benefit from PCL reconstruction.
- Nonoperative approach chronic PCL tears: warn that return to athletics carries uncertain prognosis, joint arthrosis may eventually ensue.
- Consider bone scan, MRI cartilage sequences.
- Initiate rehabilitation, patient education, avoid high knee flexion activities.

MRI, magnetic resonance imaging; PCL, posterior cruciate ligament.

important role in determining whether an abnormal increase of 10 mm or more exists, indicating loss of PCL function. Partial ligament tears are treated conservatively with an extension brace and posterior calf pad to allow for potential PCL healing.

The treatment rationale for patients with acute PCL ruptures is shown in Figure 21–12. The algorithm is divided into three major sections based on the PCL tear (partial, complete, or combined with other ligament ruptures). The 10-mm division is somewhat arbitrary. As discussed, stress radiography is helpful in determining the exact increase in posterior tibial translation. The rules to treat partial or acute isolated PCL tears are

1. Immobilize for 4 weeks in a full-knee extension brace or bivalved cylinder cast to maintain tibiofemoral reduction. Use quadriceps isometrics, electrical muscle stimulation, leg raises, and 25% weight-bearing.
2. Obtain a lateral radiograph to verify that no posterior tibial subluxation exists, which can occur in up to 50% of knees.
3. At 2 weeks, the therapist initiates 0° to 90° of motion, maintaining an anterior tibial translation load. The patient must sleep in the brace and is not allowed unsupervised knee motion to prevent posterior tibial subluxation.
4. At 4 weeks, the patient is allowed to perform active quadriceps extension out of the brace, 50% weight-bearing, crutch support and maintains brace protection.
5. At 5 to 6 weeks, the patient is weaned from the brace and crutch support, full knee flexion is allowed, and the rehabilitation protocol described in Chapter 23, Rehabilitation of Posterior Cruciate Ligament and Posterolateral Reconstructive Procedures, is followed to protect the healing PCL fibers.

In the authors' experience, 4 weeks of protection to allow initial healing of a complete PCL rupture will frequently restore partial PCL function, with less than 10 mm residual posterior tibial subluxation. The initial PCL healing process involves a low tensile strength and an additional 4 to 6 weeks of protection is recommended, including avoiding athletics, running, walking on downhill grades, walking down stairs, or other high knee flexion activities that load the PCL. Even in knees with a complete PCL tear and more than 10 mm of increased posterior tibial displacement, healing of the disrupted PCL fibers may still occur, although a residual posterior tibial subluxation of a few millimeters (with a hard endpoint) will remain. These knees in which partial PCL function has been restored should be followed and repeat stress radiographs obtained at 6 months and over the next few years to determine PCL function. These partial PCL tears seldom require reconstruction. However, Shelbourne and associates[136,137] described that one third or more of patients in this group have abnormal knee scores and pain with athletic activities owing usually to concomitant articular cartilage damage. A repeat MRI with fast-spin-echo cartilage sequences[122] helps determine the integrity of the articular cartilage and provides important information for counseling the patient on athletic activities to decrease the risk of future joint arthritis.

In cases of complete isolated midsubstance PCL ruptures that have more than 10 mm of increased posterior tibial displacement in which the patient is seen late after the injury and the previously discussed program cannot be instituted, one treatment approach in athletes and those in strenuous high-risk

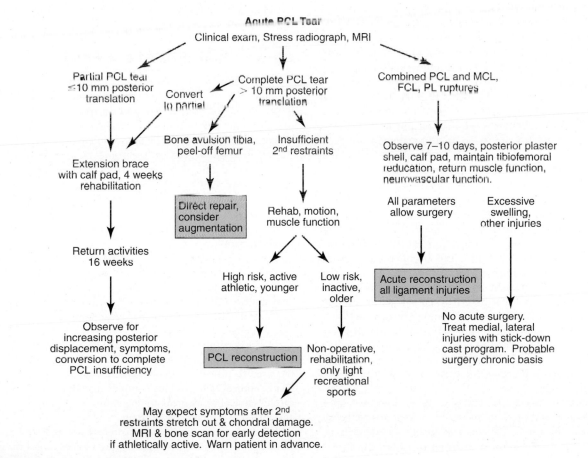

FIGURE 21–12. Treatment algorithm for acute PCL ruptures.

occupations is PCL graft reconstruction before the secondary restraints stretch out with subsequent reinjury. The authors believe that, in athletic individuals, PCL reconstructive procedures have advanced to the point at which more predictable results can be expected to restore sufficient PCL function to prevent gross posterior tibial subluxation. Studies have demonstrated, at least in the short term, that the majority of patients with acute PCL ruptures treated with reconstruction are able to return to various levels of sports activities.[95] Additional factors to be weighed in the decision to perform early surgery on an isolated PCL rupture (with > 10 mm posterior displacement, 90° flexion) include athletic goals, body weight, medial meniscus or tibiofemoral joint damage, patellofemoral joint damage, and varus malalignment; these factors add to the effects of the residual posterior subluxation in increasing knee joint loads and subsequent joint deterioration. Future long-term clinical studies will confirm the importance of these factors in the operative decision of early restoration of PCL function in active younger individuals who subject their knee to high forces in sports or work activities. Sedentary patients with a complete PCL rupture and more than 10 mm of posterior translation (90° flexion) are not considered surgical candidates; however, they are followed as previously described.

Patients with a PCL disruption and other ligament injuries have an obvious posterior tibial dropback without a firm endpoint on posterior drawer testing, and 10 mm or more of posterior tibial subluxation. In almost all of these knees, some increase in medial or lateral joint opening or external tibial rotation can be detected, although the findings may be subtle. There may be physiologic laxity of other ligament structures without a true injury (see Chapter 3, The Scientific Basis for Examination and Classification of Knee Ligament Injuries) that allows for the gross posterior tibial subluxation.

In knees that present with acute disruption of the PCL and medial or posterolateral structures, reconstruction should be delayed until the neurovascular status and other injuries are resolved and major knee ligament surgery can be safely performed. In knees that have associated posterolateral ruptures, acute anatomic repair is required within 14 days before scarring occurs and the ability to anatomically restore these structures is lost (see Chapter 22, Posterolateral Ligament Injuries: Diagnosis, Operative Techniques, and Clinical Outcomes). A similar situation exists for the medial ligament structures; however, these tissues are easier to reconstruct later if surgery cannot be performed in the ideal time period for anatomic repair. There may exist a displaced meniscus tear requiring early treatment. As a word of caution, a displaced meniscus should be reduced into the tibiofemoral joint by 3 weeks to prevent meniscus shortening and scarring that compromises a future repair and results in loss of meniscus function. Even in knees that have marked soft tissue swelling and edema, and in which major ligament reconstruction is contraindicated, a meniscus repair procedure using all-inside techniques can be performed to reduce the meniscus to a normal tibiofemoral position. The mistake is to wait until 6 weeks or later, expecting that the meniscus repair can be performed at that time.

Too frequently, major ligament surgery in dislocated knees performed under acute conditions results in joint arthrofibrosis, compromising the result. Patients should be carefully selected for acute multiligament repairs, realizing that there are proven techniques for reconstruction of the ruptured ligaments performed later under more ideal conditions. When surgery is performed on acute combined PCL and posterolateral ruptures, the procedure includes the use of appropriate grafts to restore lateral stability and allow an early protected range of knee motion program, described in Chapter 22, Posterolateral Ligament Injuries: Diagnosis, Operative Techniques, and Clinical Outcomes. The majority of acute knee dislocations should be treated in a staged approach by first treating the acute injury and then determining whether a ligament reconstruction should be performed either within the 10- to 14-day envelope or delayed. When early surgery is not advisable, the knee is protected for the first 4 weeks to prevent posterior tibial subluxation, as already described for acute isolated PCL ruptures. A lateral radiograph is obtained with the knee placed in a posterior plaster shell and a soft bolster positioned beneath the calf to prevent posterior tibial subluxation. The capsular tissues heal in 7 to 10 days to provide enough stability to prevent recurrence of dislocation.

If a nonoperative approach is selected with associated MCL and posteromedial capsular disruptions, the same program is followed with the lower limb placed in a cylinder cast to allow "stick-down" of the medial soft tissues. Plaster immobilization is required because a soft hinged brace, even if maintained at 0° of extension, does not provide sufficient protection to maintain medial joint line closure to allow the disrupted medial tissues to heal. At 7 to 10 days, the cylinder cast is split into an anterior and a posterior shell and the therapist assists the patient with range of motion from 0 to 90° in a figure-four position with the hip joint externally rotated to protect the healing medial tissues. This program of "aggressive" nonoperative treatment of associated medial ligament injuries is described in further detail in Chapter 25, Rehabilitation of Medial Ligament Injuries.

Chronic Ruptures of the PCL

The algorithm for the treatment of chronic PCL ruptures is shown in Figure 21–13. The symptoms and clinical examination determine the functional limitations, particularly the component of symptoms due to medial tibiofemoral or patellofemoral arthritis because these problems are likely to persist after surgical stabilization. Knees with chronic PCL ruptures are arbitrarily divided into three categories; those with varus osseous malalignment (and, rarely, valgus malalignment) in which an osteotomy must be considered, those with an isolated PCL rupture in which reconstruction may or may not be necessary, and those with significant combined ligament injuries that require reconstruction.

Patients are entered into a formal rehabilitation program to correct muscular weakness and gait-related problems (hyperextension) when required. The amount of joint arthritis must be determined with accuracy. Radiographs (merchant, standing PA at 45°) and MRI articular cartilage fast-spin-echo sequences provide valuable information.

In knees with no or only mild articular cartilage damage, an assessment of the patient's goals and athletic desires may indicate the need to proceed with PCL reconstruction. Combined ligament ruptures that produce complex instability patterns require careful clinical assessment to detect all of the joint subluxations and ligament deficiencies present.

Knees that have advanced arthritis are not expected to benefit from ligament reconstruction. In these knees, areas of exposed bone are frequently encountered in the medial tibiofemoral

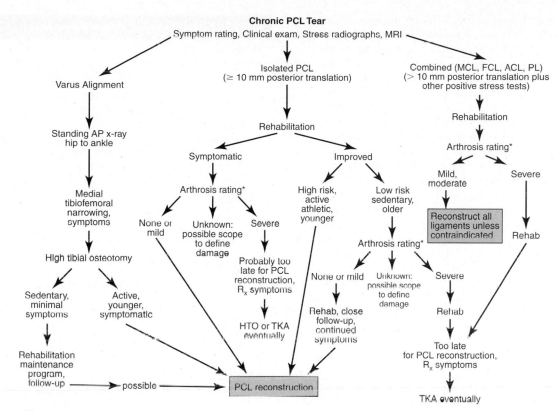

FIGURE 21-13. Treatment algorithm for chronic PCL ruptures. *Arthrosis rating: standing 45° tibiofemoral and patellofemoral views or magnetic resonance imaging special cartilage sequences.

compartment, along with diffuse cartilage fragmentation in the patellofemoral joint. In these individuals, even mildly strenuous exercises aggravate the joint arthritis symptoms and cannot be performed. The patients' initial experience with rehabilitation, and the inability to perform the required rehabilitation exercises, provides important information regarding the amount of joint arthritis present and joint symptoms that are likely permanent.

If a nonoperative approach is elected, the clinician should warn the patient that the return to athletic activities may carry an uncertain prognosis, and that although sports may be resumed in the short term, some form of joint arthritis will eventually ensue. It is therefore important to follow the patient at regular intervals. A bone scan may be used to provide some indication of abnormal blood flow dynamics; however, it is the authors' experience that the onset of pain and swelling usually indicates more advanced joint damage and a poor prognosis after PCL reconstruction. An MRI with fast-spin-echo sequences[122] provides a baseline for repeated studies at 1- to 2-year intervals. The nonoperative treatment protocol of chronic PCL injuries involves educating the patient to avoid activities such as lunges and other high knee flexion activities that increase posterior tibial subluxation.

INTRAOPERATIVE EVALUATION

The patient is instructed to use a soap scrub of the operative limb ("toes to groin") the evening before and the morning of surgery. Lower extremity hair is removed by clippers, not a shaver. Antibiotic infusion is begun 1 hour before surgery. A nonsteroidal anti-inflammatory drug (NSAID) is given to the patient with a sip of water upon arising the morning of surgery (which is continued until the 5th postoperative day unless there

Critical Points INTRAOPERATIVE EVALUATION

- Patient and staff identification of surgical procedure, "time-out," operative site signed by surgeon and patient.
- Repeat all knee ligament subluxation tests under anesthesia, both limbs.
- Bore all articular cartilage surfaces
  - ○ Normal.
  - ○ Grade 1, softening.
  - ○ Grade 2A, fissuring & fragmentation < ½ depth of the articular surface.
  - ○ Grade 2B, fissuring & fragmentation > ½ depth of the articular surface.
  - ○ Grade 3, subchondral bone exposed.
- Medial and lateral gap test at arthroscopy
  - ○ Knee 30° flexion.
  - ○ Measure millimeters of tibiofemoral compartment opening with calibrated nerve hook.

are specific contraindications to the medicine). The use of an NSAID and a postoperative firm double-cotton, double-Ace compression dressing for 72 hours (cotton, Ace, cotton, Ace layered dressing) has proved very effective in diminishing soft tissue swelling and is used in all knee surgery cases. In complex multiligament surgery, the antibiotic is repeated at 4 hours and continued for 24 hours. A urinary indwelling catheter is not used unless there are specific indications. The patients' urinary output and total fluids are carefully monitored during the procedure and in the recovery room. The knee skin area is initialed by both the patient and the surgeon before entering the operating room, with a nurse observing the procedure. The identification process is repeated with all operative personnel with a "time out" before surgery to verify the knee undergoing surgery, procedure, allergies, antibiotic infusion, and special precautions that apply. All personnel provide verbal agreement.

All knee ligament subluxation tests are performed after the induction of anesthesia in both the injured and the contralateral limbs. The amount of increased anterior tibial translation, posterior tibial translation, lateral joint opening, medial joint opening, and external tibial rotation is documented. In acute knee injuries, arthroscopic pressure is maintained at a low setting with adequate outflow at all times to prevent fluid extravasation. A thorough arthroscopic examination should be conducted, documenting articular cartilage surface abnormalities[112] and the condition of the menisci.

The medial and lateral tibiofemoral gap test is done during the arthroscopic examination (see Fig. 22–2).[103] The knee is flexed 30° and a varus and valgus load of approximately 89 N is applied. A calibrated nerve hook is used to measure the amount of lateral and medial tibiofemoral compartment opening. Twelve millimeters or more of joint opening at the periphery of the compartment indicates the need for a combined lateral or medial ligament reconstructive procedure to protect and unload the PCL reconstruction. The goal is to restore the function of all ligament structures to normal or nearly normal and not leave a knee with a residual ligament insufficiency. This also applies to the ACL, which is reconstructed at the time of PCL surgery, if deficient.

Appropriate arthroscopic procedures are performed as indicated including meniscus repairs or partial excision, débridement, and articular cartilage procedures.

OPERATIVE TECHNIQUES

PCL operative techniques continue to evolve, and clinical outcome studies remain limited to allow precise decision making. This chapter describes the senior author's recommended surgical approach and relative advantages and disadvantages of each procedure, realizing that this is an evolving treatment approach (Table 21–5).

First, the surgical approach of either the all-inside or the tibial inlay technique is chosen. The factors to consider regarding these two approaches are discussed in detail. An all-inside approach is described that places the bone portion of the PCL graft directly at the posterior tibial attachment, simulating the tibial inlay approach. In the authors' experience, soft tissue grafts placed through a large tibial tunnel have an increased risk of failure owing to delayed graft incorporation. A sclerotic line often forms about the graft periphery, with limited or delayed bone ingrowth into the central regions of the graft. When a soft

---

TABLE 21–5   Recommended Surgical Approaches
All-Inside
Single-Tunnel Tibial Approach
• Bone plug in tunnel at posterior PCL attachment (same as inlay except tunnel)
• Avoids posterior dissection, increased operative time
• Projected results similar to tibial inlay
Two-Tunnel Femoral Approach
• Provides better anatomic positioning along oval PCL attachment
• Advantage graft incorporation over single large-diameter graft
• Outside-in tunnel, graft interference screw with suture post
• Second option: single femoral tunnel for multiligament reconstruction where time, operative complexity warrant single tunnel
Tibial Inlay
• Reserved for revision knees to bypass misplaced tibial tunnel (staged bone graft may be required)
Graft Selection
Isolated PCL Rupture
• Quadriceps tendon–patellar bone autograft, ipsilateral (rarely contralateral)
• Bone–patellar tendon–bone allograft
• Achilles tendon–bone allograft
PCL Combined Other Ligament Rupture
• Use allograft listed previously
• Avoid large-diameter soft tissue allograft through tibial tunnel
• Bone plug placed at posterior tibial tunnel
• No autograft harvest same knee

---

tissue graft is placed at the tibia, the use of two tibial tunnels is preferred to allow better graft-tunnel healing, although sometimes this is not possible in smaller knees. From an antidotal standpoint, it has been the authors' experience that an increased success rate of PCL reconstruction occurs when the bone portion of the graft is placed at the tibia (tunnel or inlay), with one or two collagenous graft strands placed at the femoral site. Still, many publications describe the somewhat historical technique of placing the bone plug at the femoral site (inside-out or outside-in tunnel) and the collagenous portion through a single tibial tunnel, with an Achilles tendon–bone (AT-B) allograft used most frequently. This technique is perhaps the easiest to master and can be used when surgical time is an issue, because it is sometimes more difficult to pass the bone portion of the graft through the tibial tunnel. The authors' publication of this technique is discussed in the "Authors' Clinical Studies" section.

Second, a large graft must be selected that will fill the majority of the anatomic femoral and tibial footprints. At the femoral attachment, either a two-tunnel or a single rectangular bone plug placement will fulfill this requirement. A single large-diameter femoral tunnel may also be used; however, from a theoretical standpoint, this is considered less than ideal because portions of the graft may be outside the femoral footprint.

A third principle in selecting autografts or allografts is to use a bone-tendon-bone or bone-tendon graft for the advantage of more secure fixation and superior healing of a bone plug than that provided by a soft tissue graft without bone plugs. It is important that high-strength graft fixation methods be used to withstand the large forces expected postoperatively. For example, the use of a single soft tissue interference screw to hold a PCL graft strand provides weak fixation strength, requiring a backup procedure with sutures for added graft fixation strength.

A fourth principle is to select an autogenous graft in isolated PCL surgical procedures if possible owing to a higher success

---

Critical Points AUTHORS' PREFERRED OPERATIVE TECHNIQUES
• Choose surgical approach: all-inside or tibial inlay technique.
• Select large graft that will fill majority of anatomic femoral and tibial footprints.
• Bone-tendon or bone-tendon-bone grafts provide more secure fixation, superior healing than soft tissue grafts.
• Graft fixation: use high-strength methods.
• Use autografts whenever possible, avoid same knee autograft harvest (quadriceps, patellar tendon) in multiligament reconstructions.

rate and healing compared with allografts. In multiligament knee injuries, it is usually necessary to use allograft tissue, although an autogenous graft may be harvested from the contralateral side in select conditions. In combined ligament reconstructions, a quadriceps tendon–patellar bone (QT-PB) autograft is not removed from the same knee, because this adds to the morbidity of the operative procedure.

Selection of Tibial Attachment Techniques: Arthroscopic All-Inside versus Open Tibial Inlay Approach

The arthroscopic-assisted placement of the tibial tunnel avoids the added operative time and complexity of the posteromedial tibial inlay approach. The surgeon must have extensive arthroscopic experience to safely perform this procedure in order to identify the PCL posterior tibial attachment site, avoid penetration into the posterior capsule and subsequent damage to the neurovascular structures, and place the tibial tunnel into the anatomic PCL tibial footprint. Specially designed instruments, drill guides with safety stops for guide pins, and drills are available to lessen the serious risk of inadvertent penetration of instruments posteriorly and damage to neurovascular structures.

The all-inside arthroscopic technique is particularly advantageous in knees with multiple ligament ruptures that require repair and reconstruction. In these knees, high-strength grafts are used to reconstruct the PCL and ACL, which are appropriately tensioned and fixed to reduce the tibiofemoral joint to its normal AP position. Medial or lateral operative approaches are used for concurrent medial and posterolateral ligament and soft tissue repairs or reconstructions. A combined ACL/PCL/MCL injury involves an all arthroscopic approach for the ACL and PCL, followed by a limited medial dissection for repair of the medial tissues and meniscus attachments.

Combined ligament injuries, particularly those involving medial ligament and muscle tissues, have a high rate of postoperative motion problems and arthrofibrosis. In these knees, an open posterior tibial inlay procedure and popliteal dissection may be avoided by using the all inside arthroscopic approach. One exception is a PCL avulsion fracture from the tibial attachment. Another exception is a PCL revision knee in which a prior tibial tunnel was used and a tibial inlay graft is required to bypass this tunnel. In these cases, loss of the normal bony architecture about the posterior tibial PCL attachment may exist and

a tibial inlay bone graft is required. In other PCL revision cases that have enlarged tibial tunnels, a staged bone graft procedure may be indicated with the preference to use autogenous bone (limited iliac crest graft; see Chapter 31, Primary, Double, and Triple Varus Knee Syndromes: Diagnosis, Osteotomy Techniques, and Clinical Outcomes), supplemented with allograft bone when required. The bone grafting of the enlarged or misplaced tibial tunnel is first done from an anterior approach. After the tunnel has healed, either a tibial tunnel or a tibial inlay PCL reconstruction may be performed as indicated.

The posteromedial tibial inlay technique places a tibial inlay graft securely into the posterior PCL tibial attachment site. This approach is often selected when only the PCL requires reconstruction. The tibial inlay graft provides ideal graft fixation and early healing. A two-strand autogenous QT-PB graft with two femoral tunnels is described and results have been published.[92,93]

The all-inside technique has the theoretical disadvantage of the collagenous portion of the graft abrading against the angulated posterior tibial tunnel. There are operative techniques designed to diminish this problem. These include creating a more oblique tibial tunnel drilled through the anterolateral tibia and carefully chamfering the tunnel exit. Collagen grafts with a large cross-sectional area and diameter are favored over those with a smaller area and diameter in which any abrasion compromises graft strength. To decrease soft tissue graft abrasion at the tibial tunnel, the bone portion of the graft is placed in a tibial tunnel directly adjacent to the tunnel exit. The intent is to match the beneficial effect of the tibial inlay procedure allowing prompt osseous healing.

Biomechanical studies of PCL reconstructions also show the potential for graft abrasion and failure at the femoral attachment.[134] Operative techniques to protect against graft failure and abrasion are necessary at both tibial and femoral attachment sites.

Selection of PCL Femoral Attachment Techniques: Two-Tunnel versus Single-Tunnel Options

It is not difficult from a technical standpoint to use two well placed femoral tunnels within the PCL femoral footprint from outside-in, and this is the most ideal technique to master. When the tibia inlay or tibial tunnel bone plug two-strand graft procedure is selected, two femoral tunnels are created using the outside-in technique with a limited anteromedial subvastus

---

Critical Points SELECTION OF TIBIAL ATTACHMENT TECHNIQUES: ARTHROSCOPIC ALL-INSIDE VERSUS OPEN TIBIAL INLAY APPROACH

- Requires advanced arthroscopic experience to identify PCL posterior tibial attachment, avoid penetration posterior capsule, damage to neurovascular structures.
- Specially designed instruments, drill guides with safety stops for guide pins, and drills available.
- All-inside arthroscopic technique advantageous in dislocations, multiple ligament reconstructions.
- Combined ACL + PCL injury: all-arthroscopic approach ACL and PCL; limited dissection for medial or lateral repairs.
- Tibial inlay approach often selected isolated PCL reconstruction.

ACL, anterior cruciate ligament; PCL, posterior cruciate ligament.

Critical Points SELECTION OF POSTERIOR CRUCIATE LIGAMENT FEMORAL ATTACHMENT TECHNIQUE: TWO-TUNNEL VERSUS SINGLE-TUNNEL OPTIONS

- Two well-placed femoral tunnels within PCL femoral footprint from outside-in most ideal technique to master.
- Alternative technique: bone portion of graft placed at femoral site, rectangular femoral slot technique preferred.
- Single femoral tunnel from inside-out approach more difficult because of narrow intercondylar notch, proximity of lateral femoral condyle.
- Outside-in approach allows graft sutures and a suture post.
- Advantageous to select graft fixation methods that provide for maximum tensile strength of graft construct.

approach, described later. This allows graft tensioning, a long femoral tunnel for graft incorporation, and graft fixation with a suture post. This is the author's preferred technique with either an autograft or an allograft (see Table 21–5).

The 4 o'clock posterior PCL graft strand is shorter by at least 15 mm than the 1 o'clock anterior graft strand. The outside-in tunnel approach allows accurate tensioning, fixation, and visualization of the graft length change during knee flexion. This allows the surgeon to determine the ideal knee flexion position for graft fixation.

In the alternative technique in which the bone portion of the graft is placed at the femoral site, a rectangular femoral slot technique is preferred. The bone plug is fixated with an inside-out arthroscopic technique. The rectangular slot technique places the bone within the PCL femoral footprint, which is more ideal than a single large-diameter tunnel, although either technique may be used. One or two tibial tunnels are used for the collagenous portion of the graft, described later. In a PCL revision procedure, a misplaced femoral tunnel may exist in which the bone portion of the graft is preferred over one or two soft tissue femoral graft tunnels.

A single femoral tunnel drilled from an inside-out anterolateral portal is more difficult because of the narrow intercondylar notch, the proximity of the lateral femoral condyle, the placement of the tunnel within the PCL footprint, and the need to avoid too proximal (deep) placement of the tunnel with portions of the graft outside of the PCL footprint. For these reasons, the outside-in drilling approach for a single large-diameter femoral graft tunnel is recommended for surgeons using this technique.

The options for femoral and tibial fixation for a bone–patellar tendon–bone (B-PT-B) graft are shown in Tables 21–6 and 21–7, respectively.[14] Techniques are available for inside-out drilling of tunnels and fixation of soft tissue grafts at the femoral attachment site using interference screws (similar to that performed in ACL reconstructions).[61] However, these techniques result in lower attachment strength. The outside-in approach allows graft sutures and a suture post to be incorporated (Tables 21–8 and 21–9). PCL reconstructions are under high in vivo loads (see Chapter 20, Function of the Posterior Cruciate Ligament and Posterolateral Ligament Structures) and it is advantageous to select graft fixation methods that provide for maximum tensile strength of the graft construct.[17,82,142]

Selection of Single-Strand versus Two-Strand PCL Graft Constructs

The advantages and disadvantages of one- and two-strand PCL graft techniques are summarized in Table 21–10. The goal of adding a second strand is to place additional collagenous tissue within the PCL footprint to increase the cross-sectional area of the graft and more closely replicate the native PCL attachment. This theoretical advantage is sometimes referred to as the *mass action effect* of adding additional collagen within the PCL footprint. The improved stability and clinical success of a two-strand graft construct over those of a single-strand graft have not been proved from a clinical standpoint. Some clinical studies show that a single graft strand obtains results similar to those of a two-strand procedure.

TABLE 21–6 Femoral Fixation Options for Bone–Patellar Tendon–Bone Graft Plug in a Bone Tunnel

Construct	Failure (*N*)	Stiffness (N/mm)	Failure Mode
Metal interference screw*	710 ± 224	298 ± 36	Not reported
Metal interference screw†	640 ± 201	Not reported	Pull-out and bone block fracture
Endoscopic interference screw‡	588 ± 282	33 ± 14	Bone plug fractured, femoral screw pull-out, bone tendon rupture
Biodegradable interference screw§	565	Not reported	Failure between the cortical and the cancellous bone of the bone plug
Metal endoscopic interference screw‖	558 ± 68	Not reported	Femoral fixation failure, fracture of bone plug, tearing of graft
EndoButton¶	554 ± 276	27 ± 13	Tibial bone block fracture or suture breakage, tibial side fixation failure
BioScrew endoscopic interference screw‖	552 ± 56	Not reported	Femoral fixation failure, fracture of bone plug, tearing of graft
Mitek device¶	511 ± 350	18 ± 8	Patellar tendon failure, fracture of tibial bone block, sutures tore through bone block
Metal interference screw§	436	Not reported	Failure between the cortical and the cancellous bone of the bone plug
Interference screw from outside-in‡	423 ± 175	46 ± 24	Pull-out around the screw
BioScrew interference screw†	418 ± 118	Not reported	Bone block pull-out
Press-fit¶	350 ± 48	37 ± 16.3	Tibial bone plug pull-out, fracture of tibial bone block, patellar tendon failed
Endoscopic interference screw**	256 ± 130	70 ± 29	Bone block pull-out, bone block fracture
Interference screw outside-in**	235 ± 124	83 ± 30	Bone block pull-out, bone block fracture

*Martin, S. D.; Martin, T. L.; Brown, C. H.: Anterior cruciate ligament graft fixation. *Orthop Clin North Am* 33:685–696, 2002.

†Pena, F.; Grøntvedt, T.; Brown, G. A.; et al.: Comparison of failure strength between metallic and absorbable interference screws. Influence of insertion torque, tunnel-bone block gap, bone mineral density, and interference. *Am J Sports Med* 24:329–334, 1996.

‡Steiner, M. E.; Koskinen, S. K.; Brown, C. H.; Johnston, J.: Anterior cruciate ligament graft fixation. Comparison of hamstring and patellar tendon grafts. *Am J Sports Med* 22:240–247, 1994.

§Johnson, L. L.; vanDyk, G. E.: Metal and biodegradable interference screws: comparison of failure strength. *Arthroscopy* 12:452–456, 1996.

¶Modified from Brand, J., Jr.; Weiler, A.; Caborn, D. N.; et al.: Graft fixation in cruciate ligament reconstruction. *Am J Sports Med* 28:761–774, 2000.

‖Caborn, D. N. M.; Urban, W. P.; Johnson, D. L.; et al.: Biomechanical comparison between BioScrew and titanium alloy interference screws for bone–patellar tendon–bone graft fixation in anterior cruciate ligament reconstruction. *Arthroscopy* 13:229–232, 1997.

**Brown, C. H., Jr.; Hecker, A. T.; Hipp, J. A.; et al.: The biomechanics of interference screw fixation of patellar tendon anterior cruciate ligament grafts. *Am J Sports Med* 21:880–886, 1993.

Authors' note: Cadaveric studies have varying results, particularly when older specimens are used, with osteopenia compromising fixation strength.

TABLE 21-7   Tibial Fixation Options for Bone–Patellar Tendon–Bone Graft Plug in a Bone Tunnel

Construct	Failure (*N*)	Stiffness (N/mm)	Failure Mode
9- × 30-mm interference screw[a]	758 ± 139	49 ± 2	Tendon tearing or bone plug slippage
9-mm interference screw[†]	678	68	Tendon tearing, slipping of the bone plug
Interference screw and suture with a post[‡]	674 ± 206	50 ± 21	Bone plug fractured, pull-out around tibial screw and suture rupture
Doubled staples on patella tendon in a trough*	588 ± 62	86 ± 16	Graft slipped under staple, 27% bone block breakage
9-mm interference screw[§]	476 ± 111	58 ± 4	Grafts pulled out of the tunnel
7-mm interference screw[†]	461	47	Tendon tearing, slipping of the bone plug
Suture and post[‡]	396 ± 124	27 ± 13	Bone-tendon rupture, bone plug fracture, tibial post pull-out
9- × 25-mm biodegradable screw[‖]	293	42	Bone plug slipped, tendon tearing
Suture (No. 5) to button[§]	248 ± 40	13 ± 2	Button failed, suture pulled through the bone plug
6.5-mm AO interference screw[§]	215 ± 39	23 ± 3	Grafts pulled out of the tunnel
Staple patellar tendon[§]	129 ± 16	11 ± 2	Graft slipped under the staple

*Gerich, T. G.; Cassim, A.; Lattermann, C.; Lobenhoffer, H. P.: Pullout strength of tibial graft fixation in anterior cruciate ligament replacement with a patellar tendon graft: Interference screw versus staple fixation in human knees. *Knee Surg Sports Traumatol Arthrosc* 5:84–89, 1997.

[†]Kohn, D.; Rose, C.: Primary stability of interference screw fixation. Influence of screw diameter and insertion torque. *Am J Sports Med* 22:334–338, 1994.

[‡]Steiner, M. E.; Koskinen, S. K.; Brown, C. H.; Johnston, J.: Anterior cruciate ligament graft fixation. Comparison of hamstring and patellar tendon grafts. *Am J Sports Med* 22:240–247, 1994.

[§]Kurosaka, M.; Yoshiya, S.; Andrish, J. T.: A biomechanical comparison of different surgical techniques of graft fixation anterior cruciate ligament reconstruction. *Am J Sports Med* 15:225–229, 1987.

[‖]Brand, J. C.: Comparison of interference fixation of tendon and bone plug for the quadriceps tendon in cruciate ligament reconstruction. *Arthroscopy* 15.58, 1999.

Authors' note: Cadaveric studies have varying results, particularly when older specimens are used, with osteopenia compromising fixation strength.

AO, ankle orthosis.

TABLE 21-8   Femoral Fixation Options for a Soft Tissue Graft Plug in a Bone Tunnel

Construct	Failure (*N*)	Stiffness (N/mm)	Failure Mode
QHT with EndoButton and three No. #5 sutures*	699 ± 210	30.2 ± 8.5	Implant pulled through bone, tibial fixation failure, suture failure, tendon failure
QHT with EndoButton and Endotape[†]	644 ± 91	182 ± 20	Tape broke
QHT with EndoButton and continuous loop 20 mm[†]	1345 ± 179	179 ± 39	Tape broke
Semitendinosus fixed with EndoButton and tibial post[‡]	612 ± 73	47 ± 19	Not reported
QHT with Bone Mulch[†]	977 ± 238	257 ± 50	Tip bending at junction with screw
QHT BioScrew, 0.5 mm graft sleeve[§]	530 ± 186	Not reported	Graft slipped
QHT with Trans-Fix[†]	934 ± 296	240 ± 74	Cross-pin toggled cancellous bone, pin bending, tendon slipped off
QHT with an EndoButton Mersilene tape[‡]	320 ± 50	34.8 ± 22.3	Tape broke
QHT BioScrew[‖]	485 ± 224	71 ± 28	Pull-out from bone tunnel
QHT with Mitek[‖]	687 ± 129	230 ± 32	Breaking at junction of eyelet pin
QHT with RCI titanium screw[‖]	246 ± 99	29 ± 12	Pull-out from bone tunnel
QHT with BioScrew[¶]	341 ± 163	Not reported	Graft slipped
QHT with RCI titanium screw[¶]	242 ± 90.7	Not reported	Graft slipped

*Modified from Brand, J., Weiler, A.; Caborn, D. N., et al: Graft fixation in cruciate ligament reconstruction. *Am J Sports Med* 28:761–774, 2000.

[†]Martin, S. D.; Martin, T. L.; Brown, C. H.: Anterior cruciate ligament graft fixation. *Orthop Clin North Am* 33:685–696, 2002.

[‡]Rowden, N. J.; Sher, D.; Rogers, G. J.; Schindhelm, K.: Anterior cruciate ligament graft fixation: initial comparison of patellar tendon and semitendinosus autografts in young fresh cadavers. *Am J Sports Med* 25:472–478, 1997.

[§]Steenlage, E.; Brand, J. C., Jr.; Caborn, D. N.: Interference screw fixation of a quadrupled hamstring graft is improved with precise match of tunnel to graft diameter. *Arthroscopy* 15:59, 1999.

[‖]Brand, J., Jr.; Nyland, J.; Caborn, D. N.; Johnson, D. L.: Soft-tissue interference fixation: bioabsorbable screw versus metal screw. *Arthroscopy* 21:911–916, 2005.

[¶]Caborn, D. N. M.; Coen, M.; Neef, R.; et al: Quadrupled semitendinosus-gracilis autograft fixation in the femoral tunnel: a comparison between a metal and a bioabsorbable interference screw. *Arthroscopy* 14:241–245, 1998.

Authors' note: Cadaveric studies have varying results particularly when older specimens are used, with osteopenia compromising fixation strength.

QHT, quadrupled hamstring graft.

The incorporation of a second graft strand has the theoretical advantage of providing additional collagen tissue for load-sharing, which decreases stress in the collagen fibers, increases graft strength, and reduces cyclic fatigue of the graft construct.[134,159] The two graft strands are tensioned at surgery to share loads, which decreases the loads compared with those of a single PCL graft construct. This has been shown in a majority, but not all,[81] biomechanical studies that compared single- and two-strand graft constructs.

Studies report that the two graft strands placed in the distal two thirds of the PCL femoral footprint will function to resist posterior tibial translation with increasing knee flexion (see Chapter 20, Function of the Posterior Cruciate Ligament and Posterolateral Ligament Structures). Alternatively, when two graft strands are placed in a proximal and distal (deep and shallow) portion of the PCL footprint, graft loading is in a reciprocal manner and the graft strands are under higher loads, which is less ideal. As previously

TABLE 21–9 Tibial Fixation Options for a Soft Tissue Graft Plug in a Bone Tunnel

Construct	Failure (N)	Stiffness (N/mm)	Failure Mode
QHT with washerplate*	905 ± 291	273 ± 56	Not reported
QHT with tapered 35-mm screw[†]	825	76	Graft slipped past screw in tunnel
Doubled tibialis anterior allograft with bioabsorbable interference screw[‡]	825 ± 124	71 ± 18	Tunnel pull-out
QHT with screw and a soft tissue washer[§]	821 ± 219	29 ± 7	Tendon stretch or tibial screw pull-out
QHT with Intrafix device[‖]	796 ± 193	49 ± 22	Pull-out from tibial tunnel
QHT with tapered bioabsorbable interference screw[‖]	647 ± 269	65 ± 22	Tunnel pull-out
QHT with 28-mm screw[†]	595	66	Graft slipped past screw in tunnel
QHT with suture and post[§]	573 ± 109	18 ± 5	Suture tendon stretches, post pull-out
QHT with RCI titanium screw*	350 ± 134	248 ± 52	Not reported
QHT with biodegradable interference screw ½-mm graft sleeves[¶]	308 ± 207	Not reported	Graft slipped around tibial screw
QHT with BioScrew**	289 ± 205	40 ± 33	Pull-out from bone tunnel
QHT with RCI titanium interference screw**	252 ± 88	32 ± 15	Pull-out from bone tunnel
QHT with biodegradable interference screw 1-mm graft sleeves[¶]	222 ± 75	Not reported	Graft slipped around tibial screw
QHT with RCI titanium screw[††]	214 ± 79	9 ± 7	Tendon pull-out or slip
Stapled semitendinosus[‡‡]	137 ± 23	9 ± 1	Tendon pulled out of staple

*Magen, H. E.; Howell, S. M.; Hull, M. L.: Structural properties of six tibial fixation methods for anterior cruciate ligament soft tissue grafts. *Am J Sports Med* 27:35–43, 1999.

[†]Selby, J. B.; Johnson, D. L.; Hester, P.; Caborn, D. M.: Effect of screw length on bioabsorbable interference screw fixation in a tibial bone tunnel. *Am J Sports Med* 29: 614–619, 2001.

[‡]Nyland, J.; Kocabey, Y.; Caborn, D. N.: Insertion torque pullout strength relationship of soft tissue tendon graft tibia tunnel fixation with a bioabsorbable interference screw. *Arthroscopy* 20: 379–384, 2004.

[§]Steiner, M. E.; Koskinen, S. K.; Brown, C. H.; Johnston, J.: Anterior cruciate ligament graft fixation. Comparison of hamstring and patellar tendon grafts. *Am J Sports Med* 22:240–247, 1994.

[‖]Caborn, D. N. M.; Brand, J. C., Jr.; Nyland, J.; Kocabey, Y.: A biomechanical comparison of initial soft tissue tibial fixation devices: the Intrafix versus a tapered 35-mm bioabsorbable interference screw. *Am J Sports Med* 32:956–961, 2004.

[¶]Steenlage, E.; Brand, J. C., Jr.; Caborn, D. N.: Interference screw fixation of a quadrupled hamstring graft is improved with precise match of tunnel to graft diameter. *Arthroscopy* 15:59, 1999.

**Brand, J. C., Jr.; Nyland, J. Caborn, D. N.; Johnson, D. L.: Soft-tissue interference fixation: bioabsorbable screw versus metal screw. *Arthroscopy* 21:911–916, 2005.

[††]Modified from Brand, J.; Weiler, A.; Caborn, D. N.: Graft fixation in cruciate ligament reconstruction. *Am J Sports Med* 28:761–774, 2000.

[‡‡]Kurosaka, M.; Yoshiya, S.; Andrish, J. T.: A biomechanical comparison of different surgical techniques of graft fixation anterior cruciate ligament reconstruction. *Am J Sports Med* 15:225–229, 1987.

Authors' note: Cadaveric studies have varying results, particularly when older specimens are used, with osteopenia compromising fixation strength.

QHT, quadrupled hamstring graft.

Critical Points SELECTION OF SINGLE-STRAND VERSUS TWO-STRAND POSTERIOR CRUCIATE LIGAMENT GRAFT CONSTRUCTS

- Goal of second strand: place additional collagenous tissue within PCL footprint, increase cross-sectional area of graft, more closely replicate native PCL attachment. Decreases stress in collagen fibers, increases graft strength, reduces cyclic fatigue of graft construct.
- Second strand placed further posterior in the femoral footprint. Graft placed in distal two thirds of footprint functions to resist posterior tibial translation with increasing knee flexion.
- Biomechanical studies justify two-strand reconstruction restores posterior tibial translation to normal values.
- Clinical studies report residual posterior tibial drop-back at high knee flexion angles in majority of single-strand PCL reconstructions.
- Two-strand graft constructs
  o QT-PB, bone plug placed femoral or tibial attachment. Tendon split into two strands, tensioned separately.
  o Two separate grafts placed into two separate femoral and tibial tunnels.
- Controversy exists between well-placed single-strand and two-strand grafts owing to inadequate clinical data.
- Authors' opinion: sound theoretical reasons exist to warrant two-strand PCL reconstruction when clinically feasible.

PCL, posterior cruciate ligament; QT-PB, quadriceps tendon–patellar bone.

TABLE 21–10 Basis for the Selection of One- Versus Two-Strand Posterior Cruciate Ligament Reconstruction

	Single-Strand	Two-Strand
Greater area	–	+
Load-sharing (decreased tensile forces in each graft strand)	–	+
Operative complexity	+	–
Cyclic fatigue	–	+
Clinical results (residual posterior tibial translation)*	Unknown	Unknown

*Proven by objective measurements, including stress radiography at 90° of knee flexion.

+ Denotes relative advantage; – denotes relative disadvantage.

noted, the length and tension changes in grafts is governed for the most part by the femoral attachment, and any graft fibers in the distal two thirds are subjected to increasing tension and elongation with knee flexion.[53,140]

In Chapter 20, Function of the Posterior Cruciate Ligament and Posterolateral Ligament Structures, the function of PCL grafts is described in detail. The usual description of a posteromedial bundle that resists tension with knee extension and an anterolateral bundle that resists tension with knee flexion represents an oversimplification and an inaccurate representation of PCL fiber behaviors. In this chapter, the rule of thirds (see Fig. 21–8) is used to describe PCL fiber and graft function.

In a cadaveric study, Bergfeld and coworkers[10] reported that both single- and two-strand PCL reconstruction restored translation after PCL sectioning, and suggested that the additional strand may have no benefit. The same-diameter Achilles graft was used so that additional graft material was not added by the second strand. However, the graft forces were not measured and it was not determined whether the second strand resulted in a decrease in graft tensile forces. Studies show that a single graft will restore posterior translation limits to normal after PCL sectioning[11,77,135]; however, commonly at the expense of high graft tensile forces. Therefore, the theoretical advantage of the second graft strand is to lower the high graft forces placed on a single graft strand and decrease graft failure from cyclic loading (see Chapter 20, Function of the Posterior Cruciate Ligament and Posterolateral Ligament Structures).

In a cadaveric study, Harner and associates[56] reported that a single-strand PCL reconstruction did not restore normal posterior tibial translation or joint kinematics. These investigators found that a two-strand PCL reconstruction did restore posterior tibial translation to normal values. The difference found between the single- and the two-strand constructs may have been due to inadequate tensioning of the grafts. The single-strand grafts were tensioned to 88 N at 90° of knee flexion. The tension required to restore posterior tibial translation was not measured and would have required higher graft loads. The added 67-N tensioning of the second posterolateral graft strand provided the additional resistance to restore the tibia to a normal posterior position. Thus, the authors did not truly compare the single- and two-strand PCL graft constructs under the same loading conditions.

A justification to add a second PCL graft stand is the frequent notation in clinical studies that at high knee flexion angles, there is a residual posterior tibial drop-back in the majority of PCL reconstructions.[95] There is no question that current PCL surgical procedures are not uniformly accomplishing a functional restoration of normal joint kinematics and stability postoperatively. This is further discussed in detail in the "Authors' Clinical Studies" section of this chapter. The concern is that residual posterior tibial displacement decreases the ability of the medial meniscus, and perhaps the lateral meniscus as well, to function,[110] thereby increasing tibiofemoral contact pressures.[72,141] Increases in patellofemoral contact pressures have also been reported.[50]

There are two types of two-strand PCL graft constructs. One example is the QT-PB graft with the bone plug placed at the femoral or tibial attachment and the tendon split into two strands, which are tensioned separately and ideally placed in two separate tunnels. The other type of PCL two-strand graft construct consists of two separate grafts placed into two separate femoral and tibial tunnels. For purposes of load-sharing between graft strands with knee flexion, it is not known whether there is any difference between a single bone attachment and two separate bone attachments. In the authors' opinion, there is no functional difference between these two graft constructs that can be measured.

A technique is available to pass two bone plugs through a single tibial tunnel in which one bone plug is sutured to the tendon just proximal to the other bone plug, placing two bone plugs in series. Sutures are placed into each bone plug, and an interference screw is added in the tibial tunnel. It is difficult to pass the double graft construct into the tibial bone tunnel, which is drilled 1 to 2 mm larger in diameter. This technique is not recommended; a larger-diameter single tibial tunnel with an appropriate-sized single bone plug is preferred.

When an AT-B allograft is selected, it is important that the graft be inspected to discard those that have a narrow tendon section just adjacent to the bone attachment. A QT-PB allograft is a more suitable PCL substitute owing to the larger cross-sectional area of the tendon; however, this graft is more difficult to obtain from tissue banks.

Multicenter randomized, controlled trials of one- and two-strand PCL reconstructions are required in the future to provide a more scientific basis for selection of one type of graft procedure over another. The surgeon is currently faced with small clinical trials with level 4 evidence, described later this chapter. For this reason, more than one PCL technique is described with recommendations regarding the technical issues to maximize the clinical result. The authors' preferred PCL graft procedures are provided along with the justification and rationale for these selections. In addition, it is necessary to use a case-by-case basis for selecting the appropriate surgical procedure in multiligament knee injuries.

In summary, there appear to be sound theoretical reasons to warrant a two-strand PCL reconstruction when clinically feasible. These conditions include isolated PCL reconstructions when the added time required to perform a two-strand PCL graft does not represent a contraindication in terms of operative time and complexity. In multiligament reconstructions, the primary goal is to repair and reconstruct all ruptured ligaments. Adding a second femoral tunnel, and tensioning and securing two graft strands, may be time consuming in an already complex surgical reconstruction. Therefore, the surgeon should be prepared, based on the operative findings, to modify the preoperative plan when required. In certain multiligament-injured knees, a single-strand PCL graft construct may offer a reasonable opportunity to restore functional stability (Fig. 21–14).[81]

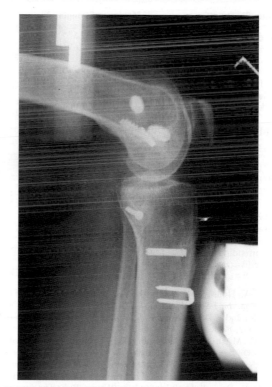

FIGURE 21–14. Posterior stress radiograph of a patient 2 years after a single-strand PCL quadriceps tendon–patellar bone (QT-PB) autograft shows only 2 mm of increased posterior tibial translation. The patient had sustained a knee dislocation and also underwent an anterior cruciate ligament (ACL) bone–patellar tendon–bone (B-PT-B) allograft reconstruction, and an anatomic posterolateral reconstruction with a fibular collateral ligament (FCL) B-PT-B allograft.

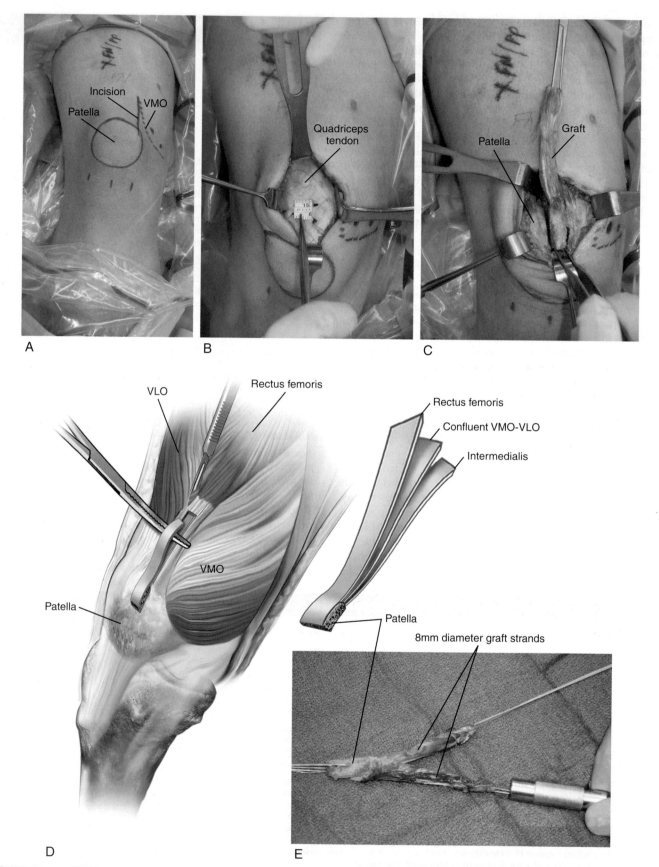

FIGURE 21–15. QT-PB autograft harvest. **A,** Medial incision. **B,** The quadriceps tendon is carefully marked to remove only 30% of its width and not extend to the musculotendinosus junction. **C,** A central 11- to 12-mm-wide full-thickness quadriceps tendon graft is harvested. The defect is later closed to maintain arthroscopic joint distention. **D,** Illustration of graft harvest. **E,** Two-strand 8-mm tendon graft with patellar bone is prepared.

- Incision just medial to superior pole of patella, extend proximally 5–6 cm.
- Cosmetic approach, subcutaneous dissection circumferentially about skin incision.
- Quadriceps tendon $\geq$ 70 mm, not counting the patellar bone plug, to be a suitable graft.
- Graft is taken from central tendon, 10–11 mm in width and thickness.
- Incise prepatellar retinaculum in midline, dissect to width of graft, protected for later closure over bone-grafted patella defect.
- Match patella bone block width to quadriceps width. Bone block length 22–24 mm, depth 8–10 mm.
- Graft prepared based on whether one- or two-strand technique is selected.
- Graft strands sutured in meticulous manner using three nonabsorbable 2-0 sutures.
- Tibial inlay, one graft strand, single femoral tunnel: all three tendon layers sutured together for tendon passage into the femoral tunnel.
- Close quadriceps tendon and synovium to provide a fluid tight closure, allows joint distention.
- Bone-graft patella bone defect with bone obtained by coring reamer, close proximal tendon defect.

is to not harvest the deep layer or to allow the blade to assume an oblique plane rather than a perpendicular plane. A curved instrument is placed behind the three tendon layers at the proximal aspect of the tendon harvest site to protect the underlying joint synovium. If the synovium is entered, it is closed along with the remaining quadriceps tendon closure to maintain joint distention for the arthroscopic procedure.

An Ellis clamp is placed about the three ends of the tendon to maintain tension. Care is taken at the quadriceps tendon attachment to the patella, because the tendon attachment is located at the proximal and anterior third of the proximal patella. A plane is established at this point just behind the quadriceps tendon attachment to preserve the posterior underlying synovial attachment and adjacent soft tissues. These tissues provide a superior buttress for the bone grafting of the patella to close the defect and secure the bone graft.

The patella bone block matches the quadriceps width, which is usually 10 to 11 mm wide. The bone block length is 22 to 24 mm and the depth is 8 to 10 mm. A thin powered saw blade is marked with a Steri-Strip to a depth of 10 mm to prevent a deep penetration. The saw is kept perpendicular to the patella for all cuts. After the anterior bone cuts are made, the quadriceps tendon is lifted superiorly at its attachment site. The inferior portion of the bone block is cut in a perpendicular manner beneath the quadriceps tendon attachment to a depth of 8 to 10 mm. This allows the bone block to be gently removed for graft preparation. The tourniquet is deflated and hemostasis obtained.

The graft is prepared based on whether the one-strand or two-strand technique is selected. The tendon graft strands are sutured in a meticulous manner using three nonabsorbable 2-0 sutures with two or three whipstitches beginning and exiting at the end of the graft strand. In the tibial inlay technique with one graft strand and a single femoral tunnel, all three tendon layers are sutured together for tendon passage into the femoral tunnel. The graft diameter is sized for the appropriate tunnel

to be drilled. In the tibial inlay or posterior tibial bone plug technique with two femoral tunnels (authors' preference), the tendon is split in a longitudinal manner and two graft strands are fashioned. A blood-soaked sponge from the wound site is wrapped around the graft to provide protection, keep the tissues moist, and potentially maintain cell viability.

In the optional all-inside technique with the patellar bone block placed into the PCL femoral attachment, either a one-strand or a two-strand technique may be selected for the graft strands placed though the tibial tunnel. When a single tibial tunnel is selected, there is still the advantage of tensioning the two graft strands separately.

The quadriceps tendon and synovium are closed to provide a fluid tight closure allowing joint distention. The quadriceps tendon defect is loosely closed with nonabsorbable 0 sutures. The tendon is closed in a Z-plasty manner, in which portions of the quadriceps tendon layers are brought together to avoid the use of circumferential tight sutures placed through all three tendon layers to decrease medial-to-lateral tension in the extensor mechanism.

The patellar bone defect is later bone-grafted in a meticulous manner with bone obtained with a coring reamer during preparation of the femoral graft tunnels. It is important to obtain a bone graft that completely fills the defect, because bone shavings from the tunnel preparations are insufficient. Postoperatively, a bone defect that was meticulously grafted heals without a palpable patella defect and decreases the incidence of graft harvest site pain.

Preparation of AT-B Allograft

The preparation of an AT-B allograft is performed in a manner similar to that of the QT-PB autograft, already described. The only difference is that it is necessary to tube each portion of the single- or double-strand graft because the tendon has a wide proximal fan shape. Care is taken when performing the incision of the tendon into two strands close to the bone attachment, because the tendon narrows in this area. For these reasons, the AT-B graft is generally used for single tibial and femoral tunnel applications, with the bone plug placed in a posterior tibial tunnel location. In the optional technique described, the bone plug is placed into a rectangular femoral site for all inside placement, or a 10- to 11-mm-diameter graft for a single femoral tunnel is placed using an outside-in technique through a VMO muscle-splitting approach.

Surgical Technique for Anteromedial Approach and Outside-In Femoral Tunnels

This approach is selected when two femoral tunnels are used and is less traumatic than a muscle-splitting approach, because it is necessary to split the VMO for 5 to 6 cm for proper visualization, which is traumatic to the muscle tissue. In addition, this approach allows for good visualization of the graft and suture post fixation. When a single femoral tunnel is selected, this

- Each portion of single or double-strand graft is tubed, Achilles tendon has a wide fan shape at its proximal aspect.
- AT-B graft used for single tibial and femoral tunnel applications.

TABLE 21–14   Posterior Cruciate Ligament All-Inside Procedures—Cont'd

Surgical Procedure	Advantages	Disadvantages	Options
B-PT-B allograft-autograft, separate tunnels 	Secure bone fixation each graft end Large allograft size Replaces femoral footprint Tensioning two strands	Allograft delayed remodeling Added time femoral and tibial tunnels Not used for multiligamentous surgery No distinct advantage two tibial tunnels vs. single with bone plug	All autograft approach B-PT-B + STG
Posterior tibial, Achilles tendon allograft without bone plug 	All-inside Tensioning two strands femur Single tibial tunnel	Allograft No bone plug • Delayed graft healing • Weaker fixation (Not recommended by authors)	EndoButton replaces suture post femoral site Femoral sockets Lateral-tibial tunnel Single femoral tunnel
QT-PB two-strand autograft tibial inlay 	Ideal autograft revision knees Replaces femoral footprint Secure fixation Tensioning two strands	Open posteromedial approach, time, multiligament surgery Posterior neurovascular injury (rare) Autograft harvest Added time, postoperative pain	Single femoral tunnel (not recommended) No femoral suture post, all-inside (not recommended) QT-PB, AT-B allografts

*Authors' preference.

AT-B, Achilles tendon–bone; B-PT-B, bone–patellar tendon–bone; PCL, posterior cruciate ligament; QT-PB, quadriceps tendon–patellar bone; STG, semitendinosus-gracilis tendons.

Patient Positioning and Setup

An examination under anesthesia is performed to confirm the diagnosis and carefully compare the injured knee with the opposite normal knee, as already described. It is important to palpate the medial tibiofemoral step-off at 90° of flexion in both knees. At surgery, the PCL grafts will be tensioned in knee flexion and the medial tibiofemoral step-off used as verification that the abnormal posterior translation has been corrected. In multiligament operative procedures, the patient is in a supine position with appropriate padding under all extremities with an Alverado foot and leg holder or similar device used to flex the knee joint to 60° to 70° (Fig. 21–17). This allows the lower limb to be secured and positioned throughout the operative procedures. After appropriate cruciate ligament surgery, any associated medial or lateral ligament procedure is performed with the knee flexion angle adjusted as necessary.

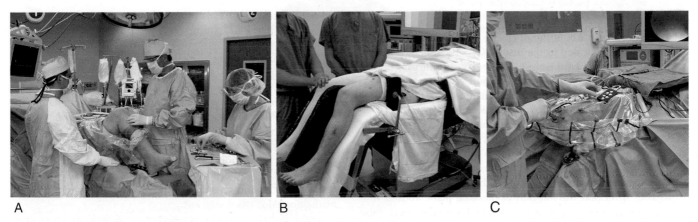

A   B   C

FIGURE 21–17. A, Patient position used in multiligament surgery with the foot in a leg holder and the knee flexed to 70°. **B** and **C,** Patient position with the knee flexed to 70° as an alternative position. Note the bed is flexed to maintain hip flexion. There is no pressure against the posterior popliteal space. The opposite leg is well padded.

Critical Points POSTERIOR CRUCIATE LIGAMENT ALL-INSIDE TECHNIQUE: PATIENT POSITIONING AND SETUP

- Palpate medial tibiofemoral step-off (90° flexion) in both knees, will be used to verify correction of abnormal posterior translation at end of procedure.
- Multiligament procedures: patient supine position, padding under all extremities, device used to flex knee to 60°–70°, 4-inch flat padded bolster is placed underneath the operative thigh.
- Begin arthroscopy with pressure regulated pump: required to maintain joint distention.
- Routine arthroscopic anteromedial, anterolateral, and superolateral portals.
- Measure lateral and medial joint opening 20° flexion with gap test.

An alternative approach is used with isolated PCL surgery. The patient is placed supine on the operating table with appropriate padding. The operating table is placed in a 15° reflexed position to prevent hyperextension of the spine and produce mild flexion of the hip in order to relieve undue tension on the right and left femoral nerves. The knee portion of the bed is flexed to 60°. A thigh tourniquet is placed over cast padding. The opposite limb is positioned in a foam leg holder with the hip slightly flexed. A thigh-high compression hose is placed on the opposite extremity. After appropriate draping, a 4-inch flat padded bolster is placed underneath the operative thigh to protect the tissues and allow for knee flexion during the operative procedure. The operative procedure is performed with the knee flexed from 60° to 90°; however, further knee flexion is possible by adjusting the operative table or using an additional thigh bolster. It is important that no undue pressure is placed against the posterior thigh and sciatic nerve during the operative procedure. For this reason, an arthroscopic thigh holder is not used. In prolonged surgical cases, abnormal pressures on the posterior thigh may exist that compromise the neurovascular structures. As a result, posterior thigh muscle ischemia and peroneal tibial nerve damage (although rare) may occur.

When a meniscus repair is required, an arthroscopic thigh holder is initially used to allow for adequate joint opening for an inside-out meniscus repair using the previously discussed patient and limb positioning. The knee position of the bed is flexed as required. After the meniscus repair is performed, the thigh holder is removed and appropriate posterior thigh padding placed as necessary.

Arthroscopy of the knee begins with a pressure-regulated pump that is adjusted to provide mild joint distention and prevent fluid extravasation. The pump is required to maintain joint distention, particularly during the drilling of the tibial tunnel, so that the fluid expands the posterior capsule out of the operative field. Modern pressure- and volume-regulated pumps allow for a controlled inflow and outflow that maintains a safe pressure. In addition, sufficient fluid inflow is maintained so a tourniquet is not required during the operative procedure.

Routine arthroscopic anteromedial, anterolateral, and superolateral portals are created (Fig. 21–18). During the PCL reconstruction, a transpatellar central portal is required. The posteromedial portal to débride the PCL tibial fibers is not required and avoids inadvertent fluid extravasation into the popliteal fossa that would limit posterior capsule distention and posterior joint arthroscopic visualization.

A standard arthroscopic examination is performed. The gap test is used to assess lateral and medial joint opening at 20° knee flexion with a varus and valgus stress as discussed. Any meniscus repairs or partial resections, débridement, or other arthroscopic procedures are performed. The PCL graft harvest procedure on the operative or contralateral limb is performed as required.

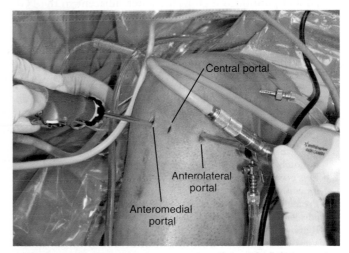

Central portal

Anterolateral portal

Anteromedial portal

FIGURE 21–18. Arthroscopic preparation of the tibial and femoral PCL graft sites through anteromedial, central, and anterolateral portals.

tunnel to be started just lateral to the tibial tubercle to produce less posterior tunnel graft angulation. However, either tunnel location is acceptable. The senior author usually prefers an entrance medial to the tibial tubercle. When an ACL reconstruction is also performed with a medial tunnel, the PCL graft is placed through a tunnel lateral to the tibial tubercle.

The arthroscope is placed in the anteromedial portal and positioned high in the notch to view the posterior aspect of the tibial PCL attachment to the capsular attachment. In the majority of cases, the 30° scope provides an excellent view. On occasion, a 70° scope is required. An alternative approach is to place the arthroscope in a posteromedial portal and view the drill guide placed through the anteromedial portal. However, this is not recommended owing to the potential for posterior fluid extravasation.

The drilling of the tibial tunnel is shown in Figure 21–21. The drill guide is placed through the transpatellar portal. The tip of the guide is placed at the desired position of the tunnel as far distal as possible, which is to the level of the posterior capsule insertion on the tibia just before the posterior tibial step-off. The distal placement of the guide pin is a critical step for success; an error is to place the guide pin too proximal in the PCL fossa, which produces a near-vertical PCL graft with limited ability to resist posterior tibial subluxation. The tip of the guide rests on the distal posterior capsule attachment with the guide pin target just 5 mm proximal to the tip. This prevents the drill from proceeding too far distally beyond the posterior tibial step-off where the drill tip would not be visualized and could penetrate neurovascular structures. The goal is to place the guide pin in the distal central portion of the PCL fossa, 20 to 25 mm from the proximal entrance of the PCL fossa. This leaves 15 mm of the posterior fossa to retain the posterior graft position and prevent a vertical PCL graft. This is a key step of the procedure. The drill guide is angled 50° to 55° to produce an oblique tibial tunnel that will decrease graft angulation effects.

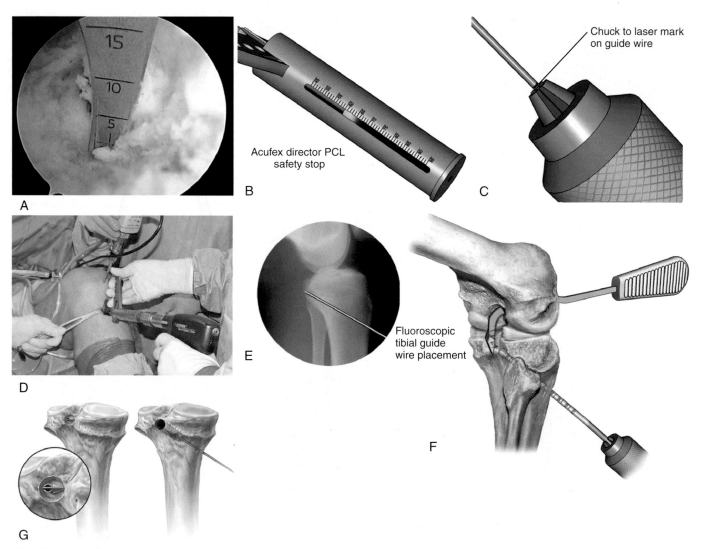

FIGURE 21–21. Drilling of tibial tunnel. **A,** Drill guide at the distal PCL attachment adjacent to the posterior capsule insertion. **B,** Acufex guide pin safety stop is attached to the drill guide. **C,** The guidewire is chucked on the power drill to the laser mark, which is the maximum length from the safety stop to the drill guide tip. This prevents the guidewire from being advanced beyond the drill guide after passing through the posterior cortex. **D,** Placement of the guide pin using the drill guide system at surgery. **E,** Fluoroscopy verifies guidewire placement. **F,** Tibial tunnel drilling with PCL Elevator/Wire Catcher to protect posterior neurovascular structures. **G,** Alternative technique using a "flip-drill" to make a posterior tibial socket for the PCL graft bone plug. Four fiberwire sutures placed through the plug are passed to the anterior tibia for graft fixation.

The next step involves use of the drill guide Safety Stop system (Acufex). The guide pin is chucked to a fixed distance with the safety stop mounted on the drill guide. The safety stop controls the depth of guide pin penetration into the tibia irrespective of the angle or position of the PCL tibial aimer and prevents the guide pin from passing beyond the guide tip and damaging neurovascular structures.

The guide pin is drilled into the selected tibial tunnel location. The depth of the guide pin is measured and used during the drilling process to determine the depth of drill penetration. The final position of the guide pin(s) is viewed and again confirmed that the guide pin is distal in the PCL fossa. Fluoroscopic confirmation of the guide pin position is recommended.

The tibial tunnel is drilled to the desired diameter using safety procedures, to be described. A commercially available PCL guide pin protector (Acufex) has a wide shape with a central recess 5 mm from its tip to engage the tibial guide pin before and during the drilling procedure. The tip of the pin is viewed at all times during the drilling process. The instrument prevents posterior migration of the pin and drill bit. The drilling process involves use of a drill with a drill tip and not a drill twist extending the length of the drill. The drill tip extends only 10 mm with a smooth shank. The drill is advanced in a slow manner. The depth of drill penetration is measured by the calibrated drill and prior drill guide pin measurements. As the drill tip reaches the posterior cortex, there is a noticeable resistance. At this point, the drill is slowly advanced without sudden penetration. A second option is to remove the power and place a hand chuck over the drill bit to complete the tunnel through the posterior tibial cortex.

When the flip-drill technique is selected, a 4-mm drill is initially used to establish the tibial tunnel. The flip-drill is then advanced under arthroscopic visualization to exit the posterior tibial tunnel. The drill is flipped and held against the posterior tibial cortex, and the tunnel is carefully drilled in a retrograde manner to the desired depth, which is determined by the measured length of the flip-drill (see Fig. 21–21). The PCL dilator remains in place posteriorly at all times to displace the posterior capsule away from the drilling procedure and prevent inadvertent capsule penetration.

To summarize, specific safety procedures are built into this technique to protect the neurovascular structures: (1) the drill guide system with the Safety Stop and controlled depth of guide pin penetration, with the guide pin placed 5 mm proximal to the distal posterior capsule insertion; (2) placement of the guide pin protector and slow drill penetration with direct viewing of the guide pin; (3) the final drill penetration of the posterior tibial cortex with complete protection posteriorly to prevent inadvertent deep drill penetration.

The proximal edge of the tibial tunnel is carefully chamfered with a rasp to limit graft abrasion effects (Fig. 21–22). Any remaining PCL fibers are removed so that the tibial tunnel entrance does not have soft tissue that would limit graft passage and to ensure the graft will lie flat against PCL tibial fossa. Again, it is necessary to have 15 mm of the posterior tibial fossa and an intact posterior intraspinous area proximal to the tunnel to maintain the normal angulation of the PCL tibial attachment to prevent a vertical PCL graft and to decrease graft tunnel enlargement (windshield-wiper effect). The most common technical mistake is to place the tibial tunnel at the proximal entrance of the PCL fossa, which is proximal to the native PCL tibial attachment.

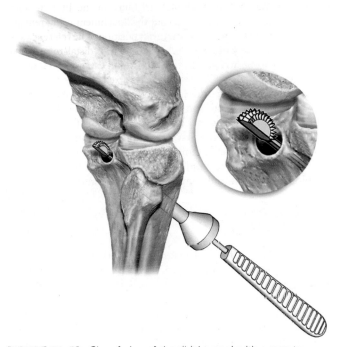

FIGURE 21–22. Chamfering of the tibial tunnel with a rasp to decrease graft abrasion effects. It is necessary to have 15 mm of bone retained in the posterior tibial fossa above the PCL footprint to prevent the graft from migrating through the tibia.

PCL Femoral Graft Technique

An important aspect of a successful PCL reconstruction is to have a clear understanding of PCL anatomy and changes in fiber-length and tension with knee flexion, as already described. The anatomic rule of thirds to describe the PCL attachment assists the surgeon in defining the anterior-to-posterior plane and the proximal-to-distal plane of the native PCL (see Fig. 21–8A and B).

As described previously, the PCL attachment is elliptical in shape, extending from high in the notch over the lateral aspect of the distal medial condyle from an approximate 11:30 to 5 o'clock position (left knee). The PCL footprint follows the articular cartilage, with the anterior portion within 2 to 3 mm of its edge depending on the reference system used as previously discussed.[87] At the 4 o'clock position, the PCL attachment is approximately 4 mm from the articular cartilage edge.[129] However, if the aMFL is present, the footprint will appear to be 1 to 2 mm from the cartilage edge. There is anatomic variability in the normal proximal-to-distal width of the PCL, and in some knees, a more oval appearance exists owing to an increased width of the middle third of the PCL

Critical Points POSTERIOR CRUCIATE LIGAMENT ALL-INSIDE TECHNIQUE: POSTERIOR CRUCIATE LIGAMENT FEMORAL GRAFT TECHNIQUE

- Anatomic rule of thirds used to define anterior-to-posterior and proximal-to-distal planes of native PCL.
- PCL footprint follows articular cartilage, anterior portion within 2–4 mm of its edge.
- At 4 o'clock position, PCL attachment is 4 mm from articular cartilage edge.
- If anterior meniscofemoral ligament present, footprint appears to be 1–2 mm from cartilage edge.

PCL, posterior cruciate ligament.

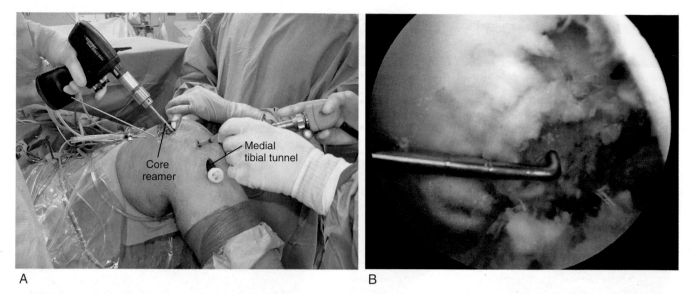

FIGURE 21–24. A, Use of the core reamer to obtain the bone graft for a patellar bone defect. **B,** Arthroscopic view shows final appearance of two femoral graft tunnels.

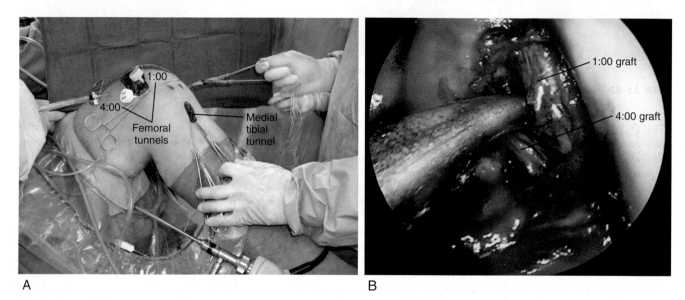

FIGURE 21–25. A, Passage of the quadriceps-bone two-strand graft through the enlarged anterolateral portal. **B,** Final appearance of the two-strand graft within the femoral tunnels.

Graft Tensioning and Fixation for All-Inside Grafts. The graft tensioning and fixation steps are the same for all grafts. For grafts with the bone block in the tibial tunnel, initial fixation is performed at the tibia (as already described) and final tensioning and fixation are performed at the femoral site. For bone blocks placed at the femoral site, fixation is first performed at the femoral site and final tensioning and fixation performed at the tibial site (Fig. 21–27).

After the initial fixation of the graft at either the femoral or the tibial site, the knee is taken through a full range of motion with an assistant displacing the tibia forward to correct for the weight of the leg and maintain joint reduction.

The knee flexion position for graft fixation is checked by determining the flexion angle at which the graft strand is the longest (functional zone) to ensure that the graft is not tensioned in its shortest position, which would overconstrain the joint and produce graft failure. A nonserrated hemostat is placed on each set of graft strand sutures exiting from either the femoral or the tibial tunnel(s) and circumferentially wound onto the clamp. The clamp is used to apply 10 pounds (44 N) of load to each graft. The grafts are conditioned by taking the knee joint through 0° to 120° of flexion. The knee is placed at 90° flexion and a normal medial tibiofemoral step-off is palpated and confirmed. This is done with the assistant placing approximately 10 pounds (44 N) of pressure against the calf to apply an anterior tibial force (assuming the ACL is intact). The knee is again taken through a full range of motion and the change in length of both graft strands noted. With increasing knee flexion, there will be increased tension and a pulling of the sutures and clamp into the tunnel of only 0 to 2 mm as the 90° position is reached.

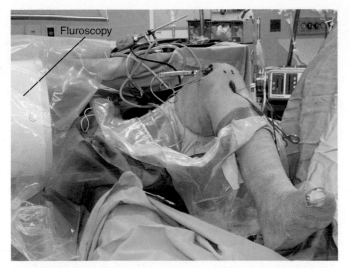

FIGURE 21–26. Fluoroscopy confirms that the patellar bone plug is directly at the posterior tibial tunnel exit.

The graft is longest at high knee flexion angles, which is the position selected for graft fixation. In most knees, the 70° flexion angle has the same graft length behavior as 90° and this position is selected. Commercial graft-tensioning devices[42] are available (as used in ACL reconstructions) that provide measurable length-tension data and may be used for measurement of graft-tensioning loads. The sutures for each graft stand are tied over a femoral or tibial post, maintaining the 10 pounds of graft load and 10 pounds of anterior tibial load.

The final position of the medial tibiofemoral joint is again verified. An absorbable interference screw is added to the

fixation. The arthroscope is again placed and with a nerve hook, the tension in the PCL graft(s) is confirmed. The knee is taken through 0° to 110° flexion.

Whereas techniques for the second posterior tunnel to be placed in a deeper, more proximal position have been described in the literature, the authors recommend placing the tunnels in the middle

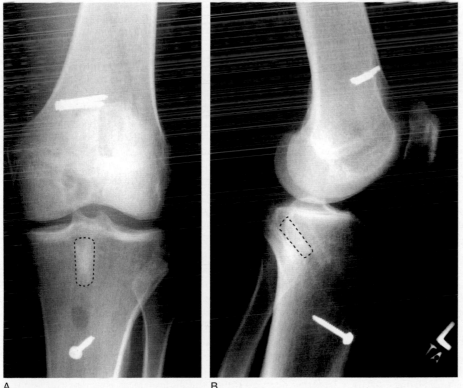

FIGURE 21–27. Anteroposterior (**A**) and lateral (**B**) radiographs of a PCL two-strand QT-PB reconstruction using a single tibial tunnel with the bone plug (*dotted*) placed in the posterior tunnel exit with fixation by an absorbable interference screw and suture post. Femoral tendon fixation is with a separate absorbable interference screw in each tunnel and a suture post (staple).

A   B

and distal two thirds of the PCL attachment, as described. This allows both graft strands to share the loading, and therefore, tensioning is at the 70° flexion position for both grafts.

It should be noted that if one or both femoral tunnels are too proximal (deep in the notch), the graft strand length decreases with knee flexion (allowing posterior subluxation) because the graft strand is longest closer to full extension. In this situation, the final graft fixation is done at the more extended position. The more proximal graft will function in a reciprocal manner and the desired load-sharing between grafts will not be achieved.

Alternatively, if the graft tibiofemoral attachment length is longer at 45° to 60° of knee flexion, as the graft is pulled into the tunnel with knee flexion, the femoral tunnels are too distal (shallow). This is not an acceptable position and the femoral tunnel is reconfigured, removing 5 mm of the proximal aspect of the tunnel to allow the graft to assume a deeper and more correct position. The interference femoral screws are placed distal in the femoral tunnels to secure the grafts in a more proximal (deep) position. With the technique described in the placement of the femoral tunnels, it would be rare for this graft tunnel adjustment to be performed.

In knees that undergo ACL reconstruction, it is important to determine as accurately as possible the neutral AP position of the medial and lateral tibiofemoral joints (without added internal or external tibial rotation). There is a tendency to displace the tibia into an abnormal anterior position by overtensioning the PCL graft. When the ACL is intact, the graft forces displace the tibial anteriorly, loading the ACL under low loads. When the ACL is insufficient, the following steps are performed to prevent anterior tibial subluxation:

1. Place the knee at full extension with a 10-pound (44 N) force on each graft (or 20 lb for a single graft) and 10 pounds anterior force on the calf to overcome gravity weight effects of the leg. This achieves a reduced tibiofemoral joint position when one or both of the medial or the fibular collateral ligaments (FCLs) are present.
2. Flex the knee to 90°, maintaining the same approximate graft load and anteriorly directed load on the calf. An anteriorly subluxated tibia at 90° (compared with 0°) will have abnormally increased tibiofemoral attachment site distances, and the graft can be observed to piston into the tibial tunnel. In essence, the graft should be nearly similar in its tibial position at both 0° and 90° of flexion.
3. Palpate for a normal tibiofemoral step-off and arthroscopically visualize a normal anterior relationship of the anterior portion of the medial and lateral meniscus in relationship to the respective femoral condyles. If there is any question, a lateral fluoroscope or radiograph may be obtained intraoperatively. This is especially helpful in large limbs in which the neutral AP position is difficult to determine with accuracy.

Femoral Placement of a Single Tunnel: Outside-in Technique

The drill guide is introduced into the anteromedial portal and the desired femoral tunnel position is located. The arthroscope is placed in the anterolateral portal. The goal is to place the tunnel into the anterior half of the PCL attachment, avoiding too proximal a placement. The entrance of the guide pin is at the 2 o'clock position and approximately 7 to 8 mm from the articular cartilage edge. This should produce a tunnel that is 2 to

---

Critical Points POSTERIOR CRUCIATE LIGAMENT ALL-INSIDE TECHNIQUE: FEMORAL PLACEMENT OF A SINGLE TUNNEL: OUTSIDE-IN TECHNIQUE

- Drill guide in anteromedial portal, locate desired femoral tunnel position.
- Entrance of guide pin: 2 o'clock position, 7–8 mm from articular cartilage edge.
- Tunnel size: 10 mm in most knees, 11 mm in larger knees.
- Small skin incision, VMO muscle-splitting approach.
- Over-ream guide pin or use coring reamer to harvest bone graft.
- Chamfer tunnel entrance into knee joint.
- Graft passage: inside-out or outside-in.
- Femoral graft fixation outside-in, interference screw.
- Prior to graft fixation, adjust graft in length to place the bone block adjacent to femoral attachment.
- All grafts at tibia have double fixation with a cancellous interference screw and suture post.
- Use single-tunnel technique when operative time limited, less technically demanding approach necessary.

VMO, vastus medialis obliquus.

---

3 mm from the articular cartilage edge. A note of caution is that there is a tendency to place the drill tunnel too proximal (deep in femoral notch) and out of the PCL femoral footprint, producing a graft that functions only at low flexion angles. The ability to carefully determine the native PCL footprint in the patient's knee is important for correct tunnel placement. The preference is for a tunnel of 10 mm in most knees and 11 mm in larger knees. If the drill diameter is larger, portions of the graft will be too deep in the notch and outside of the normal PCL footprint.

The entrance position of the guide pin in the outside-in technique is midway between the femoral epicondyle and the trochlea, at least 12 mm proximal to the articular cartilage edge. A more proximally placed guide pin would increase the tunnel angulation entering the joint and potentially increase graft abrasion effects.

A small skin incision and VMO muscle-splitting incision are made. A larger incision is not required because the bone block fixation is done with a cancellous screw without an added fixation device. The guide pin is over-reamed, or alternatively, a coring reamer may be used to harvest a bone graft. The tunnel entrance into the knee joint is chamfered to limit graft abrasion effects. A modification of this technique is used with a B-PT-B allograft in which a flip-drill is placed from outside-in instead of the guide pin and the femoral socket drilled from outside-in. This is an easier technique than placing the femoral tunnel from inside-out, as already described. When a femoral or tibial socket is placed with the flip-drill, the technique involves overdrilling the socket depth so that graft position and tensioning are possible.

At the time of graft passage, either an inside-out passage (enlarged anterolateral portal used for graft passage into the knee) or an outside-in passage (retrograde guidewire from tibial tunnel out through femoral tunnel) is used. Femoral graft fixation is easily performed in an outside-in manner with an interference screw of the surgeon's preference. Newer absorbable interference screws provide stable fixation. Prior to graft fixation, the graft is adjusted in length to place the bone block adjacent to the femoral attachment to limit fiber abrasion. The surgeon uses a headlight and adequate exposure to advance an interference screw into the anterolateral aspect of the femoral tunnel for graft fixation. Arthroscopic examination confirms that the screw is not advanced into the knee joint. The final graft conditioning, tensioning, and fixation are the same as previously described. All grafts at the tibia have double fixation with a cancellous interference screw and suture post.

Publications describe the all-inside drilling of a large single tunnel at the femoral attachment. However, the outside-in approach is preferred for large-diameter tunnels. From a technical standpoint, the drilling of a large-diameter tunnel is difficult owing to the proximity of the lateral condylar articular cartilage and the ACL, and the tendency exists to have a tunnel entrance that is markedly angled distally. In the authors' experience, a more precise and less angulated tunnel is obtained with the outside-in approach. The single femoral tunnel technique is used when operative time must be limited because this approach is the least technically demanding of all approaches for PCL femoral graft fixation.

Alternative PCL All-Inside Techniques

Femoral Placement of Rectangular (Oval) Tunnel for Bone Plug

An all-inside technique using the QT-PB autograft or B-PT-B or AT-B allograft is described in which the bone plug is placed at the femoral site and the soft tissue graft is placed through a tibial tunnel. This procedure has the advantage of easy passage

---

Critical Points ALTERNATIVE POSTERIOR CRUCIATE LIGAMENT ALL-INSIDE TECHNIQUES: FEMORAL PLACEMENT OF RECTANGULAR (OVAL) TUNNEL FOR BONE PLUG

- Bone plug placed at femoral site using rectangular femoral slot or femoral tunnel, soft tissue graft placed through tibial tunnel.
- Use when operative time is a factor, revision knees
- Goal: create 8- × 12-mm rectangular slot extends from 1 to 4 o'clock in distal two thirds of PCL attachment.
- Mark 12 o'clock, 4 o'clock positions on medial femoral condyle.
- 2.4-mm guide pin placed through anterolateral portal, knee flexed 90°, advance through medial femoral condyle 25 mm in depth.
- Place second guide pin, over-ream with endoscopic drill.
- Avoid lateral femoral condyle articular cartilage as the drill is introduced into knee joint.
- Use PCL Dilator to dilate attachment into oval 9- × 13-mm shape.
- Chamfer and rasp distal aspect femoral oval opening.
- 22-gauge wire passed through tibial tunnel, bring out through anterolateral portal.
- Pass soft tissue ends of graft through enlarged anterolateral portal.
- Use nerve hook through anteromedial portal to assist graft passage.
- Pass guide pin through anterolateral portal into rectangular femoral slot to exit anterior and proximal to medial femoral epicondyle.
- Pass bone block with sutures into the knee joint. Arthroscopically visualize bone block to ensure cancellous surface is flush at femoral attachment.
- Femoral fixation: interference screw, knee flexed 110°.
- Tibial fixation: interference screw and suture post.

PCL, posterior cruciate ligament.

---

of the soft tissue graft through the posterior tibial tunnel. This is used in select knees in which operative time is a factor. In addition, in revision knees, there may be displaced femoral tunnels in which the bone plug provides a more stable fixation at the femoral site. As already discussed, the senior author has a preference to reverse the graft with the bone plug at the posterior tibial tunnel. It is unknown from a clinical standpoint which procedure provides the best outcome related to return of joint stability.

The patient positioning and initial surgical approach are similar to the all-inside technique just described. The posterior PCL stump is removed and PCL tibial attachment prepared for one or two tibial tunnels.

When a two-strand PCL reconstruction is selected with the collagen graft strands placed in a tibial tunnel, using two tibial tunnels is advantageous owing to the smaller-diameter tunnel required. This avoids creating a large-diameter single tunnel in which both graft strands are passed. Two smaller-diameter tunnels provide for better healing potential and in-growth into the graft than a single large-diameter tunnel as already described. The two tibial tunnels are placed on the medial and lateral aspects of the tibial tubercle. The only knees in which two tunnels are difficult to drill are small knees in which the width of the PCL attachment is narrow and a single tunnel is required. Otherwise, it is possible to place two 7- or 8-mm tunnels side by-side at the distal PCL attachment site and avoid the posterior meniscus attachments. In multiligament reconstructions when operative time is a factor, a single tibial tunnel is selected. The single tibial tunnel (or double tunnels) is drilled with the technique previously described.

The technique for the femoral PCL graft attachment of the bone portion of the graft involves using either a rectangular femoral slot or a femoral tunnel. The all-inside technique for the rectangular slot is preferred to place a greater portion of the graft within the PCL femoral footprint, in which approximately three fourths of the footprint is occupied by the graft. A single circular tunnel of 10 to 11 mm replicates only the anterior and middle portions of the PCL attachment and is less ideal from a theoretical standpoint.

The goal is to create an 8- × 12-mm rectangular slot that extends from 1 o'clock to 4 o'clock in the distal two thirds of the PCL footprint. The 12 o'clock and 4 o'clock marks are made on the medial femoral condyle. Again, the guide pin mark is 6 and 8 mm from the articular cartilage of the medial femoral condyle for the anterior and posterior tunnels (Fig. 21–28), verified by observing the PCL footprint and that the two tunnels are in the distal two thirds of the footprint. Use a small curet or awl to penetrate and define the pilot hole for each tunnel. A 2.4-mm guide pin is placed through the anterolateral portal into the anterior tunnel location, the knee flexed to 90°, and the guide pin advanced through the medial femoral condyle approximately 25 mm in depth based on the patellar bone length.

The second guide pin is placed into the second marked position. The guide pins are over-reamed with an endoscopic drill (Fig. 21–29) to form an oblong tunnel entrance to a depth corresponding to the graft bone. Care is taken to avoid the lateral femoral condyle articular cartilage as the drill is introduced into the knee joint. The remaining central bone bridge is removed with a curet or bur.

The PCL Dilator (Fig. 21–30) dilates the attachment into an oval 9- × 13-mm shape that is approximately 1 mm larger than the bone portion of the graft. Care is taken at this point to use

FIGURE 21–28. A and **B,** All-inside femoral tunnel. The PCL Femoral Template is placed through the anteromedial portal with the arthroscope in the central portal and defines the position of two overlapping 7- or 8-mm tunnels. The top edge of the template is placed 2 mm from the articular margin and the bottom edge is 4 mm from the articular margin. This places the center of the anterior tunnel 6 mm from the articular cartilage margin and the center of the posterior tunnel 8 mm from the articular cartilage margin.

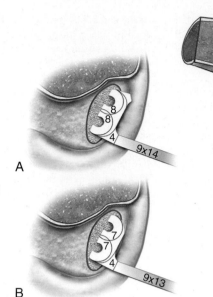

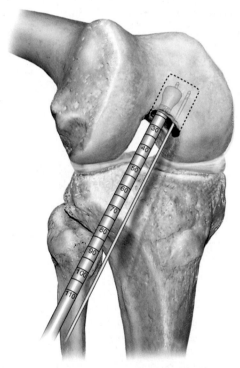

FIGURE 21–29. The guide pins are placed and then over-reamed with an endoscopic drill to a depth of 25 mm, avoiding passage of the drill through the femoral cortex. The central bone bridge is removed with a curet and bur.

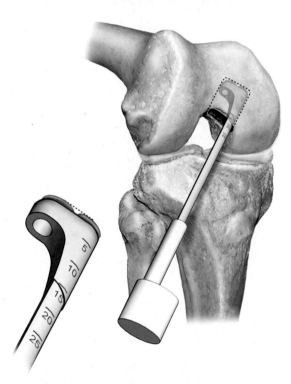

FIGURE 21–30. The PCL Dilator is used to gently conform the femoral oval footprint to 9 × 13 mm and to an appropriate depth. There is a matching oval opening in the PCL Dilator handle of 9 × 13 mm to size the bone block.

low forces in dilating the rectangular slot to avoid fracture of the femoral condyle. In the authors' experience, this has not been reported; however, it is worth a cautionary note. The PCL Dilator has a graft-sizing slot on the handle for a 9- × 13-mm bone block to assist in preparation of the graft.

The distal aspect of the femoral oval opening is chamfered and rasped to create a gentle slope to limit graft abrasion.

It should be noted that the femoral tunnel is oval in the final appearance, approximating two thirds or more of the PCL attachment site. The bone portion of the graft is rectangular, although the graft corners may be contoured to a more oval shape for easier passage into the femoral tunnel.

The passage of the graft begins with the passage of a 22-gauge wire through the tibial tunnel, which is grasped with a nerve hook and brought out through the anterolateral portal (Fig. 21–31). The tendon graft strands are passed through the enlarged anterolateral portal, which is increased 2 to 3 cm in length to prevent soft tissues from impeding graft passage.

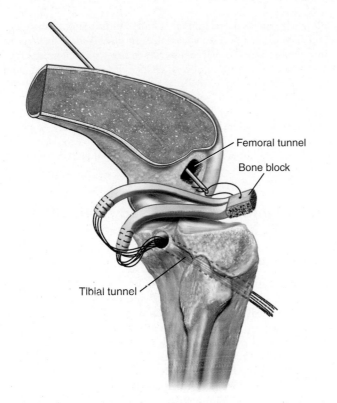

When a two-tunnel tibial technique is used, two wires are passed and the graft strands marked for the 1 o'clock graft to the lateral tunnel and the second 4 o'clock graft to the medial tibial tunnel. A towel clip or suture is used to close the anterolateral portal after graft passage to maintain joint distention.

The graft strands are viewed through the anterolateral portal adjacent to the ACL (when present), and a nerve hook through the central portal is used to gently assist and angulate the graft to enter into the respective tibial tunnel. It is easier to first pass the medial graft strand and then the lateral graft strand, maintaining the orientation of the bone portion of the graft so the lateral tibial strand corresponds to the 1 o'clock femoral position and the medial tibial strand corresponds to the 4 o'clock femoral position.

A guide pin (with an end to carry the sutures) is passed through the anterolateral portal into the rectangular femoral slot to exit anterior and proximal to the medial femoral epicondyle. The bone block with sutures is passed into the knee joint. The arthroscope views the bone block and the orientation is controlled with the cancellous surface oriented proximal (deep) in the rectangular slot. The bone block is positioned flush (not recessed) at the femoral attachment. Fixation is performed with an interference screw passed through the anterolateral portal with the knee flexed to 110° (Fig. 21–32). The interference screw is placed anterior to the bone block and snugly secures the graft.

The conditioning and graft tensioning is the same as described for the all-inside technique, except the final fixation is performed at the tibial site with an interference screw and suture post.

Two Separate Femoral and Tibial Tunnels and Two Separate Grafts

This technique uses two separate B-PT-B grafts, one autograft and one allograft. The tibial and femoral outside-in tunnels are

FIGURE 21–31. All inside graft passage. A 20-gauge wire is passed through the tibial tunnel and grasped anteriorly through the anterolateral arthrotomy. The tibial portion of the graft is passed through the single tibial tunnel. The pin is then passed through the anterolateral portal into the femoral tunnel. The bone block is passed through the enlarged anterolateral portal and carefully oriented into the correct position with the cancellous bone surface oriented deep in the oval opening.

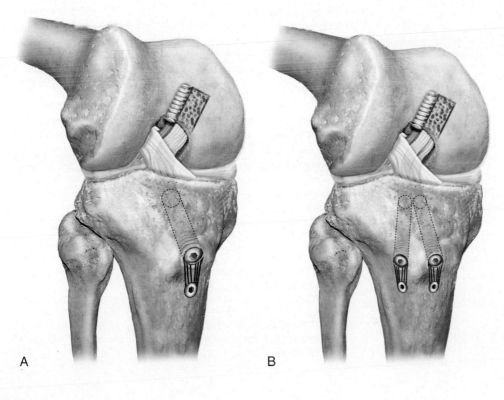

FIGURE 21–32. The final configuration of the single (**A**) or alternative two-tunnel (**B**) technique.

A   B

placed and drilled as already described. The passage of the two bone grafts is technically more demanding when the ACL is present and requires patience. Two tibial tunnel guidewires are passed and brought out the anterolateral portal. The medial tibial (4 o'clock) femoral graft is first passed with the tibial portion gently eased into the tibial tunnel. The femoral bone plug with a 4-cm loop lead suture is advanced through the anterolateral portal into the knee joint. A suture retrieval instrument is used at the posterior 4 o'clock femoral tunnel to grasp the suture and gently lift the bone block into the tunnel, assisted with a nerve hook. The scope is placed in the central or anterolateral portal to view correct placement of the femoral bone. The procedure is repeated for the lateral tibial 1 o'clock femoral graft. It is important in the preparation of the femoral tunnel that all soft tissues in the posterior aspect of the notch behind the PCL femoral attachment be removed to allow for the graft to pass and to provide sufficient visualization.

Through the anteromedial approach for the VMO, the outside aspects of the femoral tunnels are visualized. Through the arthroscope, the bone block is placed flush with the femoral tunnel opening within the joint. Each bone block is fixed with an absorbable interference screw. The visualization of the bone block deep in the tunnel is facilitated by use of the surgeon's headlight and graft position verified by arthroscopy. In revision knees or when obvious femoral bone osteopenia is present and the fixation compromised, a suture post is used for added fixation with the sutures placed in each bone block.

In the all-inside placement of the two femoral tunnels for two separate bone plugs when a B-PT-B graft is used, the graft passage is in the same order except the femoral portion of the graft is advanced through the anterolateral portal by a guidewire–suture carrier placed through the respective femoral tunnel. Interference screw fixation is performed through the anterolateral portal for each graft strand with the knee flexed to 110°. The final placement of the bone block in the femoral tunnel is more ideal (less graft angulation) when the cancellous side of the bone block is posterior (deep) and the bone advanced

flush with the femoral tunnel. Graft conditioning, tensioning, and fixation are performed as already described. The femoral interference screw is placed anterior to the 1 o'clock graft strand and distal (shallow) to the 4 o'clock graft strand, and after appropriate tensioning, the final fixation is performed at the tibial site with an interference screw and suture post.

The senior author has used this technique, and publications occasionally reference this procedure using a variety of grafts. The recommendation provided in this chapter is to use a single tibial tunnel with a bone plug without the added complexity of two tibial tunnels.

PCL Arthroscopic-Assisted Open Tibial Inlay Technique

Patient Positioning and Setup

An examination under anesthesia of both knees is performed to confirm the preoperative diagnosis and detect any subtle instability. The medial tibiofemoral step-off at 90° flexion with a posterior tibial load is noted and the joint reduced to normal and compared with the uninvolved knee. The reduced position and normal medial tibiofemoral step-off will later be reproduced with graft tensioning. Varus-valgus and tibial rotation tests for joint subluxation are performed as already described and compared between involved and uninvolved knees because concurrent ligament injuries, particularly to the posterolateral structures, are frequent and require reconstruction.

The patient is placed in a supine position on an inflatable beanbag (Fig. 21–33). The distal end of the beanbag is placed at the gluteal crease so it does not interfere with the tourniquet and the external rotation of the lower limb during the posteromedial tibial inlay approach. The beanbag is inflated and contoured to the patient's thorax and pelvis. A safety belt and kidney rest are placed to further secure the patient to the operating table when it is externally rotated (operative side down) during the posteromedial approach. A thigh tourniquet is placed over cast padding and used only intermittently for short periods during graft harvest and the posteromedial approach. The table is reflexed at its midpoint to decrease spine hyperextension, produce mild hip flexion, and prevent tension on the femoral nerve from a hip hyperextension position. The

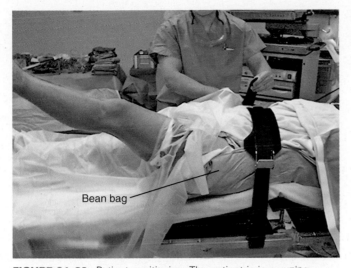

FIGURE 21–33. Patient positioning. The patient is in a supine position with an inflatable beanbag, safety belt, and kidney rest (not shown) to secure the patient to the operating table.

Critical Points POSTERIOR CRUCIATE LIGAMENT ARTHROSCOPIC-ASSISTED OPEN TIBIAL INLAY TECHNIQUE: IDENTIFICATION OF FEMORAL PCL ATTACHMENT: VASTUS MEDIALIS OBLIQUUS APPROACH

• Identify PCL femoral attachment, graft location as in all-inside technique.
• Use VMO approach for femoral tunnels with outside-in technique.
• Place guide pin 12 mm proximal to the articular cartilage for both tunnels.
• Start 1 o'clock guide pin just medial to femoral trochlea in an anterior position, begin 4 o'clock tunnel just anterior to femoral epicondyle.
• Alternative technique: use core reamer to harvest bone graft for patella defect. Replace guide pin with core reamer guide pin, visualize during drilling process.
• Chamfer two femoral tunnel entrances into the joint.
• Pass 22-gauge wire through femoral tunnels into the posterior aspect of the knee adjacent to PCL fossa for later graft passage.

PCL, posterior cruciate ligament; VMO, vastus medialis obliquus.

opposite extremity is placed in a thigh-high compression hose and posterior padded leg support to avoid hip hyperextension or abnormal pressures on the posterior thigh during the operative procedure.

The correct positioning of the operative extremity deserves special emphasis as described. During prolonged arthroscopic-assisted procedures, pressure on the posterior thigh may interfere with the vascular supply of the biceps muscle and peroneal nerve, and although rare, muscle necrosis and nerve injury have been reported. A leg holder is not used unless a meniscus repair is required, at which time, the leg holder is used initially to allow adequate tibiofemoral joint opening and is then removed for the remainder of the operative procedure.

General anesthesia is used and a urinary catheter placed when multiple operative procedures will be performed and the anesthesia time prolonged. Even though all dislocated knees have vascular consultation and ankle/brachial index studies, if there is any question of diminished pulses or vascular supply, the foot is draped in a sterile plastic bag to allow palpation of pulses and observation of color during the operative procedure.

The initial arthroscopic procedure is performed to thoroughly examine the knee joint including patellofemoral tracking, articular cartilage lesions, and medial and lateral tibiofemoral joint opening gap tests to exclude associated ligament injuries. At this time, débridement or meniscus procedures are performed as required. A pressure-regulated inflow and outflow arthroscopic pump is necessary, and joint distention is monitored continuously by the surgeon. The arthroscopic pump is set to the lowest pressure and volume for visualization, which avoids the requirement of a tourniquet.

The autograft harvest procedure or preparation of the allograft is completed as described.

Identification of the Femoral PCL Attachment: VMO Approach

The identification of the femoral PCL attachment has been described in the previous all-inside two-tunnel technique section and this section is only briefly summarized. The 1 o'clock and 4 o'clock positions within the PCL footprint are identified with the guide pin usually placed at 6 mm and 8 mm, respectively, perpendicular to the articular cartilage for an 8-mm-diameter tunnel. A separate VMO approach is used for the femoral tunnels with an outside-in technique, which allows a long femoral tunnel for graft incorporation and tensioning and fixation of the two graft strands at the femoral site. The guide pin is placed for both tunnels 12 mm proximal to the articular cartilage to prevent a potential fracture of the distal medial femoral condyle. The 1 o'clock guide pin is begun just medial to the femoral trochlea in an anterior position, and the 4 o'clock tunnel is begun just anterior to the femoral epicondyle. This provides 15 to 20 mm between the two tunnels at their outside entrance. The synovium is entered at this location; however, the adjacent tissues still provide for the fluid expansion of the joint. The position of the drill tip as it enters the joint is visualized and care taken not to displace the drill tip out of the selected region.

A curet is used over the guide pin to protect the ACL. If there is any need to adjust the tunnel a few millimeters, it is possible to start with a 6-mm drill and progressively enlarge the tunnel. This is sometimes required to protect the 2- to 3-mm bone bridge between the two tunnels.

An alternative technique is used when it is determined that the core reamer is required to harvest a bone graft from the femoral tunnel site for later grafting of the patella defect. This is required when a QT-PB autograft is harvested. The guide pin is replaced with the core reamer guide pin usually at the 1 o'clock tunnel, and its position carefully visualized during the drilling process to maintain the correct position of the two tunnels. This provides a long cancellous bone graft for grafting the patellar graft defect. A curet is placed over the guide pin to protect the ACL.

The two femoral tunnel entrances into the joint are carefully chamfered by a rasp to round the tunnel edges to limit abrasion effects against the collagenous portion of the graft. A 22-gauge wire is passed through the 1 o'clock and 4 o'clock femoral tunnels into the posterior aspect of the knee adjacent to the PCL fossa. The wire is sutured to tissues adjacent to the femoral tunnel entrance so that the guidewires do not displace during the posteromedial approach. The wire is later retrieved through the posteromedial approach for graft passage.

Posteromedial Approach[91,102,110]

With the patient in a supine position, the posteromedial aspect of the knee is viewed by rolling the table 25° with the operative side in the down position. The tourniquet is inflated. A partial figure-four knee position is assumed (45° external hip rotation, 45° knee flexion). The operative limb is elevated and the foot placed on a padded (pillow) Mayo stand to lift the knee away from the table. An assistant externally rotates the foot and controls the lower limb position on the Mayo stand during the procedure. The surgeon and assistant are seated at the side of the operative table directly viewing the entire posteromedial aspect of the knee. Operative headlights are used.

An alternative approach is for the surgeon to be seated between the patient's lower extremities by flexing the knee portion of the table and elevating the nonoperative limb into a flexed and abducted position. The senior author has not found it necessary to use this position. In either of the two limb positions, one person must be dedicated to maintain the operative limb in a safe elevated and externally rotated position supported by the padded Mayo stand.

Numerous surgical approaches that provide access to the popliteal fossa PCL tibial attachment have been described.[1,8,9,15,86,89,152] These approaches use an S-shaped popliteal incision,[8] an L-shaped popliteal incision,[15,89] or a medial incision.[71,90] The senior author recommends a medial incision as described to avoid the popliteal neurovascular structures.

A 7- to 8-cm longitudinal incision, beginning approximately 2 cm proximal to the flexion crease of the knee, is carried distally over the medial head of the gastrocnemius and the posterior border of the semitendinosus tendon (Fig. 21–34). The straight posteromedial incision, compared with an S-popliteal incision, avoids the horizontal popliteal skin crease with less skin retraction necessary and possible wound breakdown.[89]

Dissection is carried down sharply through the skin and subcutaneous tissues. Care is taken to protect the saphenous nerve posterior to the sartorius muscle and the infrapatellar branches that cross the sartorius superficially. The long saphenous vein and the saphenous branch of the descending genicular artery follow the course of the saphenous nerve and are protected as well. The gracilis and semitendinosus lie deep to the sartorius and are palpated.

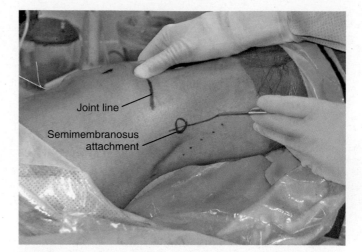

FIGURE 21–34. Intraoperative photograph of the left knee with the lower extremity in a figure-four position. The longitudinal incision begins approximately 2 cm proximal to the flexion crease of the knee. The incision is carried distally over the medial head of the gastrocnemius and the posterior border of the semitendinosus tendon. *(From Noyes, F. R.; Medvecky, M. J.; Bhargava, M.: Arthroscopically assisted quadriceps double-bundle tibial inlay posterior cruciate ligament reconstruction: an analysis of techniques and a safe operative approach to the popliteal fossa. Arthroscopy 19:894–905, 2003.)*

The first key to the approach is to incise the fascia[157] along the posterior border of semitendinosus tendon adjacent to the medial border of the gastrocnemius muscle. The three pes tendons are then retracted anteriorly (taking the saphenous nerve) and the semimembranosus tendon is visualized (Fig. 21–35).

The second key to the procedure is the dissection between the semimembranosus muscle and the gastrocnemius tendon. Understanding the anatomy of the posteromedial corner of the knee and the semimembranosus is important to obtain good exposure by mobilization of the semimembranosus tendon for the next portion of the dissection. The dissection uses the interval between the medial border of the gastrocnemius and the posterior border of the common semimembranosus tendon. In order to mobilize the semimembranosus medially and improve exposure, the tendon sheath extensions are incised to allow full mobilization of the semimembranosus tendon (Fig. 21–36). Anterior to the semimembranosus, the posterior oblique ligament is partially incised from the attachment to the semimembranosus tendon to improve exposure. These capsular attachments are later repaired at the end of the procedure. With lateral retraction of the medial gastrocnemius, the inferolateral semimembranosus tendon sheath expansion to the popliteus is visualized and dissected from its attachment to the posterior border of the common semimembranosus tendon. In this way, the insertion of tendon directly onto the posteromedial tibia is exposed.

The third key is maintaining the posterior exposure and avoiding undue retraction forces on the gastrocnemius and underlying neuromuscular structures. An S-shaped retractor is placed extra-articularly between the semimembranosus tendon and the medial femoral condyle and levered anteriorly, allowing for anterior retraction of the semimembranosus and pes anserinus tendons and muscle bellies. The medial head of the gastrocnemius is carefully retracted laterally with a Richardson retractor, allowing for exposure of the popliteus muscle belly

---

Critical Points POSTERIOR CRUCIATE LIGAMENT ARTHROSCOPIC-ASSISTED OPEN TIBIAL INLAY TECHNIQUE: POSTEROMEDIAL APPROACH

- Patient supine, partial figure-four knee position (45° external hip rotation, 45° knee flexion).
- 7- to 8-cm longitudinal incision, 2 cm proximal to knee flexion crease, distally over medial head of gastrocnemius, posterior border of semitendinosus tendon.
- Protect saphenous nerve, posterior to the sartorius muscle and the infrapatellar branches, crossing the sartorius superficially.
- Incise fascia along posterior border of semitendinosus tendon and medial border of the gastrocnemius.
- Dissect between semimembranosus muscle and gastrocnemius tendon.
- Maintain posterior exposure, avoid undue retraction forces on gastrocnemius and underlying neuromuscular structures.
- Subperiosteal dissection popliteus muscle.

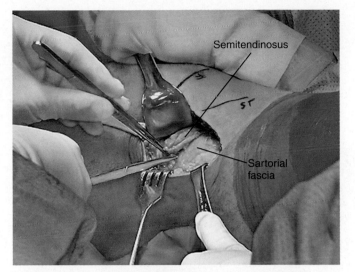

FIGURE 21–35. Surgical exposure of the left knee shows the development of the interval between the semitendinosus (ST) tendon and the gastrocnemius muscle belly. The sartorial fascia is incised along the posterior border of the ST tendon. The forceps is on the ST tendon. During the superficial dissection, care is taken to protect the main trunk as well as superficial branches of the saphenous nerve. The infrapatellar branch of the saphenous nerve is vulnerable as it superficially crosses the sartorius. *(From Noyes, F. R.; Medvecky, M. J.; Bhargava, M.: Arthroscopically assisted quadriceps double-bundle tibial inlay posterior cruciate ligament reconstruction: an analysis of techniques and a safe operative approach to the popliteal fossa. Arthroscopy 19:894–905, 2003.)*

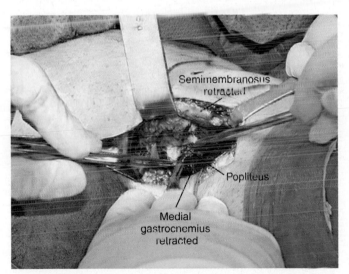

FIGURE 21–36. Surgical exposure shows the popliteus muscle exposure. The gastrocnemius muscle belly is retraced laterally and the pes tendons and the semimembranosus muscle are retracted by an S-shaped retractor away from the popliteal space, exposing the PCL fossa. Caution must be exercised with the lateral retraction of the gastrocnemius muscle because the neurovascular structures are not fully protected and the retractor should not be placed deep to the gastrocnemius muscle belly. *(From Noyes, F. R.; Medvecky, M. J.; Bhargava, M.: Arthroscopically assisted quadriceps double-bundle tibial inlay posterior cruciate ligament reconstruction: an analysis of techniques and a safe operative approach to the popliteal fossa. Arthroscopy 19:894–905, 2003.)*

on the posterior tibia. Care must be exercised at this juncture in the procedure, because undue retraction can avulse branches off the popliteal artery.

The neurovascular structures are not visualized and remain medial to the gastrocnemius muscle (medial head). The anterior tibial artery may lie directly on the popliteal muscle over the PCL fossa or pierce the popliteal muscle just distal to the PCL fossa as already described (see Fig. 21–9).

The fourth key to the procedure is the subperiosteal dissection of the popliteus muscle. Care is taken to gently dissect the popliteal muscle superior border in a distal direction to allow better subperiosteal exposure to the posterior tibia and PCL fossa for later placement of the tibial inlay graft. The inferior medial genicular artery and vein are at the superior border of the popliteus muscle and are easily identified and protected during this step, because the dissection is in a subperiosteal plane anterior and deep to the genicular artery.

Identification of Posterior Tibial PCL Attachment for Inlay Procedure

The PCL tibial attachment site is palpated as a midline depression in the proximal tibial metaphysis, between the two tibial condyles. The width of the PCL is approximately 15 mm[51] and the distal extent of the PCL is marked by a small ridge (posterior tibial step-off) that coincides with the proximal border of the popliteus.[123]

The fifth key to the exposure is to enter the joint proximal and just behind the semimembranosus tendon, avoiding the medial meniscus attachments. The posterior slope of the proximal tibia and the PCL fossa are palpated and the posterior capsule and OPL incised sharply, starting proximal and superior on the lateral aspect of the medial femoral condyle. The posterior portion of the medial femoral condyle is easily palpated. The posterior capsule just lateral to the medial femoral condyle is incised. The joint is entered directly over the inner aspect of the medial femoral condyle to establish from proximal-to-distal a safe plane of dissection (Fig. 21–37; see also Fig. 21–36). The dissection of the capsule is performed in the midline directly over the PCL fossa with care at the joint line to avoid injury to the posterior medial meniscus tibial attachment. This

---

Critical Points POSTERIOR CRUCIATE LIGAMENT ARTHROSCOPIC-ASSISTED OPEN TIBIAL INLAY TECHNIQUE: IDENTIFICATION OF POSTERIOR TIBIAL POSTERIOR CRUCIATE LIGAMENT ATTACHMENT FOR INLAY PROCEDURE

- Enter joint proximal and just behind semimembranosus tendon, avoiding medial meniscus attachments.
- Use Richardson retractor to retract medial gastrocnemius muscle. Replace with two Steinmann pins placed just lateral and distal to PCL fossa.
- Remove posterior tibial slot for inlay procedure.
- Placement, adjustment of position of PCL graft.
- Guidewires retrieved, strands passed beginning with 1 o'clock strand.
- Graft strands brought out respective femoral tunnels, positions adjusted proximal-distal direction.
- Tibial fixation graft bone with two 4.0 mm cannulated cancellous screws.

PCL, posterior cruciate ligament.

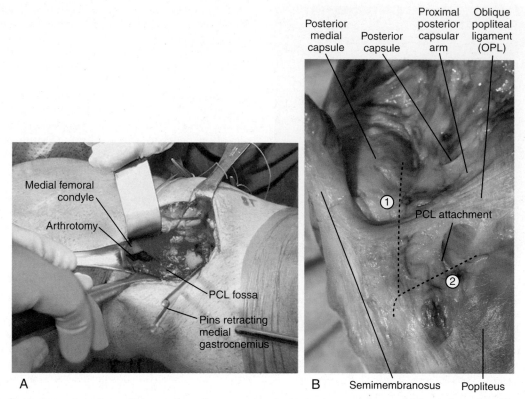

FIGURE 21–37. Surgical exposure shows the posterior arthrotomy over the inner aspect of the medial femoral condyle. The suture-passing wires are retrieved from within the joint. Care is taken during the arthrotomy to avoid injury to the medial meniscus. The subperiosteal dissection is carried to the lateral ridge of the PCL fossa to allow for creation of the tibial slot at the anatomic PCL attachment site. An S-shaped retractor assists in positioning the ST out of the operative field, allowing for better visualization of the PCL fossa. The creation of the subperiosteal popliteus flap adds an additional layer of protection and provides a safer exposure, because vascular anatomic variations may exist. Two Steinmann pins allow for retraction of the popliteus and gastrocnemius muscle. **B,** Anatomic specimen shows line of incision into posteromedial capsule and superior to popliteal muscle to expose PCL tibial attachment. (**A,** *From Noyes, F. R.; Medvecky, M. J.; Bhargava, M.: Arthroscopically assisted quadriceps double-bundle tibial inlay posterior cruciate ligament reconstruction: an analysis of techniques and a safe operative approach to the popliteal fossa.* Arthroscopy *19:894–905, 2003.*)

capsular incision is extended distally and connected to the popliteus subperiosteal exposure, which will be closed at the conclusion of the procedure. The entire PCL tibial attachment site is easily identified. The remaining PCL stump is removed.

The sixth key to the exposure involves the Richardson retractor, used to retract the medial gastrocnemius muscle, that is replaced with two Steinmann pins placed under direct vision just lateral and distal to the PCL fossa. The pins allow for excellent exposure during the tibial inlay procedure and avoid undue lateral retraction and pressure against the neurovascular structures by the surgical assistant.

The seventh key is the removal of the posterior tibial slot for the inlay procedure. A 10-mm osteotome is used to cut a rectangular slot into the PCL fossa at the proximal tibia. The slot is started 1 cm distal to the normal PCL attachment, which allows for the proximal bone block and collagenous portion of the graft to assume a normal anatomic position and preserve the proximal 15 mm of the PCL fossa. The posterior interspinous tibial bone just proximal to the PCL fossa is preserved to prevent a vertical PCL graft orientation. The rectangular bone block of the graft is placed flush into the inlay, avoiding too deep a slot, which would produce a vertical PCL graft.

The eighth key is the placement and adjustment of the position of the PCL graft. The previously positioned guidewires are retrieved from the posteromedial capsular recess within the

joint. The two strands of the sagittally split graft are identified (lateral arm, 1 o'clock tunnel; medial arm, 3 o'clock tunnel) and are passed individually starting with the 1 o'clock graft strand (Fig. 21–38). Care is taken that there is no soft tissue or native PCL fibers so the graft strands lie directly against the posterior tibia PCL fossa in a normal anatomic position.

The two graft strands are brought out of their respective femoral tunnels, and the position of the overall graft position is adjusted 5 to 10 mm by observing the graft strand in the femoral tunnel (VMO approach). The graft position is adjusted in a proximal-to-distal direction to ensure the collagen graft strands have the appropriate length for the femoral tunnels. In the alternative procedure, when a B-PT-B graft is used (rather than a QT-PB graft), too proximal a placement of the tibia inlay allows the bone plug to protrude out of the femoral tunnel proximally, compromising interference screw fixation. Too distal a placement of the tibial inlay shortens the graft in the femoral tunnels, also compromising femoral graft fixation. Visualization of both strands of the graft with an outside-in femoral tunnel approach allows for proximal-to-distal graft positioning and final fixation.

Tibial fixation of the graft bone is achieved with two 4.0-mm cannulated cancellous screws. The guidewires for the cannulated drill bit are angled distally to avoid intra-articular penetration, especially as the knee is positioned in a flexed position. A lateral radiograph may be taken intraoperatively to confirm the

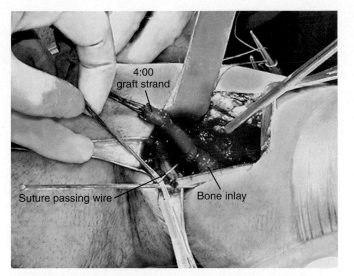

FIGURE 21–38. Surgical exposure shows placement of the quadriceps tendon autograft. The rectangular bone portion of the graft has been fixated to the proximal tibia with two 4.0-mm partially threaded cancellous screws. The sutures on the medial and lateral graft strands will be pulled intra-articularly with the suture-passing wires. The graft strands lie directly against the posterior tibia re-creating the normal anatomic PCL tibial attachments. *(From Noyes, F. R., Medvecky, M. J., Bhargava, M.: Arthroscopically assisted quadriceps double-bundle tibial inlay posterior cruciate ligament reconstruction: an analysis of techniques and a safe operative approach to the popliteal fossa. Arthroscopy 19:894–905, 2003.)*

inferior medial genicular artery or other bleeding sources be identified. The subcutaneous tissues and wound are not closed at this stage to allow for any extravasation of fluid during the final arthroscopic portion of the procedure. After graft fixation, the posteromedial wound is closed in a routine fashion.

Graft Conditioning, Tensioning, and Fixation

Arthroscopic visualization of the graft confirms proper placement of both strands prior to fixation. The graft tensioning and fixation steps have been previously described in detail in the "All-Inside Technique" section. A staple post is placed proximal to the femoral tunnels. Fixation is accomplished by tying each suture with approximately 10 pounds (44 N) on each graft strand, at 70° to 90° flexion, and 10 pounds (44 N) anterior tibial load to produce a normal medial tibiofemoral step-off, which is confirmed. A soft tissue absorbable interference screw is added for each tunnel (Fig. 21–40). Arthroscopic evaluation of the graft confirms tension, fixation, and return of stability.

The patella defect is carefully grafted with bone from the core reamer as described. The anteromedial and posterolateral approaches are closed. The knee is carefully padded in a sterile compression dressing. The lower extremity is placed in a soft hinged knee brace locked at 5° flexion, with a 3-inch cotton roll placed behind the proximal calf to prevent posterior sagging of the tibia. The neurovascular status is confirmed to be normal before leaving the operating room.

position of the screws. The length of the screws is usually 30 to 35 mm for adequate purchase.

The capsulotomy is closed, the Steinmann pins removed, and the posteromedial capsule incision and oblique popliteal ligament repaired (Fig. 21–39). The tourniquet is deflated and hemostasis verified. Vascular clips are available should the

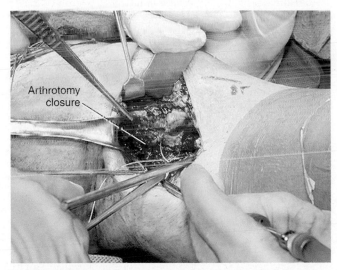

FIGURE 21–39. Surgical exposure shows the closure of the semimembranosus sheath and posterior arthrotomy. The skin incision is only partially closed at this point to allow for potential fluid extravasation during the final arthroscopic portion of the procedure. *(From Noyes, F. R.; Medvecky, M. J.; Bhargava, M.: Arthroscopically assisted quadriceps double-bundle tibial inlay posterior cruciate ligament reconstruction: an analysis of techniques and a safe operative approach to the popliteal fossa. Arthroscopy 19:894–905, 2003.)*

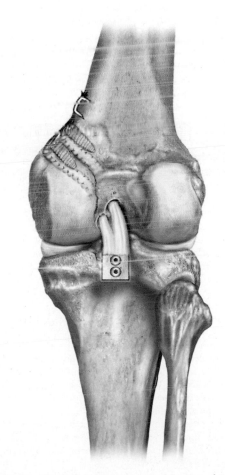

FIGURE 21–40. The final tibial and femoral fixation of the QT-PB two-strand graft.

PCL Avulsion Fractures

Avulsion fractures of the PCL are rare, and treatment options depend on the type and size of the fracture, displacement, comminution, and orientation of the fragment.[52,88] These injuries typically occur at the tibial attachment and may encompass either a small area at the posterior region of the attachment or a large area that extends anteriorly and outside of the PCL attachment. Griffith and colleagues[52] reported that the entire insertion area was avulsed in all 19 skeletally mature patients in their series of PCL avulsion fractures. The avulsion fracture is usually obvious on routine radiographs. Occasionally, a computed tomography scan is required to define the extent of the fracture pattern in major avulsion fractures extending into the joint.[16,52] Clanton and coworkers[25] reported on the importance of the diagnosis of ligament injuries in children and noted two PCL avulsions from the femur that underwent open operative reduction and fixation with sutures. Mayer and Micheli[85]

PCL, posterior cruciate ligament.

reported on one case of a PCL femoral attachment avulsion associated with posterolateral instability due to a hyperextension injury mechanism. These authors reported that avulsion or peel-off PCL injuries at the femoral site were rare in the literature.

Patients who have small, partial PCL avulsion fractures, with a negative posterior translation test at 90° knee flexion, are kept in a brace locked in full extension and remain partial weight-bearing for 4 weeks to allow healing. The brace is removed for gentle range of motion (avoiding posterior tibial translation) and quadriceps exercises as described in Chapter 23, Rehabilitation of Posterior Cruciate Ligament and Posterolateral Reconstructive Procedures. Overall, the prognosis for healing and PCL function is good to excellent in these cases.[163]

Complete avulsion of the PCL attachment at the tibia and, less frequently, at the femoral attachment[121,127] (peel-off avulsion) with posterior tibial subluxation, is an indication for surgical repair. Numerous authors have reported favorable clinical results with the open reduction and internal fixation of PCL avulsion fractures at the tibial insertion site.[62,88,150] Inoue and associates[62] reported on 31 patients followed for 2 to 8 years with good results and low side-to-side differences (<5 mm, KT-2000) after surgery. The authors reported that the majority of knees showed mild residual posterior knee displacement (mean, 3.0 mm). Along with the tibial avulsion, an abnormal MRI signal intensity may be observed within the PCL fibers, indicating partial tearing.

A number of arthroscopic techniques have been reported for PCL tibial avulsion injuries.[16,32,69,139] Kim and colleagues[69] reported the outcome of 14 knees with an avulsion fracture of the PCL at the tibial attachment. The arthroscope was placed through the posteromedial portal and a plastic sheath with waterproof diaphragm passed through the posterolateral portal. The anteromedial portal was used as required. A large bone fragment was fixed by one or two transtibial cannulated screws placed from the anterior tibia after the bony fragment had been reduced and held by pins. Small bony fragments were fixed with multiple sutures through single or double tibial tunnels. The postoperative program involved a long-leg hinged brace locked at full extension for 3 weeks. Range of knee motion was then initiated with the brace locked in full extension for walking. The brace was removed at 8 weeks. The authors reported all avulsion fractures healed. The 12 knees that underwent operative reduction and fixation operation in the acute phase showed only a trace posterior instability with stress radiographs measuring between 1.2 to 3.5 mm of residual posterior displacement at 90° knee flexion. In 2 patients who had delayed surgery, the residual displacement was 3.3 and 4.1 mm.

Shino and coworkers[139] reported on six knees that had arthroscopic fixation of a PCL tibial bone avulsion. Fixation was achieved with a single cannulated screw or by suture fixation with comminuted injuries. A pull-out button was introduced through the posteromedial portal and the sutures passed through two tibial drill holes and tied at the anterior aspect of the tibia.

In Kim and colleagues' study,[69] postoperative arthrofibrosis developed in 3 of 14 knees, which compromised the final result. The authors concluded that PCL avulsion fractures are amendable for fixation by arthroscopic methods. They speculated that an early range of motion program might be beneficial to prevent arthrofibrosis.

The concept of immediate motion is addressed in detail in Chapter 23, Rehabilitation of Posterior Cruciate Ligament and Posterolateral Reconstructive Procedures. The therapist initiates early and protected knee motion within the 1st postoperative week, applying an anteriorly directed load to protect the relatively weak suture fixation. The use of a posterior calf pad and careful positioning in the brace is required for the first 4 postoperative weeks until suitable healing has occurred. Knees with suture or pin fixation have relatively low tensile strength repairs and require expert postoperative rehabilitation.

The surgeon should select either an arthroscopic or an open technique for tibial avulsion fractures based on experience. In general, it is relatively straightforward to use an arthroscopic approach for cannulated screw fixation for large and medium avulsion fractures. For PCL tibial avulsions with small bony fragments that require a combination of sutures and bone fixation, an open posterior tibial approach is favored by the senior author because it provides good exposure and allows for secure fixation.

A peel-off type of PCL rupture from the femoral attachment has been described as a hyperextension knee injury, such as that reported by Mayer and Micheli[85] in a child while jumping on a trampoline or in patients suffering from trauma from a motor vehicle accident.[25,115] This type of PCL rupture directly at the femoral attachment may occur at the fibrocartilagenous junction with minor associated damage to the bulk of the PCL fibers. The PCL attachment is easily repaired with sutures passed through small drill holes, avoiding the proximal physeal growth plate.

Ross and associates[127] described an arthroscopic approach for repair of acute femoral peel-off tears. Three No. 2 nonabsorbable sutures are passed through the PCL substance, through a femoral tunnel at the PCL footprint, and tied over the medial cortex. Park and Kim[115] reported an arthroscopic technique that used two transfemoral tunnels for the anterior strand and two posterior tunnels for suture repair of the posterior strand. These authors noted that femoral avulsion injuries were exceedingly rare.

The senior authors' preferred technique for femoral peel-off or proximal PCL repairs is to use an arthroscopic assisted approach in which two or three guide pin tunnels (small diameter for sutures) are placed at the anterior and posterior aspects of the PCL footprint distal to the physis to fan out the PCL fiber attachment.

A VMO-sparing approach is used as previously described and respective suture passers brought into the knee joint. Through a limited medial arthrotomy and under direct visualization using a headlight, the surgeon places multiple nonabsorbable baseball looped sutures at appropriate sites in the PCL fibers to approximate the broad elliptical femoral PCL attachment. The miniarthrotomy has limited morbidity and allows the surgeon to carefully place multiple sutures into the broad PCL fibers. Secure fixation is achieved along with anatomic placement of disrupted PCL fibers.

The decision is made at this point whether a tendon augmentation of the repair through separate femoral and tibial drill holes is required. In such cases, the arthroscopically assisted tendon augmentation drill holes are first placed in the respective tibial and femoral sites, the graft is passed, and the tibiofemoral joint reduced. A nonirradiated tendon allograft is the senior author's first choice in skeletally immature patients, and the second choice is a doubled semitendinosus autograft.

The sutures in the proximal PCL stump are placed and brought out through anterior and posterior placed femoral drill holes. In children, the physis is not crossed at either the tibial or the femoral site and the augmentation tunnel is 4 to 5 mm in diameter. In most cases of a peel-off fracture, a tendon

augmentation is not necessary because the bulk of the PCL fibers can be brought back to the PCL femoral attachment.

In PCL injuries that extend away from the femoral attachment and involve the proximal third of the PCL fibers, an augmentation is favored. The postoperative protocol for a direct suture repair should take into account the low repair tensile strength requiring maximum protection. The knee is maintained in full extension and the therapist assists in gentle range of knee motion for the first 4 weeks postoperatively. Only toe-touch weight-bearing is permitted during this time period. Then, the patient may progress to 50% weight-bearing in the brace locked at full extension. At 6 weeks postoperative, weight-bearing is progressed in the brace. Knee motion is advanced to 0° to 90°. The brace is removed at 8 weeks.

PCL Augmentation Approaches and Techniques

In select knees, an acute tear of the PCL may occur at the proximal third femoral attachment (and not through the midsubstance). A considerable bulk of the PCL attachment still exists and may be repaired to the femoral attachment, as discussed for the peel-off type of tear. In these cases, it is worthwhile to add a graft augmentation to the attachment site, which may be performed in an arthroscopic-assisted manner. A 7- to 8-mm femoral tunnel is placed at the desired site where the PCL fibers require a graft augmentation, usually in the more proximal aspect of the femoral attachment.

Sutures are used to repair the more distal fibers to the femoral attachment as already described. The placement of a 7-mm tibial tunnel must be well chosen and not interfere with the PCL attachment site. The tunnel is placed just medial to the tibial PCL attachment, carefully avoiding the medial and lateral meniscus attachments. A lateral tibial tunnel is not used because PCL fibers attach in part to the posterolateral meniscus tibial attachment. The authors agree with Wang and colleagues[156] and prefer a three- or four-strand semitendinosus-gracilis (STG) autogenous graft, although an allograft may also be considered.[3,63] Suture fixation to a femoral or tibial post and an absorbable interference tibial and femoral screw in adults is required.

In skeletally immature knees, a small-diameter graft may be placed through the distal femoral and proximal epiphysis,

---

Critical Points POSTERIOR CRUCIATE LIGAMENT AUGMENTATION APPROACHES AND TECHNIQUES

- Indications: acute PCL tear at proximal one third femoral attachment. Considerable bulk of PCL attachment still exists, may be repaired.
- Prefer three- to four-strand semitendinosus-gracilis autograft.
- 7- to 8-mm femoral tunnel placed, usually in proximal aspect of femoral attachment. 7-mm tibial tunnel placed just medial to tibial PCL attachment.
- Skeletally immature knees: small-diameter graft placed through distal femoral and proximal epiphysis, avoid physeal plate, suture fixation only.
- Rare cases chronic PCL with normal appearing PCL on MRI, residual PCL elongation: distal advancement similar to tibial inlay.

MRI, magnetic resonance imaging; PCL, posterior cruciate ligament.

avoiding the physeal plate with suture fixation only (no interference screws) as previously described. An augmentation graft has the distinct advantage of maintaining tibiofemoral reduction and preventing posterior tibial subluxation in the early postoperative healing period. As such, the augmentation graft should always be considered when an area of disrupted PCL fibers exists that would benefit from this approach.

In very select knees with a prior PCL rupture and abnormal posterior tibial subluxation, the remaining PCL fibers may appear healed and intact, although with a residual elongation. Rarely, the senior author has performed a distal advancement of the tibial PCL attachment; this is considered only when the MRI shows a normal signal to the PCL fibers and arthroscopic examination also shows a normal-appearing PCL. The operative approach is similar to a tibial inlay procedure, except the native PCL tibial bone attachment is advanced distally the required amount to restore posterior stability. A proximal advancement (recession) at the femoral insertion is avoided owing to the marked influence of the PCL femoral attachment on PCL fiber function previously described.

AUTHORS' CLINICAL STUDIES

In this section, the analyses of 130 knees with PCL deficiency that were placed into clinical investigations are reported. All of the studies involved a prospective consecutive patient enrollment, with the study design using the validated CKRS. The minimum follow-up of each study was 24 months, and the results were evaluated by a clinical research staff and not the surgeon performing the surgery. All patients were entered into the study and then tracked with sequential follow-up appointments. More specific clinical outcome details are provided in the publications; this section provides a brief summary of the results and conclusions.

PCL Two-Strand QT-PB Autograft Tibial Inlay Technique

In a prospective study, the authors[93] followed 20 consecutive knees in 20 patients treated with a two-strand PCL QT-PB autograft reconstruction with a tibial inlay technique for a chronic, complete PCL rupture. All patients were included in the investigation except for 1 who lived outside the United States and who could not return for follow-up. Therefore, the study group consisted of 19 patients who were followed a mean of 35 months (range, 24–84 mo) postoperatively. The PCL reconstructions were done a mean of 43 months (range, 4–216 mo) after the original knee injury. In 9 knees, prior PCL procedures had been done elsewhere and failed.

Associated procedures were common and included posterolateral procedures in 5 knees, ACL reconstruction in 2 knees, MCL STG reconstruction in 2 knees, and meniscus transplantation[104] in 1 knee.

The results were determined with stress radiography, knee arthrometer testing, and two validated knee rating instruments (CKRS[6] and International Knee Documentations Committee [IKDC] rating system[59]).

For all 19 knees, the mean increase in posterior tibial translation (compared with the contralateral knee) on stress radiography improved from 11.6 ± 2.9 mm preoperatively to 5.0 ± 2.6 mm at follow-up (mean ± standard deviation; $P < .0001$). Preoperatively, all knees were graded C or D according the stress radiographic data. At follow-up, 2 knees (10%) were

---

> **Critical Points** AUTHORS' CLINICAL STUDIES: POSTERIOR CRUCIATE LIGAMENT TWO-STRAND QUADRICEPS TENDON–PATELLAR BONE AUTOGRAFT TIBIAL INLAY TECHNIQUE
>
> - $N = 19$ consecutive knees followed mean 35 mo (range, 24–84 mo) postoperatively.
> - PCL reconstructions mean 43 mo (range, 4–216 mo) after original knee injury.
> - Prior PCL procedures done elsewhere had failed in 9 knees.
> - Associated procedures: 5 posterolateral procedures, 2 ACL reconstructions, 2 MCL reconstructions, 1 meniscus transplant.
> - Outcome assessment: stress radiography, KT-2000 testing, Cincinnati Knee Rating System, IKDC rating system.
> - Stress radiographs: mean preoperative, 11.6 ± 2.9; follow-up, 5.0 ± 2.6 ($P < .0001$).
> - KT-2000 (70°): mean preoperative, 10.4 ± 2.9; follow-up, 2.3 ± 2.2 ($P = .004$).
> - Preoperatively, all knees graded C or D on IKDC rating.
> - At follow-up, 2 knees (10%) graded A; 12 knees (63%), B; 3 knees (16%), C; 2 knees (10%), D.
> - Pain with ADL: preoperative, 58%; follow-up, 5%
> - 58% returned mostly low-impact sports.
> - Abnormal articular cartilage surfaces in 42%.
> - Difference between patients with normal cartilage and those with abnormal cartilage in mean scores for patient rating of the overall knee condition, squatting, running.
> - No infections, permanent limitations of knee motion, donor site problems, patellar fractures.
> - 74% compounding problems articular cartilage damage, prior meniscectomy, additional ligament procedures, or osteotomy. Recommend early operative treatment be considered for PCL ruptures.
> - Objective assessment of posterior stability demonstrated superior results compared with the single-bundle PCL allografts.
> - Tibial inlay often required in PCL revision knees where prior tibial tunnel must be avoided.

ACL, anterior cruciate ligament; ADL, activities of daily living; IKDC, International Knee Documentation Committee; MCL, medial collatearal ligament; PCL, posterior cruciate ligament.

---

graded A, 12 knees (63%) were graded B, 3 knees (16%) were graded C, and 2 knees (10%) were graded D (Fig. 21–41).

The mean increase in AP displacement (compared with the contralateral knee) on arthrometer testing improved from 10.8 ± 3.0 mm preoperatively to 2.0 ± 2.2 mm at follow-up ($P = .005$) at 20° of flexion; and from 10.4 ± 2.9 mm preoperatively to 2.3 ± 2.2 mm at follow-up ($P = .004$) at 70° of flexion (Fig. 21–42).

All of the associated knee ligament procedures received an IKDC rating of A or B at follow-up. The 2 ACL reconstructions were graded as B, 1 MCL reconstruction was graded as A and 1 as B, and all 5 FCL and posterolateral ligament procedures were rated as A.

Before surgery, 11 patients (58%) had pain with daily activities, but only 1 (5%) had such pain at follow-up. Eighteen patients (95%) rated the condition of the knee as improved, and 1 patient rated the knee condition as worse. Significant improvements were noted for symptoms and limitations with daily and sports activities (Table 21–15). Eleven patients (58%) were participating in low-impact sports at follow-up without problems, and 2 were participating in more strenuous sports without problems. Two patients were participating with symptoms against advice. Three patients did not return to sports because of the knee condition, and 1 patient did not return to sports because of reasons not related to the knee condition.

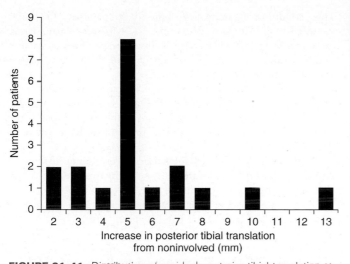

FIGURE 21–41. Distribution of residual posterior tibial translation at 90° of knee flexion on stress radiography a mean of 35 mo after PCL QT-PB two-strand autograft reconstruction with a tibial inlay technique. *(From Noyes, F. R.; Barber-Westin, S. D.: Posterior cruciate ligament replacement with a two-strand quadriceps tendon–patellar bone autograft and a tibial inlay technique. J Bone Joint Surg Am 87:1241–1262, 2005.)*

TABLE 21–15 Symptoms and Functional Limitations before and after Posterior Cruciate Ligament Quadriceps Tendon–Patellar Bone Two-Strand Reconstruction with a Tibial Inlay Technique in 19 Knees				
Factor	**Point Scale**	**Preoperative***	**Follow-up***	**P Value**
Pain	0–10	3.4 ± 1.8	6.6 ± 2.6	<.0001
Swelling	0–10	4.3 ± 2.3	7.4 ± 2.4	<.001
Full giving-way	0–10	5.6 ± 3.1	8.3 ± 2.6	<.001
Patient perception	1–10	3.2 ± 1.2	6.5 ± 2.1	.0001
Walking	0–40	29 ± 8	37 ± 9	<.01
Stair-climbing	0–40	29 ± 7	34 ± 10	<.05
Kneeling, squatting	0–40	10 ± 14	21 ± 16	.05
Running	40–100	44 ± 11	72 ± 25	<.001
Jumping	40–100	43 ± 10	62 ± 25	<.01
Twisting, turning	40–100	44 ± 11	64 ± 26	<.01

*Mean ± standard deviation

From Noyes, F. R.; Barber-Westin, S. D.: Posterior cruciate ligament replacement with a two-strand quadriceps tendon–patellar bone autograft and a tibial inlay technique. *J Bone Joint Surg Am* 87:1241–1262, 2005.

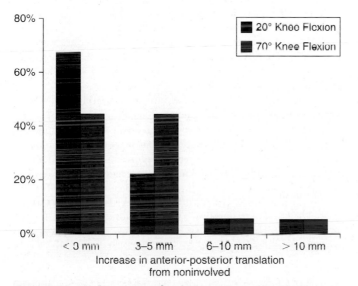

FIGURE 21–42. Distribution of residual total anterior posterior translation on KT-2000 testing a mean of 35 mo after PCL QT-PB two-strand autograft reconstruction with a tibial inlay technique. *(From Noyes, F. R.; Barber-Westin, S. D.: Posterior cruciate ligament replacement with a two-strand quadriceps tendon–patellar bone autograft and a tibial inlay technique. J Bone Joint Surg Am 87:1241–1262, 2005.)*

Abnormal articular cartilage surfaces were found during the operation in 8 knees, which were located in 1 compartment in 3 knees and in multiple compartments in 5 knees. The areas of cartilage damage were the patellofemoral compartment in 2 knees, the medial tibiofemoral compartment in 7 knees, and the lateral tibiofemoral compartment in 1 knee.

A difference was noted between patients with normal cartilage and those with abnormal cartilage surfaces in the mean scores in the patient rating of the overall knee condition (7.3 ± 1.5 and 5.4 ± 2.2 points, respectively; $P = .05$), squatting (29 ± 11 and 10 ± 14 points, respectively; $P = .005$), and running (82 ± 21 and 57 ± 25 points, respectively; $P < .05$).

Eleven patients had an isolated PCL replacement, and 8 had an additional knee ligament reconstruction. There was no difference in the mean millimeters of posterior tibial translation measured on stress radiography between these subgroups. Seven knees in the isolated replacement subgroup were graded B in the overall IKDC rating at the latest follow-up, 3 knees were graded C, and 1 knee was graded D. In the additional ligament reconstruction subgroup, 7 knees were graded B, and 1 knee was graded D. There also appeared to be no difference in the mean pain or patient perception scores at follow-up between the subgroups.

There were no infections, permanent limitations of knee motion, donor site problems, or patellar fractures. Three patients (2 who had an isolated replacement and 1 who had a combined ligament reconstruction) had a gentle manipulation under anesthesia between the 4th and the 8th postoperative week for a limitation of knee motion. One patient required an arthroscopic lysis of adhesions for a limitation of knee motion. All knees had a normal range of motion at follow-up.

All patients except 1 rated their knee condition as improved. Still, the residual symptoms prevented the majority from returning to strenuous sports. Fourteen knees (74%) had compounding problems of articular cartilage damage, prior meniscectomy, additional ligament procedures, or osteotomy.

The results affirmed the recommendation that early operative treatment be considered for PCL ruptures, because by the time surgical reconstruction is necessary for symptoms with daily activities, knee symptoms may not be improved by reconstruction owing to the arthritic joint damage.

The objective assessment of posterior stability at 70° of knee flexion in this study demonstrated superior results compared with the authors' single-strand PCL allograft study.[95] Stress radiography revealed that 68% of the knees had no more than a 5-mm increase in posterior tibial displacement compared with 37% of the knees in the allograft population (who had chronic PCL ruptures). Still, in acute injury situations, or in dislocated knees that require multiple ligament reconstructive procedures, allografts may be more suitable, as previously discussed.

The tibial inlay method is often required in PCL revision knees in which a prior tibial tunnel must be avoided to achieve graft fixation. In this study, 8 knees represented revision cases that had prior tunnels that were avoided and bone grafting was not required.

PCL Two-Strand QT-PB Autograft Tibial Tunnel Technique

Twenty-nine knees (in 29 patients) were treated with a two-strand PCL QT-PB autograft reconstruction with an all-inside tibial tunnel technique for a complete PCL rupture.[101] All patients were prospectively followed a mean of 43 months (range, 24–84 mo) postoperatively. Eighteen patients had the PCL reconstruction for chronic ruptures, and 11 for acute injuries.

Six patients had prior PCL reconstructions that had failed; 4 of these were done by direct suture repair and 2 were graft reconstructions in which the tibial tunnels had been inadequately placed. Fifteen knees required an associated ligament reconstruction, including ACL reconstruction in 9 knees, MCL repair or reconstruction in 6, posterolateral procedures in 5, and meniscus allograft in 1.

The mean increase in posterior tibial translation measured with stress radiography improved from 10.5 ± 2.9 mm preoperatively to 6.5 ± 4.3 mm at follow-up ($P = .06$). Preoperatively, all knees received an IKDC rating of C or D according the stress radiographic data. At follow-up, 3 knees (10%) were rated A; 7 knees (24%) as B; 17 knees (59%) as C; and 2 knees (7%) as D.

Preoperatively, the KT-2000 total AP displacement values were 9.6 ± 3.9 mm at 20° of flexion and 9.8 ± 3.1 at 70° of flexion. At follow-up, the total AP displacement at 20° of flexion was 2.2 ± 2.0 mm ($P < .0001$), and at 70° of flexion, 3.3 ± 2.9 ($P = .0001$).

Before surgery, 87% of the patients with chronic PCL ruptures had pain with daily activities, but only 11% had such pain at follow-up. Statistically significant improvements were noted for pain, swelling, giving-way, walking, stairs, running, jumping, and twisting/turning ($P < .01$). Ninety-four percent rated the knee condition as improved. For all 29 patients, 15 (52%) returned to low-impact sports and 7 (24%) were participating in strenuous sports without problems. One patient was participating with symptoms against advice, and 6 patients did not return owing to their knee condition.

Five of the associated ACL reconstructions received an IKDC rating of A, 3 were rated B, and 1 was rated C. Four of the MCL procedures were rated as A and 2 as B. Four of the FCL and posterolateral ligament procedures were rated as A and 1 as B.

Abnormal articular cartilage surfaces were found during the operation in 11 knees, located in one compartment in 5 knees and in multiple compartments in 6 knees.

There were no infections or patellar fractures. Two patients reported residual pain at the patellar donor site.

Analysis of the Causes of Failure of PCL Reconstruction

A study was conducted to analyze the potential factors that contributed to the failure of PCL operations.[96] Between June 1989 and July 2003, 41 knees in 40 patients were referred to the authors' center for treatment after 52 failed PCL operative procedures. The patients were evaluated a mean of 41 months (range, 1–285 mo) after the failed PCL procedures. There were 24 males and 16 females whose mean age at the initial PCL procedure was 30 years (range, 11–51 yr). The initial PCL procedures were done for an acute knee injury in 15 knees and for chronic deficiency in 26 knees.

A total of 155 operative procedures had been done in the 41 knees. PCL graft reconstructions had been done in 31 cases; primary repairs in 14; synthetic replacements in 4; and thermoplasties in 3. A single PCL procedure had been done in 32 knees; two procedures in 7 knees; three procedures in 1 knee; and 4 procedures in 1 knee. Only 4 knees (10%) had an isolated PCL reconstruction with no associated or further surgery performed.

Reconstruction of other knee ligaments had been done in 27 knees (66%). These involved 21 FCL or posterolateral complex procedures in 14 knees, 19 ACL reconstruction in 16 knees, and 9 MCL procedures in 9 knees.

Critical Points AUTHORS' CLINICAL STUDIES: POSTERIOR CRUCIATE LIGAMENT TWO-STRAND QUADRICEPS TENDON–PATELLAR BONE AUTOGRAFT TIBIAL TUNNEL TECHNIQUE

- $N = 29$ followed mean 43 mo (range, 24–84 mo) postoperatively.
- PCL chronic 18, acute 11.
- Associated procedures: 9 ACL reconstructions; 6 MCL repairs, reconstructions; 5 posterolateral procedures; 1 meniscus transplant.
- Stress radiographs: Mean preoperative, 10.5 ± 2.9; follow-up, 6.5 ± 4.3 ($P = .06$).
- Preoperatively, all knees rated C or D on IKDC scale.
- At follow-up, 3 knees (10%) graded A; 7 knees (24%), B; 17 knees (59%), C; 2 knees (7%), D.
- KT-2000 (79°): mean preoperative, 9.8 ± 3.1; follow-up, 3.3 ± 2.9 ($P = .0001$).
- Pain ADL: preoperative, 87%; follow-up, 11%.
- 94% rated knee improved.
- 52% returned low-impact sports, 24% returned strenuous sports.

ACL, anterior cruciate ligament; ADL, activities of daily living; IKDC, International Knee Documentation Committee; MCL, medial collateral ligament; PCL, posterior cruciate ligament.

Critical Points AUTHORS' CLINICAL STUDIES: ANALYSIS OF THE CAUSES OF FAILURE OF POSTERIOR CRUCIATE LIGAMENT RECONSTRUCTION

- $N = 40$ patients with 52 failed PCL operations.
- Patients evaluated mean 41 mo (range, 1–285 mo) after failed PCL procedures.
- Total 155 prior PCL operative procedures: 31 graft reconstructions, 14 primary repairs, 4 synthetic replacements, 3 thermoplasties.
- Other ligament procedures: 21 posterolateral (16 failed), 19 ACL (9 failed), 9 MCL.
- Most common probable causes of failure: associated posterolateral deficiency (40%), improper graft tunnel placement (33%), associated varus malalignment (31%), primary suture repair (25%).
- 71% pain with ADL.
- 75% no sports possible.

ACL, anterior cruciate ligament; ADL, activities of daily living; MCL, medial collateral ligament; PCL, posterior cruciate ligament.

Medical records, operative notes, radiographs, and MRI scans were reviewed and a comprehensive knee examination performed.

A single factor that caused the operations to fail was identified in 23 of the 52 operations (44%), and multiple factors were identified in 29 (56%; Table 21–16). The most common probable causes of failure were associated posterolateral deficiency (40%), improper graft tunnel placement (33%), associated varus malalignment (31%), and primary suture repair (25%).

Sixteen of 21 (76%) prior posterolateral procedures had failed, as had 9 of 19 (47%) prior ACL reconstructions. Twenty-nine knees (71%) presented with pain with activities of daily living. Thirty-four knees (83%) had compounding problems of joint arthritis, prior meniscectomy, associated ligament deficiencies, or varus malalignment.

In the patients' rating of their own knee condition, 20 (49%) rated the knee as poor; 12 (29%) as fair; and 9 (22%) as good. Thirty-one patients (75%) had given up sports activities completely, and 10 were participating with significant limitations and symptoms. Significant functional limitations were found with walking in 19 patients (46%) and during squatting in 37 (90%) patients.

In 22 knees (54%), a PCL revision reconstruction was performed. In 19 knees (46%), revision was not performed. Eleven of these 19 knees had developed advanced knee joint arthritis with significant loss of joint space on radiographs (with only a few millimeters remaining in the tibiofemoral joint) that contraindicated PCL revision. Eight patients declined further operative treatment.

Failure to restore associated ligament instabilities and incorrect tunnel placement were major factors contributing to surgical failure of PCL operative procedures. The results suggest the need for greater emphasis on the initial reconstruction in graft tunnel placement, correction of associated ligament instabilities, and correction of varus osseous malalignment. Failure of concurrent posterolateral complex reconstructions was frequently encountered, suggesting the need for higher-strength augmentation procedures or anatomic graft replacement, as discussed in Chapter 22, Posterolateral Ligament Structures: Diagnosis, Operative Techniques, and Clinical Outcomes.

Revision PCL Two-Strand QT-PB Autograft Reconstruction

From June 1995 until January 2002, a PCL revision reconstruction with a two-strand QT-PB autograft was performed in 15 knees referred after prior failed procedures.[97] There were 10 males and 5 females whose mean age at the time of PCL revision was 29 years (range, 17–49 yr). All patients were followed a mean of 44 months (range, 23–84 mo) postoperatively.

A total of 21 prior failed PCL operations had been done in these 15 knees, including 12 graft reconstructions, 5 primary repairs, 2 synthetic graft replacements, and 2 thermoplasties. A single PCL procedure had been done in 11 knees, and 2 or more PCL procedures had been done in 4 knees.

A mean of 46 months (range, 4–187 mo) had elapsed between the failed PCL procedures and the revision. The possible causes of failure of PCL reconstructions were previously presented in a larger series of knees described earlier; these 15 knees were a subgroup of that study.

Reconstruction of other knee ligaments had been done in 9 knees: ACL in 7 knees; FCL or posterolateral complex procedures in 3 knees; and MCL procedures in 3 knees. Before the PCL revision reconstruction, a staged HTO was required in 3 knees, and an autogenous bone grafting of prior graft tunnels was done in 1.

TABLE 21–16   Factors Contributing to Failure of 52 Posterior Cruciate Ligament Operations Referred to Our Center for Treatment

	Single Factor (23/52 Procedures)	Multiple Factors (29/52 Procedures)	Total
Deficiency of other knee ligaments			
Fibular collateral, posterolateral	1	20	21
Anterior cruciate	0	12	12
Medial collateral	0	3	3
Misplaced tunnels			
Posterior femoral tunnel	1	6	7
Anterior tibial tunnel	2	4	6
Proximal femoral and anterior tibial	0	4	4
Varus osseous malalignment	1	15	16
Primary repair	7	6	13
Synthetic graft, thermoplasty	1	6	7
Obesity	0	7	7
Traumatic reinjury	1	4	5
Tunnel osteolysis (allograft)	0	4	4
Postoperative infection	0	3	3
Fixation failure, tibial osteopenia	0	2	2
Failure revascularization, allograft removed	0	1	1
Unknown			1

From Noyes, F. R.; Barber-Westin, S. D.: Posterior cruciate ligament revision reconstruction, part I. Causes of surgical failure in 52 consecutive operations. *Am J Sports Med* 33:646–654, 2005.

Critical Points AUTHORS' CLINICAL STUDIES: REVISION POSTERIOR CRUCIATE LIGAMENT TWO-STRAND QUADRICEPS TENDON–PATELLAR BONE AUTOGRAFT RECONSTRUCTION

- $N = 15$ followed mean 44 mo (range, 23–84 mo) postoperatively.
- Mean 46 mo (range, 4–187 mo) between failed PCL procedures and revision.
- Staged HTO required in 3 knees, autogenous bone grafting of prior graft tunnels in 1 knee before PCL revision.
- Tibial inlay 9 knees, tibial tunnel 6 knees.
- Concomitant procedures: 4 ACL reconstruction, 4 posterolateral, 1 MCL reconstruction.
- Stress radiographs: mean preoperative, 11.7 ± 3.0; follow-up, 5.1 ± 2.4 ($P < .001$).
- KT-2000 (70°): mean preoperative, 8.9 ± 2.5; follow-up, 3.3 ± 3.9 ($P < .01$).
- Before revision, all knees rated C or D according to IKDC system.
- At follow-up, 1 knee, A; 9 knees, B; 4 knees, C; and 1 knee, D.
- 87% rated knee condition improved.
- 53% returned low-impact sports.
- 80% improved pain, 87% improved patient perception scores.
- Results inferior to primary PCL reconstructions, majority salvage knees.

ACL, anterior cruciate ligament; HTO, high tibial osteotomy; IKDC, International Knee Documentation Committee; MCL, medial collateral ligament; PCL, posterior cruciate ligament.

RESULTS FROM OTHER CLINICAL STUDIES

Single-Strand Reconstructions

Inconsistent results have been reported after various single-strand PCL reconstructive methods in restoration of normal posterior tibial displacement (Tables 21–19 and 21–20).

Two-Strand Reconstructions

Whereas many authors have described variations of a two-strand PCL reconstruction,[19,21,24,68,120,126,133,144] only a few investigators outside of the authors' center have reported on the outcome of two-strand PCL reconstruction using objective measuring instruments (Tables 21–21 and 21–22). Most of these studies used the KT-2000, and not stress radiography, to quantify the results of the

TABLE 21–19 Stability Results of Single-Strand Posterior Cruciate Ligament Reconstructions

Reference	N, Acute, Chronic, Follow-up	Type PCL Reconstruction	Other Ligament Reconstructions	Knee Arthrometer, Stress X-ray Methods	Knee Arthrometer Results (mm)	Stress X-ray Results (mm)
Wu et al., 2007[162]	N = 22 Chronic 60–76 mo	QT-PB autograft	None	KT: 70°, manual maximum	<3: 10 (45%) 3–5: 8 (36%) >5: 4 (18%)	Not done
Chan et al., 2006[18]	N = 20 Chronic 36–50 mo	ST autograft	None	KT: flexion angle NA, 89 N	<3: 50% 3–5: 35% >5: 15%	Not done
MacGillivray et al., 2006[75]	N = 20 Chronic 2–15 yr	Tibial tunnel: B-PT-B autograft (9) B-PT-B allograft (2) AT allograft (2) Tibial inlay: B-PT-B allograft (5) B-PT-B autograft (2)	None	KT: flexion angle NA, corrected posterior tibial translation	Transtibial: <3: 33% 3–5: 25% >5: 42% Tibial inlay: <3: 14% 3–5: 43% >5: 43%	Not done
Chen et al., 2006[23]	N = 52 Acute & chronic 48–70 mo	STG autograft	Posterolateral reconstruction (12)	KT: 70°, 134 N	<3: 62% 3–5: 19% >5: 19%	Not done
Jung, 2004[64]	N = 11 Acute & chronic 24–80 mo	B-PT-B autograft Tibial inlay	None	KT: 70°, manual maximum X-ray: 70°, 150 N	<3: 64% 3–5: 36%	<3: 36% 3–5: 45% >5: 18% Mean 3.4 ± 2.4
Cooper & Stewart, 2004[27]	N = 41 Acute & chronic Avg 39.4 mo	B-PT-B allograft (25) B-PT-B autograft (16) Tibial inlay Primary (35) Revision (6)	ACL (17) MCL (11) PCL/PLC (17)	X-ray: 70°, 245 N	Not done	<3: 34% 4–5: 39% 6–8: 15% 10: 12% Mean 4.11
Harner et al., 2004[57]	N = 31 Acute & chronic Dislocated knees 2–6 yr	AT allograft Tibial tunnel	All multiple ligament reconstructions	KT: 70°, quadriceps neutral angle, corrected posterior tibial translation, N = 25 tested	<3: 60% 3–5: 28% >5: 12%	Not done
Chen et al., 2004[22]	N = 29 Acute & chronic 36–70 mo	QT-PB autograft Tibial tunnel	PLC ST autograft (6)	KT: 70°, 134 N total AP translation	<3: 41% 3–5: 45% >5: 14%	Not done
Fanelli & Edson, 2004[38]	N = 41 Chronic 2–10 yr	AT allograft Tibial tunnel	PCL biceps tendon (41)	KT: Corrected anterior, posterior, PCL screen X-ray: 90°, 142 N	Mean screen: 1.80 mm Mean posterior: 2.11 mm	Mean 2.26 mm (range, –1– +7 mm)
Ohkoshi et al., 2003[114]	N = 51 Acute & chronic 25 ± 15 mo two-incision 19 ± 8 mo endoscopic	STG autograft Two-incision (22) Endoscopic (29) Tibial tunnel	None	KT: 70°, manual maximum total AP translation	Two-incision mean 3.95 ± 1.96 Endoscopic mean 2.38 ± 1.42	Not done

TABLE 21–19   Stability Results of Single-Strand Posterior Cruciate Ligament Reconstructions—Cont'd

Reference	N, Acute, Chronic, Follow-up	Type PCL Reconstruction	Other Ligament Reconstructions	Knee Arthrometer, Stress X-ray Methods	Knee Arthrometer Results (mm)	Stress X-ray Results (mm)
Deehan et al., 2003[33]	N = 23 Chronic 24–64 mo	STG autograft Tibial tunnel	MCL repair (2)	KT: 70°, 89 N, quadriceps neutral angle, total AP translation	0–2: 74% 3–4: 26%	Not done
Aglietti et al., 2002[2]	N = 18 Chronic 2–5.5 yr	QT-PB autograft Tibial inlay	FCL (6) MCL (2)	X-ray: 70°, 147 N	Not done	0–2: 17% 3–5: 61% 6–7: 11% 8–10: 11%
Fanelli & Edson, 2002[38]	N = 35, Acute & chronic 24–120 mo	AT allograft (26) B-PT-B autograft (7) STG autograft (2) Tibial tunnel	ACL (34) PLC (25)	KT: Corrected anterior, posterior, PCL screen X-ray: 90°, 142 N	Mean anterior: 3.4 (0–6.5) Mean posterior: 2.6 (0–9.0) Mean screen: 2.7 (0–7.0)	0–3: 52% 4–5: 24% 6–10: 19%
Chen et al., 2002[20]	N = 49 Acute & chronic 24–36 mo	QT-PB autograft (24) STG autograft (27) Tibial tunnel	None	KT: Manual maximum, total AP translation, flexion angle not given	QT-PB 0–2: 32% 3–5: 59% 6–10: 9% STG 0–2: 29% 3–5: 56% 6–10: 15%	Not done
Mariani et al., 2001[80]	N = 14 Acute & chronic 24–56 mo	B-PT-B autograft Tibial tunnel	All ACL STG	KT: 20°, 134 N and 70°, 89 N quadriceps neutral angle X-ray: 90°, posterior active test	20° <3: 64% 3–5: 29% >5: 7% 70° <3: 71% 3–5: 21% >5: 7%	Mean posterior translation: Lateral tibial plateau 5.8 ± 1.1 Medial tibial plateau 7.3 ± 1.5
Mariani et al., 1997[79]	N = 24 Chronic 24–53 mo	B-PT-B autograft Tibial tunnel	None	KT: 70°, 89 N quadriceps neutral angle	<3: 25% 3–5: 54% >5: 21%	Not done
Fanelli et al., 1996[11]	N = 21 Acute & chronic 24–54 mo	AT allograft (15) B-PT-B autograft (6) Tibial tunnel	PLC biceps transfer (21)	KT: 90° screen 70° corrected anterior, posterior	Screen avg. 1.6 (−0.5–+6.0) Posterior average 2.3 (0.5–9)	Not done
Barrett & Savoie, 1991[7]	N = 18 Acute 5–7.5 yr	ST (7) ST + Dacron (4) Direct repair (7)	ACL MCL PLC	Stryker 90°	ST: <5: 5 >5: 2 ST + Dacron: <3: 4 Repair <5: 5 >5: 2	Not done
Roth et al., 1988[128]	N = 31 Acute & chronic 53 mo	Medial gastrocnemius tendon transfer	Lateral reconstruction (4) Medial reconstruction (7)	KT: 30°, total AP translation 70° quadriceps active drawer	30° average 4.7 ± 4.1 70° average 3.7 ± 3.7	Not done

ACL, anterior cruciate ligament; AP, anteroposterior; AT, Achilles tendon; B-PT-B, bone–patellar tendon–bone; FCL, fibular collateral ligament; MCL, medial collateral ligament; NA, not available; PCL, posterior cruciate ligament; PLC, posterolateral complex; QT-PB, quadriceps tendon–patellar bone; ST, semitendinosus tendon; STG, semitendinosus-gracilis tendons.

operations.[113,145] Whereas the knee arthrometer is a valid tool for the measurement of total AP translation at 20° of knee flexion, it underestimates the true amount of posterior tibial translation in PCL-deficient and reconstructed knees at 70° of knee flexion. To date, only three investigations[48,97,101] used stress radiography to ascertain the results of PCL reconstruction (see Table 21–22). The range of patients with 5 mm or less of increased posterior tibial

translation in these studies was 34% to 73%. The number of patients in each study is too small to perform valid comparisons. Therefore, to date, too little evidence-based data remain to determine the indications for a two-strand versus a single-strand technique, the most advantageous graft to select for different circumstances, and the failure rate for autografts and allografts. There is an important need for well-designed level I multicenter

TABLE 21-20   Subjective and Functional Results of Single-Strand Posterior Cruciate Ligament Reconstructions

Reference	Patients	Rating Systems	Function	Symptoms	Sports	Overall IKDC	Results Other Scales
Wu et al., 2007[162]	N = 22 Chronic QT-PB autograft	IKDC Lysholm Tegner	IKDC 82% normal or nearly normal	82% no pain with moderate or strenuous activities	82% strenuous or moderate IKDC activity levels	A & B: 82% C & D: 18%	Lysholm mean score preoperative 67, F/U 89
Chan et al., 2006[18]	N = 20 Chronic ST autograft	IKDC Lysholm Tegner	IKDC 85% normal or nearly normal	95% no pain with moderate or strenuous activities	90% strenuous or moderate IKDC activity levels	A: 5 (25%) B: 12 (60%) C: 2 (10%) D: 1 (5%)	Lysholm mean score preoperative 63, F/U 93
MacGillivray et al., 2006[75]	N = 20 Chronic B-PT-B autograft, allograft, AT allograft	AAOS Lysholm Tegner	92% transtibial group satisfied 86% tibial inlay group satisfied	54% transtibial group no giving-way 43% tibial inlay group no giving-way	Mean Tegner score, 6 points for both groups	Not given	Mean Lysholm F/U 81 transtibial group, 76 tibial inlay group. Mean AAOS score 90 transtibial group, 77 tibial inlay group.
Chen et al., 2006[23]	N = 52 Acute & chronic STG autograft	IKDC Lysholm	IKDC 83% normal or nearly normal	13% pain, 10% swelling, 8% full giving-way with moderate or strenuous activities	58% strenuous or moderate, 25% light, 12% sedentary IKDC activity levels	A: 58% B: 23% C: 15% D: 4%	Lysholm mean score preoperative 54, F/U 91
Jung et al., 2004[64]	N = 21 Acute & chronic B-PT-B autograft	IKDC OAK	Not given	Not given	Not given	A: 4 (36%) B: 7 (64%) C: 0 D: 0	OAK preoperative mean 72, F/U mean 92.5 points (P <.01)
Cooper & Stewart, 2004[27]	N = 41 Acute & chronic B-PT-B allograft, autograft	IKDC Subjective	Mean 75.1 points (range, 22–100 points) All patients rated knee improved	Not given	Not given	Not given	None
Harner et al., 2004[57]	N = 31 Acute & chronic Dislocated AT allograft	IKDC Lysholm Myers Knee Outcome Survey	ADL mean score F/U 89 points (64–99 points). Acute mean 91, chronic mean 84 (P =.07)	Not given	Sports Activities mean score F/U 82 points (0–100 points). Acute mean 89, chronic mean 69 (P <.05)	A: 0 B: 11 (35%) C: 12 (39%) D: 8 (26%)	Lysholm mean F/U. score 91 acutes, 80 chronics (P =.07). Myers: 10 excellent, 13 good, 5 fair, 3 poor
Chen et al., 2004[22]	N = 20 Acute & chronic QT-PB autograft	IKDC Lysholm	IKDC Normal/near normal: 25 (86%) Abnormal: 3 86% patients rated knee function normal/near normal	Normal/near normal: Pain: 24 (86%) Swelling: 25 (86%) Full giving-way: 26 (90%)	Strenuous (I): 48% Moderate (II): 17% Light (III): 21% None (IV): 14%	A: 10 (34%) B: 14 (48%) C: 3 (10%) D: 2 (7%)	Lysholm mean score preoperative 57, F/U 90 (P <.01)
Fanelli & Edson, 2004[39]	N = 41 Chronic All with biceps tendon transfer AT allograft	Lysholm Tegner HSS	Lysholm mean score: Preoperative: 65.48 Postoperative: 91.67 HSS mean score: Preoperative: 50.48 Postop: 88.69	Not given	Tegner mean score: Preoperative: 2.7 Postoperative: 4.9 All return to "desired level of activity"	Not given	None

Study	Patients / Graft	Rating systems						Outcome
Ohkoshi et al., 2003[114]	N = 51 Acute & chronic STG autograft	IKDC	Not given	Not given	Not given	Not given	Two-incision group: A: 32% B: 50% C: 14% D: 4% Endoscopic group: A: 45% B: 52% C: 3% D: 0%	None
Deehan et al., 2003[33]	N = 23 Chronic STG autograft	IKDC Lysholm	A: 15 (65%) B: 10 (37%) C: 1 (4%) D: 1 (4%)	S.S. improvements pain, swelling, giving-way	17 (63%) returned moderate-to-strenuous activities	A: 4 (17%) B: 12 (50%) C: 7 (29%) D: 1 (4%)		Lysholm mean score preoperative 64, F/U. 94 (P <.01)
Aglietti et al., 2002[2]	N = 18 Chronic QT-PB autograft	IKDC	All patients rated knee function normal/nearly normal	Normal/near normal: Pain: 17 (94%) Swelling: 18 (100%) Full giving-way: 17 (94%)	Strenuous (I): 0% Moderate (II): 28% Light (III): 67% None (IV): 5%	A: 3 (17%) B: 9 (50%) C: 6 (33%) D: 0		None
Fanelli & Edson, 2002[38]	N = 35 Acute & chronic AT allograft, B-PT-B autograft, STG autograft	Lysholm Tegner HSS	Not given	Not given	Tegner preoperative mean 1.4, postoperative mean 5.3 (P = .001). Means only given	Not given		Lysholm mean score preoperative 32, F/U 91 (P <.001). HSS mean score preoperative 20, F/U 87 (P = .001).
Chen et al., 2002[20]	N = 49 Acute & chronic QT-PB autograft, STG autograft	IKDC Lysholm	QT-PB group: 36% patients rated knee function normal, nearly normal Hamstring group: 85% patients rated knee function normal, nearly NL	Normal/near normal: QT-PB group: Fair: 19 (86%) Swelling: 20 (91%) Full giving-way: 21 (95%) Hamstring group: Pain: 23 (85%) Swelling: 23 (85%) Full giving-way: 26 (96%)	QT-PB group: Strenuous (I): 41% Moderate (II): 14% Light (III): 27% None (IV): 18% Hamstring group: Strenuous (I): 44% Moderate (II): 15% Light (III): 22% None (IV): 19%	QT-PB group: A: 5 (23%) B: 13 (59%) C: 3 (13%) D: 1 (5%) Hamstring group: A: 7 (26%) B: 15 (55%) C: 4 (15%) D: 1 (4%)		Lysholm mean score F/U QT-PB group 90.63, hamstring group 91.44.
Mariani et al., 2001[80]	N = 14 Acute & chronic B-PT-B autograft	IKDC HSS Lysholm Tegner	Not given	IKDC Subjective A: 5 B: 7 C: 2 D: 0	Tegner: 50% returned preinjury level, 50% decreased level	Not given		Lysholm mean score preoperative 65, F/U 95 (P <.0001). HSS mean score preoperative 32, F/U 90 (P <.001);
Wascher et al., 1999[158]	N = 13 Acute & chronic Dislocated knees AT & B-PT-B allograft	IKDC Lysholm Tegner	92% satisfied	Not given	Returned, no symptoms 46% Playing with symptoms 31% No sports 23%	A: 0% B: 54% C: 45% D: 1%		Lysholm mean F/U 88 Meyers: 6 excellent, 5 good, 1 fair, 1 poor
Mariani et al., 1997[79]	N = 24 Chronic B-PT-B autograft	IKDC Lysholm Tegner	IKDC: A: 50% B: 50%	IKDC: A: 62% B: 38%	Tegner mean preoperative 34, F/U 5.4 50% returned preinjury activities	A: 25% B: 54% C: 13% D: 8%		Lysholm mean preoperative 56, F/U 94

Continued

TABLE 21-20   Subjective and Functional Results of Single-Strand Posterior Cruciate Ligament Reconstructions—Cont'd

Reference	Patients	Rating Systems	Function	Symptoms	Sports	Overall IKDC	Results Other Scales
Fanelli et al., 1996[41]	N = 21 Acute & chronic AT allograft, B-PT-B autograft	Lysholm Tegner HSS	Not given	Not given	Tegner mean preoperative 2.2, F/U 5.1	Not done	Lysholm mean preoperative 52, F/U 91 HSS mean preoperative 38, F/U 87.5
Barrett & Savoie, 1991[7]	N = 18 Acute ST, ST + Dacron, Direct repair	Clancy Hughston	94% satisfied	1 severe pain ADL 3 pain ADL 4 pain strenuous sports 28% swelling	4 preinjury level 14 decreased activity level	Not done	Clancy: 44% satisfactory, 44% fair, 2 failures Hughston: 55% good, 28% fair, 3 failures
Roth et al., 1988[28]	N = 31 Acute & chronic Medial gastrocnemius tendon transfer	Authors' own	19% unstable with walking 22% unstable with running 38% unstable with pivoting	60% swelling 16% pain ADL 25% pain with sports	1 preinjury level 18 recreational sports 13 no sports	Not done	None

AAOS, American Academy of Orthopaedic Surgeons; ADL, activities of daily living; AT, Achilles tendon; B-PT-B, bone–patellar tendon–bone; F/U, follow-up; HSS, Hospital for Special Surgery; IKDC, International Knee Documentations Committee; OAK, Orthopädische Arbeitsgruppe Knie; QT-PB, quadriceps tendon–patellar bone; S.S., statistically significant; ST, semitendinosus; STG, semitendinosus-gracilis tendons.

TABLE 21–21 Subjective and Functional Results of Two-Strand Posterior Cruciate Ligament Reconstructions

Reference	Patients	Rating Systems	Function	Symptoms	Sports	Overall IKDC	Results Other Scales
Noyes, 2006[92]; Noyes & Barber-Westin, 2005[101]	N = 48, Acute & chronic, Tibial tunnel (29), Tibial inlay (19), QT-PB autograft	Cincinnati, IKDC	Tunnel Group: S.S. improvements walking, stairs, running, jumping, twisting, turning. Inlay group: S.S. improvements walking, stairs, squatting, running, jumping, twisting, turning	Tunnel group: S.S. improvements pain, swelling, giving-way, patient perception. 37% chronics pain ADL preoperative, reduced to 5% at F/U. 94% patients rated knee condition improved. Inlay group: S.S. improvements pain, swelling, giving-way, patient perception. 58% pain ADL preoperative, reduced to 5% at F/U. 95% patients rated knee condition improved	Tunnel group: 24% strenuous sports, 52% low-impact sports, 3% sports, symptoms, 21% no sports. Inlay Group: 10% strenuous sports, 58% low-impact sports, 10% sports, symptoms, 21% no sports	Tunnel group A: 1 (3%) B: 7 (24%) C: 18 (62%) D: 3 (10%) Inlay group A: 0 B: 14 (74%) C: 3 (16%) D: 2 (10%)	
Garofalo et al., 2006[48]	N = 15, Chronic, Isolated, B-PT-B and ST autografts	IKDC, Tegner, Lysholm, HSS	S.S. improvement IKDC subjective knee score 93% rated knee improved	Not done	None able to resume preinjury sports level	Preop mean 36.6 F/U mean 66.3	S.S. improvement all rating scores
Noyes & Barber-Westin, 2005[56]	N = 15, Revisions, QT-PB autograft	Cincinnati, IKDC	S.S. improvements walking, stairs, squatting, running	S.S. improvements pain, swelling, giving-way, patient perception. 67% pair ADL preoperative, reduced to 13% at F/U. 87% patients rated knee condition improved	53% low-impact sports, 13% sports, symptoms, 26% no sports	A: 1 (7%) B: 7 (47%) C: 6 (40%) D: 1 (7%)	
Houe & Jorgensen, 2004[61]	N = 6 single-strand, N = 10 two-strand, Chronic, Tibial tunnel, B-PT-B, STG autografts	Lysholm, Tegner	Not done	Not done	Not done	Not done	Lysholm preoperative 68, F/U 97.5. Tegner preoperative 2.5, F/U 6. No difference between groups

Continued

trials, because one individual center does not have sufficient PCL cases for statistical analysis and definitive recommendations.

Stannard and coworkers[145] used a two-strand AT-B allograft in 29 patients who sustained acute traumatic multiligament injuries. The technique used a combination of two femoral tunnels and a tibial inlay technique. One femoral tunnel (anterolateral) was located approximately 8 mm from the articular surface within the PCL femoral footprint at the top of the notch, and the second tunnel was placed posterior and inferior (posteromedial). A 4-mm bone bridge existed between the two tunnels. Fixation of the graft on the posterior tibia was accomplished with a 4.5-mm cannulated screw and washer. The anterolateral strand was tensioned at 70° of knee flexion, and the posteromedial strand was tensioned at 20° of flexion. Both strands were secured with absorbable interference screws.

Fourteen patients also sustained ipsilateral lower extremity fractures, ACL, or posterolateral complex injuries were reconstructed approximately 8 weeks after the PCL reconstruction, although the number of patients who required these additional procedures was not provided. The clinical follow-up ranged from 15 to 39 months postoperatively. The authors reported that 20% of the patients had a 1+ posterior laxity and 80% had no increased posterior laxity at follow-up. However, 40% of the patients developed some degree of arthrofibrosis and required a manipulation or arthroscopic lysis of adhesions. Four knees (14%) had a loss of 5° to 10° of extension and 9 knees (31%) had less than 120° of flexion at follow-up. The KT-2000 data showed that 50% of the operated knees had less posterior tibial displacement at 70° of flexion than the contralateral knees. Stress radiographs were not performed. No data were provided for the outcome of the additional ligament reconstructions. Fifty-five percent returned to their preinjury level of activities, 41% returned to a lower level, and 3% did not return to sports.

Nyland and associates[113] reported the short-term (27 ± 2 mo) clinical results of a two-strand anterior tibialis allograft reconstruction in 19 knees with chronic PCL injuries. The technique used two femoral tunnels and a single tibial tunnel. One femoral tunnel was located at the 3 o'clock position, 12 mm posterior to the anterior articular edge, and the second tunnel was placed at 1 o'clock, 5 mm posterior to the anterior cartilage edge. Both femoral strands were secured with the knee flexion to 80° to 90° of knee flexion with interference screws. The authors attempted to re-create the reciprocating function of the two strands as described by Mannor and associates.[77]

Postoperatively, KT-1000 testing revealed a mean of 2.4 ± 2 mm posterior displacement. The authors[113] did not provide the knee flexion angle at which the arthrometer testing was performed or the range of values recorded. Stress radiographs were not performed. Posterior drawer testing showed normal (11 knees) or nearly normal (8 knees) test results. All but 1 patient had normal or nearly normal external rotation, and all but 2 patients had normal or nearly normal lateral joint opening. The authors[113] hypothesized that the two-strand technique reduced the mild to moderate posterolateral complex instability, believing that the reestablishment of the normal reciprocating function of the PCL fibers helped to restore lateral knee stability. Seventeen patients were graded as normal or nearly normal in the overall IKDC score, 1 was graded as abnormal, and 1 as severely abnormal.

Garofalo and associates[48] used two autografts (B-PT-B and semitendinosus tendon) to reconstruct chronic PCL ruptures in 15 patients. The B-PT-B graft was used to replace the posteromedial strand and the semitendinosus graft was used for the anterolateral strand. A single transtibial tunnel and two femoral tunnels were used, one of which was placed at the 11 o'clock position, 8 mm proximal from the cartilage edge, and the other at the 9 o'clock position (left knee). The anterolateral strand was tensioned and fixed at 70° of flexion, and the posteromedial strand was fixed at 30° of flexion. At follow-up, 2 to 5 years postoperatively, 40% of the patients had 6 mm or more of increased posterior tibial translation on stress radiographs. These authors concluded that the procedure offered no advantage over that of single-strand constructs in terms of restoration of normal posterior translation.

ILLUSTRATIVE CASES

Case 1.   A 16-year-old female high school athlete injured her left knee playing soccer. A PCL thermoplasty was performed, which failed, and she was referred to the authors' center 9 months later for consideration of reconstruction. The patient complained of functional limitations with all athletics and had not been able to return to soccer. Physical examination revealed 10 mm of increased posterior tibial translation, 7 mm of increased lateral joint opening, and 30° of increased external tibial rotation. Posterior stress radiographs demonstrated 11 mm of increased posterior tibial translation. The patient was a potential collegiate soccer scholarship candidate.

The patient underwent a two-strand QT-PB PCL reconstruction with a tibial inlay technique (Fig. 21–44). The posterolateral deficiency was treated with a proximal advancement of the posterolateral complex. The *arrows* in Figure 21–44A show the location of the two tunnels in the medial femoral condyle.

The patient was able to return to soccer without problems. Two years postoperatively, she had 4 mm of increased posterior tibial translation on stress radiographs at 90° flexion, no increase on KT-2000 testing at 20° of flexion, and no increase in lateral joint opening or external tibial rotation. She rated the overall condition of her knee as very good.

Case 2.   A 45-year-old man sustained a complete PCL rupture during a recreational basketball game and underwent a PCL AT-B

allograft reconstruction. He presented to the authors' center 1 year later with complaints of moderate pain with daily activities and severe difficulty with walking, stair-climbing, and squatting. He was disabled from his occupation. Radiographs demonstrated proximal and anterior placement of the tibial tunnel and enlargement of both tunnels (Fig. 21–45) with an obvious posterior tibial subluxation. Physical examination showed 10 mm of increased posterior tibial translation, 6 mm of increased lateral joint opening, and moderate patellofemoral crepitus. The patient had a tibial nerve palsy, which was improving. Stress radiographs revealed 12 mm of increased posterior tibial translation.

The treatment recommendation was a staged autogenous femoral bone graft procedure followed by a two-strand PCL revision reconstruction using a tibial inlay technique. The patient declined further operative treatment.

Authors' comment: Inadequate placement of the primary PCL graft represents one of the most common causes of failure, particularly with an anterior tibial placement that produces a vertical PCL graft.

Case 3.   A 36-year-old woman sustained a work-related injury and underwent a single-strand PCL patellar tendon allograft reconstruction. The patient's surgical history also included an MCL reconstruction

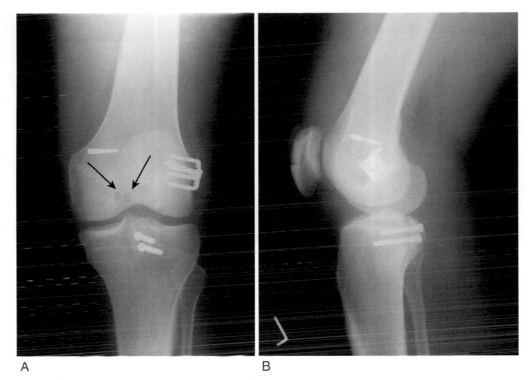

A   B

FIGURE 21–44. Case #1. (From Noyes, F. R.; Barber-Westin, S. D.: Posterior cruciate ligament replacement with a two-strand quadriceps tendon–patellar bone autograft and a tibial inlay technique. J Bone Joint Surg Am 87:1241–1262, 2005.)

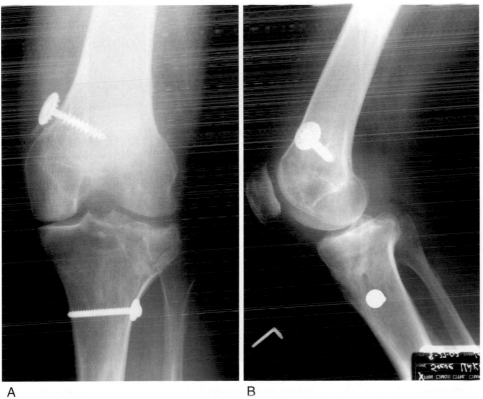

A   B

FIGURE 21-45. Case #2. (From Noyes, F. R.; Barber-Westin, S. D.: Posterior cruciate ligament revision reconstruction, part I. Causes of surgical failure in 52 consecutive operations. Am J Sports Med 33:646–654, 2005.)

149. Torg, J. S.; Barton, T. M.; Pavlov, H.; Stine, R.: Natural history of the posterior cruciate ligament–deficient knee. *Clin Orthop Relat Res* 246:208–216, 1989.

150. Torisu, T.: Avulsion fracture of the tibial attachment of the posterior cruciate ligament. Indications and results of delayed repair. *Clin Orthop Relat Res* 143:107–114, 1979.

151. Trickey, E. L.: Injuries to the posterior cruciate ligament: diagnosis and treatment of early injuries and reconstruction of late instabilty. *Clin Orthop Relat Res* 147:76–81, 1980.

152. Trickey, E. L.: Rupture of the posterior cruciate ligament of the knee. *J Bone Joint Surg Br* 50:334–341, 1968.

153. Trotter, M.: The level of termination of the popliteal artery in the white and the negro. *Am J Phys Anthrop* 27:109–118, 1940.

154. Van Dijk, R.: The anatomy of the cruciate ligaments. In *The Behavior of the Cruciate Ligaments in the Human Knee*. Amsterdam: Rodopi, 1983; pp. 5–37.

155. Van Dommelen, B. A.; Fowler, P. J.: Anatomy of the posterior cruciate ligament. A review. *Am J Sports Med* 17:24–29, 1989.

156. Wang, C. J.; Chan, Y. S.; Weng, L. H.: Posterior cruciate ligament reconstruction using hamstring tendon graft with remnant augmentation. *Arthroscopy* 21:1401, 2005.

156a. Wang, C. J.; Weng, L. H.; Hsu, C. C.; Chan, Y. S.: Arthroscopic single- versus double-bundle posterior cruciate ligament reconstruction using hamstring autograft. *Injury* 35:1293–1299, 2004.

157. Warren, L. F.; Marshall, J. L.: The supporting structures and layers on the medial side of the knee: an anatomical analysis. *J Bone Joint Surg Am* 61:56–62, 1979.

158. Wascher, D. C.; Becker, J. R.; Dexter, J. G.; Blevins, F. T.: Reconstruction of the anterior and posterior cruciate ligaments after knee dislocation. Results using fresh-frozen nonirradiated allografts. *Am J Sports Med* 27:189–196, 1999.

159. Whiddon, D. R.; Zehms, C. T.; Miller, M. D.; et al.: Double compared with single-bundle open inlay posterior cruciate ligament reconstruction in a cadaver model. *J Bone Joint Surg Am* 90:1820–1829, 2008.

160. Wind, W. M., Jr.; Bergfeld, J. A.; Parker, R. D.: Evaluation and treatment of posterior cruciate ligament injuries: revisited. *Am J Sports Med* 32:1765–1775, 2004.

161. Woo, S. L.-Y.; Hollis, J. M.; Adams, D. J.; et al.: Tensile properties of the human femur–anterior cruciate ligament–tibia complex. The effects of specimen age and orientation. *Am J Sports Med* 19:217–225, 1991.

162. Wu, C. H.; Chen, A. C.; Yuan, L. J.; et al.: Arthroscopic reconstruction of the posterior cruciate ligament by using a quadriceps tendon autograft: a minimum 5-year follow-up. *Arthroscopy* 23:420–427, 2007.

163. Zhao, J.; He, Y.; Wang, J.: Arthroscopic treatment of acute tibial avulsion fracture of the posterior cruciate ligament with suture fixation technique through Y-shaped bone tunnels. *Arthroscopy* 22:172–181, 2006.

Chapter 22

Posterolateral Ligament Injuries: Diagnosis, Operative Techniques, and Clinical Outcomes

Frank R. Noyes, MD ■ *Sue D. Barber-Westin*, BS

INDICATIONS

The primary soft tissue stabilizing structures of the lateral and posterolateral (PL) aspect of the knee joint are the fibular collateral ligament (FCL) and popliteus muscle-tendon-ligament unit (PMTL), including the popliteofibular ligament (PFL) and posterolateral capsule (PLC) shown in Figure 22–1. These structures function together to resist lateral joint opening (LJO),

---

Critical Points INDICATIONS

- 6–10 mm increased lateral tibiofemoral joint opening 20° flexion.
- ≥15° increased external tibial rotation 30°, 90° flexion.
- ± Varus recurvatum, standing and supine.
- ± Hyperextension gait abnormality.
- Double or triple varus knee, after osteotomy.
- Acute injuries, bony avulsions amenable to internal fixation.

---

posterior subluxation of the lateral tibial plateau with tibial rotation, knee hyperextension, and varus recurvatum.[11,12,31,32,47,54]

The mechanism of injury may be contact or noncontact and usually involves a combined varus and hyperextension joint displacement. The proper management of injuries involving the PL structures requires knowledge of the complex anatomy and potential variations that may exist, the function of the major soft tissue stabilizers, appropriate diagnostic techniques, and surgical options for reconstruction. Isolated PL injuries are rare; however, on occasion, an avulsion fracture at the femoral attachment occurs requiring internal fixation.[24] PL injuries are frequently accompanied by anterior cruciate ligament (ACL) or posterior cruciate ligament (PCL) ruptures.[1,8,23]

Although the incidence of PL injury is unknown (owing to misdiagnosis or failure to detect the injury), the consequences of untreated PL ruptures are readily apparent. Chronic deficiency of the PL structures may be a factor in the failure of cruciate reconstructions[34,36,42] and may also play a role in the development of gait abnormalities and giving-way.[43,45,51] The

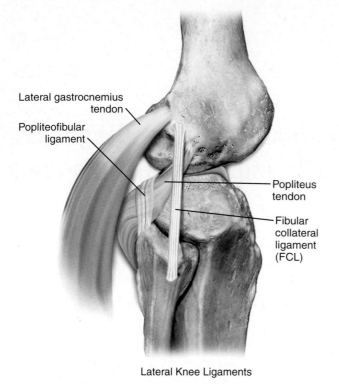

Lateral gastrocnemius tendon

Popliteofibular ligament

Popliteus tendon

Fibular collateral ligament (FCL)

Lateral Knee Ligaments

FIGURE 22–1. The anatomic relationships of the posterolateral (PL) structures.

detection and proper treatment of these problems is critical, because failure to properly treat all of the abnormalities may result in a poor outcome. The patient will complain of a varus type of instability with LJO during stance phase and show either a neutral or a valgus alignment. The abnormal LJO during stance phase is always greater than that detected on the varus stress test. The patient may demonstrate the abnormal LJO by producing a varus loading at the knee joint while standing.

Knees that fulfill the double or triple varus diagnosis criteria (varus osseous malalignment with increased LJO, external tibial rotation, varus recurvatum, and knee hyperextension [see Chapter 31, Primary, Double, and Triple Varus Knee Syndrome: Diagnosis, Osteotomy Techniques, and Clinical Outcomes])[40] require high tibial osteotomy (HTO) first, followed approximately 6 months later with an appropriate PL reconstruction. In many instances, an ACL or PCL deficiency also exists, which is corrected at the time of the PL reconstruction.

Different surgical options are available for acute knee injuries, dislocated knees with multiple ligament ruptures, chronic knees, and revision knees. The decision making process for determining the appropriate PL procedure is discussed in detail under "Operative Treatment of Acute PL Ruptures" and "Operative Treatment of Chronic PL Ruptures" later in this chapter.

CONTRAINDICATIONS

Contraindications to PL reconstruction are findings of less than 5 mm of increased lateral tibiofemoral joint opening and less than 10° of increased external tibial rotation. These findings are frequently noted in knees with associated varus osseous malalignment (double varus knees) that are candidates for HTO (see Chapter 31, Primary, Double, and Triple Varus Knee Syndromes: Diagnosis, Osteotomy Techniques, and Clinical Outcomes).[33] Correction of the varus malalignment promotes physiologic remodeling and shortening of the PL structures, decreasing the abnormal LJO and external tibial rotation and thus negating the need for a PL operative procedure.

Patients with varus malalignment who do not undergo HTO and have associated chronic insufficiency of the PL structures are not candidates for a PL procedure. Untreated varus osseous malalignment is a cause of failure of PL reconstructions.[39] In many cases, a knee hyperextension gait abnormality also exists that must be corrected before surgery with a specific gait-retraining program described in Chapter 34, Correction of Hyperextension Gait Abnormalities: Preoperative and Postoperative Techniques.[43] Failure to correct a hyperextension gait abnormality places PL reconstructions at risk for failure owing to the excessively high tensile forces placed on the PL soft tissues upon weight-bearing after surgery. Gait retraining usually decreases abnormally high knee extension and adduction moments to normal values.[43]

Patients with a history of prior joint infection or who are obese (body mass index > 30) are not candidates for PL reconstruction. Patients with muscle atrophy of the lower extremity undergo preoperative rehabilitation before PL reconstruction.

Knees that demonstrate a loss of lateral tibiofemoral compartment joint space, with less than 2 mm remaining on 45° posteroanterior (PA) weight-bearing radiographs, are usually not candidates for PL reconstruction.

CLINICAL EVALUATION

The PL structures are injured when excessive varus, external tibial rotation, and hyperextension forces are applied to the lower extremity. A blow to the anteromedial tibia during sports participation appears to be one of the most common injury mechanisms. These injuries frequently involve rupture of other knee ligament structures, complicating the diagnosis. An isolated complete PL rupture is rare because, usually, the injury is accompanied by an ACL or PCL rupture. In some cases, the PL structures are only partially disrupted and do not require surgical restoration. It is important to correctly determine the increases in LJO, external tibial rotation, and knee hyperextension of the injured knee (compared with the contralateral knee) preoperatively and intraoperatively. The decision of whether surgical restoration of the PL structures is indicated is

Critical Points CLINICAL EVALUATION

History

- Common injury mechanism blow to anteromedial tibia causing excessive knee hyperextension, external tibial rotation, lateral tibiofemoral joint opening.
- Most PL injuries occur with ACL or PCL ruptures.

Physical Examination

- Knee flexion, extension.
- Joint effusion.
- Patellofemoral (medial and lateral subluxation, Q-angle, crepitus, compression pain).
- Tibiofemoral crepitus, joint line pain, compression pain.
- Recurvatum (standing, supine).
- Gait (severe hyperextension stance phase).
- Muscle strength.

Tibiofemoral Rotation Dial Test

- Diagnosis PL injury based on final position lateral tibial plateau.
- Assess position medial and lateral tibial plateaus separately, neutral tibial rotation, 30°, 90° knee flexion.
- Produce maximal tibial external rotation, determine change in position of medial and lateral tibial plateaus separately.
- Qualitatively determine whether anterior or posterior subluxation occurred each tibial plateau.

Diagnostic Clinical Tests

- External rotation recurvatum.
- Lateral and medial tibiofemoral joint opening 5°, 20° flexion.
- Pivot shift, Lachman.
- Reverse pivot shift.
- Posterior drawer, 90° flexion.
- KT-2000 20° flexion, 134 N.

Radiographs

- Anteroposterior.
- Lateral, 30° flexion.
- Posteroanterior, weight-bearing, 45° flexion.
- Patellofemoral axial.
- Lateral stress, neutral tibial rotation.
- PCL ruptures: posterior stress lateral, 90° flexion, neutral tibial rotation.
- Varus malalignment: full standing radiographs, mechanical axis and weight bearing line.

Cincinnati Knee Rating System

- Sports Activity and Function Form.
- Occupational Rating Form.
- Symptom Rating Form.

ACL, anterior cruciate ligament; PCL, posterior cruciate ligament; PL, posterolateral.

based on the abnormal knee motion limits, joint subluxations, and the tissue disruption.

One frequent patient presentation is a failed ACL or PCL reconstruction owing to untreated PL insufficiency. Another patient presentation is a chronic varus osseous malalignment and underlying ACL insufficiency in which, over time, interstitial stretching and slackening of the PL structures occurred.[33,40] In these cases, HTO unloads the PL soft tissues to the extent at which physiologic remodeling and shortening occur and PL reconstruction is not required.[40]

A comprehensive physical examination is required, including assessment of knee flexion and extension, patellofemoral indices, tibiofemoral crepitus, tibiofemoral joint line pain, and gait abnormalities. Pain in the medial tibiofemoral compartment occurs owing to increased compressive forces related to varus osseous malalignment. Pain in the PL soft tissues may occur from increased soft tissue tensile forces due to a varus thrusting gait pattern. The abnormal knee hyperextension involves increased extension in the sagittal plane and is often accompanied by a varus alignment in the coronal plane, which has been described as a varus recurvatum alignment. Together with a varus osseous malalignment, this is referred to as a *triple varus knee* (see Chapter 31, Primary, Double, and Triple Varus Knee Syndromes: Diagnosis, Osteotomy Techniques, and Clinical Outcomes). Patients with chronic PL insufficiency have varying amounts of altered gait mechanics and knee hyperextension. Some individuals may present with a markedly abnormal gait that is severely disabling and limits ambulation. Other patients may have a less noticeable alteration because the abnormal knee hyperextension occurs only after prolonged walking and muscle fatigue. The abnormal gait pattern is characterized by excessive knee hyperextension during the stance phase, which does respond to gait retraining that initiates normal stance phase flexion (see Chapter 34, Correction of Hyperextension Gait

Abnormalities: Preoperative and Postoperative Techniques). Subjective complaints of giving-way during routine daily activities, along with severe quadriceps atrophy, often accompany this gait abnormality.

The surgeon must determine all of the abnormal translations and rotations in the knee joint. The ligament injuries that result in knee hyperextension and varus recurvatum frequently involve not only the PL structures but also other ligament and capsular structures. The biomechanical and kinematic studies that form the basis for the interpretation and diagnosis of the manual stress tests are described in Chapter 20, Function of the Posterior Cruciate Ligament and Posterolateral Ligament Structures.

The increases in LJO and external tibial rotation shown in Table 22-1 are only approximations of what would be expected with clinical injury to the PL structures. Importantly, an increase of only a few millimeters (2–5 mm) in LJO occurs with complete rupture of the FCL, whereas an increase of 5 to 9 mm occurs with complete rupture of all the PL structures (FCL, PMTL, PFL). These values are based on biomechanical studies discussed in Chapter 20, Function of the Posterior Cruciate Ligament and Posterolateral Ligament Structures, under moderate varus loads (20 Nm). LaPrade and colleagues[20] conducted a cadaveric study in which lateral stress radiography was applied at 12 Nm (on an experimental apparatus) and the increase in LJO over the intact state was compared with that measured during a clinician-applied load after an isolated FCL rupture and a combined FCL, PMTL, PFL rupture. Compared with the intact state, LJO induced by the clinician-applied load increased by 2.7 mm (isolated FCL rupture) and 4.0 mm (combined PL rupture). However, the mean values showed a wide standard deviation and variation between specimens, making extrapolation to the clinical setting difficult. In addition, the lateral joint space measurement showed wide confidence intervals. For an isolated

TABLE 22–1   Comprehensive Knee Examination

Examination	Technique	Illustration	Grading	Significance
Dial test 30°	Supine position, palpate anterior tibial prominence, medial and lateral joint, maximum external rotation, posterior position, lateral tibia (PL) subluxation, anterior position medial tibia (anteromedial subluxation).	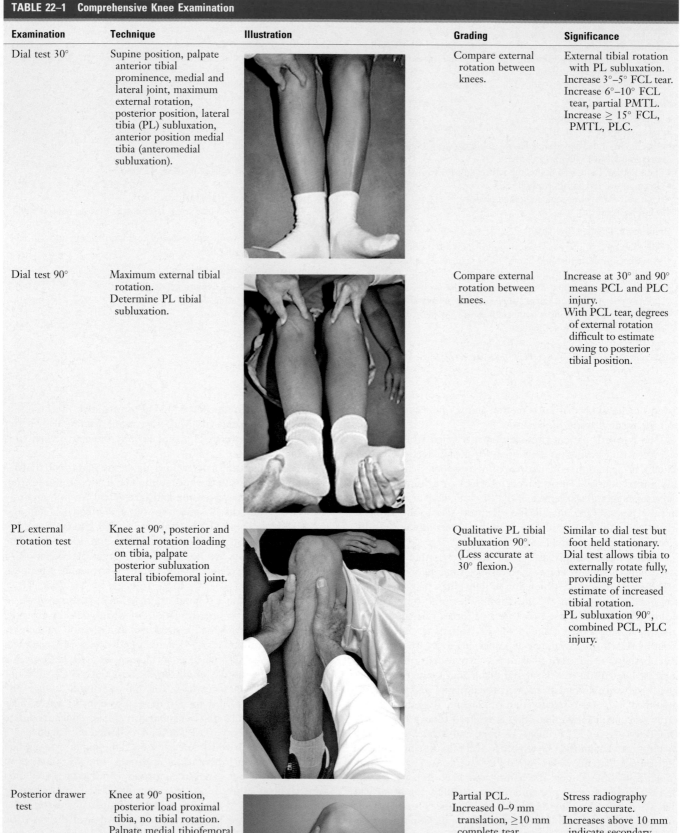	Compare external rotation between knees.	External tibial rotation with PL subluxation. Increase 3°–5° FCL tear. Increase 6°–10° FCL tear, partial PMTL. Increase ≥ 15° FCL, PMTL, PLC.
Dial test 90°	Maximum external tibial rotation. Determine PL tibial subluxation.		Compare external rotation between knees.	Increase at 30° and 90° means PCL and PLC injury. With PCL tear, degrees of external rotation difficult to estimate owing to posterior tibial position.
PL external rotation test	Knee at 90°, posterior and external rotation loading on tibia, palpate posterior subluxation lateral tibiofemoral joint.		Qualitative PL tibial subluxation 90°. (Less accurate at 30° flexion.)	Similar to dial test but foot held stationary. Dial test allows tibia to externally rotate fully, providing better estimate of increased tibial rotation. PL subluxation 90°, combined PCL, PLC injury.
Posterior drawer test	Knee at 90° position, posterior load proximal tibia, no tibial rotation. Palpate medial tibiofemoral step-off.	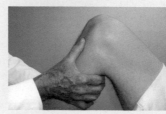	Partial PCL. Increased 0–9 mm translation, ≥10 mm complete tear.	Stress radiography more accurate. Increases above 10 mm indicate secondary restraints torn or physiologic slack (combined injury).

TABLE 22–1   Comprehensive Knee Examination—Cont'd

Examination	Technique	Illustration	Grading	Significance
Quadriceps active test	Knee position at 70°–90°. Foot stabilized by examiner, patient activates quadriceps by pushing foot against table or attempting to extend knee.		Qualitative. Observe, palpate tibiofemoral position.	Confirms posterior tibial subluxation, PCL injury at resting position. Quadriceps contraction produces anterior translation knee position ≥ 70°.
Lachman (anterior drawer, 30° flexion)	Anterior load. Proximal tibia. Compare translation between knees.		Observe anterior translation tibia. Estimate increase translation in millimeters. Soft endpoint.	Soft endpoint, ACL not resisting anterior translation, indicates ACL tear. Increase 3–5 mm ACL tear. >5 mm ACL plus secondary restraints.
Pivot shift	Knee position 10°–30° flexion. Anterior load tibia, gentle internal tibial rotation (subluxation) followed by posterior load, gentle external rotation (reduction).		Qualitative. Grade: I slipping II thud, clunk with reduction III gross anterior subluxation lateral tibiofemoral joint, anterior impingement tibia limits reduction event.	Grade I physiologic laxity, no or partial ACL tear. II ACL tear. III ACL tear + secondary restraints lax.
Reverse pivot shift test	Similar loading as pivot shift.		PL subluxation with external rotation confused for reduction in pivot shift. No abnormal anterior tibial subluxation.	Observe obvious PL tibial subluxation with posterior and external rotation loading. Dial test more accurate.
Varus stress testing	Thigh supported on examination table. Knee position 0°, 30°. Varus load with no external-internal tibial rotation. Palpate lateral joint line opening.		Subtle 30° increase LJO. 2–4 mm complete FCL tear, further increase LJO with PLC injury.	Stress radiography more accurate. 30° flexion Increase 2–4 mm FCL tear. Increase 5–9 mm complete PLC tear (also perform valgus stress test).

Continued

FCL rupture, the mean lateral gap distance was 10.99 mm (confidence interval [CI], 7.8–14.3 mm) and for the combined PL rupture, the mean distance was 12.2 mm (CI, 9.3–15.2 mm). This amount of overlap indicates that it would not be possible to accurately separate an FCL rupture alone from a combined PL injury. The measurements are important and useful in providing the clinician with a baseline in interpreting lateral stress radiographs. The gap test measurement at arthroscopy described extensively in this book is based also on these types of approximations. The gap test is based on the joint separation

TABLE 22–1   Comprehensive Knee Examination—Cont'd

Examination	Technique	Illustration	Grading	Significance
External rotation recurvatum test	Grasp and hold both feet above table, allow gravity knee hyperextension.		Qualitative. Tibia externally rotates, varus position due to PL joint opening, knee.	Hyperextension, indicates PLC injury, >10° frequently associated ligament injury (ACL, PCL).
Standing recurvatum test	Patient stands, feet together pushes knees backward into hyperextension, compare knees.		Qualitative, observe varus hyperextension position (can be measured with goniometer). Increased loading over supine recurvatum test brings out deformity.	10° hyperextension with varus alignment PLC disruption, lateral, PL joint abnormal opening, often combined PLC, ACL tear, confirm with other tests.
Standing frontal alignment	Standing 0°–5° flexion. Avoid hyperextension.	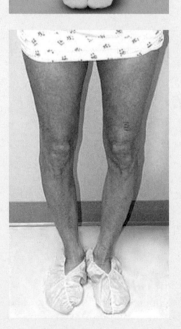	Confirm varus alignment. Hip-knee-ankle radiographs 0°–5° flexion.	Classify primary, double, triple varus based on all tests (see Chapter 31, Primary, Double, and Triple Varus Knee Syndrome: Diagnosis, Osteotomy Techniques, and Clinical Outcomes).

TABLE 22–1   Comprehensive Knee Examination—Cont'd

Examination	Technique	Illustration	Grading	Significance
Knee hyperextension gait or varus thrust	Observe gait walking to and from examiner.		Qualitative. Knee goes into hyperextension on stance phase. Knee has varus thrust without hyperextension.	Two hyperextension patterns (see Chapter 34, Correction of Hyperextension Gait Abnormalities: Preoperative and Postoperative Techniques). Forward trunk position, loss of quadriceps control, ankle dorsiflexion push-off, requires gait retraining. Varus thrust increases medial compartment loads and tensile forces lateral ligaments, osteotomy may be required.
Range of motion	Perform passive flexion-extension.		Normal 3°–0°–135° Hyperextension to neutral to flexion	10° hyperextension posterior capsule possible ACL or PCL injury. ≥15° multiple ligament injury.
Effusion, soft tissue swelling, pain	Palpate joint for effusion, tenderness, meniscus, ligament attachments.		Qualitative. Complex examination necessary + meniscus tests	Partial to complete tears PLC. FCL local tenderness, pain varus, dial tests.
Patellofemoral examination	Comprehensive examination. All tests. Alignment, PF crepitus, medial/lateral translation, patella height.		See Chapter 47, Articular Cartilage Rating Systems.	Increased external tibial rotation 30°, PLC tear, produces abnormal lateral shifting tibial tubercle, increases Q-angle.

Continued

TABLE 22–1   Comprehensive Knee Examination—Cont'd

Examination	Technique	Illustration	Grading	Significance
Neurovascular examination	Complete examination. Both lower extremities, PT, DP pulses, lower extremity muscle function.			Peroneal nerve injuries associated with severe PLC disruption (10%–30%). Arterial studies indicated multiple ligament injuries, dislocations.

ACL, anterior cruciate ligament; DP, dorsalis pedis; FCL, fibular collateral ligament; LJO, lateral joint opening; PCL, posterior cruciate ligament; PF, patellofemoral; PL, posterolateral; PLC, posterolateral capsule; PMTL, popliteus muscle-tendon-ligament; PT, posterior tibial.

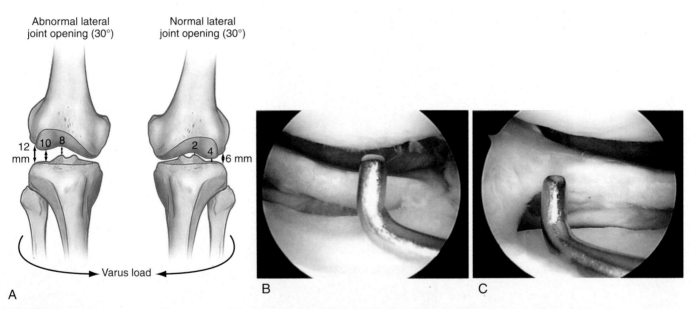

FIGURE 22–2. The gap test. **A,** The amount of lateral tibiofemoral joint opening is measured with the knee at 25° of flexion. Knees with insufficiency of the PL structures will demonstrate 12 mm of joint opening at the periphery of the lateral tibiofemoral compartment, 10 mm at the midportion of the compartment, and 8 mm at the innermost medial edge. **B,** Normal gap test. **C,** Abnormal gap test.

between articular cartilage seen at arthroscopy, and not the cortical separation on a stress radiograph. Even so, the measurements are somewhat equivalent as to the increase in the amount of millimeters with PL injuries. For example, Figure 22–2 shows an approximately normal lateral gap of 4 mm at the closest point of the lateral compartment at arthroscopy. An increase of only 6 mm results in 10 mm of absolute opening at the closest point, or 12 mm at the periphery, which is viewed as a positive gap test and indicative of injury to the PL structures. Fortunately, in most knees, these are the lesser values and it is more common that the lateral gap exceeds these measurements, indicating that concurrent PL reconstruction is necessary.

An increase in external tibial rotation may occur with anterior subluxation of the medial tibial plateau, posterior subluxation of the lateral tibial plateau, or a combination of both subluxations. The dial or spin rotation test, which the senior author developed, allows a diagnosis of tibial rotatory subluxations of the medial and lateral tibiofemoral compartments at 30° and 90° of knee flexion (see Table 22–1). Other variations of this test have been described.[6,44,55]

The position of the medial and lateral tibial plateau is assessed at the starting position (neutral tibial rotation) with the knee flexed to 30° and 90° and at the final position with the tibia in maximal external rotation. The examiner palpates the position of the medial and lateral tibial plateau, which is compared with the normal knee to assess whether a subluxation (anterior or posterior) of the medial or lateral tibial plateau is present. An increase in internal tibial rotation occurs with medial ligament and PCL disruption (see Chapter 20, Function of the Posterior Cruciate Ligament and Posterolateral Ligament Structures). The axis of tibial rotation is observed in the involved knee and compared with the normal knee to detect a shift in the medial or lateral tibiofemoral compartment during tibial rotation. It is not recommended that this test be performed in the prone position because the tibiofemoral joint cannot be accurately palpated to distinguish an anteromedial from a PL tibial subluxation.

It is not usually possible to determine the actual millimeters of translation of the medial and lateral tibial plateaus in reference to the femoral condyle. Thus, a qualitative determination of whether the reference tibial plateau is anteriorly or posteriorly subluxated from the lateral or medial femoral condyle is performed. The extent of lateral deviation of the tibial tubercle compared with the opposite knee with external tibial rotation may be increased.

The use of the dial test in knees with PCL ruptures requires maintenance of a normal anatomic tibiofemoral position. This is accomplished by applying a gentle anterior translation, loading the ACL in both limbs, during the external tibial rotation. It is still necessary to use the supine position so that the examiner can palpate the tibiofemoral position.[52] The dial test is less accurate with a PCL rupture, because it is difficult to compare limbs, and other tests to be described (LJO, gap test at arthroscopy, varus recurvatum) for the integrity of the PL structures need to be carefully assessed.

When a posterior subluxation of the lateral tibial plateau is positively identified by the tibiofemoral rotation test, additional tests must be conducted to determine the integrity of other ligament structures. The amount of LJO at 5° and 20° of knee flexion should be determined to further assess the integrity of the FCL and other secondary ligament restraints. The posterior tibial subluxation of the central tibial and medial tibiofemoral joint determines the amount of increased translation due to a PCL injury, which adds to the maximum posterior subluxation to the lateral compartment with external tibial rotation.

The presence of a varus recurvatum in both the supine and the standing positions must be carefully assessed. Often, the varus recurvatum reaches its maximum position when the patient is standing and asked to maximally hyperextend both knees.

The appropriate tests to determine the integrity of the ACL and PCL are performed, including KT-2000 arthrometer testing at 20° of flexion (134 N) to quantify total anteroposterior (AP) displacement. The pivot shift test is recorded on a scale of 0 to III (grade 0, no pivot shift; grade I, slip or glide; grade II, jerk or clunk; grade III, gross subluxation with impingement of the PL aspect of the tibial plateau against the femoral condyle). A misdiagnosis of a positive pivot shift test may occur with PL injuries as the lateral tibial plateau is brought to a reduced position (starting from a posterior subluxated position) with knee extension and then posteriorly subluxates with knee flexion (reverse pivot shift test). The medial posterior tibiofemoral step-off on the posterior drawer test is done at 90° of flexion.

Radiographs taken during the initial examination include AP, lateral at 30° of knee flexion, weight-bearing PA at 45° of knee flexion, and patellofemoral axial views. Lateral stress radiographs may be required of both knees (20° flexion, neutral tibial rotation, 67 N varus force). A comparison is made of the millimeters of lateral tibiofemoral compartment opening between knees.

A lateral radiograph is used to determine the approximate length required for FCL anatomic grafts. The distance from the anatomic femoral insertion site to the anatomic fibular insertion site is measured and adjusted for magnification. A measurement of the patellar tendon length is also made when a bone–patellar tendon–bone (B-PT-B) FCL autograft is planned.

Posterior stress radiographs are obtained in patients with PCL ruptures, especially those in which the distinction of a partial versus a complete PCL deficiency is difficult to determine on clinical examination.[14] A lateral PCL stress radiograph is taken of each knee at 90° of flexion. The limb is placed in neutral rotation with the tibia unconstrained and the quadriceps relaxed, and 89 N force applied to the proximal tibia. Measurement is made of the millimeters of posterior tibial translation in both knees. Knees with 10 mm or more of increased posterior tibial translation are considered candidates for PCL reconstruction.

Full standing radiographs of both lower extremities, from the femoral heads to the ankle joints, are done in knees with varus lower extremity alignment. The mechanical axis and weight-bearing line are measured to determine whether HTO is indicated.[10]

Patients complete questionnaires and are interviewed for the assessment of symptoms, functional limitations, sports and occupational activity levels, and their perception of the overall knee condition according to the Cincinnati Knee Rating System (CKRS; see Chapter 44, The Cincinnati Knee Rating System).[2]

CLASSIFICATION AND TREATMENT OF PARTIAL TO COMPLETE PL INJURIES

The classification and treatment of first-, second-, and third-degree acute PL injuries is detailed in Table 22–2. It is important to diagnose partial tears of the PL structures, with a mild to moderate increase in LJO and external tibial rotation, to allow protection and maintain lateral tibiofemoral joint closure in the initial 3 weeks to allow "stick-down" and healing of lateral soft tissues. This program is similar to that recommended for medial ligament ruptures (see Chapter 24, Medial and Posteromedial Ligament Injuries: Diagnosis, Operative Techniques, and Clinical Outcomes).

PREOPERATIVE PLANNING: TIMING OF SURGERY

Acute Injuries

There is a distinct advantage for repairing completely disrupted PL structures and meniscal attachments in acute injuries (Fig. 22-3). At the time of surgery, extensive disruption of these structures is observed. Careful dissection is required to identify anatomic tissue

TABLE 22–2   Diagnosis and Classification of Acute Posterolateral Injuries

	First Degree	Second Degree		Third Degree*		
Anatomic lesion	Minor tearing fibers	Partial tears, one third to two third fibers	1. FCL tear†		2. FCL tear Partial tear PMTL PL capsule	3. FCL tear, PMTL tear, PL capsule tear
Signs	Minor tenderness and swelling	Tenderness and swelling lateral tissues			Tenderness and swelling lateral tissues	
Increase in lateral joint opening‡						
30°	None	None	2–3 mm		2–5 mm	5–9 mm
0°	None	None	None		None	3–5 mm
Increase in external tibial rotation (dial test, 30°)‡	None	None	3°–5°		6°–10°	15°
Treatment	**Progress per symptoms, no crutches**	**Progress per symptoms, soft support brace**	**Bivalved cylinder cast 3 wk ROM 0°–90° 2nd wk Support brace 3–6 wk Wean crutches 3–6 wk**			**Operative repair, reconstruction Usually associated ACL, PCL**

*Avulsion FCL, popliteus tendon: surgical indication to reattach.

†Even though FCL shows complete tear, adjacent lateral tissues maintain ligament continuity for healing. Bivalved cylinder cast with protected motion, maintain lateral tibiofemoral joint closure.

‡See Chapter 20, Function of the Posterior Cruciate Ligament and Posterolateral Ligament Structures. Increases related to degrees of knee flexion, minor opening may be less under clinical conditions with lower joint loading.

ACL, anterior cruciate ligament; FCL, fibular collateral ligament; PCL, posterior cruciate ligament; PL, posterolateral; PMTL, popliteus muscle-tendon-ligament; ROM, range of motion.

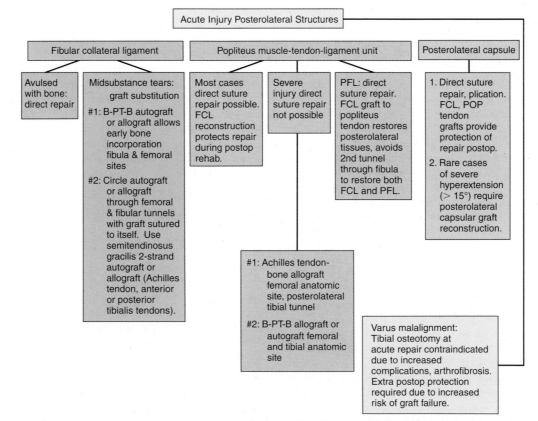

FIGURE 22–3. Algorithm for treatment of acute injuries to the PL structures. B-PT-B, bone–patellar tendon–bone; FCL, fibular collateral ligament; PFL, popliteofibular ligament; POP, popliteus.

planes and maintain an intact vascular and neural supply. The so-called golden period to perform an acute surgical repair is within 7 to 14 days of the injury. After this time, scar tissue will obliterate tissue planes and make the dissection and repair difficult.

A lower extremity venous ultrasound is obtained before surgery in acute multiligament knee injuries that have swelling and soft tissue damage to detect occult venous thrombosis that requires urgent treatment and contraindicates surgery. An initial

Acute Injuries

- Golden period acute surgical repair: 7–14 days after injury.
- Lower extremity venous ultrasound, vascular consult for multiple ligament ruptures.
- Delay surgery 5–7 days, observe neurovascular status, soft tissue swelling, skin integrity.
- Soft hinged full-leg brace, well-padded compression dressing.
- PCL rupture: bivalved cast with posterior plaster shell, posterior calf pad.
- Verify tibiofemoral reduction with lateral radiograph in multiligament injuries.
- MRI for location of major ligament disruptions.
- Protected knee motion, patellar mobilization, isometrics.
- Contraindications to acute surgery in dislocated knees: excessive soft tissue swelling, hemorrhage, edema. Delay reconstruction until swelling resolved, muscle function and knee motion restored.

Chronic Injuries

- Muscle atrophy requires preoperative rehabilitation.
- Hyperextension gait abnormality requires gait-retraining program before PL reconstruction.
- Varus osseous malalignment requires osteotomy before PL reconstruction.
- Absent lateral meniscus, early tibiofemoral arthritis, consider lateral meniscus transplant

Cruciate Reconstruction

- Ensure B-PT-B, Achilles tendon allografts available.
- Determine appropriate grafts for ACL or PCL reconstruction.

ACL, anterior cruciate ligament; B-PT-B, bone–patellar tendon–bone; MRI, magnetic resonance imaging; PCL, posterior cruciate ligament; PL, posterolateral.

delay in surgery for 5 to 7 days allows for observation of the neurovascular status, soft tissue swelling, skin integrity, and some clearing of hemorrhage in soft tissues in the injured extremity.

During this time, the lower extremity is supported in a soft hinged full-leg brace in extension with a well-padded compression dressing. In knees with extensive damage to the PL structures and PCL, a bivalved cylinder cast with a posterior plaster shell and posterior foam calf pad may be required to provide added stability and prevent posterior tibial subluxation. Reduction of the tibiofemoral joint is verified by a lateral radiograph. Lower limb elevation, ice, and compression are important. The physical therapist initiates early protected knee motion, patellar mobilization, active quadriceps function, and electrical muscle stimulation. Dislocated knees scheduled for surgery require vascular consultation, ankle/brachial studies (ankle/brachial index ≥ 90%), and possible arteriography to exclude arterial injuries, even when intact peripheral pulses are present.

Contraindications to acute surgical repair are excessive soft tissue swelling, hemorrhage, and edema that are frequently present in dislocated knees with multiple ligament ruptures. The operative procedure adds to the injury by increasing edema and soft tissue swelling, risk of infection, vascular problems (including compartment syndromes), and skin flap necrosis. In these cases, it is preferable to treat the acute injury and perform ligament reconstructive procedures later after tissue swelling is resolved and muscle function and knee motion have been restored.

In addition, there is a significant incidence of knee arthrofibrosis after acute surgical treatment of knee dislocations, which is lessened with a staged approach. In the authors' experience, only approximately one in four dislocated knees with associated PL ruptures are candidates for acute surgical procedures. A delay in surgical reconstruction results in a decreased incidence of knee arthrofibrosis and markedly improves surgical outcomes. Other obvious contraindications include open wounds and skin abrasions.

Magnetic resonance imaging (MRI) provides important information regarding ligament ruptures, articular cartilage damage, and meniscus tears. Frequently, the sites of rupture to the FCL, popliteus muscle and tendon, PFL, and meniscal attachments may be identified before surgery. One note of caution is that the tendency exists, owing to edema and swelling in the PL tissues, to misinterpret the MRI and conclude that there is greater tissue damage and disruption than is actually encountered at surgery.

Chronic Injuries

Patients with chronic knee injuries that present with severe muscle atrophy require several months of preoperative rehabilitation. Patients with a hyperextension gait abnormality must complete a gait-retraining program,[43] described in detail in Chapter 34, Correction of Hyperextension Gait Abnormalities: Preoperative and Postoperative Techniques. This program is done in addition to lower extremity muscle strengthening exercises. In the authors' experience, patients will convert to a more normal gait pattern after 4 to 6 weeks of training. More time is required for severe quadriceps atrophy before surgical intervention.

Varus osseous malalignment must be corrected before chronic PL reconstruction, as described previously. Failure to address this malalignment will greatly increase the risk of failure of any PL procedure (Fig. 22-4). In some cases in which the PL deficiency is due to interstitial stretching of the tissues and not a traumatic rupture, a simplified proximal advancement of the PL structures may be performed with the HTO. In anatomic PL reconstructions, the ligament surgery is staged after healing of the HTO. The indications for the various PL procedures are described in detail under the "Operative Treatment of Acute PL Ruptures" and "Operative Treatment of Chronic PL Ruptures" sections.

Patients who have undergone prior lateral meniscectomy and who demonstrate early tibiofemoral arthritis are considered for lateral meniscus transplantation.[41]

Cruciate Graft Reconstruction

The majority of patients who undergo PL reconstruction require a concomitant ACL or PCL reconstruction (Fig. 22-5). The appropriate grafts for the cruciate procedures should be determined; autogenous tissues with bony fixation are preferred. However, the surgeon should ensure that B-PT-B and Achilles tendon–bone (AT-B) allografts are available the day of surgery. These will be required if autogenous tissue is unavailable or not suitable for the PL or cruciate procedures.

INTRAOPERATIVE EVALUATION

All knee ligament tests are performed after the induction of anesthesia in both the injured and the contralateral limbs. The amount of increased anterior tibial translation, posterior tibial translation, LJO, and external tibial rotation is documented. A thorough

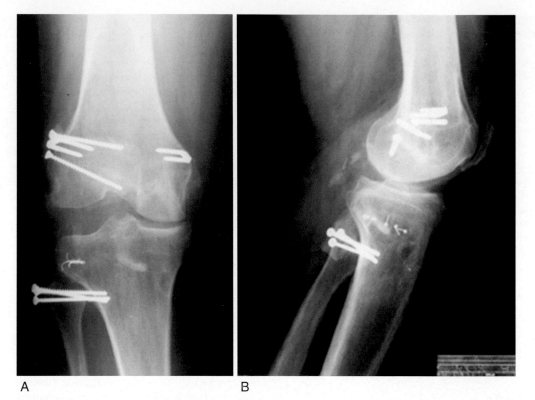

A   B

FIGURE 22–4. Standing anteroposterior (AP; **A**) and lateral (**B**) radiographs of a 28-year-old man referred to the authors' center 14 months after failure of an acute repair of the PL structures and posterior cruciate ligament (PCL) allograft reconstruction. The patient had underlying varus osseous malalignment, which likely was a factor in the failure of the ligament reconstructions. This malalignment requires correction before revision surgery. (**A** and **B**, *From Noyes, F. R.; Barber-Westin, S. D.: Posterior cruciate ligament revision reconstruction, part 1: causes of surgical failure in 52 consecutive operations. Am J Sports Med 33:646–654, 2005.*)

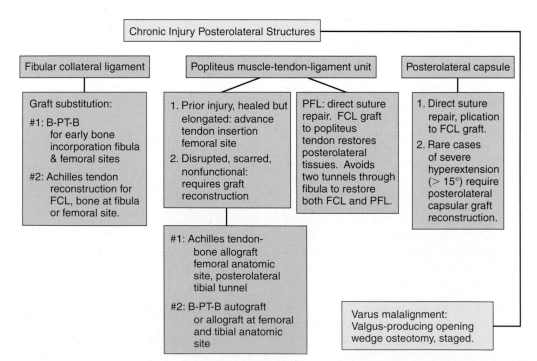

FIGURE 22–5. Algorithm for treatment of chronic injuries to the PL structures. B-PT-B, bone–patellar tendon–bone; FCL, fibular collateral ligament; PFL, popliteofibular ligament.

- Repeat all knee ligament tests under anesthesia, both limbs.
- Rate all articular cartilage surfaces for abnormalities, size of lesion
  - Normal.
  - Grade 1, softening.
  - Grade 2A, fissuring and fragmentation < 50% depth of the articular surface.
  - Grade 2B, fissuring and fragmentation > 50% depth of the articular surface.
  - Grade 3, subchondral bone exposed.
- Gap test at arthroscopy
  - Knee 30° flexion.
  - Varus load.
  - Measure millimeters lateral tibiofemoral opening with calibrated nerve hook.
- Surgical exposure inspection

  - FCL, fibular and femoral attachments.
  - PMTL, PLC, PFL.
  - Popliteus muscle, tendon attachments.
  - Meniscus attachments.

FCL, fibular collateral ligament; PFL, popliteofibular ligament; PLC, posterolateral capsule; PMTL, popliteus muscle-tendon-ligament.

arthroscopic examination is conducted, documenting articular cartilage surface abnormalities (see Chapter 47, Articular Cartilage Rating Systems) and the condition of the menisci.[46]

The gap test is done during the arthroscopic examination.[40] The knee is flexed to 30° and a varus load applied. A calibrated nerve hook is used to measure the amount of lateral tibiofemoral compartment opening (see Fig. 22–2). Knees that have 12 mm or more of joint opening at the periphery of the lateral tibiofemoral compartment require a PL reconstructive procedure.

In knees that undergo ACL reconstruction, the millimeters of joint opening at the intercondylar area at the site of the ACL graft is the critical distance in the gap test. Increases in LJO will occur postoperatively, allowing increases in ACL graft length. This space is normally 3 to 5 mm under varus loading.

After the surgical exposure (see "Operative Treatment of Acute PL Ruptures" and Operative Treatment of Chronic PL Ruptures"), the FCL and its fibular head and femoral attachment sites, the PMTL, PL capsule, and PFL are inspected. The distal popliteal tibia and fibula attachments of the popliteus tendon are identified and inspected to determine the appropriate surgical treatment. All of the lateral and PL structures, including meniscus attachments, are inspected in a stepwise manner. The peroneal nerve is identified and protected at all times.

OPERATIVE TREATMENT OF ACUTE PL RUPTURES

Operative Setup and Patient Positioning

The patient is instructed to use a soap scrub of the operative limb ("toes to groin") the evening before and the morning of surgery. Lower extremity hair is removed by clippers, not a shaver. Antibiotic infusion is begun 1 hour before surgery. A nonsteroidal anti-inflammatory drug (NSAID) is given to the patient with a sip of water upon arising the morning of surgery (which is continued until the 5th postoperative day unless there

- "Time out" before surgery: verify knee undergoing surgery, procedure, allergies, antibiotic infusion, special precautions.
- Complete examination of knee joint under anesthesia, compare with opposite knee.
- Acute dislocation or questionable vascular status: drape entire lower limb free to check anterior and posterior tibial pulses at the foot during procedure.
- Arthroscopic examination under low pressures with free or controlled open outflow to prevent fluid extravasation. Confirm damage to intra-articular structures, photograph injury.
- Place tourniquet at proximal thigh with appropriate padding. Inflate (275–300 mm Hg) during initial exploration, identify common peroneal nerve. Deflate for surgical repair, reconstruction

are specific contraindications to the medicine). The use of a NSAID and a postoperative firm double-cotton, double-Ace compression dressing for 72 hours (cotton, Ace, cotton, Ace layered dressing) has proved very effective in diminishing soft tissue swelling and is used in all knee surgery cases. In complex multiligament surgery, the antibiotic is repeated at 4 hours and continued for 24 hours. A urinary indwelling catheter is not used unless there are specific indications. The patients' urinary output and total fluids are carefully monitored during the procedure and in the recovery room. The knee skin area is initialed by both the patient and the surgeon before entering the operating room, with a nurse observing the procedure. The identification process is repeated with all operative personnel with a "time out" before surgery to verify the knee undergoing surgery, procedure, allergies, antibiotic infusion, and special precautions that apply. All personnel provide verbal agreement.

The patient is placed supine on the operative table and appropriately padded. The knee portion of the table is flexed 20°, and the table is tilted into a mild Trendelenburg position. A posterior thigh pad is placed behind the proximal thigh to suspend the knee joint at 20° to 30° of flexion. No pressure is exerted on the posterior popliteal space, allowing the posterior neurovascular tissues and popliteal tissues to drop posteriorly away from the operative approach. A common mistake is to place a posterior bolster in the popliteal space that pushes the posterior neurovascular structures into the operative dissection.

In cases of acute dislocation or any questionable vascular status, the entire lower limb is draped free to allow vascular checks of the anterior and posterior tibial pulses at the foot during the operative procedure.

An initial arthroscopic examination is performed under low-pressure conditions with a free or controlled open outflow to prevent fluid extravasation. The arthroscopic examination confirms damage to intra-articular structures and allows photographic documentation of the injury. Appropriate meniscus surgery is performed as required with the exception that lateral meniscus repairs are done after the open exposure. If a leg holder is used, it is removed for the open surgery.

The tourniquet is placed at the proximal portion of the thigh with appropriate padding. The tourniquet is inflated (275–300 mm Hg) during the initial exploration of the ligamentous injury and identification of the common peroneal nerve (CPN). The tourniquet is deflated for the remainder of the procedure. The surgeon may elect to be seated, directly facing the lateral aspect of the knee, with a headlight in place that allows for careful dissection of the lateral soft tissues including the CPN.

Identification of Ligament and Soft Tissue Rupture Pattern

A 10- to 12-cm skin incision is made in a straight line centered over the joint line and 1 cm posterior to the iliotibial band (ITB) attachment at the tibia (Fig. 22–6A). After careful mobilization of the skin flaps, the ITB, biceps tendon, and lateral structures are encountered.

Prior to dissection of the lateral aspect of the knee, the location of the CPN must be identified. If the CPN cannot be easily palpated and its course determined, then it is necessary at this point to expose and identify the nerve, which is discussed in the next section.

In the majority of knees, the ITB will be intact or demonstrate only partial tearing. In select cases, the ITB will be completely disrupted at the joint line or avulsed off its tibial attachment at Gerdy's tubercle. Posteriorly, there are capsular attachments of the ITB, including fascial attachments to the short head of the biceps femoris, which are identified for later repair if torn. If the ITB is intact, an incision is made along its posterior border to allow visualization of all of the underlying structures (see Fig. 22–6B).

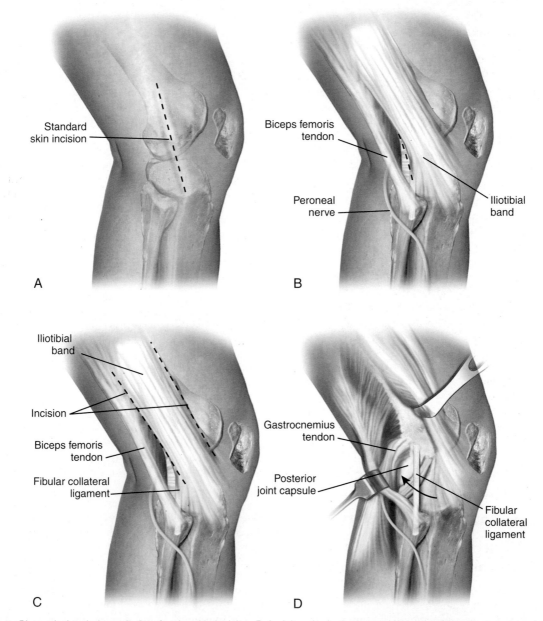

FIGURE 22–6. PL surgical technique. **A,** Site for the skin incision. **B,** Incision site in the interval between the posterior edge of the iliotibial band (ITB) and the anterior edge of the biceps tendon. **C,** In chronic cases with severe scarring, it may be necessary to add an anterior incision and displace the ITB posteriorly during the reconstructive procedure to allow better exposure. **D,** With the ITB retracted anteriorly, the interval between the lateral head of the gastrocnemius and the PL aspect of the capsule is opened bluntly, just proximal to the fibular head, without entering the joint capsule proximally.

The lateral capsular tissues and meniscal attachments are the next structures visualized. A vertical incision is made into the anterior third of the capsule and extended to the lateral meniscus just anterior to the popliteus tendon attachment. The popliteus tendon and meniscus attachments at the femoral popliteal recess are identified. Frequently, it is necessary to repair the superior and inferior meniscal fasciculi (Fig. 22–7) to restore meniscal attachments to the lateral meniscus. Careful varus stress is placed on the knee joint to allow inspection of the lateral meniscus attachments and tibiofemoral articular cartilage. On occasion, an additional anterior incision is required for visualization of underlying anatomy (see Fig. 22–6C).

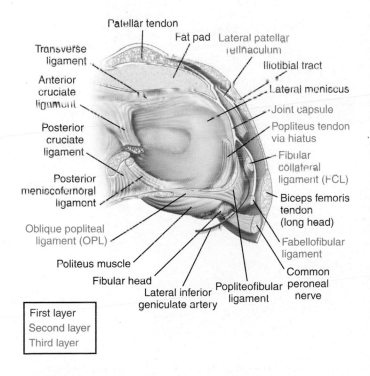

FIGURE 22–7. Illustration of the popliteus tendon and its surrounding popliteomeniscal fascicles and lateral meniscus attachments that are frequently disrupted, requiring repair.

Labels in figure:
Patellar tendon
Transverse ligament
Fat pad
Lateral patellar retinaculum
Anterior cruciate ligament
Iliotibial tract
Lateral meniscus
Joint capsule
Posterior cruciate ligament
Popliteus tendon via hiatus
Fibular collateral ligament (FCL)
Posterior meniscofemoral ligament
Biceps femoris tendon (long head)
Oblique popliteal ligament (OPL)
Fabellofibular ligament
Popliteus muscle
Fibular head
Lateral inferior geniculate artery
Popliteofibular ligament
Common peroneal nerve

First layer
Second layer
Third layer

The fibular head and attachments of the biceps femoris short and long head are the next structures visualized, which have been described in detail in Chapter 2, Lateral, Posterior, and Cruciate Knee Anatomy. The two tendinous components (direct and anterior arms) and one of the fascial components (lateral aponeurotic expansion) make up the key portion of the long head anatomy. The other fascial components are the reflected arm and the anterior aponeurotic expansion.

The most proximal component is the reflected arm. It originates just proximal to the fibular head and ascends anteriorly to insert on the posterior edge of the ITB. The direct arm inserts onto the PL edge of the fibula just distal to the tip of the styloid. A portion of the anterior arm inserts onto the lateral aspect of the fibular head, and the rest continues distally just lateral to the FCL. Portions of the anterior arm ascend anteriorly forming the lateral aponeurotic expansion that attach to the posterior and lateral aspects of the FCL. Here, a small bursa separates the anterior arm from the distal fourth of the FCL. The anterior arm thus forms the lateral wall of this bursa (see Fig. 2–12). This is an important surgical landmark, because a small horizontal incision can be made here, 1 cm proximal to the fibular head, to enter this bursa and locate the insertion of the FCL into the fibular head. The anterior arm then continues distally over the FCL, forming the anterior aponeurosis, which covers the anterior compartment of the leg. The primary areas of injury are tendon avulsions off of the fibula, which often have a major osseous component that can be repaired. In addition, the fascial extensions anteriorly and laterally are repaired.

The short head of the biceps courses just deep (or medial) and anterior to the long head tendon, sending a majority of its proximal muscular fibers to the long head tendon itself.[53] It has six distal attachments, described in detail in Chapter 2, Lateral, Posterior, and Cruciate Knee Anatomy. The most important attachments are that of the direct arm, the anterior arm, and the capsular arm.

The capsular arm originates just prior to the short head reaching the fibula and continues deep to the FCL to insert onto the PL knee capsule and fabella. Here the fibers of the capsular arm continue distally as the fabellofibular ligament. Just distal to the capsular arm, a capsulo-osseous layer forms a fascial confluence with the ITB (the biceps–capsulo-osseous iliotibial tract confluent). The direct arm of the short head inserts onto the fibular head just posterior and proximal to the direct arm of the long head tendon. The anterior arm then continues medial or deep to the FCL, partially blends with the anterior tibiofibular ligament, and inserts onto the tibia 1 cm posterior to Gerdy's tubercle. This site is also the attachment of the midthird lateral knee capsule. The lateral aponeurotic expansion of the short head inserts onto the medial aspect of the FCL. The FCL may be torn at its femoral attachment or within its substance or avulsed along with the biceps attachment at the fibula.

Proceeding posteriorly, the next structure encountered is the lateral gastrocnemius muscle tendinous attachment to the femur. The proximal third of the posterior capsule attaches to the proximal portion of the gastrocnemius muscle and fabellum (osseous or cartilagenous analog).

The interval between the posterior capsule and the gastrocnemius tendon is entered just above the fibula, similar to the exposure for a lateral meniscus repair. This exposes the popliteus muscle tibial attachments, popliteus muscle-tendon junction, PFL, popliteus tendon attachment at the femur, and fabellofibular ligament (extension of short head biceps attachments) (see Fig. 22–6D).

In dissection studies, LaPrade and coworkers[19] described a fabellum (osseous or cartilagenous) present in all specimens. This structure forms an attachment for the oblique popliteal ligament and fabellofibular ligament, which along with the posterior capsule, are important restraints for limiting knee hyperextension. Although individual capsular components and structures are difficult to discern with extensive capsular ruptures, it is important to repair disrupted posterior capsular tissues after completion of the initial dissection.

Peroneal Nerve Identification

It is important at the initial stages of the dissection to palpate and determine the location of the CPN. To expose the CPN, it is safest to begin in the proximal aspect of the operative exposure. A large retractor is used to elevate the muscular portion of the biceps femoris, placing the fascial tissues beneath the biceps muscle under gentle tension. This gentle upward displacement of the biceps muscle is key to visualize and dissect the CPN, because its normal curviform undulations are removed and it assumes a straighter appearance (Fig. 22–8A). The investing crural fascia is incised over the CPN to the fibula.

The CPN and its branches are not removed from their normal anatomic position to avoid damaging the delicate blood supply, particularly in the region where the CPN approaches and then passes around the fibular neck. Kadiyala and associates[16] reported measurements in cadaveric specimens of the blood supply to the CPN in the popliteal fossa and fibular neck region. These authors hypothesized that the susceptibility of the CPN to injury or lack of a response to operative treatment when injured may be related to deficiencies in intraneural and extraneural vascular supply and anastomoses.

The most common source of blood supply to the proximal portion of the CPN is a direct branch of the popliteal artery. This branch divides into proximal and distal anastomotic vessels that run in the connective tissue sheath of the nerve and anastomoses with the anterior recurrent tibial artery. The vessels, located in the epineurium, give rise to many small vessels of fine caliber, which extend 20 to 30 mm within the substance of CPN. It is important not to disturb this blood supply. Kadiyala and associates[16] noted that the blood supply of the CPN was somewhat sparse with poor vascularization. A connection of the vasa nervorum was not found from the geniculate arteries, but occasional contributions from muscular branches were recognized (Fig. 22–9).

Bottomley and colleagues[3] reviewed the anatomic position of the CPN in 54 patients who had damage to the PL structures. The CPN was noted to be displaced out of its normal position in 16 of 18 patients who had biceps avulsions or associated fibular head fractures. These authors advised that the surgeon should expect an abnormal nerve position on surgical exploration in knees with bone or soft tissue avulsion from the fibular head and the potential for iatrogenic damage.

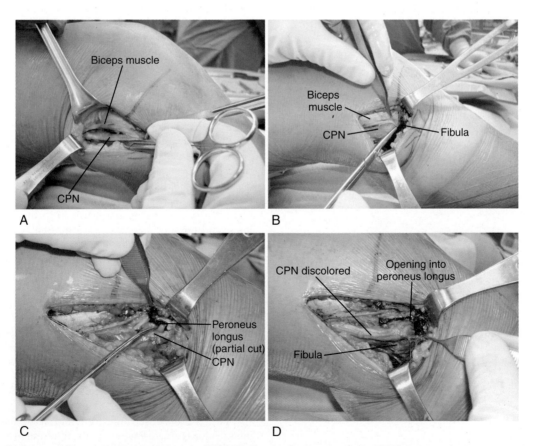

FIGURE 22–8. Exposure of the common peroneal nerve (CPN). **A,** Proximal exposure of the CPN inferior to the long head of the biceps tendon. **B,** The superficial fascia over the peroneus longus is incised. **C,** The peroneus longus muscle at the fibular neck is partially incised adjacent to the CPN. **D,** Complete exposure of the CPN entering into the anterolateral compartment. In this knee, the CPN is shown to be distinctly abnormal and edematous at this site. The CPN is not displaced from its normal anatomic site to protect the vascular supply.

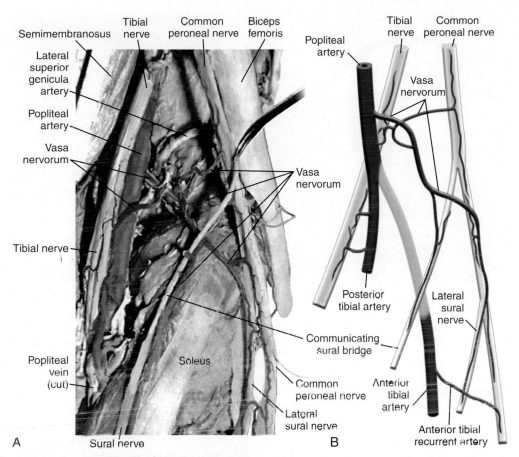

FIGURE 22–9. A, Gross dissection of the popliteal fossa of the right leg. The vessel branching from the popliteal artery gives rise to vasa nervorum to the tibial nerve and CPN and a branch that bifurcates into a vessel accompanying the sural nerve and the epineurial vessel running with the CPN. **B**, The major vascular arrangements supplying the CPN in the popliteal fossa. (**A** and **B**, Adapted from Kauliyala, H. K.; Ramirez, A.; Taylor, A. E.; et al.: The blood supply of the common peroneal nerve in the popliteal fossa. J Bone Joint Surg Br 87:337–342, 2005.)

Rubel and coworkers[49] conducted an anatomic investigation of the CPN in 31 cadaveric limbs by dissecting the CPN to its intramuscular branches. The authors described Gerdy's safe zone as the area where the CPN and anterior recurrent branch defined an arc with an average radius of 45 mm. The distance between the fibular head and Gerdy's tubercle was used to determine the radius of the safe zone. Therefore, this region in the proximal aspect of the tibia is advantageous for surgical exploration, because damage to the peroneal nerve and its branches is avoided (Fig. 22–10). The CPN divides into three branches as it enters the anterolateral musculature, with the anterior recurrent branch more proximal to the superficial and deep peroneal branches.

Dellon and associates[9] reported on the anatomic variations of the CPN at the fibular head in 29 cadavers (bilaterally) and 65 patients treated with a CPN decompression for symptoms. Three possible anatomic variants were described that require attention and decompression in chronic neuropathies for a successful outcome. First, the superficial fascia of the superficial head of the peroneus longus muscle is divided by a proximal and distal transection of the fascia (found in 30% of cadavers and 78% of patients; see Fig. 22–8B). Second, when the peroneus longus muscle at the fibular neck is partially incised adjacent and superior to the CPN and the peroneus muscle lifted anteriorly, a fibrous band may be found that requires release (soft tissue restriction found in 43% of cadavers and 20% of

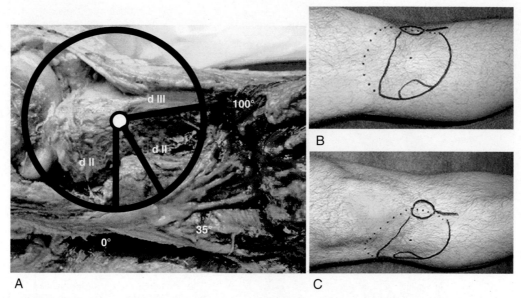

FIGURE 22-10. A, Cadaveric dissection of a fresh tissue specimen shows the circumferential area free of neural structures at the level of the proximal aspect of the tibia. The center of this circumference is located at Gerdy's tubercle with an average radius (and standard deviation) of 45.32 ± 2.6 mm. d II, distance from the most prominent aspect of Gerdy's tubercle to the starting point of the superficial branch of the CPN; d III, distance from the most prominent aspect of Gerdy's tubercle to the anterior recurrent branch of the nerve. **B,** Gerdy's safe zone marked preoperatively. Note how the marking follows the contour of the surface in a three-dimensional fashion on the lateral (**B**) and frontal (**C**) photographs. *(A–C, From Rubel, I. F.; Schwarzbard, I.; Leonard, A.; Cece, D.: Anatomic location of the peroneal nerve at the level of the proximal aspect of the tibia: Gerdy's safe zone. J Bone Joint Surg Am 86:1625–1628, 2004.)*

patients; see Fig. 22–8C). Third, there may be a fibrous connection between the peroneus longus and the soleus muscle requiring division (found in 9% of cadavers and 6% of patients). These authors advise that after CPN decompression, the surgeon's index finger should be able to gently pass along the CPN and into the anterolateral compartment (see Fig. 22–8D).

In cases of partial to complete peroneal nerve injury, it is important that added trauma to neural tissues be avoided. The goal is to identify the nerve pathway to avoid further damage during the ligament reconstructive procedure. The CPN passage into the lateral and anterolateral compartment at the entrance of the peroneal longus muscle at the fibular neck is a potential area for nerve compression. This area requires identification and division of variant fascial tissue bands, as previously described. Further CPN dissection is avoided.

Surgical Repair and Reconstruction of Acutely Disrupted Ligaments and Soft Tissues

The key to restore function to the disrupted PL structures, muscle attachments, and lateral meniscus attachments is a meticulous dissection, identification of damaged tissues, and repair of all injured structures. There does exist an unacceptably high risk of failure of primary repairs of disrupted PL structures, particularly the FCL, owing to high lateral tensile forces exerted on these tissues postoperatively.[50] Therefore, it is necessary to reconstruct one or more disrupted PL structures with an autograft or allograft, as is described. This adds tissue integrity and sufficient repair strength to resist LJO and external tibial rotation in the initial healing period of 4 to 6 postoperative weeks.

> **Critical Points** OPERATIVE TREATMENT OF ACUTE POSTEROLATERAL RUPTURES: SURGICAL REPAIR AND RECONSTRUCTION OF ACUTELY DISRUPTED LIGAMENT AND SOFT TISSUES
>
> - Unacceptably high risk of failure of primary repairs of disrupted PL structures owing to high lateral tensile forces postoperatively.
> - Less severe injuries: FCL reconstructed, other PL soft tissues and PMTL repaired.
> - Severe injuries: graft reconstruction FCL and PMTL may be necessary.
> - Surgical approach, order of repair
>   ○ Prefer B-PT-B autograft or allograft replacement of FCL.
>   ○ Graft provides secure bone fixation, prevents abnormal joint displacements, allows early protected knee motion.
>   ○ Graft provides the cornerstone for repair of other PL structures.
>   ○ Operative repair starts with deep structures and proceeds to superficial structures.
>
> B-PT-B, bone–patellar tendon–bone; FCL, fibular collateral ligament; PL, posterolateral; PMTL, popliteus muscle-tendon-ligament.

In less severe injuries, the FCL is reconstructed and the other PL soft tissues and PMTL are treated by primary repair. The FCL graft reconstruction resists lateral tibiofemoral compartment opening and PL subluxation, protecting the overall repair process during the initial healing stage. In more severe injuries, a graft reconstruction of both the FCL and the PMTL may be necessary. The reconstruction procedures are discussed in detail under "Operative Treatment of Chronic Ruptures," later in this chapter.

Surgical Approach and Order of Surgical Repair

The surgical approach favored is a graft reconstruction of the FCL with either a B-PT-B autograft or allograft or an AT-B allograft. The authors were the first to describe a femoral-fibular reconstruction,[37] which is a second option and is described later in this chapter. The FCL fibers (unless directly avulsed at their insertion) are too disrupted to perform a primary repair. The FCL reconstruction provides for secure fixation, prevents abnormal joint displacements in the immediate postoperative period, and allows for early protected knee motion. These procedures are not difficult because the attachment sites on the femur and fibula are easily identifiable. Importantly, the graft provides the cornerstone about which the remainder of the soft tissue repair of the PL structures is performed. A B-PT-B graft requires an appropriate length graft, which may not always be obtained. Alternative graft options are AT-B or quadriceps tendon- patellar bone (QT-PB). The bone portion of these grafts may be placed at either the FCL fibular attachment or the FCL femoral attachment, and the tendon may be placed within a tunnel at the other attachment site. If a soft tissue tendon graft is selected, the graft is passed through a fibular tunnel (anterior-to-posterior), the tendon is sutured back upon itself, and a soft tissue interference fibular screw may be added.

After all of the anatomic structures and rupture sites are identified and carefully exposed, the order of the operative repair starts with deeper structures and proceeds to superficial structures. Examples of an acute operative repair are shown in Figures 22–11 and 22–12.

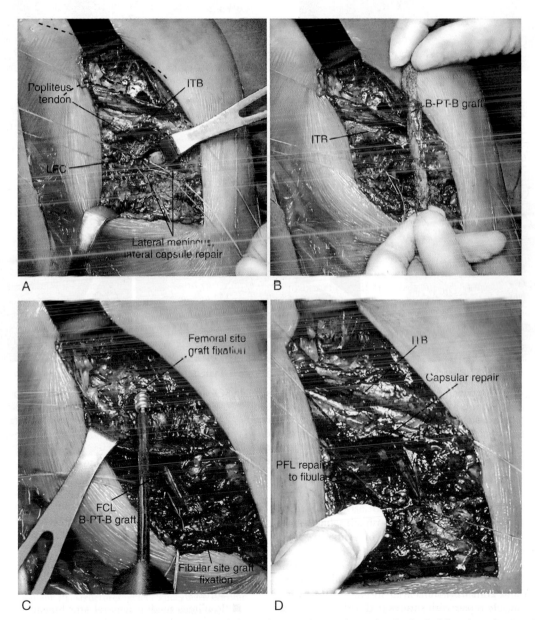

FIGURE 22–11. Acute repair of rupture to the PL structures. **A**, Lateral approach; anterior and posterior incisions have been made into the ITB. Sutures are placed to repair the lateral meniscus tibial attachments. **B**, FCL reconstruction with a B-PT-B allograft and suture of the PFL to the fibula. The popliteus tendon attachment at the femur was intact. **C**, Fixation of the FCL graft at the femoral and tibial anatomic attachments. **D**, Repair of PL capsule, biceps attachments, and posterior ITB.

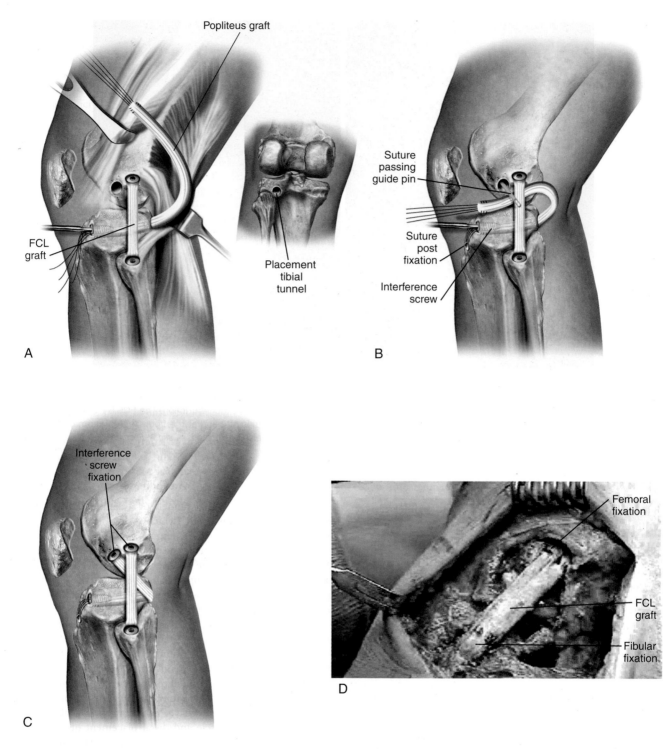

FIGURE 22–15. Anatomic popliteus muscle-tendon-ligament reconstruction and FCL reconstruction with B-PT-B autograft or allograft. **A,** Location of PL tibial tunnel and graft passage. A soft tissue interference screw and suture post are used for tibial fixation of the popliteus graft. **B,** Passage of popliteus graft beneath the FCL B-PT-B graft. **C–E,** Final fixation of the popliteus and FCL graft reconstructions.

(Continued)

knee flexion and extension, and fixation is performed with an absorbable interference screw in the tibial tunnel with the leg at 30° of knee flexion, neutral tibial rotation, and approximately 5 pounds (22 N) of tension placed on the graft. A backup suture

fixation post with a screw is used on the anterolateral aspect of the tibia.

A final assessment of the graft is done to determine that it is under adequate tension and is blocking abnormal external tibial

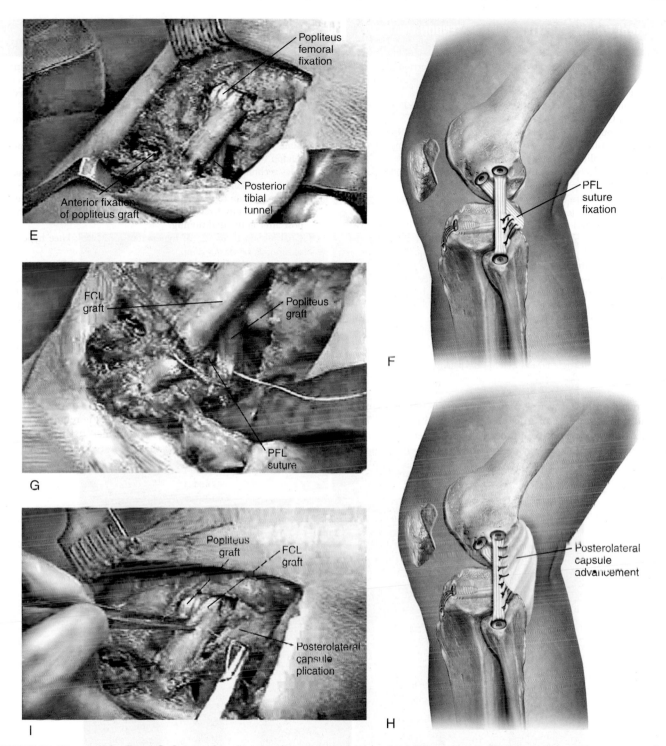

FIGURE 22–15—cont'd. F and **G**, Suture of popliteus graft to posterior margin of the FCL graft at the fibular attachment site to restore the PFL. **H** and **I**, Suture plication of the PL capsule to posterior margin of the FCL graft.

rotation and knee hyperextension. With graft reconstructions of both the FCL and the PMT, it is not necessary to add additional drill holes to the fibula to perform a graft reconstruction of the PMTL. Rather, a direct suture of the PMT graft to the FCL graft at the level of the fibular head is performed (see Fig. 22–15F and G). A plication procedure is performed of the PLC at 10° of flexion, avoiding overtension, which would limit normal extension (see Fig. 22–15H and I).

PLC Graft Reconstruction for Severe Varus Recurvatum and Hyperextension

In patients who demonstrate 15° or more of knee hyperextension, severe deficiency exists of the entire posterior capsule and oblique popliteal ligament in addition to possible cruciate, FCL, and PMTL damage (Fig. 22–16). In these severe knee injuries, a PMTL reconstruction alone will not block a severe

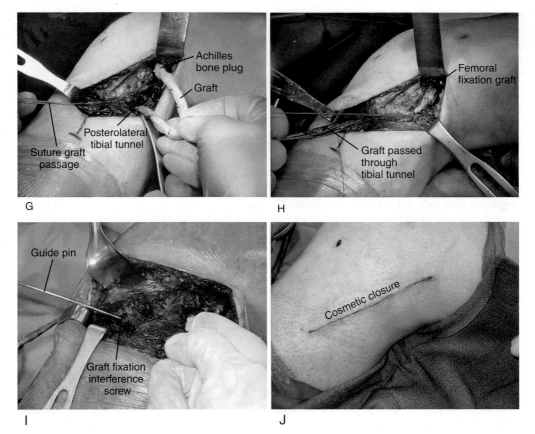

FIGURE 22–17—cont'd.   G, Placement of the Achilles tendon allograft with bone plug at femoral site. **H**, Fixation at the femoral site and graft conditioning with tension of distal graft. **I**, Graft fixation at the tibia with interference screw and suture post. **J**, Cosmetic closure.

FIGURE 22–18. AP (**A**) and lateral (**B**) radiographs show fixation of PL capsular reconstruction with two 4.0-mm cancellous screws at the femoral site and an absorbable interference tibial screw and suture post. At the femoral site, either a bone inlay or a tunnel may be selected.

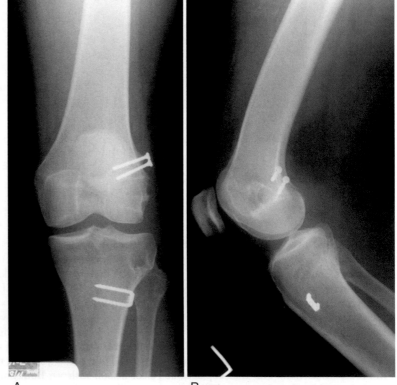

described and then fixed by sutures to a single tibial post. A soft tissue interference screw is used at the tibial tunnel after graft suture post fixation.

Femoral-Fibular Reconstruction

The nonanatomic femoral-fibular graft reconstruction is indicated when the FCL is deficient, as already described. This technique is contraindicated when a combined PMTL graft reconstruction is required. In these knees, an anatomic FCL and PMTL reconstruction is performed.

The femoral-fibular reconstruction provides a large graft reconstruction of the FCL and a posterior graft arm to augment the PL structures. The PLC reconstruction is performed by a plication procedure. The popliteus tendon is plicated to the fibular FCL reconstruction to restore the PFL. The procedure is termed a *nonanatomic reconstruction* because the femoral-fibular graft is placed adjacent but not directly at the FCL femoral and fibular anatomic attachment sites.

The FCL femoral-fibular reconstruction does have several advantages. The graft placement (by drilling a tunnel anterior and posterior to the FCL femoral and fibular attachment sites) is relatively simple and allows a large doubled graft to be placed at the lateral side of the knee joint. Direct suture of the graft to itself provides lateral stability in acute operative repairs to initiate immediate protected knee motion postoperatively.

Critical Points FEMORAL-FIBULAR RECONSTRUCTION

- Indicated when FCL is deficient, contraindicated when PMTL graft reconstruction required.
- Provides large graft reconstruction of FCL and posterior graft arm to augment PL structures. PL capsule plicated.
- FCL graft provides cornerstone for plication or repair of the other PL structures. In global knee ligament reconstructions, procedure provides lateral stability with less operative time and complexity than anatomic reconstruction of FCL, PMTL.
- Straight lateral incision, approximately 15 cm in length, centered over lateral joint line.
- Inferior incision along posterior aspect of ITB and attachments overlying the biceps muscle.
- CPN identified, protected.
- Proximal fibular head exposed anteriorly and posteriorly 12–15 mm by subperiosteal dissection.
- 6-mm drill hole anteriorly and posteriorly center of fibular head.
- 6-mm drill hole anterior-to-posterior beneath FCL femoral insertion.
- Curved curet used to make bone tunnel underneath FCL femoral insertion without removing excess bone.
- Autograft or allograft, 6–8 mm in diameter, prepared with sufficient length (19–20 cm) for proximal and distal posterior arms to overlap posteriorly.
- Graft inserted through bony tunnels in femur and fibula with stretched and slack FCL between graft arms.
- Interrupted sutures through anterior-posterior arms of graft.
- Popliteus tendon, PFL sutured to graft to restore PFL.
- PL capsule plication or advancement performed under sufficient tension to allow 0° of extension without hyperextension.
- Knee taken through 0°–90°, normal internal-external rotation determined at 30° flexion to avoid overconstraining joint.

CPN, common peroneal nerve; FCL, fibular collateral ligament; ITB, iliotibial band; PFL, popliteofibular ligament; PL, posterolateral; PMTL, popliteus muscle-tendon-ligament.

The double-strand FCL graft provides a cornerstone for plication or repair of the other disrupted PL structures. In global chronic knee ligament reconstructions when considerable operative time is necessary, the femoral-fibular reconstruction has less operative time and complexity than anatomic reconstruction of the FCL and PMTL.

A femoral-fibular reconstruction has disadvantages. In cadaver studies, a femoral-fibular graft was found not to unload a concurrent PCL graft reconstruction in the same manner as a combined FCL and PMTL graft reconstruction.[29] In addition, although a single femoral-fibular graft stabilizes the knee at time zero, this graft may stretch out in the long term when there is loss of the PMTL, which does not participate in load sharing. Therefore, all the load is transferred to the single graft. The goal of PL reconstruction is to restore the function of all the PL structures and not just the femoral-fibular component. A modification of a femoral-fibular technique is to cross the graft, placing the anterior femoral portion to the posterior fibula to restore PFL function. However, whether this option is superior to two parallel femoral-fibular graft arms is not known.

A straight lateral incision, approximately 12 cm in length, is used centered over the lateral joint line. The surgical approach already described is followed. The incision is extended distally to allow exposure of the fibular head and peroneal nerve and proximally to allow exposure of the attachment of the FCL to the femur. The skin flaps are mobilized beneath the subcutaneous tissue and fascia to protect the vascular and neural supply to the skin. The attachment of the ITB is identified.

An inferior incision is made along the posterior aspect of the ITB and the attachments overlying the biceps muscle. This allows the ITB to be reflected anteriorly so that the anatomy of the PL aspect of the knee is easily visualized. A second anterior ITB incision may also be required.

The CPN is carefully protected throughout the surgical procedure for the drill hole made through the proximal fibula for placement of the FCL graft. It is usually not necessary to dissect the peroneal nerve when its course can be identified.

The fibular head is exposed anteriorly and posteriorly by subperiosteal dissection. Only 12 to 15 mm of the proximal fibula is exposed. A 6-mm drill hole is carefully made anteriorly and posteriorly in the center of the fibular head; a drill guide is used to ensure that soft tissues are protected. A straight curet is used to dilate the 6-mm cortical hole from anterior to posterior, compressing the cancellous bone. Care is taken not to disturb the tibiofibular joint capsule, thereby preserving joint stability.

At the femoral attachment of the FCL, a 6-mm drill hole is made anterior-to-posterior to the FCL insertion. The drill hole is deepened, leaving approximately 8 to 10 mm of cortex between the anterior and the posterior tunnels. This step requires care to preserve the lateral femoral cortex at the FCL attachment site. A curved curet is used to make a bony tunnel underneath the ligament insertion without removing excess bone, which would weaken the insertion site.

A tendon allograft or autograft, 6 to 8 mm in diameter, is prepared. The graft is measured to allow sufficient length (19–20 cm) for the anterior and posterior arms of the circle graft to overlap posteriorly, which provides additional collagenous tissue to the PL aspect of the joint (Fig. 22–19A and B). Two interlocking closed loop (baseball) sutures of No. 2 nonabsorbable suture are placed into both ends of the graft. The graft is initially stretched for 15 minutes under an 89-N load with a ligament-tensioning device. A four-strand STG autograft or comparable allograft may be used.

(IKDC ratings, LJO and external tibial rotation) in all knees. Twelve patients had required a concomitant ACL reconstruction that were rated as normal or nearly normal in 8 and abnormal in 4.

Because of the increased failure rate, which was attributed to including patients with poor PL tissues and prior failed PL procedures, the authors now recommend anatomic PL reconstruction. A femoral-fibular procedure is used only in chronic knees in which the PMTL is functional and the goal is to augment a deficient FCL. This operation is also useful in acute PL disruptions to restore FCL function, along with a primary repair of the remaining PL tissues.

Proximal Advancement of PL Structures

A proximal advancement of the PL structures was done in conjunction with a cruciate ligament reconstruction in 23 consecutive patients.[38] One patient was lost to follow-up. A second patient had an early failure and required a revision PL reconstruction; this result was included in the study's overall failure rate.

Therefore, 21 patients made up the study group and were evaluated 2 to 6.1 years postoperatively. The ACL was also reconstructed in 9 knees, the PCL was reconstructed in 11 knees, and both cruciates were reconstructed in 1 knee.

At follow-up, 20 knees (91%) had normal or nearly normal LJO and external tibial rotation, and 2 (9%) failed. At least 0° to 135° of knee motion was found in 16 patients. Two patients had mild limitations (between 1° and 5°) in both extension and flexion, 1 patient had a mild limitation of extension only, and 2 patients had mild limitations in flexion only. No further operations were performed for losses of knee motion.

Before the operation, 8 patients had pain with daily activities, 8 had pain with any sports activity, and 5 could participate in light sports but had pain with moderate sports (running, twisting, turning activities). At follow-up, 2 patients had pain with daily activities, 9 patients had pain with any sports activity, and 10 were able to participate in low-impact sports without pain. Overall, 71% of patients showed improvement in the pain score or had no symptoms with light sports.

Before the operation, all patients either had given up sports activities or were participating with symptoms and functional limitations. At follow-up, 62% had returned to mostly low-impact activities without symptoms. The other patients did not return owing to their knee condition. At the time of the operation, 52% of the patients had abnormal articular cartilage lesions (grade 2A, 2B, or 3A > 15 mm, CKRS).

This study shows the advantage of this operation in properly selected patients who have interstitial stretching of the PL structures without prior traumatic disruption, allowing advancement to restore normal tension.

Causes of Failure of PL Operative Procedures

The potential causes of failure of 57 operative procedures (30 index and 27 revisions) to the PL structures of the knee were studied in a consecutive series of 30 knees that were referred to the authors' center.[39] The index PL procedures were done for an acute knee injury in 13 knees (mean, 3 wk; range, 1–11 wk after the injury) and for chronic deficiency in 17 knees a mean of 56 months (range, 4–312 mo) after the original injury.

The review of medical records in all cases was done by an independent surgeon not involved in the care of the patients. Upon the initial evaluation, a comprehensive knee examination and lateral stress radiographs were performed. KT-2000 testing was done in knees with ACL ruptures, and posterior stress radiographs were done in knees with PCL ruptures.

Overall, for all 57 failed PL operations, nonanatomic graft procedures had been done in 23 knees (77%; Table 22–3). The definition of an anatomic reconstruction was a graft placed in anatomic ligament attachment sites with secure internal fixation. Therefore, suture repairs, extra-articular ITB augmentations, and biceps tendon rerouting methods (Fig. 22–23) were not considered anatomic procedures.

Untreated varus malalignment was identified in 21 failed PL procedures (37%) or in 10 of 30 knees (Tables 22–4 and 22–5). Patients who presented with PL deficiency and varus osseous malalignment were diagnosed with triple varus knees. Associated ACL, PCL, or bicruciate deficiency was identified in 27 knees (93%). ACL deficiency was identified in 41 of the 57 (72%) failed PL procedures and associated PCL deficiency was noted in 15 of the 57 (26%) failed PL procedures.

Critical Points AUTHORS' CLINICAL STUDIES: PROXIMAL ADVANCEMENT POSTEROLATERAL STRUCTURES

- $N = 21$ followed 2–6.1 yr.
- ACL reconstructed in 8 knees, PCL reconstructed in 10 knees, ACL and PCL reconstructed in 4 knees.
- Evaluation: comprehensive knee examination, lateral stress x-ray, KT-2000, 20°, 134 N, IKDC, Cincinnati Knee Rating System.
- Results
  ○ 91% normal/nearly normal lateral tibiofemoral joint opening, external tibial rotation.
  ○ ACL normal/nearly normal in 92%.
  ○ 62% patients returned to low-impact sports without problems.

ACL, anterior cruciate ligament; IKDC, International Knee Documentation Committee; PCL, posterior cruciate ligament.

Critical Points AUTHORS' CLINICAL STUDIES: CAUSES OF FAILURE OF POSTEROLATERAL OPERATIVE PROCEDURES

- $N = 57$ failed PL procedures in 30 knees.
- Evaluation: review of medical records by an independent surgeon, comprehensive knee examination, lateral stress x-ray, KT-2000, 20°, 134 N, PCL stress x-ray, IKDC, Cincinnati Knee Rating System.
- Causes of PL failure
  ○ 93% associated cruciate deficiency (either untreated or failed reconstruction).
  ○ 77% nonanatomic PL procedures (suture repair, iliotibial band augmentations, biceps tendon rerouting).
  ○ 37% untreated varus osseous malalignment (triple varus knee).
- Conclusions
  ○ Emphasis during index operation on anatomic PL reconstruction, concurrent reconstruction all torn cruciate ligaments.
  ○ If varus osseous malalignment exists, correct with osteotomy before PL reconstruction.

IKDC, International Knee Documentation Committee; PL, posterolateral.

TABLE 22–3   Factors Contributing to Failure of 57 Posterolateral Procedures

	Acute Subgroup		Chronic Subgroup	
Factor	Index PL Procedure* Knees (*N*)	Revision PL Procedures† (*N*)	Index PL Procedure‡ Knees (*N*)	Revision PL Procedures§ (*N*)
Untreated varus malalignment	4	3	6	8
Nonanatomic graft reconstruction	10	4	7	14
Inadequate internal fixation	0	2	1	3
Infection	4	1	0	0
Primary repair chronically deficient tissues	0	0	8	1
Traumatic reinjury	1	0	1	0
Unknown	0	1	0	1
ACL rupture‖	6	2	9	14
PCL rupture‖	2	1	3	0
ACL and PCL ruptures‖	4	0	3	2

*5 of 13 knees had more than one factor identified.
†3 knees had more than one factor identified.
‡7 of 17 knees had more than one factor identified.
§8 knees had more than one factor identified.
‖Either not treated or not adequately surgically restored, procedure failed.
ACL, anterior cruciate ligament; PCL, posterior cruciate ligament; PL, posterolateral.

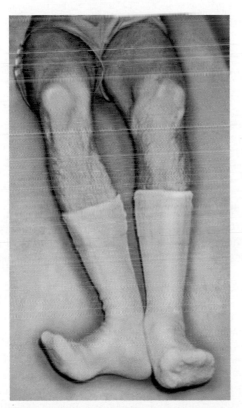

FIGURE 22–23. A patient with a failed biceps femoris tenodesis for PL instability was unable to actively rotate the left tibia externally. This procedure is not recommended.

PL deficiency subjects ACL and PCL grafts to excessive tensile loading owing to the abnormal lateral tibiofemoral joint opening that occurs with activity. Several in vitro studies reported significantly increased forces on ACL and PCL grafts in knees with sectioned PL structures (see Chapter 20, Function of the Posterior Cruciate Ligament and Posterolateral Structures), providing further evidence of the deleterious effects of FCL and PMTL insufficiency after ACL or PCL reconstruction.

Limitations of this study were similar to those of other investigations in which the potential causes of ligament reconstruction failure were defined. It is difficult to determine in a retrospective manner the exact causes of failure. Several theoretical factors exist that cannot always be detected or measured. These include failure of grafts to fully remodel or heal, poor tissue quality due to extensive disruption to the popliteus and FCL, limited healing potential of soft tissues due to repeated operations and diminished blood supply, osteopenic bone preventing appropriate fixation, and gait hyperextension abnormalities that may have occurred postoperatively without the knowledge of the investigators.

In addition, because the study period extended over 2 decades, the evolution of the diagnosis and management of PL injuries and associated abnormalities has altered the treatment of these problems. Some of the procedures in this series represent operations that are no longer routinely performed. Even so, the results of this study suggest greater emphasis during the index operation for anatomic graft reconstruction of one or more of the PL structures as necessary, restoration of all ruptured cruciate ligaments, and correction of varus malalignment. The authors have long advocated anatomic PL reconstruction over suture repair in patients who sustain acute high-energy injuries and extensive disruption of the PL structures. Usually, at least one component of the PL structures requires graft reconstruction, which is the FCL in nearly all cases.

OTHER OPERATIVE TECHNIQUES AND RESULTS

Several authors have reported clinical outcome data from PL reconstructive procedures (Table 22–6).[4,5,7,13,15,26,50,56] Stannard and colleagues[50] followed 57 patients who received either a primary repair of acutely ruptured PL structures or a graft reconstruction of chronically deficient FCL, PFL, and popliteus

TABLE 22–4 Analysis of Treatment of Associated Cruciate Ligament Ruptures and Varus Malalignment in 21 Failed Posterolateral Procedures in Knees Treated for Acute Injuries

Failed PL Procedure	Number Cruciates Ruptured	Cruciate Ligaments			Varus Malalignment	
		Ruptured or Deficient, Not Treated	Reconstructed with PL Procedure, Subsequently Failed	Reconstructed with PL Procedure, Functional	Not Treated	HTO
Index ($N = 13$)	18*	5	11	2	4	0
First revision ($N = 6$)	7†	3	0	4	2	1
Second revision ($N = 2$)	2	0	0	2	1	0
Total	27	8	11	8	7	1

*Bicruciate ruptures in 5 patients coded for treatment of ACL and PCL separately.
†Bicruciate ruptures in 1 patient coded for treatment of ACL and PCL separately.
ACL, anterior cruciate ligament; HTO, high tibial osteotomy; PCL, posterior cruciate ligament; PL, posterolateral.

TABLE 22–5 Analysis of Treatment of Associated Cruciate Ligament Ruptures and Varus Malalignment in 36 Failed Posterolateral Procedures in Knees Treated for Chronic Injuries

Failed PL Procedure	Number Cruciates Ruptured	Cruciate Ligaments			Varus Malalignment	
		Ruptured or Deficient, Not Treated	Reconstructed with PL Procedure, Subsequently Failed	Reconstructed with PL Procedure, Functional	Not Treated	HTO
Index ($N = 17$)	20*	3	15	2	6	0
First revision ($N = 10$)	12†	5	4	3	3	1
Second revision ($N = 6$)	5	4	1	0	2	0
Third revision ($N = 2$)	2	1	1	0	0	2
Fourth revision ($N = 1$)	1	1	0	0	1	0
Total	40	14	21	5	12	3

*Bicruciate ruptures in 3 patients coded for treatment of ACL and PCL separately.
†Bicruciate ruptures in 2 patients coded for treatment of ACL and PCL separately.
ACL, anterior cruciate ligament; HTO, high tibial osteotomy; PCL, posterior cruciate ligament; PL, posterolateral.

tendon structures. At an average of 33 months postoperatively, 37% of the primary repair procedures had failed, compared with 9% of the graft reconstructions. The authors concluded that primary repair of the FCL is indicated only for bony avulsions that are amenable to internal fixation. Otherwise, graft reconstruction of the FCL is recommended, especially if an immediate knee motion program is to be used postoperatively.

Harner and coworkers[13] and Chhabra and associates[5] illustrated an FCL–Achilles tendon allograft reconstructive procedure and a PFL reconstruction. The FCL reconstruction was performed in 7 patients with knee dislocations, 2 of which failed to restore normal LJO. Buzzi and colleagues[4] described an FCL reconstruction using a semitendinosus tendon autograft. In a group of 13 patients studied, all had normal or nearly normal restoration of LJO and external tibial rotation postoperatively.

Cooper and Stewart[7] presented two operative options for PL ruptures. One consisted of a combined FCL and PFL reconstruction (with a semitendinosus tendon autograft) with capsular imbrication. The second option consisted of reconstruction of the PFL only in knees with an intact FCL. In a group of 19 patients with combined PCL and PL ruptures, no patient had greater than 10° of external rotation or more than 1+ increase in LJO postoperatively.

Latimer and coworkers[26] described an anatomic FCL replacement using a B-PT-B allograft. In a cohort of 10 patients,

all but 1 had restoration of normal or nearly normal LJO and external tibial rotation an average of 28 months postoperatively.

LaPrade and coworkers[21] described an anatomic PL reconstruction (Fig. 22–24A and B). Biomechanical testing of this technique demonstrated restoration of normal knee motion limits to external tibial rotation and LJO. Clinical results of this technique are pending. The operation restores the anatomic attachment sites for the FCL and popliteus tendon, which as discussed in this chapter, allows load sharing between these two structures, which appears to have a distinct advantage over a single femoral-fibular graft reconstruction. The PL technique described by Larson and Belfie[25] that uses a semitendinosus autograft is shown in Figure 22–24C. The operative procedure is designed to restore FCL function, as in acute operative cases. However, it does not restore the PMTL unit, which may be required in chronic PL reconstructions. A technique demonstrated in Figure 22–24D avoids creating two femoral tunnels that may potentially weaken the lateral femoral condyle. This procedure is considered advantageous in knees that have prior tunnels as in ACL revision surgery and the surgeon wishes to avoid an additional tunnel and, instead, use a single bone inlay technique for femoral graft fixation. An alternative technique using a single graft to replace the FCL and popliteus tendon described by Kim and associates[17] is illustrated in Figure 22–24E.

TABLE 22-6 Clinical Outcome Data of Posterolateral Reconstructions

Reference	Number, Acute or Chronic, Follow-up	Posterolateral Operative Procedure	Other Ligament Procedures	Objective Rating Criteria	External Tibial Rotation Results*	Lateral Joint Opening Results*	Other Ligaments Results
Jung, 2008[15a]	N = 39, chronic Mean 35.3 mo (range, 24–70 mo)	Group 1: PL transtibial tunnel with either STG or Achilles tendon allograft Group 2: fibular tunnel method with either STG or Achilles tendon allograft	FCL single-strand STG autograft in all	Posterior stress x-ray 90° KT-1000 manual maximum 70°	30° & 90° flexion: Group 1: <5° 63% "lax" 37% Group 2: <5°: 85% "lax" 15%	Group 1: 0 mm: 84% <5 mm: 11% 5–10 mm: 5% Group 2: 0 mm: 95% <5 mm: 5%	PCL stress x-ray: Group 1: 2.1 ± 1.1 Group 2: 2.2 ± 0.9
Zhao et al., 2006[56]	N = 28, chronic Range, 2–4 yr	Biceps tendon slip used to reconstruct FCL, PFL, PMT	PCL STG autograft: N = 18 ACL ST autograft: N = 3 ACL & PCL: STG autograft: N = 6 ACL & PCL & PMC STG autograft: N = 1	External rotation device (Magnetic Angle Finder)	30° flexion: 0°: 25 <3°: 3	Varus rotation: 0° flexion: All patients 0° 30° flexion: 0°: 25 <5°: 2 7°: 1	Not given. Overall IKDC ratings: A: 19 B: 11 C: 3
Stannard et al., 2005[50]	N = 57, acute and chronic combined Mean 33 mo (range, 24–59 mo)	Primary repair PL N = 35 Allograft (tibialis anterior or tibialis posterior) reconstruction of FCL, PFL, popliteus N = 22	ACL & PCL N = 35 ACL N = 14 PCL N = 4 Type of grafts NA	KT-2000 30°, 70° Total AP	Repair group: <5°: 21 5°–10°: 2 10°–15°: 5 >15°: 7 Reconstruction group: <5°: 19 5°–10°: 1 >15°: 2	Repair group: 0 mm: 19 5 mm: 4 10 mm: 5 >10 mm: 7 Reconstruction group: 0 mm: 14 5 mm: 6 10 mm: 1 >10 mm: 1	Not given for ACL, PCL Failure rates for PL: 37% repair 9% reconstruction
Harner et al., 2004[13]	N = 31, acute and chronic combined Mean 44 mo (range, 2–6 yr)	AT allograft and repair of avulsed FCL N = 7 Direct repair FCL N = 1	PCL AT allograft N = 8 ACL B-PT-B allograft N = 20 MCL primary repair N = 13 MCL ratomic ST autograft or AT allograft N = 1	KT-2000 90° corrected	Not given	0–2 mm: 20 3–5 mm: 9 6–10 mm: 2 (both FCL reconstructions)	ACL 0–2 mm: 13 3–5 mm: 16 PCL 0–2 mm: 0 3–5 mm: 20 6–10 mm: 8 MCL 0–2 mm: 5 3–5 mm: 4 6–10 mm: 2
Buzzi et al., 2004[4]	N = 13, all chronic Mean 60 mo (range, 38–93 mo)	ST autograft FCL PFL not injured, no procedure required	PCL CT autograft, single bundle, tibial inlay N = 7 ACL B-PT-B autograft N = 6	Stress x-rays for FCL (5°) and PCL (70°)	ACL group: 30° <5°: 4 5°: 2 PCL group: 30° <5°: 4 5°: 2 10°: 1	ACL group: 5° 0–2 mm: 5 4 mm: 1 PCL group: 5° 0–2 mm: 6 4 mm: 1 Functional: 77% Partial: 23%	ACL <3 mm: 5 3–5 mm: 1 PCL <3 mm: 2 3–5 mm: 5

Continued

Reference	Number, Acute or Chronic, Follow-up	Posterolateral Operative Procedure	Other Ligament Procedures	Objective Rating Criteria	External Tibial Rotation Results*	Lateral Joint Opening Results*	Other Ligaments Results
Fanelli & Edson, 2004[10a]	N = 41, all chronic Range, 24–120 mo	Split biceps tendon transfer & PL capsular plication	PCL AT allograft, single bundle, tibial tunnel	Stress x-rays for PCL (90°)	30° & 90° flexion: Tighter 29 (71%) Equal 11 (27%) Greater 1 (2%)	Normal in 98% 1 failure (2%)	**PCL:** Mean stress F/U 2.26 mm (−1−+7) 1 patient grade II PD
Kim et al., 2003[17]	N = 46, acute and chronic combined Mean 40 mo, 2 yr minimum	PL isolated N = 21 PL + PCL modified Clancy (isometric placement biceps tendon) N = 25	PCL B-PT-B autograft or allograft, single bundle, tibial tunnel	Stress x-ray 30°	33% overconstrained immediately postoperative 8 (17%) failed	Mean 2–4 mm	**PCL:** grade 0 or 1: 22 grade 2: 3
Wang et al., 2002[55a]	N = 25, all chronic Mean 40 mo (range, 32–60 mo)	Popliteofemoral ligament reconstruction ITB and popliteofibular ligament reconstruction with biceps tendon N = 10 FCL advancement N = 8 PT reconstruction + FCL advancement N = 7	PCL allograft or autograft, single bundle, tibial tunnel		Mean only given 3.4 ± 5.5°	0 mm: 11 (44%) 5 mm: 10 (40%) 10 mm: 4 (16%)	**PCL:** 0 mm: 11 (44%) 5 mm: 9 (36%) 10 mm: 5 (20%)
Fanelli et al., 2002[10b]	N = 35 acute and chronic combined Range, 24–120 mo	ACL/PCL/PL: N = 19 ACL/PCL/MCL: N = 9 ACL/PCL/PL/MCL: N = 6 ACL/PCL: N = 1 Split biceps tendon transfer + PL capsular shift N = 25	PCL: allografts & autografts, single bundle, tibial tunnel ACL: allografts & autografts MCL: AT allograft & STG autograft (N = 7)	Stress x-rays for PCL KT-1000	Less than normal knee: 76% Equal to normal knee: 24%	Equal to normal knee: 88% Grade 1: 12%	**ACL** 94% normal Lachman **PCL** 0–3 mm: 52% 4–5 mm: 24% 6–10 mm: 19% **MCL** 0 mm: 100%
Latimer et al., 1998[26]	N = 10, all chronic Mean 28 mo (range, 24–38 mo)	FCL B-PT-B allograft	ACL B-PT-B allograft, autograft N = 6 PCL AT allograft, single bundle, tibial tunnel N = 5	KT-1000	30° flexion (−) 5°: 1 0°: 8 5°: 1 90° flexion 0°: 9 5°: 1	0 mm: 6 5 mm: 4	**ACL** 0 mm: 4 5 mm: 2 **PCL** 0 mm: 0 5 mm: 5

*All data involved knee – noninvolved knee.

ACL, anterior cruciate ligament; AP, anteroposterior; AT, Achilles tendon; B-PT-B, bone-patellar tendon-bone; FCL, fibular collateral ligament; F/U, follow-up; IKDC, International Knee Documentations Committee; ITB, iliotibial band; MCL, medial collateral ligament; NA, not available; PCL, posterior cruciate ligament; PD, posterior drawer; PFL, popliteofibular ligament; PL, posterolateral; PMT, popliteus muscle tendon; QT, quadriceps tendon; ST, semitendinosus; STG, semitendinosus gracilis.

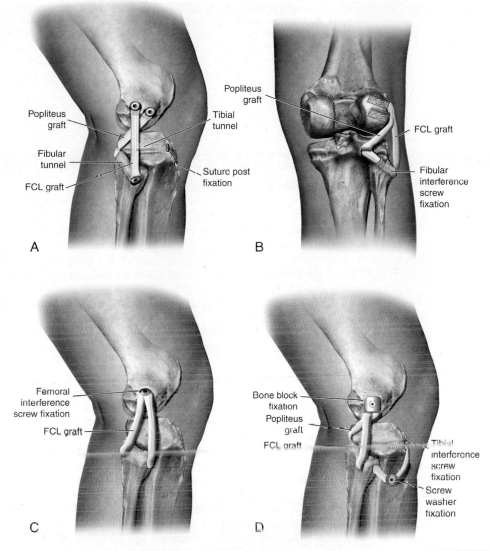

Popliteus graft

Tibial tunnel

Popliteus graft

Fibular tunnel

Suture post fixation

FCL graft

A

FCL graft

Fibular interference screw fixation

B

Femoral interference screw fixation

FCL graft

C

Bone block fixation

Popliteus graft

FCL graft

Tibial interference screw fixation

Screw washer fixation

D

Front view

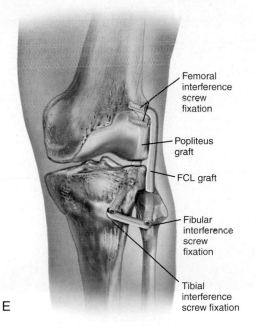

Femoral interference screw fixation

Popliteus graft

FCL graft

Fibular interference screw fixation

Tibial interference screw fixation

E

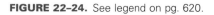

FIGURE 22–24. See legend on pg. 620.

graft (see Fig. 22–26C). At the latest follow-up evaluation, 53 months postoperative, there was no increase in LJO or external tibial rotation and the pivot shift test was negative. The patient had returned to work and light recreational sports without problems.

Authors' comment: This case demonstrates the increased failure rate when a PL reconstruction is performed in a varus-angulated knee. The vertical ACL graft was placed on the femoral notch roof outside of the normal ACL femoral attachment.

Case 3 Treatment of Prior Multiple Failed PL Procedure in a Dislocated Knee.

A 21-year-old man was referred 2 years after a knee dislocation sustained during football. He had undergone three failed PL operative procedures, including a biceps tendon reconstruction, an FCL allograft reconstruction, and a popliteal tendon allograft reconstruction. The deficient ACL had not been surgically treated. The MCL was repaired during the first operative procedure.

Physical examination revealed a grade III pivot shift, 8 mm of increased AP displacement on KT-2000 testing, 12 mm of increased LJO, and 20° of increased external tibial rotation. Stress radiographs demonstrated a severe increase in LJO (Fig. 22–27A). The patient also had 5 mm of increased medial joint opening and 5 mm of increased posterior tibial translation. He complained of pain and giving-way with daily activities and rated the overall condition of his knee as poor.

The patient underwent an anatomic FCL B-PT-B autograft reconstruction (harvested from the contralateral knee) and a proximal advancement of the PL structures and popliteus tendon. An ACL QT-PB autograft was placed at the anatomic tibial and femoral attachment sites (see Fig. 22–27B). Fissuring and fragmentation (grade 2A damage) were noted in all three compartments.

At the most recent follow-up examination, 13.7 years postoperatively, the patient had no increase in LJO or external tibial rotation and 3 mm of increased AP displacement on KT-2000 testing. He was participating in low-impact activities without symptoms.

Authors' comment: In revision PL cases, it is necessary to address all PL structures as described. In this knee, after failure of three prior PL procedures, a contralateral B-PT-B autograft provided stability. The contralateral patellar tendon autograft is reserved for revision of these types of severe cases of instability.

Case 4.

A 50-year-old male physician presented 5 months after a right knee dislocation sustained while attempting a side tackle playing soccer. The injury had been treated conservatively and the patient was experiencing increasing symptoms with daily and work activities. Physical examination revealed a lower limb varus malalignment with a mechanical axis of 5° varus, a grade III pivot shift, 12 mm of increased LJO, and 10 mm of increased posterior tibial translation. The patient desired surgical reconstruction to return to his active lifestyle, which included skiing and mountain climbing.

An opening wedge HTO was performed, followed 5 months later with a multiligament reconstruction that included an ACL B-PT-B allograft, a two-strand PCL QT-PB autograft, an FCL B-PT-B allograft, and a primary repair of the popliteus tendon. The lateral meniscus was repaired. The patient had noteworthy articular cartilage damage (grade 2B) on the patella undersurface and in the medial tibiofemoral compartment.

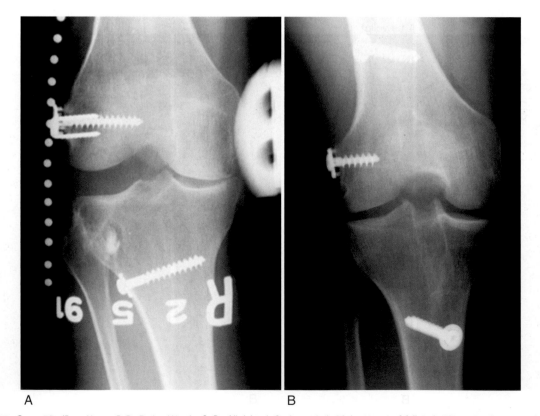

A   B

FIGURE 22–27. Case #3. *(From Noyes, F. R.; Barber-Westin, S. D.; Albright, J. C.: An analysis of the causes of failure in 57 consecutive posterolateral operative procedures. Am J Sports Med 34:1419–1430, 2006.)*

At follow-up, 4 years postoperative, the patient had a full range of knee motion, no effusion, a grade 0 pivot shift, an increase of 5 mm of AP displacement on KT-2000 testing (at 20° of knee flexion), 2 mm of increase in posterior tibial translation on posterior stress radiographs (Fig. 22–28A and B), and no increase in lateral tibiofemoral opening on lateral stress radiographs (see Fig. 22–28C and D). He had successfully returned to skiing and mountain climbing without symptoms, had run a marathon, and rated the overall condition of his knee as very good.

Case 5. A 15-year-old male presented 2 weeks after a contact injury to his right knee sustained while playing football. Physical examination revealed a moderate effusion, knee motion from 0° to 110°, moderate lateral joint line tenderness, a grade II pivot shift, 12 mm of increased LJO, and 5 mm of increased posterior tibial displacement. MRI demonstrated a complete rupture of the FCL, popliteal tendon, and ACL and a partial disruption of the PCL.

After an initial week of rehabilitation and protected knee motion, the patient underwent an ACL B-PT-B autograft (harvested from the contralateral knee), an FCL B-PT-B autograft, a direct repair of the PMTL and PLC, and a lateral meniscus repair.

At follow-up, 4 years postoperative, the patient had a normal range of knee motion, an increase of 3 mm in AP displacement

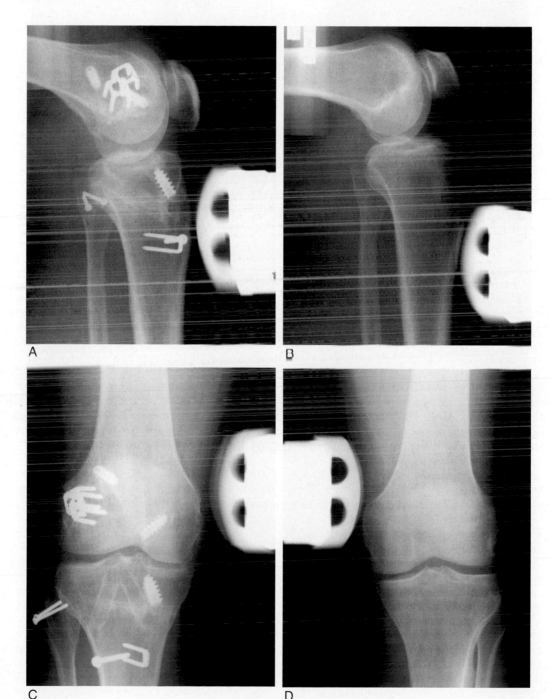

A   B

C   D

FIGURE 22–28. Case #4.

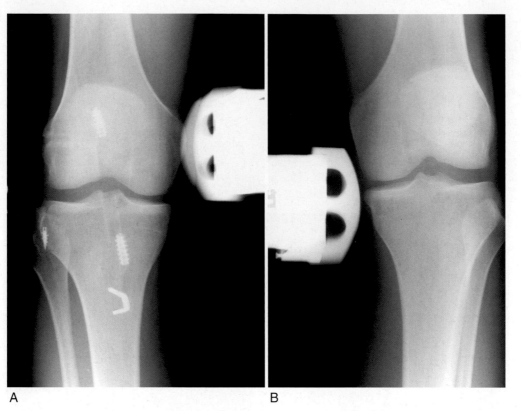

FIGURE 22–29. Case #5.

on KT-2000 testing, no increase in LJO on stress radiographs (Fig. 22–29A and B), and a grade 0 pivot shift. He had returned to basketball, baseball, and football without symptoms or limitations and rated the overall condition of his knee as normal.

Case 6. A 35-year-old man presented 2 years after bilateral knee injuries sustained during a motor vehicle accident. The right knee was initially treated with an ACL B-PT-B autograft reconstruction, an MCL repair, and a medial meniscus repair. The left knee was initially treated with a primary repair of the ACL and FCL. A second surgery involved a left ACL STG autograft and an FCL B-PT-B autograft reconstruction. A third surgery involved a left HTO and biceps tendon transfer. The patient presented with left knee symptoms of moderate pain, swelling, and lateral giving-way with daily activities and was unable to work.

Physical examination of the left knee demonstrated no effusion, a normal range of motion, a grade II pivot shift, 25 mm of increased LJO, and 10° of increased external tibial rotation. The patient's left lower limb was in valgus malalignment with a weight-bearing line of 74%; however, he drifted into varus in the unloaded position secondary to the lateral instability. The biceps femoris muscle was nonfunctional.

The patient was treated first with a biceps femoris muscle reconstruction and neurolysis of the peroneal nerve. At this operation, arthroscopy showed grade 2A articular cartilage lesions noted on the undersurface of the patella, trochlea, and medial femoral condyle. Five months later, he underwent an ACL B-PT-B allograft, an anatomic FCL B-PT-B autograft, proximal advancement of the PLC, and distal advancement of the ITB.

At follow-up, 12 years postoperative, the patient had a normal range of knee motion, no effusion, 4 mm of increased AP displacement on KT-2000 testing, 2 mm of increase in LJO on stress radiographs on the involved left knee (Fig. 22–30A) compared with the right knee (see Fig. 22–30B), and a grade 0 pivot shift. Weight-bearing PA radiographs showed preservation of tibiofemoral joint space in both compartments compared with the contralateral limb (see Fig. 22–30C). He had no symptoms with low-impact athletic activities or with his occupation and rated the overall condition of his knee as good.

Case 7. A 15-year-old female presented 1 year after an injury sustained to her right knee while jumping over a fence. The patient had undergone a bovine ACL reconstruction elsewhere, followed by a lateral ITB extra-articular procedure, both of which had failed. She complained of constant symptoms with daily activities. Physical examination demonstrated a grade III pivot shift, 10 mm of increased LJO, and 15° of increased external tibial rotation.

The patient underwent a multiligament reconstruction consisting of an ACL B-PT-B allograft, a femoral-fibular FCL Achilles tendon allograft, a proximal advancement of the PLC, and a repair of a complex medial meniscus tear. She did well, but sustained a reinjury 16 years later that required a medial meniscus repair. At the most recent follow-up, 19 years postoperative, the patient had a normal range of knee motion, no tibiofemoral compartment pain, an increase of 3 mm of AP displacement on KT-2000 testing, a grade I pivot shift, and 2 mm of increase in LJO on stress radiographs (Fig. 22–31A) compared with the contralateral

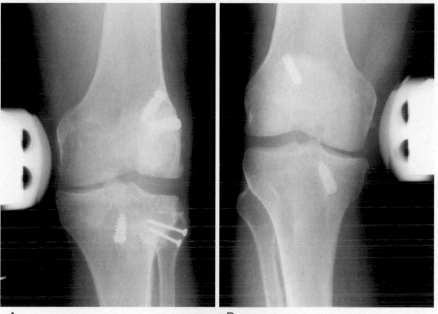

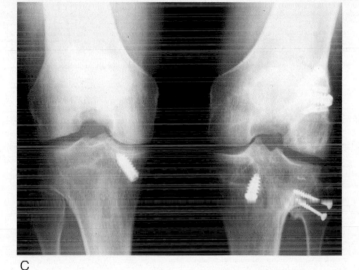

FIGURE 22–30. Case #6.

limb (see Fig. 22–31B). She had no symptoms with low-impact athletic activities and rated the overall condition of her knee as good.

Authors' comment: This surgical procedure with a 19-year follow-up was done at a time when the femoral-fibular technique was used for PL reconstruction. An anatomic technique as described in this chapter has proved in the authors' experience to have a higher success rate even though the femoral-fibular was successful in this patient.

Case 8. A 15-year-old male presented 5 weeks after a contact injury to his right knee sustained during football. He had undergone an arthroscopy and partial lateral meniscectomy elsewhere. The patient had moderate pain with daily activities and had not been able to return to sports activities. Physical examination revealed a slight effusion, normal range of knee motion, 13 mm

of increased AP displacement on KT-2000 testing, a grade III pivot shift, 10 mm of increased LJO, 10 mm of increased medial joint opening, and 15° of increased external tibial rotation.

The patient underwent 6 weeks of physical therapy and was then treated with an ACL B-PT-B allograft reconstruction, a primary repair of the MCL, and a femoral-fibular FCL Achilles tendon reconstruction. The patellar undersurface had bone exposed and there was also marked articular cartilage deterioration (grade 2B) on the medial femoral condyle.

At follow-up, 18 years postoperative, the patient had a normal range of knee motion, no tibiofemoral compartment pain, 4 mm of increased AP displacement on KT-2000 testing, no increase in medial joint opening, and no increase in LJO on stress radiographs on the right knee (Fig. 22–32A) compared with the left knee (see Fig. 22–32B). He had returned to basketball and construction work without limitations and rated the overall condition of his knee as normal.

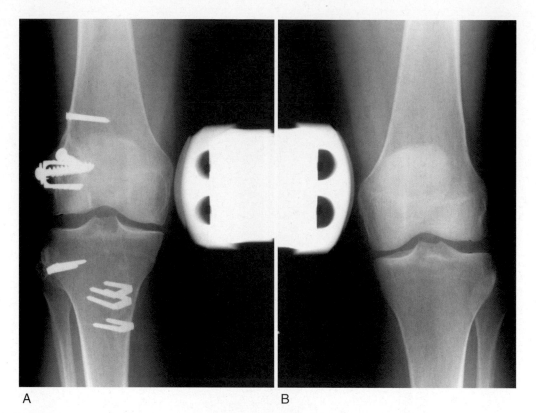

A   B

FIGURE 22–31. Case #7.

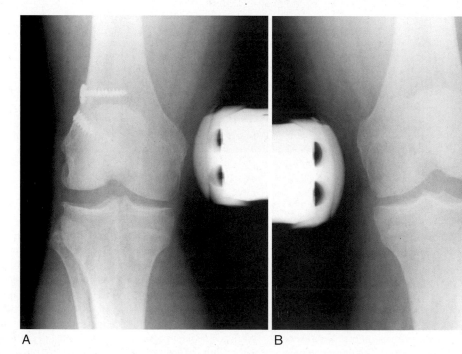

A   B

FIGURE 22–32. Case #8.

Authors' comment: This case demonstrates an unexpected good functional outcome despite articular cartilage damage at the index procedure. This patient was part of a prospective study initiated 18 years previously on ACL allografts. An autograft approach discussed in Chapter 7, Anterior Cruciate Ligament Primary and Revision Reconstruction: Diagnosis, Operative Techniques, and Clinical Outcomes, has proved to have a higher success rate, and as a result, ACL allografts are used only under select situations.

Case 9. A 19-year-old male presented 3 months after a left knee hyperextension injury sustained during long jumping. He had been treated elsewhere with a primary repair of the biceps tendon, PLC and FCL, followed by 6 weeks of casting. The patient was unable to bear weight during his initial consultation. Physical examination demonstrated a moderate effusion, a range of knee motion of 20° to 90°, marked quadriceps atrophy, a grade III pivot shift, 10 mm of increase in LJO, 5 mm of increase in medial joint opening, and 10° increase in external tibial rotation.

The patient underwent intensive physical therapy to regain joint motion and muscle function for 1 year, and then was treated with a ligament reconstruction owing to advancing symptoms of pain and giving-way. The procedure consisted of an ACL B-PT-B allograft, advancement of the MCL, advancement of the posterior medial capsule, femoral-fibular FCL Achilles tendon reconstruction, and advancement of the PL structures. The menisci and articular cartilage surfaces were normal.

At follow-up, 16 years postoperative, the patient had no effusion, a normal range of knee motion, 1 mm of increase in AP displacement on KT-2000 testing, a grade 1 pivot shift, 5 mm of increase in LJO on stress radiographs on the left knee (Fig. 22–33A) compared with the right knee (see Fig. 22–33B), and no increase in medial joint opening. He had no symptoms or limitations with basketball, running, and his occupation as a chef and rated the overall condition of his knee as very good.

Authors' comment: As already discussed, femoral-fibular reconstructions have a reasonable success rate, although the authors prefer anatomic procedures owing to the increased success rate.

Case 10. A 15-year-old male presented 3 weeks after a knee dislocation sustained during football. The patient was placed into an immobilizer but had not undergone any further medical treatment for his injury. Physical examination revealed moderate swelling, only 20° of knee motion, a loss of sensation over the lateral aspect of the leg as well as the dorsum of the foot, and a complete foot drop with 0 to 5 dorsiflexion and 0 to 5 extension of the great toe. His vascular status was intact. MRI revealed a torn ACL, PCL, FLC, and PL structures. He underwent 2 months of supervised physical therapy. A staged global reconstruction was then performed involving first an ACL B-PT-B allograft and arthroscopic PCL two-strand B-PT-B allograft reconstruction. One week later, an FCL B-PT-B allograft reconstruction and a PFL and popliteus tendon reconstruction were done (Fig. 22–34A and B).

Three years postoperative, the patient had a negative pivot shift, no increase in anterior tibial translation, no increase in external tibial rotation, and no increase in medial or LJO. He had a neurovascularly intact lower extremity and a full range of knee motion. Lateral (see Fig. 22–34C) and posterior (see Fig. 22–34D) stress radiographs showed no increase in LJO or posterior tibial translation. The patient had returned to recreational basketball and running without symptoms. He rated the overall condition of his knee as normal.

Authors' comment: This patient had an arthroscopic ACL and PCL reconstruction, at which time the decision was made, owing to operative time, to later stage by 1 week the anatomic PL reconstruction. During that week, it is required that no abnormal LJO occurs that would place the ACL and PCL grafts at risk for stretching or failure.

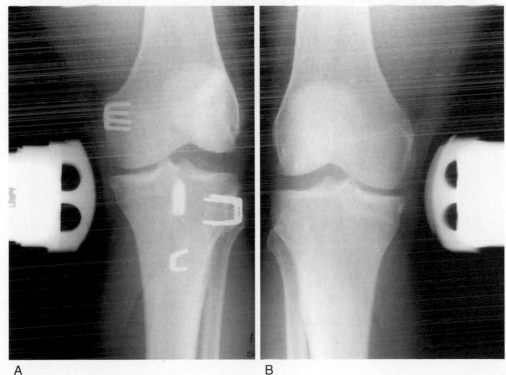

A   B

FIGURE 22–33. Case #9.

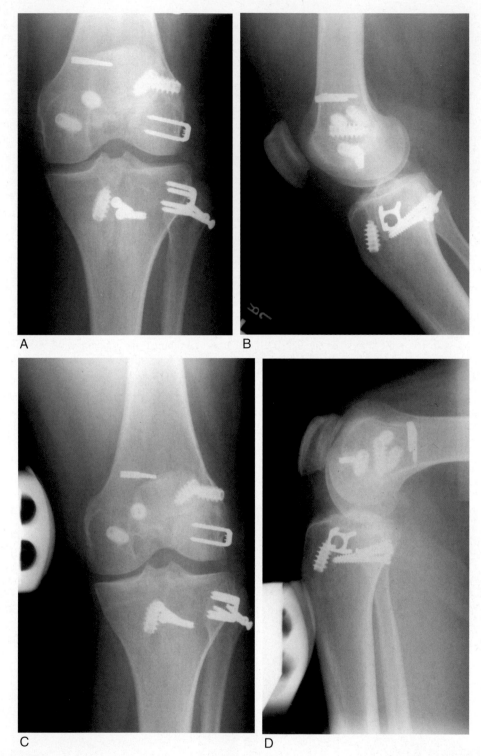

FIGURE 22–34. Case #10.

REFERENCES

1. Baker, C. L., Jr.; Norwood, L. A.; Hughston, J. C.: Acute posterolateral rotatory instability of the knee. *J Bone Joint Surg Am* 65:614–618, 1983.
2. Barber-Westin, S. D.; Noyes, F. R.; McCloskey, J. W.: Rigorous statistical reliability, validity, and responsiveness testing of the Cincinnati Knee Rating System in 350 subjects with uninjured, injured, or anterior cruciate ligament reconstructed knees. *Am J Sports Med* 27:402–416, 1999.
3. Bottomley, N.; Williams, A.; Birch, R.; et al.: Displacement of the common peroneal nerve in posterolateral corner injuries of the knee. *J Bone Joint Surg Br* 87:1225–1226, 2005.
4. Buzzi, R.; Aglietti, P.; Vena, L. M.; Giron, F.: Lateral collateral ligament reconstruction using a semitendinosus graft. *Knee Surg Sports Traumatol Arthrosc* 12:36–42, 2004.
5. Chhabra, A.; Cha, P. S.; Rihn, J. A.; et al.: Surgical management of knee dislocations. Surgical technique. *J Bone Joint Surg Am* 87 (suppl 1 pt 1):1–21, 2005.
6. Cooper, D. E.: Tests for posterolateral instability of the knee in normal subjects. Results of examination under anesthesia. *J Bone Joint Surg Am* 73:30–36, 1991.
7. Cooper, D. E.; Stewart, D.: Posterior cruciate ligament reconstruction using single-bundle patella tendon graft with tibial inlay fixation: 2- to 10-year follow-up. *Am J Sports Med* 32:346–360, 2004.
8. DeLee, J. C.; Riley, M. B.; Rockwood, C. A., Jr.: Acute posterolateral rotatory instability of the knee. *Am J Sports Med* 11:199–207, 1983.
9. Dellon, A. L.; Ebmer, J.; Swier, P.: Anatomic variations related to decompression of the common peroneal nerve at the fibular head. *Ann Plast Surg* 48:30–34, 2002.
10. Dugdale, T. W.; Noyes, F. R.; Styer, D.: Preoperative planning for high tibial osteotomy: the effect of lateral tibiofemoral separation and tibiofemoral length. *Clin Orthop Relat Res* 274:248–264, 1992.
10a. Fanelli, G. C.; Edson, C. J.: Arthroscopically assisted combined anterior and posterior cruciate ligament reconstruction in the multiple ligament injured knee: 2- to 10-year follow-up. *Arthroscopy* 18:703–714, 2002.
10b. Fanelli, G. C.; Edson, C. J.: Combined posterior cruciate ligament-posterolateral reconstructions with Achilles tendon allograft and biceps femoris tendon tenodesis: 2- to 10-year follow-up. *Arthroscopy* 20:339–345, 2004.
11. Gollehon, D. L.; Torzilli, P. A.; Warren, R. F.: The role of the posterolateral and cruciate ligaments in the stability of the human knee. A biomechanical study. *J Bone Joint Surg Am* 69:233–242, 1987.
12. Grood, E. S.; Noyes, F. R.; Butler, D. L.; Suntay, W. J.: Ligamentous and capsular restraints preventing straight medial and lateral laxity in intact human cadaver knees. *J Bone Joint Surg Am* 63:1257–1269, 1981.
13. Harner, C. D.; Waltrip, R. L.; Bennett, C. H.; et al.: Surgical management of knee dislocations. *J Bone Joint Surg Am* 86:262–273, 2004.
14. Hewett, T. E.; Noyes, F. R.; Lee, M. D.: Diagnosis of complete and partial posterior cruciate ligament ruptures. Stress radiography compared with KT-1000 arthrometer and posterior drawer testing. *Am J Sports Med* 25:648–655, 1997.
15. Jung, Y. B.; Tae, S. K.; Jung, H. J.; Lee, K. H.: Replacement of the torn posterior cruciate ligament with a mid-third patellar tendon graft with use of a modified tibial inlay method. *J Bone Joint Surg Am* 86:1878–1883, 2004.
15a. Jung, Y. B.; Jung, H. J.; Kim, S. J.; et al.: Posterolateral corner reconstruction for posterolateral rotatory instability combined with posterior cruciate ligament injuries: comparison between fibular tunnel and tibial tunnel techniques. *Knee Surg Sports Traumatol Arthrosc* 16:239–248, 2008.
16. Kadiyala, R. K.; Ramirez, A.; Taylor, A. E.; et al.: The blood supply of the common peroneal nerve in the popliteal fossa. *J Bone Joint Surg Br* 87:337–342, 2005.
17. Kim, S. J.; Park, I. S.; Cheon, Y. M.; Ryu, S. W.: New technique for chronic posterolateral instability of the knee: posterolateral reconstruction using the tibialis posterior tendon allograft. *Arthroscopy* 20(suppl 2):195–200, 2004.
18. LaPrade, R. F.: Anatomic reconstruction of the posterolateral aspect of the knee. *J Knee Surg* 18:167–171, 2005.
19. LaPrade, R. F. (ed): Posterolateral Knee Injuries. Anatomy, Evaluation, and Treatment. New York: Thieme, 2006; p. 238.
20. LaPrade, R. F.; Heikes, C.; Bakker, A. J.; Jakobsen, R. B.: The reproducibility and repeatability of varus stress radiographs in the assessment of isolated fibular collateral ligament and grade-III posterolateral knee injuries. An in vitro biomechanical study. *J Bone Joint Surg Am* 90:2069–2076, 2008.
21. LaPrade, R. F.; Johansen, S.; Wentorf, F. A.; et al.: An analysis of an anatomical posterolateral knee reconstruction: an in vitro biomechanical study and development of a surgical technique. *Am J Sports Med* 32:1405–1414, 2004.
22. LaPrade, R. F.; Ly, T. V.; Wentorf, F. A.; Engebretsen, L.: The posterolateral attachments of the knee: a qualitative and quantitative morphologic analysis of the fibular collateral ligament, popliteus tendon, popliteofibular ligament, and lateral gastrocnemius tendon. *Am J Sports Med* 31:854–860, 2003.
23. LaPrade, R. F.; Terry, G. C.: Injuries to the posterolateral aspect of the knee. Association of anatomic injury patterns with clinical instability. *Am J Sports Med* 25:433–438, 1997.
24. LaPrade, R. F.; Wentorf, F. A.; Fritts, H.; et al.: A prospective magnetic resonance imaging study of the incidence of posterolateral and multiple ligament injuries in acute knee injuries presenting with a hemarthrosis. *Arthroscopy* 23:1341–1347, 2007.
25. Larson, R. V.; Belfie, D. J.: Lateral collateral ligament reconstruction utilizing semitendinosus tendon. *Tech Knee Surg* 2:190–199, 2003.
26. Latimer, H. A.; Tibone, J. E.; ElAttrache, N. S.; McMahon, P. J.: Reconstruction of the lateral collateral ligament of the knee with patellar tendon allograft. Report of a new technique in combined ligament injuries. *Am J Sports Med* 26:656–662, 1998.
27. Malinin, T. I.; Levitt, R. L.; Bashore, C.; et al.: A study of retrieved allografts used to replace anterior cruciate ligaments. *Arthroscopy* 18:163–170, 2002.
28. Markolf, K. L.; Graves, B. R.; Sigward, S. M.; et al.: Effects of posterolateral reconstructions on external tibial rotation and forces in a posterior cruciate ligament graft. *J Bone Joint Surg Am* 89:2351–2358, 2007.
29. Markolf, K. L.; Graves, B. R.; Sigward, S. M.; et al.: How well do anatomical reconstructions of the posterolateral corner restore varus stability to the posterior cruciate ligament-reconstructed knee? *Am J Sports Med* 35:1117–1122, 2007.
30. Markolf, K. L.; Graves, B. R.; Sigward, S. M.; et al.: Popliteus bypass and popliteofibular ligament reconstructions reduce posterior tibial translations and forces in a posterior cruciate ligament graft. *Arthroscopy* 23:482–487, 2007.
31. Nielsen, S.; Ovesen, J.; Rasmussen, O.: The posterior cruciate ligament and rotatory knee instability. An experimental study. *Arch Orthop Trauma Surg* 104:53–56, 1985.
32. Nielsen, S.; Rasmussen, O.; Ovesen, J.; Andersen, K.: Rotatory instability of cadaver knees after transection of collateral ligaments and capsule. *Arch Orthop Trauma Surg* 103:165–169, 1984.
33. Noyes, F. R.; Barber, S. D.; Simon, R.: High tibial osteotomy and ligament reconstruction in varus-angulated, anterior cruciate ligament-deficient knees. A two- to seven-year follow-up study. *Am J Sports Med* 21:2–12, 1993.
34. Noyes, F. R.; Barber-Westin, S. D.: Posterior cruciate ligament revision reconstruction, part 1: causes of surgical failure in 52 consecutive operations. *Am J Sports Med* 33:646–654, 2005.
35. Noyes, F. R.; Barber-Westin, S. D.: Posterolateral knee reconstruction with an anatomical bone–patellar tendon–bone reconstruction of the fibular collateral ligament. *Am J Sports Med* 35:259–273, 2007.
36. Noyes, F. R.; Barber-Westin, S. D.: Revision anterior cruciate surgery with use of bone–patellar tendon–bone autogenous grafts. *J Bone Joint Surg Am* 83:1131–1143, 2001.
37. Noyes, F. R.; Barber-Westin, S. D.: Surgical reconstruction of severe chronic posterolateral complex injuries of the knee using allograft tissues. *Am J Sports Med* 23:2–12, 1995.
38. Noyes, F. R.; Barber-Westin, S. D.: Surgical restoration to treat chronic deficiency of the posterolateral complex and cruciate ligaments of the knee joint. *Am J Sports Med* 24:415–426, 1996.
39. Noyes, F. R.; Barber-Westin, S. D.; Albright, J. C.: An analysis of the causes of failure in 57 consecutive posterolateral operative procedures. *Am J Sports Med* 34:1419–1430, 2006.

40. Noyes, F. R.; Barber-Westin, S. D.; Hewett, T. E.: High tibial osteotomy and ligament reconstruction for varus-angulated anterior cruciate ligament–deficient knees. *Am J Sports Med* 28:282–296, 2000.

41. Noyes, F. R.; Barber-Westin, S. D.; Rankin, M.: Meniscal transplantation in symptomatic patients less than fifty years old. *J Bone Joint Surg Am* 86:1392–1404, 2004.

42. Noyes, F. R.; Barber-Westin, S. D.; Roberts, C. S.: Use of allografts after failed treatment of rupture of the anterior cruciate ligament. *J Bone Joint Surg Am* 76:1019–1031, 1994.

43. Noyes, F. R.; Dunworth, L. A.; Andriacchi, T. P.; et al.: Knee hyperextension gait abnormalities in unstable knees. Recognition and preoperative gait retraining. *Am J Sports Med* 24:35–45, 1996.

44. Noyes, F. R.; Grood, E. S.; Torzilli, P. A.: Current concepts review. The definitions of terms for motion and position of the knee and injuries of the ligaments. *J Bone Joint Surg Am* 71:465–472, 1989.

45. Noyes, F. R.; Schipplein, O. D.; Andriacchi, T. P.; et al.: The anterior cruciate ligament–deficient knee with varus alignment. An analysis of gait adaptations and dynamic joint loadings. *Am J Sports Med* 20:707–716, 1992.

46. Noyes, F. R.; Stabler, C. L.: A system for grading articular cartilage lesions at arthroscopy. *Am J Sports Med* 17:505–513, 1989.

47. Pasque, C.; Noyes, F. R.; Gibbons, M.; et al.: The role of the popliteofibular ligament and the tendon of popliteus in providing stability in the human knee. *J Bone Joint Surg Br* 85:292–298, 2003.

48. Rodeo, S. A.; Arnoczky, S. P.; Torzilli, P. A.; et al.: Tendon-healing in a bone tunnel. A biomechanical and histological study in the dog. *J Bone Joint Surg Am* 75:1795–1803, 1993.

49. Rubel, I. F.; Schwarzbard, I.; Leonard, A.; Cece, D.: Anatomic location of the peroneal nerve at the level of the proximal aspect of the tibia: Gerdy's safe zone. *J Bone Joint Surg Am* 86:1625–1628, 2004.

50. Stannard, J. P.; Brown, S. L.; Farris, R. C.; et al.: The posterolateral corner of the knee: repair versus reconstruction. *Am J Sports Med* 33:881–888, 2005.

51. Staubli, H. U.: Posteromedial and posterolateral capsular injuries associated with posterior cruciate ligament insufficiency. *Sports Med Arthrosc Rev* 2:146–164, 1994.

52. Strauss, E. J.; Ishak, C.; Inzerillo, C.; et al.: Effect of tibial positioning on the diagnosis of posterolateral rotatory instability in the posterior cruciate ligament-deficient knee. *Br J Sports Med* 41:481–485; discussion 485, 2007.

53. Terry, G. C.; LaPrade, R. F.: The biceps femoris muscle complex at the knee. Its anatomy and injury patterns associated with acute anterolateral-anteromedial rotatory instability. *Am J Sports Med* 24:2–8, 1996.

54. Veltri, D. M.; Deng, X. H.; Torzilli, P. A.; et al.: The role of the cruciate and posterolateral ligaments in stability of the knee. A biomechanical study. *Am J Sports Med* 23:436–443, 1995.

55. Veltri, D. M.; Warren, R. F.: Anatomy, biomechanics, and physical findings in posterolateral knee instability. *Clin Sports Med* 13:599–614, 1994.

55a. Wang, C. J.; Chen, H. S.; Huang, T. W.; Yuan, L. J.: Outcome of surgical reconstruction for posterior cruciate and posterolateral instabilities of the knee. *Injury* 33:815–821, 2002.

56. Zhao, J.; He, Y.; Wang, J.: Anatomical reconstruction of knee posterolateral complex with the tendon of the long head of biceps femoris. *Am J Sports Med* 34:1615–1622, 2006.

Rehabilitation of Posterior Cruciate Ligament and Posterolateral Reconstructive Procedures

Frank R. Noyes, MD ▪ *Sue D. Barber-Westin*, BS ▪ *Timothy P. Heckmann*, PT, ATC

CLINICAL CONCEPTS

A paucity of information exists in the literature concerning rehabilitation after reconstruction of the posterior cruciate ligament (PCL) and posterolateral structures. The posterolateral structures comprise the fibular collateral ligament and popliteus muscle-tendon-ligament unit, including the popliteofibular ligament and posterolateral capsule.

The rehabilitation protocols described in this chapter consist of a careful incorporation of exercise concepts supported by scientific data and clinical experience.[3,14,15,17] The goal is to progress a patient on a rate that takes into account athletic and occupational goals, condition of the articular surfaces and menisci, return of muscle function and lower limb control, postoperative graft healing, and graft remodeling. Modifications to the postoperative exercise program may be required if noteworthy articular cartilage deterioration is found during surgery.

The protocol for PCL reconstruction was developed for a high-strength two-strand graft (quadriceps tendon–bone, bone–patellar tendon–bone). The protocol for posterolateral reconstruction may be used after the various operative options described in detail in Chapter 22, including anatomic and proximal advancement techniques of the posterolateral structures and nonanatomic femoral-fibular reconstruction.

The supervised rehabilitation programs are supplemented with home exercises performed daily. The therapist must routinely examine the patient in the clinic in order to implement and progress the appropriate protocol. Therapeutic procedures and modalities are used as required for successful rehabilitation. For the majority of patients, a range of 11 to 21 postoperative physical therapy visits is expected to produce a desirable result. A few more visits may be required for advanced training between the 6th and the 12th postoperative month for certain patients who desire to return to strenuous activities.

For all patients, joint swelling, pain, gait pattern, knee motion, patellar mobility, muscle strength, and flexibility are continually monitored postoperatively.

Patients are warned to avoid any exercises or activities that place high posterior shear forces on the tibia such as walking down inclines or squatting for the first 6 postoperative months. In addition, patients are cautioned that an early return to strenuous activities postoperatively carries a risk of a repeat injury or the potential of compounding the original injury. These risks cannot always be scientifically predicted, and patients are cautioned to avoid strenuous activities for 9 to 12 postoperative months and to avoid activities that produce pain, swelling, or a feeling of instability. These patients are monitored after surgery with posterior drawer testing and stress radiography if an increase in posterior tibial displacement is detected.

Patients with posterolateral reconstruction are warned specifically at the 4th to 8th postoperative weeks that, with resumption of weight-bearing and weaning of crutches, to avoid a varus or internal tibial rotation position that could place high tensile forces on the posterolateral structures.[13,16] It is important that the patient demonstrates good lower extremity control with suitable muscle strength to maintain tibiofemoral compensation and avoid a lift-off of the lateral tibiofemoral joint, which may disrupt the posterolateral reconstruction.

PCL CLINICAL BIOMECHANICS

Kaufman and coworkers[8] used a three-dimensional biomechanical model to predict dynamic patellofemoral and tibiofemoral forces generated during isokinetic exercises at 60°/sec and 180°/sec. During isokinetic extension, posterior shear forces were detected at knee flexion angles of 40° and greater. The maximum posterior shear force occurred at 70° to 80° of knee flexion and measured 0.5 ± 0.1 body weight at 60°/sec and 0.6 ± 0.1 body weight at 180°/sec.

A posterior shear force occurred throughout the entire flexion exercise at all knee flexion angles, reaching a peak at 75° of knee flexion of 1.7 ± 0.8 body weight (60°/sec) to 1.4 ± 0.5 body weight (180°/sec). The authors concluded that isokinetic exercise exerted moderate posterior shear forces and should be used cautiously after PCL rupture and reconstruction.

Ohkoshi and associates[19] used a two-dimensional model to calculate shear force exerted on the tibia during standing at various knee flexion angles in 21 healthy subjects. Posterior shear forces were found in the upright position of the trunk and at knee flexion angles of 15° to 90° (Fig. 23–1). At 30° and 60°, the posterior drawer force was significantly increased by anterior flexion of the trunk.

Castle and colleagues[4] measured posterior tibial subluxation during a static double-legged squat in patients with PCL-deficient knees. The results revealed a statistically significant mean increase of 5.9 mm in posterior tibial translation ($P < .05$) of the injured knee compared with the contralateral knee at high knee flexion angles. At low flexion angles, the magnitude of increase in mean posterior tibial translation was only 2.1 mm. Tibiofemoral shear forces were small compared with tibiofemoral joint compression forces.

Berchuck and coworkers[2] calculated large posterior shear forces during gait analysis for the activities of jogging, ascending stairs, and descending stairs (Fig. 23–2) in five normal subjects. Lutz and associates[9] evaluated tibiofemoral joint shear and

---

Critical Points POSTERIOR CRUCIATE LIGAMENT CLINICAL BIOMECHANICS

- Isokinetic flexion exercise exerts moderate posterior shear forces, use cautiously after PCL reconstruction.
- Posterior shear forces significantly increased during standing by anterior flexion of the trunk.
- Static squat: Significant increase in posterior tibial translation occurs at high knee flexion angles.
- Large posterior shear forces exist during jogging, ascending and descending stairs.
- OKC flexion exercise produces posterior shear forces beyond 30° of knee flexion.
- CKC leg press produces significantly less posterior shear forces than OKC flexion. Co-contraction of quadriceps and hamstrings occurs during CKC, greatest at 30° and 60° of knee flexion.
- Posterior shear forces during CKC squat exercise are relatively low from 0° to 45° of knee flexion. Co-contraction of quadriceps and hamstrings occurs from 0° to 30° of flexion.
- OKC knee extension produces posterior shear forces from 60° to 100° of knee flexion, but these forces are lower than those measured during CKC leg press and squat exercises.
- Leg press induces minimal hamstring muscle activity.
- In situ forces in the PCL significantly increase with knee flexion in response to an isolated hamstrings load, reaching a maximum at 90° of flexion. A simulated co-contraction of the quadriceps and hamstrings reduces the in situ forces in the PCL.
- Isokinetic extension exercise at knee flexion angles less than 70° is safe early postoperatively.
- Isokinetic flexion and deep squats should be avoided early after PCL reconstruction.
- Hamstrings load significantly increases PCL force from 15° to 120° of knee flexion
- The application of tibial torque in either an anterior or a posterior direction when the knee is flexed greater than 60° increases PCL force. Isolated hamstrings activity (with tibial torque) further increases PCL force.

CKC, closed kinetic chain; OKC, open kinetic chain; PCL, posterior cruciate ligament.

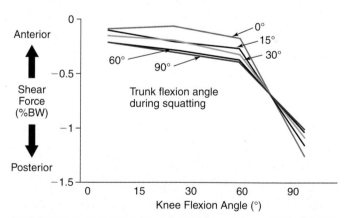

FIGURE 23–1. Calculated shear force (kilograms) per body weight (kilograms) while standing on both legs at various flexion angles of the knee and trunk. *(From Ohkoshi, Y.; Yasuda, K.; Kaneda, K.; et al.: Biomechanical analysis of rehabilitation in the standing position.* Am J Sports Med *19:605–611, 1991.)*

compressive shear forces using a two-dimensional biomechanical model and electromyographic (EMG) activity of hamstrings and quadriceps muscle activity during a closed kinetic chain (CKC) leg press exercise, an isometric open kinetic chain (OKC)

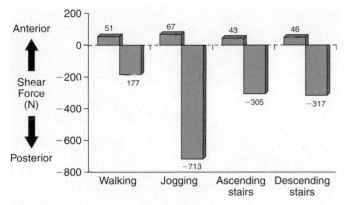

FIGURE 23–2. Calculated tibiofemoral shear forces during activities.

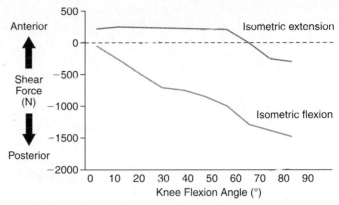

FIGURE 23–4. Calculated tibiofemoral shear forces during isometric knee extension and flexion.

exercise, and an OKC flexion exercise. Measurements of maximum muscle contractions were obtained at 30°, 60°, and 90° of knee flexion. The OKC isometric flexion exercise produced posterior shear forces at all knee flexion angles (Fig. 23–3), ranging from –939 ± 174 N at 30° of knee flexion to a maximum of –1780 ± 699 N at 90° of knee flexion. The CKC exercises produced significantly less posterior shear forces at 60° and 90° of flexion (–538 N; $P < .05$). These findings were similar to those reported by Smidt[21] during isometric knee extension and flexion exercises (Fig. 23–4). Maximum hamstrings EMG activity was detected during the OKC exercise at 90° of flexion (82 ± 15% of maximum contraction). The antagonistic muscle activity was minimal during this exercise at all knee flexion angles. In contrast, co-contraction of the quadriceps and hamstrings was observed during the CKC exercise, which was greatest at 30° and 60° of flexion. The authors concluded that CKC exercise produced significantly less tibiofemoral shear forces compared with OKC exercise ($P < .05$).

Wilk and colleagues[23] evaluated tibiofemoral shear forces and EMG activity of the quadriceps, hamstrings, and gastrocnemius muscles during OKC extension and CKC leg press and squat exercises. Both CKC exercises produced posterior shear forces. However, during the squat, these forces were relatively low (245–565 N) from 0° to 45° of knee flexion. A rapid increase in posterior shear forces was detected from 45° to 72° of flexion. In addition, co-contraction of the quadriceps and hamstrings occurred from 0° to 30° of flexion. The authors concluded that

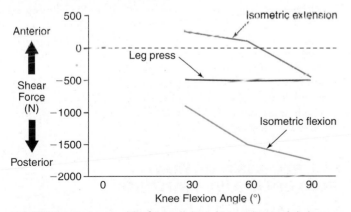

FIGURE 23–3. Average tibiofemoral shear forces observed during the closed kinetic chain leg press, the open kinetic chain extension, and the open kinetic chain flexion exercise. *(From Lutz, G. F.; Palmitier, R. A.; An, K. N.; Chao, E. Y.: Comparison of tibiofemoral joint forces during open-kinetic-chain and closed-kinetic-chain exercises. J Bone Joint Surg Am 75:732–739, 1993.)*

vertical squats from 0° to 45° of flexion should not be performed in knees in the early stages of PCL reconstruction rehabilitation.

Wilk and colleagues[23] also found that the knee extension exercise produced posterior shear forces from 60° to 100° of knee flexion; however, these forces were lower than those measured during both CKC exercises. The leg press induced minimal hamstring muscle activity.

Hoher and coworkers[7] reported that the in situ forces in the PCL significantly increased with knee flexion in response to an isolated hamstrings load, reaching a maximum at 90° of flexion. These findings were in agreement with other authors[5,24] who also reported increased strain in the PCL with knee flexion. The addition of a 200-N quadriceps load (simulating co-contraction of the quadriceps and hamstrings) reduced the in situ forces in the PCL.

Toutoungi and associates[22] combined noninvasive experimental measurements with geometrical modeling of the lower extremity to calculate ligament forces during isometric, isokinetic, and squat exercises. The data indicated that isokinetic extension at knee flexion angles less than 70° should be safe in the early postoperative period after PCL reconstruction. However, isokinetic flexion and deep squats should be avoided. During isokinetic flexion, only the PCL is loaded and peak forces may reach over 4 times the patient's body weight at 90° of knee flexion. During squatting, PCL forces may reach 3.5 times body weight at high knee flexion angles. Shallow squats with knee flexion angles kept below 50° may be considered.

Markolf and colleagues[10] studied the effects of muscle loads on cruciate force levels when the knee was subjected to external forces and moments. Load cells were installed into cadaveric knees to record forces in the ACL and PCL under five loading conditions. These force measurements were repeated with a 100-N load applied to the quadriceps tendon and with a combined 50-N load applied to both the biceps and the semimembranosus-semitendinosus tendons.

With no applied tibial force, application of hamstrings load significantly increased mean PCL force from 15° to 120° of knee flexion (Fig. 23–5; $P < .05$). With the application of a 100-N posterior tibial force, the addition of hamstrings load significantly increased mean PCL force between 30° and 105° of flexion (Fig. 23–6; $P < .05$). When a 5-Nm external tibial torque was applied, the addition of hamstrings load significantly increased mean PCL force beyond 75° of knee flexion ($P < .05$). Under a 5-Nm internal tibial torque, application of hamstrings load also significantly increased mean PCL force

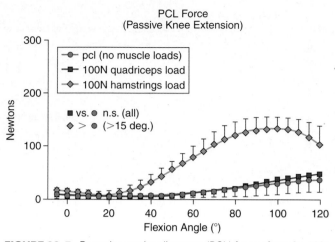

PCL Force
(Passive Knee Extension)

FIGURE 23–5. Posterior cruciate ligament (PCL) forces from 0°–120° of knee flexion with no tibial force. Application of a 100-N hamstrings load significantly increased mean PCL force at flexion angles greater than 15°. *(From Markolf, K. L.; O'Neill, G.; Jackson, S. R.; McAllister, D. R.: Effects of applied quadriceps and hamstrings muscle loads on forces in the anterior and posterior cruciate ligaments. Am J Sports Med 32:1144–1149, 2004.)*

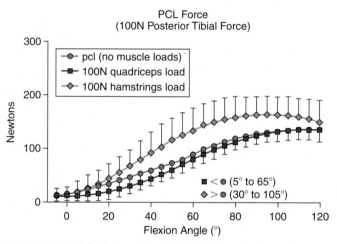

PCL Force
(100N Posterior Tibial Force)

FIGURE 23–6. PCL forces from 0°–120° of knee flexion under a constant 100-N posterior tibial force. Application of a 100-N hamstrings load significantly increased mean PCL force at flexion angles between 30° and 105°. *(From Markolf, K. L.; O'Neill, G.; Jackson, S. R.; McAllister, D. R.: Effects of applied quadriceps and hamstrings muscle loads on forces in the anterior and posterior cruciate ligaments. Am J Sports Med 32:1144–1149, 2004.)*

between 60° and 100° of flexion ($P < .05$). The authors concluded that, in general, the hamstrings were more effective in producing changes in cruciate force levels. Application of tibial torque in either an anterior or a posterior direction when the knee was flexed greater than 60° increased PCL force, and isolated hamstrings activity (with tibial torque) further increased PCL force.

PROTOCOL FOR PARTIAL OR ACUTE ISOLATED PCL RUPTURES

This program does not apply to PCL avulsions in which surgery may be indicated and partial tears with 5 mm or less of increased posterior tibial translation. The goal with complete

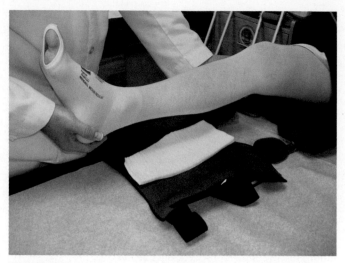

FIGURE 23–7. Knee extension brace with posterior calf pad to maintain tibiofemoral reduction.

PCL disruptions (8–10 mm of increased posterior tibial translation at 90° flexion) is to allow PCL healing and possibly reduce some of the posterior tibial translation. Importantly, this includes maintaining normal tibiofemoral contact at full knee extension or with knee flexion. An anterior drawer produced by the therapist during motion will allow for healing of PCL fibers with the least amount of residual abnormal PCL elongation and posterior tibial translation. Although clinical data are not available, the empirical favorable experience of the authors warrants the program described below.

The rules to treat partial or acute isolated PCL tears are

1. Protect for 6 weeks in full knee extension with a brace and posterior calf pad (Fig. 23–7) or bivalved cylinder cast to maintain tibiofemoral reduction. Use quadriceps isometrics, electrical muscle stimulation (EMS), leg raises, and 25% weight-bearing.
2. Obtain a lateral radiograph to verify that no posterior tibial subluxation exists, which can occur in up to 50% of knees.
3. At 2 weeks, the therapist initiates 0° to 90° of motion, maintaining anterior tibial translation load during knee motion exercises. The patient must sleep in the brace and is not allowed unsupervised knee motion. Only passive flexion is permitted.
4. At 4 weeks, the patient is allowed to perform active quadriceps extension out of the brace, use 50% weight-bearing with crutch support, and continue brace protection.
5. At 5 to 6 weeks, the patient is weaned from the brace and crutch support, active full knee flexion is allowed, and the rehabilitation protocol described later beginning at this time period is followed.

PCL RECONSTRUCTION POSTOPERATIVE PROTOCOL

Immediate Postoperative Management

Patients present to physical therapy the 1st day after surgery on bilateral axillary crutches in a postoperative dressing with a long-leg brace locked in full extension (Table 23–1). The

Critical Points IMMEDIATE POSTOPERATIVE
MANAGEMENT

Postoperative compression dressing, long-leg brace, compression stockings, cryotherapy, lower limb elevation, pain management.

Common Complications

- Excessive pain/swelling.
- Quadriceps shutdown.
- Limitation knee flexion, extension.

  Early detection and treatment complications critical.

Brace Support

- PCL reconstruction
  - Long-leg hinged brace 8 wk.
  - Functional PCL brace return to higher level occupational or sports.
- PCL reconstruction with posterolateral procedure
  - Bivalved cast 4 postoperative wk.
  - Lower extremity, hinged, double-upright brace applied locked at 10° of extension 4–6 wk.
  - Brace unlocked 6 wk to allow flexion.
  - Custom medial unloading brace at 8 wk.

Range of Knee Motion

- Passive flexion, passive & active-assisted extension exercises 1st day postoperative, 0°–120°
- Advance flexion slowly, limit total number daily knee cycles to 60 for first 4 wk.
- Flexion is passive for first 12 wk, avoid hamstring activation.
- 135° allowed 7–8 wk.

  Begin ROM overpressure program 1 wk postoperative if 0° not achieved.

Weight-Bearing

- Partial weight-bearing first 6 wk, full 7–8 wk.
- Weight-bearing progressed using normal gait technique, avoid locked-knee position, encourage normal flexion throughout gait cycle.
- Warn avoid squatting, walking down hills or ramps, any sudden deceleration movements for at least 6 mo.

PCL, posterior cruciate ligament; ROM, range of motion

postoperative bandage and dressing are changed to allow the application of thigh high compression stockings and a compression bandage. Early control of postoperative effusion is essential for pain management and early quadriceps reeducation. In addition to compression, cryotherapy is important in this time period.

Patients are instructed to keep the lower limb elevated as frequently as possible during the 1st week. The initial response to surgery and progression during the first 2 weeks sets the tone for the initial phases of the rehabilitation program. Common postoperative complications include excessive pain or swelling, quadriceps shutdown, and range of motion (ROM) limitations. Early recognition and treatment of these problems are critical for a successful outcome.

Modalities

Therapeutic modalities after PCL reconstruction are used as required by the evaluation. If the patient demonstrates a fair or poor rating of the quadriceps or vastus medialis obliquus (VMO) musculature, then EMS is initiated. Electrodes are placed over the VMO and on the central to lateral aspect of the upper one third of the quadriceps muscle belly. The patient actively contracts the quadriceps muscle simultaneously with the machine's stimulation. Treatment sessions last for 20 minutes. A portable neuromuscular electric stimulator such as the EMPI PV 300 (EMPI, St. Paul, MN) may be helpful in individuals whose muscle rating is poor. This device is used six times per day, 15 minutes per session, until the muscle grade is rated as good.

Biofeedback therapy is also quite useful in facilitating quadriceps muscle contractions. The surface electrode is placed over the selected muscle component to provide information to the patient and clinician regarding the quality of active or voluntary quadriceps contraction. This modality can enhance relaxation of the hamstring musculature if the patient has difficulty achieving full knee extension owing to knee pain or muscle spasm. The electrode is placed over the belly of the hamstring muscle while the patient performs ROM exercises.

Cryotherapy is begun in the recovery room after surgery. Several different modalities are available for use in both the clinic and the home settings. Clinically, devices such as the Game Ready (Game Ready, Berkeley, CA) cryotherapy machine are used to provide compression simultaneously with the cold program. For most patients, cryotherapy is accomplished with an ice bag or commercial cold pack. Patients also receive a commercial cooling unit, which is used six to eight times daily at home. Other commercially available cold therapy units include motorized cooler units that maintain a constant temperature and circulation of ice water through a pad that provides excellent pain control. Gravity-flow units also provide effective pain management; however, the maintenance of a constant temperature is more difficult with these devices. The temperature can be controlled by using gravity to backflow and drain the water, refilling the cuff with fresh ice water as required. Standard treatment times are 20 minutes in length, performed from three times a day to every waking hour depending upon the extent of pain and swelling. In some cases, the treatment time can be extended based on the thickness of the buffer used between the skin and the device. Cryotherapy is typically used after exercise or when required for pain and swelling control and is maintained throughout the entire postoperative rehabilitation protocol.

Brace Support

For patients who undergo PCL reconstruction without a concurrent posterolateral procedure, a long-leg hinged postoperative brace with a posterior calf pad is worn for the first 6 weeks postoperatively. The brace is worn 24 hours a day, including during sleep, to avoid sudden knee flexion motions that may occur. Initially, the brace is worn in full extension for the first 3 to 4 weeks and is then opened to 0° to 90°. For individuals evaluated with physiologic joint laxity or poor muscle control of the lower limb, the brace is used for up to 12 weeks postoperatively.

During this phase, the patient may also be measured for a functional PCL brace, which is indicated for higher-level occupational or sports activities. For patients who return to lower levels of activity, or who develop patellofemoral symptoms, a patellofemoral knee sleeve may be indicated for prolonged standing and walking activities.

A standard soft-hinged brace is not considered adequate for protection of complex reconstructions that involve both the PCL and the posterolateral structures. These braces do not prevent excessive lateral forces (joint opening) that place the posterolateral reconstruction at risk in the initial 4 weeks postoperatively. In these knees, a bivalved cast is used to limit lateral joint opening during

TABLE 23–1　Rehabilitation Protocol after Posterior Cruciate Ligament Reconstruction

	Postoperative Weeks					Postoperative Months			
	1–2	3–4	5–6	7–8	9–12	4	5	6	7–12
Hinged long-leg postoperative brace	X	X	X						
Patellar knee sleeve				X	X	X	X		
Functional brace								X	X
ROM minimum goals									
0°–90°	X								
0°–110°		X							
0°–120°			X						
0°–135°				X					
Weight-bearing									
25% body weight	X								
50% body weight		X							
Full			X						
Patella mobilization	X	X	X	X					
Modalities									
EMS	X	X	X	X	X				
Pain/edema management (cryotherapy)	X	X	X	X	X	X	X	X	X
Stretching									
Hamstring, gastrocnemius-soleus, iliotibial band, quadriceps	X	X	X	X	X	X	X	X	X
Strengthening									
Quadriceps isometrics, straight leg raises, active knee extension	X	X	X	X	X				
Closed chain: gait retraining, toe-raises, wall-sits, mini-squats			X	X	X	X	X	X	
Knee flexion hamstring curls (90°–0°)					X	X	X	X	X
Knee extension quadriceps (90°–30°)		X	X	X	X	X	X	X	X
Hip abduction-adduction, multihip		X	X	X	X	X	X	X	X
Leg press (70°–10°)			X	X	X	X	X	X	X
Balance/proprioceptive training									
Weight-shifting, cup-walking, BBS			X	X					
BBS, BAPS, perturbation training, balance board, minitrampoline			X	X	X	X	X	X	X
Conditioning									
UBC	X	X	X	X	X				
Bike (stationary)			X	X	X	X	X	X	X
Aquatic program					X	X	X	X	X
Swimming (kicking)						X	X	X	X
Walking					X	X	X	X	X
Stair-climbing machine					X	X	X	X	X
Ski machine					X	X	X	X	X
Running: straight								X	
Cutting: lateral carioca, figure-eights									X
Plyometric training									X
Full sports									X

PHASE 1. WEEKS 1 TO 2 (VISITS: 2–4)

General Observation	Toe-touch to 25% weight-bearing	
	Brace	
Evaluation		**Goals**
	Pain	Controlled
	Hemarthrosis	Mild
	Patellar mobility	Good
	ROM minimum	0°–90°
	Quadriceps contraction & patella migration	Good
	Soft tissue contracture	None
Frequency		**Duration**
3–4 x/day	**ROM**	
10 min	ROM 0°–90° (active extension/passive flexion with 10 lb. anterior drawer)	20 cycles
		10 x/30 sec
	Patella mobilization	
	Ankle pumps (plantar flexion with resistance band)	
	Hamstring, gastrocnemius-soleus stretches	5 reps x 30 sec

3 x/day 15 min	**Strengthening** Straight leg raises (flexion, 0–5 lb ankle weight) Active quadriceps isometrics Knee extension (active-assisted, 70°–0°, 0–7.5 lb weight)	3 sets x 10 reps 1 set x 10 reps 3 sets x 10 reps
2 x/day 10 min	**Aerobic conditioning** UBC	
As required	**Modalities** EMS Cryotherapy	20 min 20 min
While sleeping	**Activities of daily living** Knee brace to avoid sudden knee flexion while asleep	
Goals	ROM 0°–90° Adequate quadriceps contraction Control inflammation, effusion Prevent tissue contracture Protect ligament reconstruction at insertion site	

PHASE 2. WEEKS 3 TO 4 (VISITS: 2–4)

General Observation	50% weight-bearing when: • Pain controlled • Hemarthrosis controlled • Muscle control throughout ROM Brace	
Evaluation		**Goals**
	Pain	Controlled
	Effusion	Mild
	Patellar mobility	Good
	ROM minimum	0°–110°
	Quadriceps contraction & patella migration	Good
	Soft tissue contracture	None
Frequency		**Duration**
3–4 x/day 10 min	**ROM** ROM (passive, 0°–110°, 10# anterior drawer) Patella mobilization Ankle pumps (plantar flexion with resistance band) Hamstring, gastrocnemius-soleus stretches	20 cycles 10 x, 30 sec 5 reps x 30 sec
2–3 x/day 20 min	**Strengthening** Straight leg raises (flexion, adduction, abduction) Isometric training: multi-angle (0°–60°) Knee extension (active-assisted, 90°–0°, 0–7.5 lb weight)	3 sets x 10 reps 1 set x 10 reps 3 sets x 10 reps
2 x/day 10 min	**Aerobic conditioning** UBC	
As required	**Modalities** EMS Cryotherapy	20 min 20 min
While sleeping	**Activities of daily living** Knee brace to avoid sudden knee flexion while asleep	
Goals	ROM 0°–110° Control inflammation, effusion Muscle control Prevent soft tissue contracture Protect ligament reconstruction at insertion sites	

PHASE 3. WEEKS 5 TO 6 (VISITS: 1–2)

General Observation	Full weight bearing when • Pain controlled without narcotics • Hemarthrosis controlled • Muscle control throughout ROM Brace

Continued

Evaluation		Goals
	Pain	Mild/no RSD
	Effusion	Minimal
	Patellar mobility	Good
	ROM	0°–120°
	Muscle control	3/5
	Inflammatory response	None
	Joint arthrometer (6 wk), 20° 89 N and 70° 89 N	<3 mm

Frequency		Duration
3–4 x/day		
10 min	**ROM**	
	ROM (passive, 0°–120°)	
	Patella mobilization	
	Hamstring, gastrocnemius-soleus stretches	5 reps x 30 sec
3 x/day	**Strengthening**	
15 min	Straight leg raises (ankle weight, not to exceed 10% of body weight)	3 sets x 10 reps
	Isometric training: multiangle (90°, 60°, 30°)	2 sets x 10 reps
	Knee extension (active, 90°–0°)	3 sets x 10 reps
	Closed chain	3 sets x 10 reps
	• Heel-raise/toe-raise	3 sets x 10 reps
	• Wall-sits	5 reps
	Multihip machine (flexion, extension, abduction, adduction)	3 sets x 10 reps
	Leg press (50°–10°)	3 sets x 10 reps
3 x/day	**Balance training**	
5 min	Weight shift side/side and forward/back	5 sets x 10 reps
	Balance board/two-legged	
	Cup-walking	
	Single-leg stance	
2 x/day	**Aerobic conditioning** (patellofemoral precautions)	
10 min	UBC	
	Stationary bicycling	
As required	**Modalities**	
	EMS	20 min
	Cryotherapy	20 min
While sleeping	**Activities of daily living**	
	Knee brace to avoid sudden knee flexion while asleep	
Goals	ROM 0°–120°	
	Control inflammation, effusion	
	Muscle control	
	Early recognition complications (motion loss, RSD, increased AP displacement, patellofemoral)	

General Observation		
	Full weight-bearing	
	Brace	

Evaluation		Goals
	Pain	Mild/no RSD
	Effusion	Minimal
	Patellar mobility	Good
	ROM	0°–135°
	Muscle control	4/5
	Inflammatory response	None
	Joint arthrometer (8 wk), 20° 89 N and 70° 89 N	<3 mm

Frequency		Duration
3–4 x/day		
10 min	**ROM**	
	ROM (passive, 0°–135°)	
	Patellar mobilization	
	Hamstring, gastrocnemius-soleus stretches	5 reps x 30 sec
3 x/day	**Strengthening**	
15 min	Straight leg raises (flexion, abduction, adduction)	3 sets x 10 reps
	Straight leg raises, rubber tubing	3 sets x 30 reps
	Knee extension (active, 90°–0°)	3 sets x 10 reps
	Knee flexion (active, 0°–90°)	3 sets x 10 reps
	Leg press (50°–10°)	3 sets x 10 reps

	Closed-chain	
	• Wall-sits	5 reps
	• Mini-squats (rubber tubing, 0°–30°)	3 sets x 20 reps
	Multi-hip machine (flexion, extension, abduction, adduction)	3 sets x 10 reps
3 x/day 5 min	**Balance training** Balance board/two-legged Single-leg stance	
2 x/day 10–15 min	**Aerobic conditioning** UBC Stationary bicycling	
As required	**Modalities** EMS Cryotherapy	20 min 20 min
While sleeping	**Activities of daily living** Knee brace to avoid sudden knee flexion while asleep	
Goals	Full weight-bearing, normal gait Control inflammation, effusion Muscle control ROM 0°–135°	

PHASE 5. WEEKS 9 TO 12 (VISITS: 1–2)

General Observation

No effusion, painless ROM, joint stability
Performs activities of daily living without pain
ROM 0°–135°
Brace optional

Evaluation

		Goals
Pain		Minimal/no RSD
Manual muscle test		4/5
Quadriceps, hip abductors/adductors/flexors/extensors		
Swelling		Minimal
Joint arthrometer (12 wk) 20° 134 N and 70° 89 N		3 mm
Patellar mobility		Good
Crepitus		None/slight
Gait		Symmetrical

Frequency		**Duration**
3–4 x/day 10 min	**ROM** Hamstring, gastrocnemius-soleus, quadriceps, ITB stretches	5 reps x 30 sec

3 x/day
15–20 min
	Strengthening
	  Straight leg raises (add extension)
	  Straight leg raises, rubber tubing
	  Hamstring curls
	  Knee extension with resistance (90°–30°)
	  Knee flexion (active, 0°–90°)
	  Leg press (50°–10°)
	  Closed chain
	    • Wall sits
	    • Mini-squats (0°–40°)
	    • Lateral step-ups (2"–4" block)
	  Multi-hip machine (flexion, extension, abduction, adduction)
		3 sets x 10 reps
		3 sets x 30 reps
		3 sets x 10 reps
		3 sets x 10 reps
		3 sets x 10 reps
		3 sets x 10 reps
		
		To fatigue x 3 reps
		3 sets x 20 reps
		3 sets x 10 reps
		3 sets x 10 reps

3 x/day 5 min	**Balance training** Balance board/two-legged Single-leg stance	

1 x/day
15–20 min
	Aerobic conditioning (patellofemoral precautions)
	  Stationary bicycling
	  Water-walking
	  UBC
	  Stair machine (low resistance, low stroke)
	  Ski machine (short stride, level, low resistance)	

As required	**Modalities** EMS Cryotherapy	20 min 20 min

Continued

hanging weight away from the proximal tibia to avoid posterior shear stresses. Zero degrees of knee extension should be obtained by the 3rd to 6th postoperative weeks. If this is not accomplished, or if the clinician notes a firm end feel, a serial casting program may be required (see Chapter 41, Prevention and Treatment of Knee Arthrofibrosis). Hyperextension is avoided to protect the healing PCL graft.

Passive knee flexion exercises are performed in the seated position, using an anterior manual force to provide proximal tibial support to prevent posterior drop-back. A 10-pound anterior drawer is maintained on the proximal tibia during passive knee flexion (Fig. 23–9) because PCL forces significantly increase after 70° of flexion. Knee flexion exercises are primarily passive for the first 6 weeks and are then active for the next 6 weeks. Care must be taken to avoid activating the hamstrings. Other overpressure techniques to assist in gaining flexion include chair-rolling (Fig. 23–10), wall-sliding using the opposite extremity (Fig. 23–11), commercial devices (Fig. 23–12), and passive quadriceps-stretching exercises.

Weight-Bearing

Patients are allowed to bear 25% of their body weight during the first 1 to 2 postoperative weeks. Weight-bearing is then slowly progressed and crutches are usually discontinued at postoperative week 6. Weight-bearing is progressed using a normal gait technique, avoiding a locked-knee position and encouraging normal flexion throughout the gait cycle. This allows for

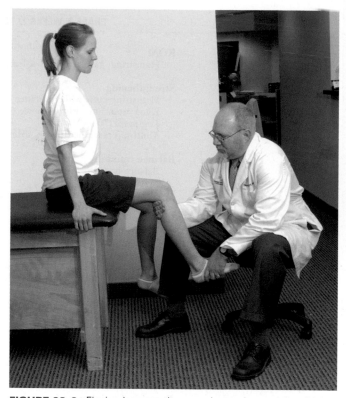

FIGURE 23–9. Flexion knee motion exercises using anterior tibial pressure to prevent posterior tibial drop-back.

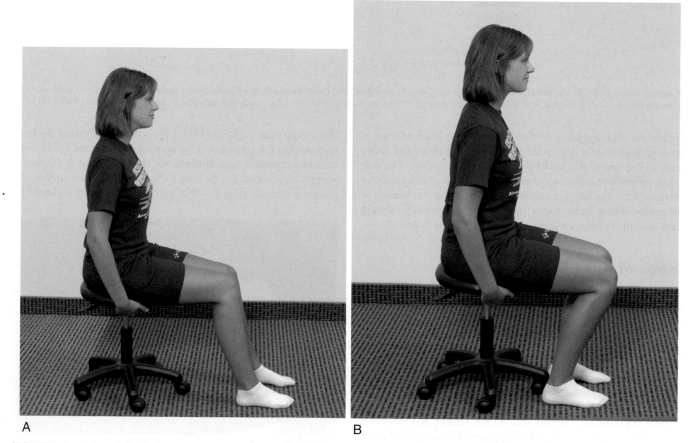

A   B

FIGURE 23–10. A and **B,** Flexion overpressure using a rolling stool.

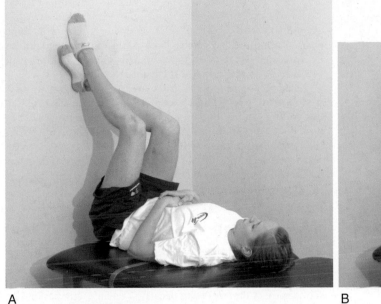 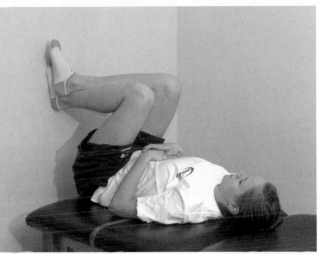

A   B

FIGURE 23–11. A and **B,** Flexion overpressure using a wall-slide technique.

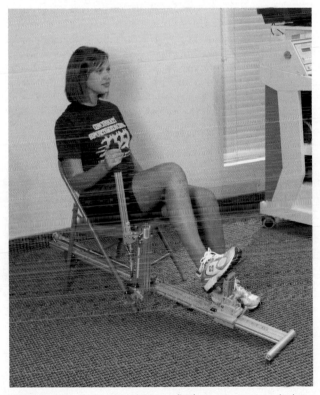

FIGURE 23–12. A commercial knee flexion overpressure device.

normal patterning of heel-to-toe ambulation, quadriceps contraction during midstance, and hip and knee flexion during the gait cycle. The locked-knee position is avoided owing to the potential of the development of a quadriceps-avoidance gait pattern.

Once patients are full weight-bearing, they are warned to avoid squatting, walking down hills or ramps, or any sudden deceleration movements that may place high forces on the PCL graft. These precautions are maintained for at least the first 6 postoperative months.

Patellar Mobilization

Patellar mobilization is important in the promotion of a full range of knee motion. The loss of patellar mobility is often associated with knee motion complications and, in extreme cases, the development of patella infera.[18] Patellar glides are performed in all four planes (superior, inferior, medial, and lateral) with sustained pressure applied to the appropriate patellar border for at least 10 seconds (Fig 23–13). This exercise is performed for 5 minutes before ROM exercises are completed. Caution is warranted if an extensor lag is detected, because this may be associated with poor superior migration of the patella, indicating the need for additional emphasis on this exercise.

Critical Points PATELLAR MOBILIZATION, MODALITIES, FLEXIBILITY

Patellar Mobilization Paramount to Achieving Full Knee Motion
- Superior, inferior, medial, lateral directions—5 min—when ROM exercises are performed.
- Extensor lag may be associated with poor superior patellar migration.

Modalities
- EMS if quadriceps rated fair or poor.
- Biofeedback for quadriceps activation.
- Cryotherapy, entire rehabilitation period.

Flexibility
- Hamstring, gastrocnemius-soleus begun 1st day
  - Modified hurdler.
  - Towel-pull.
- Quadriceps, iliotibial band begun 9th wk.

EMS, electrical muscle stimulation; ROM, range of motion.

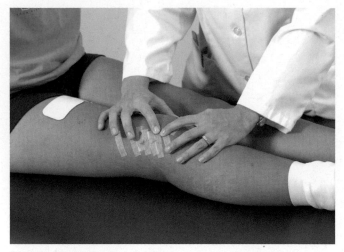

FIGURE 23–13. Patellar mobilization.

Patellar mobilization is performed for approximately 8 weeks postoperatively.

Flexibility

Hamstring and gastrocnemius-soleus flexibility exercises are begun the 1st postoperative day. A sustained static stretch is held for 30 seconds and repeated five times. The modified hurdler stretch is the most common hamstring exercise, and the towel-pull is the most common gastrocnemius-soleus stretch. These exercises assist in controlling pain that occurs because of the reflex response created in the hamstrings when the knee is kept in the flexed position. As well, the towel-pulling exercise can

help lessen discomfort in the calf, Achilles tendon, and ankle. These stretches represent critical components of the ROM program, because the ability to relax these muscle groups is imperative to achieving full passive knee extension. The patient must be instructed not to perform harsh, aggressive stretching, which could result in activation of the hamstring muscles.

Quadriceps and iliotibial band stretches are begun at the 9th postoperative week. These exercises assist in achieving full knee flexion and controlling lateral hip and thigh tightness. When designing a flexibility program, the therapist should determine the particular sport or activity the individual wishes to return to, as well as the position or physical requirements of that activity. The flexibility program should be continued after the patient is discharged from formal care.

Strengthening

The strengthening program is begun on the first postoperative visit. Early emphasis on the quadriceps muscle group is critical for a safe return to functional activities and to prevent posterior subluxation of the tibia from occurring during activities in which the knee is flexed greater than 50°. In this phase of rehabilitation, initiation of a good voluntary quadriceps contraction sets the tone for the progression of the strengthening program.

Isometric quadriceps contractions are done every hour following the repetition rules of 10-second holds, 10 repetitions, 10 times per day. Evaluation of the contraction by both the therapist and the patient is critical. The patient can monitor contractions by visual or manual means, comparing the quality of the contractions to those achieved by the contralateral limb. She or he can also assess the superior migration of the patella during the contraction, which should be approximately 1 cm, and the inferior migration of the patella during the initial relaxation of the contraction.

Critical Points STRENGTHENING

1–2 Wk Postoperative
- Quadriceps isometrics
- Straight leg raises (flexion)
- Active-assisted knee extension, 0°–70°

3–4 Wk Postoperative
- Multi-angle quadriceps isometrics 0°, 60°
- Straight leg raises (flexion, adduction)
- Active-assisted knee extension 0°–90°

5–6 Wk Postoperative
- Multiangle quadriceps isometrics 30°, 60°, 90°
- Straight leg raises (flexion, adduction)
- Active-assisted knee extension 0°–90°
- Heel-raise/toe-raise
- Wall-sits
- Multi-hip machine
- Leg press 50°–10°

7–8 Wk Postoperative
- Straight leg raises (flexion, adduction, abduction), rubber tubing
- Active knee extension 0°–90°
- Mini-squats 0°–30°, rubber tubing
- Wall-sits
- Multi-hip machine
- Leg press 50°–10°

9–12 Wk Postoperative
- Straight leg raises (flexion, adduction, abduction, extension), rubber tubing
- Hamstring curls 0°–90°
- Active knee extension 0°–90°
- Mini-squats 0°–40°, rubber tubing
- Wall-sits
- Lateral step-ups 2"–4" block
- Multi-hip machine
- Leg press 50°–10°

13–26 Wk Postoperative
- Hamstring curls 0°–90°
- Knee extension with resistance 30°–90°
- Mini-squats 0°–40°, rubber tubing
- Wall sits
- Lateral step-ups 2"–4" block
- Multi-hip machine
- Leg press 50°–10°

27–52 Wk Postoperative
- Hamstring curls with resistance 0°–90°
- Knee extension with resistance 30°–90°
- Multi-hip machine
- Leg press 70°–10°

Other exercises performed immediately postoperatively are supine straight leg raises and active-assisted knee extension (70°–0° postoperative wk 1 and 2, then 90°–0°). The patient must achieve a sufficient isometric quadriceps contraction with the leg raises to benefit the quadriceps. Initially, 1- to 2-pound ankle weights are used; and eventually, an ankle weight up to 10 pounds is used as long as this does not represent more than 10% of the patient's body weight.

Active-assisted ROM facilitates the quadriceps muscle if poor tone is observed during isometric contractions. At postoperative weeks 3 to 4, adduction and abduction straight leg raises are incorporated. The exceptions are in knees that undergo concomitant posterolateral procedures, for which abduction leg raises are delayed until postoperative weeks 7 to 8. Extension leg raises are initiated at postoperative week 9. These exercises are continued through at least postoperative week 12, at which time emphasis is placed on controlling pain and swelling, regaining full ROM, achieving quadriceps control and proximal hip stabilization, and resuming a normal gait pattern.

Once partial weight-bearing is initiated, CKC exercises are begun. The first CKC exercise is cup-walking, an activity designed to facilitate adequate quadriceps control during midstance of gait to prevent knee hyperextension from occurring (Fig. 23–14). When the patient progresses to 50% to 75% weight-bearing, toe-raises for gastrocnemius-soleus strengthening, wall-sitting isometrics for quadriceps control, and mini-squats for quadriceps strengthening are begun. The goal of wall-sitting is to improve quadriceps contraction by performing the exercise to muscle exhaustion. This

exercise may be modified to decrease patellar pain or place additional stress on the quadriceps muscle. Patellar pain may be decreased by either altering the knee flexion angle of the sit or subtly changing the toe-out/toe-in angle by no more than 10°.

Additional stress to the quadriceps can be accomplished by several methods. First, the patient can voluntarily set the quadriceps muscle once he or she reaches his or her maximum knee flexion angle, which is typically between 30° and 45°. This contraction and knee flexion position is held until muscle fatigue occurs, and the exercise is repeated two to three times, for eight repetitions per day. In a second modification, the patient performs a hip adduction contraction by squeezing a ball between the distal thighs. This modification promotes a stronger VMO contraction. In a third variation, the patient holds dumbbell weights in his or her hands to increase body weight, which promotes an even-stronger quadriceps contraction. Finally, the patient can shift his or her body weight over the involved side to stimulate a single-leg contraction. These exercises are highly beneficial and result in the patient experiencing a true muscle burn as each repetition is held to maximum quadriceps muscle fatigue, which is not achieved at this point with other exercises. The sets should be performed ideally twice each and repeated five to six times a day.

The last CKC exercise is the mini-squat. Initially, the patient's body weight is used as resistance. Gradually, TheraBand or surgical tubing is employed as a resistance mechanism (Fig. 23–15). The depth of the squat is controlled to protect the patellofemoral joint. Quick, smooth, rhythmic squats are performed to a high-set/high-repetition cadence to promote muscle fatigue. Hip position is

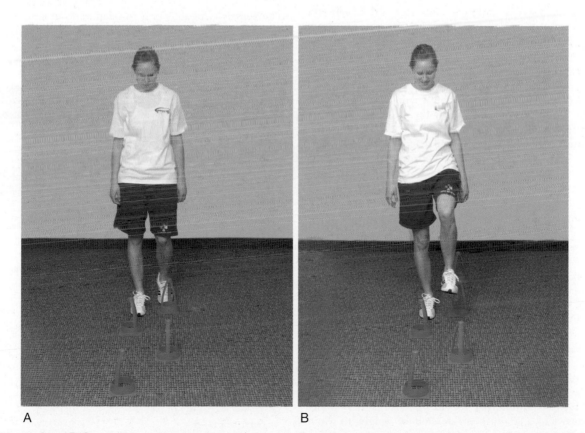

A   B

FIGURE 23–14. A and **B,** Cup-walking used early postoperatively to develop symmetry between the surgical and the contralateral limbs, hip and knee flexion, quadriceps control during midstance, hip and pelvic control during midstance, and adequate gastrocnemius-soleus control during push-off.

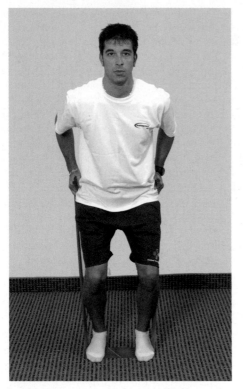

FIGURE 23–15. Mini-squats made more difficult with TheraBand.

important to monitor in order to emphasize the quadriceps. Increased trunk flexion facilitates increased hamstring contractions[19] and, therefore, must be carefully monitored to avoid forceful hamstring contractions for a minimum of 3 to 6 months.

OKC exercises are included in the rehabilitation program owing to the advantage of muscle group isolation provided by weight machines. Initially, if the lightest amount of weight on the machine is too heavy to be lifted by the involved limb alone, the patient is instructed to lift the weight with both legs and lower it with the involved side. Eccentric contractions can also be used in the advanced stages of strength training if tendinitis or overuse syndromes develop. Weight training is used in the latter stages of rehabilitation and continues after the patient has returned to activity.

The timing of the initiation of extension, hip, leg press, and hamstring curl OKC exercises is shown in Table 23–1. Knee flexion hamstring curls are delayed until the 12th postoperative week to avoid excessive posterior shear forces incurred with this activity. Leg press (range, 50°–0°) and hip abduction-adduction exercises are allowed at the 4th postoperative week. Caution is warranted owing to the potential problems knee extension OKC exercises may create for the healing graft and the patellofemoral joint. Many patients have an unsatisfactory outcome based on persistent anterior or patellofemoral knee pain, which can occur owing to improper training in the terminal phase of extension (0°–30°). Therefore, recommendations for knee extension exercises include emphasis on patellofemoral protection (monitoring for changes in pain, swelling, and crepitus) and a gradual progression of weight to avoid overuse syndromes.

A full lower extremity–strengthening program is critical for long-term success of the rehabilitation program.

Gastrocnemius-soleus strength is a key component for both early ambulation and running. In addition, an upper extremity and core strength program is important for safe return to work or sports. These exercises are included as part of general conditioning and general strength-training concepts are emphasized. Sports and position specificity are taken into account when devising the program to maximize its benefits.

Balance, Proprioceptive, and Perturbation Training

Balance and proprioceptive training are initiated at approximately 4 to 6 weeks postoperatively when the patient is partial weight-bearing. The first exercise involves weight-shifting from side-to-side and front-to-back. This activity assists patient confidence in the leg's ability to withstand the pressures of weight-bearing and initiates the stimulus to knee joint position sense. A second exercise is cup-walking, which is designed to both promote strength and develop symmetry between the surgical and the uninvolved limbs. Cup-walking helps develop hip and knee flexion, quadriceps control during midstance, hip and pelvic control during midstance, and adequate gastrocnemius-soleus control during push-off and controls hip hiking.

Another helpful activity for balance control is the single-leg balance exercise. The stance position is key to making this exercise beneficial. The patient is instructed to point the foot straight ahead, flex the knee approximately 20° to 30°, extend the arms outward to horizontal, and position the torso upright with the shoulders above the hips and the hips above the ankles. The object of this activity is to stand in position until balance is disturbed. A minitrampoline or unstable surface can be used to make this exercise more challenging. The unstable position

---

Critical Points BALANCE/PROPRIOCEPTIVE/PLYOMETRIC TRAINING

Begin Balance Training 5–6 Wk Postoperative

- Side-to-side and front-to-back weight-shifting.
- Cup-walking.
- Single-leg balance.
- Styrofoam half and whole rolls.
- BAPS board, double-leg & single-leg stance.
- Balance systems.
- Computerized stability systems.

Plyometric Training

- Begin 6–9 mo postoperative, no more than 20% deficit on quadriceps and hamstrings isokinetic testing.
- Level surface box hopping on four-square grid
  - ○ Double-leg hop initially, land in flexion.
  - ○ Complete four levels.
  - ○ Single-leg hops.
- Vertical box hopping.

Plyometric Training Considerations

- Surface: Firm but forgiving such as wooden gym floor. Avoid hard surfaces such as concrete.
- Footwear: Cross-training or running shoe. Check wear patterns, outer sole wear.
- Warm-up: Include light cardiovascular workout.

BAPS, Biomechanical Ankle Platform System.

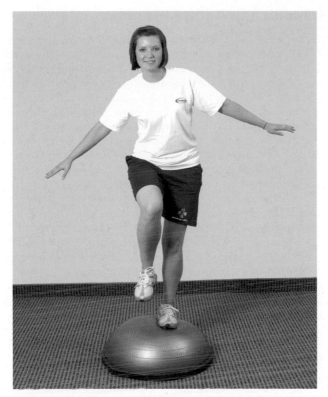

FIGURE 23–16. Single-leg stance on an unstable platform.

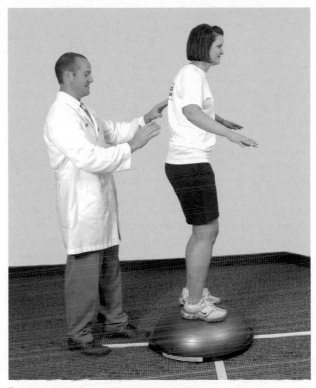

FIGURE 23–17. Perturbation technique. The therapist stands behind the patient and intermittently touches the patient's back to disturb balance.

created with the soft surface requires greater dynamic limb control than that used to stand on a flat surface (Fig. 23–16).

In the early phases of full, unassisted weight-bearing, half foam rolls are used as part of the gait-retraining program. Walking on half rolls helps the patient develop balance and dynamic muscular control required to maintain an upright position and be able to walk from one end of the roll to the other. Developing a center of balance, limb symmetry, quadriceps control in midstance, and postural positioning are benefits obtained from this type of training.

Perturbation-training techniques are initiated at approximately the 7th to 8th postoperative weeks. The therapist stands behind the patient and disrupts her or his body posture and position periodically to enhance dynamic knee stability. The techniques involve either direct contact with the patient (Fig. 23–17) or disruption of the platform the patient is standing on (Fig. 23–18).

Another effective proprioceptive exercise is a balance board with the patient assuming first a double-leg stance and eventually a single-leg stance as strength and balance improve. To provide a greater functional challenge, patients may assume the single-leg stance position and throw/catch a weighted ball against an inverted minitrampoline until fatigue occurs.

The use of more sophisticated devices adds another dimension to the proprioception program, because certain units objectively attempt to document balance and dynamic control. Many balance systems are available, with a wide cost variance. Two of the more common units include Biodex's Balance System (Biodex Medical Systems, Inc., Shirley, NY) and Neurocom's Balance System (Neurocom, Clackamas, OR). Whereas these systems may provide objective information, more research is required to justify the cost and reliability of each unit.

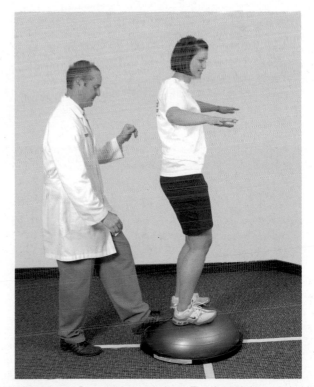

FIGURE 23–18. Perturbation technique. The therapist stands behind the patient and intermittently taps the unstable platform to disturb balance.

Conditioning

The primary consideration for the conditioning program throughout the rehabilitation protocol is to stress the cardiovascular system without compromising the joint. Depending on accessibility, a cardiovascular program may be initiated at approximately the 3rd to 4th postoperative weeks with an upper extremity ergometer. The surgical limb should be elevated to minimize lower extremity swelling. This exercise is performed to tolerance.

Stationary bicycling is begun at postoperative weeks 5 to 6. During bicycling, the seat height is adjusted to its highest level based on patient body size and a low resistance level is used during the workout. Toe clips should be avoided to decrease hamstring involvement. Gradually, between the 9th and the 12th postoperative weeks, cross-country skiing, elliptical cross-trainer, and stair-climbing machines are incorporated. Protection against high stresses to the patellofemoral joint is strongly advocated in patients with symptoms or articular cartilage deterioration. If a stair-climbing machine is tolerated, a short step and lower resistance levels should be encouraged. Monitoring heart rate will ensure that work levels are sufficient to improve cardiovascular fitness.

The goals of early conditioning exercises include facilitation of full ROM, gait retraining, and cardiovascular reconditioning. In order to improve cardiovascular endurance, the program should be performed at least three times per week for 20 to 30 minutes, and the exercise performed to at least 60% to 85% of maximal heart rate. It is generally regarded that performing in the higher levels of percentage of maximal heart rate achieves greater cardiovascular efficiency and endurance.

A complete cardiovascular exercise program is an important component of the latter phases of rehabilitation. In addition to the previously described exercises, an aquatic program that includes lap work using freestyle or flutter kicking, water-walking, water aerobics, and deep-water running is initiated. Determining which cardiovascular exercises are appropriate is based on each individual patient. Factors to assess include concomitant operative procedures, secondary injuries, access to specific equipment, individual preferences, and prior experience.

Running and Agility Program

Current studies do not allow a prediction of return of strength of PCL grafts; hence, conservative estimates regarding return to strenuous activities are warranted. In order to initiate the running program, the patient must demonstrate no more than a 30% deficit in average torque for the quadriceps and hamstrings on isometric testing, have no more than 3 mm of increase in anteroposterior displacement on arthrometer testing, and be at least 6 months postoperative. The running program in an elite athlete under ideal conditions described after a quadriceps tendon–patellar bone autograft has been found in the authors' clinic to be safe and not result in graft stretching or an increase in posterior tibial translation. However, most recreational athletes do not start the program until 9 to 12 months after surgery. The rules for when to introduce more strenuous running and cutting activities for allografts have not been scientifically established. In general, a prudent rule is to provide additional time for graft healing and remodeling and wait until 12 months, although it is recognized that allograft healing is delayed even further. The running program is designed based on the sport the patient desires to return to, as well as the particular position or physical requirements of the activity. For instance, an individual returning back to short-duration, high-intensity activities participates in a sprinting program rather than a long-distance endurance program.

The beginning level running program is first performed with a straight-ahead walk/run combination. Running distances are 20, 40, 60, and 100 yards (18, 37, 55, and 91 m) in both forward and backward directions. Initially, running speed is approximately one fourth to one half of the patient's normal speed, and gradually progresses to three fourths and full speed. An interval training–rest approach is applied in which the rest phase is two to three times the length of the training phase. The running program is performed three times per week, on opposite days of the strength program. Because the running program may not reach aerobic levels initially, a cross-training program is used to facilitate cardiovascular fitness. The cross-training program is performed on the same day as the strength workout.

After the patient is able to run straight ahead at full speed, the program progresses to include lateral running and crossover

---

Critical Points CONDITIONING

3–4 Wk Postoperative
- UBC.

5–6 Wk Postoperative
- Stationary bicycling (patellofemoral joint precautions).

9–12 Wk Postoperative
- Stationary bicycling.
- Water-walking.
- Stair-climbing machine.
- Cross-country ski machine.

13 Wk and Beyond
- Add swimming, walking.

    Cardio program done 3 times/wk, 20- to 30-min sessions.
    Exercise level should be at least 60%–85% of maximal heart rate.

UBC, upper body cycle.

Critical Points RUNNING PROGRAM, RETURN TO SPORTS ACTIVITIES

Running Program
- Begin 6 mo postoperative if no more than 30% deficit on quadriceps & hamstrings peak torque on isometric testing.
- Use walk/run program initially, 3 times/wk
  - 18, 37, 55, 91 m.
  - 25%–50% normal running speed, straight.
  - Progress to 100% speed.
- Add lateral, crossover maneuvers, 18 m.
- Figure-eight running drills, 18 m initially, decrease to 9 m.
- Cutting patterns, directional change at 45° and 90°.

Return to Sports Activities
- Sports-specific drills done based on patient goals.
- No more than 10% deficit quadriceps & hamstrings peak torque on isokinetic testing.
- Successful completion running and functional training.
- Trial of function recommended, monitor for overuse symptoms.

maneuvers. Short distances, such as 20 yards (18 m), are used to work on speed and agility. Side-to-side running over cups may be used to facilitate proprioception. At this time, sports-specific equipment is introduced to enhance skill development (e.g., a soccer ball for a soccer player to work on dribbling and passing activities). These variations are useful to motivate the patient and minimize training boredom.

The third level of the running program incorporates figure-eight running drills. These drills begin with long and wide movement patterns to encourage subtle cutting. The training distance initially is 20 yards (18 m); as speed and confidence improve, the distance is decreased to approximately 10 yards (9 m). Progression through this phase is similar to that used in the lateral side-to-side program just described. Speed and agility are emphasized, and as well, equipment is introduced to develop sports-specific skills.

The fourth phase in the running program introduces cutting patterns. These patterns include directional changes at 45° and 90° angles that allow the patient to progress from subtle to sharp cuts.

Plyometric Training

Plyometric training is begun upon successful completion of the running program in order to minimize bilateral alterations in neuromuscular function and proprioception. This training begins after the 9th postoperative month for patients who desire to return to strenuous athletics. Again, this training should be delayed on an empirical basis to 12 months when PCL allografts are used. The patient should demonstrate no more than a 20% deficit for the quadriceps and hamstrings on isokinetic testing. Important parameters when performing plyometric exercises are surface, footwear, and warm-up. The jump drills should be done on a firm, yet forgiving surface such as a wooden gym floor. Very hard surfaces like concrete should be avoided. A cross-training or running shoe should be worn to provide adequate shock absorption as well as adequate stability to the foot. Checking wear patterns and outer sole wear will help avoid overuse injuries.

During the jumps, the patient is instructed to keep the body weight on the balls of the feet and to jump and land with the knees flexed and a shoulder-width apart to avoid knee hyperextension and an overall valgus lower limb position (Fig. 23-19), as described in detail in Chapter 19, Decreasing the Risk of Anterior Cruciate Ligament Injuries in Female Athletes. The patient should understand that the exercises are reaction and agility drills and, although speed is emphasized, correct body posture must be maintained throughout the drills.

The first exercise is level surface box-hopping using both legs. A four-square grid of four equally sized boxes is created with tape on the floor. The patient is instructed to first hop from box 1 to box 3 (front-to-back) and then from box 1 to box 2 (side-to-side). The second level incorporates both of these directions into one sequence and also includes hopping in both right and left directions (e.g., box 1 to box 2 to box 4 to box 2 to box 1). Level-three progresses to diagonal hops, and level four includes pivot hops in 90° and 180° directions. Once the patient can perform level four double-leg hops, the same exercises are done on a single leg. The next phase incorporates vertical box hops.

It is important to stress that plyometric exercise is intense and adequate rest must be included in the program. Individual sessions can be performed in a manner similar to that for interval training. Initially, the rest period lasts two to three times the length of the exercise period and is gradually decreased to one to

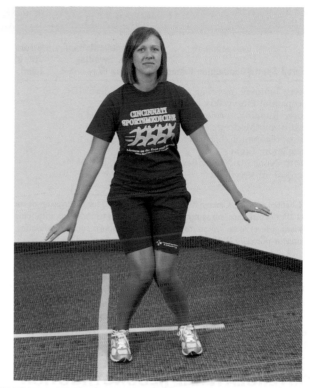

FIGURE 23-19. An improper, overall valgus lower limb position on landing a plyometric jumping exercise.

two times the length of the exercise period. Plyometric training is performed two to three times weekly.

Improvement is measured by counting the number of hops in a defined time period. The initial exercise time period is 15 seconds. The patient is asked to complete as many hops between the squares as possible in 15 seconds. Three sets are performed for both directions and the number of hops recorded. The program is progressed as the number of hops increases, along with patient confidence.

Return to Sports Activities

Discharge criteria after PCL reconstruction is based on patient goals for athletics and occupations and the rating of symptoms, stress radiography (90° flexion), KT-2000 testing, muscle strength testing, and function testing (Table 23-2). First, patients complete the Cincinnati Sports Activity Scale and Occupational Rating Scale[1] to provide sports and occupational levels that are desired after surgery. Upon completion of the protocol, pain, swelling, and giving-way are rated on the Cincinnati Symptom Rating Scale.[1] The patient must not experience these symptoms at the level of activity that he or she wishes to participate in prior to discharge.

Stress radiography is performed as described previously,[6] and the difference between knees must be within 5 mm prior to recommendation of return to strenuous activities.

Muscle strength testing is performed with a Biodex isokinetic dynamometer (Biodex Corporation, Shirley, NY) to ensure that adequate strength exists prior to the initiation of the plyometric, running, and cutting programs. At least two function tests are completed and limb symmetry calculated as previously described[11] prior to the final discharge.

A trial of function is encouraged in which the patient is monitored for overuse symptoms or giving-way episodes. Upon

PHASE 1. WEEKS 1 TO 2 (VISITS: 2–4)—Cont'd

Frequency		Duration
3–4 x/day	**ROM**	
10 min	ROM (passive, 0°–90°)	
	Patella mobilization	
	Ankle pumps (plantar flexion with resistance band)	
	Hamstring, gastrocnemius-soleus stretches	5 reps x 30 sec
3 x/day	**Strengthening**	
15 min	Straight leg raises (flexion)	3 sets x 10 reps
	Active quadriceps isometrics	1 set x 10 reps
	Knee extension (active-assisted, 90°–30°, per quadriceps control)	3 sets x 10 reps
As required	**Modalities**	
	EMS	20 min
	Cryotherapy	20 min
Goals	ROM 0°–90°	
	Adequate quadriceps contraction	
	Control inflammation, effusion	

PHASE 2. WEEKS 3 TO 4 (VISITS: 2–4)

General Observation	Non–weight-bearing, maximum protection	
	Bivalved cylinder cast	
	Must avoid hyperextension, varus loads, lateral joint opening	

Evaluation		Goals
	Pain	Controlled
	Effusion	Mild
	Patellar mobility	Good
	ROM minimum	0°–90°
	Quadriceps contraction & patella migration	Good
	Soft tissue contracture	None

Frequency		Duration
3–4 x/day	**ROM**	
10 min	ROM (passive, 0°–90°)	
	Patella mobilization	
	Ankle pumps (plantar flexion with resistance band)	
	Hamstring, gastrocnemius-soleus stretches	5 reps x 30 sec
2–3 x/day	**Strengthening**	
20 min	Straight leg raises (flexion)	3 sets x 10 reps
	Isometric training: multiangle (0°, 60°)	1 set x 10 reps
	Knee extension (active-assisted, 90°–30°, per quadriceps control)	3 sets x 10 reps
2 x/day	**Aerobic conditioning**	
10 min	UBC	
As required	**Modalities**	
	EMS	20 min
	Cryotherapy	20 min
Goals	ROM 0°–90°	
	Control inflammation, effusion	
	Muscle control	

PHASE 3. WEEKS 5 TO 6 (VISITS: 1–2)

General Observation	Partial (25%–50%) weight-bearing when	
	• Pain controlled without narcotics	
	• Hemarthrosis controlled	
	• ROM 0°–100°	
	• Muscle control throughout ROM	
	Custom medial unloader brace or hinged soft tissue brace	
	Avoid hyperextension, varus loads	

Evaluation		Goals
	Pain	Mild/No RSD
	Effusion	Minimal
	Patellar mobility	Good
	ROM	0°–110°
	Muscle control	3/5
	Inflammatory response	None

PHASE 3. WEEKS 5 TO 6 (VISITS: 1–2)—Cont'd

Frequency		Duration
3 x/day 10 min	**ROM** ROM (passive, 0°–110°) Patella mobilization Hamstring, gastrocnemius-soleus stretches	5 reps x 30 sec
2 x/day 20 min	**Strengthening** Straight leg raises (flexion: ankle weight, <10% of body weight) Isometric training: multiangle (90°, 60°, 30°) Closed chain • Mini-squats Knee extension (active, 90°–30°)	3 sets x 10 reps 2 sets x 10 reps 3 sets x 20 reps 3 sets x 10 reps
2 x/day 10 min	**Aerobic conditioning** (patellofemoral precautions) UBC Stationary bicycling **Gait retraining** (high risk for stretching reconstruction with resumption of weight-bearing) Muscle control quadriceps & hamstrings Walk with toe-out gait, avoid toe-in varus position Observe gait for any varus thrust or hyperextension Smooth stance-phase flexion pattern	
As required	**Modalities** EMS Cryotherapy	20 min 20 min
Goals	ROM 0°–110° Control inflammation, effusion Muscle control Early recognition complications (motion, RSD, patellofemoral) 50% weight bearing	

PHASE 4. WEEKS 7 TO 8 (VISITS: 1–2)

General Observation	Full weight bearing with cane when • Pain controlled • Hemarthrosis controlled • ROM 0°–120° • Voluntary quadriceps contraction achieved Custom medial unloader brace or hinged soft tissue brace	

Evaluation		Goals
	Pain	Mild/No RSD
	Effusion	Minimal
	Patellar mobility	Good
	ROM	0°–120°
	Muscle control	4/5
	Inflammatory response	None

Frequency		Duration
2 x/day 10 min	**ROM** ROM (0°–120°) Patella mobilization Hamstring, gastrocnemius-soleus stretches	5 reps x 30 sec
2 x/day 20 min	**Strengthening** Straight leg raises (flexion, extension, abduction, adduction) Straight leg raises, rubber tubing Knee extension (active, 90°–30°) Closed chain • Wall sits • Mini-squats (rubber tubing, 0°–30°)	3 sets x 10 reps 3 sets x 30 reps 3 sets x 10 reps To fatigue x 3 3 sets x 20 reps
3 x/day 5 min	**Balance training** Cup-walking	
1–2 x/day 15 min	**Aerobic conditioning** UBC Stationary bicycling	

Continued

	PHASE 4. WEEKS 7 TO 8 (VISITS: 1–2)—Cont'd	
	Gait retraining	
	Progress program	
	Continue to observe for varus thrust, hyperextension	
As required	**Modalities**	
	EMS	20 min
	Cryotherapy	20 min
Goals	Full weight-bearing	
	Muscle control	
	Control inflammation, effusion	
	ROM 0°–120°	

	PHASE 5. WEEKS 9 TO 12 (VISITS: 1–2)	
General Observation	Full weight-bearing (wk 12) when	
	• Pain, effusion controlled	
	• Muscle control throughout ROM	
	ROM 0°–135°	
	Custom medial unloader brace or hinged soft tissue brace	

Evaluation		**Goals**
	Pain	Minimal/No RSD
	Manual muscle test (hamstrings, quadriceps, hip abductors/adductors/flexors/extensors)	4/5
	Swelling	Minimal
	Patellar mobility	Good
	Crepitus	None/slight
	Gait	Symmetrical

Frequency		**Duration**
2 x/day	**ROM**	
10 min	Hamstring, gastrocnemius-soleus, quadriceps, ITB stretches	5 reps x 30 sec
2 x/day	**Strengthening**	
20 min	Straight leg raises	3 sets x 10 reps
	Straight leg raises, rubber tubing	3 sets x 30 reps
	Hamstring curls (wk 12, active, 0°–90°)	3 sets x 10 reps
	Knee extension with resistance (90°–30°)	3 sets x 10 reps
	Leg press (70°–10°)	3 sets x 10 reps
	Closed chain	
	• Wall-sits	To fatigue x 3
	• Mini-squats (rubber tubing, 0°–40°)	3 sets x 20 reps
	• Lateral step-ups (2"–4" block)	3 sets x 10 reps
	Multi-hip machine (flexion, extension, abduction, adduction)	3 sets x 10 reps
3 x/day	**Balance training**	
5 min	Cup-walking	
1 x/day	**Aerobic conditioning** (patellofemoral precautions)	
15–20 min	Water-walking	
	Swimming (straight leg kicking)	
	Stationary bicycling	
	Stair machine (low resistance, low stroke)	
As required	**Modalities**	
	Cryotherapy	20 min
Goals	Increase strength and endurance	
	ROM 0°–130°	
	Normal gait without varus, hyperextension	

	PHASE 6. WEEKS 13 TO 26 (VISITS: 2–3)	
General Observation	No effusion, painless ROM, joint stability	
	Performs activities of daily living, can walk 20 min without pain	
	ROM 0°–130°	
	Custom medial unloader brace or hinged soft tissue brace	

Evaluation		**Goals**
	Pain	Minimal/No RSD
	Manual muscle test	4/5
	Swelling	Minimal

PHASE 6. WEEKS 13 TO 26 (VISITS: 2–3)—Cont'd

	Patellar mobility	Good
	Crepitus	None/slight
	Gait	Symmetrical

Frequency		**Duration**
2 x/day 10 min	**ROM** Hamstring, gastrocnemius-soleus, quadriceps, ITB stretches	5 reps x 30 sec

2 x/day
20 min
	Strengthening
	   Straight leg raises, rubber tubing (high speed)
	   Hamstring curls (active, 0°–90°)
	   Knee extension with resistance (90°–30°)
	   Leg press (70°–10°)
	   Multi-hip machine (flexion, extension, abduction, adduction)
	   Closed chain
	      • Mini-squats (rubber tubing, 0°–40°)
		3 sets x 30 reps
		3 sets x 10 reps
		3 sets x 10 reps
		3 sets x 10 reps
		3 sets x 10 reps
		
		3 sets x 20 reps

1–3 x/day
5 min
	Balance training
	   Balance board/two-legged
	   Single-leg stance	

3 x/week
20 min
	Aerobic conditioning (patellofemoral precautions)
	   Stationary bicycling
	   Water-walking
	   Swimming (kicking)
	   Walking
	   Stair machine (low resistance, low stroke)
	   Ski machine (short stride, level, low resistance)	

As required	**Modalities** Cryotherapy	20 min
Goals	Increase strength and endurance	

PHASE 7. WEEKS 27 TO 52 (VISITS: 2–3)

General Observation	No effusion, painless ROM, joint stability Performs activities of daily living, can walk 20 min without pain Custom medial unloader brace or hinged soft tissue brace	

Evaluation		**Goals**
	Isometric test (% difference between quadriceps & hamstrings) Swelling Patellar mobility Crepitus	10–15 None Good None/slight

Frequency		**Duration**
2 x/day 10 min	**ROM** Hamstring, gastrocnemius-soleus, quadriceps, ITB stretches	5 reps x 30 sec

1 x/day
20–30 min
	Strengthening
	   Straight leg raises, rubber tubing (high speed)
	   Hamstring curls (0°–90°)
	   Knee extension with resistance (90°–30°)
	   Leg press (70°–10°)
	   Multi-hip machine (flexion, extension, abduction, adduction)
	   Closed chain
	      • Mini-squats (rubber tubing, 0°–40°)
		3 sets x 30 reps
		3 sets x 10 reps
		3 sets x 10 reps
		3 sets x 10 reps
		3 sets x 10 reps
		
		3 sets x 20 reps

1–3 x/day
5 min
	Balance training
	   Balance board/two-legged
	   Single-leg stance	

3 x/wk
20–30 min
	Aerobic conditioning (patellofemoral precautions)
	   Stationary bicycling
	   Water-walking
	   Swimming (kicking)
	   Walking
	   Stair machine (low resistance, low stroke)
	   Ski machine (short stride, level, low resistance)	

Continued

PHASE 7. WEEKS 27 TO 52 (VISITS: 2–3)—Cont'd		
3 x/wk 15–20 min	**Running program** (9 mo. minimum, straight, 30% deficit isometric test)	
	Jog	¼ mile
	Walk	¼ mile
	Backward run	20 yd
3 x/wk	**Cutting program** (12 mo minimum, 20% deficit isometric test)	
	Lateral, carioca, figure-eights	20 yd
3 x/wk	**Functional training** (12 mo minimum)	
	Plyometric training: box hops, level, double-leg	15 sec,
	Sports-specific drills (10–15% deficit isometric test)	4–6 sets
As required	**Modalities**	
	Cryotherapy	20 min
Goals	Increase function Return to previous activity level Maintain strength, endurance	

BAPS, Biomechanical Ankle Platform System (Camp, Jackson, MI); BBS, Biodex Balance System (Biodex Medical Systems, Inc., Shirley, NY); EMS, electrical muscle stimulation; ITB, iliotibial band; ROM, range of motion; RSD, reflex sympathetic dystrophy; UBC, upper body cycle (Biodex Medical Systems, Inc., Shirley, NY).

the bivalved cylinder cast is contraindicated. There are commercially available soft tissue hinged braces that have a design in which the hinge support and medial-lateral arms are more rigid that provide (when properly applied) a resistance to prevent abnormal lateral joint opening with ambulation. A more-flexible hinged soft tissue brace is not advised. The surgeon provides information on the expected strength of the posterolateral reconstruction. For example, a double-graft anatomic reconstruction provides considerable strength to allow a soft-hinged brace. A single femorofibular graft reconstruction has less strength, and more postoperative protection is required for the first 4 weeks.

At 7 to 8 weeks, a custom medial unloading brace is applied as weight-bearing progresses to full and flexion is advanced to 120°. The brace is also used to provide protection against knee hyperextension and excessive varus loads as patients return to activity.

Patients are allowed 0° to 90° immediately postoperatively. Flexion is slowly advanced to 110° by postoperative week 5, 120° by week 8, and 130° by week 12. Patients are cautioned to avoid varus tensioning when performing knee flexion exercises. They are taught (and the assistance of a partner is encouraged) to place a hand on the lateral aspect of the knee and create a 10-pound valgus load to protect the posterolateral structures.

Patients are not allowed to bear weight for the first 2 postoperative weeks. Then, partial weight-bearing (25% of the patient's body weight) is begun at postoperative weeks 3 to 4, with slow advancement to full by week 8 with cane or crutch support, which is used for approximately another 3 to 4 weeks. Patients are warned to avoid knee hyperextension and activities that would incur varus loading, external tibial rotation, or lateral joint opening.

Patellar mobilization, flexibility exercises, modality usage, and the strengthening and conditioning programs are all similar to those described in the PCL reconstruction protocol.

In select athletes, a running program is begun at approximately the 9th postoperative month, and plyometric- and sports-specific–training programs are initiated at the 12th postoperative month. However, the majority of patients who require multiple ligament reconstructive procedures do not desire to return to high-impact sports, and therefore, this advanced conditioning and training is usually not required. Patients who have articular cartilage damage are advised to return to only low-impact activities to protect the knee joint.

Discharge criteria after lateral and posterolateral graft reconstructions is based on patient goals for athletics and occupations and the rating of symptoms, lateral joint opening, muscle strength testing, and function testing (Table 23–4). Lateral joint opening is assessed by either stress radiography or manual testing at 20° of flexion. The remainder of the assessment is performed as previously described for PCL reconstructions.

TABLE 23–4   Discharge Rehabilitation Criteria after Posterolateral Reconstruction

Desired Sports/Occupation Rating*	Symptom Rating[†] Pain, Swelling, Giving-Way	Lateral Joint Opening (20°, I-N, mm)	Biodex Isometric Test (% deficit I-N)	Function Testing Limb Symmetry (%)
Sports: Jumping, pivoting, cutting Occupation: Heavy/very heavy	None, level 10	None	≤15	>85
Sports: Running, turning, twisting Occupation: Moderate	None, level 8	<3	≤20	≥85
Sports: Swimming, bicycling Occupation: Light	None, level 6	3–5	≤30	≥75
Sports: None, daily activities only Occupation: Very light	None, level 4	3–5	≥30	≥75

*See Chapter 44, The Cincinnati Knee Rating System, on Knee Rating Outcome Instruments for description of sports and occupational rating levels.
[†]Level 10, normal knee, no symptoms with strenuous work/sports with jumping, hard pivoting; level 8, no symptoms with moderate work/sports with running, turning, twisting; level 6, no symptoms with light work/sports such as swimming, bicycling; level 4, no symptoms with daily activities.
I-N, involved limb minus noninvolved limb.

REFERENCES

1. Barber-Westin, S. D.; Noyes, F. R.; McCloskey, J. W.: Rigorous statistical reliability, validity, and responsiveness testing of the Cincinnati Knee Rating System in 350 subjects with uninjured, injured, or anterior cruciate ligament–reconstructed knees. *Am J Sports Med* 27:402–416, 1999.

2. Berchuck, M.; Andriacchi, T. P.; Bach, B. R.; Reider, B.: Gait adaptations by patients who have a deficient anterior cruciate ligament. *J Bone Joint Surg Am* 72:871–877, 1990.

3. Butler, D. L.; Noyes, F. R.; Grood, E. S.: Ligamentous restraints to anterior-posterior drawer in the human knee. A biomechanical study. *J Bone Joint Surg Am* 62:259–270, 1980.

4. Castle, T. H., Jr.; Noyes, F. R.; Grood, E. S.: Posterior tibial subluxation of the posterior cruciate–deficient knee. *Clin Orthop* 284:193–202, 1992.

5. Durselen, L.; Claes, L.; Kiefer, H.: The influence of muscle forces and external loads on cruciate ligament strain. *Am J Sports Med* 23:129–136, 1995.

6. Hewett, T. E.; Noyes, F. R.; Lee, M. D.: Diagnosis of complete and partial posterior cruciate ligament ruptures. Stress radiography compared with KT-1000 arthrometer and posterior drawer testing. *Am J Sports Med* 25:648–655, 1997.

7. Hoher, J.; Vogrin, T. M.; Woo, S. L.; et al.: In situ forces in the human posterior cruciate ligament in response to muscle loads: a cadaveric study. *J Orthop Res* 17:763–768, 1999.

8. Kaufman, K. R.; An, K. N.; Litchy, W. J.; et al.: Dynamic joint forces during knee isokinetic exercise. *Am J Sports Med* 19:305–316, 1991.

9. Lutz, G. E.; Palmitier, R. A.; An, K. N.; Chao, E. Y.: Comparison of tibiofemoral joint forces during open-kinetic-chain and closed-kinetic-chain exercises. *J Bone Joint Surg Am* 75:732–739, 1993.

10. Markolf, K. L.; O'Neill, G.; Jackson, S. R.; McAllister, D. R.: Effects of applied quadriceps and hamstrings muscle loads on forces in the anterior and posterior cruciate ligaments. *Am J Sports Med* 32:1144–1149, 2004.

11. Noyes, F. R.; Barber, S. D.; Mangine, R. E.: Abnormal lower limb symmetry determined by function hop tests after anterior cruciate ligament rupture. *Am J Sports Med* 19:513–518, 1991.

12. Noyes, F. R.; Barber-Westin, S.: Posterior cruciate ligament replacement with a two-strand quadriceps tendon–patellar bone autograft and a tibial inlay technique. *J Bone Joint Surg Am* 87:1241–1252, 2005.

13. Noyes, F. R.; Dunworth, L. A.; Andriacchi, T. P.; et al.: Knee hyperextension gait abnormalities in unstable knees. Recognition and preoperative gait retraining. *Am J Sports Med* 24:35–45, 1996.

14. Noyes, F. R.; Grood, E. S.: Diagnosis of knee ligament injuries: five concepts. In Feagin, J. (ed.): *The Crucial Ligaments*. New York: Churchill Livingstone, 1988.

15. Noyes, F. R.; Heckmann, T. P.; Barber-Westin, S. D.: Posterior cruciate ligament and posterolateral reconstruction. In Ellenbecker, T. S. (ed.): *Knee Ligament Rehabilitation*. Philadelphia: Churchill Livingstone, 2000; pp. 167–185.

16. Noyes, F. R.; Schipplein, O. D.; Andriacchi, T. P.; et al.: The anterior cruciate ligament–deficient knee with varus alignment. An analysis of gait adaptations and dynamic joint loadings. *Am J Sports Med* 20:707–716, 1992.

17. Noyes, F. R.; Stowers, S. F.; Grood, E. S.; et al.: Posterior subluxations of the medial and lateral tibiofemoral compartments. An in vitro ligament sectioning study in cadaveric knees. *Am J Sports Med* 21:407–414, 1993.

18. Noyes, F. R.; Wojtys, E. M.; Marshall, M. T.: The early diagnosis and treatment of developmental patella infera syndrome. *Clin Orthop* 265:241–252, 1991.

19. Ohkoshi, Y.; Yasuda, K.; Kaneda, K.; et al.: Biomechanical analysis of rehabilitation in the standing position. *Am J Sports Med* 19:605–611, 1991.

20. Shearn, J. T.; Grood, E. S.; Noyes, F. R.; Levy, M. S.: One- and two-strand posterior cruciate ligament reconstructions: cyclic fatigue testing. *J Orthop Res* 23:958–963, 2005.

21. Smidt, G. L.: Biomechanical analysis of knee flexion and extension. *J Biomech* 6:79–92, 1973.

22. Toutoungi, D. E.; Lu, T. W.; Leardini, A.; et al.: Cruciate ligament forces in the human knee during rehabilitation exercises. *Clin Biomech (Bristol, Avon)* 15:176–187, 2000.

23. Wilk, K. E.; Escamilla, R. F.; Fleisig, G. S.; et al.: A comparison of tibiofemoral joint forces and electromyographic activity during open and closed kinetic chain exercises. *Am J Sports Med* 24:518–527, 1996.

24. Zavatsky, A. B.; Beard, D. J.; O'Connor, J. J.: Cruciate ligament loading during isometric muscle contractions. A theoretical basis for rehabilitation. *Am J Sports Med* 22:418–423, 1994.

Medial Collateral Ligament

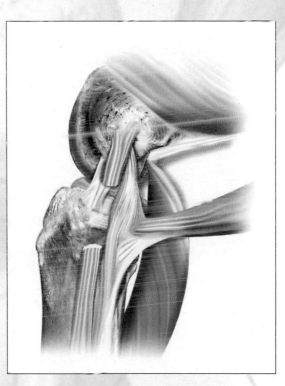

Medial and Posteromedial Ligament Injuries: Diagnosis, Operative Techniques, and Clinical Outcomes

Frank R. Noyes, MD ▪ *Sue D. Barber-Westin*, BS

INDICATIONS

Medial ligament injuries are among the most frequently treated problems of the knee joint, with the majority not requiring operative intervention. Whereas isolated superficial medial collateral ligament (SMCL) ruptures are common, concomitant damage to the anterior cruciate ligament (ACL) also occurs in many cases, especially in young and active patients.[6,11,14,28,33]

Overall, there are four types of SMCL injury patterns: (1) SMCL alone, (2) associated posteromedial capsular (PMC) tears (posterior oblique ligament [POL]), (3) associated ACL or posterior cruciate ligament (PCL) tears with patterns 1 or 2, and (4) multiple ligament injuries or knee dislocations.

The mechanism of injury to the medial ligaments involves a valgus stress with usually a combined external tibial rotation component from either a noncontact (pivoting or cutting) or a contact injury (direct blow to the lateral side of the thigh or knee). The decision process regarding the appropriate treatment of medial ligament injuries involves determining the severity of the injury to the entire knee, including the other knee ligaments, and the specific injury pattern of the medial structures and menisci.

Critical Points INDICATIONS

- Medial ligament injuries are among the most frequently treated problems of the knee joint, with the majority not requiring operative intervention.
- Decision regarding treatment involves determining the severity of injury to the entire knee, including all of the medial structures and other knee ligaments.
- Medial structures identified for surgical treatment are the superficial medial collateral ligament (SMCL), deep medial collateral ligament (DMCL; including meniscus attachments), and the posteromedial capsule (PMC; including the posterior oblique ligament [POL] and semimembranosus attachments).
- Majority acute injuries that involve damage to the SMCL alone, or SMCL and PMC, are treated conservatively.
- Knees with gross major disruption of all of the medial structures alone or in addition to the anterior cruciate ligament (ACL) or posterior cruciate ligament (PCL) tears may require surgery.
- Chronic medial injuries: determine complaints of giving-way and the levels of activity at which these symptoms occur as an indication for reconstruction.

The medial structures identified for purposes of surgical treatment consist of the SMCL, deep medial collateral ligament (DMCL, including meniscus attachments), and the PMC, which includes the structures referred to as the POL and semimembranosus attachments.[22,44] The key to the diagnosis and treatment of medial ligament injuries relies on a comprehensive understanding of the intricate anatomy on the medial side of the knee. This is presented in detail in Chapter 1, Medial and Anterior Knee Anatomy. In Figure 24–1, the osseous attachments of the medial structures are shown. Figure 24–2 shows the medial and posteromedial ligament structures, which are discussed in detail. Figure 24–3 shows the relationship of the semimembranosus muscle attachments to the posteromedial structures and POL. These include the bifurcation of the semimembranosus tendon into a direct and anterior area just distal to the joint line and a minor attachment of the direct arm to the medial coronary ligament along the posterior horn of the medial meniscus. The semimembranosus tendon sheath makes up a distal tibial expansion that includes a medial and lateral division. A major attachment of the semimembranosus forms the oblique popliteal ligament, which is a broad fascial band that courses laterally attaching to the fabella, posterolateral capsule, and plantaris (see Chapter 1, Medial and Anterior Knee Anatomy, Figs. 1–4 to 1–10).

It is important to understand and classify the soft tissue injury of all the medial structures. The majority of acute medial ligament injuries that involve damage to the SMCL alone, or SMCL and PMC, are treated conservatively. The nonoperative treatment algorithm is shown in Figure 24–4 and discussed later in more detail. Gross major disruption of all of the medial structures alone or in addition to the ACL or PCL tears involve a group of select knees. The treatment of these gross ligament disruptions is discussed in a later section of this chapter.

In cases of chronic injury to the medial ligaments, it is important to obtain a complete history and objective and functional rating. The authors' use the Cincinnati Knee Rating System (CKRS) for this analysis (see Chapter 44, The Cincinnati Knee Rating System) to determine patient complaints of giving-way and the levels of activity at which this symptom occurs as an indication for surgical stabilization procedures. In this chapter, *instability* refers to an increase in abnormal motion limits as detected on the physical examination, and is not used to indicate giving-way events.

CONTRAINDICATIONS

Patients that have medial ligament tears classified as first, second, or third degree that demonstrate either no increase or a mild to moderate increase in medial joint opening at 0° and 30° of flexion do not require acute medial ligament reconstruction.

A valgus malalignment and valgus thrust on walking contraindicates a medial ligament reconstruction in chronic cases without first performing an osteotomy to correct the lower limb malalignment. Alternatively, a genu varus provides a theoretical benefit of decreased tensile loads on the medial ligament structures.

In chronic cases of disruption of the medial ligaments, particularly associated with ACL or PCL tears, joint arthritis and associated pain and swelling may exist that contraindicate a soft tissue reconstruction. The patient goals and anticipated symptoms from the preexisting arthrosis are carefully considered.

FIGURE 24–1. The medial capsule, ligament, and muscle bone attachments are shown. A key to surgical repair and reconstruction of medial injuries is to restore normal anatomy and attachment locations.

MEDIAL KNEE ATTACHMENTS

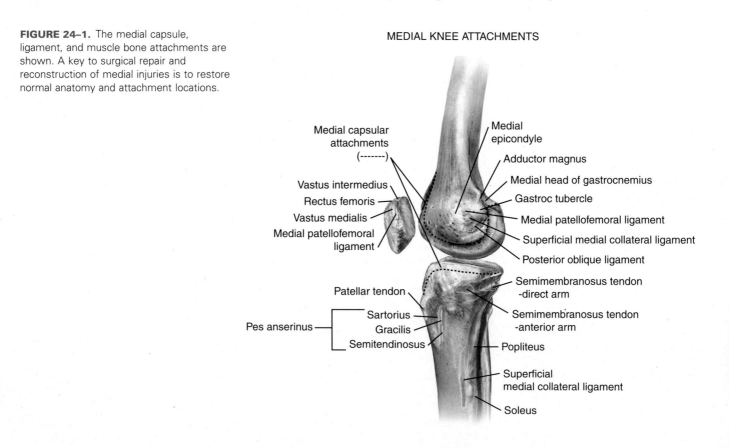

Medial capsular attachments (-------)
Vastus intermedius
Rectus femoris
Vastus medialis
Medial patellofemoral ligament
Patellar tendon
Pes anserinus
Sartorius
Gracilis
Semitendinosus
Medial epicondyle
Adductor magnus
Medial head of gastrocnemius
Gastroc tubercle
Medial patellofemoral ligament
Superficial medial collateral ligament
Posterior oblique ligament
Semimembranosus tendon -direct arm
Semimembranosus tendon -anterior arm
Popliteus
Superficial medial collateral ligament
Soleus

POSTERIOR OBLIQUE LIGAMENT (POL)

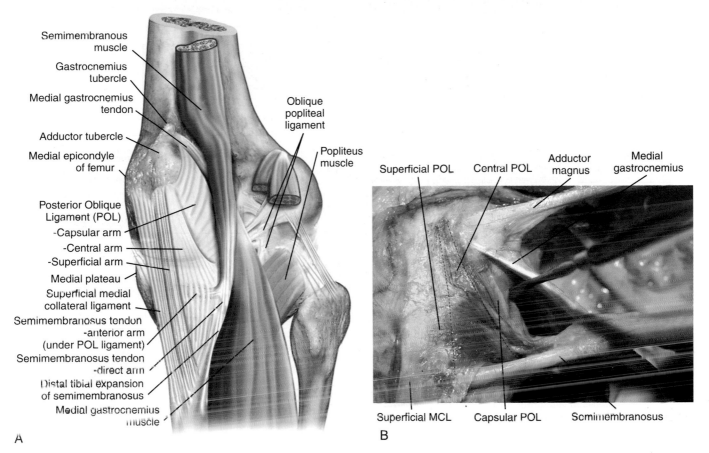

Semimembranous muscle

Gastrocnemius tubercle

Medial gastrocnemius tendon

Adductor tubercle

Medial epicondyle of femur

Posterior Oblique Ligament (POL)
-Capsular arm
-Central arm
-Superficial arm

Medial plateau

Superficial medial collateral ligament

Semimembranosus tendon
-anterior arm
(under POL ligament)

Semimembranosus tendon
-direct arm

Distal tibial expansion of semimembranosus

Medial gastrocnemius muscle

Oblique popliteal ligament

Popliteus muscle

A

Superficial POL   Central POL   Adductor magnus   Medial gastrocnemius

Superficial MCL   Capsular POL   Semimembranosus

B

FIGURE 24–2. A and **B**, The anatomy of the medial and posteromedial aspect of the knee. The posteromedial capsule is shown divided into three functional regions, commonly designated as the *posterior oblique ligament (POL)*.

MEDIAL KNEE LIGAMENTS

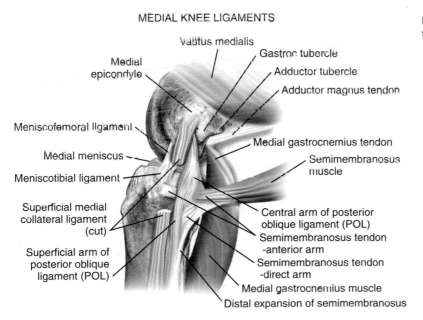

Vastus medialis

Medial epicondyle

Meniscofemoral ligament

Medial meniscus

Meniscotibial ligament

Superficial medial collateral ligament (cut)

Superficial arm of posterior oblique ligament (POL)

Gastroc tubercle

Adductor tubercle

Adductor magnus tendon

Medial gastrocnemius tendon

Semimembranosus muscle

Central arm of posterior oblique ligament (POL)

Semimembranosus tendon
-anterior arm

Semimembranosus tendon
-direct arm

Medial gastrocnemius muscle

Distal expansion of semimembranosus

FIGURE 24–3. Semimembranosus muscle attachments to the posteromedial structures.

examination (see Chapter 21, Posterior Cruciate Ligament: Diagnosis, Operative Techniques, and Clinical Outcomes).[16] Lateral stress radiographs may be required in knees with lateral ligament injury (see Chapter 22, Posterolateral Ligament Injuries: Diagnosis, Operative Techniques, and Clinical Outcomes). Full standing radiographs of both lower extremities, from the femoral heads to the ankle joints, are done in knees with varus or valgus lower extremity malalignment (see Chapter 31, Primary, Double, and Triple Varus Knee Syndrome: Diagnosis, Operative Techniques, and Clinical Outcomes). The mechanical axis and weight-bearing line are measured.[7] Of concern is to exclude a knee with lower extremity valgus alignment and increased medial soft tissue tensile forces with a valgus thrust, indicating the need for a corrective osteotomy in chronic medial injuries.

MRI is helpful to reveal the location of ligament anatomic disruptions, bone contusions, other ligament ruptures, and meniscus tears (Fig. 24–9). A high rate of concurrent lateral meniscus tears has been reported with MCL ruptures, making MRI an important adjunct for an accurate diagnosis.[30,41] Ligament avulsion or osteochondral injuries requiring treatment within the initial 7- to 10-day period after injury may exist.

CONSERVATIVE VERSUS OPERATIVE TREATMENT RULES AND PLANNING

Acute Medial and Posteromedial Ligament Ruptures

The treatment rationale for patients with acute medial ligament ruptures is shown in Figure 24–4. The algorithm is divided into three major sections based on the extent of injury to the SMCL and PMC/POL. The first- and second-degree injuries are treated initially with a functional brace, weight-bearing as tolerated, and rehabilitation as detailed in Chapter 25, Rehabilitation of Medial Ligament Injuries. Some second-degree injuries may have considerable medial pain and swelling; in these cases, an extension brace is used for the initial 1 to 2 weeks after the injury.

The rule for conservative treatment of all third-degree medial ligament injuries involves the necessity for short-term immobilization to allow the medial ligament structures to heal with the least elongation or laxity by limiting medial joint opening and external tibial rotation. In addition, meniscotibial attachment tears requiring protection for healing may exist. The lower limb is placed in a cylinder cast to allow "stick-down" of the disrupted medial soft tissues. Plaster

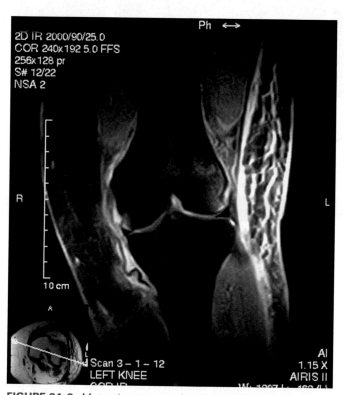

FIGURE 24–9. Magnetic resonance imaging (MRI) demonstrates extensive damage to the medial ligamentous structures. The superficial medial collateral ligament (SMCL) is disrupted from its proximal attachment and there is disruption of meniscus attachments and the POL. MRI provides important information on the injury severity. The finding of a coiled lax SMCL, particularly close to an attachment site, is a relative indication for surgery, because immobilization would not be expected to allow for approximation of the SMCL/POL injury. An open operative repair was performed in this athlete, along with an ACL reconstruction.

Critical Points CONSERVATIVE VERSUS OPERATIVE TREATMENT RULES AND PLANNING

Acute Injuries

- First- and second-degree injuries treated with a functional brace, weight-bearing as tolerated, rehabilitation.
- Third-degree injuries treated with short-term (10 days) immobilization, cylinder cast, to allow the medial ligament structures to heal. Toe-touch weight-bearing, quadriceps isometrics hourly, electrical muscle stimulation.
- 10 days, cast split into anterior/posterior shell, patient performs range of motion 0°–90° in figure-of-four position. 3 wk later, brace replaces cast.

Operative Treatment

- Injury rehabilitated for 7 days. If motion to 90° and initial quadriceps muscle function are restored, and the joint and extremity soft tissue swelling is in the mild range.
- Indications

  ○ Displaced meniscus tear.
  ○ High-performance athletes with complete disruption of SMCL and POL.
  ○ PCL tears with gross disruption of the SMCL and POL, all-inside arthroscopic PCL reconstruction and open medial repair.

Knee Dislocations

- Treat injury with stick-down conservative program; manage associated injuries at a later time period.
- Add posterior calf pad to cylinder cast to maintain gentle posterior loading, prevent posterior tibial subluxation.
- Lateral radiograph to verify tibiofemoral reduction.
- Vascular consultation indicated.
- Operative repair considered in athletic patients.

Chronic Injuries

- Patients with severe muscle atrophy require preoperative rehabilitation, patient education before consideration of reconstruction.
- Appropriate grafts for cruciate procedures determined preoperatively.

immobilization is required because a soft hinged or functional brace, even if maintained at 0° of extension, does not provide sufficient protection to maintain medial joint line closure to allow close approximation of the disrupted medial ligament and meniscus attachment soft tissues. Patients are allowed toe-touch weight-bearing and perform quadriceps isometrics every hour, palpating the muscle tension and increase in thigh volume with their hand. Electrical muscle stimulation is also used. These modalities are important because thigh atrophy can occur even with short-term immobilization.

At 7 days, the cylinder cast is split into an anterior and a posterior shell (Fig. 24–10) and the therapist assists the patient with ROM from 0° to 90° in a figure-of-four position (Fig. 24–11) with the hip joint externally rotated to protect the healing medial tissues, described in detail in Chapter 41, Prevention and Treatment of Knee Arthrosis. This protected ROM program is taught to the patient and performed three to four times a day. The split-cylinder cast protection in extension is maintained for 3 weeks, followed by a soft hinged brace. The rehabilitation and crutch-weaning program is detailed in Chapter 25, Rehabilitation of Medial Ligament Injuries. It must be stressed that the senior author has commonly encountered knees referred for treatment in which a complete SMCL injury (and partial-to-complete POL injury) was treated with a soft functional brace in which the golden period of the first few weeks after the injury was lost. A residual symptomatic increased medial joint opening

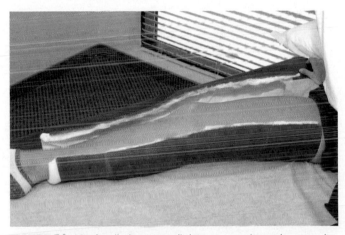

FIGURE 24–10. A cylinder cast split into an anterior and a posterior shell to allow the patient to perform range of motion exercises.

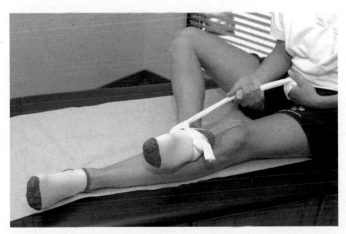

FIGURE 24–11. Flexion overpressure exercise in a figure-of-four position.

and external tibial rotation required a chronic medial and posteromedial reconstruction.

It is possible to treat almost all medial ligament injuries (with or without concomitant ACL ruptures) using this conservative stick-down program. Operative treatment is recommended for select cases, as discussed next. A displaced meniscus tear on MRI would indicate the necessity to perform a meniscus repair. When there is an associated ACL tear, an ACL reconstruction is performed at an elective time, or under ideal conditions (minimal swelling, early motion), an ACL procedure is performed along with the meniscus repair. In high-performance athletes with gross disruption of the SMCL and POL (with or without ACL tear), the senior author prefers to perform an anatomic repair to restore anatomic continuity and function. In addition, in these gross medial disruptions, the repair of the medial meniscus attachments is always required. In select knees with acute SMCL, POL, and ACL injuries, the medial meniscus may be partially dislodged from the joint, and the distal SMCL so extensively displaced or coiled, that there is a reduced chance that protected immobilization would result in functional medial ligament structures (see Fig. 24–9). An example is the illustrative case described later in this chapter. In the authors' experience, these knees do better with operative repair. A four-strand semitendinosus-gracilis (STG) autograft may be selected if there is an indication to decrease the morbidity of a bone-patellar tendon-bone (B-PT-B) autograft. The authors prefer an autograft over allografts for reasons discussed in detail in Chapter 7, Anterior Cruciate Ligament Primary and Revision Reconstruction: Diagnosis, Operative Techniques, and Clinical Outcomes.

In select acute PCL tears with gross disruption of the SMCL and POL that do not have excessive soft tissue swelling and edema, the senior author prefers an all-inside arthroscopic PCL reconstruction and open medial repair. These knees have a gross amount of medial joint opening and posterior subluxation; surgical stabilization is preferred in younger active patients. Sedentary patients are treated with the stick-down cast program, with a posterior calf pad added to prevent posterior subluxation (confirmed with a lateral radiograph). An SMCL femoral or tibial avulsion may exist in which operative reattachment is indicated through a limited medial approach.

In knees considered for operative intervention, the knee is rehabilitated for 7 days, motion to 90° is obtained, and early quadriceps muscle function is restored. The joint and extremity soft tissue swelling must not be excessive. A routine venous ultrasound is conducted before surgery. In acute medial injuries, it is usually not necessary to perform an augmentation of the repair (described later for chronic reconstructions), because the suture fixation methods restore ligament continuity and healing after surgery is prompt. These knees are treated with an immediate ROM program as detailed in Chapter 25, Rehabilitation of Medial Ligament Injuries. Proximal medial ligament disruptions with extensive edema and soft tissue swelling are at risk for ectopic calcification and limitation of joint motion in the first 2 to 3 weeks after surgery. Indomethacin (Indocin) treatment is not routinely administered; however, observation is warranted because indomethacin is only effective if given within the early postoperative course.

Acute Medial Ligament Ruptures with Knee Dislocation

A traumatic knee dislocation with involvement of the medial ligament structures along with the ACL and PCL represents a difficult treatment entity. Too often, these knees have a high incidence of arthrofibrosis after surgery. In the authors' opinion, it is prudent to treat these knees with the stick-down conservative program and manage the associated injuries at a later time. A posterior calf pad is added to the cylinder cast to maintain a gentle posterior loading and prevent posterior tibial subluxation. Again, a lateral radiograph is obtained to verify tibiofemoral reduction. It is possible for the physical therapist to begin a careful ROM program with the bivalved cylinder cast at the 2nd week as detailed in Chapter 41, Prevention and Treatment of Knee Arthrofibrosis. In select athletes, under ideal circumstances, operative intervention may be considered; these knee injuries are evaluated and treated on a case-by-case basis. Issues related to evaluation of the vascular system are discussed in Chapter 27, Management of Acute Knee Dislocations before Surgical Intervention. The surgery is delayed for 7 days and the initial rehabilitation program begun, as previously discussed. Consultation is always obtained with exclusion of a vascular injury by repeated evaluation and appropriate diagnostic tests including ankle-brachial indices, MRI, and arteriography as indicated. A venous ultrasound is obtained. At surgery, the foot and ankle are positioned to allow vascular checks including Doppler, and tourniquet use is limited to only the initial open exploration to define the injury pattern, then deflated for the repair procedure.

Chronic Medial and Posteromedial Ruptures

Patients with chronic knee injuries that present with severe muscle atrophy require preoperative rehabilitation and patient education before consideration of surgical reconstruction. Frequently, patients who undergo MCL reconstruction (Fig. 24–12) require a concomitant ACL or PCL reconstruction. The appropriate grafts for the cruciate procedures should be determined, as detailed in separate chapters, and autogenous tissues are preferred. However, the surgeon should ensure that B-PT-B and Achilles tendon–bone allografts are available in multiligament reconstructions if needed and advise the patient of this possible choice.

INTRAOPERATIVE EVALUATION

All knee ligament subluxation tests are performed after the induction of anesthesia in both the injured and the contralateral limbs. The amount of increased anterior tibial translation, posterior tibial translation, lateral joint opening, medial joint opening, and external-internal tibial rotation is documented. With ACL and/or SMCL/POL disruptions, the lower portion of the bed is flexed and flexion of the knee is performed as required for the arthroscopic and open approaches (Fig. 24–13A).

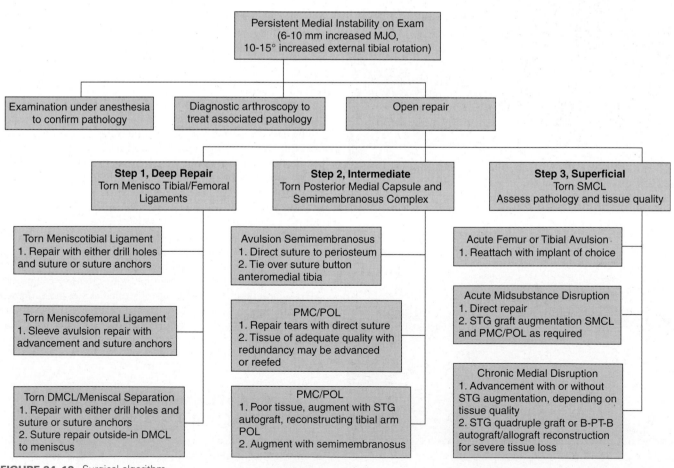

FIGURE 24–12. Surgical algorithm.

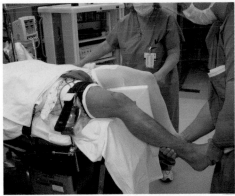

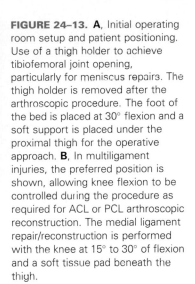

FIGURE 24–13. A, Initial operating room setup and patient positioning. Use of a thigh holder to achieve tibiofemoral joint opening, particularly for meniscus repairs. The thigh holder is removed after the arthroscopic procedure. The foot of the bed is placed at 30° flexion and a soft support is placed under the proximal thigh for the operative approach. **B**, In multiligament injuries, the preferred position is shown, allowing knee flexion to be controlled during the procedure as required for ACL or PCL arthroscopic reconstruction. The medial ligament repair/reconstruction is performed with the knee at 15° to 30° of flexion and a soft tissue pad beneath the thigh.

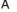

Critical Points INTRAOPERATIVE EVALUATION

- All knee ligament subluxation tests performed after induction of anesthesia in both limbs.
- Leg holder used for initial arthroscopic procedure, meniscus procedures, then removed.
- Arthroscopic pressure maintained at low setting with adequate outflow at all times.
- Thorough arthroscopic examination is conducted, procedures performed as indicated.
- Medial and lateral tibiofemoral gap test done: knees ≥ 12 mm or more of absolute joint opening at the periphery of a tibiofemoral compartment indicate gross disruption of all the ligament structures.

A leg holder is used for the initial arthroscopic and meniscus procedures and then removed. An alternative approach used in multiligament and PCL disruptions is to position the lower extremity with the foot in an Alvardo holder or thigh post and foot rest to allow the desired amount of knee flexion during surgery (see Fig. 24–13B). The arthroscopic pressure is maintained at a low setting with adequate outflow at all times to prevent fluid extravasation and popliteal and calf swelling, which is documented throughout the case. A thorough arthroscopic examination is conducted, documenting articular cartilage surface abnormalities and the condition of the menisci. It is rare to have the complication of fluid extravasation if these precautions are taken; however, if extravasation occurs, an open approach is used throughout the remainder of the procedure.

Medial and lateral tibiofemoral gap tests are done during the arthroscopic examination. The knee is flexed to 30° and a varus and valgus load of approximately 89 N applied. A calibrated nerve hook is used to measure the amount of lateral and medial tibiofemoral compartment opening. Knees that have 12 mm or more of absolute joint opening at the periphery of the medial or lateral tibiofemoral compartment indicate gross disruption of all the ligament structures. An absolute opening of 10 mm (~7 mm increase over the contralateral limb) also indicates significant injury to the SMCL and PMC and, along with increased

external tibial rotation, may represent a problem for athletic patients in twisting and cutting activities.

Appropriate arthroscopic procedures are performed as indicated including meniscus repairs or partial excision, débridement, and articular cartilage procedures.

OPERATIVE TREATMENT

Acute Medial and Posteromedial Ligament Repairs

The key to the operative procedure is a thorough understanding of the medial anatomy (see Figs. 24–1 to 24–3), because the integrity and injury to the SMCL, POL, semimembranosus attachments, and meniscus attachments (DMCL) need to be identified. The goal is to restore normal anatomy and function

---

Critical Points OPERATIVE TREATMENT

Acute Medial and Posteromedial Ligament Repairs

- Integrity, injury to SMCL, POL, semimembranosus attachments, meniscus attachments (DMCL) identified.
- Operative steps outlined in Table 24–3.
- Tourniquet used for initial exploration, then deflated during repair procedure.
- Limited cosmetic incision along the anteromedial aspect of the tibia preferred.
- First goal: restore normal anatomy, attachment sites.
- Second goal: perform meticulous anatomic repair of sufficient strength to allow immediate knee motion.

Chronic Medial and Posteromedial Ligament Repairs

- Operative steps outlined in Table 24–4.
- Use remaining SMCL as a part of the reconstruction by femoral or tibial advancement based on the site of the prior tears.
- Augment the SMCL reconstruction with semitendinosus-gracilis tendons.
- Bone-patellar tendon-bone allograft used when no remaining medial ligamentous tissues are present.
- In most knees, the POL can be reattached to a prior disrupted femoral or tibial site and plicated as necessary to the posterior edge of the SMCL graft.

of all of these structures. The surgical dissection uses a layered approach[45] following the description provided in Chapter 1, Medial and Anterior Knee Anatomy (Fig. 24–14).

Before surgery, the operative extremity is signed by the patient and surgeon with nursing personnel present. A time-out is performed with the patient's name, procedure, allergies, preoperative antibiotics, special precautions given and agreed upon by the surgeon, anesthetist, and nursing personnel.

The operative steps are outlined in Table 24–3. It is important to perform a careful limited dissection to avoid further disruption of the neurovascular supply of tissues (Fig. 24–15).

Based on preoperative MRI and limited medial dissection, it is possible to identify the tear site of most of the soft tissue structures for the operative repair. A tourniquet is used for the initial exploration and then deflated during the repair portion of the procedure. A limited cosmetic incision along the anteromedial aspect of the tibia provides good exposure for both ACL and medial repairs and is favored over a two-incision approach (Fig. 24–16).

During the initial dissection, an incision is made into the sartorius fascia just anterior to the SMCL and the fascia and pes tendons are reflected posteriorly to allow identification of the medial

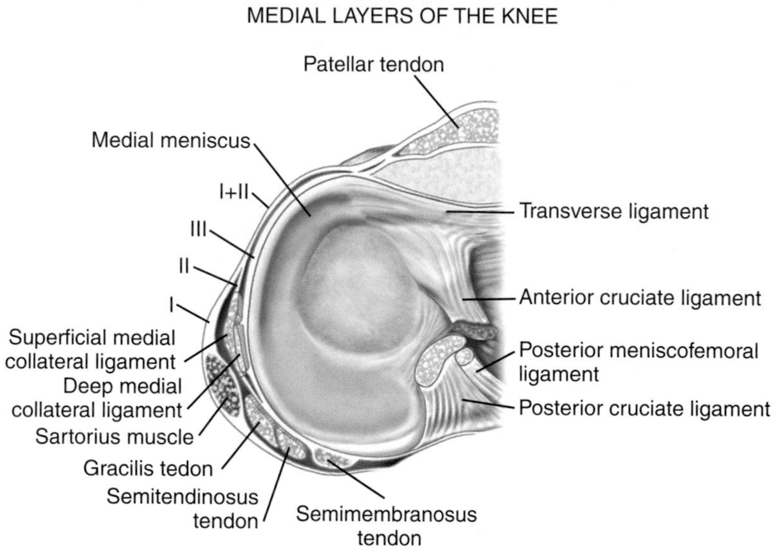

FIGURE 24–14. Medial layers of the knee. The gracilis and semitendinosus lie between layers 1 and 2.

MEDIAL LAYERS OF THE KNEE

TABLE 24–3 **Operative Steps for Acute Medial Ligamentous Ruptures**

1. Use a limited medial approach, dissect skin flaps beneath fascia and not in subcutaneous tissue to preserve blood supply to overlying skin.
2. Approach carefully avoids superficial nerve structures, protects infrapatellar nerve branches to limit postoperative neuroma or loss of cutaneous sensation.
3. Incision anterior sartorial fascia extending from adductor tubercle to anterior border of SMCL, identify pes bursae, posterior retraction of pes tendons.
4. Limited medial dissection at site of injury, but not beyond, with preservation of vascular and nerve supply.
5. Identification of site of SMCL tear preoperatively on MRI and confirmation at surgery including medial patellofemoral ligament, which may require repair.
6. Identification of site of PMC tear on MRI and operatively using anatomic attachments shown in Figures 24–2 and 24–3. There may be interstitial tear or disruption at femoral or tibial attachments.
7. Identification of semimembranosus attachments and particularly tears at POL, meniscus attachments.
8. Identification of deep MCL and meniscal attachments requiring repair.
9. Appropriate repair of all disrupted structures using nonabsorbable and absorbable sutures to decrease overall suture load. Initial repair proceeds deep to superficial with meniscus attachments meticulously first repaired, usually by suture anchors.
10. SMCL repairs performed next to provide stable medial column. Repair frequently requires baseball-type sutures fixed to suture post at attachment site, which provides high-tensile strength for immediate postoperative motion. Avulsion at femur or tibia fixed by screw and soft tissue washer. Suture anchors may be used to supplement repair.
11. Avoid shortening SMCL at tibial attachment site by fixation too proximal, goal is to restore normal anatomic attachment locations.
12. Avoid placement of tibial staples or other large metallic fixation devices, which frequently are painful and require subsequent repeat surgery.
13. POL repair performed next, frequently requires suture anchor fixation at respective tear site. Anterior portion of POL sutured to posterior SMCL after femoral or tibial attachment repaired. Avoid constraint to full knee extension, which is tested after POL repair.
14. Perform final full knee extension and flexion at operative table to make sure that suture fixation of all soft tissue structures has not constrained normal joint motion.
15. Medial patellofemoral ligament and retinaculum closed with knee at 20°, avoiding overtensioning with normal lateral patellar glide of approximately one quadrant (25% patellar width) to avoid "capture" of patellofemoral joint and limited knee flexion.
16. Close partial fascia over SMCL, medial repair.
17. Meticulous hemostasis and closure of dead spaces beneath skin flaps to avoid hematoma.
18. Routine closure, double compression bandage with cotton, ice bladder, soft-hinged postoperative brace.

MCL, medial collateral ligament; MRI, magnetic resonance imaging; PMC, posteromedial capsule; POL, posterior oblique ligament; SMCL, superficial medial collateral ligament.

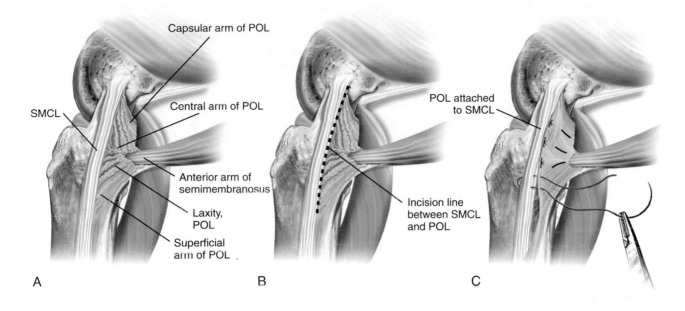

FIGURE 24–15 Surgical plication procedure for POL. **A,** Identification of laxity and redundant POL that involves all three components. In the majority of knees, there will exist concurrent laxity of the SMCL, which also requires surgical reconstruction as described (not shown). **B,** Incision into the POL just behind the SMCL, avoiding the medial meniscus tibial attachments. **C,** Suture plication vest-over-pants technique to restore tension in the POL, performed at 20° flexion in order to avoid overtensioning that would limit full knee extension.

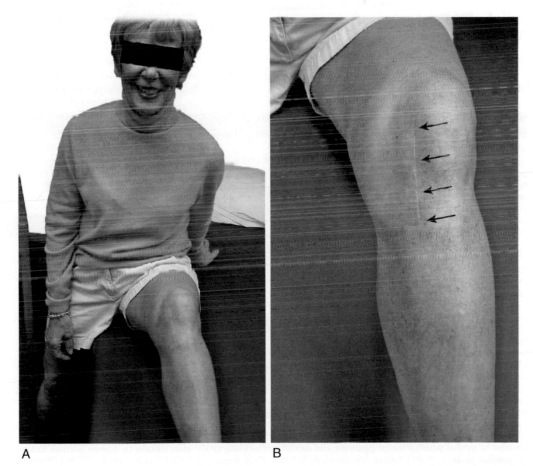

FIGURE 24–16. **A** and **B,** Cosmetic skin incision of the knee joint in an expert skier, 6 months after bone–patellar tendon–bone (B-PT-B) ACL autograft and SMCL, POL, and displaced medial meniscus repair followed by an immediate motion program. In this knee with a gross medial disruption and a medial meniscus that was displaced into the joint, the decision was made to proceed with a combined arthroscopic and open repair of all structures. An ACL autograft (semitendinosus-gracilis [STG], B-PT-B) reconstruction is preferred over an allograft.

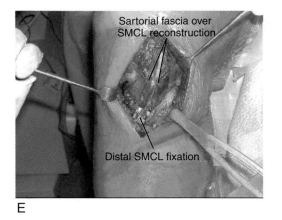

E

FIGURE 24–18—cont'd. E, Final closure, sartorius attachments closed over SMCL that has been advanced distally with STG tendon reconstruction.

required. The Achilles tendon is an alternative allograft, with the bone portion placed at the native SMCL femoral attachment and the full-thickness tendon fixed by a screw and soft tissue washer with additional baseball sutures at the native tibial attachment. The correct attachment points for the SMCL graft are at the native femoral and tibial attachments. If there is any question, the graft attachment is verified by placing a K-wire at the femoral site, attaching suture to the tibial site, and taking the knee through a full ROM. The POL is reattached to its native femoral or tibial site when disruption has occurred. For capsular redundancy, a plication procedure is performed to the posterior edge of the SMCL graft, which provides the stable medial column for the capsular reconstruction.

COMPLICATIONS

The most frequent complication of medial and posteromedial ligament surgery relates to the approximately 25% of operated knees that will have initial limitations in regaining normal flexion and extension. It is necessary at surgery not to overtighten the POL plication or repair. The repair is performed at 10° to 15° of flexion, and the knee is taken to full extension at the end of the procedure. The SMCL augmentation or replacement is fixated at native femoral and tibial attachments and not overtensioned in order not to constrain the knee joint. The treatment

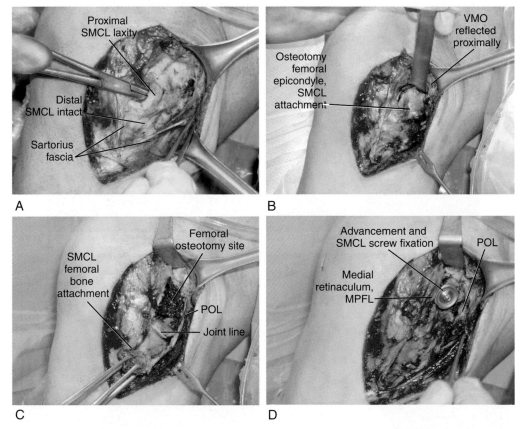

FIGURE 24–19. Demonstration of chronic medial ligament disruption treated with a proximal advancement of SMCL and PMC capsular plication. **A**, On initial exploration, the overlying sartorius retinaculum is split to expose the SMCL. An incision at the anterior border shows SMCL fibers, somewhat thickened, but without scar tissue replacement and suitable for an advancement procedure. If there is any question as to the integrity or future function of the SMCL, an STG graft is added, which is usually required, but not necessary in this case. **B**, The vastus medialis obliquus (VMO) attachment is incised and reflected proximally with dissection carried beneath the muscle without entering the knee joint. Osteotomy of the proximal SMCL attachment is performed. **C**, The SMCL with a 20- x 20-mm proximal bone attachment. Further inspection of the SMCL confirms that it is of a normal appearance with healthy collagen fibers and a tendon augmentation is not needed. The meniscus tibial attachments are intact and do not require fixation. **D**, Proximal fixation of the SMCL with screw and washer. The POL is shown and has been dissected to prove its proximal and distal attachments are intact.

Continued

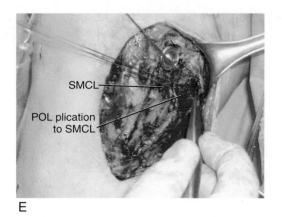

E

FIGURE 24–19—cont'd. E, POL plication to the posterior edge of the SMCL with suture tension adjusted to allow full knee extension. The SMCL and medial retinaculum were closed to the anterior SMCL edge at 30° flexion, allowing a normal lateral patellar glide.

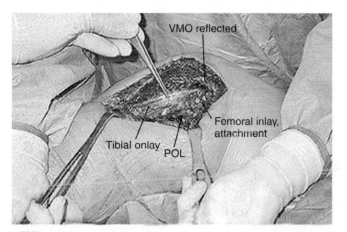

FIGURE 24–20. Demonstration of the use of a long B-PT-B allograft for a severe medial ligament disruption in which no remaining SMCL was present. The bone portions of the graft are placed as an inlay on the femur and as an onlay on the tibia and fixated with cancellous and small fragment screws, respectively. A POL plication was performed (see Table 24–4 for operative steps).

Critical Points COMPLICATIONS

- Most frequent: limitation of knee motion. Do not overtighten POL plication or repair. Begin immediate knee motion.
- Five-day course maximum dose nonsteroidal anti-inflammatory medication, begun the night before surgery.
- Ultrasound all acutely injured knees before surgery and postoperatively if warranted.

of knee motion limitations, principles of patellofemoral mobilization, and muscle rehabilitation exercises are covered in detail in Chapter 25, Rehabilitation of Medial Ligament Injuries.

The authors use a 5-day course of maximum-dose nonsteroidal anti-inflammatory medication, which is begun the night before surgery. A firm double compression wrap and cotton dressing, ice delivery system, and elevation are used for the 1st week after surgery. Patients are carefully examined

preoperatively and postoperatively for deep venous thrombosis, with ultrasound used on all acutely injured knees before surgery and postoperatively if warranted. After surgery, patients use calf compression venous return devices, and ankle pumps are performed hourly.

The complication of infection is rare with the use of preoperative intravenous antibiotics at appropriate doses, careful handling of tissues, and other precautions as detailed in Chapter 7, Anterior Cruciate Ligament Primary and Revision Reconstruction: Diagnosis, Operative Techniques, and Clinical Outcomes.

AUTHORS' CLINICAL STUDY

A prospective study was conducted to determine the outcome of 46 knees with acute ACL-MCL ruptures in which all patients received an ACL reconstruction and either conservative or operative management of the medial ligament injury, based on the extent of the injury.[30] The inclusionary criteria were a complete rupture of the ACL, rupture to a portion or all of the medial ligamentous structures, no rupture to the other knee ligaments, and reconstruction performed within 10 weeks of the original knee injury.

Group I comprised 34 patients who sustained a complete rupture to all of the medial ligament structures (SMCL and PMC), which were repaired at the time of ACL reconstruction. There were 14 male and 20 female patients, mean age of 26 years (range, 13–51 yr), all but 3 of whom were injured during athletic activities. Surgery was delayed for at least 7 days in all patients to allow initiation of quadriceps muscle and ROM exercises and resolution of knee pain and effusion. All patients were treated with an irradiated ACL allograft, because this graft

Critical Points AUTHORS' CLINICAL STUDY

46 knees with acute ACL-MCL ruptures:
- Group I: 34 patients complete rupture all of medial ligament structures (SMCL and PMC), which were repaired at the time of ACL reconstruction. Followed mean 69 months (range, 24–107 mo) postoperatively.
- Group II: 12 patients who sustained a complete rupture to the SMCL only, underwent ACL reconstruction alone. All treated with initial nonoperative program of at least 4 wk to allow SMCL to heal. Followed mean 50 months (range, 28–68 mo) postoperatively.

Meniscus repairs done in 23 (68%) of group I and in 11 (92%) of group II.

At follow-up, no patient in either group had more than 2–3 mm of increase in medial joint space opening.

ACL reconstructions rated as normal in 61% in group I and in 82% in group II; nearly normal in 21% in group I and in 18% in group II; and failed in 18% of group I.

7 patients in group I had significant difficulty squatting or kneeling. More patients in group I had swelling and pain with sports activities than those in group II.

Overall rating scores:
- Group I: 58% excellent or good, 42% fair or poor.
- Group II: 91% excellent or good, 9% fair.

Treatment program of knee motion limitations required in 26% of group I, 17% of group II.

Study resulted in the conservative treatment recommendations described in this chapter for ACL/MCL ruptures.

source was under prospective investigation at the authors' center at the time of this study. All patients completed questionnaires from the CKRS a mean of 69 months (range, 24–107 mo) postoperatively, and all but 1 returned for a comprehensive clinical evaluation.

Group II comprised 12 patients who sustained a complete rupture to the SMCL only. The PMC structures were considered functional, because little to no increase was demonstrated in medial joint space opening on clinical valgus stress testing at 0°. There were 7 male and 5 female patients, with a mean age of 21 years (range, 16–33 yr), and all but 1 sustained the injury during sports activities. These patients underwent an initial nonoperative treatment program of at least 4 weeks of protection from valgus joint loads in a hinged knee brace locked at 0° of extension. The brace was removed three to four times a day for knee motion and exercises. After a period of rehabilitation of the medial ligament injury, an ACL reconstruction was performed. All of these patients completed questionnaires from the CKRS a mean of 50 months (range, 28–68 mo) postoperatively, and all but 1 returned for a comprehensive clinical evaluation.

In group I, a direct repair of the ruptured MCL was performed with two to four baseball-type sutures either to internally fixate the disrupted ligament back to the insertion site or to approximate the ligament ends. The sutures were tied over a soft tissue washer or staple. The capsular tissues were also repaired using multiple sutures. In 2 patients, the midsubstance rupture of the MCL was so severe that a semitendinosus autograft was incorporated into the repair.

Meniscus tears were common in both groups of patients, occurring in 23 patients (68%) in group I and in 11 patients (92%) in group II. The lateral meniscus was torn in 61% of the knees and the medial meniscus was torn in 33%. In group I, the medial meniscus was repaired in 12 knees and the lateral meniscus was repaired in 7 knees using techniques described in Chapter 28, Meniscus Tears, Diagnosis, Operative Techniques, and Clinical Outcomes.[38,39] Thirteen other lateral meniscus tears required partial resection. In group II, the medial meniscus was repaired in 3 knees and the lateral meniscus was repaired in 6 knees. Four other lateral meniscus tears required partial resection.

At follow-up, no patient in either group had more than 2 to 3 mm of increase in medial joint space opening (Table 24–5). Moderate patellofemoral crepitus was detected in 7 patients in group I and severe crepitus was found in 1 patient. One patient in group II had moderate patellofemoral crepitus. The crepitus was symptomatic with sports activities in 2 of these 9 patients. The ACL reconstructions were rated (based on knee arthrometer and pivot shift testing) as normal in 61% in group I and in 82% in group II; nearly normal in 21% in group I and in 18% in group II; and failed in 18% of group I.

Before the injury, all patients except 1 were participating in sports activities (Table 24–6). At follow-up, all except 3 patients in group I had returned to athletics, although over half had returned to a lower level of participation. No patient in either group had problems with walking or stair climbing. However, 7 patients in group I had significant difficulty squatting or kneeling. More patients in group I had swelling and pain with sports activities than those in group II (Fig. 24–21).

TABLE 24–5   Medial Joint Opening to Manual Valgus Stress Testing at 5° and 25° of Knee Flexion (mm)

Difference Involved – Noninvolved (mm)	Group I (*N*)				Group II (*N*)			
	Preoperative 5° flexion	Preoperative 25° flexion	Follow-up 5° flexion	Follow-up 25° flexion	Preoperative 5° flexion	Preoperative 25° flexion	Follow-up 5° flexion	Follow-up 25° flexion
0–3	0	0	33	33	12	3	11	11
4–5	19	2	0	0	0	6	0	0
6–10	15	27	0	0	0	3	0	0
11–15	0	5	0	0	0	0	0	0

From Noyes, F. R.; Barber-Westin, S. D.: The treatment of acute combined ruptures of the anterior cruciate and medial ligaments of the knee. *Am J Sports Med* 23:380–391, 1995.

TABLE 24–6   Sports Activities before the Injury and a Follow-up

Type of Sport	Preoperative		Follow-up	
	Group I *N* (%)	Group II *N* (%)	Group I *N* (%)	Group II *N* (%)
Jumping, pivoting, cutting	21 (62)	8 (67)	9 (26)	4 (33)
Running, twisting, turning	9 (26)	4 (33)	10 (29)	5 (42)
Swimming, cycling	3 (9)	0	12 (35)	3 (25)
None	1 (3)	0	3 (10)	0
Change in sports activities				
Same level, no symptoms			8 (23)	3 (25)
Decreased level, no symptoms, knee-related			17 (50)	6 (50)
Decreased level, no symptoms, non–knee-related			3 (9)	3 (25)
Participating with symptoms			3 (9)	0
No sports, knee-related			3 (9)	0
No sports, non–knee-related			0	0

From Noyes, F. R.; Barber-Westin, S. D.: The treatment of acute combined ruptures of the anterior cruciate and medial ligaments of the knee. *Am J Sports Med* 23:380–391, 1995.

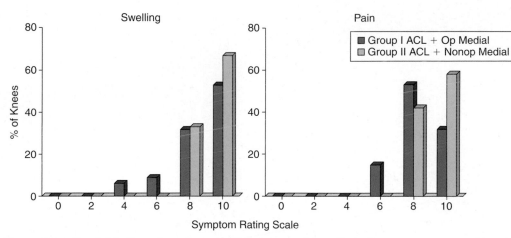

FIGURE 24–21. The postoperative distributions of swelling and pain scores are shown. Scale: 0, severe symptoms with activities of daily living; 2, moderate symptoms with activities of daily living; 4, no symptoms with activities of daily living but symptoms with sports; 6, no symptoms with swimming or cycling but symptoms with other sports activities; 8, no symptoms with running, twisting, or turning, but symptoms with jumping, hard pivoting, or cutting; 10, no symptoms with jumping, hard pivoting, or cutting. *(From Noyes, F. R.; Barber-Westin, S. D.: The treatment of acute combined ruptures of the anterior cruciate and medial ligaments of the knee. Am J Sports Med 23:380–391, 1995.)*

The overall rating scores for group I, based on the CKRS, were excellent in 2 patients, good in 17, fair in 7, and poor in 7. Therefore, 58% in this group were rated as excellent or good, and 42% were rated as fair or poor. For group II, the overall ratings were excellent in 1 patient, good in 9, and fair in 1. Therefore, 91% in this group were rated as excellent or good, whereas 9% were rated as fair.

In this investigation, 74% of the patients sustained meniscus tears and 20% had noteworthy articular cartilage deterioration, and therefore, the results should not be compared with those of isolated ACL reconstruction studies. At an average of 5 years postoperatively, no patient demonstrated more than 2 to 3 mm of increase in medial joint opening at either 0° or 25° of knee flexion. Healing was therefore demonstrated in both the surgically repaired complete medial ligament disruptions and the conservatively treated knees with SMCL disruption.

The rehabilitation program and early treatment of knee motion limitations successfully restored at least 0° to 135° of knee motion in 96% of the patients. The treatment program of knee motion limitations, described in Chapter 41, Prevention and Treatment of Knee Arthrofibrosis, was instituted in 24% of the knees (26% of group I and 17% of group II). This program is most successful if begun early postoperatively, as early as 3 to 4 weeks if the initial motion goals have not been obtained. Patients with ruptures at or proximal to the medial joint line had a higher incidence of motion complications (7 of 15 patients, 47%) than those with ruptures located distal to the joint line (2 of 18 patients, 11%). Similar findings were reported by Robins and associates.[34]

The strict overall rating system used in this investigation resulted in 14 patients receiving a fair or poor score. Seven of these 14 patients received this rating, in part, owing to failure of the ACL allograft and the authors advocate autogenous B-PT-B grafts for ACL reconstruction. At the time of the study, the authors used irradiated allografts, and as discussed in Chapter 7, Anterior Cruciate Ligament Primary and Revision Reconstruction: Diagnosis, Operative Techniques, and Clinical Outcomes, the irradiation process appeared to increase the rate of failure compared with other studies in which fresh-frozen allografts were selected. Patellofemoral joint symptoms

accounted for the low ratings in 4 knees, and postoperative motion complications accounted for the ratings in 3 knees. This study was also conducted at a time in which complete disruptions of ACL and medial ligaments were more often treated by operative intervention.

The results of this study, along with other investigations,[4,27,29,32,43] promoted a worthwhile reevaluation of the operative recommendation for combined ACL and medial ligament injuries, resulting in the conservative recommendations in this chapter, which have now been used for many years.

RESULTS FROM OTHER CLINICAL STUDIES

Since the early 1990s, several studies have been published that presented various treatment options and outcomes for isolated MCL injuries and combined ACL-MCL ruptures. As shown in Tables 24–7 and 24–8, the severity of the medial ligamentous injuries varies and, in many instances, is difficult to interpret

Critical Points RESULTS FROM OTHER CLINICAL STUDIES

- Problems exist in studies with terminology, lack of data medial joint opening both 30° and 0°, lack of objective stress radiography pre- and postoperative, consistent treatment protocol.
- Majority studies SMCL primary suture repair, only 2 studies used graft for chronic ruptures.
- Only 1 study[14] to date randomized grade 3 medial ruptures to primary repair or conservative protocol. Conclusion: SMCL ruptures do not require operative treatment when a concomitant ACL rupture is reconstructed early following injury.
- Several studies document successful management of isolated MCL injuries in athletes with nonoperative treatment as long as there are no other ligament or meniscus injuries and the knees are stable to valgus stress testing in full extension.
- Higher incidence of knee motion complications and poorer subjective scores noted in knees that undergo early ACL reconstruction compared with those in whom the ACL reconstruction is delayed.

TABLE 24–7 Results of Treatment of Isolated Medial Collateral Ligament Ruptures

Reference	Number of Cases, Time Followed after Injury	Pretreatment MCL Grade, Medial Joint Opening	Treatment of MCL	Follow-up Medial Joint Opening	Follow-up Symptoms, Function, Activity Level	Reinjuries	Recommendations
Petermann, 1993[31a]	N = 102, 86 followed mean 44 mo	30°; 1+ (≤5 mm): 39; 2+ (6–10 mm): 41; 3+ (>10 mm): 6	Cast brace 4 wk, ROM 10°–90°, weight-bearing as tolerated, return to activity 8 wk	No increase in all except 2 knees that had 2+ injuries, persistent 1+ instability at follow-up	97% returned to previous activity level	None	Isolated MCL injuries can be successfully managed nonoperatively.
Reider, 1994[33a]	N = 36, 34 completed questionnaires, 30 reexamined 2.5–8 yr	Grade III (tenderness over MCL, abnormally increased valgus laxity, soft endpoint in flexion). Millimeters of increase not given.	Lateral hinged brace, weight-bearing as tolerated, ROM, supervised therapy program	No increase: 8; <5 mm: 17; 6–9 mm: 5	23 patients had at least one residual symptom. 18 patients had mild pain. 11 patients had feeling of looseness. All returned to preinjury sports, 7 at a lower level.	7 sustained new traumatic knee injuries, 6 during football.	Early functional rehabilitation isolated grade III MCL injuries effective, but residual symptoms common. Unknown correlation with reinjuries; longer follow-up required.
Indelicato et al., 1990[24]	N = 28 football players, 21 followed 18–72 mo	Grade III (>10 mm medial opening 30°, soft endpoint).	Immobilized 2 wk, 4 wk brace 30°–90°, weight-bearing as tolerated, rehabilitation	No increase: 8; 1+ (<5 mm): 13	18 returned to contact drills mean 9.2 wk	None	Grade III MCL tears successful conservative management as long as there is no damage to ACL or menisci.
Jones, 1986[25a]	N = 22 football players followed mean 6 mo	Grade III (millimeters of increase not given)	Immobilized 1 wk in brace, then ROM allowed with weight-bearing as tolerated, supervised rehabilitation as required.	All 0–1+	All returned football 24–38 days after injury	None; 1 ACL rupture missed at initial diagnosis	Conservative management isolated grade III MCL injuries satisfactory short-term results.
Indelicato, 1983[23]	N = 36 followed 1.9–4.3 yr	Grade III (no valgus instability in full extension.)	Group I (N = 16): MCL primary repair, 6 wk cast, rehabilitation; Group II (N = 20): MCL no operation, cast 2 wk, cast brace 4 wk, rehabilitation	Group I: 94% no or mild instability (<5 mm 30°); 6% moderate instability (5–10 mm 30°); Group II: 85% no or mild instability, 15% moderate instability	Group I: 88% good to excellent, 12% fair; Group II: 90% good to excellent, 10% fair. Fair results due to patellofemoral symptoms, recurrent effusions	None	Nonoperative management isolated MCL tears provides good to excellent results, no benefit for surgery. Important that there is no associated damage to ACL or menisci.
Holden et al., 1983[18]	N = 51	Grade I: 17 knees (no instability, stable in extension); Grade II: 34 knees (10°–15° instability, firm endpoint)	No immobilization, 4-wk formal rehabilitation program.	Not given	80% returned to full sports participation mean 21 days (range, 9–32 days).	9 knees required surgery. 4 patients reinjured knee. ACL ruptures in 6 missed upon initial diagnosis	Conservative management isolated grades I and II MCL ruptures provides satisfactory results.
Hastings, 1980[15]	N = 26	5–12 mm increase 20°	Immobilization 5–6 wk, then changed protocol to 2 wk in cast followed by 4 wk in cast brace, return to activity in brace	1 patient "slight" medial laxity. 3 patients "objective medial laxity" (no subjective instability). 22 patients no significant laxity.	All but 1 returned previous activity level.	2 reinjuries.	MCL tears in absence of ACL tear may be managed effectively nonoperatively.

ACL, anterior cruciate ligament; MCL, medial collateral ligament; ROM, range of motion.

TABLE 24–8 Results of Treatment of Combined Medial Collateral Ligament–Anterior Collateral Ligament Injuries

Reference	Number, Follow-up, Acute/Chronic	Preoperative Ligament Ruptures	Treatment of Ligament Ruptures	Follow-up Medial Joint Opening	Follow-up Data Other Reconstructed Ligaments	Follow-up IKDC Ratings*	Follow-up Symptoms, Function, Activity Level	Complications	Recommendations
Halinen et al., 2006[14]	N = 47, all followed mean, 27 mo (range, 20-37 mo). All acute, operations done 4-23 days after injury.	MCL: 25°: >10 mm 5°: Subtle increase ACL: Complete rupture in all	MCL: Randomized repair (group 1) vs. nonoperative (group 2) MCL repairs either suture anchors or sutured through bone tunnels ACL: B-PT-B autograft	Stress x-ray (flexion angle NA) mean I-N: Group 1: 0.9 (range, -0.8–3.6) Group 2: 1.7 (range, -0.5–+6.4) No difference between groups.	KT-1000: 77% <3 mm 21% 3-5 mm 2% 6-10 mm No difference between groups.	Overall: Group 1: 70% A, B Group 2: 83% A, B C, D ratings due to pair with activities, not ligament outcome	Lysholm: 83% in both groups excellent/good scores	1 infection. No further operations for knee motion problems. 4 reoperations for meniscus tears.	Method of treatment of MCL rupture did not affect outcome. Patients' older age (group 1 mean, 40 yr; group 2 mean, 38 yr) might have affected results. MCL repair not required if ACL reconstructed acutely.
Yoshiya, 2005[47]	N = 27, 24 followed mean 27 mo (range, 24-48 mo) All chronic, operations done 4-204 mo after injury.	MCL: Gross medial instability with no firm endpoint. 12 + ACL 7 + PCL 3 + ACL & PCL	MCL: STG reconstruction ACL/PCL: contralateral B-PT-B or QT autograft	Stress x-ray 20 mean I-N: Preoperative: 4.1 mm (range, 3-6 mm) Postoperative: 0.2 mm (range, -1–+2)	KT-1000 ACL: 7 <3 mm 5 3-5 mm PCL (stress x-ray): 1 <3 mm 4 3-5 mm 2 >5 mm	Symptoms: 21 A, B 3 C	3 patients pain & instability with light activities	None	Procedure effective, but only restores anterior longitudinal portion of the superficial MCL.
Millett et al., 2004[27]	N = 19 followed mean 45 mo (range, 24-98 mo) All acute, operations done mean 7.5 days (range, 0-20 days) after injury.	MCL: 7: Grade II (5-10 mm, 30°) 12: Grade III (>10 mm, 30°). All complete ACL	ACL B-PT-B or STG autograft Brace 6 wk postoperative to protect from valgus loads	No valgus instability in any patient.	KT-1000 data on 13 patients mean 15 mo postoperative: mean 2.3 mm No positive pivot shift in any patient	NA	Mean Lysholm 94.5 points, mean Tegner 8.4 points	1 scope for arthrofibrosis	Early ACL reconstruction (within 6 wk of injury) and conservative treatment of MCL rupture lead to acceptable results.
Nakamura et al., 2003[29]	N = 17 followed 5 yr All treated first with brace protection for 6 wk	MCL: Grade III (clinically unstable valgus stress test 0°, 30°, no endpoint) All complete ACL	MCL: Advancement or reconstruction with fascia lata autograft or allograft superficial layer in patients with >4 mm increase medial joint opening 0° (N = 5) ACL STG autograft	MCL operative: 75% <3 mm 5% 3-5 mm ACL nonoperative: 78% <3 mm 22% 3-5 mm	KT mean: MCL operative (N = 6) 2.25 ± 1.39 mm MCL nonoperative 1.33 ± 1.32 mm	Patient grade knee condition: MCL operative 50% normal, 40% nearly normal MCL nonoperative 64% normal, 36% nearly normal	NA	None	MRI grading system according to location of superficial MCL injury useful to determine treatment. Restoration valgus stability correlated with location of superficial fiber damage.

Continued

TABLE 24–8 Results of Treatment of Combined Medial Collateral Ligament–Anterior Collateral Ligament Injuries—Cont'd

Reference	Number, Follow-up, Acute/Chronic	Preoperative Ligament Ruptures	Treatment of Ligament Ruptures	Follow-up Medial Joint Opening	Follow-up Data Other Reconstructed Ligaments	Follow-up IKDC Ratings*	Follow-up Symptoms, Function, Activity Level	Complications	Recommendations
Shelbourne & Baele, 1988[40]	N = 27 followed mean 33 mo. All but 2 acute (<6 wk).	MCL: Grade not given ACL: Ruptured in all	Group 1: MCL primary repair, ACL B-PT-B autograft in 13 knees. 6 knees casted 6 weeks, 7 knees used CPM on day 3 for 2–3 wk. Partial weight-bearing 6 wk. Group 2: ACL B-PT-B autograft in 14 knees. All CPM, earlier weight-bearing, more aggressive ROM protocol than group 1.	MCL: Trace to 1+ with firm endpoint in all patients (millimeters of increase medial joint opening not given)	ACL: Firm endpoint on Lachman testing. No further data provided.	NA	NA	Group 1: Mean ROM 3 mo 12°–95° Group 2: Mean ROM 3 mo 0°–125° More rapid return strength than group 1 patients (data not provided).	Treat MCL injuries conservatively first, followed by ACL reconstruction.
Kannus, 1988[26]	N = 81 followed mean 8.6 yr	MCL: Grade II: 54 (1+ or 2+ abduction instability, hard endpoint, 30°) Grade III: 27 (3+ abduction instability, soft endpoint 30°, mild 1+ abduction instability 0°). ACL: None detected	MCL: Immobilized mean 3.6 wk Grade II, mean 4.9 wk Grade III. Weight-bearing as tolerated after 2–4 wk, supervised rehabilitation 6 mo.	Grade II group: Grade 0: 5 Grade 1+: 13 Grade 2+: 25 Grade 3+: 11 Grade III group: Grade 2+: 2 Grade 3+: 12 Grade 4+: 13	Grade II group: Anterior instability Grade 1+: 12 Grade 2+: 9 Grade 3+: 4 Grade III group: Anterior instability Grade 1+: 3 Grade 2+: 8 Grade 3+: 8 Grade 4+: 8		Grade II group: all returned preinjury level function. Lysholm score excellent Grade III group: 63% decreased sports activities, 22% giving way episodes 63% x-ray evidence post-traumatic osteoarthritis	Grade II group: 14 patients reinjured knee Grade III group: 7 patients reinjured knee	Grade II MCL satisfactory results conservative treatment. Grade III MCL poor results, due in part to untreated ACL ruptures. Recommend operative management grade 3 ruptures.
Jokl et al., 1984[25]	N = 28 followed mean 3 yr (range, 8 mo–11 yr).	MCL: Grade not given, stress x-ray > 15 mm increase medial joint opening 20° flexion ACL: complete rupture in all	No surgery. Immobilized 3–7 days, ROM begun 1–2 wk, rehabilitation, running 2–6 wk, return full activity mean 4 mo.	Not given	Not given	NA	68% returned preinjury sports activity. Poorest function in older, nonathletic patients.	6 patients reinjured knee	Recommend conservative treatment acute ACL-MCL tears unless initial result is unsatisfactory.

*A, normal; B, nearly normal; C, abnormal; D, severely abnormal.

ACL, anterior cruciate ligament; ADL, activities of daily living; B-PT-B, bone-patellar tendon-bone; CPM, continuous passive motion; IKDC, International Knee Documentation Committee; I-N, involved to uninvolved; MCL, medial collateral ligament; MJO, medial joint opening; MRI, magnetic resonance imaging; NA, not available; PCL, posterior cruciate ligament; PL, peroneus longus tendon; POL, posterior oblique ligament; QT, quadriceps tendon; ROM, range of motion; ST, semitendinosus; STG, semitendinosus-gracilis.

owing to both the ambiguous terminology used to describe the degree or grade of the injury and the lack of data on the estimated (or measured) millimeters of medial joint opening at both 30° and 0° of knee flexion before and after treatment. Even fewer investigators use stress radiography to objectively measure medial joint opening before and after treatment. Therefore, the exact structures that are ruptured (and those that remain intact) in most studies are unknown. Future investigations should provide these data to enable clinicians to understand the exact anatomic structures involved and form rationale treatment decisions regarding which structures require operative restoration and the appropriate timing of those procedures.

In knees with combined ACL-MCL ruptures, additional problems in the published literature arise from the wide variety of treatment methods proposed and compared, including

1. Repair or reconstruction of both the MCL and the ACL.[2,9,34,46]
2. Repair of the MCL, no reconstruction of the ACL.[12,19]
3. Repair or reconstruction of both the MCL and the ACL versus conservative management of the MCL and reconstruction of the ACL.[14,17,40]
4. Repair or reconstruction of both the MCL and the ACL versus repair of the MCL and conservative management of the ACL.[3]
5. Conservative management of the MCL, ACL reconstructed.[4,27,29,32,43]
6. Conservative management of both the MCL and the ACL.[25,26]

The majority of clinical studies that have described the outcome of operative management of SMCL ruptures used primary suture repair procedures, some of which were combined with advancement of the PMC, for acute knee injuries.[2,3,12,14,17,19,34,40] Only two series to date described the use of a graft to reconstruct chronic SMCL ruptures; both involved knees with multiligament injuries. Yoshiya and colleagues[16] followed 24 patients who underwent an STG SMCL reconstruction. The SMCL ruptures were classified as having gross medial instability with no firm endpoint. It is noted in this study that preoperative valgus stress radiographs measured only a mean of 4.1 mm (range, 3–6 mm) of increased medial joint opening and, therefore, it would appear that these knees would be in the category in which conservative treatment is usually recommended. Twelve patients had a concomitant ACL reconstruction, 7 had a concomitant PCL reconstruction, and 3 had a concomitant bicruciate reconstruction. At an average of 27 months postoperatively, stress radiographs revealed a mean of 0.2 mm (range, –1–+2 mm) increase in medial joint opening. The authors cautioned that, although the procedure was effective, it restored only the anterior longitudinal portion of the SMCL.

Fanelli and Edson[9] described a procedure to reconstruct the SMCL in patients with "high-grade" SMCL ruptures using either an Achilles tendon allograft or a semitendinosus tendon autograft. The millimeters of increased medial joint opening at 0° and 30° of flexion that were present before surgery were not provided. The PMC was advanced and sutured into the graft. In a small series of 7 patients followed 2 to 10 years postoperatively, no increase was noted on manual valgus testing at 30° of knee flexion.

Halinen and coworkers[14] published to date the only study of acute grade III medial ruptures (defined by the authors as > 10 mm increase in medial joint opening at 25° of flexion and a "subtle" increase at 5° of flexion) that were randomized to either a primary repair or a conservative management group.

All 47 patients in the study also had complete ACL ruptures, which were reconstructed with a B-PT-B autograft. The reconstructions were performed between 4 and 23 days after the injury. At follow-up, a mean of 27 months postoperatively, stress radiographs (25° flexion) revealed a mean increase in medial joint opening of 0.9 mm (range, –0.8–+3.6 mm) in the SMCL operatively treated group, and 1.7 mm (range, –0.5–+ 6.4 mm) in the SMCL conservatively treated group. The authors concluded the SMCL ruptures do not require operative treatment when a concomitant ACL rupture is reconstructed early after injury.

Conservative management of SMCL ruptures has been recommended by many authors following the early investigations of Ellsasser and associates[8] and Fetto and Marshall.[11] Ellsasser and associates[8] reported successful management of isolated MCL injuries in athletes with nonoperative treatment as long as there were no other ligament or meniscus injuries and the knees were stable to valgus stress testing in full extension after the injury. Fetto and Marshall's series[11] included patients with medial joint opening in full extension (termed grade III), and the authors noted that 80% of grade III medial ruptures had concomitant cruciate ligament damage. An excellent or good result in these knees was related to the recovery of ACL stability and not to residual medial joint opening. Many subsequently published studies verified the importance of an intact or reconstructed ACL in the successful nonoperative management of SMCL ruptures.[4,15,18,23,24,26,27,32,43]

The question of the appropriate timing of ACL reconstruction in knees with concomitant SMCL tears has been addressed by a few investigations. Millett and colleagues[27] followed 18 patients who had an ACL reconstruction (B-PT-B or STG autograft) performed a mean of 7.5 days (range, 0–20 days) after an acute ACL-MCL injury. Seven patients had a grade II SMCL injury (5–10 mm medial joint opening at 30° flexion) and 12 had a grade III injury (>10 mm at 30° flexion). Postoperatively, the patients were kept in a brace to protect from excessive valgus loads. At follow-up, a mean of 45 months postoperatively, no valgus instability (at 30° flexion) or positive pivot shift test was detected in any patient. One patient required an arthroscopic procedure for arthrofibrosis. The authors did not provide data regarding the number of patients who returned to preinjury levels of activity or symptoms and functional limitations. They concluded that early ACL reconstruction did not increase the risk of complications, but acknowledged that it is unknown whether this treatment strategy provides superior results over those from a delayed ACL reconstruction approach.

Peterson and Laprell[32] found a higher incidence of knee motion complications and poorer subjective scores in knees that underwent early ACL reconstruction (1–21 days after injury) compared with those in whom the ACL reconstruction was delayed (10–12 wk after injury). All patients in their series received a B-PT-B autograft and all had a grade III medial ligament rupture (defined as a positive valgus stress test without an endpoint). Postoperative rehabilitation included no brace in the ACL delayed group, a brace in the early ACL group with limits set from 0° to 100°, full weight-bearing within 1 week for all patients, and intensive therapy training for 2 to 3 months. The authors did not provide preoperative data on muscle strength or range of knee motion for either group. Speculation was made that the motion limitations were due to the postoperative brace worn in the early ACL group, although the amount of time the brace was worn was not provided.

Shelbourne and Patel[42] reported that patients with acute combined ACL-SMCL ruptures treated with only ACL reconstruction had more rapid return of knee motion and muscle strength than those treated with ACL reconstruction and SMCL repair. However, 6 of the 13 knees in the combined ACL-SMCL repair group underwent 6 weeks of casting postoperatively whereas the remainder of the knees in the series initiated continuous passive motion on the 3rd postoperative day. The authors did not assess the effect of casting on the study's outcome. In addition, the severity of the SMCL ruptures was unknown, as no data were provided on the millimeters of medial joint opening at either 30° or 0° of knee flexion before or after surgery. The authors later recommended that all MCL injuries be treated conservatively, regardless of the severity of the injury.[42]

ILLUSTRATIVE CASE

Case 1. Acute Combined ACL, SMCL, POL Ligament Disruption with Dislodged Bucket-Handle Lateral Meniscus Tear in the Femoral Notch.

A 16-year-old male sustained a twisting injury to his left knee while water skiing. He was evaluated 5 days after the injury. MRI showed a coiled, disrupted distal MCL rupture, meniscotibial attachment tears, a displaced lateral meniscus within the femoral notch, and an ACL midsubstance rupture (Fig. 24–22A). The physical examination showed 10 mm of increased medial joint opening at 30° of flexion and 5 mm increase at 0°, a positive

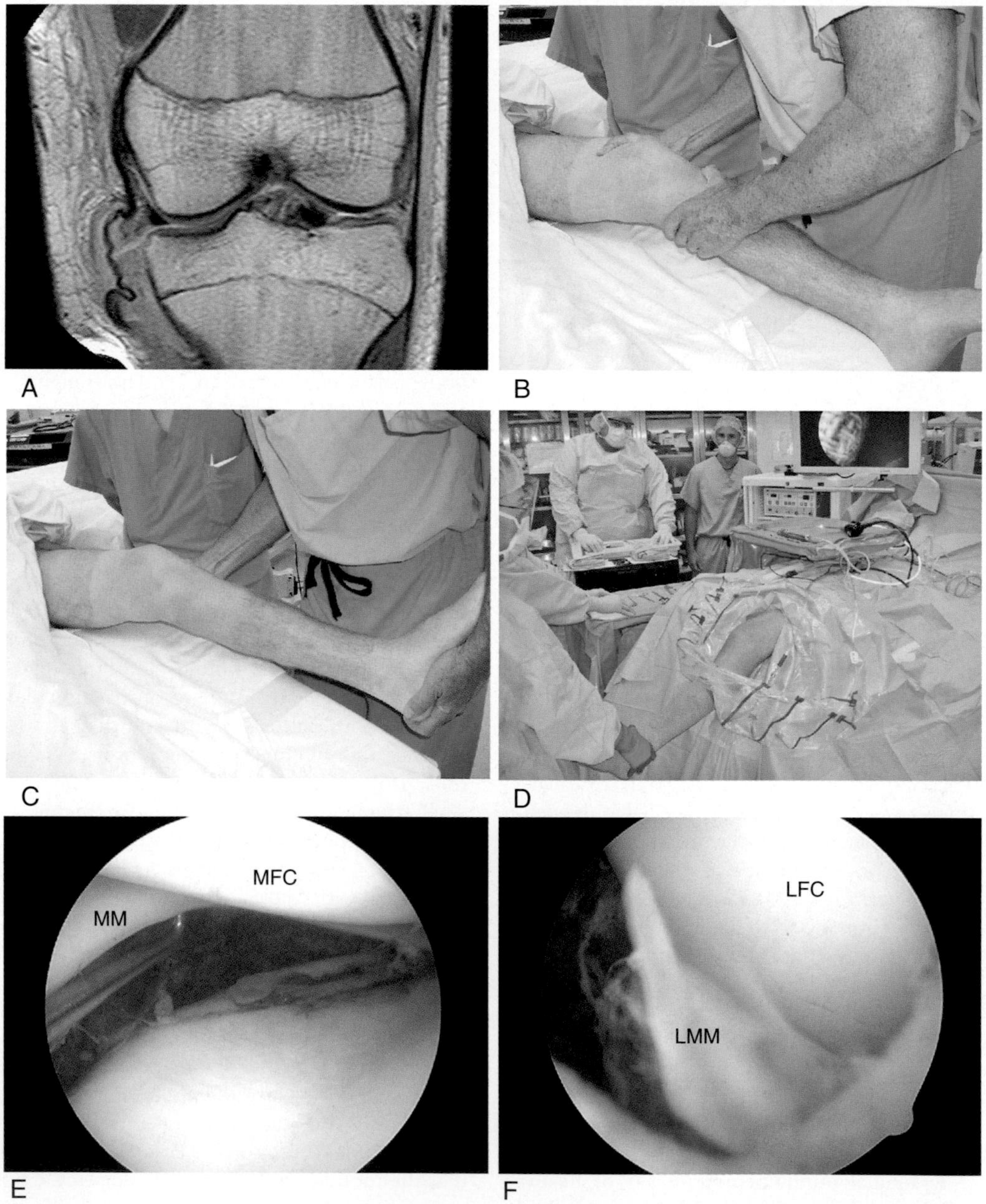

FIGURE 24–22. Illustrative case, acute combined ACL-SMCL, POL ligament disruption with dislodged bucket-handle lateral meniscus tear in the femoral notch, see text.

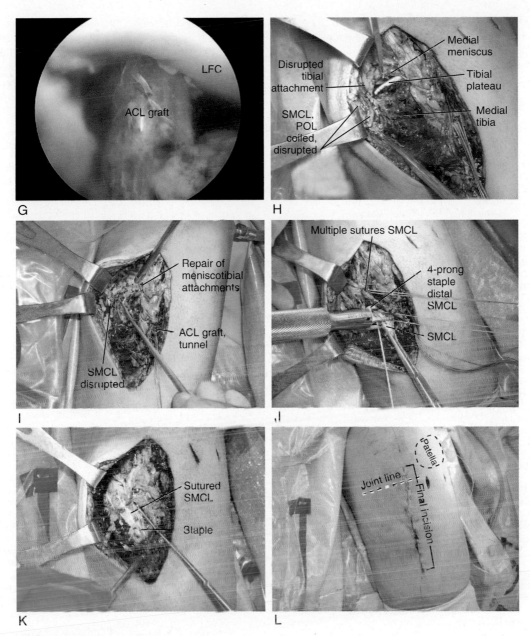

FIGURE 24–22—cont'd.

Lachman test, and a grade III pivot shift test. Surgery was indicated to reduce and repair the lateral meniscus bucket-handle tear. Because the patient had minimal swelling, restoration of motion, and early return of quadriceps function, the decision was made to proceed with a combined ACL-MCL reconstruction.

Under anesthesia, the increases in medial joint opening and external tibial rotation were noted (see Fig. 24–22B), along with a positive Lachman test (see Fig. 24–22C). The operative setup allowed for full flexion and extension, with a leg holder used initially for the lateral meniscus repair (see Fig. 24–22D). At arthroscopy, the tearing of the meniscotibial attachments and a 12-mm increase in the medial gap test were noted. The meniscus had a normal relationship with the femoral condyle, indicating a distal attachment tear (see Fig. 24–22E). The lateral meniscus was displaced into the notch, which was reduced and repaired with multiple

vertical divergent sutures placed with an inside-out technique through an accessory posterolateral incision (see Fig. 24–22F). An ACL four-strand STG reconstruction was performed using a two-incision technique to achieve anatomic central tibial and femoral attachment locations (see Chapter 7, Anterior Cruciate Ligament Primary and Revision Reconstruction: Diagnosis, Operative Techniques, and Clinical Outcomes). The distal ACL attachment was fixed after the MCL repair (see Fig. 24–22G).

The medial exploration through the medial incision showed a meniscotibial attachment tear, increased medial joint opening, and disrupted distal SMCL and POL at the tibial attachment (see Fig. 24–22H). The procedure was begun deep with the medial meniscotibial attachment repair using multiple sutures (see Fig. 24–22I). In this case, suture anchors were not required. The entire SMCL and POL tibial attachment sleeve was reattached with three No. 2 baseball sutures placed in the posterior, middle, and anterior portions. A four-prong low-profile staple was used for distal SMCL fixation and as a suture post (see Fig. 24–22J). The combined suture and staple fixation provided

secure fixation to allow immediate knee motion (see Fig. 24–22K). The final appearance of the incision is shown in Figure 24–22L, which extended from the midpoint of the patella 10 cm to the point adjacent to the tibial tubercle.

REFERENCES

1. Council on Scientific Affairs Standard Nomenclature of Athletic Injuries. Chicago, American Medical Association, 1966.
2. Aglietti, P.; Buzzi, R.; Zaccherotti, G.; D'Andria, S.: Operative treatment of acute complete lesions of the anterior cruciate and medial collateral ligaments. A 4- to 7-year follow-up study. *Am J Knee Surg* 4:186–194, 1991.
3. Andersson, C.; Gillquist, J.: Treatment of acute isolated and combined ruptures of the anterior cruciate ligament. A long-term follow-up study. *Am J Sports Med* 20:7–12, 1992.
4. Ballmer, P. M.; Ballmer, F. T.; Jakob, R. P.: Reconstruction of the anterior cruciate ligament alone in the treatment of a combined instability with complete rupture of the medial collateral ligament. A prospective study. *Arch Orthop Trauma Surg* 110:139–141, 1991.
5. Bergfeld, J.: First-, second-, and third-degree sprains. *Am Sports Med* 7:207–209, 1979.
6. Deibert, M. C.; Aronsson, D. D.; Johnson, R. J.; et al.: Skiing injuries in children, adolescents, and adults. *J Bone Joint Surg Am* 80:25–32, 1998.
7. Dugdale, T. W.; Noyes, F. R.; Styer, D.: Preoperative planning for high tibial osteotomy: the effect of lateral tibiofemoral separation and tibiofemoral length. *Clin Orthop Relat Res* 274:248–264, 1992.
8. Ellsasser, J. C.; Reynolds, F. C.; Omohundro, J. R.: The nonoperative treatment of collateral ligament injuries of the knee in professional football players. An analysis of seventy-four injuries treated non-operatively and twenty-four injuries treated surgically. *J Bone Joint Surg Am* 56:1185–1190, 1974.
9. Fanelli, G. C.; Edson, C. J.: Arthroscopically assisted combined anterior and posterior cruciate ligament reconstruction in the multiple ligament injured knee: 2- to 10-year follow-up. *Arthroscopy* 18:703–714, 2002.
10. Fanelli, G. C.; Harris, J. D.: Late medial collateral ligament reconstruction. *Tech Knee Surg* 6:99–105, 2007.
11. Fetto, J. F.; Marshall, J. L.: Medial collateral ligament injuries of the knee: a rationale for treatment. *Clin Orthop Relat Res* 132:206–218, 1978.
12. Frolke, J. P.; Oskam, J.; Vierhout, P. A.: Primary reconstruction of the medial collateral ligament in combined injury of the medial collateral and anterior cruciate ligaments. Short-term results. *Knee Surg Sports Traumatol Arthrosc* 6:103–106, 1998.
13. Garrick, J. G. (ed): Orthopaedic Knowledge Update: Sports Medicine 3. Rosemont, IL: American Academy of Orthopaedic Surgeons, 2004; p. 466.
14. Halinen, J.; Lindahl, J.; Hirvensalo, E.; Santavirta, S.: Operative and nonoperative treatments of medial collateral ligament rupture with early anterior cruciate ligament reconstruction: a prospective randomized study. *Am J Sports Med* 34:1134–1140, 2006.
15. Hastings, D. E.: The non-operative management of collateral ligament injuries of the knee joint. *Clin Orthop Relat Res* 147:22–28, 1980.
16. Hewett, T. E.; Noyes, F. R.; Lee, M. D.: Diagnosis of complete and partial posterior cruciate ligament ruptures. Stress radiography compared with KT-1000 arthrometer and posterior drawer testing. *Am J Sports Med* 25:648–655, 1997.
17. Hillard-Sembell, D.; Daniel, D. M.; Stone, M. L.; et al.: Combined injuries of the anterior cruciate and medial collateral ligaments of the knee. Effect of treatment on stability and function of the joint. *J Bone Joint Surg Am* 78:169–176, 1996.
18. Holden, D. L.; Eggert, A. W.; Butler, J. E.: The nonoperative treatment of grade I and II medial collateral ligament injuries to the knee. *Am J Sports Med* 11:340–344, 1983.
19. Hughston, J. C.: The importance of the posterior oblique ligament in repairs of acute tears of the medial ligaments in knees with and without an associated rupture of the anterior cruciate ligament. Results of long-term follow-up. *J Bone Joint Surg Am* 76:1328–1344, 1994.
20. Hughston, J. C.; Andrews, J. R.; Cross, M. J.; Moschi, A.: Classification of knee ligament instabilities. Part I. The medial compartment and cruciate ligaments. *J Bone Joint Surg Am* 58:159–172, 1976.
21. Hughston, J. C.; Barrett, G. R.: Acute anteromedial rotatory instability. Long-term results of surgical repair. *J Bone Joint Surg Am* 65:145–153, 1983.
22. Hughston, J. C.; Eilers, A. F.: The role of the posterior oblique ligament in repairs of acute medial (collateral) ligament tears of the knee. *J Bone Joint Surg Am* 55:923–940, 1973.
23. Indelicato, P. A.: Non-operative treatment of complete tears of the medial collateral ligament of the knee. *J Bone Joint Surg Am* 65:323–329, 1983.
24. Indelicato, P. A.; Hermansdorfer, J.; Huegel, M.: Nonoperative management of complete tears of the medial collateral ligament of the knee in intercollegiate football players. *Clin Orthop Relat Res* 256:174–177, 1990.
25. Jokl, P.; Kaplan, N.; Stovell, P.; Keggi, K.: Non-operative treatment of severe injuries to the medial and anterior cruciate ligaments of the knee. *J Bone Joint Surg Am* 66:741–744, 1984.
25a. Jones, R. E.; Henley, M. B.; Francis, P.: Nonoperative management of isolated grade III collateral ligament injury in high school football players. *Clin Orthop Rel Res* 213:137–140, 1986.
26. Kannus, P.: Long-term results of conservatively treated medial collateral ligament injuries of the knee joint. *Clin Orthop Relat Res* 226:103–112, 1988.
27. Millett, P. J.; Pennock, A. T.; Sterett, W. I.; Steadman, J. R.: Early ACL reconstruction in combined ACL-MCL injuries. *J Knee Surg* 17:94–98, 2004.
28. Najibi, S.; Albright, J. P.: The use of knee braces, part 1: prophylactic knee braces in contact sports. *Am J Sports Med* 33:602–611, 2005.
29. Nakamura, N.; Horibe, S.; Toritsuka, Y.; et al.: Acute grade III medial collateral ligament injury of the knee associated with anterior cruciate ligament tear. The usefulness of magnetic resonance imaging in determining a treatment regimen. *Am J Sports Med* 31:261–267, 2003.
30. Noyes, F. R.; Barber-Westin, S. D.: The treatment of acute combined ruptures of the anterior cruciate and medial ligaments of the knee. *Am J Sports Med* 23:380–389, 1995.
31. Noyes, F. R.; Grood, E. S.; Torzilli, P. A.: Current concepts review. The definitions of terms for motion and position of the knee and injuries of the ligaments. *J Bone Joint Surg Am* 71:465–472, 1989.
31a. Petermann, J.; von Garrel, T.; Gotzen, L.: Non-operative treatment of acute medial collateral ligament lesions of the knee joint. *Knee Surg Sports Traumatol Arthosc* 1:93–96, 1993.
32. Petersen, W.; Laprell, H.: Combined injuries of the medial collateral ligament and the anterior cruciate ligament. Early ACL reconstruction versus late ACL reconstruction. *Arch Orthop Trauma Surg* 119:258–262, 1999.
33. Peterson, L.; Junge, A.; Chomiak, J.; et al.: Incidence of football injuries and complaints in different age groups and skill-level groups. *Am J Sports Med* 28(5 suppl):S51–S57, 2000.
33a. Reider, B.; Sathy, M. R.; Talkington, J.; et al.: Treatment of isolated medial collateral ligament injuries in athletes with early functional rehabilitation. A five-year follow-up study. *Am J Sports Med* 22:470–477, 1994.
34. Robins, A. J.; Newman, A. P.; Burks, R. T.: Postoperative return of motion in anterior cruciate ligament and medial collateral ligament injuries. The effect of medial collateral ligament rupture location. *Am J Sports Med* 21:20–25, 1993.
35. Robinson, J. R.; Bull, A. M.; Amis, A. A.: Structural properties of the medial collateral ligament complex of the human knee. *J Biomech* 38:1067–1074, 2005.
36. Robinson, J. R.; Bull, A. M.; Thomas, R. R.; Amis, A. A.: The role of the medial collateral ligament and posteromedial capsule in controlling knee laxity. *Am J Sports Med* 34:1815–1823, 2006.

37. Robinson, J. R.; Sanchez-Ballester, J.; Bull, A. M.; et al.: The posteromedial corner revisited. An anatomical description of the passive restraining structures of the medial aspect of the human knee. *J Bone Joint Surg Br* 86:674–681, 2004.

38. Rubman, M. H.; Noyes, F. R.; Barber-Westin, S. D.: Arthroscopic repair of meniscal tears that extend into the avascular zone. A review of 198 single and complex tears. *Am J Sports Med* 26:87–95, 1998.

39. Rubman, M. H.; Noyes, F. R.; Barber-Westin, S. D.: Technical considerations in the management of complex meniscus tears. *Clin Sports Med* 15:511–530, 1996.

40. Shelbourne, K. D.; Baele, J. R.: Treatment of combined anterior cruciate ligament and medial collateral ligament injuries. *Am J Knee Surg* 1:56–58, 1988.

41. Shelbourne, K. D.; Nitz, P. A.: The O'Donoghue triad revisited. Combined knee injuries involving anterior cruciate and medial collateral ligament tears. *Am J Sports Med* 19:474–477, 1991.

42. Shelbourne, K. D.; Patel, D. V.: Management of combined injuries of the anterior cruciate and medial collateral ligaments. *J Bone Joint Surg Am* 77:800–806, 1995.

43. Shelbourne, K. D.; Porter, D. A.: Anterior cruciate ligament–medial collateral ligament injury: nonoperative management of medial collateral ligament tears with anterior cruciate ligament reconstruction. A preliminary report. *Am J Sports Med* 20:283–286, 1992.

44. Sims, W. F.; Jacobson, K. E.: The posteromedial corner of the knee: medial-sided injury patterns revisited. *Am J Sports Med* 32:337–345, 2004.

45. Warren, L. F.; Marshall, J. L.: The supporting structures and layers on the medial side of the knee: an anatomical analysis. *J Bone Joint Surg Am* 61:56–62, 1979.

46. Yoshiya, S.; Kuroda, R.; Mizuno, K.; et al.: Medial collateral ligament reconstruction using autogenous hamstring tendons: technique and results in initial cases. *Am J Sports Med* 33:1380–1385, 2005.

47. Yoshiya, S.; Kuroda, R.; Mizuno, K.; et al.: Medial collateral ligament reconstruction using autogenous hamstring tendons: technique and results in initial cases. *Am J Sports Med* 33:1380–1385, 2005.

Chapter 25

Rehabilitation of Medial Ligament Injuries

Timothy P. Heckmann, PT, ATC ■ *Sue D. Barber-Westin*, BS ■ *Frank R. Noyes*, MD

CLINICAL CONCEPTS

Medial ligament injuries are among the most frequently treated problems of the knee joint. Whereas isolated superficial medial collateral ligament (SMCL) ruptures are common, concomitant damage to the anterior cruciate ligament (ACL) occurs in many cases, especially in young and active patients.[1–4,9] The majority of isolated acute injuries that involve damage to the SMCL alone, or to the SMCL and posteromedial capsule (PMC), do not require surgery. Patients who have medial ligament tears classified as first degree (tear involving a few fibers), second degree (partial tear, no instability, ≤3 mm of increased medial joint opening), or third degree (complete rupture) who demonstrate either a mild to moderate increase in medial joint opening at 30° of flexion and no increase at 0° do not require acute medial ligament reconstruction. These knees are treated with the conservative rehabilitation program, and if concomitant injury exists to other ligaments, the decision of whether to reconstruct those structures is based on the extent of the injury, patient goals, and other issues addressed for the ACL in Chapter 7, Anterior Cruciate Ligament Primary and Revision Reconstruction: Diagnosis, Operative Techniques, and Clinical Outcomes, the posterior cruciate ligament (PCL) in Chapter 21, Posterior Cruciate Ligament: Diagnosis, Operative Techniques, and Clinical Outcomes, and the posterolateral ligament structures in Chapter 22, Posterolateral Ligament Injuries: Diagnosis, Operative Techniques, and Clinical Outcomes.

Critical Points CLINICAL CONCEPTS

- Majority of isolated acute medial ligament injuries do not require surgery
  - Treated with conservative rehabilitation.
  - If concomitant injury exists to other ligaments, the decision of whether to reconstruct those structures is based on the extent of the injury, patient goals, and other issues.
- Acute third-degree injury of all of the medial structures, either alone or in combination with cruciate ligament tears, often require surgery.
- Chronic deficiency of the medial ligament structures that causes partial giving-way during athletic activities may require reconstruction.

An acute third-degree injury consisting of gross major disruption of all of the medial structures (SMCL, deep medial collateral ligament, meniscus attachments, PMC, posterior oblique ligament [POL], and semimembranosus attachments), either alone or in combination with cruciate ligament tears, often require surgical intervention. In these knees, large increases in medial joint opening are present at 30° of flexion, and at least 5 mm of increased medial joint opening exists at 0°. In addition, repair of medial meniscus attachments is indicated to retain meniscus function. Chronic deficiency of the medial ligament structures that causes partial giving-way during athletic activities may require reconstruction. In these knees, partial or complete ACL deficiency is frequently noted. The indications for medial ligament surgery and the appropriate candidates are discussed in detail in Chapter 24, Medial and Posteromedial Ligament Injuries: Diagnosis, Operative Techniques, and Clinical Outcomes.

CONSERVATIVE TREATMENT OF MEDIAL LIGAMENT INJURIES

The goals of rehabilitation of medial ligament injuries are to

- Provide appropriate protection initially after the injury to allow the disrupted medial ligament structures to "stick-down" and heal with the least amount of residual ligament elongation or abnormal medial joint opening.
- Control of joint pain, swelling, and hemarthrosis.
- Regain a normal range of knee motion.
- Restore a normal gait pattern and neuromuscular stability for ambulation.
- Recover normal lower limb muscle strength.
- Regain normal proprioception, balance, coordination, and neuromuscular control for desired activities.
- Achieve optimal functional outcome based on orthopaedic and patient goals.

The treatment rationale for patients with acute medial ligament ruptures is shown in Figure 25–1. The algorithm is divided into three major sections based on the extent of injury to the SMCL and PMC/POL. The first- and second-degree injuries are treated initially with a functional brace, weight-bearing as tolerated, and the rehabilitation program summarized in Tables 25–1 and 25–2. Some second-degree injuries may have considerable medial pain and swelling, and in these cases, an extension brace and assistive ambulatory devices are used for the initial 1 to 2 weeks after the injury. The type of functional brace varies from a medial/lateral hinge elastic type to a long leg postoperative brace in select cases in which more support is required.

Third-Degree Injuries: Weeks 1 to 3

The treatment of third-degree medial ligament injuries involves short-term immobilization to allow the medial ligament structures time to heal with the least elongation or laxity by limiting medial joint opening and external tibial rotation. The lower limb is placed in a cylinder cast positioned in slight varus and internal rotation for 1 week to allow the disrupted medial soft tissues to "stick-down." Plaster immobilization is required because a soft hinged or functional brace, even if locked at 0°, does not provide sufficient protection to maintain medial joint line closure to allow close approximation of the disrupted medial ligament and meniscus attachment soft tissues. The patient is instructed to maintain the leg in an elevated position with the limb supported in order to control lower extremity swelling. The patient is also instructed to stay off of the lower limb as much as possible. In addition, ankle-pumping exercises are performed to maintain lower extremity circulation, and quadriceps isometrics are done hourly. Electrical muscle stimulation (EMS) is used to augment the voluntary quadriceps contraction. Windows may be cut into the cast in order to observe the electrodes to ensure that they do not irritate the skin or to determine whether they need to be replaced. EMS is used approximately six times per day for 15-minute sessions. A co-contraction should occur between the stimulator and the patient's voluntary contraction. Hamstring and gastrocnemius flexibility exercises are also encouraged to promote posterior muscle relaxation.

At 7 to 10 days, the cylinder cast is split into an anterior and a posterior shell (Fig. 25–2) to permit the patient to begin passive range of motion (ROM) exercises, which are initially assisted by the therapist. The cast is used for an additional 2 weeks to allow for early stick-down of the medial ligament structures. The patient is allowed to bear 25% of her or his body weight as long as the cast is in place. ROM exercises are initiated in a figure-four position from 0° to 90° in order to avoid valgus and external rotation loads on the healing ligaments (Fig. 25–3). A 4-inch

---

Critical Points CONSERVATIVE TREATMENT OF MEDIAL LIGAMENT INJURIES

- First- and second-degree medial ligament injuries treated initially with a functional brace, weight-bearing as tolerated, and the rehabilitation program summarized in Tables 25-1 and 25-2.
- Third-degree medial ligament injuries require short-term immobilization to allow structures time to heal.
- Weeks 1–3
  - Cylinder cast 7–10 days.
  - Cast bivalved into anterior, posterior shell, worn 2 more wk. Knee motion done in figure-four position, 3–4 times/day.
  - Quadriceps isometrics, flexion straight leg raises.
- Weeks 4–6
  - Cast discontinued, functional brace worn.
  - Weight-bearing progressed 25%/wk, discontinue crutches by 6th wk.
  - Straight leg raises, closed-chain exercises.
  - Emphasis on ligament protection during gait and exercise.
- Weeks 7–9
  - Gait and range of motion normal or nearly normal.
  - Emphasis on returning lower extremity strength to normal.
- Begin cross-training for cardiovascular endurance.
- Balance, proprioception exercises.
- Weeks 10–12
  - Focus on return to activity.
  - Gait, knee motion, activities of daily living, symptoms should be within normal limits.
  - Isokinetic muscle strength parameters within 70% and 90% for straight-ahead running and more strenuous turning/cutting drills, respectively.
  - Full running program, sports-specific training.
- Concomitant anterior cruciate ligament (ACL) rupture and third-degree medial ligament rupture requires initial stick-down program and treatment described. 3–6 wk of conservative management before ACL reconstruction.
- Concomitant posterior cruciate ligament rupture and medial ligament rupture requires initial stick-down program with a posterior calf pad to prevent posterior tibial subluxation. Hamstrings contractions not allowed for 6 wk, then permitted in the active mode only for an additional 6 wk.

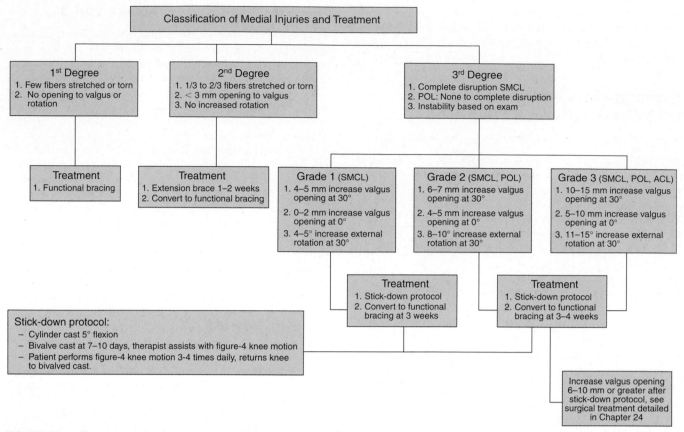

Classification of Medial Injuries and Treatment

1st Degree
1. Few fibers stretched or torn
2. No opening to valgus or rotation

2nd Degree
1. 1/3 to 2/3 fibers stretched or torn
2. < 3 mm opening to valgus
3. No increased rotation

3rd Degree
1. Complete disruption SMCL
2. POL: None to complete disruption
3. Instability based on exam

Treatment
1. Functional bracing

Treatment
1. Extension brace 1–2 weeks
2. Convert to functional bracing

Grade 1 (SMCL)
1. 4–5 mm increase valgus opening at 30°
2. 0–2 mm increase valgus opening at 0°
3. 4–5° increase external rotation at 30°

Grade 2 (SMCL, POL)
1. 6–7 mm increase valgus opening at 30°
2. 4–5 mm increase valgus opening at 0°
3. 8–10° increase external rotation at 30°

Grade 3 (SMCL, POL, ACL)
1. 10–15 mm increase valgus opening at 30°
2. 5–10 mm increase valgus opening at 0°
3. 11–15° increase external rotation at 30°

Treatment
1. Stick-down protocol
2. Convert to functional bracing at 3 weeks

Treatment
1. Stick-down protocol
2. Convert to functional bracing at 3–4 weeks

Stick-down protocol:
– Cylinder cast 5° flexion
– Bivalve cast at 7–10 days, therapist assists with figure-4 knee motion
– Patient performs figure-4 knee motion 3-4 times daily, returns knee to bivalved cast.

Increase valgus opening 6–10 mm or greater after stick-down protocol, see surgical treatment detailed in Chapter 24

FIGURE 25–1. Treatment rationale for patients with acute medial ligament ruptures.

TABLE 25–1   Conservative Management of First-Degree Medial Ligament Injuries

- Weight-bearing as tolerated with assistive device if required.
- Functional brace for protection for 3–4 wk postinjury.
- Active ROM exercises to achieve full ROM as tolerated.
- Strengthening exercises: open and closed kinetic chain as tolerated.
- Progress to agility, proprioceptive, neuromuscular, sports-specific activities as tolerated.
- Return to full activities when strength is equal to the opposite side, all symptoms resolved.

ROM, range of motion.

TABLE 25–2   Conservative Management of Second-Degree Medial Ligament Injuries

- Weight-bearing as tolerated with assistive device if required.
- Extension brace for 1–2 wk postinjury if excessive medial compartment pain, swelling.
- Functional brace for next 4–6 wk.
- Active ROM exercises to achieve full ROM as tolerated.
- Electrical muscle stimulation, straight leg raises begun immediately.
- Strengthening exercises: open and closed kinetic chain as tolerated.
- Progress to agility, proprioceptive, neuromuscular, sports-specific activities upon resumption of full weight-bearing as tolerated.
- Return to full activities when strength is equal to the opposite side, all symptoms resolved.

ROM, range of motion.

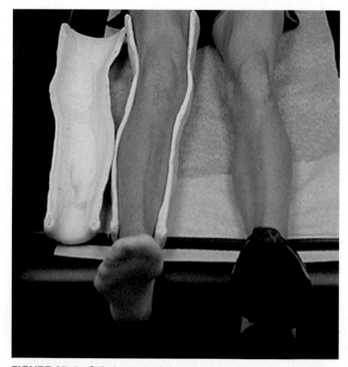

FIGURE 25–2. Cylinder cast split into an anterior and a posterior shell.

tubular stocking is double-wrapped around the foot and ankle to allow the patient under her or his own power to flex the knee. This protected ROM program is performed three to four times a day for 10 to 15 minutes per session. Quadriceps strengthening exercises including isometrics and flexion straight leg raises are emphasized. TheraBand resistance for plantar flexion is used to maintain gastrocnemius tone. Ice, compression, and elevation are used for pain and swelling control.

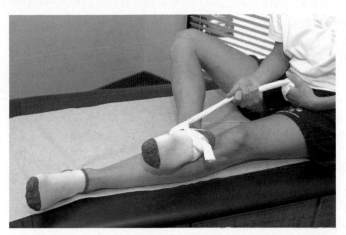

FIGURE 25–3. Patient performs range of motion (ROM) exercises from 0° to 90° in a figure-four position with the hip joint externally rotated to protect the healing medial tissues.

Third-Degree Injuries: Weeks 4 to 6

At the end of the first 3 to 4 weeks, the bivalved cast is discontinued and the patient is placed into either a functional knee brace (for medial ligament unloading) or a long-leg ROM brace depending on the extent of the knee effusion and residual tenderness to medial soft tissue pressure. A functional osteoarthritis brace is encouraged in order to avoid the expense of a transitional brace; however, this determination is based on each individual patient. Weight-bearing is progressed approximately 25% each week in order to discontinue crutches by the 6th week. Gait retraining is encouraged to allow for return of the normal reciprocal gait pattern (sufficient push-off during toe-off, midstance quadriceps contraction, hip and knee flexion during swing, and an upright posture).

Cryotherapy and EMS are continued in order to maintain control of pain and swelling as well as quadriceps reeducation. Exercises include quadriceps isometrics and straight leg raises in the flexion and prone positions through the 4th week. Abduction and adduction leg raises may then be initiated as long as there is sufficient quadriceps control to limit varus/valgus loading. Any resistance in a side-to-side fashion is kept above the knee through at least the 6th week. Closed-chain exercises such as standing calf raises and wall-sitting isometrics are encouraged. ROM is progressed with figure-four protection continued through the 4th to 6th week.

Emphasis during this time period focuses on ligament protection during gait and exercise. The progression of exercise allows knee motion to be restored within normal limits. Muscle strengthening includes both closed-chain and table exercises (straight leg raises). Emphasis is placed on hip and core control plus progression of quadriceps strengthening (Table 25-3).

TABLE 25–3 Cincinnati Sportsmedicine and Orthopaedic Center Rehabilitation Protocol for Medial Ligament Repair or Reconstruction									
	Postoperative Weeks					**Postoperative Months**			
	1–2	3–4	5–6	7–8	9–12	4	5	6	7–12
Brace									
Long-leg postoperative	X	X	X						
Custom unloading if required				X	X	X	X	X	X
ROM minimum goals									
0°–90°	X								
0°–110°		X							
0°–120°			X						
0°–130°				X					
Weight-bearing									
None	X								
Toe touch ~25% body weight		X							
25%–50% body weight			X						
100% body weight				X					
Patella mobilization	X	X	X	X	X				
Modalities									
EMS	X	X	X	X					
Pain/edema management (cryotherapy)	X	X	X	X	X	X	X	X	X
Stretching									
Hamstring, gastrocnemius-soleus, ITB, quadriceps	X	X	X	X	X	X	X	X	X
Strengthening									
Quadriceps isometrics, straight leg raises	X	X	X	X	X				
Active knee extension		X	X	X	X				
Closed-chain: gait retraining, toe-raises, wall-sits, mini-squats	X	X	X	X	X	X	X	X	
Knee flexion hamstring curls (90°)					X	X	X	X	X
Knee extension quads (90°–30°)		X	X	X	X	X	X	X	X
Hip abduction-adduction, multi-hip					X	X	X	X	X
Leg press (70°–10°)				X	X	X	X	X	X
Balance/proprioceptive training									
Weight-shifting, cup-walking, BBS			X	X					
BBS, BAPS, perturbation training, balance board, mini-trampoline					X	X	X	X	X

Continued

TABLE 25–3 Cincinnati Sportsmedicine and Orthopaedic Center Rehabilitation Protocol for Medial Ligament Repair or Reconstruction—Cont'd

	Postoperative Weeks					Postoperative Months			
	1–2	3–4	5–6	7–8	9–12	4	5	6	7–12
Conditioning									
UBC		X	X	X					
Bike (stationary)			X	X	X	X	X	X	X
Aquatic program					X	X	X	X	X
Elliptical machine					X	X	X	X	X
Swimming (kicking)					X	X	X	X	X
Walking					X	X	X	X	X
Stair-climbing machine					X	X	X	X	X
Ski machine						X	X	X	X
Running: straight								X	X
Cutting: lateral carioca, figure-eights									X
Plyometric training									X
Full sports									X

PHASE 1. WEEKS 1 TO 2 (VISITS 2–4)

General Observation	Non–weight-bearing, maximum protection	
	Brace locked at 0° (motion exercises 3–4 times/day)	
	Avoid valgus loads, abnormal external tibial rotation	
Evaluation		**Goals**
	Pain	Controlled
	Hemarthrosis	Mild
	Patellar mobility	Good
	ROM minimum	0°–90°
	Quadriceps contraction & patella migration	Good
	Soft tissue contracture	None
Frequency		**Duration**
3–4 x/day	**ROM**	
10 min	• ROM (passive, 0°–90°)	
	• Patella mobilization	
	• Ankle pumps (plantar flexion with resistance band)	
	• Hamstring, gastrocnemius-soleus stretches	5 reps x 30 sec
3 x/day	**Strengthening**	
15 min	Straight leg raises (flexion)	3 sets x 10 reps
	Active quadriceps isometrics	1 set x 10 reps
	Knee extension (active-assisted, 90°–30°, per quadriceps control)	3 sets x 10 reps
As required	**Modalities**	
	EMS	20 min
	Cryotherapy	20 min
Goals	ROM 0°–90°	
	Adequate quadriceps contraction	
	Control inflammation, effusion	

PHASE 2. WEEKS 3 TO 4 (VISITS 2–4)

General Observation	Partial weight bearing: toe touch to 25% body weight	
	Brace locked at 0° (motion exercises 3–4 times/day)	
	Avoid valgus loads, abnormal external tibial rotation	
Evaluation		**Goals**
	Pain	Controlled
	Effusion	Mild
	Patellar mobility	Good
	ROM minimum	0°–90°
	Quadriceps contraction & patella migration	Good
	Soft tissue contracture	None
Frequency		**Duration**
3–4 x/day	**ROM**	
10 min	• ROM (passive, 0°–110°)	
	• Patella mobilization	
	• Ankle pumps (plantar flexion with resistance band)	
	• Hamstring, gastrocnemius-soleus stretches	5 reps x 30 sec
2–3 x/day	**Strengthening**	
20 min	Straight leg raises (flexion)	3 sets x 10 reps
	Isometric training: multi-angle (0°, 60°)	1 set x 10 reps
	Knee extension (active, 90°–30°, per quadriceps control)	3 sets x 10 reps
2 x/day	**Aerobic conditioning**	
10 min	UBC	

As required	**Modalities**	
	EMS	20 min
	Cryotherapy	20 min
Goals	ROM 0°–110°	
	Control inflammation, effusion	
	Muscle control	

PHASE 3. WEEKS 5 TO 6 (VISITS 1–2)

General Observation

Partial (25%–50%) weight-bearing when
- Pain controlled without narcotics
- Hemarthrosis controlled
- Muscle control throughout ROM
- ROM 0°–120°
- Custom unloading brace
- Avoid valgus loads

Evaluation

	Goals
Pain	Mild/no RSD
Effusion	Minimal
Patellar mobility	Good
ROM	0°–120°
Muscle control	3/5
Inflammatory response	None

Frequency		**Duration**
3 x/day	**ROM**	
10 min	ROM (passive, 0°–120°)	
	Patella mobilization	
	Hamstring, gastrocnemius-soleus stretches	5 reps x 30 sec
2 x/day	**Strengthening**	
20 min	Straight leg raises (ankle weight, not to exceed 10% of body weight)	3 sets x 10 reps
	Isometric training: multiangle (90°, 60°, 30°)	2 sets x 10 reps
	Closed-chain	
	• Mini-squats	3 sets x 20 reps
	Knee extension (active, 90°–30°)	3 sets x 10 reps
2 x/day	**Aerobic conditioning**	
10 min	UBC	
	Stationary bicycling	
	Gait retraining	
	Muscle control quadriceps & hamstrings	
	Walk with toe-in gait, avoid toe-out valgus position	
	Observe gait for any tendency for valgus thrust or external tibial rotation	
	Smooth stance phase flexion pattern	
As required	**Modalities**	
	EMS	20 min
	Cryotherapy	20 min
Goals	ROM 0°–10°	
	Control inflammation, effusion	
	Muscle control	
	Early recognition complications (motion, RSD, patellofemoral)	
	50% weight bearing	

PHASE 4. WEEKS 7 TO 8 (VISITS 1–2)

General Observation

Full weight-bearing
Custom unloading brace
ROM 0°–130°

Evaluation

	Goals
Pain	Mild/no RSD
Effusion	Minimal
Patellar mobility	Good
ROM	0°–130°
Muscle control	4/5
Inflammatory response	None

Frequency		**Duration**
2 x/day	**ROM**	
10 min	ROM (0°–120°)	
	Hamstring, gastrocnemius-soleus stretches	5 reps x 30 sec
	Patellar mobility	
2 x/day	**Strengthening**	
20 min	Straight leg raises (flexion, extension, abduction, adduction)	3 sets x 10 reps
	Straight leg raises, rubber tubing	3 sets x 30 reps
	Knee extension (active, 90°–30°)	3 sets x 10 reps
	Closed-chain	
	• Wall sits	To fatigue x 3
	• Mini-squats (rubber tubing, 0°–30°)	3 sets x 20 reps
	Leg press (70°–10°)	3 sets x 10 reps

Continued

3 x/day
5 min
	Balance training
	    Cup-walking
	    BBS	

1–2 x/day
15 min
	Aerobic conditioning
	    UBC
	    Stationary bicycling	

	Gait retraining
	    Progress program
	    Continue to observe for valgus thrust, external tibial rotation	

As required	**Modalities**
	    EMS
	    Cryotherapy
		20 min
		20 min

Goals	Full weight-bearing Muscle control Control inflammation, effusion ROM 0°–130°	

PHASE 5. WEEKS 9 TO 12 (VISITS 1–2)

General Observation	Full weight-bearing ROM 0°–130° Custom unloading brace	
Evaluation		**Goals**
	Pain	Minimal/no RSD
	Manual muscle test: hamstrings, quadriceps, hip abductors/adductors/flexors/ extensors	4/5
	Swelling	Minimal
	Patellar mobility	Good
	Crepitus	None/slight
	Gait	Symmetrical
Frequency		**Duration**

2 x/day
10 min
	ROM
	    Hamstring, gastrocnemius-soleus, quadriceps, ITB stretches
	    Patellar mobility
		5 reps x 30 sec

2 x/day
20 min
	Strengthening
	    Straight leg raises
	    Straight leg raises, rubber tubing
	    Hamstring curls (wk 12, active, 0°–90°)
	    Knee extension with resistance (90°–30°)
	    Leg press (70°–10°)
	    Closed-chain
	        • Wall-sits
	        • Mini-squats (rubber tubing, 0°–40°)
	        • Lateral step-ups (2"–4" block)
	    Multi-hip machine (flexion, extension, abduction, adduction)
		3 sets x 10 reps
		3 sets x 30 reps
		3 sets x 10 reps
		3 sets x 10 reps
		3 sets x 10 reps
		
		To fatigue x 3
		3 sets x 20 reps
		3 sets x 10 reps
		3 sets x 10 reps

3 x/day 5 min	**Balance training** Cup-walking, BBS, BAPS, perturbation training	

1 x/day
15–20 min
	Aerobic conditioning (patellofemoral precautions)
	    Water-walking
	    Elliptical machine
	    Stationary bicycling
	    Stair machine (low resistance, low stroke)
	    Swimming (kicking)
	    Walking	

As required	**Modalities** Cryotherapy	20 min
Goals	Increase strength and endurance ROM 0°–130° Normal gait without valgus, external tibial rotation	

PHASE 6. WEEKS 13 TO 26 (VISITS 2–3)

General Observation	No effusion, painless ROM, joint stability Performs activities of daily living, can walk 20 min without pain ROM 0°–130° Custom unloading brace	
Evaluation		**Goals**
	Pain	Minimal/no RSD
	Manual muscle test	4/5
	Swelling	Minimal
	Patellar mobility	Good
	Crepitus	None/slight
	Gait	Symmetrical

Frequency		Duration
2 x/day	**ROM**	
10 min	Hamstring, gastrocnemius-soleus, quadriceps, ITB stretches	5 reps x 30 sec
2 x/day	**Strengthening**	
20 min	Straight leg raises, rubber tubing (high speed)	3 sets x 30 reps
	Hamstring curls (active, 0°–90°)	3 sets x 10 reps
	Knee extension with resistance (90°–30°)	3 sets x 10 reps
	Leg press (70°–10°)	3 sets x 10 reps
	Multi-hip machine (flexion, extension, abduction, adduction)	3 sets x 10 reps
	Closed-chain: mini-squats (rubber tubing, 0°–40°)	3 sets x 20 reps
1–3 x/day	**Balance training**	
5 min	Balance board/two-legged	
	Single-leg stance	
3 x/wk	**Aerobic conditioning (patellofemoral precautions)**	
20 min	Stationary bicycling	
	Water-walking	
	Swimming (kicking)	
	Walking	
	Elliptical machine	
	Stair machine (low resistance, low stroke)	
	Ski machine (short stride, level, low resistance)	
As required	**Modalities**	
	Cryotherapy	20 min
Goals	Increase strength and endurance	

PHASE 7. WEEKS 27 TO 52 (VISITS 2–3)

General Observation	No effusion, painless ROM, joint stability	
	Performs activities of daily living, can walk 20 min without pain	
	Custom unloading brace	
Evaluation		**Goals**
	Isometric test (% difference quadriceps & hamstrings)	10–15
	Swelling	None
	Patellar mobility	Good
	Crepitus	None/slight
Frequency		Duration
2 x/day	**ROM**	
10 min	Hamstring, gastrocnemius-soleus, quadriceps, ITB stretches	5 reps x 30 sec
1 x/day	**Strengthening**	
20–30 min	Straight leg raises, rubber tubing (high speed)	3 sets x 30 reps
	Hamstring curls (0°–90°)	3 sets x 10 reps
	Knee extension with resistance (90°–30°)	3 sets x 10 reps
	Leg press (70°–10°)	3 sets x 10 reps
	Multi-hip machine (flexion, extension, abduction, adduction)	3 sets x 10 reps
	Closed-chain: mini-squats (rubber tubing, 0°–40°)	3 sets x 20 reps
1–3 x/day	**Balance training**	
5 min	Balance board/two-legged	
	Single-leg stance	
3 x/wk	**Aerobic conditioning (patellofemoral precautions)**	
20–30 min	Stationary bicycling	
	Water-walking	
	Swimming (kicking)	
	Walking	
	Elliptical machine	
	Stair machine (low resistance, low stroke)	
	Ski machine (short stride, level, low resistance)	
3 x/wk	**Running program** (9 mo minimum, straight, 30% deficit isometric test)	
15–20 min	Jog	¼ mile
	Walk	⅛ mile
	Backward run	20 yd
3 x/wk	**Cutting program** (12 mo minimum, 20% deficit isometric test)—lateral, carioca, figure-eights	20 yd
3 x/wk	**Functional training** (12 mo minimum)	15 sec,
	Plyometric training: box hops, level, double-leg	4–6 sets
	Sports-specific drills (10%–15% deficit isometric test)	
As required	**Modalities**	
	Cryotherapy	20 min
Goals	Increase function	
	Maintain strength, endurance	
	Return to previous activity level	

BAPS, Biomechanical Ankle Platform System (Camp, Jackson, MI); BBS, Biodex Balance System (Biodex Medical Systems, Inc., Shirley, NY); EMS, electrical muscle stimulation; ITB, iliotibial band; ROM, range of motion; RSD, reflex sympathetic dystrophy; UBC, upper body cycle (Biodex Medical Systems, Inc., Shirley, NY).

Third-Degree Injuries: Weeks 7 to 9

If a long-leg brace was used in the previous phase, a functional brace is now initiated. Patients who already have a functional brace maintain its usage for ambulation. Gait and ROM should be normal or nearly normal, with restoration to normal as soon as possible. Pain and swelling should be within normal limits. Emphasis during this phase of treatment is on returning lower extremity strength to normal and to begin cross-training for cardiovascular endurance. Balance and proprioception exercises are also important components of this phase (see Chapter 13, Rehabilitation of Primary and Revision Anterior Cruciate Ligament Reconstructions).

Straight leg raises in multiple planes with ankle weights are used for hip control. Ten pounds of resistance represents the target goal for these exercises. Progression of the closed-chain program includes performing calf raises off of the edge of a step or with weight added for resistance. Isometric wall-sits are done with a gradual increase in hold time and then with handheld weights added. TheraBand resistance is used with mini-squats and terminal knee extension. Gait retraining is done with a heavy elastic band positioned about the thighs. In addition, the patient is progressed to a machine-oriented program for leg-press (80°–10°), knee extension (90°–30°), seated hamstring curls (0°–90°), hip abduction/adduction, and calf presses.

Endurance training includes a stationary bicycle, elliptical cross-trainer, and/or aquatics for 20 to 30 minutes at least three times per week. Activities such as cutting or twisting that place valgus and external rotation torques on the lower extremity are still limited. Proprioception and balance training includes unidirectional exercises balancing on a rocker board and multidirectional activities such as a wobble board or balance board. Balance activities at home progress from tandem balance positioning to single-leg stance. Isokinetic testing is performed to measure quadriceps and hamstrings muscle strength. The goals for initiating a running program are at least 70% bilateral comparison for quadriceps and hamstrings torque–to–body weight ratios (based on age and gender) and a hamstring-quadriceps ratio of 60%.

Third-Degree Injuries: Weeks 10 to 12

The focus of this final phase is on return to activity. By this time period, gait, ROM, activities of daily living, and symptoms should be within normal limits. The exercise progression advocates return of isokinetic muscle strength parameters within 70% and 90% for straight-ahead running and more strenuous turning/cutting drills, respectively. The cross-training program is advanced to a full running program that then allows for sports-specific training. Distance and direction-specific running and agility drills are incorporated. Heavy strength training occurs on opposite days of the running program. Injury prevention and neuromuscular retraining programs include jump-training activities with emphasis on technique, position, alignment, and repetition as discussed in detail in Chapter 19, Decreasing the Risk of Anterior Cruciate Ligament Injuries in Female Athletes. Isokinetic testing is performed, with the goal of achieving a 90% bilateral comparison for quadriceps and hamstrings torque–to–body weight ratios (corrected for age and gender), and a hamstring-to-quadriceps ratio of 60% at 120°/sec. Patients continue brace use for activity only. Follow-up treatment is based on the need for symptom control and/or functional progression for unrestricted return to activity.

Concomitant Cruciate Ligament Injuries

Patients who have a concomitant ACL rupture and third-degree medial ligament rupture undergo the initial stick-down program and treatment described. According to the severity of the medial collateral ligament (MCL) injury, sufficient time is required to stick down the medial structures, allow for figure-four ROM, protect with partial weight-bearing, and initiate early quadriceps exercises. Initial knee motion goals are 0° to 90°. Normally, 3 to 6 weeks of conservative management is required before the patient undergoes ACL reconstruction. The progression of exercises and weight-bearing is consistent with that described earlier.

Patients who have a concomitant PCL rupture and medial ligament rupture also undergo the initial stick-down program with a posterior calf pad to prevent posterior tibial subluxation. The cast is used for 4 weeks, followed with a long-leg brace with a posterior pad, which is used for 4 weeks. Then, weight-bearing, range of knee motion, and quadriceps exercises are progressed. Figure-four ROM exercises with an anterior drawer support allow for protection of both ligaments. The initial knee motion goal is 0° to 90°, which is then gradually progressed to full 6 weeks after cast wear. Full weight-bearing is permitted after 6 weeks, with emphasis on quadriceps control. Hamstrings contractions are not allowed for the initial 6 weeks and are then permitted in the active mode only for an additional 6 weeks. The patient's gait, knee motion, quadriceps control, and symptoms should be back to normal limits in order to consider surgical intervention. Knee injuries with combined third-degree medial ligament ruptures and PCL ruptures often require operative repair; the postoperative course is described in Chapter 23, Rehabilitation of Posterior Cruciate Ligament and Posterolateral Reconstructive Procedures.

POSTOPERATIVE REHABILITATION OF MEDIAL LIGAMENT REPAIRS/ RECONSTRUCTIONS

The surgical treatment of acute third-degree medial ligament ruptures involves anatomic repair to restore continuity and function, including repair of the medial meniscus attachments. Knees with chronic deficiency of the medial ligament ruptures often require a graft reconstruction using a semitendinosus-gracilis autograft or allograft, discussed in Chapter 24, Medial and Posteromedial Ligament Injuries: Diagnosis, Operative Techniques, and Clinical Outcomes. The operative procedure is designed to provide sufficient tensile strength to the reconstructed medial tissues to allow immediate knee motion and restore early limb function. The goal is to provide 4 weeks of maximum protection, using a long-leg postoperative brace. After this period, the rehabilitation program progresses, as soft tissue healing provides sufficient strength for ambulatory activities.

The postoperative protocol (see Table 25–3) is divided into seven phases according to the time period postoperatively (e.g., phase I comprises postoperative wk 1–2). Each phase has four main categories that describe the factors evaluated by the therapist and exercises performed by the patient:

■ General observation of the patient's condition.
■ Evaluation and measurement of specific variables, with goals identified for each variable.
■ Treatment and exercise program according to frequency and duration.
■ Rehabilitation goals that must be achieved to enter the next phase.

Critical Points POSTOPERATIVE REHABILITATION OF MEDIAL LIGAMENT REPAIRS/RECONSTRUCTIONS

- Surgical treatment acute third-degree medial ligament ruptures involves anatomic repair to restore continuity and function, including repair of the medial meniscus attachments.
- Chronic deficiency of the medial ligament ruptures often requires semitendinosus-gracilis autograft or allograft.
- Protocol incorporates a home self-management program, along with an estimated number of formal physical therapy visits.
- First postoperative wk critical in regard to control of knee joint pain and swelling, return of adequate quadriceps muscle contraction, initiation of immediate knee motion exercises from 0° to 90°, and maintenance of adequate limb elevation.
- Modalities
  - ○ EMS.
  - ○ Biofeedback.
  - ○ Cryotherapy.
- Bracing
  - ○ Long-leg postoperative brace locked 0° for 2 wk.
  - ○ Brace unlocked, worn another 4–6 wk.
  - ○ Off-the-shelf brace or custom medial unloading brace for extensive repairs.
- Weight-bearing
  - ○ None for first 2 wk.
  - ○ Toe touch to 25% wk 3–4.
  - ○ Slowly progressed to full wk 7–8.
- Range of knee motion: begin 1st postoperative day
  - ○ Goal: 0°–90° 1st postoperative wk.
  - ○ Exercises done 4–6 times/day.
  - ○ Use overpressure exercises if goals not met.
- Patellar mobilization
  - ○ Begin 1st postoperative day, perform with range of motion exercises.
- Flexibility
  - ○ Hamstring, gastrocnemius-soleus 1st postoperative day.
  - ○ Quadriceps, iliotibial band begun wk 9.

- Strengthening
  - ○ Begin 1st postoperative day quadriceps isometrics, straight leg raises, hip flexion.
- Closed kinetic chain exercises when 50% weight-bearing tolerated
  - ○ Hamstring curls wk 9–12.
  - ○ Open kinetic chain exercises within 1st few weeks, patellofemoral precautions.
  - ○ Full lower extremity program, include upper extremity and core.
- Balance, proprioception
  - ○ Begin when 50% weight-bearing tolerated.
  - ○ Weight-shifting.
  - ○ Cup-walking.
  - ○ Double-, single-leg balance.
  - ○ Perturbation training
  - ○ Walking half foam rolls.
- Conditioning
  - ○ Stationary bicycling 5–6 wk.
  - ○ Water-walking, swimming, elliptical machine 9–12 wk.
  - ○ Perform 3 times/wk for 20–30 min.
- Running and agility
  - ○ Running criteria: ≤30% deficit average torque quadriceps and hamstrings on isokinetic testing, ≤3 mm increased medial joint opening (30° flexion). Majority of patients are at least 6 mo postoperative.
  - ○ Program based on patient goals, done 3 times/wk opposite days of strength program.
- Plyometric training
  - ○ Begin after completion of running program.
  - ○ Footwear, surface important.
  - ○ Jump and land with knees flexed and shoulder-width apart to avoid knee hyperextension and an overall valgus lower limb position.

Specific criteria are evaluated throughout the rehabilitation program to determine whether the patient is ready to progress from one phase to the next. The protocol incorporates a home self-management program, along with an estimated number of formal physical therapy visits. For most patients, 11 to 21 postoperative visits are expected to produce a desirable result.

The following signs are continually monitored postoperatively: joint swelling, pain, gait pattern, knee motion, patellar mobility, muscle strength, flexibility, and medial tibiofemoral compartment opening. Any individual who experiences difficulty progressing through the protocol or who develops a complication is expected to require additional supervision in the formal clinic setting.

The 1st postoperative week represents a critical time period in regard to control of knee joint pain and swelling, return of adequate quadriceps muscle contraction, initiation of immediate knee motion exercises from 0° to 90°, and maintenance of adequate limb elevation. A bulky compression dressing is used for 48 hours and then converted to compression stockings with an additional compression bandage if necessary. Patients are encouraged to stay in bed and elevate the limb above their heart for the first 5 to 7 days, rising only to perform exercises and attend to personal bathing issues. Prophylaxis against deep venous thrombosis includes one aspirin a day for 10 days, ambulation (with crutch support) six to eight times a day for short periods of time, ankle pumping every hour that the patient is awake, and close observation of the lower limb by the therapist and surgeon. Knee joint

hemarthroses require aspiration. Nonsteroidal anti-inflammatories are used for 5 days postoperative. Appropriate pain medication is prescribed to provide relief and allow the immediate exercise protocol described later to be performed.

Modalities

In the immediate postoperative period, knee effusion must be controlled to avoid the quadriceps inhibition phenomenon. Electrogalvanic stimulation or high-voltage EMS may be used along with ice, compression, and elevation to control swelling. Treatment duration is approximately 30 minutes, the intensity is set to patient tolerance, and the treatment frequency is three to six times per day.

Once joint effusion is controlled, functional EMS is used for quadriceps muscle reeducation based on the evaluation of quadriceps muscle tone. One electrode is placed over the vastus medialis oblique (VMO) and a second electrode is placed on the central to lateral aspect of the upper third of the quadriceps muscle belly. The treatment duration is 20 minutes. The patient actively contracts the quadriceps muscle simultaneously with the machine's stimulation.

Biofeedback therapy is important to facilitate an adequate quadriceps muscle contraction early postoperatively. The surface electrode is placed over the selected muscle component to provide feedback to the patient and clinician regarding the quality of active or voluntary quadriceps contraction. Biofeedback is also useful in enhancing hamstring relaxation if the patient has difficulty achieving full knee extension owing to knee pain or muscle spasm. The electrode is placed over the belly of the hamstring muscle while the patient performs ROM exercises.

Cryotherapy is begun in the recovery room after surgery. The standard method of cold therapy is an ice bag or commercial cold pack, which is kept in the freezer until required. Empirically, patients prefer motorized cooler units. These units maintain a constant temperature and circulation of ice water through a pad, which provides excellent pain control. Cryotherapy is used from three times a day to every waking hour for 20 minutes at a time depending upon the extent of pain and swelling. Cold therapy is typically done after exercise or when required for pain and swelling control and is maintained throughout the entire postoperative rehabilitation protocol.

Postoperative Bracing

Immediately after surgery, patients are placed into a long-leg postoperative brace that is locked at 0° extension for 2 weeks until the initial postoperative pain has receded and return of lower limb muscle control occurs. At this time, the brace is unlocked and the patient taught to resume a normal gait, with flexion during the stance phase, under 25% of body weight. After 6 weeks, the long-leg brace is stopped and a functional off-the-shelf brace is used. In select knees in which extensive surgery was performed and additional protection indicated, a custom medial unloading brace is prescribed for at least the 1st year postoperative.

Weight-Bearing

Patients are kept non–weight-bearing for the first 2 weeks. Then, toe-touch to 25% of the patient's body weight is permitted from weeks 3 to 4. Partial weight-bearing is allowed as long as pain and swelling are controlled and a voluntary quadriceps contraction is demonstrated. The patient is taught to walk with a toe-in gait and avoid a toe-out valgus position. The therapist should observe the gait cycle for any tendency for a valgus thrust or external tibial rotation, which requires immediate correction to avoid placing excessive loads on the MCL repair or graft reconstruction. Weight-bearing is slowly progressed to full by the 7th to 8th week.

Range of Knee Motion

The goal in the 1st postoperative week is to obtain 0° to 90°. A continuous passive motion machine is not required. Patients perform passive and active ROM exercises in a seated position for 10 minutes a session, approximately four to six times per day. Initially, the therapist performs this exercise by applying a mild amount of varus and internal tibial rotation stress during flexion to unload the medial compartment (Fig. 25–4). Full passive knee extension must be obtained immediately to avoid excessive scarring in the intercondylar notch and posterior capsular tissues. It is important to note that patients undergoing SMCL repair or reconstruction are at an increased risk for developing a knee motion problem postoperatively.[5] Supervision and close monitoring of the patient's progress by the therapist is essential to avoid a potential arthrofibrotic response. If the patient has difficulty regaining at least 0° by the 7th postoperative day, an overpressure program is begun as described in detail in Chapters 13, Rehabilitation of Primary and Revision Anterior Cruciate Ligament Reconstruction, and 41, Prevention and Treatment of Knee Arthrosis. Overpressure exercises and modalities include hanging weight, extension board, and a drop-out cast (Fig. 25–5).

Knee flexion is gradually increased to 130° by the 7th to 8th postoperative week. Passive knee flexion exercises are performed initially in the figure-four position. Other methods to assist in

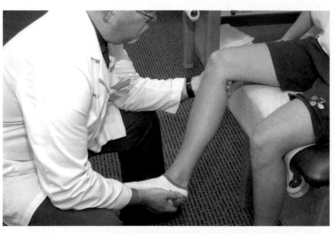

FIGURE 25–4. Early postoperatively, the therapist performs knee motion exercises by applying a mild amount of varus and internal tibial rotation stress during flexion to unload the medial compartment.

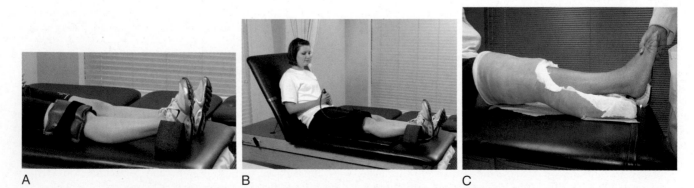

A   B   C

FIGURE 25–5. Extension overpressure exercises. **A,** Hanging weight. **B,** Extension board. **C,** Drop-out cast.

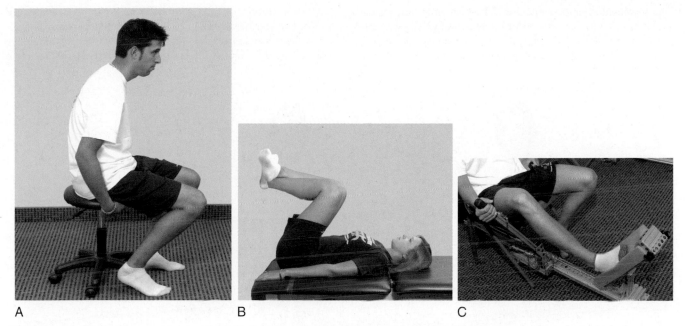

FIGURE 25–6. Flexion overpressure exercises. **A,** Rolling stool. **B,** Wall-slides. **C,** Commercial device.

achieving flexion include chair-rolling, wall-slides, commercial devices (Fig. 25–6), and passive quadriceps stretching exercises.

Patellar Mobilization

Maintaining normal patellar mobility is critical to regain a normal range of knee motion. The loss of patellar mobility is often associated with arthrofibrosis and, in extreme cases, the development of patella infera.[6,8] Patellar glides are performed beginning the 1st postoperative day in all four planes (superior, inferior, medial, and lateral) with sustained pressure applied to the appropriate patellar border for at least 10 seconds (Fig. 25–7). This exercise is performed for 5 minutes before ROM exercises. Caution is warranted if an extensor lag is detected, because this may be associated with poor superior migration of the patella, indicating the need for additional emphasis on this exercise. Patellar mobilization is performed for approximately 12 weeks postoperatively.

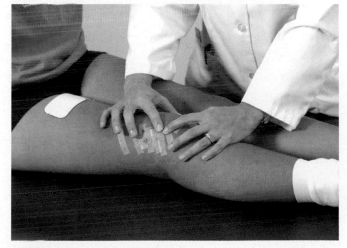

FIGURE 25–7. Patellar mobilization.

Flexibility

Hamstring and gastrocnemius-soleus flexibility exercises are begun the 1st day postoperatively. A sustained static stretch is held for 30 seconds and repeated five times. These exercises help control pain due to the reflex response created in the hamstrings when the knee is kept in the flexed position. As well, the gastrocnemius-soleus towel-pulling exercise can help lessen discomfort in the calf, Achilles tendon, and ankle. Quadriceps and iliotibial band flexibility exercises are initiated at week 9. The flexibility program is maintained throughout the course of the rehabilitation program.

Strengthening

The strengthening program is begun on the 1st postoperative day. Early emphasis on the generation of a good voluntary quadriceps contraction is critical for a successful and safe return to functional activity. Isometric quadriceps contractions are completed hourly following the rules of 10-second holds, 10 repetitions, 10 times per day. Adequate evaluation of the quadriceps contraction by both the therapist and the patient is critical. If necessary, biofeedback can also be used to reinforce a good quadriceps contraction.

Straight leg raises are initiated the 1st postoperative day in the hip flexion plane. At weeks 7 to 8, the other three planes (adduction, abduction, and extension) are added to this exercise. As leg-raises become easy to perform, ankle weights are added to progress muscle strengthening. Initially, 1 to 2 pounds of weight are used and eventually; up to 10 pounds may be added as long as this is not more than 10% of the patient's body weight.

Active-assisted ROM can also be used to facilitate the quadriceps muscle if poor tone is observed during isometric contractions. These exercises are primarily used during the first 8 postoperative weeks in which emphasis is placed on controlling pain and swelling, regaining full ROM, achieving early quadriceps control and proximal stabilization, and resuming a normal gait pattern.

Closed kinetic chain exercises are begun when partial weight-bearing of at least 50% is tolerated. Patients are instructed to avoid valgus loading during these exercises. These activities initially consist of mini-squats from 0° to 45°, toe-raises, and wall-sits. During the wall-sitting exercise, the patient may squeeze a ball between the distal thighs, inducing a hip adduction contraction and a stronger VMO contraction, or hold dumbbell weights in his or her hands to increase body weight (Fig. 25–8). The patient can also shift his or her body weight over the involved side to stimulate a single-leg contraction. The wall-sitting position should be held to a maximum

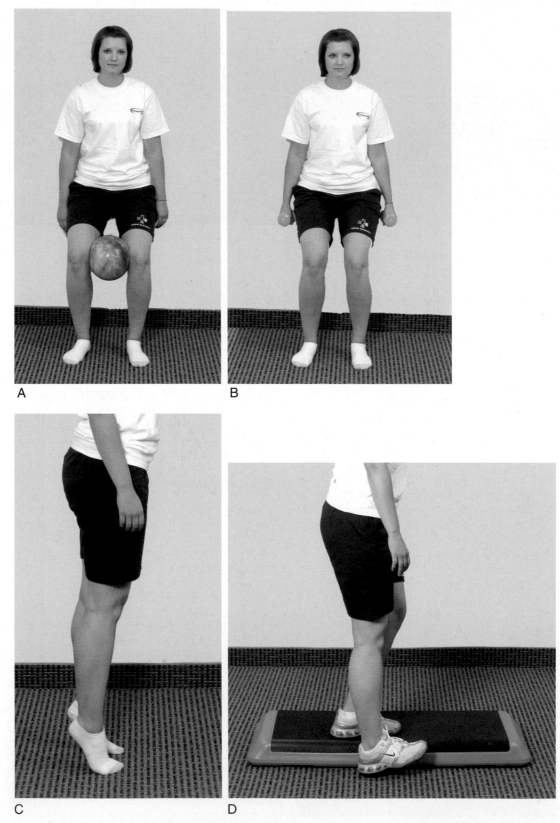

A

B

C

D

FIGURE 25–8. Strengthening exercises. **A,** Wall-sitting while squeezing a ball between the thighs. **B,** Wall-sitting while holding hand weights. **C,** Toe-raises. **D,** Lateral step-ups.

burning of the quadriceps and repeated. This is an excellent exercise to mimic a stationary leg-press, achieve quadriceps muscle fiber recruitment, and induce muscle fatigue to build strength.

Lateral step-ups are begun when the patient has achieved full weight-bearing. The height of the step is gradually increased based on patient tolerance from 2 to 8 inches.

Hamstring curls are begun with Velcro ankle weights between weeks 9 and 12 and eventually advanced to weight machines. The patient exercises the involved limb alone, as well as both limbs together. Weight training is used throughout the program and continues in the return to activity and maintenance phases of rehabilitation.

Open kinetic chain extension exercises are incorporated within the first few weeks to further develop quadriceps muscle strength. Caution is warranted owing to the potential problems these exercises may create for the patellofemoral joint. Resisted knee extension is begun with Velcro ankle weights from 90° to 30° at postoperative weeks 3 to 4. The terminal phase of extension is avoided owing to the forces placed on the patellofemoral joint. The patellofemoral joint must be monitored for pain, swelling, and crepitus to avoid a conversion in which painful patellofemoral crepitus develops with articular cartilage damage. The surgeon should advise the therapist if patellofemoral joint damage was observed at surgery. The therapist should palpate the patellofemoral joint during active knee extension every therapy session to detect pain or an onset of joint crepitus. A patellofemoral conversion to a symptomatic state will occur in select knees, especially those with preexisting patellofemoral joint damage. In these knees, modification of the entire rehabilitation program is required.

A full lower extremity strengthening program is critical for early and long-term success of the rehabilitation program. Other muscle groups included in this routine are the hip abductors, hip adductors, hip flexors, and hip extensors. These muscle groups may be exercised on either a multi-hip or cable system machine or a hip abductor-adductor machine. Gastrocnemius-soleus strength is a key component for both early ambulation and the running program. In addition, upper extremity and core strengthening are important for a safe and effective return to work or sports.

Balance, Proprioceptive, and Perturbation Training

Balance and proprioceptive training are initiated when the patient achieves 50% weight-bearing. Initially, the patient stands and shifts weight from side-to-side and front-to-back. This activity promotes confidence in the leg's ability to withstand the pressures of weight-bearing and initiates the stimulus to knee joint position sense. Cup walking is begun when the patient achieves full weight-bearing to promote symmetry between the surgical and the uninvolved limbs (Fig. 25–9).

Double- and single-leg balance exercises in the stance position are beneficial and initiated during phases 5 to 6, depending on patient tolerance. During the single-leg exercise, the foot is pointed straight ahead, the knee flexed 20° to 30°, the arms extended outward to horizontal, and the torso positioned upright with the shoulders above the hips and the hips above the ankles. The patient remains in this position until balance is disturbed. A minitrampoline or unstable platform makes this exercise more challenging. The patient may assume the single-leg stance position and throw/catch a weighted ball against an inverted minitrampoline until fatigue occurs.

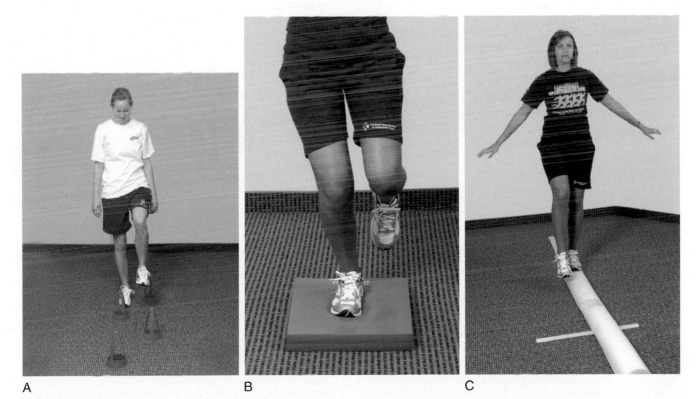

FIGURE 25–9. Balance and proprioceptive training. **A,** Cup- (or cone-) walking. **B,** Single-leg balancing on an unstable platform. **C,** Walking on half foam rolls.

A   B   C

Perturbation training techniques are initiated during balance exercises. The therapist stands behind the patient and disrupts her or his body posture and position periodically to enhance dynamic knee stability. The techniques involve either direct contact with the patient or disruption of the platform the patient is standing on.

Walking on half foam rolls is also used in the gait retraining and balance program. This activity helps the patient develop balance and dynamic muscular control required to maintain an upright position and be able to walk from one end of the roll to the other. Developing a center of balance, limb symmetry, quadriceps control in midstance, and postural positioning are benefits obtained from this type of training.

Conditioning

Depending on accessibility, a cardiovascular program is begun as soon as the patient can sufficiently tolerate the upright position with an upper extremity ergometer. The surgical limb should be elevated to minimize lower extremity swelling. This exercise is performed as tolerated. Stationary bicycling is begun in the 5th to 6th postoperative week

Water-walking, swimming, and the use of an elliptical machine are allowed during the 9th to 12th postoperative weeks. Then, cross-country ski and stair-climbing machines are permitted. Protection against high stresses to the patellofemoral joint is strongly advocated. During bicycling, the seat height is adjusted to its highest level based on patient body size and a low-resistance level is used initially. Stair-climbing machines are adjusted to produce a short step and low resistance.

In order to improve cardiovascular endurance, the program should be performed at least three times per week for 20 to 30 minutes, and the exercise performed to at least 60% to 85% of maximal heart rate. It is generally regarded that performing in the higher levels of percentage of maximal heart rate achieves greater cardiovascular efficiency and endurance.

Running and Agility Program

In order to initiate the running program, the patient must demonstrate no more than a 30% deficit in average torque for the quadriceps and hamstrings on isokinetic testing and have no more than 3 mm of increase in medial joint opening (30° flexion). The majority of patients are at least 6 months postoperative.

The running program is based on the patient's athletic goals, particularly the position or physical requirements of the activity, and is described in detail in Chapter 13, Rehabilitation of Primary and Revision Anterior Cruciate Ligament Reconstructions. The program is performed three times per week, on opposite days of the strength program. Because the running program may not reach aerobic levels initially, a cross-training program is used to facilitate cardiovascular fitness. The cross-training program is performed on the same day as the strength workout.

Plyometric Training

Plyometric training is begun upon successful completion of the running program in order to minimize alterations in neuromuscular function and proprioception. Important parameters to consider when performing plyometric exercises include surface, footwear, and warm-up. The jump training should be done on a firm, yet forgiving surface such as a wooden gym floor. Very hard surfaces like concrete should be avoided. A cross-training or running shoe should be worn to provide adequate shock absorption, as well as adequate stability to the foot. Checking wear patterns and outer sole wear will help avoid overuse injuries.

During the various jumps, the patient is instructed to keep his or her body weight on the balls of the feet. He or she should jump and land with the knees flexed and shoulder-width apart to avoid knee hyperextension and an overall valgus lower limb position. The patient should understand that the exercises are reaction and agility drills, and although speed is emphasized, correct body posture must be maintained throughout the drills. This program is described in detail in Chapter 13, Rehabilitation of Primary Revision Anterior Cruciate Ligament Reconstructions.

Once the patient has completed the running and plyometric programs and strength and function testing reach normal values, return to sports is allowed. A trial of function is encouraged in which the patient is monitored for knee swelling, pain, overuse symptoms, and giving-way episodes. Some athletes will experience transient knee swelling upon return to strenuous activities and should be educated on how to recognize this problem and the importance of reducing activities until the swelling subsides. If swelling persists, the athlete is advised to reduce athletics for 2 to 6 weeks, consider use of nonsteroidal anti-inflammatories, and use ice and elevation. Upon successful return to activity, the patient is encouraged to continue with a maintenance program. During the in-season, a conditioning program of two workouts a week is recommended. In the off-season or preseason, this program should be performed three times a week to maximize gains in flexibility, strength, and cardiovascular endurance.

During the entire functional progression, the therapist and surgeon should individualize the program based on the initial injury (particularly to the menisci and articular cartilage), magnitude of the operative procedure, and healing response of the patient. Athletes with loss of a meniscus or articular cartilage damage refrain from high-impact activities and are followed yearly to detect progression of the joint injury. These patients frequently have episodes of joint swelling and pain during the functional progression and are instructed to "play smart" and not be a knee abuser.

REFERENCES

1. Deibert, M. C., Aronsson, D. D.; Johnson, R. J.; et al.: Skiing injuries in children, adolescents, and adults. *J Bone Joint Surg Am* 80:25–32, 1998.
2. Fetto, J. F.; Marshall, J. L.: Medial collateral ligament injuries of the knee: a rationale for treatment. *Clin Orthop Relat Res* 132:206–218, 1978.
3. Halinen, J.; Lindahl, J.; Hirvensalo, E.; Santavirta, S.: Operative and nonoperative treatments of medial collateral ligament rupture with early anterior cruciate ligament reconstruction: a prospective randomized study. *Am J Sports Med* 34:1134–1140, 2006.
4. Najibi, S.; Albright, J. P.: The use of knee braces, part 1: prophylactic knee braces in contact sports. *Am J Sports Med* 33:602–611, 2005.
5. Noyes, F. R.; Barber-Westin, S. D.: The treatment of acute combined ruptures of the anterior cruciate and medial ligaments of the knee. *Am J Sports Med* 23:380–389, 1995.

6. Noyes, F. R.; Wojtys, E. M.: The early recognition, diagnosis and treatment of the patella infera syndrome. In Tullos, H. S. (ed): *Instructional Course Lectures*. Rosemont, IL: American Academy of Orthopedic Surgeons, 1991; pp. 233–247.

7. Noyes, F. R.; Wojtys, E. M.; Marshall, M. T.: The early diagnosis and treatment of developmental patella infera syndrome. *Clin Orthop* 265:241–252, 1991.

8. Paulos, L. E.; Rosenberg, T. D.; Drawbert, J.; et al.: Infrapatellar contracture syndrome. An unrecognized cause of knee stiffness with patella entrapment and patella infera. *Am J Sports Med* 15:331–341, 1987.

9. Peterson, L.; Junge, A.; Chomiak, J.; et al.: Incidence of football injuries and complaints in different age groups and skill-level groups. *Am J Sports Med* 28(5 suppl):S51–S57, 2000.

Dislocated Knees and Multiple Ligament Injuries

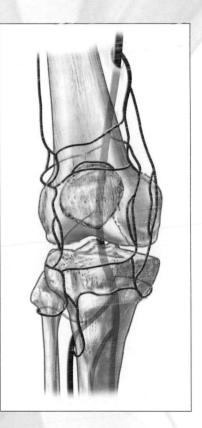

Classification of Knee Dislocations

Dustin L. Richter, BS ■ *Daniel C. Wascher*, MD ■ *Robert C. Schenck, Jr.*, MD

INTRODUCTION

The concept of a dislocated knee has changed markedly over the past few decades. In 1971, Meyers and Harvey[10] predicted that most orthopaedists would not see more than one knee dislocation in their entire career. However, evidence indicates that knee dislocations are being seen with increasing frequency for a variety of reasons. Increasing trauma, changes in automotive design, and recognition of spontaneously reduced knee dislocations have all added to the increased incidence. The increasing number of knee dislocations has created the need for a classification system that will help guide the management of these complex injuries. Classification systems should be simple and reproducible; they should give information to the clinician that will be helpful in making treatment decisions and aid in the communication of like injuries as well as in developing prognoses for injuries. This chapter reviews the shortcomings of the older classification systems of knee dislocations and presents the anatomic classification system that is simple, accurate, reproducible, and useful.[18–20,28]

DEFINITION OF KNEE DISLOCATION

Classically, a knee dislocation was defined as greater than 100% displacement of the tibiofemoral articulation. This displacement

Critical Points ASSESSMENT OF KNEE DISLOCATIONS

- Clinicians must be alert to the presence of "reduced" dislocations in order not to miss a limb-threatening arterial injury.
- Although rare, cruciate intact knee dislocations do occur, adding to the stability of the knee and changing the management of these injuries.
- A classification system for knee dislocations must take into account the presence of both "reduced" and cruciate-intact knee dislocations.

had to be present on either physical examination or radiographic imaging. Since the 1990s, several authors have recognized the existence of "reduced" knee dislocations. These are knees that present to the treating physician reduced but have multiple injured ligaments (usually including both cruciates) and gross instability on stress testing. Some of these injuries represent a spontaneous reduction of a knee dislocation, and others are dislocated knees that are reduced in the field before transport to a medical facility. The incidence of this type of reduced knee dislocation may be as high as 50% of all knee injuries classified as a dislocation.[3,28,32] A study from our institution showed that the incidence of vascular injury in the reduced dislocations was equal to that of knees that presented dislocated (Fig. 26–1).[32] In general, more recent studies have shown that the risk of arterial injury is approximately 7% to 12% with a diagnosis of a dislocated knee.[26] Clinicians must be alert to the presence of reduced dislocations in order not to miss a limb-threatening arterial injury, as shown in Figure 26–1. A multiligament-injured knee with gross instability must be treated the same as a knee that presents dislocated.

Although most knee dislocations involve tears of both cruciate ligaments (posterior cruciate ligament [PCL] and anterior cruciate ligament [ACL]), case reports of cruciate-intact knee dislocations do exist. A PCL-intact knee dislocation was first described in 1975.[11] Several authors[2,23] have reported on patients with a radiographically documented knee dislocation that, upon reduction or operative exploration, demonstrated a functioning PCL or ACL. Although some of these patients were noted to have suffered partial PCL tears, the presence of a functioning PCL provides increased stability and changes the management of these PCL-intact dislocations. In most PCL-intact knee dislocations, the tibia is perched anterior on the distal femur (Fig. 26–2). In addition to an ACL tear, there is often complete rupture of either the medial collateral ligament (MCL) or the posterolateral structures.

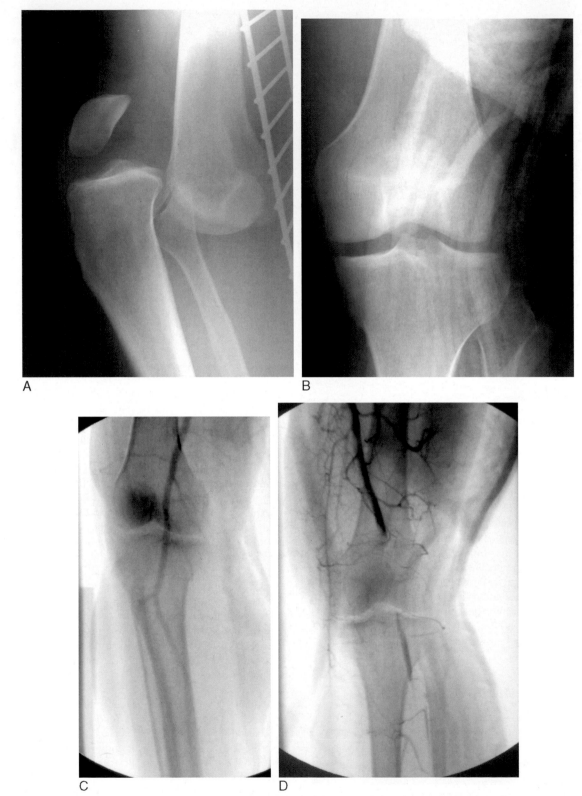

FIGURE 26–1. Bilateral knee injuries, both classified as dislocation, presenting in the same patient. **A,** A lateral radiograph of the right knee demonstrates an anterior dislocation. On examination, the patient was noted to have sustained an anterior cruciate ligament/posterior cruciate ligament/medial collateral ligament (ACL/PCL/MCL) injury (knee dislocation [KD] III-M). **B,** An anteroposterior (AP) view of the left knee on initial presentation shows that the knee is reduced. On physical examination, the injury pattern involved the ACL/PCL/fibular collateral ligament [FCL] (KD III-L-C). **C,** An arteriogram of the right knee reveals good flow through the popliteal artery. **D,** An arteriogram of the reduced left knee demonstrates complete occlusion of the left popliteal artery and hence the knee required revascularization. *(A–D, Reprinted from Wascher, D. C.: High-energy knee dislocations. In Drez, D., Jr.; DeLee, J. C. [eds]: Operative Techniques in Sports Medicine, Vol. 11. Philadelphia: W. B. Saunders, 2003; p. 237.)*

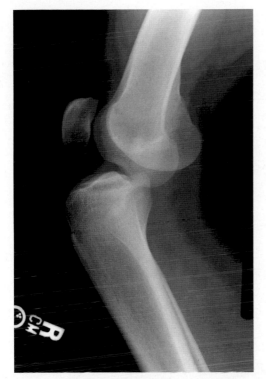

FIGURE 26–2. This patient presented with a PCL-intact knee dislocation. Note how the tibia is perched anterior on the distal femur. This type of injury would be classified as a KD I according to the anatomic classification system, to be discussed later.

Similarly, ACL-intact knee dislocations have also been reported. These are also extremely rare injuries. The tibia is perched posterior on the femur, and there is a complete tear of the PCL associated with a complete collateral ligament injury. Again, the presence of a functional ACL provides increased stability in the knee and changes the management of these injuries. A classification system for knee dislocations must take into account the presence of both reduced and cruciate-intact knee dislocations.

POSITION CLASSIFICATION SYSTEM

In 1963, Kennedy[9] was the first to classify knee dislocations. He proposed a classification system based on the tibial position with respect to the femur. For example, an anterior knee dislocation implies that the tibia is positioned anterior to the femoral condyles. He identified five types of knee dislocation: anterior, posterior, lateral, medial, and rotatory. Rotatory dislocations were further subdivided into four groups: anteromedial, anterolateral, posteromedial, and posterolateral, with posterolateral being the most frequently described type of rotatory knee dislocation.[5,6,14,15] This classification system has been widely utilized in the literature.*

The position classification system can help the physician plan a reduction maneuver for the dislocated knee. However, most knee dislocations can be easily reduced with longitudinal traction. The position classification system can also be useful to alert the clinician to the possibility of coexisting injuries.

---

*See references 4, 5, 8, 10, 11, 14–16, 22, 24, 25, 27.

For example, several studies have shown a higher incidence of popliteal artery injury in anterior dislocations.[5,8-10] However, vascular injury can occur with any position of knee dislocation; one must have a high index of suspicion for associated neurovascular injuries in any dislocated knee, regardless of position. Although knowing that an anterior dislocation carries an increased risk of vascular injury is helpful to the clinician, it does not give any information about what structures (ligamentous, neurovascular) have been injured and what treatment is required.

One example of the utility of the position classification system is the rare but important posterolateral dislocation (Fig. 26–3). The mechanism of injury is an abduction force to a flexed knee coupled with internal rotation of the tibia. This force causes the medial femoral condyle to "buttonhole" through the medial capsule and the MCL invaginates into the knee joint. The trapped condyle and MCL prevent closed reduction. The clinical hallmark of the posterolateral dislocation and irreducibility by closed means is a transverse furrow seen on the medial aspect of the knee.[6,15] Peroneal nerve palsy, theoretically resulting from a traction injury to the nerve over the lateral femoral condyle, is frequently associated with this type of dislocation. Skin necrosis secondary to pressure from the medially displaced femur has also been reported. For a posterolateral knee dislocation, the position classification system alerts the clinician to the injured structures and the means of treating the injury.

The major limitation of the position classification system is that up to half of knee dislocations are unable to be classified. Knees that present with a spontaneous reduction or that have been reduced in the field cannot be described within the structure of the position classification system. The clinician does not have any information about damaged ligaments nor of the possibility of coexisting vascular or nerve injury. Even more dangerous is the fact that by this injury not being included in the position classification system, the inexperienced physician may not recognize the reduced knee dislocation as a significant ligamentous injury and will not undertake the rigorous vascular examination required to detect a popliteal artery injury.

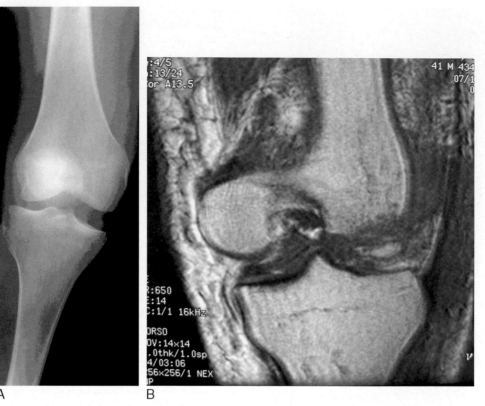

FIGURE 26–3. AP radiograph (**A**) and magnetic resonance imaging (MRI) study (**B**) of a posterolateral dislocation. The injury pattern involved the ACL/PCL/MCL and included damage to the peroneal nerve (KD III-M-N).

ENERGY OF INJURY CLASSIFICATION SYSTEM

Knee dislocations have also been classified by the degree of energy imparted to the knee joint. Most commonly, knee dislocations result from high-energy mechanisms such as motor vehicle wrecks, industrial accidents, and falls from a height (Fig. 26–4). The injury mechanisms in high-energy knee dislocations often cause significant associated head, chest, abdominal, and extremity injuries as well as soft tissue injury about the affected knee. Many of these injuries can be life-threatening, and their management

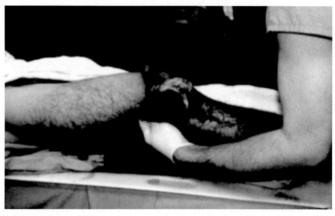

FIGURE 26–4. This patient sustained a severe dashboard injury in a high-speed car accident. He presented with a severe open knee dislocation, with rupture of the ACL, PCL, FCL, and posterolateral capsule (KD III-L). *(Reprinted from Wascher, D. C.: High-velocity knee dislocation with vascular injury: treatment principles. In Miller, M. D.; Johnson, D. L. [eds]: Clinics in Sports Medicine: The Dislocated Knee, Vol. 19. Philadelphia: W. B. Saunders, 2000; p. 467.)*

Critical Points ENERGY OF INJURY CLASSIFICATION SYSTEM

The energy of injury classification system is based on the degree of energy imparted to the knee joint.

Uses

- The energy of injury classification system often dictates management of the dislocated knee (early vs. delayed treatment).
- High-energy knee dislocations (e.g., motor vehicle accident) alert the physician to the increased risk of vascular and nerve injury, although vascular injury can occur regardless of the energy of injury.

Limitations

- The energy of injury classification system categories are somewhat arbitrary.
- The energy of injury classification system does not alert the orthopaedic surgeon as to which knee structures need to be repaired or reconstructed.

---

takes precedence over the knee ligaments. Regardless of the energy of injury, the clinician must remain vigilant about the possibility of a popliteal artery injury in any knee dislocation. The orthopaedic surgeon must be alerted to the possibility of other life-threatening trauma in a patient with a knee dislocation. Conversely, trauma surgeons must include a gross assessment of knee stability in all patients involved in high-energy injury mechanisms. The risk of vascular and nerve injury is increased in high-energy knee dislocations.[9,13,22,30]

Knee dislocations can also occur from low-energy trauma such as that seen in sports activities or in minor falls. Sports in which knee dislocations are occasionally encountered include football, rugby, horseback riding, and skiing. Patients with dislocated knees from minor falls are often obese. Patients who sustain low-energy knee dislocations rarely have associated traumatic injuries. Although the risk of vascular injury is lower in low-energy mechanisms, the physician must still be vigilant in assessing the popliteal artery in all patients with a knee dislocation. In the past, knee dislocations have been described as low- or high-velocity injuries.[22] It is our opinion that the term *energy*, rather than the term *velocity*, more accurately describes the injury mechanism.

The energy of injury system often dictates management of the dislocated knee. The associated injuries in high-energy dislocations frequently preclude early operative management of the knee ligaments. Initial management of the knee dislocation in a multiply injured patient commonly includes the use of external fixation spanning the knee joint to stabilize the knee in a reduced position and to facilitate patient transport and positioning. The use of an external fixator should be limited to 1 to 2 weeks so that an early protected range of motion program may be instituted to prevent arthrofibrosis. Delayed treatment of high-energy dislocations often requires collateral ligament reconstruction in addition to reconstruction of both cruciate ligaments. Conversely, low-energy dislocations can frequently undergo early operative intervention. The collateral ligaments can often be primarily repaired or reconstructed, yielding results superior to those obtained with delayed reconstruction.

One of the problems with the energy of injury classification system is that the categories are somewhat arbitrary. If a patient sustains a knee dislocation when hit by a slow-speed car in a parking lot, is this a high- or low-energy dislocation? What about a patient who falls off of a roof or a high tower? Although it is useful for the clinician to think in terms of the energy imparted to the knee, ultimately it is the pattern of ligament injury, the presence or absence of neurovascular injuries, and the overall clinical assessment that will dictate treatment of the knee dislocation. A morbidly obese patient with a major psychiatric illness who dislocates a knee slipping on a wet bathroom floor (low-energy dislocation) may be treated definitively with external fixation. Conversely, an athletic patient with an isolated knee dislocation from a motorcycle wreck (high-energy dislocation) might be best treated by early ligament repair and reconstruction. Finally, the energy of injury classification system does not alert the orthopaedic surgeon as to which knee structures need to be repaired or reconstructed.

ANATOMIC CLASSIFICATION SYSTEM

A classification system for knee dislocations has been described and is based on what ligamentous structures are torn.[28] The ligament anatomy of the knee is complex, with many injury patterns possible when a knee dislocation occurs.[18,20,32] Conceptually, the knee can be separated into four simply identifiable structures: the ACL, the PCL, the medial ligamentous structures, and the posterolateral corner. The medial structures include the superficial and deep MCL as well as the posteromedial capsule. The posterolateral corner is primarily composed of the fibular (lateral) collateral ligament, the popliteofibular ligament, the popliteus tendon, and the lateral joint capsule. This simplistic representation of knee anatomy can be useful to the clinician in planning treatment of a dislocated knee.

Critical Points ANATOMIC CLASSIFICATION SYSTEM

The anatomic classification system for knee dislocations is based on the anatomic structures injured.
- The anatomic classification system requires a thorough ligamentous and neurovascular assessment of the knee, consisting of three parts: an initial examination in the trauma room or office, a preoperative magnetic resonance imaging (MRI) study, and an examination under anesthesia at the time of surgery.
- The anatomic classification system describes five major ligamentous injury patterns and associated neurovascular injury (if applicable).

Advantages
- All knee dislocations can adequately be described by the anatomic classification system, even those that present "reduced."
- No judgment is required for placing a dislocated knee within a specific group.
- The anatomic classification system has the ability to help guide the clinician in treatment by simple and accurate identification of the injured structures and planning of surgical intervention.
- The anatomic classification system rapidly communicates the extent of the injuries between clinicians and allows for comparisons of like injuries in the wide spectrum of knee dislocations.
- The anatomic classification system helps the clinician predict outcomes in the treatment of dislocated knees.

In order to classify a knee dislocation by the injured anatomy, it is important to obtain a thorough assessment of the injured knee. The clinician must perform a thorough physical examination of the knee on initial presentation to the emergency room or office. At a minimum, this should include a Lachman test, a posterior drawer test, varus and valgus stress testing at 0° and 30°, and a spin or dial test at 30° and 90°. A thorough neurovascular examination must also be performed. Any vascular abnormality warrants careful evaluation, which may include serial examinations, ankle brachial index evaluation, angiography, and/or popliteal artery exploration and repair/reverse saphenous vein graft. A complete neurologic examination may be difficult in a patient with head trauma, but in most cases, a gross assessment of tibial and peroneal nerve function can and should be obtained. As soon as the patient's overall condition allows, we recommend obtaining a magnetic resonance imaging (MRI) scan of the knee to better assess the degree and location of ligament injuries. Several authors[3,17,19,41] have commented on the utility of the MRI in the evaluation of ligament injury in knee dislocations. Certain injuries (e.g., the presence of a PCL peel-off injury or a popliteus tendon avulsion) can be accurately detected preoperatively only by MRI. Knowing preoperatively which ligaments are torn and detecting the presence of avulsions can help the surgeon plan the number and types of allografts required and the fixation devices necessary to restore functional stability to the knee.[19,21,31] The final and most critical assessment of knee ligament function occurs with an examination under anesthesia (EUA) at the time of knee reconstruction. The EUA provides a final assessment of the degree of translation, the presence of an endpoint on ligament stress testing, and the overall functionality of the specific ligamentous structure. Whereas MRI can identify which ligaments are injured, the EUA gives an accurate assessment of the functional stability of the injured knee ligaments.[1,7,20,23,29] In the dislocated knee, partial ligament tears can often be treated nonoperatively. To summarize, the assessment of the dislocated knee consists of

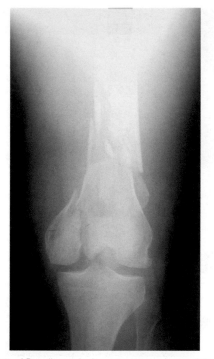

FIGURE 26–9. AP radiograph demonstrates a knee dislocation with the presence of a major periarticular fracture (KD V). In this case, the patient has a femoral-sided fracture-dislocation, which includes a fracture of the medial epicondyle. *(Courtesy of Robert C. Schenck, Jr.)*

and allows for comparisons of like injuries in the wide spectrum of knee dislocations. At our institution, residents and attending physicians quickly describe the ACL/MCL/PCL knee injury as a KD III-M. The injury diagnosis and ligamentous involvement are easily communicated. Here are a few additional examples of the usefulness of the anatomic classification system: The C subtype quickly alerts the physician to the need for urgent vascular surgery to restore flow to the ischemic limb. A KD II injury has functionally intact collateral ligaments and can be treated just as successfully with either an early or a delayed reconstruction of the cruciate ligaments. A KD IV injury identifies a knee with severe instability that may require external fixation to maintain joint reduction prior to ligament reconstruction.

Finally, the anatomic classification system will help the clinician predict outcomes in the treatment of dislocated knees. On average, knees with a higher roman numeral classification will have inferior outcome scores. Likewise, it has been shown that KD III-L injuries fare worse than KD III-M injuries.[3,28] Knee dislocations with neurovascular injuries (subtypes C or N) are also more likely to have unsatisfactory outcome measurements. KD V injuries are associated with a high complication rate related to the increased incidence of arterial injury, inadequate fracture reduction, or difficulty in achieving a satisfactory ligament reconstruction.

dislocations that present reduced can be classified after a physical examination and MRI have identified the torn ligaments and associated injuries. In contrast to the energy of injury classification system, no judgment is required for placing a dislocated knee within a specific group. If a ligament is injured and functionally incompetent, it is "torn" for the purposes of the anatomic classification system. Most important, however, is the ability of the anatomic classification system to help guide the clinician in treatment. The surgeon can readily identify the injured structures and can then proceed to plan how best to "fix what is torn." The anatomic classification system rapidly communicates between clinicians about the extent of the injuries

CONCLUSION

Successful treatment of the dislocated knee requires a thorough understanding of the knee injury. Older classification systems are not able to categorize all knee dislocations, do not guide treatment, and are not predictive of outcome. The anatomic classification system that we have used for the past 15 years readily allows the physician to classify all knee dislocations on the basis of the injured structures identified by physical examination and imaging studies. This simple system helps the surgeon plan treatment of the dislocated knee and has been predictive of outcomes in published reports. Hopefully, more widespread use and reporting of this classification system in future series of knee dislocations will yield additional insight into the optimal treatment of these uncommon yet challenging injuries.

REFERENCES

1. Almekinders, L.; Logan, T.: Results following treatment of traumatic dislocations of the knee joint. *Clin Orthop Relat Res* 284:203–207, 1992.
2. Cooper, D. E.; Speer, K. P.; Wickiewicz, T. L.; et al.: Complete knee dislocation without posterior cruciate ligament disruption: a report of four cases and review of the literature. *Clin Orthop* 284:228–233, 1992.
3. Eastlack, R. K.; Schenck, R. C., Jr.; Guarducci, C.: The dislocated knee: classification, treatment, and outcome. *US Army Med Dep J* 11(12):2–9, 1997.
4. Frassica, F. S.; Franklin, H. S.; Staeheli, J. W.; et al.: Dislocation of the knee. *Clin Orthop* 263:200–205, 1992.
5. Green, N. E.; Allen, B. L.: Vascular injuries associated with dislocation of the knee. *J Bone Joint Surg Am* 59:236–239, 1977.
6. Hill, J. A.; Rana, N. A.: Complications of posterolateral dislocation of the knee: case report and literature review. *Clin Orthop* 154:212–215, 1981.
7. Honton, J. L.; Le Rebeller, A.; Legroux, P.; et al.: Traumatic dislocation of the knee treated by early surgical repair. *Rev Chir Orthop Reparatrice Appar Mot* 64:213–219, 1978.

8. Jones, R. E.; Smith, E. C.; Bone, G. E.: Vascular and orthopaedic complications of knee dislocation. *Surg Gynecol Obstet* 149:554–558, 1979.
9. Kennedy, J. C.: Complete dislocation of the knee joint. *J Bone Joint Surg Am* 45:889–904, 1963.
10. Meyers, M.; Harvey, J. P.: Traumatic dislocation of the knee joint. *J Bone Joint Surg Am* 53:16–29, 1971.
11. Meyers, M.; Moore, T.; Harvey, J. P.: Follow-up notes on articles previously published in *The Journal*: traumatic dislocation of the knee joint. *J Bone Joint Surg Am* 57:430–433, 1975.
12. Moore, T. M.: Fracture-dislocation of the knee. *Clin Orthop* 156:128–140, 1981.
13. Muscat, J. O.; Rogers, W.; Cruz, A. B.; et al.: Arterial injuries in orthopaedics: the posteromedial approach for vascular control about the knee. *J Orthop Trauma* 10:476–480, 1996.
14. O'Donoghue, D.: *Treatment of Injuries to Athletes*, 2nd ed. Philadelphia: W. B. Saunders, 1970; pp. 508–510.
15. Quinlan, A. G.; Sharrard, W. J. W.: Posterolateral dislocation of the knee with capsular interposition. *J Bone Joint Surg Br* 40:660–663, 1958.

16. Reckling, F. W.; Peltier, L. F.: Acute knee dislocations and their complications. *J Trauma* 9:181–191, 1969.
17. Reddy, P. K.; Posteraro, R. H.; Schenck, R. C., Jr.: The role of MRI in evaluation of the cruciate ligaments in knee dislocations. *Orthopedics* 19:166–170, 1996.
18. Schenck, R. C.: Knee dislocations. *Instr Course Lect* 43:127–136, 1994.
19. Schenck, R. C.; DeCoster, T.; Wascher, D.: MRI and knee dislocations. *Sports Med Rep* 2:89–96, 2000.
20. Schenck, R. C.; Hunter, R.; Ostrum, R.; et al.: Knee dislocations. *Instr Course Lect* 48:515–522, 1999.
21. Schenck, R. C.; McGanity, P. L. J.; Heckman, J. D.: Femoral-sided fracture-dislocations of the knee. *J Orthop Trauma* 11:416–421, 1997.
22. Shelbourne, K. D.; Porter, D. A.; Clingman, J. A.; et al.: Low velocity knee dislocations. *Orthop Rev* 11:995–1004, 1991.
23. Shelbourne, K. D.; Pritchard, J.; Rettig, A. C.; et al.: Knee dislocations with intact PCL. *Orthop Rev* 21:607–611, 1992.
24. Shields, L.; Mitral, M.; Cave, E. F.: Complete dislocation of the knee: experience at the Massachusetts General Hospital. *J Trauma* 9:192–215, 1969.
25. Sisto, D. J.; Warren, R. F.: Complete knee dislocation. *Clin Orthop* 198:94–101, 1985.
26. Stannard, J. P.; Sheils, T. M.; Lopez-Ben, R. R.; et al.: Vascular injuries in knee dislocations following blunt trauma: evaluating the role of physical examination to determine the need for arteriography. *J Bone Joint Surg Am* 86:910–915, 2004.
27. Taylor, A. R.; Arden, G. P.; Rainey, H. A.: Traumatic dislocation of the knee: a report of forty-three cases with special references to conservative treatment. *J Bone Joint Surg Br* 54:96–109, 1972.
28. Walker, D. N.; Hardison, R.; Schenck, R. C.: A baker's dozen of knee dislocations. *Am J Knee Surg* 7:117–124, 1994.
29. Wascher, D. C.: High-velocity knee dislocation with vascular injury: treatment principles. *Clin Sports Med* 19:457–477, 2000.
30. Wascher, D. C.; Becker, J. R.; Dexter, J. G.; et al.: Reconstruction of the anterior and posterior cruciate ligaments after knee dislocation: results using fresh-frozen nonirradiated allografts. *Am J Sports Med* 27:189–196, 1999.
31. Wascher, D. C.; DeCoster, T. A.; Schenck, R. C.: 10 commandments of knee dislocation. *Orthopedics Spec Ed* 7(2):28–31, 2001.
32. Wascher, D. C.; Dvirnak, P. C.; DeCoster, T. A.: Knee dislocation: initial assessment and implications for treatment. *J Orthop Trauma* 11:525–529, 1997.

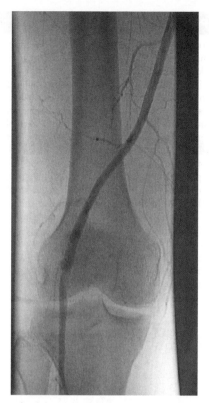

FIGURE 27–2. Angiogram demonstrates diffuse irregularity in the popliteal artery with intimal dissection.

guarantee that an arterial injury is not present. There are multiple reports of vascular occlusion or intimal tears with normal distal pulses; the incidence is reported to be 5% to 15%.[1,24,33,61] In 2004, Barnes and coworkers[4] performed a meta-analysis that included 284 multiligamentous knee injuries in seven studies. Seven of 52 patients requiring vascular surgery had normal pulses on presentation. Thirteen of 140 patients with normal pulses who underwent arteriography had nonocclusive intimal defects that were safely observed. Abnormal pulses had a sensitivity rate of 0.79 (95% confidence interval [CI], 0.64–0.89), specificity rate of 0.91 (95% CI, 0.78–0.96), positive predictive value of 0.75 (95% CI, 0.61–0.83), and a negative predictive value of 0.93 (95% CI, 0.85–0.96). The low sensitivity and specificity may be associated with hypotension in the acutely traumatized patient, as well as intimal lesions that may initially present with normal pulses.

The ABI is the second diagnostic tool to be used. ABIs are determined by measuring the systolic blood pressure for all four extremities using a Doppler probe and a standardized blood pressure cuff. For the lower extremity, the systolic pressure is measured at the posterior tibial and dorsalis pedis arteries. ABI is then calculated by dividing the highest measured pressure in the ankle or foot by the higher of the brachial arterial pressures. An ABI of less than 0.90 is considered abnormal and should prompt arteriography. In 2004, Mills and associates[37] demonstrated that 11 of 11 patients with ABIs less than 0.90 required a reverse saphenous vein graft for popliteal artery injury (3 popliteal artery transections, 6 popliteal artery occlusions, 1 common femoral and peroneal artery thrombosis, and 1 high-grade superficial femoral artery occlusion with intimal flap altering popliteal artery flow). None of the 27 patients with ABIs greater than 0.90 had evidence of vascular injury by serial examination or duplex ultrasonography. The sensitivity and specificity was 100%. In 1998, Cole and colleagues[8] evaluated 70 consecutive patients with blunt trauma and found no arterial injury with ABI greater than 0.90, whereas an ABI lower than 0.90 had a positive predictive value of 88%. Lynch and Johansen[31] studied blunt and penetrating trauma in 100 consecutive patients and found an ABI less than 0.90 predicted vascular surgery with a sensitivity of 87%, specificity of 97%, and positive predictive value of 91%.

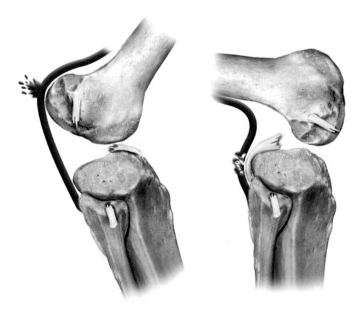

FIGURE 27–3. Left, An anterior knee dislocation demonstrates a traction injury to the popliteal artery. **Right,** A posterior dislocation demonstrates a transaction injury to the popliteal artery.

Arteriography, developed in the 1960s, has improved outcomes and reduced the number of negative explorations. Many authors have advocated routine use of arteriography to evaluate the limb after a suspected knee dislocation.[1,9,17,25,26,30,32,33,67] The routine use of arteriograms for suspected knee dislocations is justified by the relative low morbidity of the test, the high incidence of popliteal injury, and the devastating consequences of a delay in diagnosis.[46] However, clinicians should be aware that not all arterial trauma is detectable with arteriography. Stretch injuries of the intimal wall and small intimal flap tears may not be visualized on the arteriogram, but may subsequently clot and result in arterial occlusion. Those patients who worsen usually do so within the first 3 months, but more commonly, within a week after injury. McDonough and Wojtys[34] reported on three patients with normal initial arteriograms. Two patients who had loss of pulse after tourniquet release during ligament reconstruction were found to have chronic intimal flaps with thrombi at immediate revascularization. One patient developed a pseudoaneurysm, which was recognized by a second arteriorgram after there was significant postoperative swelling.[34]

Arteriograms can be performed in the operating room if there are obviously diminished pulses or if the delay in obtaining a formal arteriogram in the angiography suite would compromise limb survival. Six to 8 hours of warm ischemic time will significantly compromise a lower extremity.[17] Formal angiography is performed with a femoral artery puncture followed by insertion of a pigtail catheter. Next, a bolus of contrast is injected and an angiographic unit is used to capture images. The length of the segment to be imaged determines the number of acquisitions needed.

Intraoperative arteriogram can be performed by injecting 45 mL of contrast through an 18-gauge catheter with a single film exposure[35] or a vascular fluoroscopic unit.

Unfortunately, arteriography is not without risks, costs, and false-negative results. The complication rate has been reported to be 1.7% and includes thrombosis, arteriovenous fistulae, bleeding, renal failure, reaction to contrast material, and pseudoaneurysm formation.[3,27,37,61,66] The reported false-positive results have ranged from 2.4% to 7%, which could lead to unnecessary surgical intervention.[3,58,61,66] The cost of the arteriograms ranged from $750 to $1,500 per study in 1990; a more recent figure was $5,240 in 2003.[3,58,61]

In addition to formal angiography, new techniques such as computed tomographic angiography (CTA) and magnetic resonance angiography (MRA) are being developed. These techniques make use of readily available imaging techniques often with a bolus of contrast to define the lower extremity arterial system. Potter and coworkers[43] demonstrated 100% correlation between conventional angiography and MRA in a small cohort of patients (six patients: four normal, one intimal tear, one decreased flow).

NEUROLOGIC INJURIES

Neurologic damage occurs in 16% to 40% of knee dislocations.[2,57] This may range from a stretch injury (neurapraxia) to a complete transection (neurotmesis). The peroneal nerve is most commonly injured as it is stretched over the fibular neck during a posterolateral dislocation (Fig. 27–4).[14,47,60,62,67]

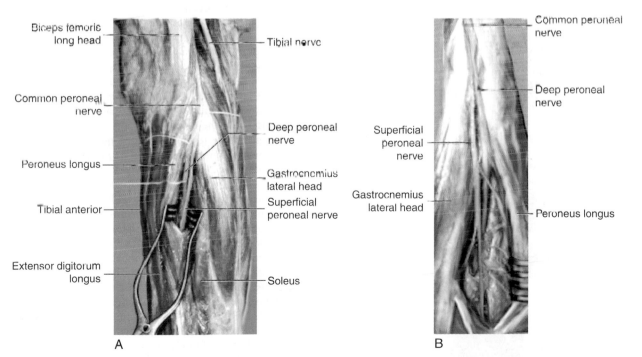

FIGURE 27–4. **A,** Posterolateral view of a left lower extremity cadaveric microdissection depicts the common peroneal nerve in the distal popliteal fossa and its branches, the superficial and deep peroneal nerves. **B,** Lateral view of a right lower extremity cadaveric microdissection shows the deep peroneal nerve muscular branches supplying the tibialis anterior, extensor digitorum longus, extensor hallucis longus, and peroneus tertius muscles. lat., lateral; N, nerve. *(Used with permission from Kim, D. H.; Murovic, J. A.; Tiel, R. L.; Kline, D. G.: Management and outcomes in 318 operative common peroneal nerve lesions at the Louisiana State University Health Sciences Center. Neurosurgery 54.1421–1428, 2004.)*

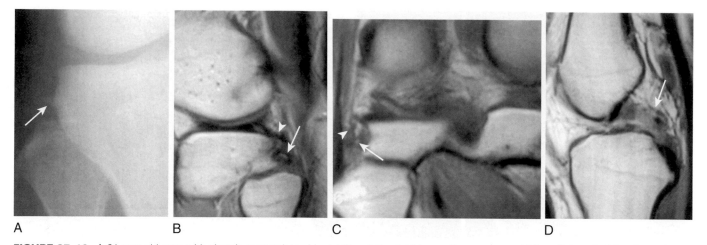

FIGURE 27–10. A 21-year-old man with chronic posterolateral instability of the right knee after a motor vehicle collision. **A,** AP radiograph reveals avulsed bone fragment of the fibular styloid process (*arrow*). **B,** Sagittal spin-echo proton density-weighted magnetic resonance image (TR/TE, 1800/20) reveals avulsed osseous fragment (*arrow*) adjacent to the popliteal tendon (*arrowhead*). **C,** Coronal spin-echo proton density-weighted magnetic resonance image (1800/20) reveals disruption of the lateral collateral ligament (*arrowhead*) and avulsed osseous fragment (*arrow*) in the corresponding course of the popliteofibular ligament. **D,** Sagittal spin-echo proton density-weighted magnetic resonance image (1800/20) obtained medial to image **B** reveals a tear of the PCL (*arrow*). (A–D, *Used with permission from Huang, G.-S.; Yu, J. S.; Munshi, M.; et al.: Avulsion fracture of the head of the fibula [the "arcuate sign"]: MR imaging findings predictive of injuries to the posterolateral ligaments and posterior cruciate ligament. AJR Am J Roentgenol 180:381–387, 2003.)*

EMERGENT SURGERY

Whereas the rationale for determining the type of treatment (surgical or nonsurgical) most appropriate for a patient with a dislocated knee is beyond the scope of this chapter, the timing of surgical procedures is dependent on the postinjury physical examination and associated injuries.

Emergent surgery is indicated for vascular injury, compartment syndrome, open injury, or irreducible dislocations.[46] Vascular reconstruction, often performed with reverse saphenous vein grafts, should be performed within 6 hours to minimize ischemia to the muscles and increase the chances for limb survival. The orthopaedic surgeon may need to stabilize the limb with an external fixator to allow access to the limb during reconstruction and for postoperative wound management. Fasciotomies are often required after revascularization to prevent compartment syndrome.

Acute compartment syndrome is a condition in which the pressure within a fascial compartment rises to a level that decreases tissue perfusion leading to cellular anoxia, muscle ischemia, and death. Diagnosis is primarily clinical with supplementation by compartment pressure measurements. Clinical signs of compartment syndrome include pain out of proportion, pain aggravated by passive stretch, paresthesias, and late signs that include pulselessness, paralysis, and pallor. Compartment

pressure measurements of 20 mm Hg below diastolic pressure or 30 mm Hg below the mean arterial blood pressure suggest muscle ischemia. Urgent restoration of perfusion and normalization of compartment pressures is accomplished by complete fasciotomy of all compartments.[39]

When open knee dislocations are encountered, wound management principles should be employed. Irrigation and débridement of the open wound should be performed urgently. The patient should be started on appropriate antibiotics. Acute ligament reconstruction is contraindicated in the face of an open wound. Soft tissue issues may delay reconstruction for several months.[46]

Irreducible dislocations, most commonly posterolateral dislocations with a dimple sign, require surgical reduction to avoid neurovascular compromise. Although possible, ligament reconstruction should be delayed until adequate imaging of the knee and appropriate resources for reconstruction have been assembled.

DEFINITIVE MANAGEMENT

Most, if not all, surgeons would agree that soft tissue dissection, ligament, and capsular repairs are easier in the acute setting, less than 2 weeks after the injury. Unfortunately, this is when the knee is usually swollen and range of motion is poor with decreased or absent muscle control of the limb. All of these factors can increase the risk of a permanently stiff knee. Even in the environment of a high-volume knee trauma center,[6,59] loss of motion with a multiple ligament reconstruction is difficult to prevent. Therefore, these decisions must take into account this risk of stiffness along with other patient factors such as complicating injuries, medical

---

Critical Points EMERGENT SURGERY

- Emergent surgery is indicated for vascular injury, compartment syndrome, open injury, or irreducible dislocations.[46]
- Acute compartment syndrome is a condition in which the pressure within a fascial compartment rises to a level that decreases tissue perfusion, leading to cellular anoxia, muscle ischemia, and death.
- Urgent restoration of perfusion and normalization of compartment pressures is accomplished by complete fasciotomy of all compartments.[39]

Critical Points DEFINITIVE MANAGEMENT

- For patients with high physical demands, optimizing the condition of the knee (muscle function, range of motion, and swelling) and relying on reconstruction rather than acute repair may yield a superior functional result.

comorbidities, participation in rehabilitation efforts, ability to maintain knee reduction, soft tissue coverage and skin condition, and patient expectations. Fortunately, reconstructive options today surpass those available even a few years ago, thereby decreasing the need for acute repair. For patients with high physical demands, optimizing the condition of the knee (muscle function, range of motion, and swelling) and relying on reconstruction rather than acute repair may yield a superior functional result. Although time from injury dictates options such as repair versus reconstruction, it is the condition of the knee that may ultimately determine stiffness and functional results.

Arthroscopically assisted surgery should usually be delayed a minimum of 10 to 14 days after the injury to allow the joint capsule to heal and therefore minimize the risk of fluid extravasation and subsequent compartment syndrome.[51] In addition, this delay allows for monitoring of the vascular status, decreased swelling, improvement in quadriceps tone, and range of motion.[7]

Shelbourne and colleagues[54] in 1991 demonstrated a significantly increased incidence of arthrofibrosis in patients undergoing ACL reconstruction within 1 week of injury compared with those delayed 21 days or more. These authors also believed that delayed surgery gave the patient the opportunity to ask questions, as well as improve her or his psychological outlook on the injury and rehabilitation. Stannard and coworkers[59] compared acute repair (within 3 wk) of the posterolateral corner with reconstruction. These investigators found significantly inferior results of repair (37% failure) to reconstruction (9% failure) in 56 patients with 57 posterolateral corner injuries at 2 years.

REFERENCES

1. Alberty, R. E.; Goodfried, G.; Boyden, A. M.: Popliteal artery injury with fractural dislocation of the knee. *Am J Surg* 142:36–40, 1981.
2. Almekinders, L. C.; Logan, T. C.: Results following treatment of traumatic dislocations of the knee joint. *Clin Orthop Relat Res* 284:203–207, 1992.
3. Applebaum, R.; Yellin, A. E.; Weaver, F. A.; et al.: Role of routine arteriography in blunt lower-extremity trauma. *Am J Surg* 160:221–224, discussion 224–225, 1990.
4. Barnes, C. J.; Pietrobon, R.; Higgins, L. D.: Does the pulse examination in patients with traumatic knee dislocation predict a surgical arterial injury? A meta-analysis. *J Trauma* 53:1109–1114, 2002.
5. Campos, J. C.; Chung, C. B.; Lektrakul, N.; et al.: Pathogenesis of the Segond fracture: anatomic and MR imaging evidence of an iliotibial tract or anterior oblique band avulsion. *Radiology* 219:381–386, 2001.
6. Chhabra, A.; Cha, P. S.; Rihn, J. A.; Cole, B.; et al.: Surgical management of knee dislocations. Surgical technique. *J Bone Joint Surg Am* 87(suppl 1 pt 1):1–21, 2005.
7. Cole, B. J.; Harner, C. D.: The multiple ligament injured knee. *Clin Sports Med* 18:241–262, 1999.
8. Cole, P. A.; Campbell, R.; Swiontkowski, M. F.; Johansen, K. H.: Doppler arterial measurements reliably exclude occult arterial injury in blunt extremity trauma. Abstract. Orthopaedic Trauma Association, October 1998.
9. Dart, C. H., Jr.; Braitman, H. E.: Popliteal artery injury following fracture or dislocation at the knee. Diagnosis and management. *Arch Surg* 112:969–973, 1977.
10. Dietz, G. W.; Wilcox, D. M.; Montgomery, J. B.: Segond tibial condyle fracture: lateral capsular ligament avulsion. *Radiology* 159:467–469, 1986.
11. Donaldson, W. F., 3rd; Warren, R. F.; Wickiewicz, T.: A comparison of acute anterior cruciate ligament examinations. Initial versus examination under anesthesia. *Am J Sports Med* 13:5–10, 1985.
12. Escobedo, E. M.; Mills, W. J.; Hunter, J. C.: The "reverse Segond" fracture: association with a tear of the posterior cruciate ligament and medial meniscus. *AJR Am J Roentgenol* 178:979–983, 2002.
13. Ferraresi, S.; Garozzo, D.; Buffatti, P.: Common peroneal nerve injuries: results with one-stage nerve repair and tendon transfer. *Neurosurg Rev* 26:175–179, 2003.
14. Goitz, R. J.; Tomaino, M. M.: Management of peroneal nerve injuries associated with knee dislocations. *Am J Orthop* 32:14–16, 2003.
15. Goldman, A. B.; Pavlov, H.; Rubenstein, D.: The Segond fracture of the proximal tibia: a small avulsion that reflects major ligamentous damage. *AJR Am J Roentgenol* 151:1163–1167, 1988.
16. Good, L.; Johnson, R. J.: The dislocated knee. *J Am Acad Orthop Surg* 3:284–292, 1995.
17. Green, N. E.; Allen, B. L.: Vascular injuries associated with dislocation of the knee. *J Bone Joint Surg Am* 59:236–239, 1977.
18. Griffith, J. F.; Antonio, G. E.; Tong, C. W.; Ming, C. K.: Cruciate ligament avulsion fractures. *Arthroscopy* 20:803–812, 2004.
19. Gruber, H.; Peer, S.; Meirer, R.; Bodner, G.: Peroneal nerve palsy associated with knee luxation: evaluation by sonography—initial experiences. *AJR Am J Roentgenol* 185:1119–1125, 2005.
20. Hoover, G. H.; Frost, H. M.: Dynamic correction of spastic rocker-bottom foot. Peroneal to anterior tibial tendon transfer and heel-cord lengthening. *Clin Orthop Relat Res* 65:175–182, 1969.
21. Hoppenfeld, S. (ed): *Physical Examination of the Spine and Extremeties.* Norwalk, CT: Appleton-Century-Crofts, 1976.
22. Huang, G. S.; Yu, J. S.; Munshi, M.; et al.: Avulsion fracture of the head of the fibula (the "arcuate" sign): MR imaging findings predictive of injuries to the posterolateral ligaments and posterior cruciate ligament. *AJR Am J Roentgenol* 180:381–387, 2003.
23. Jackson, C. T.; Weighill, F. J.: A combined peroneal tendon transfer and subtalar fusion using excised fibular bone. *Br J Clin Pract* 27:329–330, 1973.
24. Jones, R. E.; Smith, E. C.; Bone, G. E.: Vascular and orthopedic complications of knee dislocation. *Surg Gynecol Obstet* 149:554–558, 1979.
25. Kendall, R. W.; Taylor, D. C.; Salvian, A. J.; O'Brien, P. J.: The role of arteriography in assessing vascular injuries associated with dislocations of the knee. *J Trauma* 35:875–878, 1993.
26. Kennedy, J. C.: Complete dislocation of the knee joint. *J Bone Joint Surg Am* 45:889–904, 1963.
27. Kim, D. H.; Kline, D. G.: Management and results of peroneal nerve lesions. *Neurosurgery* 39:312–319, discussion 319–320, 1996.
28. Kim, D. H.; Murovic, J. A.; Tiel, R. L.; Kline, D. G.: Management and outcomes in 318 operative common peroneal nerve lesions at the Louisiana State University Health Sciences Center. *Neurosurgery* 54:1421–1428; discussion 1428–1429, 2004.
29. Kim, T. K.; Savino, R. M.; McFarland, E. G.; Cosgarea, A. J.: Neurovascular complications of knee arthroscopy. *Am J Sports Med* 30:619–629, 2002.
30. Lefrak, E. A.: Knee dislocation. An illusive cause of critical arterial occlusion. *Arch Surg* 111:1021–1024, 1976.
31. Lynch, K.; Johansen, K.: Can Doppler pressure measurement replace "exclusion" arteriography in the diagnosis of occult extremity arterial trauma? *Ann Surg* 214:737–741, 1991.
32. McCoy, G. F.; Hannon, D. G.; Barr, R. J.; Templeton, J.: Vascular injury associated with low-velocity dislocations of the knee. *J Bone Joint Surg Br* 69:285–287, 1987.
33. McCutchan, J. D.; Gillham, N. R.: Injury to the popliteal artery associated with dislocation of the knee: palpable distal pulses do not negate the requirement for arteriography. *Injury* 20:307–310, 1989.
34. McDonough, E. B.; Wojtys, E. M.: Multi-ligamentous injuries of the knee and associated vascular injuries. *Am J Sports Med* 37:156–159, 2009.
35. Merrill, K. D.: Knee dislocations with vascular injuries. *Orthop Clin North Am* 25:707–713, 1994.
36. Meyers, M. H.; Moore, T. M.; Harvey, J. P., Jr.: Traumatic dislocation of the knee joint. *J Bone Joint Surg Am* 57:430–433, 1975.

37. Mills, W. J.; Barei, D. P.; McNair, P.: The value of the ankle-brachial index for diagnosing arterial injury after knee dislocation: a prospective study. *J Trauma* 56:1261–1265, 2004.
38. Nystrom, M.; Samimi, S.; Ha'Eri, G. B.: Two cases of irreducible knee dislocation occurring simultaneously in two patients and a review of the literature. *Clin Orthop Relat Res* 277:197–200, 1992.
39. Olson, S. A.; Glasgow, R. R.: Acute compartment syndrome in lower extremity musculoskeletal trauma. *J Am Acad Orthop Surg* 13:436–444, 2005.
40. Ottolenghi, C. E.: Vascular complications in injuries about the knee joint. *Clin Orthop Relat Res* 165:148–156, 1982.
41. Peck, J. J.; Eastman, A. B.; Bergan, J. J.; et al.: Popliteal vascular trauma. A community experience. *Arch Surg* 125:1339–1343; discussion 1343–1344, 1990.
42. Pinzur, M. S.; Kett, N.; Trilla, M.: Combined anteroposterior tibial tendon transfer in post-traumatic peroneal palsy. *Foot Ankle* 8:271–275, 1988.
43. Potter, H. G.; Weinstein, M.; Allen, A. A.; et al.: Magnetic resonance imaging of the multiple-ligament injured knee. *J Orthop Trauma* 16:330–339, 2002.
44. Quinlan, A. G.: Irreducible posterolateral dislocation of the knee with button-holing of the medial femoral condyle. *J Bone Joint Surg Am* 48:1619–1621, 1966.
45. Reckling, F. W.; Peltier, L. F.: Acute knee dislocations and their complications. 1969. *Clin Orthop Relat Res* 422:135–141, 2004.
46. Rihn, J. A.; Groff, Y. J.; Harner, C. D.; Cha, P. S.: The acutely dislocated knee: evaluation and management. *J Am Acad Orthop Surg* 12:334–346, 2004.
47. Rios, A.; Villa, A.; Fahandezh, H.; et al.: Results after treatment of traumatic knee dislocations: a report of 26 cases. *J Trauma* 55:489–494, 2003.
48. Roman, P. D.; Hopson, C. N.; Zenni, E. J., Jr.: Traumatic dislocation of the knee: a report of 30 cases and literature review. *Orthop Rev* 16:917–924, 1987.
49. Samimi, S.; Shahriaree, H.: Arthroscopic view of an irreducible knee dislocation. *Arthroscopy* 9:322–326, 1993.
50. Schenck, R. C., Jr.: The dislocated knee. *Instr Course Lect* 43:127–136, 1994.
51. Schenck, R, C., Jr.; Hunter, R. E., Ostrum, R. F.; Perry, C. R.: Knee dislocations. *Instr Course Lect* 48:515–522, 1999.
52. Sedel, L.; Nizard, R. S.: Nerve grafting for traction injuries of the common peroneal nerve. A report of 17 cases. *J Bone Joint Surg Br* 75:772–774, 1993.
53. Segond P. Recherches cliniques et experimentales sur les epanchements sanguins du genou par entorse. *Prog Med* 7:297–299, 319–321, 340–341, 1879.
54. Shelbourne, K. D.; Porter, D. A.; Clingman, J. A.; et al.: Low-velocity knee dislocation. *Orthop Rev* 20:995–1004, 1991.
55. Shields, L.; Mital, M.; Cave, E. F.: Complete dislocation of the knee: experience at the Massachusetts General Hospital. *J Trauma* 9:192–215, 1969.
56. Simonka, J. A.: [Management of a foot deformity, caused by paralysis of the peroneal nerve, by transfer of the tendon of the posterior tibial muscle]. *Magy Traumatol Orthop Helyreallito Seb* 34:230–232, 1991.
57. Sisto, D. J.; Warren, R. F.: Complete knee dislocation. A follow-up study of operative treatment. *Clin Orthop Relat Res* 198:94–101, 1985.
58. Stannard, J. P.; Sheils, T. M.; Lopez-Ben, R. R.; et al.: Vascular injuries in knee dislocations: the role of physical examination in determining the need for arteriography. *J Bone Joint Surg Am* 86:910–915, 2004.
59. Stannard, J. P.; Riley, R. S.; Sheils, T. M.; et al.: Anatomic reconstruction of the posterior cruciate ligament after multiligament knee injuries. A combination of the tibial-inlay and two-femoral-tunnel techniques. *Am J Sports Med* 31:196–202, 2003.
60. Tomaino, M.; Day, C.; Papageorgiou, C.; et al.: Peroneal nerve palsy following knee dislocation: pathoanatomy and implications for treatment. *Knee Surg Sports Traumatol Arthrosc* 8:163–165, 2000.
61. Treiman, G. S.; Yellin, A. E.; Weaver, F. A.; et al.: Examination of the patient with a knee dislocation. The case for selective arteriography. *Arch Surg* 127:1056–1062; discussion 1062–1063, 1992.
62. Twaddle, B. C.; Bidwell, T. A.; Chapman, J. R.: Knee dislocations: where are the lesions? A prospective evaluation of surgical findings in 63 cases. *J Orthop Trauma* 17:198–202, 2003.
63. Vertullo, C. J.; Nunley, J. A.: Acquired flatfoot deformity following posterior tibial tendon transfer for peroneal nerve injury: a case report. *J Bone Joint Surg Am* 84:1214–1217, 2002.
64. Vigasio, A.; Marcoccio, I.; Patelli, A.; et al.: New tendon transfer for correction of drop-foot in common peroneal nerve palsy. *Clin Orthop Relat Res* 466:1454–1466, 2008. Epub 2008; April 15.
65. Wapner, K. L.; Taras, J. S.; Lin, S. S.; Chao, W.: Staged reconstruction for chronic rupture of both peroneal tendons using Hunter rod and flexor hallucis longus tendon transfer: a long-term followup study. *Foot Ankle Int* 27:591–597, 2006.
66. Wascher, D. C.: High-velocity knee dislocation with vascular injury. Treatment principles. *Clin Sports Med* 19:457–477, 2000.
67. Welling, R. E.; Kakkasseril, J.; Cranley, J. J.: Complete dislocations of the knee with popliteal vascular injury. *J Trauma* 21:450–453, 1981.

Section VIII

Meniscus

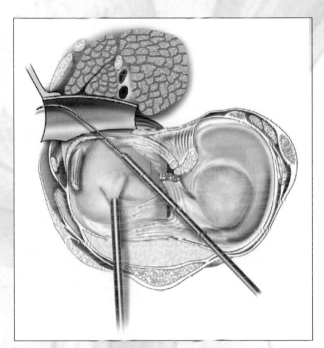

Chapter 28

Meniscus Tears: Diagnosis, Repair Techniques, and Clinical Outcomes

Frank R. Noyes, MD ■ *Sue D. Barber-Westin*, BS

INDICATIONS

The importance of the menisci in the human knee is well understood and documented. The menisci occupy 60% of the contact area between the tibial and the femoral cartilage surfaces and transmit greater than 50% of joint compression forces. After meniscectomy, the tibiofemoral contact area decreases by approximately 50% and the contact forces increase two- to threefold.[2,45,66,71,83,139] Meniscectomy frequently leads to irreparable joint damage, including articular cartilage degeneration, flattening of articular surfaces, and subchondral bone sclerosis. Poor long-term clinical results have been reported by many investigators after partial and total meniscectomy.* For instance, Scheller and coworkers[122] followed 75 knees that underwent partial lateral meniscectomy 5 to 15 years postoperatively and noted that 78% had Fairbank's signs of radiographic

---

*See references 6, 41, 56, 62, 63, 79, 85, 114, 118, 119, 122, 133, 140.

> **Critical Points INDICATIONS**
>
> - Meniscus tear with tibiofemoral joint line pain.
> - Active patient <60 yr of age.
> - Concurrent knee ligament reconstruction or osteotomy.
> - Meniscus tear reducible, good tissue integrity, normal position in the joint once repaired.
> - Meniscus tear classified by location, type of tear, integrity, damage to meniscus tissue, remaining meniscus bed.
> - Peripheral single longitudinal tears: red-red, one plane: repairable in all cases, high success rates.
> - Middle third region: red-white (vascular supply present) or white-white (no blood supply).
> - Outer third and middle third regions longitudinal, radial, horizontal tears: red-white, one plane: often repairable.
> - Outer third and middle third regions complex double or triple longitudinal, flap tears: red-white, multiple planes: repair vs. excision.

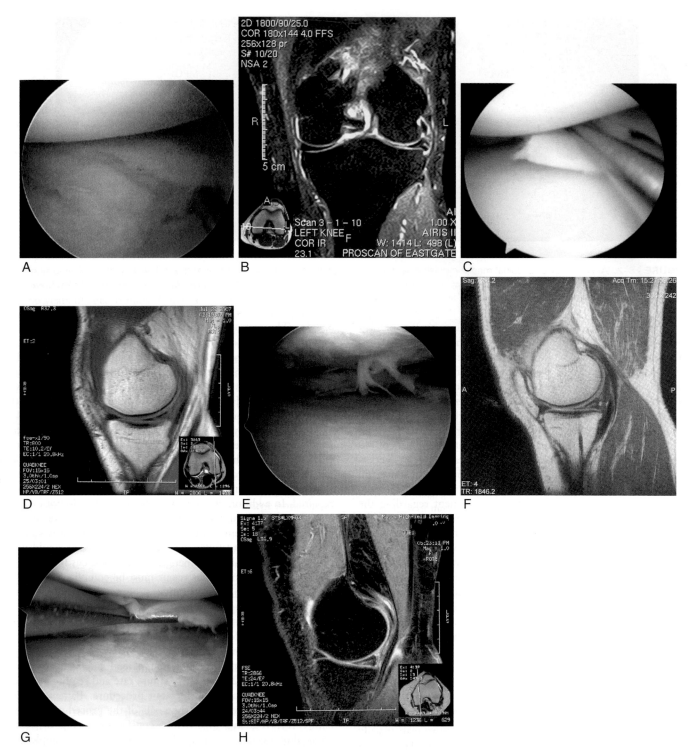

FIGURE 28–3. Examples of irreparable meniscus tears. **A** and **B**, A 40-year-old man with a complex middle third longitudinal tear of the lateral meniscus. **C** and **D**, A 39-year-old man with a complex flap tear to the posterior horn of the medial meniscus. **E** and **F**, A 43-year-old man with a degenerative tear extending to the undersurface of the medial meniscus. **G** and **H**, A 55-year-old woman with a degenerative longitudinal tear to the medial meniscus. Magnetic resonance imaging (MRI) does not provide sufficient detail of the tear and integrity of the meniscus tissue to determine whether a repair of the complex tear is possible.

to four all-inside sutures. This procedure is performed in all active patients, except older patients (>50 yr of age) who are sedentary. A complex tear that is located in both red-white and white-white regions may have a success rate of approximately 50%, and the repair of these more difficult tears is usually performed in young patients in an attempt to preserve some meniscal function. In others, a partial meniscectomy is performed.

CLINICAL BIOMECHANICS

Meniscus Function

The menisci provide several vital mechanical functions in the knee joint. They act as a spacer between the femoral condyle and the tibial plateau and, when there are no compressive weight-bearing loads across the joint, limit contact between the articular surfaces. The amount of joint narrowing due strictly to the physical absence of the menisci is in the range of 1 to 2 mm.

Under static-loading conditions, the menisci assume a significant load-bearing function in the tibiofemoral articulation.[2,26,45] At least 50% of the compressive load of the knee joint is transmitted through the menisci in 0° of extension, and approximately 85% of the load is transmitted at 90° of flexion.[2] The presence of the menisci increases the contact area to 2.5 times the size of a meniscectomized joint. The larger contact area provided by the menisci reduces the average contact stress (force/unit area) acting between the joint surfaces. Removal of as little as 15% to 34% of a meniscus increases contact pressures by more than 350%.[124]

Lee and colleagues[75] evaluated the biomechanical effects of serial meniscectomies in the posterior segment of the medial meniscus. Compared with the intact state, the medial contact area decreased from 20% (after removal of 50% of the posterior segment of the medial meniscus) to 54% (total meniscectomy). Medial contact stress increased from 24% (50% meniscectomy) to 134% (total meniscectomy). Medial peak contact stress increased from 43% (50% meniscectomy) to 136% (total meniscectomy). The peripheral portion of the medial meniscus provides a greater contribution to increasing contact area and decreasing contact stresses than the central portion. Peak contact stresses increase proportionally with the amount of meniscus removed.

Medial meniscectomy performed after sectioning of the ACL results in increased anterior translation at 20° of knee flexion compared with that measured in knees with an intact ACL.[77] Thus, the loss of the medial meniscus after an ACL rupture is problematic, especially in varus-angulated knees. In knees with posterior cruciate ligament (PCL) ruptures, the increase in posterior tibial translation allows a change in tibiofemoral contact in which the menisci posterior horns have a reduced weight-bearing function. This is sometimes referred to as a "PCL meniscectomy." The effect is greater for the medial compartment in which the middle and anterior thirds of the medial meniscus have less weight-bearing function than the lateral meniscus.

The menisci remain in constant congruity to the tibial and femoral articular surfaces throughout knee flexion and extension[135,146] and are thus believed to contribute to stability to the knee joint.[92] The lateral meniscus provides concavity to the lateral tibiofemoral joint owing to the normal posterior convexity of the lateral tibial condyle, allowing the stabilizing effect of joint weight-bearing forces to reduce lateral compartment anterior and posterior translations.[82] Total lateral meniscectomy results in a 45% to 50% decrease in total contact area and a 235% to 335% increase in peak local contact pressure.[103]

Loss of the medial meniscus results in a smaller, more medial displacement of the center of pressure. Load is subsequently transmitted through the articular cartilage and subchondral bone to the underlying cancellous bone through this more central route, thus stress-shielding the proximal aspects of the medial tibial cortex. The deleterious effects of meniscectomy on tibiofemoral compartment articular cartilage have been demonstrated in multiple experimental studies.[65,104,132,145] For these reasons, it is paramount to preserve meniscal function, if possible, in knees with varus osseous malalignment.

In addition, the menisci provide shock absorption to the knee joint during walking and are theorized to assist in overall lubrication of the articular surfaces.[92,141]

Meniscus Suture Repair Biomechanics

Various suture repair techniques and suture materials have been tested experimentally to determine initial fixation strength and performance under cyclical loading.[13,106] Suture techniques have also been compared with several meniscus repair devices.* Post and coworkers[106] compared the pull-out strength of vertical mattress, horizontal, and knot-end sutures in a porcine model using either 2-0 Ethibond, 0-polydioxanone sutures (PDS), or 1-PDS suture material. The vertical mattress technique with 1-PDS suture had significantly greater ($P < .05$) mean load-to-failure values than any other combination (146 ± 17 N). This was followed by the vertical mattress technique with 0-PDS suture material (116 ± 28 N). The vertical mattress technique had significantly greater mean load-to-failure values than the horizontal mattress technique, regardless of suture type ($P < .0001$). There was no difference in the relative strength between horizontal and knot-end suture techniques.

Asik and coworkers[13] compared the failure strengths of vertical, vertical mattress, vertical loop, horizontal mattress, and knot-end suture techniques in a bovine model. Each group consisted of four medial menisci, and 1-Prolene suture material was used in all specimens. The vertically oriented sutures showed significantly higher initial fixation strengths (mean, ~131 N) compared with the knot-end (64 N; $P < .001$) and horizontal (98 N; $P < .001$) techniques. In another study, Asik and Sener[17] compared the mean load to failure of a variety of meniscus repair devices with that of horizontal and vertically oriented sutures in a bovine model. The strongest repair method was the vertical sutures with 0 PDS (mean, 104.7 N). The mean

---

*See references 4, 16, 17, 24, 25, 37, 43, 88, 126, 143, 147, 148.

failure strengths of all of the devices were lower than both suturing techniques (range, 9.8 N for the Arthrex dart to 51.4 N for the T-Fix device).

Miller and associates[88] assessed healing rates and chondral injuries of three all-inside devices in a goat model 6 months after implantation. A 15-mm longitudinal tear was created in the peripheral 25% of the posterior-central horn and then repaired with either two Meniscal Fasteners (Mitek, Ethicon, Westwood, MA), two 10-mm BioStingers (Linvatec, Largo, FL), or two 10-mm Clearfix Meniscal Screws (Mitek). A group of goats that had undergone repair with two vertical mattress sutures for a similar lesion was used for control.[89] The authors reported that the suture group had a significantly higher rate of healing (93% completely healed, 7% no healing) than all three of the device groups ($P < .01$), which ranged from 43% to 54% complete healing and from 0% to 25% no healing. In addition, significant chondral injury was observed in the majority of animals in all three device groups.

Several investigations compared the biomechanical properties of meniscus arrows with those of vertical and horizontal sutures.[4,12,16,24,37,110,126,143] Vertical sutures are superior to both horizontal sutures and meniscus arrows in mean load-to-failure values.[12,42,143] Dervin and colleagues[37] reported that the meniscus arrow had approximately one half the failure strength of vertical sutures (30 N and 58 N, respectively; $P < .001$). Song and Lee[126] found that the maximum tensile strength of the meniscus arrows was significantly lower (38 N) than both vertical (114 N) and horizontal (75 N) sutures ($P < .05$). Walsh and coworkers[143] reported that the meniscus arrow and meniscus staple had significantly lower mean force-at-failure values (44.3 N and 17.8 N, respectively) than vertical suture (73.9 N; $P < .005$).

Rankin and associates[110] used a bovine model to compare vertical sutures, horizontal sutures, meniscus arrows, and T-Fix repairs in which three sutures or devices were used for each repair. Vertical sutures were stronger than all other repair methods and showed the smallest average residual displacement (0.21 mm). The force required to generate 2 mm of tear displacement was greatest for the vertical sutures and least for the arrow (143 N and 43.6 N, respectively; $P < .0001$). The superior strength of vertical sutures is believed to be due to the perpendicular orientation to the circumferential collagen bundles of the meniscus.[110]

Becker and colleagues[21] compared the biomechanical behavior of several biodegradable implants for meniscus repair with that of vertical and horizontal mattress sutures in response to cyclical loading and load-to-failure testing. Seventy lateral menisci were removed from patients aged 52 to 60 years prior to total knee replacement. One suture or device was used for each repair. The pull-out strength of the vertical and horizontal sutures was superior to those of the implants. Superior stiffness during load-to-failure testing and lower displacement under cyclical loading were found for the vertical sutures compared with horizontal sutures and all implants.

Nyland and associates[100] evaluated displacement (repair site gapping) of all-inside vertically or horizontally placed FasT-Fix (Smith & Nephew, Endoscopy Division, Andover, MA) devices to horizontally placed RapidLoc devices (Mitek Surgical Products, Westwood, MA) under cyclical loading conditions in human cadavers (mean age, 65 ± 7.7 yr). Two implants placed 5 mm apart were used for each repair. The vertical FasT-Fix group had significantly less displacement after 500 cycles than the other two groups ($P < .01$) and greater stiffness.

Meniscus Repair Healing

There are few published experimental studies on the strength of a healing meniscus suture repair (without cell-based therapy or growth factors) subjected to tensile loads. Newman and associates[94] measured the mechanical behavior of canine joints after repair of peripheral and radial meniscus tears. Contralateral limbs served as controls. The peripheral tears were repaired with four vertically oriented sutures, and the radial tears were repaired with two horizontally oriented sutures. Thirteen weeks later, the peripheral repairs demonstrated no statistically significant differences between the repaired and the control limb in compressive force-displacement behavior, input energy, and ratio of dissipated to input energy. All of the peripheral repairs healed, with no gapping at the repair site. However, the radial repairs showed significant differences in the structural and material properties compared with the control limb. These repairs healed with 3- to 5-mm-wide fibrovascular scars, and 10 of 17 (59%) specimens failed to refill the gap completely to the inner meniscal rim. The authors concluded that the mechanical function was restored after peripheral repairs, but not after radial repairs in this animal model.

In a rabbit model, Roeddecker and colleagues[117] studied tissue strength after repair of longitudinal meniscal lesions located in the central third region. A 3-mm lesion was created and then either left alone, repaired using one suture, or repaired with a fibrin sealant. The contralateral limb was used as a control. After 6 weeks, the mean relative strength of the healing tissues were 26% (suture) and 42.5% (fibrin glue) of the control values. These strength values remained similar after 13 weeks.

CLINICAL EVALUATION

A thorough history includes assessment of the injury mechanism, initial and residual symptoms, and functional limitations. Common injury mechanisms are a sudden twist, change in direction, or deep knee flexion. Meniscus tears are frequently encountered in knees with ACL ruptures. A comprehensive knee examination is performed, which includes assessment of knee motion, patellofemoral indices, tibiofemoral pain and crepitus, muscle strength, ligament subluxation tests, and gait abnormalities.

The presence of tibiofemoral joint line pain on joint palpation is a primary indicator of a meniscus tear. Other clinical signs include pain on forced flexion, obvious meniscal displacement during joint compression and flexion and extension, lack of full extension, and a positive McMurray test.[84] All ligament stability tests are performed and compared with the opposite knee joint. MRI may be obtained using a proton-density–weighted, high-resolution, fast-spin-echo sequence[107,108] to determine the status of the articular cartilage and menisci. This evaluation is useful in knees with suspected degenerative tears[142] and chronic ACL ruptures and to determine whether a meniscus cyst is present. A recent investigation that examined the ability of MRI to predict reparability of longitudinal full-thickness meniscus lesions reported high sensitivity and specificity rates (overall, 94% and 81%, respectively).[95]

LaPrade and Konowalchuk[73] described a figure-four test that attempts to replicate symptoms in patients with tears of the lateral meniscus popliteomeniscal attachments. The patient is placed supine, the knee flexed to approximately 90°, the foot placed over the contralateral knee, and the hip externally

Critical Points CLINICAL EVALUATION

Physical Examination

- Tibiofemoral joint line pain, compression pain.
- McMurray test.
- Knee flexion & extension.
- Joint effusion.
- Patellofemoral (medial & lateral subluxation, Q-angle, crepitus, compression pain).
- Muscle strength.

Magnetic Resonance Imaging

- Proton-density–weighted, high-resolution, fast-spin-echo sequence.

Ligament Subluxation Tests

- Pivot shift, Lachman.
- KT-2000 20° knee flexion, 134 N force.
- Posterior drawer, 90° knee flexion.
- External tibial rotation 30°, 90° knee flexion.
- Tibiofemoral rotation dial 30°, 90° knee flexion.
- External rotation recurvatum.
- Lateral tibiofemoral joint opening 5°, 20° knee flexion.
- Reverse pivot shift.
- Medial tibiofemoral joint opening 5°, 20° knee flexion.

Radiographs

- Anteroposterior.
- Lateral, 30° knee flexion.
- Posteroanterior, weight-bearing, 45° knee flexion.
- Patellofemoral axial.

Assessment of Symptoms and Functional Limitations with Activity: Cincinnati Knee Rating System

- Sports Activity and Function Form.
- Occupational Rating Form.
- Symptom Rating Form.

---

rotated. A varus loading at the knee joint increases tensile loading in the damaged posterolateral soft tissue meniscal attachments. The primary symptom from popliteomeniscal tears is lateral compartment pain with activities, especially turning and twisting with sports. MRI is frequently negative. The authors described an open approach to repair the popliteomeniscal attachments. However, these peripheral tears are amendable to an inside-out repair technique, as is described later.

The clinical examination may reveal tenderness upon palpation at the posterolateral aspect of the joint at the anatomic site of the popliteomeniscal attachments. The McMurray test is performed in maximum flexion, progressing from maximum external rotation to internal rotation and then back to external rotation. This test may produce a lateral palpable snapping sensation, representing an anterior subluxation of the posterior horn of the lateral meniscus with maximum internal rotation. The snapping is produced with external rotation as the meniscus returns to a normal position. Of interest, patients with physiologic joint laxity and increases in tibial rotation limits can commonly produce this lateral snapping sign in both knees under examination, which is not painful. Patients with tears of the popliteomeniscal attachments may have a positive snapping sign in only the symptomatic knee, which produces posterolateral joint pain.

Radiographs taken during the initial examination include lateral at 30° of knee flexion, weight-bearing PA at 45° of knee flexion, and patellofemoral axial. Axial lower limb alignment is measured using full standing hip-knee-ankle weight-bearing

radiographs in knees that demonstrate varus or valgus alignment.[38] Knees that have deficiency of the posterolateral structures may require lateral stress radiographs. Posterior stress radiographs may be used in patients with PCL ruptures.

Patients complete questionnaires and are interviewed to rate symptoms, functional limitations, sports and occupational activity levels, and patient perception of the overall knee condition according to the Cincinnati Knee Rating System.[19]

PREOPERATIVE PLANNING

Concomitant injuries should be evaluated and may include cruciate or collateral ligament rupture, extensor mechanism injury or malalignment, chondral fracture, osseous malalignment, or an overuse syndrome. The patient is informed that the rehabilitation program may require modification according to the procedures performed. Knees with ACL or PCL deficiency require concomitant ligament reconstruction with the meniscus repair to achieve knee stability and protect the repair site. Knees with varus osseous malalignment that require osteotomy may also have chronic medial meniscus tears that are occasionally repaired.

INTRAOPERATIVE EVALUATION

All knee ligament subluxation tests should be performed after the induction of anesthesia in both the injured and the contralateral limbs. The amount of increased anterior tibial translation, posterior tibial translation, lateral and medial joint opening, and internal-external tibial rotation should be documented.

A thorough arthroscopic examination is conducted, documenting articular cartilage surface abnormalities.[99] A probe inserted from the medial infrapatellar portal is used to tension the meniscus to determine the integrity of the peripheral rim and the anterior and posterior attachments. The probe is placed underneath the meniscus to visualize the entire undersurface (see Fig. 26-2). Flap tears that otherwise may not be evident may be discovered during this examination.

A 30° or 70° arthroscope is used in the anteromedial portal to examine the posteromedial meniscal region. The anteromedial portal is purposely placed immediately adjacent to the medial border of the patellar tendon. The arthroscope sheath with a blunt obturator is passed along the lateral aspect of the medial femoral condyle distal to the PCL attachment into the posteromedial compartment. The meniscal-synovial junction, the peripheral edge of the meniscus, the opening of a synovial cyst, and the posterior articular surface of the medial femoral condyle are inspected. A nerve hook is passed from the anteromedial portal and brought over the top of the meniscus into the posteromedial compartment. The peripheral attachment of the

Critical Points PREOPERATIVE PLANNING

- Knees with cruciate deficiency: plan reconstruction with meniscus repair.
- Other concomitant injuries may include collateral ligament ruptures, extensor mechanism injuries, chondral fractures.
- Associated chronic conditions may include extensor mechanism malalignment, overuse syndrome, varus osseous malalignment. Consider meniscus repair whenever possible in these knees.

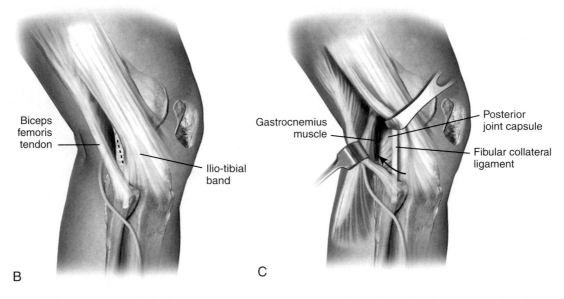

Biceps
femoris
tendon

Ilio-tibial
band

B

Gastrocnemius
muscle

Posterior
joint capsule

Fibular collateral
ligament

C

FIGURE 28–8—cont'd. B, Incision site in the interval between the posterior edge of the iliotibial band and the anterior edge of the biceps tendon. **C**, The interval between the lateral gastrocnemius and the posterolateral capsule is opened bluntly, just proximal to the fibular head, avoiding entering the joint capsule.

above the fibular head. This avoids penetrating and opening the posterior capsule. The space between the posterolateral capsule and the lateral gastrocnemius tendon is further developed bluntly with the index finger. A Henning retractor is used to push the neurovascular bundle medially (Fig. 28–9). The

inferior lateral geniculate artery may be visualized in the inferior aspect of the exposure and may be damaged and require electro-coagulation (which is avoided if possible to maintain the vascular supply to the lateral meniscus). The retractor must always be positioned anterior to the gastrocnemius muscle and tendon

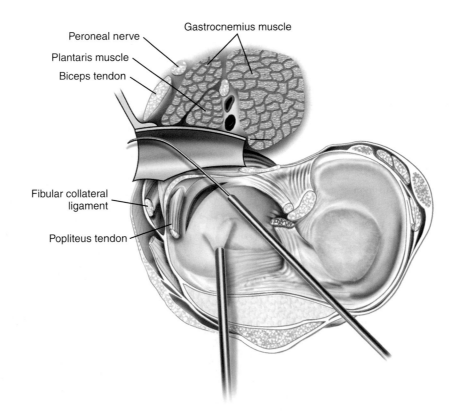

Peroneal nerve

Gastrocnemius muscle

Plantaris muscle

Biceps tendon

Fibular collateral
ligament

Popliteus tendon

FIGURE 28–9. Cross-section shows popliteal retractor between the lateral gastrocnemius and the posterior capsule. A curved suture cannula is also used to angle the needles away from the neurovascular structures.

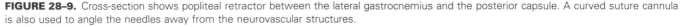

and directly posterior to the posterior capsule and posterior meniscus bed. The retractor blocks the suture needles from passing too posterior and potentially injuring the common peroneal nerve. During the meniscus suture steps, the surgeon should frequently check the position of the retractor to always ensure that it is anterior to the gastrocnemius muscle. If the retractor is mistakenly placed posterior to the gastrocnemius muscle, the peroneal nerve may be injured.

Patient Positioning and Equipment for Inside-Out Suture Repair

An assistant sits in a chair on the medial or lateral side of the knee with a headlight to visualize the posterior meniscus and capsule penetration of the inside-out–directed suture needles. The assistant has a needle holder to catch the suture needles and suture scissors. An inverted clamp is attached to the drapes to act as an instrument holder for this equipment. A scrub nurse stands opposite the surgeon to pass sutures through the single cannula, one at a time, after the surgeon has positioned the cannula. An assistant holds the lower leg with the knee at 20° to 30° of flexion and applies the force required to open the tibiofemoral compartment. The articular cartilage is carefully protected at all times to avoid damage.

Instruments required in addition to routine arthroscopic equipment are a ball-tipped rasp for synovial rasping, a Henning or similar popliteal retractor for protection of the posterior neurovascular structures, a single-barrel straight and curved cannula for suture passage, and 10-inch double-armed meniscal sutures. Nonabsorbable sutures are used for interbody tears.

Suture Repair Techniques

For medial meniscus repairs, the knee is flexed 30° and an abduction load is applied. A 30° arthroscope is positioned through the medial portal to visualize the meniscus. The cannula is positioned through the lateral portal and pointed to the exact location of suture placement. This allows the suture needle to angle away from the midline neurovascular structures. Occasionally, the tibial spines block access for the suture cannula and the surgeon must place the suture cannula in the medial portal. The suture cannula with a large radius curve is selected to angle the needle away from the neurovascular structures posteriorly. The second assistant passes a 10-inch flexible needle through the cannula. The first assistant, seated on the medial side of the knee, catches the needle with the needle holder as it exits through the exposed meniscus bed. The next suture is passed in the same manner. The first assistant catches the double-armed needles and pulls the suture through. Both needles are cut, and the suture is tied with five knots. The surgeon closely observes the reduction of the meniscus body and closure of the tear site with passage and tying of the vertical divergent sutures. The next sutures are placed in a similar fashion. Vertical divergent sutures are alternated; the sutures are placed, first, on the superior surface to reduce the meniscus and, second, on the inferior surface to close the inferior tear.

The neurovascular structures are protected throughout the procedure with the appropriate posteromedial exposure and a Henning retractor. For tears of the medial meniscus that extend entirely to the posterior horn, the surgeon must always place the needle cannula in the lateral portal to angle the sutures away from the neurovascular structures.

For lateral meniscus repairs, the first assistant is seated on the lateral side of the knee, and an adduction stress is applied to the flexed knee. Otherwise, the positioning and technique are the same as those described for the medial meniscus repair.

Multiple 2-0 braided polyester nonabsorbable sutures (Ticron, Davis and Geck Co., Danbury, CT; or Ethibond, Ethicon Inc., Somerville, NJ) are used on a 10-inch straight cutting needle to repair all meniscus tears. The sutures are inserted through the superior and inferior meniscal surfaces in an interrupted vertical fashion to close the meniscus tear both superiorly and inferiorly. The vertical placement is used owing to its higher failure strength than that of horizontally placed sutures.[111] In addition, the vertical suture orientation mimics the function of the radial collagen fibers within the meniscus, which can improve its load-carrying capacity.[29]

In addition, a single-barrel straight or curved arthroscopic cannula is used that allows for accurate placement of the sutures along the edge in tissue that will hold the stitches. A double-barrel cannula is not advocated, because the distance between the barrels is insufficient and needle control is compromised. The location of sutures depends on the tear pattern to be described.

Single and Double Longitudinal Tears

Only select double longitudinal tears are repaired; those with a peripheral meniscal-capsular disruption and those in which the second tear is at or close to the red-white junction. A tear entirely within the central meniscus third is only 6 to 7 mm in width and is not repaired. A longitudinal tear of the anterior horn of the medial or lateral meniscus that is at the periphery or extends into the red-white junction that fulfills the repair criteria is occasionally encountered. The senior author performs a mini-open direct 2- to 3-cm incision for an open repair. An outside-in placement of sutures for a simple tear is a second option.

A double-stacked suture technique is used for single and double longitudinal meniscus tears. This technique consists of two layers of sutures (Figs. 28–10 and 28–11) placed at 3- to 4-mm intervals along the length of the tear. The first layer of sutures is placed superiorly to anchor the meniscus to its bed and prevent superior migration of the meniscus during the repair. The cannula is used to hold and reduce the torn meniscus on the tibia.

The first pass of the double-armed suture is placed in the meniscal-synovial junction (periphery) of the intact portion of the meniscus. The second pass of the double-armed suture is placed through the torn portion of the meniscus in a vertical plane so that it bridges the tear (Fig. 28–12). The inferior sutures are placed next in a vertical plane, crossing the tear in the same manner as the superior sutures. The sutures are brought out through the accessory incision and tied directly over the posterior meniscal attachment and capsule. The sutures are tied as they are passed to determine the apposition of the tear surfaces. The tension in each suture is confirmed arthroscopically after the knot is tied. This double-stacked technique provides stable fixation of the meniscal tear on both sides and entirely closes the meniscus gap at the repair site (Fig. 28–13).

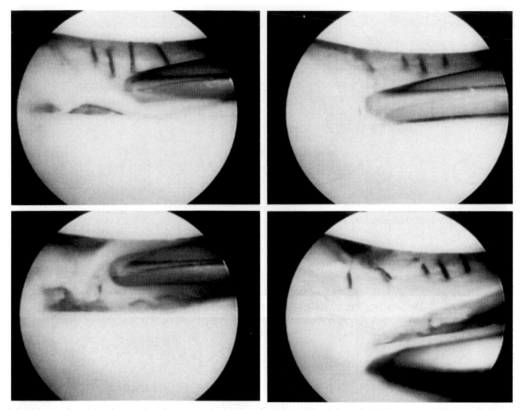

FIGURE 28–13. A longitudinal meniscal tear site demonstrates some fragmentation inferiorly. This tear required multiple superior and inferior vertical divergent sutures to achieve an anatomic reduction. *(Reprinted with permission from Noyes, F. R.; Barber-Westin, S. D.: Arthroscopic repair of meniscal tears extending into the avascular zone in patients younger than twenty years of age. Am J Sports Med 30:589–600, 2002.)*

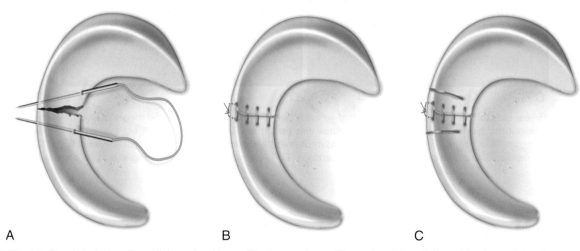

A   B   C

FIGURE 28–14. Repair technique for radial meniscal tears. The inner sutures (**A**) are placed first, followed by the peripheral sutures (**B**). The first suture needle is placed midway through the meniscus body and then used to apply a circumferential tension to reduce the tear gap, then advanced through the posterior meniscus bed. The second suture needle is placed in a similar manner. This reduces the radial gap, allowing subsequent sutures to be placed. Usually, 3 to 4 sutures are placed superiorly and two sutures, inferiorly. **C**, Occasionally, superior vertical divergent sutures are placed along the tear site to help stabilize the repair.

The initial sutures are placed first through the body using the needle to place the meniscus toward the tear site, followed by needle passage through the meniscus bed. This allows the tear site gap to be closed. Only radial tears that extend to the outer third of the meniscus body are repaired, because those that are confined to the inner and middle zones have a poor blood supply and will not heal. A radial tear that extends to the meniscus rim compromises the hoop stress and is equivalent to a total loss of meniscus function. Occasionally, the edges of the radial tear are degenerative with poor suture-holding capability and repair is not possible. Traumatic radial tears have a better chance of healing. The goal is to retain partial meniscus function, if possible, because it is rare to have successful healing of a tear in the inner aspect of the meniscus. Because only a limited number of sutures are used, the holding strength is low and a period of non–weight-bearing for 4 weeks is required to prevent disruption of the repair site. The patient is advised that this type of repair has a guarded prognosis in terms of providing function. The repair may heal, but the meniscus tear edges separate in the healing process with the interval replaced with poorly organized fibrous tissue with an elongated meniscus structure that displaces from the joint.

Lateral Radial Tears Associated with a Cyst

Because partial meniscectomy and cyst excision may remove a substantial portion of the meniscus body and disrupt its peripheral rim, a cyst should be excised through a limited open lateral exposure (Fig. 28–15). This is followed by repair of the peripheral rim of the meniscus using an open technique. Then, the radial tear and any associated horizontal tears may be repaired using the arthroscopic techniques described previously. It is not recommended to evacuate the cyst through the intra-articular radial tear site because this damages meniscus tissues and prevents repair. A lateral meniscus cyst is commonly associated with combined radial and horizontal tears that are not reparable; however, this is difficult to determine preoperatively. The mistake is to excise the meniscus in a patient 50 years of age or younger in whom a repair is possible to preserve some meniscus function where progression to lateral compartment arthritis occurs in a short time, particularly in a valgus-aligned lower extremity.

Horizontal Tears

The majority of horizontal tears are degenerative with poor tissue quality and are not reparable. These irreparable tears have thickened tissues, fatty deposition, and partial flap tears. Occasionally, a large horizontal flap tear is encountered in patients younger than 50 years of age in which the tear extends throughout the body creating superior and inferior segments, but the meniscal tissue is of good quality, has not displaced outside the tibiofemoral compartment, and can be repaired. The meniscus is rasped through the superior and inferior synovial attachments and within the horizontal tear. Minor meniscus fragments are removed. Vertical divergent

sutures are used to close the tear site. The soft Ethibond sutures are preferred that, by experience, do not damage articular cartilage. A fibrin clot may be added to the repair site, placed within the horizontal tear. However, whether or not this technique increases the repair success rate has not been scientifically proved.

Meniscus Attachment Root Tears

An important reparable meniscus tear is one in which the posterior horn is torn directly at its posterior attachment, producing a complete loss of meniscus function as it displaces under weight-bearing loads. Instruments used in shoulder rotator cuff tears can be used to pass two mattress-type sutures for firm fixation of the meniscus (Fig. 28–16). Alternatively, a suture lasso instrument can be passed through a small tibial tunnel. The suturing instrument is passed twice through the medial or lateral portal using a cannula. The mattress suture is performed rather than a single throw of the suture to increase holding strength. A leg holder is required to allow sufficient joint opening for passing and using the suture device, particularly for medial meniscus root tears. Without suturing, the tear results in complete loss of meniscus function. A 4- to 5-mm tibial tunnel using an ACL tibial guide is placed directly at the attachment site. The sutures are tied over a tibial post. Weight-bearing is restricted for 4 weeks.

Flap Tears

Two sets of sutures are required to repair flap tears (Fig. 28–17). Tension sutures are inserted first through the flap and then into the intact meniscal rim to anchor and reduce the flap into its anatomic bed. This restores the longitudinally running fibers of the meniscus and is performed in a manner similar to that for a radial tear repair. With the meniscus reduced, the remaining tear is repaired in the same fashion as a longitudinal tear, with superior and inferior vertical divergent sutures. The radial portion of the flap tear may only partially heal; however, the more peripheral longitudinal tear may heal, retaining partial meniscus function. Flap tears that represent 75% of the meniscus with the tear at the periphery or red-white junction are amenable for repair. Smaller flap tears 10 to 12 mm in length that occupy the red-white and white-white zones are not repaired.

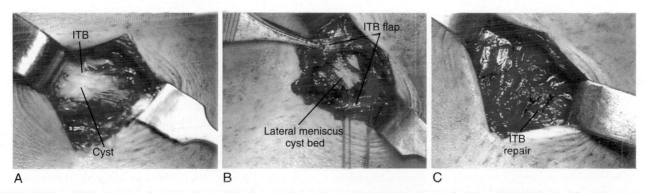

A   **B**   **C**

FIGURE 28–15. Demonstration of repair of lateral meniscus horizontal tear with a meniscal cyst. **A**, A 3-cm lateral joint incision placed directly over cyst shows the iliotibial band and an obvious protruding cyst. **B**, Iliotibial band is split in a line of fibers over the cyst and retracted, the cyst is removed, and repair is performed of the remaining meniscus to the attachments. **C**, Closure of the iliotibial band over the meniscus. Vertical sutures placed through the peripheral meniscus and iliotibial band help stabilize the repair. Then the arthroscopic inside-out repair of the meniscus body tear is performed.

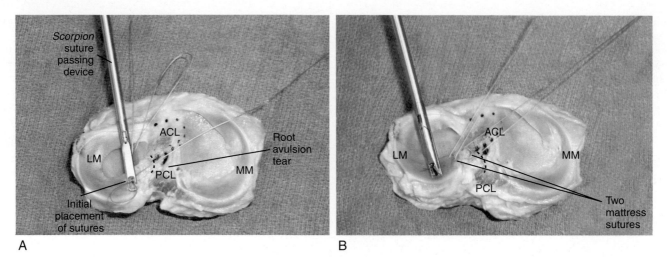

FIGURE 28–16. Posterior meniscus root attachment tear: Demonstration of the use of the Scorpion (Arthrex, Naples, FL) suture-passing device. **A**, Placement of two mattress sutures; the device can be passed in and out of the portal to place higher–holding strength mattress sutures over a single suture. **B**, Final placement of sutures brought out through a 4-mm transtibial tunnel and tied over a post to restore meniscus attachment.

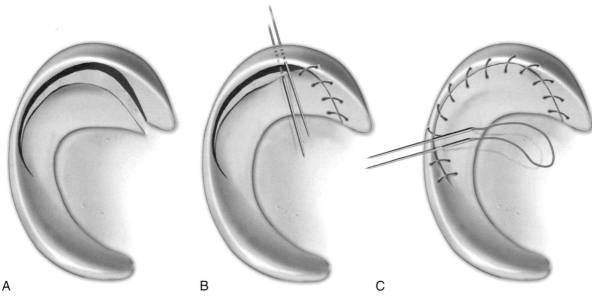

FIGURE 28–17. Repair technique for flap tears. **A**, The tear is identified and reduced. **B**, Horizontal tension sutures are placed to anchor the radial component of the tear. **C**, The longitudinal component is sutured using the double-stacked suture technique.

Repair of the Lateral Meniscus Popliteomeniscal Fascicles and Attachments

At arthroscopy, a nerve hook is placed at the superior and then inferior popliteal hiatus to displace the lateral meniscus anteriorly and superiorly. The knee joint is placed in 60° to 90° of flexion with a figure-four varus load applied to allow lateral tibiofemoral joint opening and maximum meniscus displacement (which is otherwise obstructed by the lateral femoral condyle). The posterior horn may be subluxated anteriorly 8 mm or more (usually not enough for locking into the joint) and superior "lift-off" of 10 to 12 mm is usually present, indicating laxity of the meniscotibial attachments. There is usually a tear of the meniscotibial attachments in which the normal inferior popliteal hiatus is enlarged with attenuation or tearing of the meniscus attachments.

The repair of the popliteomeniscal fascicles requires a meticulous inside-out technique with multiple sutures to obtain stability of the lateral meniscus and alleviate clinical symptoms. All-inside meniscus fixators or use of only a few sutures is not suitable to provide a stable construct and repair. The arthroscope is placed in the lateral portal and the suture cannula in the medial portal. The superior and inferior sites are rasped to encourage healing. The inside-out meniscus repair technique requires placement of multiple vertical divergent sutures, placed superiorly at the anteroinferior and posterosuperior fascicle attachments (either side of the popliteus tendon) to reduce the lateral meniscus posterior horn to a normal tibial position and restore the meniscus attachments.

The more difficult repair involves inferior vertical divergent sutures at the inferior popliteal hiatus and meniscotibial meniscus attachments. The tissues may be thin and four to six sutures must be placed through the inferior capsule at the level of the tibial attachment, and then in a vertical manner through the inferior outer third of the meniscus posterior horn. It is important that the previously placed superior vertical sutures retain the meniscus reduction so that placement of the inferior sutures does not displace the meniscus in an abnormal cephalad direction.

Techniques to Stimulate Healing of Meniscus Repairs

The initial vascular response of the meniscus to injury and tearing is characterized by the formation of a fibrin clot that is rich in inflammatory cells. This clot acts as a scaffold through which cells from the synovial membrane adjacent to the meniscus migrate.[7,8] The meniscal fibrochondrocytes may add to the intrinsic healing process.

Several experimental studies have investigated techniques to stimulate meniscus healing, including trephination or vascular ingrowth,[8,46,149,150] abrasion of the meniscal-synovial region,[51,93,112] grafting of the synovial pedicle,[47] incorporation of a fibrin clot,[93,112] and use of growth factors and cell-based therapy.* Although trephination, or creation of vascular access channels, has been demonstrated experimentally to promote healing, the creation of these channels disrupts the normal peripheral structure of the meniscus. Investigations of growth factors and cell-based therapies have all been experimental to date, with no published clinical trials to document the potential effectiveness.

The incorporation of a fibrin clot[52] at the repair site is theoretically beneficial because it provides a scaffold to support the reparative cells and provide chemotactic and mitogenic stimuli.[144] The absence of a well-defined fibrin clot in the initial healing period along with a limited vascular supply may be the most important factors limiting meniscus healing in tears located in the middle third region. The problem is that a fibrin clot inserted between the tear edges of the meniscus prevents meticulous suturing of the tear both superiorly and inferiorly. A fibrin clot may be beneficial in horizontal tears in which the clot may be placed between the superior and the inferior tear sites. The clot is prepared with a glass stirring rod. The clot is passed into the knee joint through a cannula, guided by a loop of suture placed around the clot from previously passed meniscus suture needles.

Ritchie and coworkers[112] found that abrasion of the parameniscal synovium was more effective than the incorporation of a fibrin clot in central meniscus repairs. Synovial abrasion stimulates vessels and mesenchymal cells to form a proliferate vascular pannus that migrates into the repair site.[35,50,123]

Several studies have demonstrated that an ACL reconstruction performed concomitantly with meniscal repair increases the success rate because the reconstruction protects the meniscus repair site owing to the restored knee stability and provides the beneficial healing effects of the postoperative hemarthrosis.[33,36,60,91,134] In the majority of meniscus repairs done without concomitant ACL reconstruction, the meniscal-synovial junction is abraded and a micropick used in the intercondylar notch

*See references 22, 49, 53, 54, 59, 61, 105, 129, 137, 138.

region to produce bleeding that promotes adherence of platelets and fibrin at the repair site. The meticulous suture placement described in this chapter stabilizes the tear and prevents gap formation at the repair site, allowing the subsequent repair process to progress.

The remodeling events and extent of reformation of a normal collagen architecture after meniscus repair remain unknown. Whether repaired meniscal tears in the middle third region have normal load-sharing capabilities and mechanical and material properties to prevent joint arthrosis remains unanswered. In the future, specific chemotactic and mitogenic agents may play an important role in stimulating the repair process of tears that extend into the avascular portions of the meniscus.

AUTHORS' CLINICAL STUDIES

Arthroscopic Assessment of Meniscus Repairs in the Outer and Middle Third Regions

An investigation was conducted on 66 patients who underwent a concomitant meniscus repair and ACL reconstruction, then follow-up arthroscopy 6 to 25 months postoperatively.[31] There were a total of 79 meniscus repairs; 51 were done for tears located in the outer third region (periphery) and 28 were done for complex tears that extended into the middle third avascular region. Follow-up arthroscopy was indicated for symptoms related to either tibial hardware or tibiofemoral joint pain.

All patients were placed into a postoperative rehabilitation program that included immediate knee motion exercises the 1st postoperative day. During the time period of this study (1983–1988), knee motion was limited to 20° to 90° for the first 4 weeks, with full extension then achieved by the 8th postoperative week. Early partial weight-bearing was initiated between the 1st and the 3rd postoperative weeks and was progressed to full by the 8th to 10th week. Postoperative strengthening exercises were initiated on the 2nd postoperative day and included patellar mobilization, straight leg raises, isometrics, and electrical muscle stimulation.

The arthroscopic videotapes and operative records were reviewed by a surgeon who had not been involved in the care

---

Critical Points AUTHORS' CLINICAL STUDIES: ARTHROSCOPIC ASSESSMENT OF MENISCUS REPAIRS IN THE OUTER AND MIDDLE THIRD REGIONS

- $N = 79$ meniscus repairs: 51 tears located in outer third region, 28 extended into middle third region.
- All had anterior cruciate ligament reconstruction with meniscus repair.
- Follow-up arthroscopy average 12 mo (range, 6–25 mo) after repair.
- Healing rates
  - Outer third: 94% healed, 4% partially healed, 2% failed.
  - Middle third: 54% healed, 32% partially healed, 14% failed.
- No effect on meniscus repair healing rates: length of meniscus tear, tibiofemoral compartment of repair, patient age, length of time from injury to repair, length of follow-up, arthroscopic vs. open procedure.
- Use of immediate knee motion and early weight-bearing not deleterious to healing meniscus repair.

of the patients. The rate of meniscus healing was classified as either completely healed (no visible surface defect), partially healed (at least 50% healed with meniscus stability and continuity restored), or failed (no visible healing). The effects of rim width, length of the tear, tibiofemoral compartment, patient age, length of time from injury to repair, length of follow-up, and arthroscopic versus open procedure were analyzed on the healing rates. The three healing categories were analyzed separately, and then the categories of healed and partially healed were combined and this category (retained meniscus) was compared with the failure rates.

Repairs of tears located in the outer third region were classified as completely healed in 94%, partially healed in 4%, and failed in 2% (Table 28–1). Repairs of tears that extended into the avascular region were classified as completely healed in 54%, partially healed in 32%, and failed in 14%. The other factors analyzed in this study had no significant effect on the healing rates.

The use of immediate knee motion and early weight-bearing was not deleterious to the healing meniscus repairs. Upon the completion of this study, the postoperative program was adjusted to allow full extension the 1st postoperative day in all patients undergoing meniscus repairs. This was one of the first investigations to demonstrate that repair of meniscus tears located in either the outer third or that extended into the middle third region have a satisfactory rate of healing when clinical grounds warrant the procedure.

The increase in healing of meniscus tears with concurrent ACL surgery is well appreciated. In knees that undergo meniscus repairs without ACL surgery, the femoral notch region is trephinated to induce joint bleeding and potentially aid in the deposition of blood products at the healing site for the initial fibrin clot formation.

Outcome of 198 Meniscus Repairs in the Middle Third Region

The clinical outcome of 198 meniscus tears that extended into the middle third region, or that had a rim width of 4 mm or greater, was determined in a prospective study.[121] Either a clinical examination a minimum of 2 years postoperatively or follow-up arthroscopy were used for inclusionary criteria. The 198 meniscus repairs were performed in 177 patients. Of these, 180 repairs (91%) were evaluated with a clinical examination a mean of 42 months (range, 23–116 mo) postoperatively. In addition, 91 repairs (46%) were evaluated with a follow-up arthroscopic examination a mean of 18 months (range, 2–81 mo) after the initial repair.

Seventy-six of the meniscus repairs were performed for acute or subacute tears and 122 for chronic tears. ACL ruptures also occurred in 128 patients. Of these, 126 (71%) underwent ACL reconstruction either with the meniscus repair (96 patients) or a mean of 22 weeks after the repair (30 patients). The ACL reconstructions were done with allografts in 72 knees and with bone–patellar tendon–bone (B-PT-B) autografts in 54 knees. After surgery, patients began immediate knee motion from 0° to 90°. Flexion was advanced to 125° by the 3rd postoperative week. Crutches were used for the first 4 weeks for longitudinal tears and for the first 6 weeks for horizontal, radial, or complex multiplanar tears. Squatting or deep knee flexion greater than 125° was not permitted for 4 to 6 months postoperatively. Full sports activity was restricted for 6 months.

At follow-up arthroscopy, the meniscus repairs were classified as healed if full-thickness apposition of the original tear occurred with no more than 10% of the original tear remaining. Repairs were considered partially healed if at least 50% of the original tear was healed and was stable when probed and the meniscus body was in its normal position in the tibiofemoral joint. Repairs were considered failed if more than 50% of the original tear was present or if unstable fragments required additional sutures. On clinical examination, a McMurray test was used with joint line palpation and compression to detect tibiofemoral joint symptoms.

TABLE 28–1 Effect of Six Factors on Healing Rate of Meniscal Repairs			
Factor	Complete Healing (N)	Partial Healing (N)	Failed (N)
Rim width			
Outer third (0–3 mm, N = 51)	48*	2	1
Central third (4–6 mm, N = 14)	6	5	3
Double longitudinal (N = 10)	6	4	0
Flap (N = 4)	3	0	1
Length of meniscus tear			
≤2.5 cm (N = 43)	34	7	2
>2.5 cm (N = 36)	29	4	3
Type of meniscus			
Medial (N = 51)	40	6	5
Lateral (N = 28)	23	5	0
Age of patient			
<25 yr (N = 51)	44	5	2
≥25 yr (N = 28)	19	6	3
Interval to repair			
Initial, ≤8 wk (N = 37)	33	3	1
Delayed, >8 wk (N = 42)	30	8	4
Length of follow-up			
<12 mo (N = 55)	35	5	1
≥12 mo (N = 24)	28	6	4
Open vs. scope			
Open (N = 33)	32	1	0
Scope (N = 30)	24	4	2

*P < .01

Critical Points AUTHORS' CLINICAL STUDIES: OUTCOME OF 198 MENISCUS REPAIRS IN MIDDLE THIRD REGION

- N = 198 meniscus repairs in 177 patients.
- 71% had anterior cruciate ligament reconstruction either with or after meniscus repair.
- 91% evaluated clinically 23–116 mo postoperatively.
- 46% evaluated follow-up arthroscopy 2–81 mo postoperatively.
- Advanced rehabilitation program allowed 0°–90° of knee motion immediately postoperatively.
- Deep knee flexion, full sports delayed for 6 mo to protect repair site.
- Overall reoperation rate for tibiofemoral symptoms: 20%.
- 80% asymptomatic for tibiofemoral symptoms, not interpreted as rate of healing.
- Significant differences in healing rates in menisci evaluated with follow-up arthroscopy:
  - Higher rate of retention lateral meniscus compared with medial meniscus.
  - Higher rate of healing repairs assessed ≤12 mo compared with repairs assessed >12 mo with follow-up arthroscopy.
  - Higher rate of healing in knees without tibiofemoral joint symptoms compared with those with joint line pain.
- Results support repair of meniscus tears that extend into middle avascular region, especially in patients in their 20s and 30s.

TABLE 28–2   Reoperation Rates for Meniscal Repairs due to Tibiofemoral Joint Symptoms

Type of Meniscus Tear	Total Number of Meniscus Tears in Study	Number Requiring Repeat Arthroscopy
Single longitudinal	92	11 (12%)
Double longitudinal	40	11 (28%)
Complex multiplanar	26	7 (27%)
Radial	15	4 (27%)
Horizontal	14	4 (29%)
Flap	9	2 (22%)
Triple longitudinal	2	0
Total	198	39 (20%)

TABLE 28–3   Effect of Various Factors on Healing Rates of Meniscal Repairs that Had Follow-up Arthroscopy

Factor	Healed (N)	Partially Healed (N)	Failed (N)
Tibiofemoral compartment of meniscal repair*			
Medial (N = 47)	8	15	24
Lateral (N = 44)	15	20	9
Time from meniscus repair to follow-up arthroscopy†			
≤12 mo (N = 61)	18	27	16
>12 mo (N = 30)	5	8	17
Timing of ACL reconstruction			
With meniscal repair (N = 39)	12	18	9
After meniscal repair (N = 27)	9	11	7
Presence of tibiofemoral compartment symptoms‡			
Symptomatic (N = 39)	2	13	24
Asymptomatic (N = 52)	21	22	9
Time from original knee injury to meniscal repair§			
≥10 wk (N = 33)	13	10	10
>10 wk (N = 58)	10	25	23
Patient age			
<25 yr (N = 44)	13	17	14
>25 yr (N = 47)	10	18	19

*Lateral success rate is significantly higher than medial, $P = .008$.
†Follow-up arthroscopy <12 mo postoperative success rate is significantly higher than >12 mo, $P = .02$.
‡Tibiofemoral symptoms have a higher failure rate than no symptoms, $P = .0001$.
§<10 wk from injury higher success rate, $P = .06$.

The overall reoperation rate for tibiofemoral symptoms was 20% (39 meniscus tears). All patients who had tibiofemoral pain underwent follow-up arthroscopy. The reoperation rates according to the type of tear are shown in Table 28–2. The limited number of meniscal tears in the individual classification categories precludes specific conclusions on the outcome for each tear pattern. Of the 39 menisci examined, 2 were classified as healed, 13 as partially healed, and 24 as failed. The reoperation rates for tibiofemoral joint symptoms were 12% for single longitudinal tears, 28% for double longitudinal tears, and 27% for the most difficult complex multiplanar tears.

A total of 91 meniscus repairs were evaluated by follow-up arthroscopy; the 39 described above and 52 others that underwent surgery for reasons other than tibiofemoral joint symptoms. Of these 91, 23 (25%) were classified as healed, 35 (38%) as partially healed, and 33 (36%) as failed.

The effect of six factors on healing rates of meniscal repairs was evaluated (Table 28–3). Statistically significant differences were found in the rates of healing for three factors: tibiofemoral compartment of the meniscus repair (higher healing rate in lateral meniscus repairs than in medial meniscus repairs), time from repair to follow-up arthroscopy (higher healing rate in patients evaluated ≤12 mo compared with those evaluated >12 mo postoperatively), and the presence of tibiofemoral symptoms (higher healing rate in asymptomatic patients than in symptomatic patients). A trend ($P = .06$) was observed for the factor of time from the original knee injury to the meniscus repair (higher healing rate in patients operated on ≤10 wk than in those operated on >10 wk after the injury).

Menisci examined with arthroscopy greater than 1 year postoperatively had a higher rate of tibiofemoral joint symptoms and failed repairs than those examined less than 1 year postoperatively. The average time from the repair to the follow-up arthroscopy in the 39 menisci with tibiofemoral symptoms attributed to a failed repair was 24 months (range, 3–81 mo). Of these 39, 25 (64%) had an interval longer than 12 months between procedures. Of the 33 menisci proven failed by follow-up arthroscopy, 21 (64%) had an interval of greater than 1 year between procedures: 15 were between 1 and 3 years, and 6 were between 3 and 5 years after repair.

There was no statistical difference in the rate of meniscus healing or in the percentage of menisci that required follow-up arthroscopy when an ACL reconstruction was performed concurrently or after the meniscus repair. There was also no difference between the reoperation rate and the function of the ACL graft as determined by arthrometer and pivot shift testing.

The significantly higher rate of retention of lateral meniscus repairs found in this study agrees with those of other reports.[91,120,123] The reasons for the higher failure rate of medial meniscus repairs are unknown at present. The results of this investigation support the repair of meniscus tears that extend into the middle avascular region, especially in patients in their 20s and 30s and highly competitive athletes. The study's reoperation rate should not be interpreted as the rate of meniscal healing. The long-term function and chondroprotective effects of the repaired menisci need to be determined, and this group of patients is under prospective long-term evaluation.

Outcome of Meniscus Repairs in the Middle Third Region in Patients 40 Years of Age and Older

The clinical outcome of meniscus tears that extended into the avascular region in patients 40 years of age and older was prospectively determined.[97] Thirty of 31 consecutive meniscus repairs in 29 patients were followed by either clinical examination or arthroscopy after the initial repair. A clinical evaluation was conducted in 27 patients (28 meniscus repairs) a mean of 34 months (range, 23–71 mo) postoperatively. Six repairs were evaluated with arthroscopy a mean of 24 months (range, 16–36 mo) after the repair.

ACL reconstruction was performed at the time of the meniscus repair in 21 patients (72%). Ten meniscus repairs were done for acute knee injuries (<10 wk from injury) and 20 were done for chronic injuries.

Critical Points AUTHORS' CLINICAL STUDIES: OUTCOME OF MENISCUS REPAIRS IN MIDDLE THIRD REGION IN PATIENTS 40 YEARS OF AGE AND OLDER

- $N = 30$ meniscus repairs in 29 patients.
- 72% had anterior cruciate ligament reconstruction with the meniscus repair.
- 93% evaluated clinically 23–71 mo postoperatively.
- 20% evaluated by follow-up arthroscopy 16–36 mo postoperatively.
- 87% asymptomatic for both tibiofemoral symptoms and had not required further surgery.
- No significant effect on presence of tibiofemoral pain or meniscus resection of tibiofemoral compartment of meniscus repair, chronicity of injury, concomitant anterior cruciate ligament reconstruction, condition of articular cartilage.
- Knees with chronic injuries had significant improvements in symptoms, functional limitations with sports and daily activities.
- Patient rating overall knee condition: 76% normal/very good, 12% good, 12% fair/poor.
- 76% returned to sports or regular activities with no problems, 4% returned to sports but had symptoms, 20% did not return to sports.
- Indications for meniscus repair should be based on patient's current and future desired activity level, not on age.

TABLE 28–5 Effect of Four Factors on Presence of Tibiofemoral Symptoms or Arthroscopic Second-Look Failure of Meniscal Repair

Factor	Asymptomatic	Tibiofemoral Symptoms or Arthroscopic Failure	P value
Tibiofemoral compartment of meniscal repair			
Medial ($N = 19$)	17 (89%)	2 (11%)	.55
Lateral ($N = 11$)	9 (82%)	2 (8%)	
Time from injury to meniscal repair			
≤10 wk ($N = 10$)	9 (90%)	1 (10%)	.70
>10 wk ($N = 20$)	17 (85%)	3 (15%)	
Concomitant ACL reconstruction			
Yes ($N = 22$)	20 (91%)	2 (9%)	.26
No, ACL intact ($N = 8$)	6 (75%)	2 (25%)	
Articular cartilage			
Normal ($N = 16$)	13 (81%)	3 (19%)	.35
Abnormal ($N = 14$)*	13 (93%)	1 (7%)	

*Abnormal articular cartilage was considered present if fissuring and fragmentation of more than one half of the involved surface over an area of 15 mm² were detected or subchondral bone was exposed.

ACL, anterior cruciate ligament.

At follow-up arthroscopy, the meniscus repairs were classified as healed if full-thickness apposition of the original tear occurred with no more than 10% of the original tear remaining. Repairs were considered partially healed if at least 50% of the original tear was healed, it was stable when probed, and the meniscus body was in its normal position in the tibiofemoral joint. Repairs were considered failed if more than 50% of the original tear was present or if unstable fragments required additional sutures. On clinical examination, a McMurray test was used with joint line palpation and compression to detect tibiofemoral joint symptoms.

At follow-up, 26 meniscus repairs (87%) both were asymptomatic for tibiofemoral joint symptoms and had not required further surgery (Table 28–4). There was no significant effect of the tibiofemoral compartment of the meniscus repair, chronicity of injury, concomitant ACL reconstruction, or condition of the articular cartilage on the presence of tibiofemoral pain or meniscus resection (Table 28–5).

A subjective evaluation using the Cincinnati Knee Rating System was completed at follow-up on 25 knees; 3 knees whose meniscal repairs failed and required removal at follow-up arthroscopy and 1 other knee that had follow-up arthroscopy but not a clinical evaluation 2 years postoperatively were not included. Of these 25 knees, 17 had chronic meniscal tears and 8 had acute tears before the index repair procedure. Nineteen had a concomitant ACL reconstruction.

The 17 knees with chronic symptoms had statistically significant improvements at follow-up in the mean scores for pain, swelling, and giving-way ($P < .01$). The mean preoperative pain score of 4.4 improved to 7.1, and the mean preoperative giving-way score of 5.9 improved to 8.8 (scale, 0–10). These knees also had significant improvements in the mean scores for squatting ($P < .05$), running, jumping, and cutting ($P < .0001$).

Before the meniscal repair, patients with 12 of the knees with chronic injuries had given up sports and 5 were participating with symptoms and functional limitations. At follow-up, 12 had returned to sports without problems, 1 was participating with symptoms, and 4 had not returned to sports owing to the knee condition. In the patient rating of the overall knee condition, 11 rated their knees as normal or very good; 3, good; 2, fair; and 1, poor.

TABLE 28–4 Types of Meniscal Tears and Results of Repair According to Follow-up Arthroscopy and Clinical Examination

Type of Meniscal Tear	N	Follow-up Arthroscopy Indications	Follow-up Arthroscopy Healing Classification	Clinical Evaluation Tibiofemoral Pain With Pain (N)	Follow-up Arthroscopy?
Single longitudinal ($N = 10$)	2	Reinjury,* remove hardware	Healed, partial healed	0	
Double longitudinal ($N = 4$)	1	Reinjury*	Failed	0	
Complex multiplanar ($N = 4$)	1	Remove hardware	Failed	1	No
Radial ($N = 4$)	1	Reinjury*	Partial healed	0	
Horizontal ($N = 4$)	1	Tibiofemoral symptoms	Failed	1	Yes
Flap ($N = 4$)	0			0	

*No tibiofemoral joint symptoms at site of meniscus repair.

Seven of the 8 patients with an acute injury were involved in athletics prior to their injury. The 1 patient who was not involved in athletics returned to normal activities of daily living without symptoms. Six patients returned to athletics without problems. Only 1 patient reported difficulty with squatting, and 1 patient had problems with running, jumping, and cutting. All 8 patients rated their overall knee condition as normal or very good.

There were no infections, knee motion problems, saphenous neuritis, or other major complications.

With many patients remaining active in middle age, the ability to retain the meniscus after an injury is an important goal. The treatment of tears that extend into the middle third avascular zone represents a problem in these patients. Usually, these tears are removed to the extent at which the remainder of meniscal tissue is nonfunctional. This study demonstrated that repair of complex tears in older adults is feasible and that the majority are asymptomatic for tibiofemoral joint symptoms an average of 3 years postoperatively. In athletically active patients, the indications of meniscus repair are based on current and future activity levels and the authors recommend the preservation of meniscal tissue wherever possible regardless of age. It should be noted that the majority of meniscus tears in patients over 40 years of age are degenerative and not reparable. This group of select patients had tears that were classified as amenable to repair by the criteria already provided.

Outcome of Meniscus Repairs in the Middle Third Region in Patients Younger than 20 Years of Age

A prospective study was conducted on 71 of 74 consecutive meniscus repairs (96% follow-up) that had been done in 58 patients under the age of 20 to determine the clinical outcome.[96] Sixty-seven meniscal repairs were examined clinically a mean of 51 months (range, 24–196 mo) after the operation. Thirty-six menisci in 28 knees were evaluated during follow-up arthroscopy a mean of 18 months (range, 3–60 mo) postoperatively. Of these, only 4 menisci were not examined a minimum of 2 years postoperatively.

There were 36 males and 25 females whose mean age at the time of the meniscus repair was 16 years (range, 9–19 yr). Two patients were 9 years of age and the remainder were in the second decade. Skeletal maturity, according to closed or nearly closed physes on roentgenograms of the distal femur and proximal tibia, had been reached in 54 knees (88%). The mean time from the original injury to the meniscus repair was 40 weeks (range, 1–256 wk). Forty meniscal repairs were done for an acute knee injury (1–12 wk after the injury) and 31 meniscal repairs were done for a chronic knee injury.

Forty-three meniscal repairs (61%) in 36 knees were performed concurrently with an ACL reconstruction. Fourteen meniscal repairs (20%) were done in 11 knees a mean of 34 weeks (median, 4 wk; range, 4–176 wk) prior to an ACL reconstruction. Skeletal maturity had been completed in all knees that had ACL reconstructions.

At follow-up, 53 of 71 meniscal repairs (75%) had no tibiofemoral symptoms and had not been classified as failed on follow-up arthroscopy.

Fourteen meniscal repairs (20%) developed tibiofemoral joint symptoms; all but 1 of these had follow-up arthroscopy a

---

Critical Points AUTHORS' CLINICAL STUDIES: OUTCOME OF MENISCUS REPAIRS IN MIDDLE THIRD REGION IN PATIENTS YOUNGER THAN 20 YEARS OF AGE

- $N = 71$ meniscus repairs in 58 patients.
- 61% had anterior cruciate ligament reconstruction either with or after meniscus repair.
- 94% evaluated clinically 24–196 mo postoperatively.
- 51% evaluated by follow-up arthroscopy 3–60 mo postoperatively.
- 75% had no tibiofemoral symptoms or failed meniscus repair according to arthroscopic classification.
- Reoperation rates owing to tibiofemoral joint symptoms: 8% single longitudinal tears, 33% double longitudinal tears, 14% complex multiplanar tears.
- No effect on tibiofemoral joint symptoms or arthroscopic classification of failure: tibiofemoral compartment of meniscal repair (medial vs. lateral), chronicity of injury, concomitant anterior cruciate ligament reconstruction.
- Presence of tibiofemoral pain: sensitivity rate of 57%, specificity rate of 93% in identifying repairs classified as failed at follow-up arthroscopy.
- Knees with concomitant meniscus repair and ACL reconstruction
  ○ No problems with daily activities.
  ○ 73% return to sports without problems.
  ○ 87% rated overall knee condition as normal or very good.
  ○ No complications, arthrofibrosis.
- Presence of tibiofemoral pain not always indicative of a failed meniscus repair, consider magnetic resonance imaging before arthroscopy to determine source of pain.
- Results allow recommendation of repair meniscus tears that extend into middle third region when conditions indicate that stable repair can be obtained.
- This recommendation is particularly appropriate in young active individuals in whom removal of meniscus tear that extends into middle avascular region would result in major loss of meniscus function and risk for future joint arthrosis.

---

mean of 19 months (range, 3–49 mo) postoperatively. One repair had healed and 1 had partially healed with small segments of the original tear requiring removal. Eight repairs had failed: 2 required removal at the prior repair site, 3 required near-total meniscectomy, and 2 had a repeat repair. In 1 knee that required a near-total lateral meniscectomy, a meniscus allograft was implanted.

The reoperation rates due to tibiofemoral joint symptoms were 8% for single longitudinal tears, 33% for double longitudinal tears, and 14% for complex multiplanar tears. Twenty-three other meniscal repairs had follow-up arthroscopy for reasons other than tibiofemoral symptoms a mean of 17 months postoperatively (range, 7–60 mo). Twelve of these meniscal repairs had healed. Seven repairs had partially healed; in 5, partial meniscectomy was required, and in 2, the meniscal tears were deemed stable and left intact. Four of these 23 meniscal repairs (in 3 knees) failed. A lateral and a medial meniscus allograft were implanted 40 months and 42 months, respectively, after the index repair procedure in 1 knee. A repeat meniscus repair was done in 1 knee, and a partial meniscectomy at the prior repair site was required in another knee.

There was no statistically significant effect of the tibiofemoral compartment of the meniscal repair, chronicity of injury, or concomitant ACL reconstruction on the presence of tibiofemoral joint symptoms or arthroscopic classification of failure. The presence of tibiofemoral pain on the physical

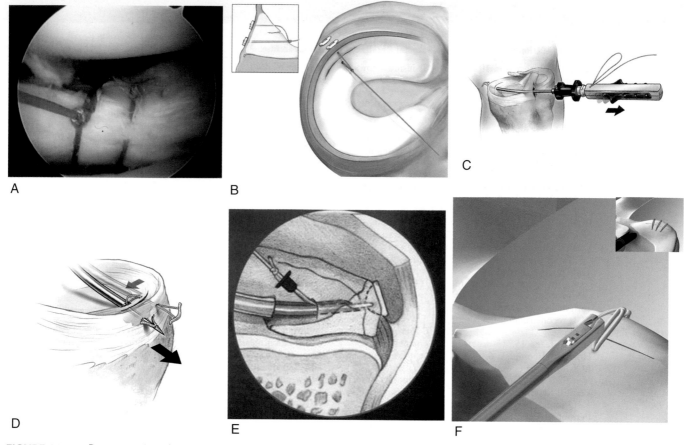

FIGURE 28–19. Demonstration of meniscus repairs using newer-generation all-inside suture-based devices that allow tensioning. See text for published results of these procedures. Careful selection of the type of meniscus tear for these techniques is required, because usually only two to four sutures are used and the fixation strength is inferior to that of multiple vertical divergent sutures. With proper selection of tears and avoidance of complex tears, there appears to be a role for these procedures in simple longitudinal tears in the red-red and red-white zones. **A** and **B**, Ultra Fast-Fix. **C** and **D**, MaxFire. **E**, RapidLoc. **F**, An inside-out posterior horn repair using the Meniscal Viper. (B, *With permission from Accufex, Smith & Nephew, Andover, MA; C and D, with permission from Biomet, Warsaw, IN; E, from Billante, M. J.; Diduch, D. R.; Lunardini, D. J.; et al.: Meniscal repair using an all-inside, rapidly absorbing, tensionable device.* Arthroscopy *24:779–785, 2008; F, with permission from Arthrex, Naples, FL.)*

6 knees (35% of the failures) and slippage of the cannula during fixator implantation with subsequent arrow breakage in 7 cases. Siebold and associates[125] reported a 28% failure rate a mean of 6 years postoperatively in 113 consecutive patients whose meniscus tears were repaired with the Meniscus Arrow. Lee and Diduch[74] reported an increasing rate of failure over time in 28 patients who underwent meniscus repair with the Meniscus Arrow and a concomitant ACL reconstruction. The initial success rate of 90.6% reported a mean of 2.3 years postoperatively decreased to 71.4% at 6.6 years. The investigators hypothesized that repair with the arrow resulted in a high rate of partial or incomplete meniscus healing, predisposing the meniscus to subsequent tearing. All failures occurred in knees in which normal or nearly normal stability had been achieved according to KT-2000 data. Complications with this device including chondral damage, cyst formation, chronic effusions, joint irritation, synovitis; device breakage and migration into the extra-articular soft tissues have been reported by several authors.[5,32,57,58,72,86,87,102,136]

The question of whether meniscal repair is effective in preventing joint deterioration remains unanswered according to published clinical data. The problem of commonly associated ACL tears or other injuries found in these knees precludes scientifically justifiable answers. However, based on the well-documented irreparable joint damage and poor results of long-term clinical studies after partial and total meniscectomy,* preservation of meniscal tissue is paramount for long-term joint function. It is the authors' opinion that the gold standard for meniscus repair procedures remains a meticulous inside-out repair with multiple vertical divergent sutures and an accessory posteromedial or posterolateral approach to tie the sutures directly posterior to the meniscus attachment. This procedure requires added time and assistants. The less ideal all-inside devices, although more time-efficient, have too high of a failure and complication rate. Revision meniscus repair procedures are often not possible and therefore, the technique with the highest success rate should be performed initially. The authors consider meniscus repair as important, if not more important, as an ACL reconstruction in regard to long-term knee function. The procedures and surgical approaches are not difficult and the anatomical approach is straightforward. There should be an exceedingly low risk of intraoperative complications such as nerve damage and arthrofibrosis if the operative procedure and rehabilitation program discussed in this and other chapters are followed.

The authors disagree with the approach of leaving a meniscus tear greater than 10 mm in length untreated at the time of ACL

---

*See references 6, 41, 56, 62, 63, 79, 85, 114, 118, 119, 122, 133, 140.

surgery. To use a conservative approach and hope for healing may risk further tearing and subsequent loss of meniscus function. Unfortunately, once a meniscectomy has been performed in a younger patient, few options exist and even meniscus transplants do not provide a dependable long-term successful solution. In patients requiring meniscus transplants, the authors have frequently observed that the original treatment of the meniscus tear was ineffective; either a large tear was left untreated, a repair was done with too few sutures or with

fixators that provided only limited stability, or a tear that extended into the middle avascular region was removed that could have been repaired.

In the future, tissue engineering may provide increased success rates of meniscus repair, especially for tears that extend into the avascular region.[1,30,34,40,131] Cell-based therapy using either meniscal fibrochondrocytes, articular chondrocytes, or mesenchymal stem cells seeded onto scaffolds offers promise,[116,130] as does the introduction of growth factors into repair sites.

ILLUSTRATIVE CASES

Case 1. A 30-year-old woman U.S. military instructor presented with complaints of pain to the lateral aspect of her right knee of 3 years' duration. The symptoms began after the patient had completed a 7-mile marathon and gradually progressed to pain with daily activities. MRI was negative for a lateral meniscus abnormality. Physical examination revealed tenderness to the lateral tibiofemoral joint, but all other tests and radiographs were normal. All meniscus tests were negative including standing single-leg rotation, McMurray flexion-rotation, and varus axial loading.

Arthroscopy was performed that initially demonstrated a normal lateral meniscus (Fig 28–20A). However, further evaluation revealed a large tear of the meniscotibial attachments (see Fig. 28–20B) with an abnormal lift-off and anterior subluxation of the posterior horn from the tibia (see Fig. 28–20C). Maximal varus loading and lateral joint opening was required to separate the tibiofemoral joint, which produced the subluxation of the posterior horn. Multiple vertical divergent sutures were placed superiorly

and inferiorly with an outside-in technique, avoiding the popliteal tendon (see Fig. 28–20D and E). The initial sutures were placed superiorly to reduce the meniscus onto the tibia. The patient recovered and returned to athletic activities 6 months postoperatively without pain. The cosmetic appearance of the 2-cm posterolateral approach is shown (see Fig. 28–20F).

Case 2. A 16-year-old male athlete presented with a chronic medial meniscus tear that had been treated conservatively. Physical examination demonstrated medial tibiofemoral joint pain, but all other tests and radiographs were normal. At arthroscopy, an unusual complex horizontal meniscal tear was found that extended throughout the entire meniscal body from the periphery to the inner meniscal margin (Fig. 28–21A). Removal of either the superior or the inferior tear component would have substantially compromised the remaining meniscal tissue and function. The body of the meniscus, between the superior and the inferior tear

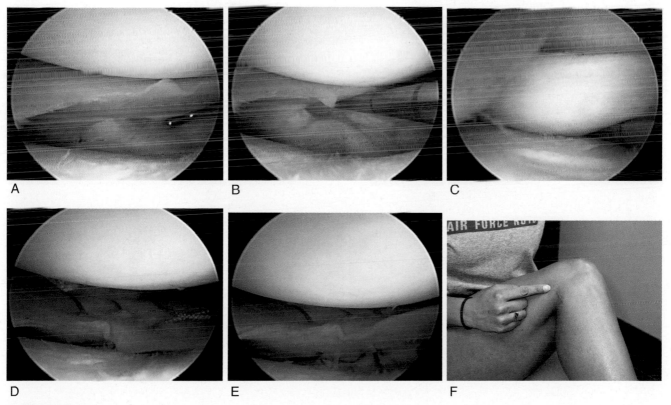

FIGURE 28–20. Case 1.

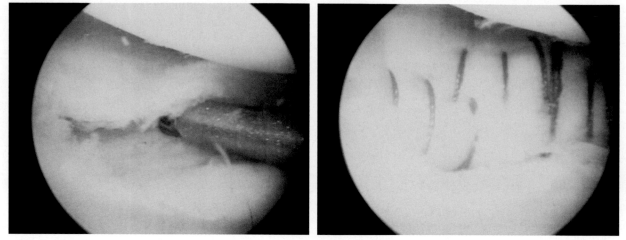

FIGURE 28–21. Case 2.

edges, was rasped. Multiple vertical divergent sutures were placed to close the gap between the superior and the inferior tear edges (see Fig. 28–21B).

At the most recent follow-up evaluation, 4 years postoperative, the patient had no symptoms and had returned to recreational athletics without problems.

Case 3. An 18-year-old Division I collegiate hockey player presented 10 months after sustaining a right knee injury in which the lateral aspect of his leg was struck with a helmet. He complained of pain with squatting, twisting, and turning activities. Examination demonstrated lateral joint line tenderness in deep flexion, but no other abnormalities. MRI was negative for a lateral

meniscus tear. The patient continued to have pain over the ensuing 5 months and elected to undergo arthroscopy for a potential hypermobile meniscus abnormality. The lateral meniscus hiatus was noted to be increased in size (Fig. 28–22A), and although the meniscus was firmly attached to the capsule, there was increased translation in the central portion of the lateral tibiofemoral compartment. In addition, the anterior rim at the meniscocapsular junction demonstrated fraying (see Fig. 28–22B). An inside-out lateral meniscus repair was performed with eight sutures under arthroscopic control, which successfully resolved the meniscus hypermobility (see Fig. 28–22C).

The patient did well and returned to collegiate hockey without problems. Three years later, he sustained a twisting injury to the

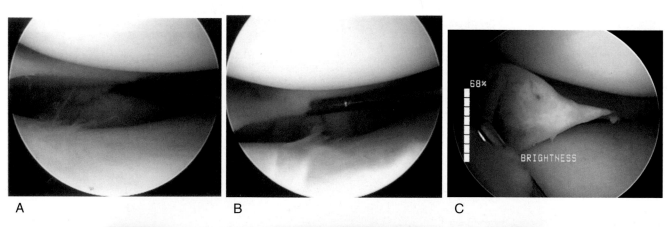

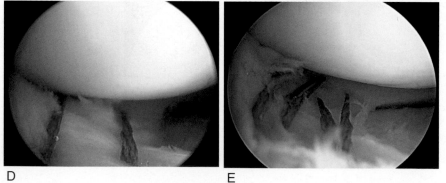

FIGURE 28–22. Case 3.

same knee and suffered a complete ACL tear and a radial lateral meniscus tear. An ACL autogenous B-PT-B reconstruction was performed. The lateral compartment demonstrated the healed prior meniscus repair in the posterior horn (see Fig. 28–22D). A new radial tear, found at the junction of the anterior and middle thirds, that extended to the capsular margin was repaired with six horizontal mattress sutures (see Fig. 28–22E). The patient recovered without complications.

Case 4. A 33-year-old man presented 1 week after a left knee injury sustained while playing basketball. Physical examination revealed 7 mm of increased anterior tibial translation and severe medial joint line tenderness. The patient had a mild effusion and 90° of knee flexion. He was referred to physical therapy for 4 weeks of rehabilitation to regain normal knee motion and muscle function. A B-PT-B ACL autograft, repair of a complex multiplanar lateral meniscus central third tear, and repair of a 15-mm single longitudinal medial meniscus central third tear were then performed (Fig. 28–23A). The patient had a chronic PCL rupture on the right knee of 12 years' duration, which had been treated conservatively.

At the latest follow-up evaluation, 15 years postoperatively, the patient had no complaints with his right knee. He had participated in basketball without symptoms and rated the overall condition of his knee as normal. Physical examination demonstrated a grade I pivot shift, a full range of knee motion, and no crepitus, swelling, or joint line pain. All meniscus tests were negative. Standing PA radiographs demonstrated only 1 mm of decrease in the lateral tibiofemoral compartment joint space compared with the opposite knee and no decrease in the medial tibiofemoral compartment joint space (see Fig. 28–23B).

Case 5. A 35-year-old man presented 19 years after a right ACL rupture (which had been treated conservatively) and 2 days after a left ACL and MCL injury. The left knee injury was treated with a B-PT-B ACL allograft reconstruction, medial collateral ligament primary repair, and a proximal patellar realignment. The patient recovered from this procedure well, but developed increasing instability symptoms with the right knee along with painful crepitus to the lateral tibiofemoral compartment. He underwent a right B-PT-B allograft ACL reconstruction and repair of bilateral peripheral medial (Fig. 28–24A) and lateral (see Fig. 28–24B) meniscus tears. Noteworthy fissuring and fragmentation were noted in the lateral femoral condyle, the medial femoral condyle, and on the undersurface of the patella.

Four years later, the patient presented with instability complaints to the left knee of a gradual onset. Physical examination revealed a positive pivot shift test, 10 mm of anterior tibial translation, crepitus in the lateral tibiofemoral compartment, and medial tibiofemoral joint line pain. He underwent a revision B-PT-B autogenous ACL reconstruction and repair of a complex medial meniscus tear at the meniscal-synovial junction.

At the most recent evaluation, 11 years postoperatively, the patient reported no knee pain or left knee instability. He participated in low-impact activities weekly without complaints. He had a normal range of knee motion, a grade I pivot shift test, and no joint line tenderness. Radiographs show preservation of the medial tibiofemoral joint space (see Fig. 28–24C).

Case 6. A 31-year-old man presented 2 months after a twisting injury to the right knee sustained during a soccer game that had been treated elsewhere with a diagnostic arthroscopy. Physical examination revealed 10 mm of increased anterior tibial translation, moderate medial tibiofemoral joint line pain, and a mild effusion. The patient underwent a B-PT-B autogenous ACL reconstruction and a repair of a 20-mm peripheral medial meniscus tear (Fig. 28–25A). Noteworthy fissuring and fragmentation were noted on the medial femoral condyle (see Fig. 28–25B). The patient recovered and was released to full sports activities 9 months later.

At the most recent follow-up evaluation, 16 years postoperative, the patient stated he had participated in competitive soccer without symptoms or functional limitations until a reinjury that had occurred 3 months prior to his examination. He underwent a partial medial meniscectomy elsewhere. Physical examination revealed 2 mm of increased anteroposterior (AP) tibial displacement on KT-2000 testing, no crepitus, a normal range of motion, and no joint line pain. The patient rated the overall condition of his knee as very good. Radiographs demonstrated preservation of the medial tibiofemoral compartment (see Fig. 28–25C). However, the patient was warned that continued high-impact activities might accelerate medial compartment joint arthrosis with the loss of the medial meniscus and preexisting damage noted on the medial femoral condyle.

Case 7. An 18-year-old male sustained a right knee injury playing basketball and presented 2 weeks later with a mild effusion, 12 mm of increased anterior tibial translation, medial joint line pain, and a nearly normal range of knee motion. He underwent a B-PT-B autogenous ACL reconstruction and bilateral meniscus repairs for double

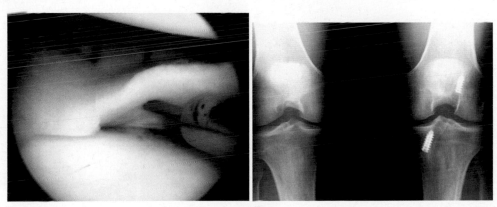

A   B

FIGURE 28–23. Case 4.

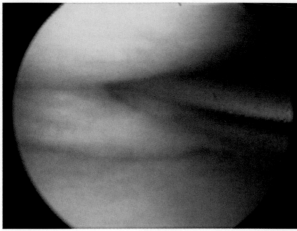

A

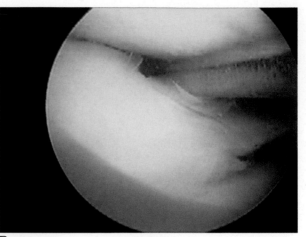

B

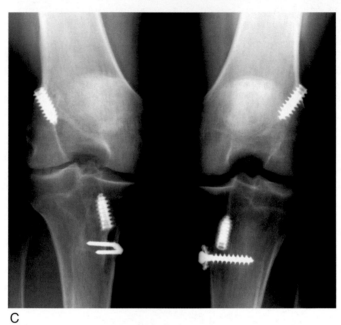

C

FIGURE 28–24. Case 5.

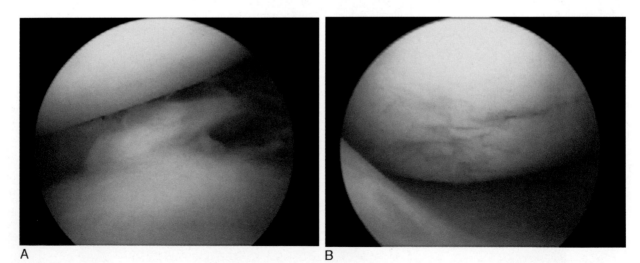

A

B

FIGURE 28–25. Case 6.

Continued

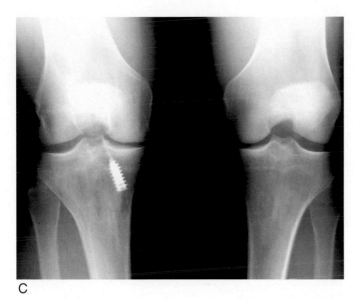

C

FIGURE 28–25—cont'd

longitudinal posterior horn tears (Fig. 28–26A). There were noteworthy fissuring and fragmentation of the medial femoral condyle (see Fig. 28–26B). He recovered well and returned to basketball for several years. The patient sustained a left knee injury 5 years later and underwent an ACL reconstruction and total medial meniscectomy elsewhere.

At the most recent follow-up evaluation, 14 years postoperative, the patient rated his right knee as nearly normal without symptoms. Physical examination of the right knee demonstrated a negative Lachman and pivot shift, no meniscus pathology, a full range of knee motion, and no joint effusion. The left knee was symptomatic for medial tibiofemoral compartment symptoms and had drifted into varus malalignment. Radiographs demonstrated preservation of the medial and lateral tibiofemoral compartment joint spaces in the right knee (see Fig. 28–26C), but loss of medial joint space in the left knee (see Fig. 28–26D). An opening wedge high tibial osteotomy was subsequently performed on the left knee.

Case 8. A 24-year-old man presented 3 days after a right knee injury sustained playing volleyball. Physical examination demonstrated a moderate effusion, range of motion from 10° to 70°,

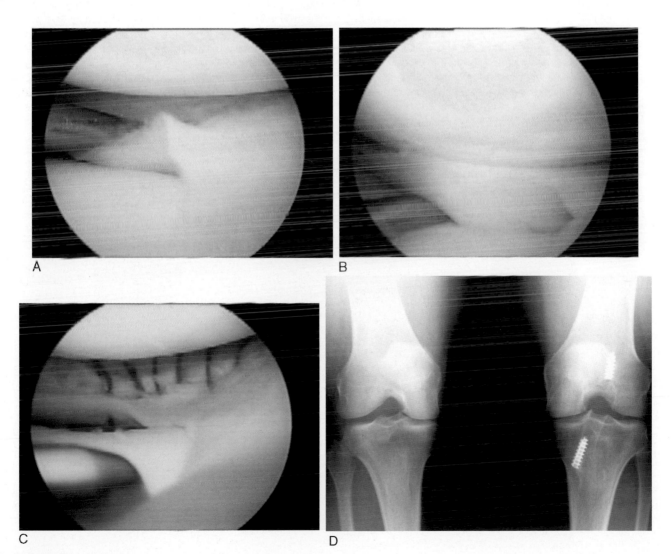

A

B

C

D

FIGURE 28–26. Case 7.

poor quadriceps contraction, moderate medial joint line pain, and 5 mm of increased anterior tibial translation. He underwent 4 weeks of physical therapy to regain knee motion and quadriceps strength. A B-PT-B autogenous ACL reconstruction and a repair of a 30-mm double longitudinal medial meniscus tear were done. Noteworthy fissuring and fragmentation were noted on the medial and lateral femoral condyles.

At the most recent follow-up evaluation, 14 years postoperative, the patient reported no symptoms, locking, or catching and rated the overall condition of his knee as normal. Physical examination demonstrated a negative pivot shift test, 3 mm of increased AP displacement on KT-2000 testing, no tibiofemoral joint line pain or crepitus, and a normal range of knee motion. The patient had a sedentary occupation and weighed 265 pounds. Radiographs detected narrowing to the medial tibiofemoral compartment and 2° of varus alignment (Fig. 28–27). MRI revealed deterioration of the medial meniscus, with only a small remnant remaining. The patient was counseled regarding the potential for a future high tibial osteotomy based on medial tibiofemoral compartment symptoms.

Case 9. A 32-year-old man sustained a left knee twisting injury and underwent arthroscopy and removal of the anteromedial bundle of the ACL elsewhere. The patient was treated conservatively for 7 years, but gradually developed symptoms and presented for treatment. MRI demonstrated a complex bucket-handle medial meniscus tear. Arthroscopy revealed a complex 20-mm longitudinal tear with an additional vertical tear component. Noteworthy fissuring and fragmentation were found on the medial femoral condyle and in the patellofemoral compartment. Repair of the meniscus tear with multiple divergent sutures was performed.

The patient did well for 1 year until he developed lateral joint line pain and catching symptoms. Repeat arthroscopy

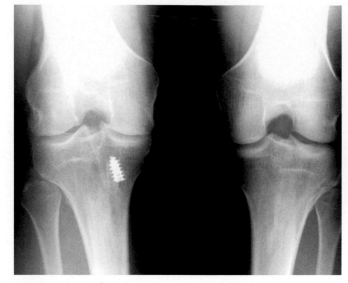

FIGURE 28–27. Case 8.

demonstrated a complex medial meniscus tear extending from the posterior horn to the midbody with horizontal and vertical longitudinal components. A revision meniscus repair was successfully performed with only a small portion of the posterior horn removed. Six years later, the patient reported no problems with light recreational sports and daily activities and rated the overall condition of the knee as good. Physical examination demonstrated a normal range of knee motion, no effusion, no tibiofemoral pain or crepitus, and no meniscus symptoms. Radiographs showed preservation of the medial tibiofemoral joint space (Fig. 28–28A and B).

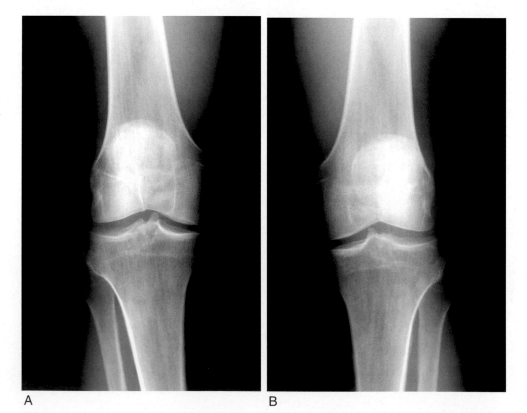

A

B

FIGURE 28–28. Case 9.

Case 10. A 14-year-old male presented 1 day after a left knee contact injury sustained while playing football. Physical examination demonstrated a severe effusion and limitation of knee motion. One week later, the patient underwent arthroscopy and repair of an interstitial tear of the posterior horn of the medial meniscus and repair of a central third tear of the posterior horn of the lateral meniscus. Six weeks later, the patient underwent an ACL B-PT-B allograft reconstruction with a ligament augmentation device. Both menisci appeared to be intact and stable. No articular cartilage damage was noted.

Two years later, the patient had an onset of medial joint line pain and locking. Arthroscopy demonstrated an incomplete tear to the medial meniscus along the inferior border posteriorly (Fig. 28–29A). No repair was deemed necessary. Articular cartilage damage (grade 2A) was noted on the undersurface of the patella, the medial femoral condyle, and the lateral femoral condyle. The patient continued to have a catching sensation and discomfort and underwent arthroscopy 6 months later. The medial meniscus was intact and the lateral meniscus was stable with the exception of a 3-mm radial tear, which was excised.

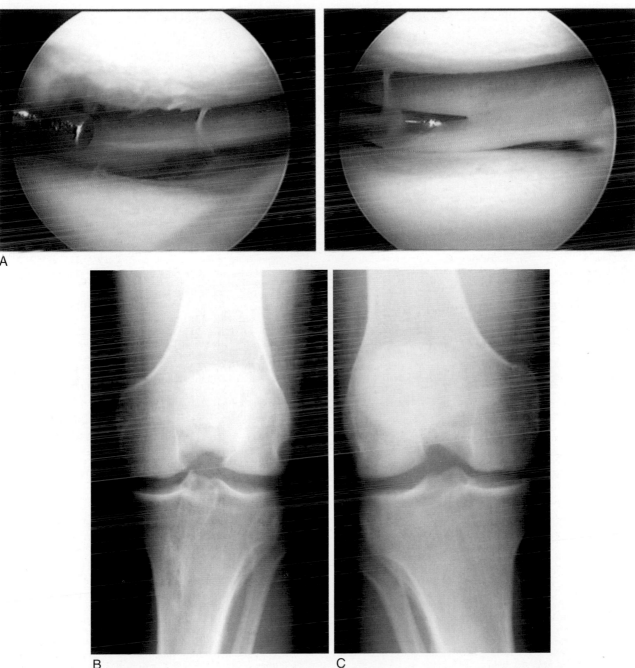

FIGURE 28–29. Case 10.

At the most recent follow-up evaluation, 19 years after the original bilateral meniscus repair procedure, the patient had no symptoms and rated the overall condition of his knee as very good. Physical examination revealed no effusion, a normal range of knee motion, a negative pivot shift test, no increase in AP displacement on KT-2000 testing, and no tibiofemoral joint line pain. Standing PA radiographs demonstrated excellent retention of the lateral and medial compartments of the involved knee (see Fig. 28–29B) compared with the contralateral knee (see Fig. 28–29C).

REFERENCES

1. Adams, S. B., Jr.; Randolph, M. A.; Gill, T. J.: Tissue engineering for meniscus repair. *J Knee Surg* 18:25–30, 2005.
2. Ahmed, A. M.; Burke, D. L.: In-vitro measurement of static pressure distribution in synovial joints—part I: tibial surface of the knee. *J Biomech Eng* 105:216–225, 1983.
3. Albrecht-Olsen, P.; Kristensen, G.; Burgaard, P.; et al.: The arrow versus horizontal suture in arthroscopic meniscus repair. A prospective randomized study with arthroscopic evaluation. *Knee Surg Sports Traumatol Arthrosc* 7:268–273, 1999.
4. Albrecht-Olsen, P.; Lind, T.; Kristensen, G.; Falkenberg, B.: Failure strength of a new meniscus arrow repair technique: biomechanical comparison with horizontal suture. *Arthroscopy* 13:183–187, 1997.
5. Albrecht-Olsen, P. M.; Bak, K.: Arthroscopic repair of the bucket-handle meniscus. 10 failures in 27 stable knees followed for 3 years. *Acta Orthop Scand* 64:446–448, 1993.
6. Andersson-Molina, H.; Karlsson, H.; Rockborn, P.: Arthroscopic partial and total meniscectomy: a long-term follow-up study with matched controls. *Arthroscopy* 18:183–189, 2002.
7. Arnoczky, S. P.; Warren, R. F.: Microvasculature of the human meniscus. *Am J Sports Med* 10:90–95, 1982.
8. Arnoczky, S. P.; Warren, R. F.: The microvasculature of the meniscus and its response to injury. An experimental study in the dog. *Am J Sports Med* 11:131–141, 1983.
9. Asahina, S.; Muneta, T.; Hoshino, A.; et al.: Intermediate-term results of meniscal repair in anterior cruciate ligament-reconstructed knees. *Am J Sports Med* 26:688–691, 1998.
10. Asahina, S.; Muneta, T.; Yamamoto, H.: Arthroscopic meniscal repair in conjunction with anterior cruciate ligament reconstruction: factors affecting the healing rate. *Arthroscopy* 12:541–545, 1996.
11. Asik, M.; Sen, C.; Erginsu, M.: Arthroscopic meniscal repair using T-fix. *Knee Surg Sports Traumatol Arthrosc* 10:284–288, 2002.
12. Asik, M.; Sener, N.: Failure strength of repair devices versus meniscus suturing techniques. *Knee Surg Sports Traumatol Arthrosc* 10:25–29, 2002.
13. Asik, M.; Sener, N.; Akpinar, S.; et al.: Strength of different meniscus suturing techniques. *Knee Surg Sports Traumatol Arthrosc* 5:80–83, 1997.
14. Barber, F. A.; Coons, D. A.: Midterm results of meniscal repair using the BioStinger meniscal repair device. *Arthroscopy* 22:400–405, 2006.
15. Barber, F. A.; Coons, D. A.; Ruiz-Suarez, M.: Meniscal repair with the RapidLoc meniscal repair device. *Arthroscopy* 22:962–966, 2006.
16. Barber, F. A.; Herbert, M. A.: Meniscal repair devices. *Arthroscopy* 16:613–618, 2000.
17. Barber, F. A.; Herbert, M. A.; Richards, D. P.: Load to failure testing of new meniscal repair devices. *Arthroscopy* 20:45–50, 2004.
18. Barber, F. A.; Johnson, D. H.; Halbrecht, J. L.: Arthroscopic meniscal repair using the BioStinger. *Arthroscopy* 21:744–750, 2005.
19. Barber-Westin, S. D.; Noyes, F. R.; McCloskey, J. W.: Rigorous statistical reliability, validity, and responsiveness testing of the Cincinnati Knee Rating System in 350 subjects with uninjured, injured, or anterior cruciate ligament–reconstructed knees. *Am J Sports Med* 27:402–416, 1999.
20. Barrett, G. R.; Treacy, S. H.; Ruff, C. G.: Preliminary results of the T-fix endoscopic meniscus repair technique in an anterior cruciate ligament reconstruction population. *Arthroscopy* 13:218–223, 1997.
21. Becker, R.; Starke, C.; Heymann, M.; Nebelung, W.: Biomechanical properties under cyclic loading of seven meniscus repair techniques. *Clin Orthop Relat Res* 400:236–245, 2002.
22. Bhargava, M. M.; Hidaka, C.; Hannafin, J. A.; et al.: Effects of hepatocyte growth factor and platelet-derived growth factor on the repair of meniscal defects in vitro. *In Vitro Cell Dev Biol Anim* 41:305–310, 2005.
23. Billante, M. J.; Diduch, D. R.; Lunardini, D. J.; et al.: Meniscal repair using an all-inside, rapidly absorbing, tensionable device. *Arthroscopy* 24:779–785, 2008.
24. Boenisch, U. W.; Faber, K. J.; Ciarelli, M.; et al.: Pull-out strength and stiffness of meniscal repair using absorbable arrows or Ti-Cron vertical and horizontal loop sutures. *Am J Sports Med* 27:626–631, 1999.
25. Borden, P.; Nyland, J.; Caborn, D. N.; Pienkowski, D.: Biomechanical comparison of the FasT-Fix meniscal repair suture system with vertical mattress sutures and meniscus arrows. *Am J Sports Med* 31:374–378, 2003.
26. Bourne, R. B.; Finlay, J. B.; Papadopoulos, P.; Andreae, P.: The effect of medial meniscectomy on strain distribution in the proximal part of the tibia. *J Bone Joint Surg Am* 66:1431–1437, 1984.
27. Boytim, M. J.; Smith, J.; Fischer, D. A.; Quick, D. C.: Arthroscopic posteromedial visualization of the knee. *Clin Orthop Relat Res* 310:82–86, 1995.
28. Bryant, D.; Dill, J.; Litchfield, R.; et al.: Effectiveness of bioabsorbable arrows compared with inside-out suturing for vertical, reparable meniscal lesions: a randomized clinical trial. *Am J Sports Med* 35:889–896, 2007.
29. Bullough, P. G.; Munuera, L.; Murphy, J.; Weinstein, A. M.: The strength of the menisci of the knee as it relates to their fine structure. *J Bone Joint Surg Br* 52:564–570, 1970.
30. Buma, P.; Ramrattan, N. N.; van Tienen, T. G.; Veth, R. P.: Tissue engineering of the meniscus. *Biomaterials* 25:1523–1532, 2004.
31. Buseck, M. S.; Noyes, F. R.: Arthroscopic evaluation of meniscal repairs after anterior cruciate ligament reconstruction and immediate motion. *Am J Sports Med* 19:489–494, 1991.
32. Calder, S. J.; Myers, P. T.: Broken arrow: a complication of meniscal repair. *Arthroscopy* 15:651–652, 1999.
33. Cannon, W. D., Jr.; Vittori, J. M.: The incidence of healing in arthroscopic meniscal repairs in anterior cruciate ligament–reconstructed knees versus stable knees. *Am J Sports Med* 20:176–181, 1992.
34. Caplan, A. I.: Adult mesenchymal stem cells for tissue engineering versus regenerative medicine. *J Cell Physiol* 213:341–347, 2007.
35. DeHaven, K. E.; Arnoczky, S. P.: Meniscal repair. Part I: basic science, indications for repair, and open repair. *J Bone Joint Surg Am* 76:140–152, 1994.
36. DeHaven, K. E.; Lohrer, W. A.; Lovelock, J. E.: Long-term results of open meniscal repair. *Am J Sports Med* 23:524–530, 1995.
37. Dervin, G. F.; Downing, K. J.; Keene, G. C.; McBride, D. G.: Failure strengths of suture versus biodegradable arrow for meniscal repair: an in vitro study. *Arthroscopy* 13:296–300, 1997.
38. Dugdale, T. W.; Noyes, F. R.; Styer, D.: Preoperative planning for high tibial osteotomy: The effect of lateral tibiofemoral separation and tibiofemoral length. *Clin Orthop Relat Res* 274:248–264, 1992.
39. Ellermann, A.; Siebold, R.; Buelow, J. U.; Sobau, C.: Clinical evaluation of meniscus repair with a bioabsorbable arrow: a 2- to 3-year follow-up study. *Knee Surg Sports Traumatol Arthrosc* 10:289–293, 2002.
40. Evans, C. H.; Ghivizzani, S. C.; Robbins, P. D.: The 2003 Nicolas Andry Award. Orthopaedic gene therapy. *Clin Orthop Relat Res* 429:316–329, 2004.
41. Fairbank, F. J.: Knee joint changes after meniscectomy. *J Bone Joint Surg Br* 30:664–670, 1948.
42. Farng, E.; Sherman, O.: Meniscal repair devices: a clinical and biomechanical literature review. *Arthroscopy* 20:273–286, 2004.
43. Fisher, S. R.; Markel, D. C.; Koman, J. D.; Atkinson, T. S.: Pull-out and shear failure strengths of arthroscopic meniscal repair systems. *Knee Surg Sports Traumatol Arthrosc* 10:294–299, 2002.

44. Fox, M. G.: MR imaging of the meniscus: review, current trends, and clinical implications. *Radiol Clin North Am* 45:1033–1053, vii, 2007.

45. Fukubayashi, T.; Kurosawa, H.: The contact area and pressure distribution pattern of the knee. A study of normal and osteoarthrotic knee joints. *Acta Orthop Scand* 51:871–879, 1980.

46. Gershuni, D. H.; Skyhar, M. J.; Danzig, L. A.; et al.: Experimental models to promote healing of tears in the avascular segment of canine knee menisci. *J Bone Joint Surg Am* 71:1363–1370, 1989.

47. Ghadially, F. N.; Wedge, J. H.; LaLonde, J.-M.: Experimental methods of repairing injured menisci. *J Bone Joint Surg Br* 68:106–110, 1986.

48. Haas, A. L.; Schepsis, A. A.; Hornstein, J.; Edgar, C. M.: Meniscal repair using the FasT-Fix all-inside meniscal repair device. *Arthroscopy* 21:167–175, 2005.

49. Hashimoto, J.; Kurosaka, M.; Yoshiya, S.; Hirohata, K.: Meniscal repair using fibrin sealant and endothelial cell growth factor. An experimental study in dogs. *Am J Sports Med* 20:537–541, 1992.

50. Heatley, F. W.: The meniscus-can it be repaired? An experimental investigation in rabbits. *J Bone Joint Surg Br* 62:397–402, 1980.

51. Henning, C. E.; Lynch, M. A.; Clark, J. R.: Vascularity for healing of meniscus repairs. *Arthroscopy* 3:13–18, 1987.

52. Henning, C. E.; Lynch, M. A.; Yearout, K. M.; et al.: Arthroscopic meniscal repair using an exogenous fibrin clot. *Clin Orthop Relat Res* 252:64–72, 1990.

53. Hoben, G. M.; Athanasiou, K. A.: Creating a spectrum of fibrocartilages through different cell sources and biochemical stimuli. *Biotechnol Bioeng* 100:587–598, 2008.

54. Hoben, G. M.; Athanasiou, K. A.: Meniscal repair with fibrocartilage engineering. *Sports Med Arthrosc* 14:129–137, 2006.

55. Horibe, S.; Shino, K.; Maeda, A.; et al.: Results of isolated meniscal repair evaluated by second-look arthroscopy. *Arthroscopy* 12:150–155, 1996.

56. Hoshikawa, Y.; Kurosawa, H.; Fukubayashi, T.; et al.: The prognosis of meniscectomy in athletes. The simple meniscus lesions without ligamentous instabilities. *Am J Sports Med* 11:8–13, 1983.

57. Hurel, C.; Mertens, F.; Verdonk, R.: Biofix resorbable meniscus arrow for meniscal ruptures: results of a 1-year follow-up. *Knee Surg Sports Traumatol Arthrosc* 8:46–52, 2000.

58. Hutchinson, M. R.; Ash, S. A.: Failure of a biodegradable meniscal arrow. A case report. *Am J Sports Med* 27:101–103, 1999.

59. Ishimura, M.; Ohgushi, H.; Habata, T.; et al.: Arthroscopic meniscal repair using fibrin glue. Part I: experimental study. *Arthroscopy* 13:551–557, 1997.

60. Jensen, N. C.; Riis, J.; Robertsen, K.; Holm, A. R.: Arthroscopic repair of the ruptured meniscus: one to 6.3 years follow-up. *Arthroscopy* 10:211–214, 1994.

61. Johns, D. E.; Athanasiou, K. A.: Growth factor effects on costal chondrocytes for tissue engineering fibrocartilage. *Cell Tissue Res* 333:439–447, 2008.

62. Johnson, R. J.; Kettelkamp, D. B.; Clark, W.; Leaverton, P.: Factors affecting late results after meniscectomy. *J Bone Joint Surg Am* 56:719–729, 1974.

63. Jorgensen, U.; Sonne-Holm, S.; Lauridsen, F.; Rosenklint, A.: Long-term follow-up of meniscectomy in athletes. A prospective longitudinal study. *J Bone Joint Surg Br* 69:80–83, 1987.

64. Kalliakmanis, A.; Zourntos, S.; Bousgas, D.; Nikolaou, P.: Comparison of arthroscopic meniscal repair results using 3 different meniscal repair devices in anterior cruciate ligament reconstruction patients. *Arthroscopy* 24:810–816, 2008.

65. Kelly, B. T.; Potter, H. G.; Deng, X. H.; et al.: Meniscal allograft transplantation in the sheep knee: evaluation of chondroprotective effects. *Am J Sports Med* 34:1464–1477, 2006.

66. Kettelkamp, D. B.; Jacobs, A. W.: Tibiofemoral contact area—determination and implications. *J Bone Joint Surg Am* 54:349–356, 1972.

67. Kocabey, Y.; Nyland, J.; Isbell, W. M.; Caborn, D. N.: Patient outcomes following T-Fix meniscal repair and a modifiable, progressive rehabilitation program, a retrospective study. *Arch Orthop Trauma Surg* 124:592–596, 2004.

68. Kotsovolos, E. S.; Hantes, M. E.; Mastrokalos, D. S.; et al.: Results of all-inside meniscal repair with the FasT-Fix meniscal repair system. *Arthroscopy* 22:3–9, 2006.

69. Krych, A. J.; McIntosh, A. L.; Voll, A. E.; et al.: Arthroscopic repair of isolated meniscal tears in patients 18 years and younger. *Am J Sports Med* 36:1283–1289, 2008.

70. Kurosaka, M.; Yoshiya, S.; Kuroda, R.; et al.: Repeat tears of repaired menisci after arthroscopic confirmation of healing. *J Bone Joint Surg Br* 84:34–37, 2002.

71. Kurosawa, H.; Fukubayashi, T.; Nakajima, H.: Load-bearing mode of the knee joint: physical behavior of the knee joint with or without menisci. *Clin Orthop Relat Res* 149:283–290, 1980.

72. Kurzweil, P. R.; Tifford, C. D.; Ignacio, E. M.: Unsatisfactory clinical results of meniscal repair using the meniscus arrow. *Arthroscopy* 21:905, 2005.

73. LaPrade, R. F.; Konowalchuk, B. K.: Popliteomeniscal fascicle tears causing symptomatic lateral compartment knee pain: diagnosis by the figure-4 test and treatment by open repair. *Am J Sports Med* 33:1231–1236, 2005.

74. Lee, G. P.; Diduch, D. R.: Deteriorating outcomes after meniscal repair using the meniscus arrow in knees undergoing concurrent anterior cruciate ligament reconstruction: increased failure rate with long-term follow-up. *Am J Sports Med* 33:1138–1141, 2005.

75. Lee, S. J.; Aadalen, K. J.; Malaviya, P.; et al.: Tibiofemoral contact mechanics after serial medial meniscectomies in the human cadaveric knee. *Am J Sports Med* 34:1334–1344, 2006.

76. Levy, A. S.; Meier, S. W.: Approach to cartilage injury in the anterior cruciate ligament–deficient knee. *Orthop Clin North Am* 34:149–167, 2003.

77. Levy, I. M.; Torzilli, P. A.; Warren, R. F.: The effect of medial meniscectomy on anterior-posterior motion of the knee. *J Bone Joint Surg Am* 64:883–888, 1982.

78. Lozano, J.; Ma, C. B.; Cannon, W. D.: All-inside meniscus repair: a systematic review. *Clin Orthop Relat Res* 455:134–141, 2007.

79. Lynch, M. A.; Henning, C. E.; Glick, K. R., Jr.: Knee joint surface changes. Long-term follow-up meniscus tear treatment in stable anterior cruciate ligament reconstructions. *Clin Orthop Relat Res* 172:148–153, 1983.

80. Majewski, M.; Stoll, R.; Widmer, H.; et al.: Midterm and long-term results after arthroscopic suture repair of isolated, longitudinal, vertical meniscal tears in stable knees. *Am J Sports Med* 34:1072–1076, 2006.

81. Mariani, P. P.; Santori, N.; Adriani, E.; Mastantuono, M.: Accelerated rehabilitation after arthroscopic meniscal repair: a clinical and magnetic resonance imaging evaluation. *Arthroscopy* 12:680–686, 1996.

82. Markolf, K. L.; Bargar, W. L.; Shoemaker, S. C.; Amstutz, H. C.: The role of joint load in knee stability. *J Bone Joint Surg Am* 63:570–585, 1981.

83. McDermott, I. D.; Lie, D. T.; Edwards, A.; et al.: The effects of lateral meniscal allograft transplantation techniques on tibiofemoral contact pressures. *Knee Surg Sports Traumatol Arthrosc* 16:553–560, 2008.

84. McMurray, T. P.: The semilunar cartilages. *Br J Surg* 29:407, 1942.

85. McNicholas, M. J.; Rowley, D. I.; McGurty, D.; et al.: Total meniscectomy in adolescence. A thirty-year follow-up. *J Bone Joint Surg Br* 82:217–221, 2000.

86. Menche, D. S.; Phillips, G. I.; Pitman, M. I.; Steiner, G. C.: Inflammatory foreign-body reaction to an arthroscopic bioabsorbable meniscal arrow repair. *Arthroscopy* 15:770–772, 1999.

87. Menetrey, J.; Seil, R.; Rupp, S.; Fritschy, D.: Chondral damage after meniscal repair with the use of a bioabsorbable implant. *Am J Sports Med* 30:896–899, 2002.

88. Miller, M. D.; Kline, A. J.; Jepsen, K. G.: "All-inside" meniscal repair devices: an experimental study in the goat model. *Am J Sports Med* 32:858–862, 2004.

89. Miller, M. D.; Ritchie, J. R.; Gomez, B. A.; et al.: Meniscal repair. An experimental study in the goat. *Am J Sports Med* 23:124–128, 1995.

90. Mintzer, C. M.; Richmond, J. C.; Taylor, J.: Meniscal repair in the young athlete. *Am J Sports Med* 26:630–633, 1998.

91. Morgan, C. D.; Wojtys, E. M.; Casscells, C. D.; Casscells, S. W.: Arthroscopic meniscal repair evaluated by second-look arthroscopy. *Am J Sports Med* 19:632–637; discussion 637–638, 1991.

92. Mow, V. C.; Ratcliffe, A.; Chern, K. Y.; Kelly, M. A.: Structure and function relationships of the menisci of the knee. In Mow, V. C.; Arnoczky, S. P.; Jackson, D. W. (eds.): *Knee Meniscus: Basic and Clinical Foundations.* New York: Raven, 1992; pp. 37–57.

93. Nakhostine, M.; Gershuni, D. H.; Danzig, L. A.: Effects of an insubstance conduit with injection of a blood clot on tears in the avascular region of the meniscus. *Acta Orthop Belg* 57:242–246, 1991.

94. Newman, A. P.; Anderson, D. R.; Daniels, A. U.; Dales, M. C.: Mechanics of the healed meniscus in a canine model. *Am J Sports Med* 17:164–175, 1989.

95. Nourissat, G.; Beaufils, P.; Charrois, O.; et al.: Magnetic resonance imaging as a tool to predict reparability of longitudinal full-thickness meniscus lesions. *Knee Surg Sports Traumatol Arthrosc* 16:482–486, 2008.

96. Noyes, F. R.; Barber-Westin, S. D.: Arthroscopic repair of meniscal tears extending into the avascular zone in patients younger than twenty years of age. *Am J Sports Med* 30:589–600, 2002.

97. Noyes, F. R.; Barber-Westin, S. D.: Arthroscopic repair of meniscus tears extending into the avascular zone with or without anterior cruciate ligament reconstruction in patients 40 years of age and older. *Arthroscopy* 16:822–829, 2000.

98. Noyes, F. R.; Bassett, R. W.; Grood, E. S.; Butler, D. L.: Arthroscopy in acute traumatic hemarthrosis of the knee. Incidence of anterior cruciate tears and other injuries. *J Bone Joint Surg Am* 62:687–695, 757, 1980.

99. Noyes, F. R.; Stabler, C. L.: A system for grading articular cartilage lesions at arthroscopy. *Am J Sports Med* 17:505–513, 1989.

100. Nyland, J.; Chang, H.; Kocabey, Y.; et al.: A cyclic testing comparison of FasT-Fix and RapidLoc devices in human cadaveric meniscus. *Arch Orthop Trauma Surg* 128:489–494, 2008.

101. O'Shea, J. J.; Shelbourne, K. D.: Repair of locked bucket-handle meniscal tears in knees with chronic anterior cruciate ligament deficiency. *Am J Sports Med* 31:216–220, 2003.

102. Oliverson, T. J.; Lintner, D. M.: Biofix arrow appearing as a subcutaneous foreign body. *Arthroscopy* 16:652–655, 2000.

103. Paletta, G. A.; Manning, T.; Snell, E.; et al.: The effect of allograft meniscal replacement on intra-articular contact area and pressures in the human knee. A biomechanical study. *Am J Sports Med* 25:692–698, 1997.

104. Pena, E.; Calvo, B.; Martinez, M. A.; et al.: Finite element analysis of the effect of meniscal tears and meniscectomies on human knee biomechanics. *Clin Biomech (Bristol, Avon)* 20:498–507, 2005.

105. Peretti, G. M.; Gill, T. J.; Xu, J. W.; et al.: Cell-based therapy for meniscal repair: a large animal study. *Am J Sports Med* 32:146–158, 2004.

106. Post, W. R.; Akers, S. R.; Kish, V.: Load to failure of common meniscal repair techniques: effects of suture technique and suture material. *Arthroscopy* 13:731–736, 1997.

107. Potter, H. G.; Linklater, J. M.; Allen, A. A.; et al.: Magnetic resonance imaging of articular cartilage in the knee. An evaluation with use of fast-spin-echo imaging. *J Bone Joint Surg Am* 80:1276–1284, 1998.

108. Potter, H. G.; Rodeo, S. A.; Wickiewicz, T. L.; Warren, R. F.: Imaging of meniscal allografts: correlation with clinical and arthroscopic outcomes. *Radiology* 198:509–514, 1996.

109. Quinby, J. S.; Golish, S. R.; Hart, J. A.; Diduch, D. R.: All-inside meniscal repair using a new flexible, tensionable device. *Am J Sports Med* 34:1281–1286, 2006.

110. Rankin, C. C.; Lintner, D. M.; Noble, P. C.; et al.: A biomechanical analysis of meniscal repair techniques. *Am J Sports Med* 30:492–497, 2002.

111. Rimmer, M. G.; Nawana, N. S.; Keene, G. C. R.; Pearcy, M. J.: Failure strengths of different meniscal suturing techniques. *Arthroscopy* 11:146–150, 1995.

112. Ritchie, J. R.; Miller, M. D.; Bents, R. T.; Smith, D. K.: Meniscal repair in the goat model. The use of healing adjuncts on central tears and the role of magnetic resonance arthrography in repair evaluation. *Am J Sports Med* 26:278–284, 1998.

113. Rockborn, P.; Gillquist, J.: Results of open meniscus repair. Long-term follow-up study with a matched uninjured control group. *J Bone Joint Surg Br* 82:494–498, 2000.

114. Rockborn, P.; Messner, K.: Long-term results of meniscus repair and meniscectomy: a 13-year functional and radiographic follow-up study. *Knee Surg Sports Traumatol Arthrosc* 8:2–10, 2000.

115. Rodeo, S. A.: Arthroscopic meniscal repair with use of the outside-in technique. *J Bone Joint Surg Am* 82:127–141, 2000.

116. Rodkey, W. G.; Steadman, J. R.; Li, S.-T.: A clinical study of collagen meniscus implants to restore the injured meniscus. *Clin Orthop Relat Res* 367(Suppl):S281–S292, 1999.

117. Roeddecker, K.; Muennich, U.; Nagelschmidt, M.: Meniscal healing: A biomechanical study. *J Surg Res* 56:20–27, 1994.

118. Roos, E. M.; Ostenberg, A.; Roos, H.; et al.: Long-term outcome of meniscectomy: symptoms, function, and performance tests in patients with or without radiographic osteoarthritis compared to matched controls. *Osteoarthritis Cartilage* 9:316–324, 2001.

119. Roos, H.; Lauren, M.; Adalberth, T.; et al.: Knee osteoarthritis after meniscectomy: prevalence of radiographic changes after twenty-one years, compared with matched controls. *Arthritis Rheum* 41:687–693, 1998.

120. Rosenberg, T. D.; Scott, S. M.; Coward, D. B.; et al.: Arthroscopic meniscal repair evaluated with repeat arthroscopy. *Arthroscopy* 2:14–20, 1986.

121. Rubman, M. H.; Noyes, F. R.; Barber-Westin, S. D.: Arthroscopic repair of meniscal tears that extend into the avascular zone. A review of 198 single and complex tears. *Am J Sports Med* 26:87–95, 1998.

122. Scheller, G.; Sobau, C.; Bulow, J. U.: Arthroscopic partial lateral meniscectomy in an otherwise normal knee: clinical, functional, and radiographic results of a long-term follow-up study. *Arthroscopy* 17:946–952, 2001.

123. Scott, G. A.; Jolly, B. L.; Henning, C. E.: Combined posterior incision and arthroscopic intra-articular repair of the meniscus: an examination of factors affecting healing. *J Bone Joint Surg Am* 68:847–861, 1986.

124. Seedhom, B. B.; Hargreaves, D. J.: Transmission of the load in the knee joint with special reference to the role of the menisci. Part II. Experimental results, discussion, and conclusions. *Eng Med* 8:220–228, 1979.

125. Siebold, R.; Dehler, C.; Boes, L.; Ellermann, A.: Arthroscopic all-inside repair using the Meniscus Arrow: long-term clinical follow-up of 113 patients. *Arthroscopy* 23:394–399, 2007.

126. Song, E. K.; Lee, K. B.: Biomechanical test comparing the load to failure of the biodegradable meniscus arrow versus meniscal suture. *Arthroscopy* 15:726–732, 1999.

127. Spindler, K. P.; McCarty, E. C.; Warren, T. A.; et al.: Prospective comparison of arthroscopic medial meniscal repair technique: inside-out suture versus entirely arthroscopic arrows. *Am J Sports Med* 31:929–934, 2003.

128. Steenbrugge, F.; Verdonk, R.; Hurel, C.; Verstraete, K.: Arthroscopic meniscus repair: inside-out technique vs. Biofix meniscus arrow. *Knee Surg Sports Traumatol Arthrosc* 12:43–49, 2004.

129. Steinert, A. F.; Palmer, G. D.; Capito, R.; et al.: Genetically enhanced engineering of meniscus tissue using ex vivo delivery of transforming growth factor-beta 1 complementary deoxyribonucleic acid. *Tissue Eng* 13:2227–2237, 2007.

130. Stone, K. R.; Rodkey, W. G.; Webber, R.; et al.: Meniscal regeneration with copolymeric collagen scaffolds. In vitro and in vivo studies evaluated clinically, histologically, and biochemically. *Am J Sports Med* 20:104–111, 1992.

131. Sweigart, M. A.; Athanasiou, K. A.: Toward tissue engineering of the knee meniscus. *Tissue Eng* 7:111–129, 2001.

132. Szomor, Z. L.; Martin, T. E.; Bonar, F.; Murrell, G. A.: The protective effects of meniscal transplantation on cartilage. An experimental study in sheep. *J Bone Joint Surg Am* 82:80–88, 2000.

133. Tapper, E. M.; Hoover, N. W.: Late results after meniscectomy. *J Bone Joint Surg Am* 51:517–526 passim, 1969.

134. Tenuta, J. J.; Arciero, R. A.: Arthroscopic evaluation of meniscal repairs. Factors that affect healing. *Am J Sports Med* 22:797–802, 1994.

135. Thompson, W. O.; Thaete, F. L.; Fu, F. H.; Dye, S. F.: Tibial meniscal dynamics using three-dimensional reconstruction of magnetic resonance images. *Am J Sports Med* 19:210–216, 1991.

136. Tingstad, E. M.; Teitz, C. C.; Simonian, P. T.: Complications associated with the use of meniscal arrows. *Am J Sports Med* 29:96–98, 2001.

137. Tumia, N. S.; Johnstone, A. J.: Promoting the proliferative and synthetic activity of knee meniscal fibrochondrocytes using basic fibroblast growth factor in vitro. *Am J Sports Med* 32:915–920, 2004.

138. Tumia, N. S.; Johnstone, A. J.: Regional regenerative potential of meniscal cartilage exposed to recombinant insulin-like growth factor-I in vitro. *J Bone Joint Surg Br* 86:1077–1081, 2004.

139. Verma, N. N.; Kolb, E.; Cole, B. J.; et al.: The effects of medial meniscal transplantation techniques on intra-articular contact pressures. *J Knee Surg* 21:20–26, 2008.

140. Veth, R. P. H.: Clinical significance of knee joint changes after meniscectomy. *Clin Orthop Relat Res* 198:56–60, 1985.
141. Voloshin, A. S.; Wosk, J.: Shock absorption of meniscectomized and painful knees: a comparative in vivo study. *J Biomed Eng* 5:157–161, 1983.
142. von Engelhardt, L. V.; Schmitz, A.; Pennekamp, P. H.; et al.: Diagnostics of degenerative meniscal tears at 3-Tesla MRI compared to arthroscopy as reference standard. *Arch Orthop Trauma Surg* 128:451–456, 2008.
143. Walsh, S. P.; Evans, S. L.; O'Doherty, D. M.; Barlow, I. W.: Failure strengths of suture vs. biodegradable arrow and staple for meniscal repair: an in vitro study. *Knee* 8:151–156, 2001.
144. Webber, R. J.; Harris, M. G.; Hough, A. J.: Cell culture of rabbit meniscal fibrochondrocytes: proliferative and synthetic response to growth factors and ascorbate. *J Orthop Res* 3:36–42, 1985.
145. Wilson, W.; van Rietbergen, B.; van Donkelaar, C. C.; Huiskes, R.: Pathways of load-induced cartilage damage causing cartilage degeneration in the knee after meniscectomy. *J Biomech* 36: 845–851, 2003.
146. Yao, J.; Lancianese, S. L.; Hovinga, K. R.; et al.: Magnetic resonance image analysis of meniscal translation and tibio-menisco-femoral contact in deep knee flexion. *J Orthop Res* 26:673–684, 2008.
147. Zantop, T.; Eggers, A. K.; Weimann, A.; et al.: Initial fixation strength of flexible all-inside meniscus suture anchors in comparison to conventional suture technique and rigid anchors: biomechanical evaluation of new meniscus refixation systems. *Am J Sports Med* 32:863–869, 2004.
148. Zantop, T.; Ruemmler, M.; Welbers, B.; et al.: Cyclic loading comparison between biodegradable interference screw fixation and biodegradable double cross-pin fixation of human bone-patellar tendon-bone grafts. *Arthroscopy* 21:934–941, 2005.
149. Zhang, Z.; Arnold, J. A.; Williams, T.; McCann, B.: Repairs by trephination and suturing of longitudinal injuries in the avascular area of the meniscus in goats. *Am J Sports Med* 23:35–41, 1995.
150. Zhang, Z. N.; Tu, K. Y.; Xu, Y. K.; et al.: Treatment of longitudinal injuries in avascular area of meniscus in dogs by trephination. *Arthroscopy* 4:151–159, 1988.

Chapter 29

Meniscus Transplantation: Diagnosis, Operative Techniques, and Clinical Outcomes

Frank R. Noyes, MD ▪ *Sue D. Barber-Westin*, BS

INDICATIONS

The meniscus provides important functions in the human knee, including load bearing, shock absorption, stability, and joint nutrition, that are vital for the integrity of the articular cartilage. Although many meniscus tears can be successfully repaired, including complex tears that extend into the central avascular region,[52,53] not all are salvageable, especially if considerable tissue damage has occurred. Transplantation of human menisci is hypothesized to restore partial load-bearing meniscus function, decrease patient symptoms, and provide some chondroprotective effects.[10,25,37,63,70] However, the procedure remains in an evolving state, as investigations of tissue-processing, secondary sterilization, and long-term function continue to evaluate its effectiveness. Clinical studies have

shown that meniscus transplantation decreases tibiofemoral joint pain in the short term. However, long-term investigations report that most transplants gradually deteriorate, tear, or shrink in size, thereby losing the ability to provide function, as is described later. Accordingly, the goal is to provide short-term benefits until a more suitable meniscus transplant is clinically available. At best, the transplant provides only partial function, and therefore, strenuous sports and high-impact activities are not advised postoperatively even though many younger patients have the desire to return to unrestricted athletics. Education of the patient and family is required so that all understand and accept these current limitations of the procedure.

The optimal candidate is a patient under the age of 50 who has had a total meniscectomy, has pain that limits daily activities, and demonstrates early articular cartilage deterioration in the involved tibiofemoral compartment. There should be no radiographic evidence of advanced tibiofemoral joint arthritis. At least 2 mm of tibiofemoral joint space should be visible on 45° weight-bearing posteroanterior (PA) radiographs.[50] Arthroscopic examination performed prior to meniscus transplantation confirms that the patient is a suitable candidate. In the most advanced cases, there should be no or only minimal bone exposed on tibiofemoral surfaces. Few treatment options are available for these individuals, especially those younger than 30 years of age, and the goal in the short-term

---

Critical Points INDICATIONS

- Prior meniscectomy.
- Age ≤50 yr.
- Pain in the meniscectomized tibiofemoral compartment.
- No radiographic evidence of advanced joint deterioration, ≥2 mm of tibiofemoral joint space on 45° weight-bearing posteroanterior radiographs.
- No or only minimal bone exposed on tibiofemoral surfaces.
- Normal axial alignment.

is to decrease pain, increase knee function, allow pain-free activities of daily living, and delay the onset of tibiofemoral arthritis. Normal axial alignment and a stable joint are required. The body mass index (BMI) must be within normal range.

CONTRAINDICATIONS

Patients who have had a meniscectomy are evaluated with 45° PA weight-bearing radiographs and magnetic resonance imaging (MRI)[45,46] to determine the status of the joint, articular cartilage, and subchondral bone edema. Advanced knee joint arthritis with flattening of the femoral condyle, concavity of the tibial plateau, and osteophytes that prevent anatomic seating of the meniscus transplant are contraindications. Clinical studies have shown poor results and high failure rates in knees with this amount of joint damage.[19,35,46,60]

Untreated lower limb malalignment is associated with failed meniscus transplantation[8,12,64,65]; therefore, the patient must be willing to first undergo a corrective osteotomy. Axial correction is recommended in knees in which the weight-bearing line is less than 45% (varus) or greater than 55% (valgus), representing a 2° to 3° change from normal alignment. Uncorrected knee joint instability, especially anterior cruciate ligament (ACL) deficiency, is also associated with poor outcomes after meniscus transplantation.[64] Patients must undergo concurrent or staged ACL reconstruction to restore normal stability to protect the meniscus transplant.

Preexisting knee arthrofibrosis, significant lower limb muscular atrophy, and a history of prior joint infection with subsequent arthritis are all contraindications for this operation. Symptomatic noteworthy patellofemoral articular cartilage deterioration (subchondral bone exposure) and obesity (BMI > 30) are also contraindications.

Prophylactic meniscus transplantation after total meniscectomy is not recommended in asymptomatic patients who do not have articular cartilage deterioration because long-term predictable success rates for transplants are not available. In addition, the operative procedure does carry a slight risk for complications that could make the patient's condition worse.

The clinical problem is often encountered involving patients younger than 30 years of age who have undergone meniscectomy years ago, do not have articular cartilage damage, and are asymptomatic. Clinical studies show that eventual deterioration of the meniscectomized tibiofemoral compartment will most likely occur. These patients are advised that there is no optimal or predictable operative procedure to replace meniscus function and that they should decrease or refrain from participating in high-impact, strenuous activities. There are sensitive and accurate MRI cartilage techniques to determine the status of the articular cartilage in the meniscectomized compartment.[44,45] When early but definite articular cartilage damage is detected, it can be logically assumed that the joint deterioration will continue over time and the opportunity exists to perform meniscus transplantation. This still represents a difficult choice for the patient in terms of undergoing surgery before the onset of major joint symptoms. In addition, the transplant may not function and further arthroscopic surgery may be required to remove the tissue. Most patients who develop early cartilage damage in the meniscectomized compartment complain of pain with strenuous athletic activities, but not with recreational or daily activities. These patients are not truly asymptomatic and desire to lessen the risk of further joint deterioration to the level at which it will affect lower intensity activities. Patient education and a conservative approach to recommendation of transplantation are important until a more dependable transplant is available.

The presence of a full-thickness femoral condylar defect with bone exposure is a relative contraindication to meniscus transplantation. Concurrent articular cartilage restorative procedures (such as osteochondral grafts or autologous chondrocyte implantation) can be successfully performed with meniscus transplantation[18,38] and expand the indications to include knees with these lesions.

CLINICAL BIOMECHANICS

Chondroprotective Effects

The deleterious effects of meniscectomy on knee joint contact pressures and tibiofemoral articular cartilage have been demonstrated in multiple experimental studies.[7,25,28,42,63,72,74] Bylski-Austrow and coworkers[7] reported that medial meniscectomy

---

Critical Points CONTRAINDICATIONS

- Advanced knee joint arthrosis with flattening of the femoral condyle, concavity of the tibial plateau, osteophytes that prevent anatomic seating of the meniscus transplant.
- Uncorrected varus or valgus axial malalignment.
- Uncorrected knee joint instability, anterior cruciate ligament deficiency.
- Knee arthrofibrosis.
- Significant muscular atrophy.
- Prior joint infection with subsequent arthrosis.
- Symptomatic noteworthy patellofemoral articular cartilage deterioration.
- Obesity (body mass index > 30).
- Prophylactic procedure (asymptomatic patient with no articular cartilage damage).

Critical Points CLINICAL BIOMECHANICS

Chondroprotective Effects

- 50% reduction in area of damage to the articular cartilage compared with meniscectomized knees in experimental large animal study.[63]
- Lateral meniscus transplants increased total contact area by 42%–65% compared with meniscectomized knees in cadaver study.[41]

Knee Joint Contact Mechanics after Meniscus Transplantation

- Allografts reduced normalized maximum and mean contact pressures by 75% compared with meniscectomized cadaver knees.
- However, the allografts did not restore normal contact mechanics and demonstrated greater variability in normalized maximum and mean pressure than the autografts.
- Lateral allografts sized > 10% of native menisci restore contact mechanics close to normal.

Effect Fixation and Location of Meniscus Transplants

- Method of fixation of meniscus transplants critical for subsequent load-bearing function and chondroprotective effects.
- Transplant with bone for fixation required. Soft tissue meniscus transplants, without bone fixation, are not recommended.
- Experimental studies show implant that has either a bony bridge or bone plug fixation of both horns produces contact area, peak contact pressure, and average central pressure results similar to those of an intact meniscus.
- Posterior horn tunnel of medial meniscus allograft should be placed as close to its anatomic position as possible, with a tolerance tighter than 5 mm medial and 5 mm posterior to this location.

caused a decrease in medial compartment contact pressures compared with intact joints of 70% by 4 months postoperatively and 42% by 8 months postoperatively in the goat model. The overall goal of meniscus transplantation is to protect the articular cartilage from subsequent deterioration.

Szomor and associates[63] conducted a study to determine the chondroprotective effects of meniscus allografts and autografts in a large animal model. Medial meniscectomy, medial meniscus autografts, and medial meniscus allografts were performed in 24 sheep. The grafts were placed into the anatomic anterior and posterior horn attachment sites and secured to the tibial plateau with three suture anchors. At 16 weeks postoperative, both the allograft and the autograft knees demonstrated a 34% to 40% reduction in the score for macroscopic damage to the articular cartilage and an approximate 50% reduction in the area of damage to the articular cartilage compared with the meniscectomized knees. However, neither graft provided complete protection, which the investigators hypothesized could have been due to nonisometric positioning and tensioning and graft fixation. Histologic analysis revealed that the allografts had fibrinoid degeneration, areas of hypocellularity, and cloning of meniscus cells.

Kelly and colleagues[25] developed a meniscus allograft surgical technique that attempted to restore the anatomic anterior tibial and posterior femoral meniscal attachments in a sheep model. Fixation of the allografts was accomplished through bone tunnels. Lateral meniscus allografts were implanted into 17 animals, and lateral meniscectomies were performed in 24 animals. Gross inspection, histologic analysis, biomechanical testing, MRI, and T_2 mapping of the central weight-bearing portion of the lateral tibial plateau performed 2 and 4 months postoperatively demonstrated protective effects of the allografts. Significantly decreased cartilage wear and increased cartilage stiffness were found in the allografted joints compared with the meniscectomized knees. However, at 4 months postoperative, the allografted knees had significantly worse values for these outcome measures than the intact knees. The authors noted the successful utilization of MRI with T_2 mapping to detect early articular cartilage degeneration. In summary, experimental studies published to date are short term and show only partial function of the meniscus transplant in terms of contact area measurements.

Knee Joint Contact Mechanics after Meniscus Transplantation

Alhalki and coworkers[2] measured the maximum pressure, mean pressure, and contact area of the medial tibial articular surface after medial meniscectomy and implantation of ipsilateral medial meniscus autografts and cryopreserved allografts in 10 cadaveric knees (mean age, 70 yr). The autografts and allografts were implanted using the same technique of bone plug fixation through anterior and posterior horn transtibial tunnels.

The allografts significantly reduced normalized maximum and mean contact pressures by 75% compared with meniscectomized knees. In addition, the maximum pressure was restricted to a small region of the contact area. The authors hypothesized that the reduction of this magnitude could reduce the rate of cartilage wear compared with that in a meniscectomized knee. However, the allografts did not restore normal contact mechanics and demonstrated greater variability in normalized maximum and mean contact pressures than the autografts. The authors

concluded that the variability in contact mechanics could have been due to poor matching of the three-dimensional geometry of the allograft to the recipient knee. Dimensions for the allograft were matched from standard anteroposterior (AP) and lateral radiographs in the transverse plane. Studies by Paletta and associates[41] and Haut and colleagues[21] revealed that measurements made in the transverse plane only weakly predict the cross-sectional shape of the meniscus.

The effect of the size of lateral meniscus allografts (in comparison with native menisci) on tibial plateau contact mechanics was investigated by Dienst and coworkers.[14] Allografts that were 17.5% larger than native menisci showed significantly higher contact pressures across the articular cartilage. Although allografts sized 10.5% smaller than native menisci had normal contact forces, increased forces in the meniscal tissue were detected that the authors hypothesized could cause early transplant failure. Allografts sized 10% larger or smaller than native menisci restored contact mechanics close to normal. The authors concluded that the surgeon should select lateral meniscus transplants (LMTs) that are slightly larger than native menisci (rather than smaller) to reduce the risk of early failure.

Paletta and associates[41] investigated the effects of lateral meniscectomy, cryopreserved lateral meniscus transplantation with bone plug fixation, and lateral meniscus transplantation without fixation of the anterior and posterior horn attachments. The study involved 10 cadaver knees less than 48 years of age. The lateral meniscal transplants increased total contact area by 42% to 65% compared with meniscectomized knees at all flexion angles (0°, 30°, and 60°). However, there remained a residual 17% to 23% decrease in contact area compared with intact knees. Release of the horn attachments resulted in contact area that was identical to meniscectomized specimens. McDermott and associates[28] assessed the effects of lateral meniscal transplantation with and without bone block fixation in eight cadaver knees. These investigators reported no difference between the two methods in peak contact pressures compared with intact knees. The cadaver specimens used in the study were aged 81 to 98 years, and all had moderate to severe degenerative changes. In addition, no formal size matching was performed with the allografts and recipient knees.

Effect Fixation and Location of Meniscus Transplants

The method of fixation of meniscus transplants to the surrounding tissues is believed to be paramount in subsequent load-bearing function and chondroprotective effects. The goal is to reproduce the normal attachment sites, allowing lateral and medial transplants to remain in their anatomic location and move normally throughout knee motion.[47,68] The use of a transplant with bone for fixation incorporated with either a central bone bridge or a two-tunnel technique (as described later in this chapter) is, in the authors' opinion, required to obtain these goals. Soft tissue meniscus transplants, without bone fixation, are not recommended. Although soft tissue transplants are far easier to prepare and implant surgically, scientific data are inadequate to support that the soft tissue ends of the meniscus implant will heal and provide the circumferential tension in the meniscus that is required for function (Fig. 29–1).

The importance of securing the anterior and posterior horns of an LMT was documented by Chen and colleagues,[9] who

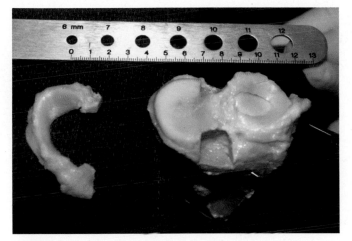

FIGURE 29–1. Visual inspection of meniscus allograft prior to implantation.

investigated a variety of surgical methods for meniscus implantation. Using an autograft cadaver model, the study revealed that a transplant that had either a bony bridge or bone plug fixation of both horns produced contact area, peak contact pressure, and average central pressure results similar to those of an intact meniscus. Procedures in which either only one horn was secured or neither horn was secured demonstrated a loss of mechanical function and subsequent expected benefit of the transplant.

Alhalki and coworkers[1] compared three fixation methods of medial meniscus autografts in cadaver knees to determine which method restored tibial contact mechanics closest to normal. The experimental design tested bone plug fixation alone, bone plug fixation combined with peripheral suturing of the transplant to the native rim, and suturing of the horns through bone tunnels combined with peripheral suturing of the transplant to the native rim. The study revealed that bone plug fixation produced contact mechanics closest to normal; however, the maximum pressure was significantly greater than that in the intact knee. There was no benefit in adding peripheral sutures to the bone plug fixation model. Importantly, fixation with sutures only did not restore normal contact mechanics and was not recommended by the investigators.

Verma and associates[77] measured medial compartment peak pressure, mean pressure, and contact area in eight cadaver knees to determine whether a difference existed between medial meniscus transplants (MMTs) implanted with a bone plug technique and those with a bone trough technique. The data indicated no difference between the two techniques for all three variables, which were restored to values similar to those measured in the intact knees. The authors cited clinical advantages with the trough technique for both medial and lateral meniscus transplantation.

The effect of variations in placement of the posterior horn attachment of an MMT were investigated by Sekaran and colleagues.[56] Using a cadaver autograft model, the posterior horn tunnel was placed either in its anatomic position or 5 mm medial or 5 mm posterior to the anatomic location. The study showed that placing the posterior horn tunnel 5 mm medial to its anatomic position caused an increase in normalized maximum pressure, a posterior shift in the location of the centroid of the contact area, and an increase in the normalized mean pressure. Placing the posterior horn tunnel 5 mm posterior was not as

detrimental; however, this location resulted in a significant shift in the centroid of contact area. The authors concluded that surgeons should place the posterior horn tunnel as close to its anatomic position as possible, with a tolerance limit of less than 5 mm medial and 5 mm posterior to this location.

CLINICAL EVALUATION

A thorough history is taken that includes assessment of prior operative records and current symptoms and functional limitations. A comprehensive knee examination is performed that includes assessment of knee flexion and extension, patellofemoral indices, tibiofemoral pain and crepitus, muscle strength, and gait abnormalities. The appropriate clinical tests for the ACL, posterior cruciate ligament (PCL), medial, and posterolateral structures are performed.

MRI is obtained using proton-density–weighted, high-resolution, fast-spin-echo sequences[45,46] to determine the status of the articular cartilage and prior meniscectomized tibiofemoral compartment. Radiographs include AP, lateral at 30° of knee flexion, weight-bearing PA at 45° of knee flexion, and patellofemoral axial views. Axial lower limb alignment is measured using double-limb standing hip-knee-ankle weight-bearing radiographs[16] in knees that demonstrate varus or valgus alignment.

Patients complete questionnaires and are interviewed for the assessment of symptoms, functional limitations, sports and

---

Critical Points CLINICAL EVALUATION

Physical Examination
- Tibiofemoral joint line pain, compression pain, crepitus
- McMurray test
- Knee flexion & extension
- Joint effusion
- Patellofemoral (medial & lateral subluxation, Q-angle, crepitus, compression pain)
- Muscle strength
- Alignment
- Gait

Ligament Subluxation Tests
- Pivot shift, Lachman
- KT-2000 20° knee flexion, 134 N force
- Posterior drawer, 90° knee flexion
- Tibiofemoral rotation dial 30°, 90° knee flexion
- External rotation recurvatum
- Lateral tibiofemoral joint opening 5°, 20° knee flexion
- Reverse pivot shift
- Medial tibiofemoral joint opening 5°, 20° knee flexion

Magnetic Resonance Imaging
- Proton-density–weighted, high-resolution, fast-spin-echo sequences

Radiographs
- Anteroposterior
- Lateral, 30° knee flexion
- Posteroanterior, weight-bearing, 45° knee flexion
- Patellofemoral axial

Assessment of Symptoms and Functional Limitations with Activity: Cincinnati Knee Rating System
- Sports Activity and Function Form
- Occupational Rating Form
- Symptom Rating Form

occupational activity levels, and patient perception of the overall knee condition according to the Cincinnati Knee Rating System (CKRS).[4]

PREOPERATIVE PLANNING

Meniscus transplants are obtained from tissue banks accredited by the American Association of Tissue Banks (AATB) and inspected by the U.S. Food and Drug Administration (FDA), in which serologic testing meets or exceeds the standards of these organizations.[67] Importantly, donor selection criteria may vary between tissue banks and the surgeon should understand the specific criteria used by the bank chosen to supply the transplant.

A variety of sterilization techniques have been described for meniscus transplants, including none (fresh-frozen), irradiated, cryopreserved, and proprietary chemical techniques. To date, no scientific data exist to select one type of graft processing method over another. Some authors[8] advocate combined secondary sterilization using low-dose irradiation (1–2 Mrads) and chemical agents.

Surgeons should be aware that so-called sterilization processes may not prevent contamination and do not guarantee a sterile graft. The authors recommend that grafts be selected that have undergone some form of sterilization to decrease the risk of bacterial infection. Prophylactic antibiotics are administered intravenously before surgery, and patients are carefully monitored postoperatively for any signs of infection. The implications of different processing techniques on graft sterility and donor selection issues, allograft harvesting techniques, and disease testing are beyond the scope of this chapter and have been discussed in detail by others.[5,10,67]

Although there is no standard protocol at present, AP and lateral radiographs are used to obtain approximate width and length measurements for the meniscus transplant.[43] A number of studies have been performed to determine the appropriate sizing method for meniscus transplants.[15,21,58,61] Shaffer and coworkers[58] found no difference between AP radiographs and MRI in terms of accuracy in measuring actual meniscus width and length. With accuracy defined as no more than a 2-mm difference between actual meniscus dimensions in cadaver specimens and that measured on the films, the accuracy rates were 33% for AP radiographs and 37% for MRI. Stone and associates[61] suggested that recipient height, weight, and gender be considered as important matching criteria when selecting meniscus transplants. These investigators measured meniscus and tibial plateau dimensions in 111 patients using MRI and correlated the dimensions with the patients' height, weight, BMI, and gender. Height correlated well with total tibial plateau width ($R = 0.7194$), and females generally had smaller meniscus dimensions than males. In addition, patients with a BMI greater than 25 had larger meniscus dimensions than patients with a lower BMI at any given height.

Donahue and colleagues[15] developed an algorithm for meniscus transplant sizing based on MRI measurements. The authors recommended that tissue banks follow the algorithm, which involves a series of six steps. These include making four transverse and six cross-sectional measurements for each transplant in the bank's inventory using a three-dimensional coordinate digitizing system, obtaining MRI of the recipient's uninjured knee and measuring nine parameters for the medial or lateral meniscus, and performing a series of calculations to determine the best match.

The problem still exists that even though an approximate size can be determined preoperatively, in many knees the tibiofemoral joint has undergone degenerative changes that produce subtle alterations in joint geometry leading to permanent alterations in the normal surface stress distribution of the joint surface.[7] A meniscus transplant does not have the ability to restore the native or normal state of the meniscectomized compartment. Future studies are required to determine the effect of subtle size and shape mismatch of the transplant on retaining articular cartilage functional properties. A chondroprotective effect of meniscus transplants has yet to be proved. This involves sophisticated questions regarding the chondrocyte function, cartilage collagen, and glycosaminoglycan homeostasis and resultant biomechanical properties.

It is preferred that the tissue bank provides a digital photograph of the transplant selected for the patient before surgery. A metric ruler is placed adjacent to the transplant in the photograph to ensure that the specimen is of adequate size and width. Certain medial menisci may have a hypoplastic anterior horn that is narrow, inserting distal to the medial tibial surface (type III[6]), and are not acceptable for implantation. The middle third of a medial or lateral meniscus may be 8 to 10 mm in width and suitable only for small patients. The lateral meniscus may have reduced anterior-to-posterior length, less than that calculated on the sagittal radiograph, and not be suitable for implantation.

Judgment is required at surgery when the meniscus bone bridge technique is performed, which requires good size matching to prevent medial or lateral meniscus extrusion. The authors prefer to take the added time to use a bone bridge or bone plug technique (bone-meniscus-bone implant), which does require a good geometric and anatomic fit. Alternative techniques are available in which the meniscus is sutured in place without bone plugs, which is not recommended.

The patient is advised that the transplant will be inspected in the operating room before the induction of anesthesia. It is rare that the operative procedure cannot be performed as planned; however, there is always the chance that the transplant will not meet the desired criteria.

Knees with associated varus osseous malalignment require a staged corrective osteotomy prior to the meniscus transplant procedure. Knees with ligament deficiency require a staged ligament reconstruction. Some studies have advocated concurrent ACL reconstruction and meniscus transplantation.[20,57,77] The normal ACL tibial attachment site and the ACL tibial graft tunnel may compromise meniscus transplant tibial fixation.

Critical Points PREOPERATIVE PLANNING

- Obtain transplants from tissue banks accredited by American Association of Tissue Banks, inspected by U.S. Food and Drug Administration.
- Anteroposterior, lateral radiographs to measure transplant size (with scale).
- Request photograph of transplant with metric ruler placed adjacent to document that size is adequate.
- Knees in varus malalignment: Perform osteotomy prior to or with meniscus transplant.
- Knees with cruciate deficiency: Perform reconstruction prior to or with meniscus transplant.

This may occur when the slot technique to be described is selected in patients whose central tibial intercondylar region is not wide enough to accommodate both the meniscus transplant slot and the ACL tibial graft tunnel. Because it is not possible in these knees to use the central slot technique, a two-tunnel procedure is selected for the MMT.

INTRAOPERATIVE EVALUATION

MMTs are not prepared until the surgeon determines whether the central bone bridge technique (which is preferred) or the two-tunnel technique (separate anterior and posterior bone attachments and tunnels) will be performed, as is described later.

LMTs are prepared before the operative procedure to determine the depth and width required for the tibial slot for the central bone bridge technique. The central bone portion of the LMT incorporates the anterior and posterior meniscal attachments and usually measures 8 mm in width in smaller patients and 9 mm in larger patients. The posterior 8 to 10 mm of tibia bone bridge that protrudes beyond the posterior horn attachment is removed to produce a buttress against the prepared bone slots in the host knee. Commercially available (Stryker Endoscopy Co., Kalamazoo, MI, and Cryolife Inc., Kennesaw, GA) sizing blocks and channel cutters are helpful for appropriate sizing, as is described later.

All knee ligament subluxation tests should be performed after the induction of anesthesia in both the injured and the contralateral limbs. The amounts of increased anterior tibial translation, posterior tibial translation, lateral and medial joint opening, and external tibial rotation should be documented. A thorough arthroscopic examination should be conducted, documenting articular cartilage surface abnormalities[39] and the condition of the menisci.

OPERATIVE TECHNIQUE: LMT

The patient is placed in a supine position on the operating room table with a tourniquet applied with a leg holder, and the table adjusted to allow 90° of knee flexion. The opposite lower extremity is placed in a thigh-high elastic stocking and is padded to maintain mild hip flexion to decrease tension on the femoral nerve. After examination under anesthesia, diagnostic arthroscopy confirms the preoperative diagnosis and articular cartilage

Critical Points INTRAOPERATIVE EVALUATION

- Inspect transplant prior to administration of anesthesia.
- Medial meniscus transplant: Choose either central bone bridge or two-tunnel technique.
- Lateral meniscus transplant: Prepare implant to determine depth and width required for tibial slot.
- Repeat all knee ligament subluxation tests under anesthesia, both injured and contralateral limbs.
- Rate all articular cartilage surfaces for abnormalities
  - Normal.
  - Grade 1, softening.
  - Grade 2A, fissuring & fragmentation < 50% depth of the articular surface.
  - Grade 2B, fissuring & fragmentation > 50% depth of the articular surface.
  - Grade 3, subchondral bone exposed.

Critical Points OPERATIVE TECHNIQUE: LATERAL MENISCUS TRANSPLANT

- Diagnostic arthroscopy confirms preoperative diagnosis, articular cartilage changes.
- Limited 3-cm lateral arthrotomy just adjacent to patellar tendon.
- Patellar tendon displaced medially to properly place tibial slot.
- Second 3-cm posterolateral incision made just behind fibular collateral ligament.
- Interval between short head of biceps muscle and iliotibial band identified.
- Inferior lateral geniculate artery identified, preserved.
- Space between posterolateral capsule and lateral head of gastrocnemius further developed bluntly.
- Width of transplant determined, template inserted into lateral compartment to determine proper placement of bone slot.
- Sizing step ensures there is no lateral overhang of the meniscal body.
- Tibial bone slot 1–2 mm wider than transplant to facilitate implantation. Anterior and posterior horns of implant placed into normal attachment locations.
- Transplant sizing block confirms transplant bone bridge is correct width, depth.
- Dovetail technique or rectangular bone technique chosen.
- Implant inserted into slot, bone portion of graft seated against posterior bone buttress to achieve correct anterior-to-posterior placement of attachment sites.
- Transplant sutured to native meniscus rim.
- Two fixation methods for the central bone attachment: two 2-0 nonabsorbable sutures placed retrograde into tibial slot, passed over the central bone bridge, tied to tibial post (preferred).
- Place a 7- × 25-mm interference screw adjacent medially to the bone bridge.
- Arthrotomy is closed, inside-out meniscal repair completed with multiple vertical divergent sutures.

changes. A meniscus bed of 3 mm is retained when possible, except at the popliteal tendon region where the native meniscus rim is removed. The meniscus bed and adjacent synovium are rasped to aid in revascularization of the transplant.

The tourniquet is inflated for only the two initial operative approaches. A limited 3-cm lateral arthrotomy is made just adjacent to the patellar tendon. Although arthroscopic techniques are available to prepare the tibial slot, the limited arthrotomy provides superior visualization and avoids incising into the patellar tendon, which must be displaced medially to properly place the tibial slot. A common mistake involves placing the central tibial slot lateral to the normal attachment of the anterior horn of the lateral meniscus.

A second 3-cm posterolateral incision is made just behind the fibular collateral ligament (FCL; Fig. 29–2), similar to that described in Chapter 28, Meniscus Tears: Diagnosis, Repair Techniques, and Clinical Outcomes, for inside-out lateral meniscus repairs.[29,53] The interval between the short head of the biceps muscle and the iliotibial band is identified and incised. The lateral head of the gastrocnemius is gently dissected with Metzenbaum scissors off the posterior capsule at the joint line just above the fibular head. Care is taken at this point because dissection that extends too far proximal to the joint line would enter the joint capsule. If this occurs, a capsular repair is required to maintain joint integrity during the inside-out meniscal repair procedure.

The inferior lateral geniculate artery, in close proximity, is identified and preserved. The space between the posterolateral

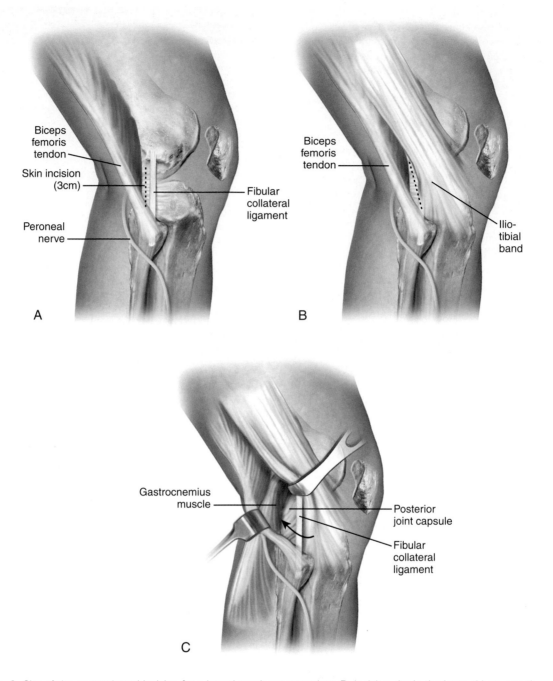

FIGURE 29–2. A, Site of the posterolateral incision for a lateral meniscus transplant. **B**, Incision site in the interval between the posterior edge of the iliotibial band and the anterior edge of the biceps tendon. **C**, The interval between the lateral gastrocnemius and the posterolateral capsule is opened bluntly, just proximal to the fibular head, avoiding entering the joint capsule proximally.

capsule and the lateral head of the gastrocnemius is further developed bluntly. An appropriately sized popliteal retractor is placed directly behind the lateral meniscus bed and anterior to the lateral gastrocnemius muscle.

The width of the transplant is determined. A template made out of aluminum foil of the transplant's width and length is cut and inserted into the lateral compartment to determine the proper placement of the bone slot. This sizing step is important to ensure that there is no lateral overhang (extrusion) of the meniscal body produced by placing the bone slot too far laterally. If there is a mismatch that results in lateral extrusion, the procedure may be converted from the bone bridge technique to

one using two separate bone plugs and bone tunnels. The posterior bone plug is located directly at the lateral meniscus attachment. The anterior bone plug is placed more medially by a few millimeters to prevent lateral extrusion. The use of the bone bridge technique does require adequate size matching, and judgment is required at surgery in using the central bridge or separate bone plug technique. This same concept applies to MMTs. A rectangular bone slot is prepared at the anterior and posterior meniscus tibial attachment sites to match the dimensions of the prepared transplant.

The sequence of steps to prepare the lateral tibial slot is shown in Figure 29–3. The tibial bone slot is 1 to 2 mm wider

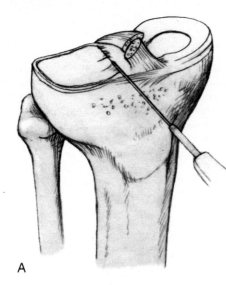

A

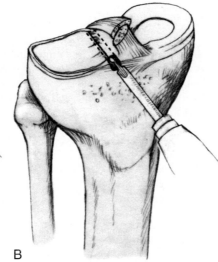

B

C

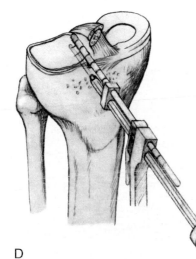

D

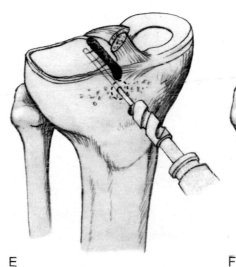

E

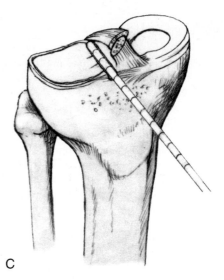

F

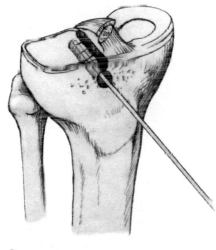

G

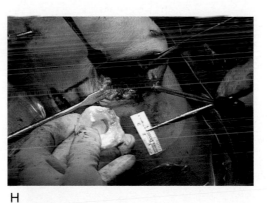

H

FIGURE 29–3. A, Tibial slot technique for lateral meniscus transplantation. The technique is shown for the lateral meniscus. An arthroscopically assisted technique or minilateral arthrotomy may be used in this procedure. The authors prefer the miniarthrotomy because it offers superior visualization and avoids incising the patellar tendon. Establish a line connecting the center of the anterior and posterior horn attachments using an electrocautery device. In the mini–open arthrotomy, a template of the meniscus coronal width is used to verify the medial-to-lateral width of the transplant to move the slot appropriately to prevent tibial overhang of the transplant. **B,** A burr removes the tibial spine and creates a 4-mm straight anterior-to-posterior reference slot along the plane of the tibial slope. **C,** This calibrated guide pin sits flush with the articular cartilage. **D,** The drill guide uses a guide pin that has been marked with a laser to set the depth of a second guide pin, allowing a drill to ream 5 mm less to retain the posterior portion of the tibial slot. **E–G,** The 8-mm drill bit with a collar at the defined depth is used, followed by use of a box cutter to create a rectangular slot of the desired depth and width. **H,** The lateral meniscus transplant with the central bone bridge technique is ready to be placed into the tibial slot. *(A–H, Reprinted with permission from Noyes, F. R.; Barber-Westin, S. D.; Rankin, M.. Meniscal transplantation in symptomatic patients less than fifty years old: surgical technique.* J Bone Joint Surg Am *87[suppl 1{pt 2}]:149–165, 2005.)*

than the transplant to facilitate implantation. The anterior and posterior horns of the transplant are placed into their normal attachment locations, adjacent to the ACL. It is important to note that a prior ACL reconstruction in which the tibial tunnel was placed in a lateral position may produce a technical problem in creating the tibial slot.

A starter chisel and finishing chisels provide an alternative technique to create and fashion the tibial slot to its final depth and width (Fig. 29–4A). A tibial slot sizing guide is used to check the length and depth (see Fig. 29–4B). A sizing block (see Fig. 29–4C) confirms that the transplant bone bridge is of the correct width and depth.

A dovetail technique may also be considered, which has the advantage of providing added stability to the fixation at the tibial bone portion of the transplant (Fig. 29–5). This procedure entails cutting a trapezoidal bone block that includes a more narrow 7-mm bone bridge. This procedure requires additional time to prepare the transplant.

The transplant is inserted into the slot, and the bone portion of the graft is seated against the posterior bone buttress to achieve correct anterior-to-posterior placement of the attachment sites. A vertical suture in the posterior meniscus body is passed posteriorly to provide tension and facilitate transplant placement. The suture is tied later in the procedure. The knee is flexed, extended, and rotated to confirm that correct placement of the transplant has been obtained. Sutures are placed into the anterior third of the meniscus, attaching it to the prepared meniscus rim under direct visualization.

Two fixation methods are available for the central bone attachment. Two 2-0 nonabsorbable sutures may be placed retrograde into the tibial slot, passed over the central bone bridge prior to transplant passage, and tied to a tibial post. The sutures hold the transplant securely in the tibial slot and, along with the peripheral sutures, provide fixation. This is the preferred technique because it is simple and effective. Another option is to place a 7- × 25-mm interference screw composed of an

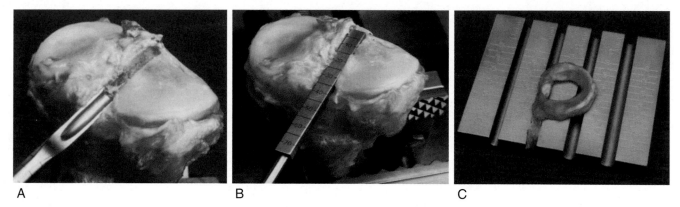

A **B** **C**

FIGURE 29–4. A, An alternative technique uses a starter chisel and finishing chisels to fashion the tibial slot to its final depth and width. **B,** A tibial slot sizing guide is used to check the length and depth. **C,** The allograft sizing block confirms that the allograft bone bridge is of the desired width and depth. *(A–C, Reprinted with permission from Noyes, F. R.; Barber-Westin, S. D.; Rankin, M.: Meniscal transplantation in symptomatic patients less than fifty years old: surgical technique. J Bone Joint Surg Am 87[suppl 1{pt 2}]:149–165, 2005.)*

FIGURE 29–5. Dovetail meniscus allograft technique. **A,** An outline of the dovetail bone block is drawn on the end of the bone plug. A transplant jig system is used to hold the meniscus transplant and produce the desired bone cuts. **B,** Final appearance shows the typical dimensions for the trapezoidal bone block prior to transplant insertion.

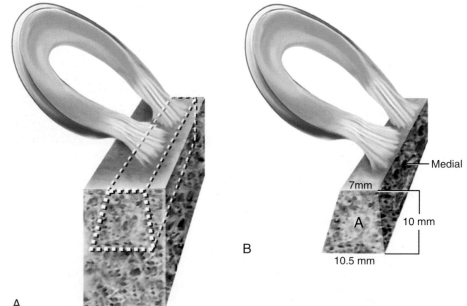

A

B

Medial

7mm

10 mm

10.5 mm

A

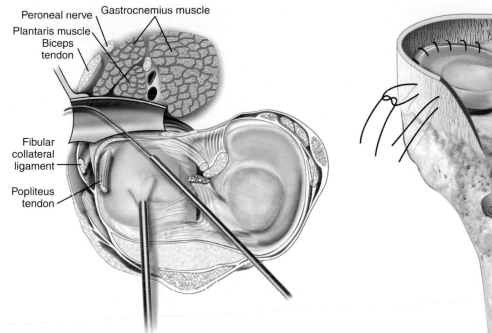

Peroneal nerve — Gastrocnemius muscle
Plantaris muscle
Biceps tendon
Fibular collateral ligament
Popliteus tendon

FIGURE 29–6. Cross-section shows a popliteal retractor between the lateral gastrocnemius and the posterior capsule. A single cannula is introduced from the adjacent portal to facilitate placement of the vertical sutures into the periphery of the meniscus transplant.

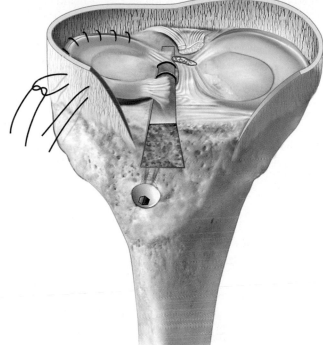

FIGURE 29–7. Lateral meniscus graft in place and sutured.

absorbable composite material adjacent medially to the bone bridge.[17] A tap is inserted over the guidewire to create a path for the interference screw with the bone bridge held in place manually. This technique is not used if there is tibial bone osteopenia or if a prior ACL graft tunnel exists because inadequate fixation will occur.

The arthrotomy is closed, and the inside-out meniscal repair completed with multiple vertical divergent sutures that are placed first superiorly to reduce the meniscus (Fig. 29–6) and then inferiorly in the outer third of the transplant. Sutures are not placed in the middle and inner thirds to avoid weakening the transplant owing to its limited healing capability in these regions (Fig. 29–7).

OPERATIVE TECHNIQUE: MMT

The patient is placed in a supine position on the operating room table with a tourniquet applied with a leg holder, and the table adjusted to allow 90° of knee flexion. The opposite lower extremity is placed in a thigh-high elastic stocking and is padded to maintain mild hip flexion to decrease tension on the femoral nerve. After knee examination and diagnostic arthroscopy, the meniscus bed is prepared by removing remaining meniscal tissue. It is important to preserve, whenever possible, a 3-mm rim to help contain the meniscus and prevent medial extrusion. Although there are techniques for suturing the meniscus implant without bone plugs, the authors prefer to take the added time to secure a bone-meniscus-bone implant and have identified on weight-bearing MRI studies (presented

later in this chapter) that this procedure results in a meniscus implant that heals without medial extrusion. The same concept applies to lateral meniscus implants. The authors are not aware of similar clinical MRI studies after meniscus implants without bone attachments to prove that early partial meniscus extrusion

Critical Points OPERATIVE TECHNIQUE: MEDIAL MENISCUS TRANSPLANT

- Diagnostic arthroscopy confirms preoperative diagnosis, articular cartilage changes.
- Tourniquet inflated only for anteromedial, posteromedial surgical approaches.
- 4-cm skin anteromedial incision adjacent to tibial tubercle and patellar tendon.
- 3-cm vertical posteromedial incision.
- Identify, avoid injury to infrapatellar branches of saphenous nerve.
- Tendon sheath of semimembranosus incised to facilitate exposure.
- Meniscus retractor placed in interval anterior to gastrocnemius tendon, directly posterior to meniscus bed, posterior capsule.
- Aluminum foil template medial meniscus transplant made, measured according to anterior-posterior, medial-lateral dimensions.
- Template inserted through anterior arthrotomy to measure medial tibial plateau.
- Position of central bone slot marked.
- Surgeon determines whether meniscus implant will be properly positioned; if so, central bone bridge technique is used.
- If implant requires adjustment for improper fit in medial compartment, two-tunnel technique is selected.

is not a problem. Biomechanical studies[1,2,9,41] support this concept and have shown that meniscus implants sutured, without additional bony fixation, do not restore normal joint contact pressures, although one study did not agree.[28] Any loss of meniscus to its bony attachment may result in loss of function. Sekaran and colleagues[56] showed that even a 5-mm malposition in the medial meniscus posterior bone plug adversely affects joint contact pressure. The meniscus bed and synovium are rasped to aid in revascularization of the transplant.

The tourniquet is inflated only for the anteromedial and posteromedial surgical approaches. A 4-cm skin anteromedial incision is made adjacent to the patellar tendon for the anterior arthrotomy. A second 3-cm vertical posteromedial incision is made, similar to that described for inside-out meniscus repairs[29]

(Fig. 29–8). The fascia is incised anterior to the sartorius muscle, and the pes anserine muscle groups are retracted posteriorly. Great care is taken to identify and avoid injury to the infrapatellar branches of the saphenous nerve. The interval between the semimembranosus tendon and the capsule is dissected. The tendon sheath of the semimembranosus is incised to facilitate exposure. The layer between the medial gastrocnemius tendon and the posterior capsule is separated with blunt dissection. A meniscus retractor is placed in the interval anterior to the gastrocnemius tendon and directly posterior to the meniscus bed and posterior capsule. The two approaches are performed with the tourniquet inflated to 275 mm and usually require less than 15 minutes; otherwise, the tourniquet is not used.

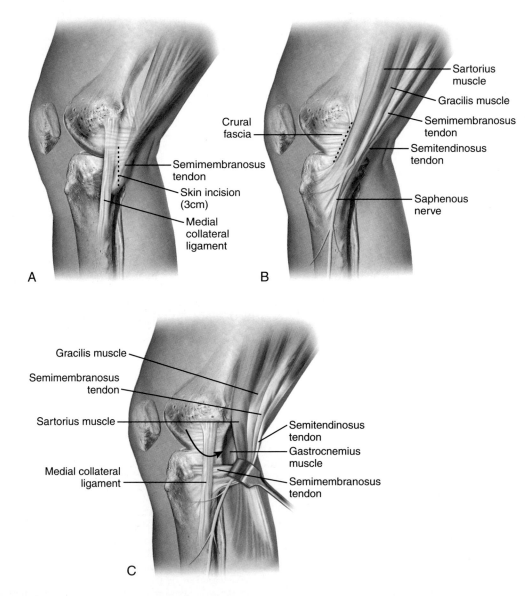

FIGURE 29–8. The accessory posteromedial approach is shown for a medial meniscus allograft. **A**, Site of the posteromedial skin incision. **B**, The incision is shown through the anterior portion of the sartorius fascia. **C**, The interval is opened between the posteromedial capsule and the gastrocnemius tendon, just proximal to the semimembranosus tendon (*arrow*). The fascia over the tendon is excised to its tibial attachment to facilitate retrieval of the meniscus sutures.

The goal of the operative procedure is to transplant the medial meniscus and bone attachments into the normal anterior and posterior attachments and to suture the transplant to maintain the desired position in the knee joint. An aluminum foil template of the MMT is measured according to its anterior-to-posterior and medial-to-lateral dimensions and is inserted through the anterior arthrotomy to measure the medial tibial plateau. This allows the position of the central bone slot to be marked and to determine whether the meniscus transplant will be properly positioned adjacent to the ACL tibial attachment without medial tibial overhang.

The anterior and posterior meniscus attachment locations are verified to be at the anatomically correct sites. The central bone bridge technique removes 4 to 6 mm of the medial intercondylar tubercle. If the transplant is suitable and no medial tibial overhang is present, the central bone bridge technique may be used. If the transplant needs to be adjusted to fit to the medial tibial plateau (by attaching the anterior horn placement further laterally), the two-tunnel technique is selected. This sizing step is critical to obtain proper placement of the MMT into the host tibia.

In many knees, the central slot technique will not be possible owing to a sizing problem that results in excessive medial displacement of the meniscus body or that would compromise the ACL tibial attachment. Once the appropriate technique has been determined, the meniscus transplant is prepared.

Medial Meniscus Central Bone Bridge Technique

The technique is similar to that already described for lateral meniscus transplantation. The meniscus transplant is prepared using either a rectangular or a dovetail technique. A reference slot is first made on the tibial plateau in the anterior-to-posterior direction. A guide pin is positioned in the slot, inferiorly on the tibia, and a cannulated drill bit is placed over the pin to drill a tunnel. An alternative technique is to use osteotomes and chisels to prepare the tibial slot. The ACL attachment is directly lateral to the tibial slot, and no more than 2 mm of its attachment may be compromised. The final tibial slot is 8 to 9 mm in width and 10 mm in depth. A rasp is used to smooth the slot to allow insertion of the transplant central bone bridge.

In the dovetail technique, the central bone bridge of the transplant is sized to a width of 7 mm (1 mm less than the dimension at the tibial site) and a depth of 10 mm.[17] The dovetail technique requires less central bone resection and, therefore, is more protective of the ACL attachment.

A vertical suture is placed through the posterior meniscus horn and advanced through the capsule to exit through the posteromedial incision. The meniscus is passed through the arthrotomy into the knee with tension placed on the posterior suture to facilitate proper positioning in the knee joint. Care is taken to align the meniscus bone bridge with the recipient tibial slot. The adjustment of the central bone bridge position is performed in the anterior-to-posterior direction to fit in the anatomically correct position relative to the femoral condyle. The knee is taken through flexion and extension and tibial rotation to align the transplant. Occasionally, there will be an osteophyte on the anterior portion of the medial tibial plateau, which must be resected to avoid meniscal transplant compression.

The fixation of the central bone bridge is accomplished with two sutures that are passed through a tunnel in the central tibial slot or with an interference absorbable screw, as already described. The anterior horn of the meniscus is sutured with vertical sutures (2-0 Ethibond) under direct visualization (Fig. 29-9). The anterior arthrotomy is closed and the inside-out vertical divergent sutures are placed, as described, to suture the meniscus to the meniscus bed, removing any transplant undulations and restoring circumferential meniscal tension.

Critical Points OPERATIVE TECHNIQUE: MEDIAL MENISCUS CENTRAL BONE BRIDGE TECHNIQUE

- Transplant prepared using rectangular or dovetail technique.
- Reference slot tibial plateau, anteroposterior direction.
- Anterior cruciate ligament attachment directly lateral to tibial slot, no more than 2 mm of its attachment may be compromised.
- Final tibial slot 8–9 mm wide, 10 mm deep.
- Dovetail technique: central bone bridge sized to a width of 7 mm (1 mm less than dimension at tibial site) and a depth of 10 mm.
- Meniscus passed through arthrotomy into knee.
- Align meniscus bone bridge with recipient tibial slot.
- Fixation: Two sutures passed through tunnel in tibial slot or an absorbable bone interference screw.
- Anterior horn sutured vertical sutures, direct visualization.
- Anterior arthrotomy closed, inside-out vertical divergent sutures placed to suture transplant to meniscus bed.

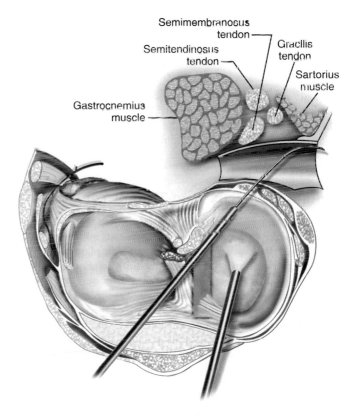

FIGURE 29-9. Cross-section shows the arthroscope, needle cannula, and popliteal retractor in place. The meniscus is passed through the arthrotomy into the knee with tension placed on the sutures to facilitate proper positioning in the knee joint. Using a single-barrel cannula, the suture is advanced through the capsule at the corresponding attachment site of the meniscus and exits through an accessory incision.

of the meniscus transplants failed and were removed before the minimum 2-year follow-up study period; these cases were included in the overall failure rate. Thirty-five patients were followed (36 meniscus transplants; 18 lateral, 16 medial, 1 bilateral) a mean of 40 months (range, 24–69 mo) postoperatively. There were 18 males and 17 females whose mean age at surgery was 30 years (range, 14–49 yr).

A mean of 139 months (range, 12–372 mo) had elapsed between the knee injury and the meniscus transplant. A total of 128 prior operative procedures had been done, including 61 partial or total meniscectomies, 13 ACL reconstructions, 4 PCL reconstructions, 1 FCL reconstruction, 5 high tibial osteotomies (HTOs), and 3 osteochondral autograft transfer procedures.

At the time of the LMT, a concurrent osteochondral autograft transfer of the lateral femoral condyle was done in 13 knees for full-thickness articular cartilage defects. Knee ligament reconstructions were done before the meniscus transplant in 4 knees and at the same time as the transplant in 4 knees. In 6 knees, ACL reconstructions were done using either bone–patellar tendon–bone or semitendinosus-gracilis autografts. A PCL two-strand quadriceps tendon autograft reconstruction[33] was done in 1 knee, and both the PCL and the ACL were reconstructed in another.

Abnormal articular cartilage surfaces (lesion > 15 mm in diameter with fissuring and fragmentation extending greater than half of the depth of the cartilage or subchondral bone exposed) were detected in the meniscectomized tibiofemoral compartment in 31 knees (88%) at the time of meniscus transplantation.

Subchondral bone exposure was found in 18 knees, and extensive fissuring and fragmentation was noted in 13 others.

A total of 29 meniscus transplants (73%) were analyzed with MRI using the research protocol previously described in detail[37,47] an average of 35 months (range, 12–67 mo) postoperatively. The films were reviewed and measured by independent orthopaedic surgeons blinded to patient information. The height, width, and displacement of the transplant were determined during full or partial weight-bearing conditions.

A subset of eight meniscus transplants in seven knees were studied 15 to 34 months postoperatively[47] in an open configuration Signa SP MRI System (General Electric Medical Systems, Milwaukee, WI). This system is a 0.5-T superconducting magnet in which the windings are located in separate but communicating cryostats. The vertical orientation of the scanner allows the patient to stand between the cryostats with the knee at isocenter (Fig. 29–13). Single-slice sagittal and coronal images were obtained on both knees at 0°, 30°, 60°, and 90° of knee flexion.

The subjective and functional results were assessed with the CKRS. A classification system of meniscus transplant characteristics was developed on the basis of MRI, clinical examination, follow-up arthroscopy (when performed), and tibiofemoral symptoms (Table 29–1). The International Knee Documentations Committee (IKDC) classification system was used to determine knee ligament graft function.

Before surgery, 27 patients (77%) had moderate to severe pain with daily activities, but at follow-up, only 2 (6%) had pain with daily activities (Fig. 29–14; $P < .0001$). All patients had pain in the meniscectomized tibiofemoral compartment preoperatively, but at follow-up, only 10 (29%) had some component of tibiofemoral pain.

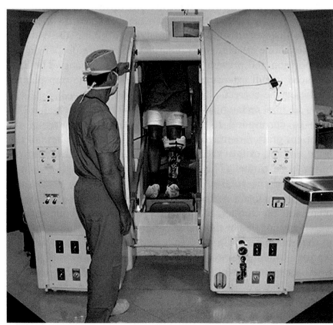

FIGURE 29–13. An open configuration 0.5-T superconducting magnet. The vertical orientation of the scanner allows the patients to stand and images are taken under full weight-bearing conditions. *(From Rankin, M.; Noyes, F. R.; Barber-Westin, S. D.; et al.: Human meniscus allografts' in vivo size and motion characteristics: magnetic resonance imaging assessment under weightbearing conditions. Am J Sports Med 34:98–107, 2006.)*

TABLE 29-1   Meniscus Allograft Classification*

Allograft Classification	Magnetic Resonance Imaging Evaluation (*N* = 29)				Clinical Examination: Tibiofemoral (*N* = 39)		Follow-up Arthroscopy (*N* =13)
	Peripheral Attachment	Position in Joint†	Signal Intensity		Meniscus Signs	Pain, Clinical Symptoms	Meniscus Tears
Normal	Healed	Normal (0%–25% of meniscus width)	None		None	None	None
Altered		Displacement (26%–50% of meniscus width)	Grades 1, 2			Mild pain, improved over preoperative	Partial meniscectomy (<⅓ removed)
Failed	Not healed	Major displacement (>50% of meniscus width)	Grade 3 (tearing, signal intensity extended to articular surface)		Obvious signs of meniscus tear	Definite pain, not improved over preoperative	Partial or total meniscectomy (>⅓ removed)

*One abnormal result = failed.
†Coronal and sagittal planes, percentage of displacement of posterior or medial plateau margin perpendicular to the joint line.
N, number of meniscus allografts.
From Noyes, F. R.; Barber-Westin, S. D.; Rankin, M.: Meniscal transplantation in symptomatic patients less than fifty years old. *J Bone Joint Surg Am* 86:1392-1404, 2004.

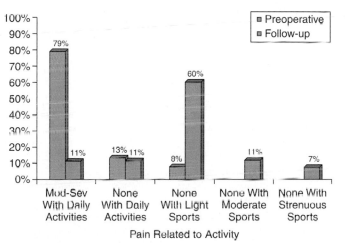

FIGURE 29-14. The pain scale shows the highest level of activity possible without the patient experiencing knee pain. The difference between preoperative and follow-up was statistically significant (*P* < .0001) Mod, moderate, Sev, severe. *(From Noyes, F. R., Barber-Westin, S. D.; Rankin, M.: Meniscal transplantation in symptomatic patients less than fifty years old. J Bone Joint Surg Am 86:1392-1404, 2004.)*

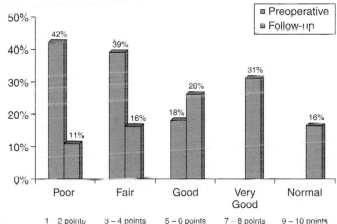

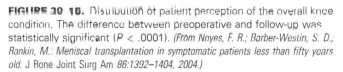

FIGURE 29-15. Distribution of patient perception of the overall knee condition. The difference between preoperative and follow-up was statistically significant (*P* < .0001). *(From Noyes, F. R.; Barber-Westin, S. D.; Rankin, M.: Meniscal transplantation in symptomatic patients less than fifty years old. J Bone Joint Surg Am 86:1392-1404, 2004.)*

Thirty-three of 35 patients (94%) stated their knee condition had improved on self-assessment ratings (Fig. 29–15). The mean preoperative patient perception score (scale, 1–10) of 3.1 points (range, 1–6 points) improved to a mean of 6.2 points (range, 1–9 points) at follow-up (Table 29–2; *P* < .0001). Preoperatively, only 1 patient was able to participate in sports without problems. At follow-up, 27 patients (77%) were participating in light, low-impact sports without problems and 1 patient was participating with symptoms against advice (Table 29–3).

Before the operation, 15 patients suffered symptoms and limitations during work activities (Table 29–4), whereas at follow-up, only 2 patients continued to have problems related to the knee condition at work.

One patient had signs of a meniscus transplant tear at follow-up. One patient had tibiofemoral joint line pain and increased palpable crepitation compared with the preoperative examination. All patients had a normal range of knee motion.

TABLE 29-2   Pain and Function Scores before and after Meniscal Transplantation

Factor/Scale	Preoperative*	Follow-up*	*P* Value†
Scale, 0–10 points			
Pain	2.5 ± 1.4	5.8 ± 2.2	.0001
Swelling	3.7 ± 2.6	5.8 ± 2.0	.0003
Full giving-way	5.8 ± 2.8	6.4 ± 2.0	NS
Scale, 1–10 points			
Patient perception	3.2 ± 1.3	6.2 ± 2.1	.0001
Scale, 0–40 points			
Walking	29 ± 9	37 ± 10	.0008
Stair-climbing	24 ± 12	30 + 14	.008
Squatting	10 ± 14	17 ± 16	.04
Scale, 40–100 points			
Running	44 ± 9	57 ± 22	.0001
Jumping	43 ± 7	51 ± 20	.01
Twisting/turning	43 ± 8	52 ± 19	.008

*Values shown are mean ± standard deviation.
†P value: paired t-test between preoperative and follow-up data.
NS, not significant.

TABLE 29–3 Sports Activity Levels of Patients before and after Meniscal Transplantation

Type of Sport	Preoperative (N)	Follow-up (N)
Jumping, hard pivoting, cutting	0	1
Running, twisting, turning	0	4
Swimming, bicycling	7	24
None	31	9
Change in sports activities		
Increased level, no symptoms	0	25
Same level, no symptoms	0	2
Decreased level, no symptoms	1	1
Playing with symptoms	6	1
No sports, knee-related reasons	31	8
No sports, non–knee-related reasons	0	1

TABLE 29–4 Occupational Levels of Patients before and after Meniscal Transplantation

Occupational Level	Preoperative (N)	Follow-up (N)
Disabled	5	3
Very light/light	12	21
Moderate	2	1
Heavy/very heavy	4	5
Student/homemaker	15	8
Change in occupational level		
Increased level, no symptoms	0	5
Same level, no symptoms	2	15
Decreased level, no symptoms	1	5
Working with symptoms	15	2
No work, knee-related reasons	5	3
No work, non–knee-related reasons	15	8

TABLE 29–5 Results of Magnetic Resonance Imaging Studies of 29 Meniscus Allografts

Structure	Imaging Plane	Height*	Width*	Displacement*
Posterior horn	Sagittal	7.7 ± 1.9	10.4 ± 2.6	1.1 ± 2.0
Anterior horn	Sagittal	7.1 ± 1.4	10.1 ± 1.8	1.2 ± 1.7
Allograft midbody	Coronal	7.8 ± 1.9	11.7 ± 3.7	2.2 ± 1.5

*All data are in millimeters, mean ± standard deviation.

the meniscus transplant for unresolved knee pain. With the 6 patients described previously and the 4 meniscus transplants that required removal early postoperatively, the reoperation rate for meniscal transplant symptoms was 25% (10 of 40 meniscus transplants).

The mean displacement of the 29 meniscus transplants examined with MRI was 2.2 ± 1.5 mm (range, 0–5 mm) in the coronal plane (Table 29–5). Seventeen transplants (59%) had no displacement, 11 had minor displacement, and 1 could not be evaluated.

In the sagittal plane, the mean displacement of the posterior horn of the transplants was 1.1 ± 2.0 mm (range, 0–9 mm). Twenty-five transplants (86%) had no displacement of the posterior horn, 3 had minor displacement, and 1 had major displacement (9 mm). The mean displacement of the anterior horn of the transplants was 1.2 ± 1.7 mm (range, 0–6 mm). Twenty-five transplants had no displacement of the anterior horn, 3 had minor displacement, and 1 had major displacement (6 mm). Intrameniscal signal intensity was normal in 1, grade 1 in 13, grade 2 in 11, grade 3 in 3, and could not be evaluated in 1.

In the subgroup of 8 transplants examined with the standing full weight-bearing MRI protocol, the mean height and width of the anterior and posterior horns of the transplants were similar to those of native menisci (Table 29–6). The millimeters of coronal displacement of motion of the midbody was also similar between the transplants and the native menisci. The anterior horn of the native medial menisci moved an average of 5 mm more (total anterior-to-posterior translation, $P < .05$) than the transplants. The posterior horn of the native medial menisci and both horns of the native lateral menisci also tended to move more than the corresponding horns of the transplanted menisci (Fig. 29–16), although this could not be confirmed statistically, given the number of menisci studied.

All knees that had an ACL reconstruction had normal or nearly normal anterior stability restored except 1 in which the reconstruction failed. The PCL reconstructions restored nearly normal function in both knees at 20° and 90° of flexion, except for 1 knee in which partial function was restored at 90° of flexion.

Five patients had follow-up arthroscopy for symptoms related to the transplant. In 3 patients, tears in the periphery of the meniscus transplant at the capsular junction were successfully repaired. In 2 patients, small tears in the transplant were resected. None of these patients had further complaints. One other patient had a total knee replacement 35 months after

TABLE 29–6 Height and Width Measurements of Eight Meniscus Allografts and Native Menisci* in the Sagittal Plane

Knee Flexion Angle	Height (mm)				Width (mm)			
	Posterior Horn		Anterior Horn		Posterior Horn		Anterior Horn	
	Allograft	Native	Allograft	Native	Allograft	Native	Allograft	Native
0°	8 ± 3	9 ± 3	7 ± 1	6 ± 1	14 ± 3	15 ± 2	12 ± 3	13 ± 2
30°	8 ± 2	7 ± 2	8 ± 1	6 ± 1	15 ± 1	15 ± 2	14 ± 4	14 ± 1
60°	8 ± 1	7 ± 1	8 ± 1	7 ± 1	14 ± 2	15 ± 2	15 ± 3	14 ± 2
90°	8 ± 1	8 ± 1	7 ± 2	8 ± 2	14 ± 3	15 ± 1	14 ± 4	14 ± 2
Change from 0°–90°	0.4 ± 2.1	0.4 ± 3.6	0.5 ± 1.5	2 ± 2	0 ± 3	−0.5 ± 1.9	1.9 ± 3.4	1.3 ± 2.7

*Medial and lateral menisci combined. Data are given as mean ± standard deviation.

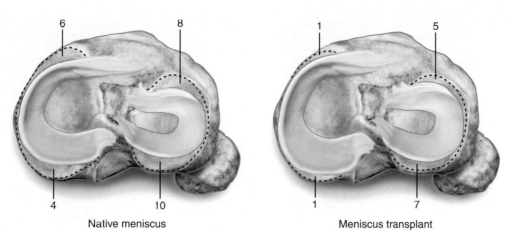

Native meniscus   Meniscus transplant

FIGURE 29–16. Illustrations in the axial plane of the native and transplanted menisci, approximating the pattern of meniscal displacement from full extension to 90° of flexion (*slashed lines*). These are not to scale. *(From Rankin, M.; Noyes, F. R.; Barber-Westin, S. D.; et al.: Human meniscus allografts' in vivo size and motion characteristics: magnetic resonance imaging assessment under weightbearing conditions. Am J Sports Med 34:98–107, 2006.)*

Seventeen of the meniscus transplants (42.5%) had normal characteristics, 12 (30%) had altered characteristics, and 11 (27.5%) failed. Of the 20 lateral menisci transplants, 9 had normal characteristics, 7 had altered characteristics, and 4 failed. Of the 20 MMTs, 8 had normal characteristics, 5 had altered characteristics, and 7 failed.

There was a correlation between the arthritis rating on MRI and the transplant characteristics ($P = .01$). Of the 16 transplants in knees with mild arthritis, 10 had normal characteristics and 6 had altered characteristics. Of the 12 transplants in knees with moderate arthritis, 3 had normal characteristics, 4 had altered characteristics, and 5 failed.

Irradiated Meniscus Transplantation

The results of 96 consecutive irradiated meniscus transplants implanted into 82 patients were previously described.[36] Twenty-eight menisci in 27 patients required early arthroscopic resection owing to lack of meniscal healing a mean of 10 months (range, 2–20 mo) postoperatively. These 28 menisci were included in the overall failure rate. In addition, 1 patient died of causes unrelated to the knee condition prior to the 2-year follow-up. This left 67 menisci (57 medial, 10 lateral) in 62 patients (63 knees) who all returned for follow-up a mean of 44 months postoperatively (range, 22–111 mo).

The patients were divided into three groups for analysis of the meniscus transplant. Group 1 had normal to mild articular cartilage arthritis on MRI, group 2 had moderate arthritis, and group 3 had severe arthritis. The meniscus transplant failure rate was 6% (1 of 18 knees) in knees with normal or only mild arthritis on MRI, 45% (14 of 31 knees) in knees with moderate arthritis, and 80% (12 of 15 knees) in knees with advanced arthritis (Fig. 29–17). The relationship between the meniscus transplant failure rate and increasing severity of joint arthritis was significant ($P < .001$).

Histologic evaluations were conducted by independent examiners on the 28 meniscus allografts that failed early postoperatively. Nine specimens (5 medial, 4 lateral) that included the peripheral meniscal-capsular junction and an intact meniscal body were critically analyzed (Fig. 29–18). These allografts had been removed a mean of 11 months (range, 2–21 mo) postoperatively and the tibiofemoral and inner-outer orientations were easily identifiable. There was no evidence of a cellular reaction suggestive of a rejection phenomenon in any of the tissues examined. The specimens consistently demonstrated minimal, if any, cellular repopulation of the femoral and tibial surfaces or central core of the meniscus (Fig. 29–19A and B). The predominant cell type was a fibrocyte (see Fig. 29–19C). Remodeling with abnormal collagen orientation was found in 6 specimens. The remodeling phenomenon resulted in a loss of the normal surface radial collagen architecture and a loss of the normal circumferential fibers within the meniscal substance (see Fig. 29–19D).

The role of low-dose irradiation (2.0–2.5 Mrads) in terms of increasing the failure rate is not scientifically known at this time in meniscus allografts. This study provided needed information on patient selection criteria for meniscus transplants. Patients with advanced arthritis or alterations in joint geometry (major tibial concavity, femoral condyle flattening) with exposed bone surfaces over the majority of the tibiofemoral compartment are not candidates for meniscus transplantation.

Critical Points AUTHORS' CLINICAL STUDIES: IRRADIATED MENISCUS TRANSPLANTS

- $N = 96$ irradiated transplants in 82 patients followed mean 44 mo (range, 22–111 mo).
- Average 8.5 yr from injury to transplant.
- Staged or concurrent anterior cruciate ligament reconstructions done in 81%.
- 92% knees had abnormal articular cartilage surfaces.
- 95% meniscus transplants assessed with MRI 18–54 mo postoperative.
- Meniscus transplant characteristics determined with classification system: MRI, clinical examination, follow-up arthroscopy (when performed)
- Correlation MRI arthrosis rating and transplant failure rate
  ○ No/mild arthrosis: 6%.
  ○ Moderate arthrosis: 45%.
  ○ Advanced arthrosis: 80%.

MRI, magnetic resonance imaging.

FIGURE 29–17. Distribution of meniscus transplants rated on magnetic resonance imaging as normal, altered, and failed for the authors' clinical investigations.

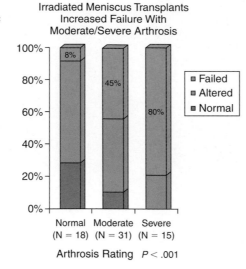

Irradiated Meniscus Transplants
Increased Failure With
Moderate/Severe Arthrosis

Arthrosis Rating $P < .001$

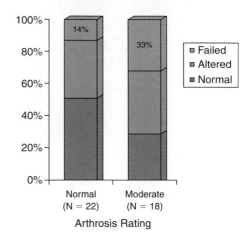

Cryopreserved Meniscus Transplants
(Excluded Severe Arthrosis)

Arthrosis Rating

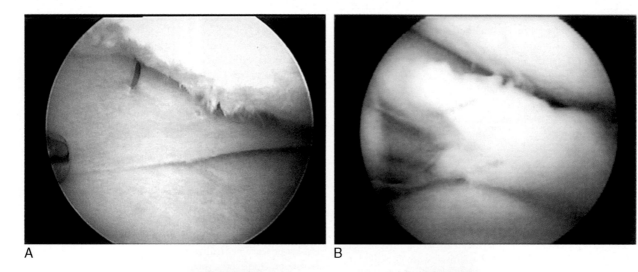

A   B

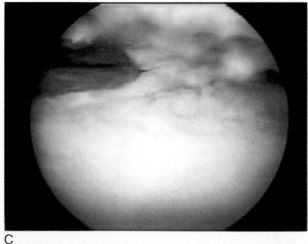

C

FIGURE 29–18. A, Irradiated medial meniscus–bone transplant upon initial implantation. **B** and **C,** At follow-up arthroscopy 7 months later, the medial meniscus transplant had torn and failed and was removed. This case was included in the histologic assessment of failed meniscus transplants.

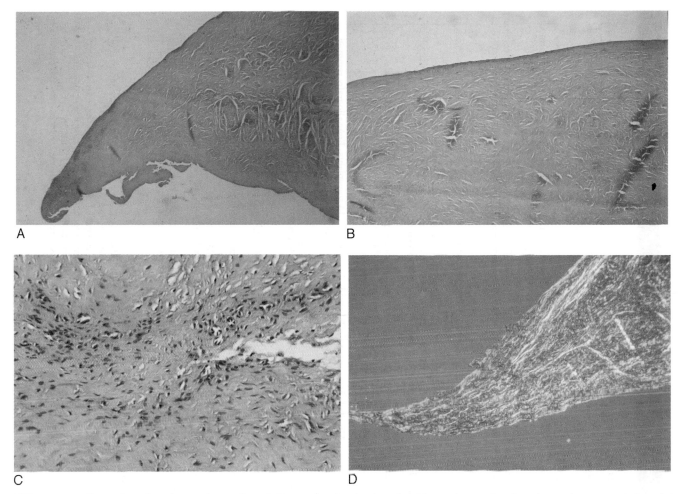

FIGURE 29-19. Coronal section of a meniscus allograft 17 months after implantation. Photomicrographs show incomplete repopulation of the femoral surface (**A**, 40x), and the remaining tissue is acellular (**B**, 40x), with some cells resembling fibrochondrocytes (**C**, 200x) **D**, Polarized light micrograph shows fibers aligned parallel to the surface, with poorly organized collagen fibers at the remodeling site. There is a loss of normal radial and circumferential collagen orientation in the body of the allograft, which has not undergone remodeling (40x).

RESULTS FROM OTHER CLINICAL STUDIES

Since 1984, over 30 clinical investigations have reported results of meniscus transplant surgery (Table 29-7).* Differences in tissue processing, secondary sterilization, preservation, operative technique, and rating schemes make comparisons between studies difficult, and others have performed lengthy reviews of these investigations.[10,27,49]

Other studies of cryopreserved meniscus transplants reveal an approximate failure rate of 30%. Stollsteimer and coworkers[60] followed 23 patients who had cryopreserved meniscal transplants 13 to 69 months postoperatively. Eight patients (35%) required a second operation for meniscal symptoms 5 to 28 months postoperatively. Although good pain relief was obtained in 18 knees, MRI in 12 knees showed some shrinkage of the transplants in that the transplants were an average of 63% the size of the contralateral normal menisci. No or only minimal transplant displacement was detected, and minor signal abnormalities were present in 5 knees.

Rath and associates[48] followed 22 cryopreserved meniscal transplants for 2 to 8 years postoperatively. Concomitant ACL reconstructions were done in 11 of the 18 patients. Eight menisci (36%) failed and were removed an average of 31 months postimplantation. Even so, all patients except 1 had significant improvements in Short-Form 36-item questionnaire (SF-36) scores. Histologic analysis of the torn transplants demonstrated greater than a 50% reduction in the number of meniscal fibrochondrocytes at the periphery compared with torn native menisci. Hommen and colleagues[22] followed 20 cryopreserved meniscus transplants for 9 to 13 years postoperatively and reported a 10-year survival rate of only 45%. The failures were identified from low Lysholm scores (<65 points), no improvement in pain, MRI, and second-look arthroscopy data.

van Arkel and coworkers[66] reported on the results of 19 cryopreserved meniscus transplants followed 14 to 55 months postoperatively with MRI, arthroscopy, and clinical examination. The authors reported 16 transplants were successful and 3 failed based on clinical findings. However, MRI criteria revealed 8 failures because 4 transplants had severe shrinkage and 4 transplants had moderate shrinkage. None of the transplants were in a normal position; 11 showed subextrusion, 6 demonstrated extrusion, and 2 had bucket-handle–like appearances. The authors did not

*See references 8, 11–13, 18–20, 22, 24, 26, 30–32, 34, 46, 48, 51, 54, 55, 59, 60, 62, 64, 66, 69–71, 73, 75–79.

and a normal range of knee motion. She rated the overall condition of her knee as good despite the lateral tibiofemoral arthritis.

Case 4. A 32-year-old woman presented with left knee medial tibiofemoral pain, locking, and instability with daily activities of 6 months' duration. She had undergone a medial meniscectomy 17 years previously and an ACL allograft reconstruction 7 years before her initial evaluation. Physical examination demonstrated

15 mm of increased anterior-to-posterior displacement compared with the contralateral knee on KT-2000 testing, no other ligament deficiencies, a marked varus recurvatum deformity, and a hyperextension gait abnormality. Full standing radiographs showed a weight-bearing line of 19%, a mechanical axis of 5° varus, and moderate narrowing of the medial tibiofemoral compartment (Fig. 29–23A). MRI demonstrated advanced articular cartilage deterioration in the medial tibiofemoral compartment. Owing

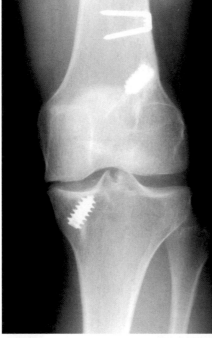

A

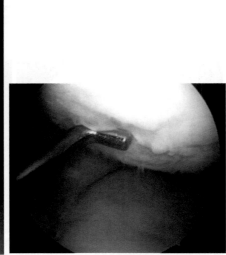

B

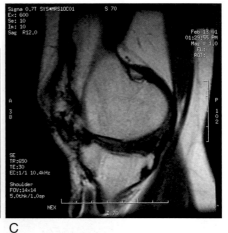

C

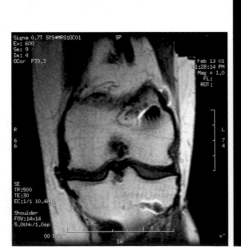

D

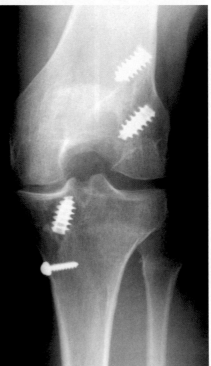

E

FIGURE 29–23. Case 4.

to the patient's age, she was not considered a candidate for a unicompartmental knee replacement. The treatment recommendation was to first correct the lower limb varus malalignment and then perform meniscus transplantation and ACL revision. The patient underwent a gait-retraining program (see Chapter 34, Correction of Hyperextension Gait Abnormalities: Preoperative and Postoperative Techniques) to correct the hyperextension abnormality before proceeding to HTO.

A closing wedge osteotomy was performed, with a small 12- to 15-mm area of grade 3A articular cartilage deterioration noted in the medial tibiofemoral compartment at the time of surgery (see Fig. 29–23B). Four months later, an MMT and osteochondral autograft transfer of the medial femoral condyle were performed. An ACL patellar tendon autogenous revision reconstruction was done 3 months later, along with removal of hardware from the osteotomy.

At the most recent follow-up evaluation, 5.5 years posttransplantation, the patient had no symptoms or limitations with daily activities. She rated the overall condition of her knee as good and had no problems with her occupation in engineering. MRI

showed an intact meniscus transplant (see Fig. 29–23C and D), still in position in the tibiofemoral joint. There was increased signal intensity noted, and some extrusion of the implant. Standing PA radiographs showed no progression of loss of the medial tibiofemoral joint space (see Fig. 29–23E). She had no increase in anterior tibial translation, a negative pivot shift test, and a normal range of knee motion.

Case 5. A 16-year-old female presented 3 years after a right lateral meniscectomy for a symptomatic discoid meniscus. She complained of pain and swelling with all sports activities of 6 months' duration. Her walking tolerance was 1 hour and she was unable to kneel or squat. Physical examination revealed a normal range of knee motion, no ligament deficiencies, moderate pain and crepitation in the lateral tibiofemoral compartment, and an overall valgus alignment. Arthroscopic examination conducted elsewhere 5 months earlier revealed noteworthy articular cartilage deterioration on the lateral tibial plateau. Owing to the patient's young age and rapid deterioration of the lateral compartment (Fig. 29–24A), she was treated with an LMT (see Fig. 29–24B). In

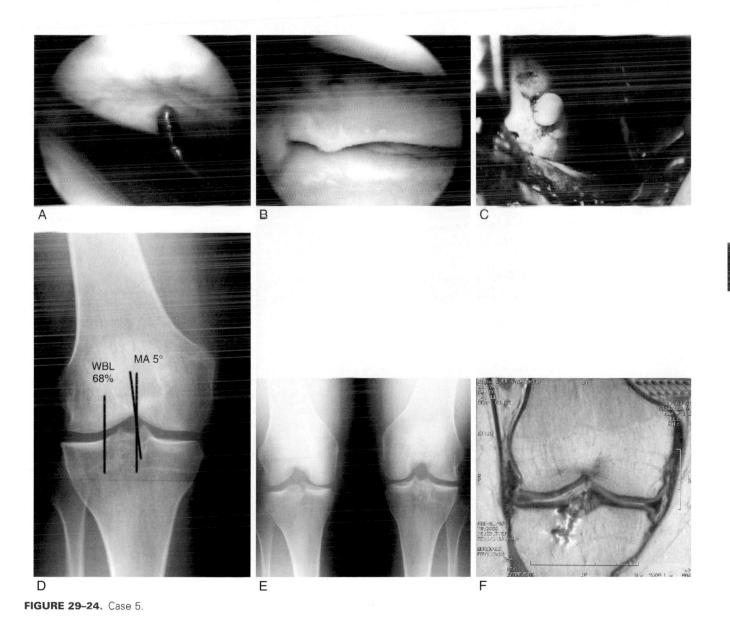

FIGURE 29–24. Case 5.

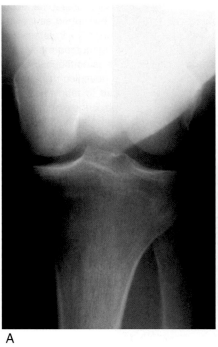

A

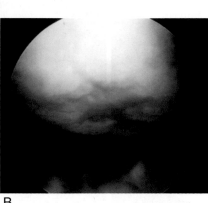

B

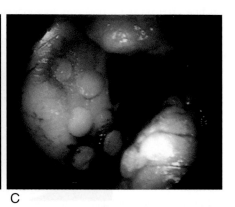

C

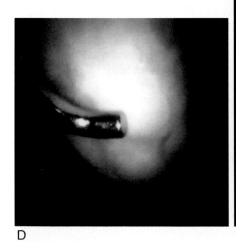

D

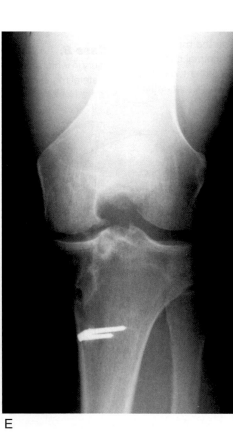

E

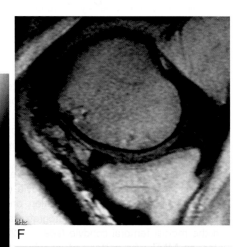

F

G

FIGURE 29–26. Case 7.

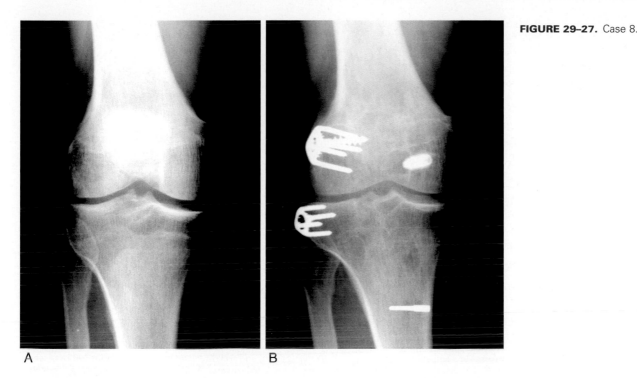

FIGURE 29–27. Case 8.

A   B

REFERENCES

1. Alhalki, M. M.; Howell, S. M.; Hull, M. L.: How three methods for fixing a medial meniscus autograft affect tibial contact mechanics. *Am J Sports Med* 27:320–328, 1999.
2. Alhalki, M. M.; Hull, M. L.; Howell, S. M.: Contact mechanics of the medial tibial plateau after implantation of a medial meniscal allograft. A human cadaveric study. *Am J Sports Med* 28:370–376, 2000.
3. Arnoczky, S. P.; DiCarlo, E. F.; O'Brien, S. J.; Warren, R. F.: Cellular repopulation of deep frozen meniscal autografts: an experimental study in the dog. *Arthroscopy* 8:428–436, 1992.
4. Barbour Wurtin, G. D.; Noyes, F. R.; McCloskey, J. W.: Rigorous statistical reliability, validity, and responsiveness testing of the Cincinnati Knee Rating System in 350 subjects with uninjured, injured, or anterior cruciate ligament–reconstructed knees. *Am J Sports Med* 27:402–416, 1999.
5. Barbour, S. A.; King, W.: The safe and effective use of allograft tissue–an update. *Am J Sports Med* 31:791–797, 2003.
6. Berlet, G. C.; Fowler, P. J.: The anterior horn of the medial meniscus. An anatomic study of its insertion. *Am J Sports Med* 26:540–543, 1998.
7. Bylski-Austrow, D. I.; Malumed, J.; Meade, T.; Grood, E. S.: Knee joint contact pressure decreases after chronic meniscectomy relative to the acutely meniscectomized joint: a mechanical study in the goat. *J Orthop Res* 11:796–804, 1993.
8. Cameron, J. C.; Saha, S.: Meniscal allograft transplantation for unicompartmental arthritis of the knee. *Clin Orthop Relat Res* 337:164–171, 1997.
9. Chen, M. I.; Branch, T. P.; Hutton, W. C.: Is it important to secure the horns during lateral meniscal transplantation? A cadaveric study. *Arthroscopy* 12:174–181, 1996.
10. Cole, B. J.; Carter, T. R.; Rodeo, S. A.: Allograft meniscal transplantation. Background, techniques, and results. *J Bone Joint Surg Am* 84:1236–1250, 2002.
11. Cole, B. J.; Dennis, M. G.; Lee, S. J.; et al.: Prospective evaluation of allograft meniscus transplantation: a minimum 2-year follow-up. *Am J Sports Med* 34:919–927, 2006.
12. De Boer, H. H.; and Koudstaal, J.: Failed meniscal transplantation. A report of three cases. *Clin Orthop Relat Res* 306:155–162, 1994.
13. De Boer, H. H.; Koudstaal, J.: The fate of meniscus cartilage after transplantation of cryopreserved nontissue-antigen–matched allograft. A case report. *Clin Orthop Relat Res* 266:145–151, 1991.
14. Dienst, M.; Greis, P. E.; Ellis, B. J.; et al.: Effect of lateral meniscal allograft sizing on contact mechanics of the lateral tibial plateau: an experimental study in human cadaveric knee joints. *Am J Sports Med* 35:34–42, 2007.
15. Donahue, T. L.; Hull, M. L.; Howell, S. M.: New algorithm for selecting meniscal allografts that best match the size and shape of the damaged meniscus. *J Orthop Res* 24:1535–1543, 2006.
16. Dugdale, T. W.; Noyes, F. R.; Styer, D.: Preoperative planning for high tibial osteotomy: the effect of lateral tibiofemoral separation and tibiofemoral length. *Clin Orthop Relat Res* 274:248–264, 1992.
17. Farr, J.; Meneghini, R. M.; Cole, B. J.: Allograft interference screw fixation in meniscus transplantation. *Arthroscopy* 20:322–327, 2004.
18. Farr, J.; Rawal, A.; Marberry, K. M.: Concomitant meniscal allograft transplantation and autologous chondrocyte implantation: minimum 2-year follow-up. *Am J Sports Med* 35:1459–1466, 2007.
19. Garrett, J. C.: Meniscal transplantation: a review of 43 cases with 2- to 7-year follow-up. *Sports Med Arthrosc Rev* 1:164–167, 1993.
20. Graf, K. W., Jr.; Sekiya, J. K.; Wojtys, E. M.: Long-term results after combined medial meniscal allograft transplantation and anterior cruciate ligament reconstruction: minimum 8.5-year follow-up study. *Arthroscopy* 20:129–140, 2004.
21. Haut, T. L.; Hull, M. L.; Howell, S. M.: Use of roentgenography and magnetic resonance imaging to predict meniscal geometry determined with a three-dimensional coordinate digitizing system. *J Orthop Res* 18:228–237, 2000.
22. Hommen, J. P.; Applegate, G. R.; Del Pizzo, W.: Meniscus allograft transplantation: ten-year results of cryopreserved allografts. *Arthroscopy* 23:388–393, 2007.
23. Jackson, D. W.; Simon, T. M.: Biology of meniscal allograft. In Mow, V. C.; Arnoczky, S. P.; Jackson, D. W. (eds.): *Knee Meniscus: Basic and Clinical Foundations.* New York: Raven, 1992; pp. 141–152.
24. Keene, G. C.; Paterson, R. S.; Teague, D. C.: Advances in arthroscopic surgery. *Clin Orthop Relat Res* 224:64–70, 1987.
25. Kelly, B. T.; Potter, H. G.; Deng, X. H.; et al.: Meniscal allograft transplantation in the sheep knee: evaluation of chondroprotective effects. *Am J Sports Med* 34:1464–1477, 2006.
26. Locht, R. C.; Gross, A. E.; Langer, R.: Late osteochondral allograft resurfacing for tibial plateau fractures. *J Bone Joint Surgery Am* 66:328–335, 1984.
27. Matava, M. J.: Meniscal allograft transplantation: a systematic review. *Clin Orthop Relat Res* 455:142–257, 2007.

28. McDermott, I. D.; Lie, D. T.; Edwards, A.; et al.: The effects of lateral meniscal allograft transplantation techniques on tibio-femoral contact pressures. *Knee Surg Sports Traumatol Arthrosc* 16:553–560, 2008.

29. McLaughlin, J. R.; Noyes, F. R.: Arthroscopic meniscus repair: Recommended surgical techniques for complex meniscal tears. *Tech Orthop* 8:129–136, 1993.

30. Meyers, M. H.; Akeson, W.; Convery, F. R.: Resurfacing of the knee with fresh osteochondral allograft. *J Bone Joint Surg Am* 71:704–713, 1989.

31. Milachowski, K. A.; Weismeier, K.; Wirth, C. J.: Homologous meniscus transplantation. *Int Orthop* 13:1–11, 1989.

32. Milachowski, K. A.; Weismeier, K.; Wirth, C. J.; Kohn, D.: Meniscus transplantation—experimental study and first clinical report. *Am J Sports Med* 15:626, 1987.

33. Noyes, F. R.; Barber-Westin, S.: Posterior cruciate ligament replacement with a two-strand quadriceps tendon–patellar bone autograft and a tibial inlay technique. *J Bone Joint Surg Am* 87:1241–1252, 2005.

34. Noyes, F. R.; Barber-Westin, S. D.: Irradiated meniscus allografts in the human knee. A two- to five-year follow-up study. *Orthop Trans* 19:417, 1995.

35. Noyes, F. R.; Barber-Westin, S. D.: Meniscus transplantation: indications, techniques, clinical outcomes. *Instr Course Lect* 54:341–353, 2005.

36. Noyes, F. R.; Barber-Westin, S. D.; Butler, D. L.; Wilkins, R. M.: The role of allografts in repair and reconstruction of knee joint ligaments and menisci. *Instr Course Lect* 47:379–396, 1998.

37. Noyes, F. R.; Barber-Westin, S. D.; Rankin, M.: Meniscal transplantation in symptomatic patients less than fifty years old. *J Bone Joint Surg Am* 86:1392–1404, 2004.

38. Noyes, F. R.; Barber-Westin, S. D.; Rankin, M.: Meniscal transplantation in symptomatic patients less than fifty years old: surgical technique. *J Bone Joint Surg Am* 87(suppl 1[pt 2]):149–165, 2005.

39. Noyes, F. R.; Stabler, C. L.: A system for grading articular cartilage lesions at arthroscopy. *Am J Sports Med* 17:505–513, 1989.

40. Outerbridge, R. E.: The etiology of chondromalacia patellae. *J Bone Joint Surg Br* 43:752–757, 1961.

41. Paletta, G. A.; Manning, T.; Snell, E.; et al.: The effect of allograft meniscal replacement on intra-articular contact area and pressures in the human knee. A biomechanical study. *Am J Sports Med* 25:692–698, 1997.

42. Pena, E.; Calvo, B.; Martinez, M. A.; et al.: Finite element analysis of the effect of meniscal tears and meniscectomies on human knee biomechanics. *Clin Biomech (Bristol, Avon)* 20:498–507, 2005.

43. Pollard, M. E.; Kang, Q.; Berg, E. E.: Radiographic sizing for meniscal transplantation. *Arthroscopy* 11:684–687, 1995.

44. Potter, H. G.; Foo, L. F.: Magnetic resonance imaging of articular cartilage: trauma, degeneration, and repair. *Am J Sports Med* 34:661–677, 2006.

45. Potter, H. G.; Linklater, J. M.; Allen, A. A.; et al.: Magnetic resonance imaging of articular cartilage in the knee. An evaluation with use of fast-spin-echo imaging. *J Bone Joint Surg Am* 80:1276–1284, 1998.

46. Potter, H. G.; Rodeo, S. A.; Wickiewicz, T. L.; Warren, R. F.: Imaging of meniscal allografts: correlation with clinical and arthroscopic outcomes. *Radiology* 198:509–514, 1996.

47. Rankin, M.; Noyes, F. R.; Barber-Westin, S. D.; et al.: Human meniscus allografts' in vivo size and motion characteristics: magnetic resonance imaging assessment under weightbearing conditions. *Am J Sports Med* 34:98–107, 2006.

48. Rath, E.; Richmond, J. C.; Yassir, W.; et al.: Meniscal allograft transplantation. Two- to eight-year results. *Am J Sports Med* 29:410–414, 2001.

49. Rodeo, S. A.: Meniscal allografts—where do we stand? *Am J Sports Med* 29:246–261, 2001.

50. Rosenberg, T. D.; Paulos, L. E.; Parker, R. D.; et al.: The forty-five-degree posteroanterior flexion weight-bearing radiograph of the knee. *J Bone Joint Surg Am* 70:1479–1483, 1988.

51. Rubins, D.; Barrett, J. P.; Hayter, R.: Arthroscopic meniscal allograft transplantation. *Arthroscopy* 9:356–357, 1993.

52. Rubman, M. H.; Noyes, F. R.; Barber-Westin, S. D.: Arthroscopic repair of meniscal tears that extend into the avascular zone. A review of 198 single and complex tears. *Am J Sports Med* 26:87–95, 1998.

53. Rubman, M. H.; Noyes, F. R.; Barber-Westin, S. D.: Technical considerations in the management of complex meniscus tears. *Clin Sports Med* 15:511–530, 1996.

54. Rueff, D.; Nyland, J.; Kocabey, Y.; et al.: Self-reported patient outcomes at a minimum of 5 years after allograft anterior cruciate ligament reconstruction with or without medial meniscus transplantation: an age-, sex-, and activity level–matched comparison in patients aged approximately 50 years. *Arthroscopy* 22:1053–1062, 2006.

55. Ryu, R. K.; Dunbar, V. W.; Morse, G. G.: Meniscal allograft replacement: a 1-year to 6-year experience. *Arthroscopy* 18:989–994, 2002.

56. Sekaran, S. V.; Hull, M. L.; Howell, S. M.: Nonanatomic location of the posterior horn of a medial meniscal autograft implanted in a cadaveric knee adversely affects the pressure distribution on the tibial plateau. *Am J Sports Med* 30:74–82, 2002.

57. Sekiya, J. K.; Giffin, J. R.; Irrgang, J. J.; et al.: Clinical outcomes after combined meniscal allograft transplantation and anterior cruciate ligament reconstruction. *Am J Sports Med* 31:896–906, 2003.

58. Shaffer, B.; Kennedy, S.; Klimkiewicz, J.; Yao, L.: Preoperative sizing of meniscal allografts in meniscus transplantation. *Am J Sports Med* 28:524–533, 2000.

59. Shelton, W. R.: Meniscal allotransplantation: an arthroscopically assisted technique. *Arthroscopy* 9:361, 1993.

60. Stollsteimer, G. T.; Shelton, W. R.; Dukes, A.; Bomboy, A. L.: Meniscal allograft transplantation: a 1- to 5-year follow-up of 22 patients. *Arthroscopy* 16:343–347, 2000.

61. Stone, K. R.; Freyer, A.; Turek, T.; et al.: Meniscal sizing based on gender, height, and weight. *Arthroscopy* 23:503–508, 2007.

62. Stone, K. R.; Walgenbach, A. W.; Turek, T. J.; et al.: Meniscus allograft survival in patients with moderate to severe unicompartmental arthritis: a 2- to 7-year follow-up. *Arthroscopy* 22:469–478, 2006.

63. Szomor, Z. L.; Martin, T. E.; Bonar, F.; Murrell, G. A.: The protective effects of meniscal transplantation on cartilage. An experimental study in sheep. *J Bone Joint Surg Am* 82:80–88, 2000.

64. van Arkel, E. R.; de Boer, H. H.: Survival analysis of human meniscal transplantations. *J Bone Joint Surg Br* 84:227–231, 2002.

65. van Arkel, E. R. A.; De Boer, H. H.: Human meniscal transplantation. Preliminary results at 2- to 5-year follow-up. *J Bone Joint Surg Br* 77:589–595, 1995.

66. van Arkel, E. R. A.; Goei, R.; de Ploeg, I.; de Boer, H. H.: Meniscal allografts: evaluation with magnetic resonance imaging and correlation with arthroscopy. *Arthroscopy* 16:517–521, 2000.

67. Vangsness, C. T., Jr.; Garcia, I. A.; Mills, C. R.; et al.: Allograft transplantation in the knee: tissue regulation, procurement, processing, and sterilization. *Am J Sports Med* 31:474–481, 2003.

68. Vedi, V.; Williams, A.; Tennant, S. J.; et al.: Meniscal movement. An in-vivo study using dynamic MRI. *J Bone Joint Surg Br* 81:37–41, 1999.

69. Veltri, D. M.; Warren, R. F.; Wickiewicz, T. L.; O'Brien, S. J.: Current status of allograft meniscal transplantation. *Clin Orthop Relat Res* 303:44–55, 1994.

70. Verdonk, P. C.; Demurie, A.; Almqvist, K. F.; et al.: Transplantation of viable meniscal allograft. Survivorship analysis and clinical outcome of one hundred cases. *J Bone Joint Surg Am* 87:715–724, 2005.

71. Verdonk, P. C.; Verstraete, K. L.; Almqvist, K. F.; et al.: Meniscal allograft transplantation: long-term clinical results with radiological and magnetic resonance imaging correlations. *Knee Surg Sports Traumatol Arthrosc* 14:694–706, 2006.

72. Verma, N. N.; Kolb, E.; Cole, B. J.; et al.: The effects of medial meniscal transplantation techniques on intra-articular contact pressures. *J Knee Surg* 21:20–26, 2008.

73. von Lewinski, G.; Milachowski, K. A.; Weismeier, K.; et al.: Twenty-year results of combined meniscal allograft transplantation, anterior cruciate ligament reconstruction and advancement of the medial collateral ligament. *Knee Surg Sports Traumatol Arthrosc* 15:1072–1082, 2007.

74. Wilson, W.; van Rietbergen, B.; van Donkelaar, C. C.; Huiskes, R.: Pathways of load-induced cartilage damage causing cartilage degeneration in the knee after meniscectomy. *J Biomech* 36:845–851, 2003.

75. Wirth, C. J.; Peters, G.; Milachowski, K. A.; et al.: Long-term results of meniscal allograft transplantation. *Am J Sports Med* 30:174–181, 2002.

76. Wojtys, E. M.; Carpenter, J. E.: Meniscal replacement—early experience. *Arthroscopy* 10:337, 1994.

77. Yoldas, E. A.; Sekiya, J. K.; Irrgang, J. J.; et al.: Arthroscopically assisted meniscal allograft transplantation with and without combined anterior cruciate ligament reconstruction. *Knee Surg Sports Traumatol Arthrosc* 11:173–182, 2003.

78. Zukor, D.; Brooks, P.; Gross, A.; Cameron, J.: Meniscal allografts—experimental and clinical study. *Orthop Rev* 17:522, 1988.

79. Zukor, D. J.; Cameron, J. C.; Brooks, P. J.; et al.: The fate of human meniscal allografts. In Ewing, J. W. (ed.): *Articular Cartilage and Knee Joint Function: Basic Science and Arthroscopy.* New York: Raven, 1990; pp. 147–152.

Chapter 30

Rehabilitation of Meniscus Repair and Transplantation Procedures

Timothy P. Heckmann, PT, ATC ■ *Frank R. Noyes*, MD ■ *Sue D. Barber-Westin*, BS

CLINICAL CONCEPTS

The postoperative program for meniscus repair and transplantation is shown in Table 30–1. The initial goal is to prevent excessive weight-bearing, because high compressive and shear forces can disrupt healing meniscus repair sites (especially radial repairs) and transplants. Variations are built into the protocol according to the type, location, and size of the meniscus repair and whether concomitant procedures (such as ligament reconstructions) are performed. The surgeon has the responsibility to inform the physical therapy team of details regarding the type of tear and the repair that was performed. Meniscus repairs with

Critical Points CLINICAL CONCEPTS

Initial rehabilitation goal: prevent excessive compressive and shear forces through limited weight-bearing.

General Postoperative Healing Expectations

• Rapid healing of peripheral meniscus repairs
• Delayed healing of complex meniscus repairs in middle third region
• Further delayed healing of meniscus transplants (1–2 yr)

Preoperative patient counseling and education entire rehabilitation program are paramount.

Premature return to high-impact loading activities (jogging, deep knee flexion, pivoting) risks repeat meniscus tear or tear to transplant.

Obtain lateral and anteroposterior x-rays 1 and 6 wk after meniscus transplantation to verify position of osseous component.

all-inside fixators have inferior holding strength, and commonly, only a few sutures are used. These repairs require more protection to allow for healing during the first 6 postoperative weeks. Inside-out meniscus repair techniques involve multiple vertical divergent sutures (see Chapter 28, Meniscus Tears: Diagnosis, Operative Techniques, and Clinical Outcomes) and have superior holding strength.

Clinicians should be aware that meniscus repairs located in the periphery (outer third region) heal rapidly, whereas complex repairs that extend into the central third region tend to heal more slowly and require greater caution. In addition, modifications to the postoperative exercise program may be required if noteworthy articular cartilage deterioration is found during the arthroscopic procedure. This rehabilitation program has been used at the authors' institution in hundreds of meniscus transplant and repair recipients, and the results of clinical investigations[3–5,7] demonstrate its safety and effectiveness in restoring normal knee motion, muscle, and gait characteristics.

Patients receive instructions before surgery regarding the postoperative protocol so they have a thorough understanding of what is expected after surgery. Patients are warned that an early return to strenuous activities including impact loading, jogging, deep knee flexion, or pivoting carries a definite risk of a repeat meniscus tear or tear to the transplant. This is particularly true in the first 4 to 6 months postoperatively.

The supervised rehabilitation program is supplemented with home exercises that are performed daily. The therapist routinely examines the patient in the clinic in order to implement and progress the appropriate protocol. Therapeutic procedures and modalities are used as required for successful rehabilitation.

TABLE 30–1   Rehabilitation Protocol Summary for Meniscus Repairs and Transplants

	Postoperative Weeks					Postoperative Months			
	1–2	3–4	5–6	7–8	9–12	4	5	6	7–12
Brace: Long-leg postoperative	X	X	X						
Range of motion minimum goals									
0°–90°	X								
0°–120°		X							
0°–135°			X						
Weight-bearing									
Toe touch to 50% body weight	P								
75% to 100% body weight		P							
Toe touch to 25% body weight	C, T								
50% to 75% body weight		C, T	C						
100% body weight			T	C					
Patella mobilization	X	X	X						
Stretching									
Hamstring, gastrocnemius-soleus, iliotibial band, quadriceps	X	X	X	X	X	X	X	X	X
Strengthening									
Quadriceps isometrics, straight leg raises, active knee extension	X	X	X	X	X	X	X	X	X
Closed-chain: gait retraining, toe raises, wall-sits, mini-squats		P	C	X	X	X	X	X	
Knee flexion hamstring curls (90°)			P	C	X	X	X	X	X
Knee extension quadriceps (90°–30°)			X	X	X	X	X	X	X
Hip abduction-adduction, multi-hip			X	X	X	X	X	X	X
Leg press (70°–10°)			P	P	X	X	X	X	X
Balance/proprioceptive training									
Weight-shifting, minitrampoline, BAPS, BBS, plyometrics		P	X	X	X	X	X	X	X
Conditioning									
Upper body ergometer		X	X	X					
Bike (stationary)					X	X	X	X	X
Aquatic program						X	X	X	X
Swimming (kicking)					P, C	X	X	X	X
Walking						X	X	X	X
Stair-climbing machine					P, C	P, C	P, C	P, C	X
Ski machine					P	P	P	C	X
*Running: straight						P	P	C	X
*Cutting: lateral carioca, figure-eights							P	P	X
*Full sports							P	P	X

*Return to running, cutting, and full sports based on multiple criteria (see text). Patients with noteworthy articular cartilage damage are advised to return to light recreational activities only.

BAPS, Biomechanical Ankle Platform System (Camp, Jackson, MI), DBS, Biodex Balance System (Shirley, NY); C, complex meniscus repairs extending into middle third region; P, peripheral meniscus repairs; T, transplants; X, all meniscus repairs and transplants.

From Heckmann, T.; Barber-Westin, S. D., Noyes, F. R.. Meniscal repair and transplantation: indications, techniques, rehabilitation, and clinical outcome. *J Orthop Sports Phys Ther* 36:795–814, 2006.

On average, patients require 11 to 16 physical therapy visits over 9 to 12 months to produce a desirable result.

Lateral and anteroposterior plain radiographs are obtained 1 week postoperatively to verify the position of the osseous component of meniscus transplants and at 6 to 8 weeks to verify healing and retention of the bony portion of the transplant within the slot or tunnels. Any onset of tibiofemoral joint line clicking or pain may indicate failure of the meniscus repair or transplant and should be noted immediately for consideration of refixation.

IMMEDIATE POSTOPERATIVE MANAGEMENT

Important early postoperative signs for the therapist to monitor include effusion, pain, gait, knee flexion and extension, patellar mobility, strength and control of the lower extremity, lower

Critical Points IMMEDIATE POSTOPERATIVE MANAGEMENT

Therapist Monitors Early Postoperatively

Knee effusion, pain, gait, flexion and extension, patellar mobility, lower extremity strength and flexibility, and tibiofemoral joint symptoms.

Use postoperative compression dressing, long-leg brace, compression stockings, cryotherapy, lower limb elevation, and pain management.

Common Complications

- Excessive pain/swelling—quadriceps shutdown
- Limitation knee flexion, extension
- Saphenous nerve irritation

Early detection and treatment of complications are critical.

TABLE 30–2   Postoperative Signs and Symptoms Requiring Prompt Treatment

Postoperative Sign and/or Symptom	Treatment Recommendations
Continued pain in the medial or lateral tibiofemoral compartment of the meniscus repair or transplant	Physician examination, assess need for refixation or re-repair
Tibiofemoral compartment clicking, or a subjective sensation by the patient of "something being loose" within the tibiofemoral joint	Physician examination, assess need for refixation or re-repair
Failure to meet knee extension and flexion goals (see text)	Overpressure program, early gentle manipulation under anesthesia if 0°–135° not met by 6 wk postoperatively
Decreased patellar mobility (indicative of early arthrofibrosis)	Aggressive knee flexion, extension overpressure program, or gentle manipulation under anesthesia to regain full ROM and normal patellar mobility
Decrease in voluntary quadriceps contraction and muscle tone, advancing muscle atrophy	Aggressive quadriceps muscle strengthening program, EMS
Persistent joint effusion, joint inflammation	Aspiration, rule out infection, close physician observation

EMS, electrical muscle stimulation; ROM, range of knee motion.

From Heckmann, T.; Barber-Westin, S. D.; Noyes, F. R.: Meniscal repair and transplantation: Indications, techniques, rehabilitation, and clinical outcome. *J Orthop Sports Phys Ther* 36:795–814, 2006.

extremity flexibility, and tibiofemoral symptoms indicative of a meniscal tear (Table 30–2).

Patients present to physical therapy on the 1st day after surgery on bilateral axillary crutches in a postoperative dressing with a long-leg brace locked in full extension. The postoperative bandage and dressing are changed to allow the application of thigh-high compression stockings and a compression bandage. Early control of postoperative effusion is essential for pain management and early quadriceps reeducation. In addition to compression, cryotherapy is critical in this time period. Patients receive a commercial cooling unit, which is used six to eight times daily at home. In the clinic, the use of various cryotherapy machines provide compression simultaneously with the cold program (Fig. 30–1).

Patients are instructed to maintain lower limb elevation as frequently as possible during the 1st week. A portable neuromuscular electric stimulator may be helpful for quadriceps reeducation and pain management (Fig. 30–2). These devices are used six times per day, 15 minutes per session, until the patient displays an excellent voluntary quadriceps contraction.

The patient's initial response to surgery and progression during the first 2 weeks sets the tone for the initial phases of the rehabilitation program. Common postoperative complications include excessive pain or swelling, quadriceps shutdown or loss

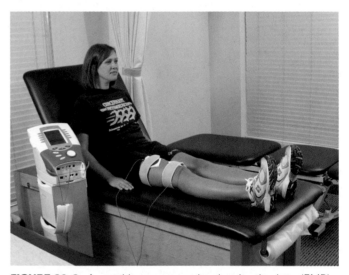

FIGURE 30–2. A portable neuromuscular electric stimulator (EMPI, St. Paul, MN) is effective for quadriceps reeducation and pain management in the early postoperative phase.

of voluntary isometric contraction, range of motion (ROM) limitations, and saphenous nerve irritations for medial repairs. It is important to monitor patient complaints of posteromedial or infrapatellar burning, posteromedial tenderness along the distal pes anserine tendons, tenderness of Hunter's canal along the medial thigh, hypersensitivity to light pressure, or hypersensitivity to temperature change. These abnormal symptoms or signs occur in early cases of complex regional pain syndrome (see Chapter 43, Diagnosis and Treatment of Complex Regional Pain Syndrome) and require immediate treatment.

BRACE AND CRUTCH SUPPORT

A long-leg postoperative brace is placed immediately after surgery following complex meniscus repairs or transplants. The brace is opened from 0° to 90°, but it is locked at 0° extension at night for the first 2 weeks. Thereafter, the brace is not routinely locked except in patients who cannot maintain 0° of extension. In these cases, the brace is locked at 0° extension as required during the day and night. The brace is used for 6 weeks. A brace is not routinely used after repair of a peripheral

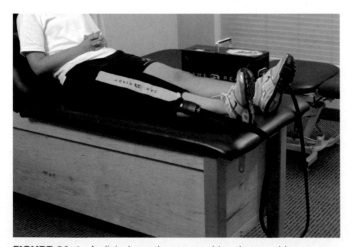

FIGURE 30–1. A clinical cryotherapy machine that provides compression with the cold program (Game Ready, Berkeley, CA) is used in the initial postoperative period.

Brace Used 6 Wk in Complex Meniscus Repairs and Transplants

- Locked 0° at night for first 2 postoperative wk
- Opened 0°–90° during the day

Brace not required in simple meniscus repairs in periphery (outer third region).

Crutch support for 4 wk postoperative. Patients weaned when normal gait demonstrated.

Crutches with partial weight-bearing are recommended for the first 4 wk in all cases.

Weight-bearing is gradually progressed as shown in Table 30–1, and patients are encouraged to use a normal gait that avoids a locked knee and assumes normal flexion throughout the gait cycle.

Begin passive flexion, passive and active-assisted extension exercises 1st day postoperative, 0°–90°.

Advance Flexion

- Goal 135° by 5–6 wk.

Begin ROM Overpressure Program 1 Wk Postoperative if 0°–90° not Achieved

- Extension: hanging weights, 10-min sessions
- Flexion: chair-rolling, wall-sliding, ERMI Knee Flexionator device

Patellar mobilization, flexibility exercises paramount to achieving full ROM.

ROM, range of motion.

---

meniscus tear unless an all-inside fixator with only a few sutures is used for added protection.

Crutches with partial weight-bearing are recommended for the first 4 weeks in all cases. Weight-bearing is gradually progressed as shown in Table 30–1, and patients are encouraged to use a normal gait that avoids a locked knee and assumes normal flexion throughout the gait cycle. Patients who had a repair of a radial meniscus tear are kept non–weight-bearing for 4 weeks to protect the repair site.

RANGE OF KNEE MOTION AND FLEXIBILITY

Passive knee flexion and passive and active/active-assisted knee extension exercises are begun the 1st day postoperatively. Active knee flexion is limited to avoid hamstring strain to the postero medial joint. ROM exercises are performed in the seated position initially from 0° to 90°. Flexion is gradually advanced to 120° by the 3rd to 4th week and 135° by the 5th to 6th week (Table 30–3). Patients who had extensive repairs may be required to limit ROM to 0° to 90° for the first 2 weeks. Knee motion exercises are performed three to four times daily until normal motion is achieved. Hyperextension is avoided in individuals who have had anterior horn meniscus repairs.

If 0° to 90° of knee motion is not easily achieved by the end of the 1st postoperative week, the patient may be at risk for a knee motion complication. Individuals who develop such a limitation are placed into a specific treatment program previously described in detail.[2,6] Overpressure exercises are usually successful in achieving the last few degrees of extension if initiated within the first few weeks after surgery. The patient props the foot and ankle on a towel to elevate the hamstrings and gastrocnemius, which allows the knee to drop into full extension. A 10-pound weight may be added to the distal thigh and knee to stretch the posterior capsule (Fig. 30–3). This program is done for 10 minutes at a time, six to eight times per day.

Flexion exercises are performed in the seated position, using the opposite lower extremity to provide overpressure (Fig. 30–4). Chair-rolling, wall-sliding, passive quadriceps stretching, and ROM devices such as the ERMI Knee Flexionator (ERMI, Atlanta, GA) are also helpful in regaining full knee flexion. It is important that no squatting exercises are performed for at least 4 months, because this places large tensile forces on posterior meniscus repairs and transplants.

ROM exercises are accompanied by patellar mobilization (in the superior, inferior, medial, and lateral directions), which is paramount to achieve full knee motion (Fig. 30–5). Flexibility

---

TABLE 30–3   Range of Motion, Flexibility, and Modality Usage after Meniscus Repair and Transplantation

Time Postoperative, Frequency	Extension-Flexion Limits	Patellar Mobilization	Flexibility (5 reps x 20 sec)	Electrical Muscle Stimulation (20 min)	Cryotherapy (20 min)
1–2 wk 3–4 x/day, 10-min sessions	0°–90°	Medial-lateral Superior-inferior	Hamstring, gastrocnemius-soleus	Yes	Yes
3–4 wk 3–4 x/day, 10-min sessions	0°–120°	Medial-lateral Superior-inferior	Hamstring, gastrocnemius-soleus	Yes	Yes
5–6 wk 3 x/day, 10-min sessions	0°–135°	Medial-lateral Superior-inferior	Hamstring, gastrocnemius-soleus	Yes	Yes
7–8 wk 2 x/day, 10-min sessions	0°–135°	(If required)	Hamstring, gastrocnemius-soleus, quadriceps, iliotibial band		Yes
9–52 wk 2 x/day, 10-min sessions	(Should be full)		Hamstring, gastrocnemius-soleus, quadriceps, iliotibial band		Yes

From Heckmann, T.; Barber-Westin, S. D.; Noyes, F. R.: Meniscal repair and transplantation: indications, techniques, rehabilitation, and clinical outcome. *J Orthop Sports Phys Ther* 36:795–814, 2006.

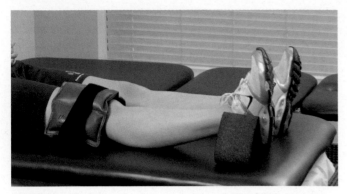

FIGURE 30–3. Extension overpressure hanging-weight exercise.

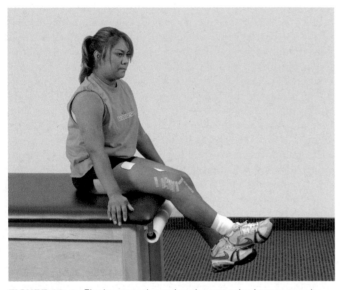

FIGURE 30–4. Flexion exercise using the opposite knee to apply pressure.

exercises, beginning with hamstring and gastrocnemius-soleus, are begun the 1st day postoperatively and are done three times per day. Quadriceps and iliotibial band flexibility exercises are incorporated at 7 to 8 weeks postoperative. Sustained static stretching is performed, with the stretch held for 30 seconds and repeated five times.

The knee motion program is effective, because no patient in the authors' clinical studies who had an isolated meniscus repair or transplant required further surgery for a knee motion complication. Only 2 of 193 patients who had meniscal repair, and 4 of 38 patients who had a transplant, required a gentle manipulation for a limitation of flexion. In these 6 patients, a major concomitant procedure, such as a cruciate ligament reconstruction, had been performed.

Close supervision and additional exercises may be required in patients who undergo combined procedures to successfully restore normal knee motion. No difference exists between medial and lateral meniscus repairs or transplants in regard to knee motion complications.

BALANCE AND PROPRIOCEPTIVE TRAINING

Balance and proprioception exercises are initiated when patients achieve partial weight-bearing, typically the 1st week after surgery. Crutches are used for support during these exercises until full weight-bearing is allowed. Initially, patients perform weight-shifting from side-to-side and front-to-back. Then, cup-walking is encouraged to develop symmetry between the surgical and the contralateral limbs, hip and knee flexion, quadriceps control during midstance, hip and pelvic control during midstance, and adequate gastrocnemius-soleus control during push-off (Fig. 30–6).

Tandem balance is begun during the partial weight-bearing phase to assist with position sense and balance. Single-leg balance exercise is also done by pointing the foot straight ahead, flexing the knee to 20° to 30°, extending the arms outward to horizontal, and positioning the torso upright with the shoulders

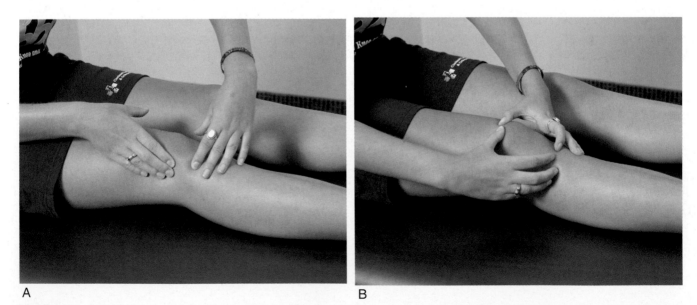

A   B

FIGURE 30–5. A and **B,** Patellar mobilization exercises (in the superior, inferior, medial, and lateral directions), paramount in regaining a full range of motion, are initiated the 1st day postoperatively.

above the hips and the hips above the ankles. The patient stands in this position until balance is disturbed. A minitrampoline is used to make this exercise more challenging after it is mastered on a hard surface.

Many devices are available to assist with balance and gait retraining, including Styrofoam half rolls and whole rolls, and the Biomechanical Ankle Platform System (BAPS, Camp, Jackson, MI). Patients walk (unassisted) on Styrofoam half rolls to develop a center of balance, quadriceps control in midstance, and postural positioning. The BAPS board is used in double-leg and single-leg stance to promote proprioception. More sophisticated devices are also available (Fig. 30-7), including Biodex's Balance System (Biodex Corporation, Shirley, NY) and Neurocom's Balance System (Neurocom, Clackamas, OR). These devices provide visual feedback to assist with a variety of balance activities.

The proprioceptive training includes plyometric exercises, which are incorporated in the end-stage of rehabilitation to provide a functional basis for return to activity for patients who desire to return to strenuous sports activities. These exercises are promoted in younger athletic patients who have an associated anterior cruciate ligament reconstruction. These exercises are described in detail later in this chapter.

STRENGTHENING

The strengthening program is begun on the 1st day postoperative with quadriceps isometrics, straight leg raises (Fig. 30-8), and active-assisted knee extension from 90° to 30° (Table 30-4). Initially, straight leg raises are performed in the flexion plane only. The patient must achieve a sufficient quadriceps contraction to eliminate an extensor lag before adding straight leg raises in the other three planes (abduction, adduction, and extension). These exercises are performed as three to five sets of 10 repetitions, and this set/repetition rule allows for systematic progression of ankle weights as tolerated.

At weeks 3 to 4, closed kinetic chain weight-bearing exercises are begun. Toe-raises for gastrocnemius-soleus strengthening, wall sits, and mini-squats for quadriceps strengthening are added when patients are 50% weight-bearing. Wall-sits (Fig. 30-9) and mini-squats (Fig. 30-10) are begun at 5 to 6 weeks postoperative after meniscal transplantation. These activities should be limited from 0° to 60° of flexion to protect the posterior horn of the meniscus.

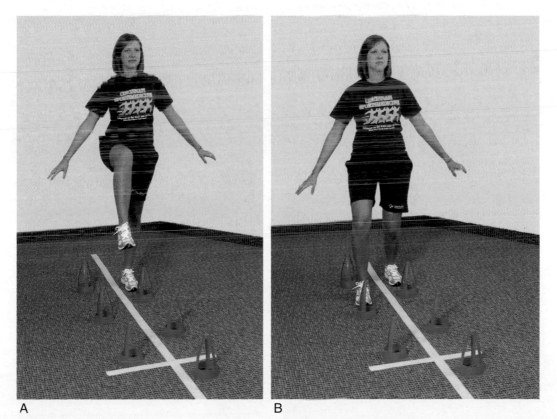

A   B

FIGURE 30-6. A and **B,** Cup-walking is used early postoperatively to develop symmetry between the surgical and the contralateral limbs, hip and knee flexion, quadriceps control during midstance, hip and pelvic control during midstance, and adequate gastrocnemius-soleus control during push-off. This exercise also facilitates quadriceps control to prevent knee hyperextension from occurring during gait.

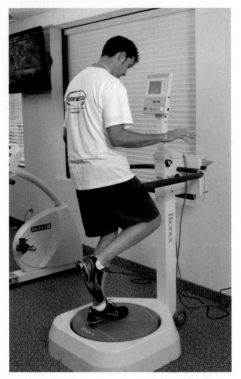

FIGURE 30–7. A sophisticated balance device (Biodex Corporation, Shirley, NY) provides visual feedback to assist with a variety of balance activities.

Critical Points STRENGTHENING

1st Day Postoperative
- Quadriceps isometrics
- Straight leg raises
- Active-assisted knee extension, 90°–30°

3-4 Wk Postoperative

Closed Kinetic Chain Exercises
- Toe-raises
- Wall-sits (0°–60°)
- Mini-squats (0°–60°)

Delay wall sits, mini-squats until 7–8 wk after meniscus transplantation.
- Open kinetic chain knee extension 90°–30°

5–6 Wk Postoperative
- Hamstring curls 0°–90° (delayed until 7–8 wk after complex meniscus repair, 9–12 wk after transplant)
- Leg press machine 70°–10° (delayed 9–12 wk after transplant)
- Multiangle hip machine

Wall-sitting isometrics can be made more challenging by modifying the exercise technique. First, the patient can voluntarily set the quadriceps muscle once he or she reaches the maximum knee flexion angle, which is typically between 30 and 45°. This contraction and knee flexion position are held until muscle fatigue occurs, and the exercise is repeated three to five times. In a second modification, designed to promote a stronger vastus lateralis obliquus contraction, the patient performs a hip adduction contraction by squeezing a ball between the distal thighs. In a third variation, the patient holds dumbbell weights in the hands to increase body weight, which promotes an even stronger quadriceps contraction. Finally, the patient

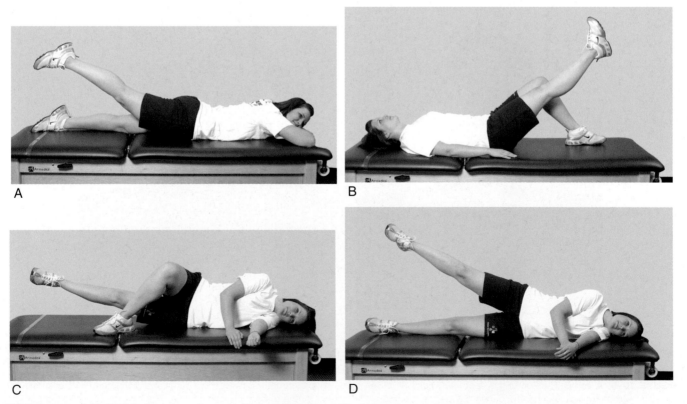

A

B

C

D

FIGURE 30–8. A–D, Straight leg raises shown in flexion, abduction, adduction, and extension planes.

TABLE 30-4 Muscle Strengthening Exercises after Meniscus Repair and Transplantation*

Time Postoperative, Frequency	Quadriceps Isometrics (Active)	Straight Leg Raises	Knee Extension (Active-Assisted; 90°-30°)	Toe Raises	Wall-Sits (To fatigue)	Mini-Squats	Lateral Step-ups (5- to 10-cm block)	Hamstring Curls (0°-90°)	Multi-hip (Flex, Ext, Abd, Add)	Leg Press (70°-10°)
1-2 wk 3 x/day 15 min	1 set x 10 reps (every hr)	Flex 3 sets x 10 reps	3 sets x 10 reps							
3-4 wk 2-3 x/day 20 min	Multiangle 0°, 60° 1 set x 10 reps each	Flex, ext, add 3 sets x 10 reps	3 sets x 10 reps	Meniscus repairs only 3 sets x 20 reps	Meniscus repairs only 3 sets	Meniscus repairs only 3 sets				
5-6 wk 2 x/day 20 min	Multiangle 30°, 60°, 90°, 2 sets x 10 reps	Add ankle weight ≤ 10% of body weight 3 sets x 10 reps	Active 3 sets x 10 reps	Meniscus repairs only Add heel-raises 3 sets x 10 reps	Transplants start 3 sets	Transplants start 3 sets		Peripheral repairs only Active, 3 sets x 10 reps	3 sets x 10 reps	Meniscus repairs only 3 sets x 10 reps
7-8 wk 2 x/day 20 min		Add abd 3 sets x 10 reps Add rubber tubing, 3 sets x 30 reps	Active 3 sets x 10 reps				3 sets x 10 reps	All meniscus repairs only Active, 3 sets x 10 reps	3 sets x 10 reps	Meniscus repairs only 3 sets x 10 reps
9-12 wk 2 x/day 20 min		3 sets x 10 reps Rubber tubing, 3 sets x 30 reps	Active 3 sets x 10 reps		3 sets	Add rubber tubing, 0°-40°, 3 sets x 20 reps	3 sets x 10 reps	Transplants start Active, 3 sets x 10 reps	3 sets x 10 reps	Transplants start 3 sets x 10 reps
13-26 wk 2 x/day 20 min		Rubber tubing, high speed, 3 sets x 30 reps	With resistance 3 sets x 10 reps			3 sets x 20 reps		Add resistance 3 sets x 10 reps	3 sets x 10 reps	3 sets x 10 reps
27-52 wk 1 x/day 20-30 min		Rubber tubing, high speed, 3 sets x 30 reps	With resistance 3 sets x 10 reps			3 sets x 20 reps		With resistance 3 sets x 10 reps	3 sets x 10 reps	3 sets x 10 reps

*Exercises done by recipients of either meniscus repair or transplantation, unless otherwise indicated.

abd, abduction; add, adduction; ext, extension; flex, flexion; reps, repetitions.

From Heckmann, T.; Barber-Westin, S. D.; Noyes, F. R.: Meniscal repair and transplantation: indications, techniques, rehabilitation, and clinical outcome. *J Orthop Sports Phys Ther* 36:795-814, 2006.

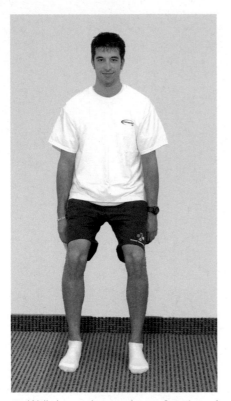

FIGURE 30–9. Wall-sit exercises are begun 3 to 4 weeks after meniscus repair and 5 to 6 weeks after meniscal transplantation. This exercises is limited from 0° to 60° of flexion to protect the posterior horn of the meniscus.

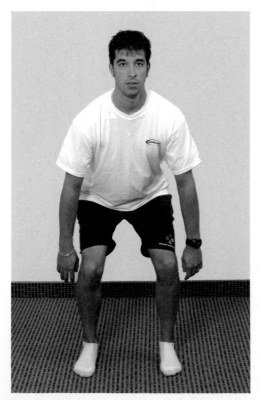

FIGURE 30–10. Mini-squats, begun 3 to 4 weeks after meniscus repair and 5 to 6 weeks after meniscal transplantation, are an effective quadriceps strengthening exercise.

can shift the body weight over the involved side to simulate a single-leg contraction.

Mini-squats are initially done using the patient's body weight as resistance. Gradually, TheraBand or surgical tubing is used as a resistance mechanism. The depth of the squat is controlled to protect the meniscus repair or transplant and the patellofemoral joint. Quick, smooth, rhythmic squats are performed to a high-set/high-repetition cadence to promote muscle fatigue. Hip position is important to monitor in order to emphasize the quadriceps.

Open kinetic chain non–weight-bearing exercises are begun 5 to 6 weeks postoperative (see Table 30–4). Knee extension progressive resistive exercises (PREs) are initiated from 90° to 30° to protect the patellofemoral joint.[1] By keeping the quadriceps exercises in this protected ROM, minimal forces will be placed along peripheral and midsubstance repair sites. Progression from ankle weights to machines occurs as the patient progresses the amount of weight in the exercise program. Quadriceps control is critical to the program progression.

Hamstring curls from 0° to 90° are initiated in patients who had peripheral meniscus repairs at the same time as the knee extension PREs. Care should be taken to avoid hyperextension, which places tension on the posterior capsule. This exercise is delayed until at least 7 to 8 weeks after a complex meniscus repair and until 9 to 12 weeks after meniscus transplantation. Isolated resisted hamstring curls are limited in complex repairs and transplants owing to the medial hamstring insertion along the posteromedial joint capsule. This limitation is designed to lessen potential traction forces being imposed onto the repair site. Initially, hamstring curls are done with Velcro ankle weights; then the exercise is progressed to weight machines.

A leg press machine is initiated in the range of 70° to 10° at 5 to 6 weeks after all meniscus repairs and at 9 to 12 weeks after transplantation. The limitation in flexion is incorporated owing to the increased load placed on the posterior horn of the meniscus after 60° to 70° of flexion.

Side-lying straight leg raises are initiated early in the rehabilitation program. Later, when patients have access to the cable column or multi-hip machines, hip flexion, extension, abduction, and adduction are also included in the exercise program. These activities are implemented at 5 to 6 weeks postoperative.

CONDITIONING

A cardiovascular program may be begun as early as 2 to 4 weeks postoperatively if the patient has access to an upper body ergometer (Table 30–5). Stationary bicycling is begun 7 to 8 weeks postoperative. The seat height is adjusted to its highest level based on patient body size, and a low-resistance level is used. A recumbent bicycle may be substituted in patients who have damage to the patellofemoral joint articular cartilage or anterior knee pain.

Water-walking may be implemented during this timeframe. Walking in waist-high water decreases the impact load to the knee by 50%. To protect the healing meniscus, swimming with straight leg kicking and dry land walking programs are initiated between the 9th and the 12th weeks. At this time, patients who had a meniscus repair may also begin using stair-climbing, elliptical cross-trainers, or cross-country ski machines. Protection against high stresses to the patellofemoral joint is required in patients with symptoms or articular cartilage damage. If a stair-climbing machine is tolerable, a short step is maintained with

TABLE 30-5 Aerobic Conditioning Exercises after Meniscus Repair and Transplantation*

Time Postoperative, Frequency	UBE	Bicycle (Stationary)	Water-Walking	Swimming	Walking	Stair Climbing Machine (Low Resistance, Low Stroke)	Ski Machine (Short Stride, Level, Low Resistance)	Running (Straight)	Cutting	Functional Training
3-4 wk 1-2 x/day	10 min									
5-6 wk 2 x/day	10 min									
7-8 wk 1-2 x/day	15 min	15 min								
9-12 wk 1 x/day (select one activity per session)		15 min	15 min	15 min	15 min	Meniscus repairs only 15 min	Meniscus repairs only 15 min			
13-26 wk 3 x/wk (select one activity per session)		20 min	20 min	20 min	20 min	Meniscus repairs only 20 min	Meniscus repairs only 20 min			
Peripheral meniscus repairs only†										
20 wk 3 x/wk								Jog ¼ mile Walk ⅛ mile Backward run 20 yd	Lateral, carioca, figure-eights, 20 yd	Plyometrics box hops, level, double-leg 15 sec, 4-6 sets Sports-specific drills 4-6 sets
27 wk and beyond 3 x/wk (select one activity per session)		20-30 min	20-30 min	20-30 min	20-30 min	20-30 min	20-30 min			
30 wk and beyond								**Complex meniscus repairs start 30 wk postoperative Advance program as needed Transplants start, with precautions**	**Complex meniscus repairs start >35 wk postoperative Advance program as needed**	**Complex meniscus repairs start >35 wk postoperative Advance program as needed**
12 mo and beyond										

*Exercises done by recipients of either meniscus repair or transplantation, unless otherwise indicated.

†Begin running program when no more than 30% deficit elicited on isokinetic testing; begin cutting program when no more than 20% deficit elicited on isokinetic testing.

UBE, upper body ergometer.

From Heckmann, T.; Barber-Westin, S. D.; Noyes, F. R.: Meniscal repair and transplantation: indications, techniques, rehabilitation, and clinical outcome. *J Orthop Sports Phys Ther* 36:795-814, 2006.

low resistance levels. The cardiovascular program should be done at least three times a week for 20 to 30 minutes, and the exercise should be performed to at least 60% to 85% of maximal heart rate.

RUNNING PROGRAM

A running program is begun at approximately 20 weeks postoperative in patients who had peripheral meniscus repairs and who have no more than a 30% deficit in average peak torque for the quadriceps and hamstrings on isometric testing performed on a Biodex dynamometer (Biodex Corp., Shirley, NY). This program is delayed until approximately 30 weeks postoperative in patients who had complex meniscus repairs and until at least 1 year postoperative in patients who had a meniscus transplant.

Isometric muscle testing is initially performed at an angle of 60° of knee flexion, which places the knee in a protected position for both the meniscus and the patella. Progression to isokinetic testing at high speeds is important, but the initial goal is to test the integrity of the quadriceps and hamstring musculatures. Other testing parameters worth evaluating include peak torque–to–body weight ratios, agonist-to-antagonist ratios, and time to peak torque values.

Patients begin with a walk/run combination program, using running distances of 18, 37, 55, and 91 meters. Initially, patients run at 25% to 50% of their normal speed. Once patients can run straight ahead at full speed, lateral and crossover maneuvers are added. Short distances (such as 18 m) are used to work on speed and agility. Side-to-side running over cups may be used to facilitate agility and proprioception. Figure-eight and carioca running drills are also useful.

PLYOMETRIC TRAINING

Progressive plyometric training is initiated upon successful completion of the running program. These activities are typically incorporated after 6 months postoperative in patients who have had a large peripheral tear or complex repair. In patients who had a radial meniscus repair, this program may be delayed until 9 months postoperative owing to the disruption that occurred in the hoop stresses of the meniscus.

Individual sessions are performed in a manner similar to that for interval training. Initially, a rest period is incorporated that lasts two to three times the length of the exercise period; this is gradually decreased to one to two times the length of the exercise period. In addition, plyometric hopping is performed two to three times each week and is incorporated into the strength and cardiovascular endurance program.

The program beings with level-surface box-hopping. A four-square grid of four equal-sized boxes is created on the floor with tape. The patient first hops from box 1 to box 3 (front-to-back), and then from box 1 to box 2 (side-to-side). This drill is initially performed using both legs, with the body weight kept on the ball of the foot.

The patient hops as fast as possible with the knees bent and lands in flexion to avoid knee hyperextension. It is important for the patient to focus on limb symmetry during this exercise.

The initial exercise time period lasts 15 seconds, with the patient completing as many hops between the squares as possible. Three sets are performed for both directions, and the number of hops is recorded. Progression of the program occurs as the number of hops, as well as patient confidence, improves. This exercise has four levels. The first level includes front-to-back and side-to-side hopping, as previously described. The second level incorporates both of the directions in level one into one sequence and also includes hopping in both right and left directions (i.e., box 1 to box 2 to box 4 to box 2 to box 1). Level three progresses to diagonal hops, and level four includes pivot hops in a 180° direction. Once the patient can perform level-four double-leg hops, similar exercises are initiated using single-leg hops. Vertical box hops are incorporated into the next phase of plyometric exercises.

Important parameters to consider when performing plyometric exercises include surface, footwear, and warm-up. This program should be performed on a surface that is firm, yet forgiving, such as a wooden gym floor. Very hard surfaces like concrete should be avoided. In addition, a cross-training or running shoe should be worn to provide adequate shock absorption as well as adequate stability to the foot. Checking wear patterns and outer sole wear will help avoid overuse injuries. Finally, an adequate warm-up should include exercises and a light cardiovascular workout.

RETURN TO SPORTS ACTIVITIES

Sports-specific drills and cutting patterns of 45° and 90° angles may be implemented, based on the patient's athletic goals. Repeat isokinetic testing is typically performed monthly, progressing from isometric testing for the first 6 months to isokinetic testing at speeds of 180° and 300° per second. This testing not only provides the patient with feedback on performance but also serves to assist the clinician with program progression. Goals for testing should be at least 70% to begin running and 90% for full activity for the bilateral torque comparisons and approximately 60% for agonist-to-antagonist ratios. Torque-to–body weight ratios are based on age, sex, and body weight parameters.

Critical Points RETURN TO SPORTS ACTIVITIES

- Sports-specific drills completed based on patient goals
- No more than 10% deficit in quadriceps and hamstrings peak torque on isokinetic testing
- Successful completion of running and functional training
- Trial of function recommended, monitor for overuse symptoms
- Majority meniscus transplant patients are not candidates owing to joint damage; encourage low-impact activities, weight control

Return to sports activities is based on successful completion of the running and functional-training program. Muscle and functional testing should be within normal limits, and a trial of function is encouraged, during which time the patient is monitored for overuse symptoms. The majority of patients who undergo meniscal transplantation have noteworthy articular cartilage deterioration and are not candidates for strenuous plyometric training or sports activities. Return to low-impact activities is therefore recommended.

ACKNOWLEDGMENT

The authors have no commercial relationship with any of the orthopaedic manufacturers mentioned in this chapter or shown in the figures. The manufacturers are provided for the benefit of the reader.

REFERENCES

1. Grood, E. S.; Suntay, W. J.; Noyes, F. R.; Butler, D. L.: Biomechanics of the knee-extension exercise. Effect of cutting the anterior cruciate ligament. J Bone Joint Surg Am 66:725–734, 1984.
2. Heckmann, T. P.; Noyes, F. R.; Barber-Westin, S. D.: Autogeneic and allogeneic anterior cruciate ligament rehabilitation. In Ellenbecker, T. S. (ed.): Knee Ligament Rehabilitation. Philadelphia: Churchill Livingstone, 2000; pp. 132–150.
3. Noyes, F. R.; Barber-Westin, S. D.: Arthroscopic repair of meniscal tears extending into the avascular zone in patients younger than twenty years of age. Am J Sports Med 30:589–600, 2002.
4. Noyes, F. R.; Barber-Westin, S. D.: Arthroscopic repair of meniscus tears extending into the avascular zone with or without anterior cruciate ligament reconstruction in patients 40 years of age and older. Arthroscopy 16:822–829, 2000.
5. Noyes, F. R.; Barber-Westin, S. D.; Rankin, M.: Meniscal transplantation in symptomatic patients less than fifty years old. J Bone Joint Surg Am 86:1392–1404, 2004.
6. Noyes, F. R.; Berrios-Torres, S.; Barber-Westin, S. D.; Heckmann, T. P.: Prevention of permanent arthrofibrosis after anterior cruciate ligament reconstruction alone or combined with associated procedures: a prospective study in 443 knees. Knee Surg Sports Traumatol Arthrosc 8:196–206, 2000.
7. Rubman, M. H.; Noyes, F. R.; Barber-Westin, S. D.: Arthroscopic repair of meniscal tears that extend into the avascular zone. A review of 198 single and complex tears. Am J Sports Med 26:87–95, 1998.

Lower Extremity Osseous Malalignment

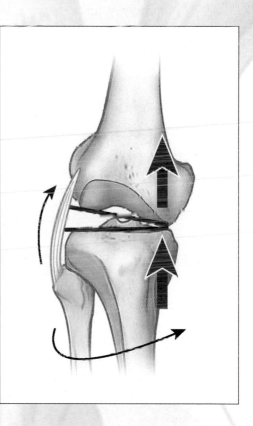

Chapter 31

Primary, Double, and Triple Varus Knee Syndromes: Diagnosis, Osteotomy Techniques, and Clinical Outcomes

Frank R. Noyes, MD ■ *Sue D. Barber-Westin,* BS

INDICATIONS

High tibial osteotomy (HTO) has gained wide acceptance as a treatment option for patients with medial tibiofemoral osteoarthritis and varus deformity of the lower extremity. Most candidates are in their 3rd to 5th decade and wish to remain active and avoid unicompartmental or total knee replacement. The recommendations for this procedure are derived from a careful evaluation of subjective symptoms, findings on physical examination, radiographic evidence of malalignment and arthritis, and gait analysis when available.

The predominant indication for HTO is lower limb osseous malalignment (Fig. 31–1) in younger patients who have medial tibiofemoral joint pain and wish to maintain an active lifestyle. The goal is to correct the mechanical abnormality of excessive loading of the medial tibiofemoral compartment by redistributing weight-bearing loads onto the lateral compartment. Varus malalignment is present when the weight-bearing line (WBL) crosses less than 50% of the mediolateral transverse width of the tibial plateau.

Unfortunately, a prior medial meniscectomy is a major risk factor for progression of arthritis in these knees. Because any underlying arthritis is expected to progress, it is advisable to perform HTO while the joint damage is in the early stages before the development of severe articular cartilage deterioration and loss of tibiofemoral joint space.[52,113]

One advantage of performing HTO in young patients who have early medial tibiofemoral arthritis after medial meniscectomy is the opportunity to also perform a meniscus transplant and a cartilage restoration procedure if indicated.

The appropriate level of physical activity that can be recommended after HTO remains questionable. Patient education is important so that activity limitations to be followed postoperatively are well understood. The goal of the osteotomy is to allow an active, pain-free lifestyle that includes low-impact recreational pursuits, but not high-loading activities such as twisting, turning, jumping, and pivoting.

The majority of patients who undergo HTO are 50 years of age or younger with varus malalignment and mild to moderate medial tibiofemoral joint arthritis. Many patients have had a prior medial meniscectomy. Patients older than 60 years are usually candidates for partial or total joint replacement. The difficult decision is the treatment recommendation for patients between 50 and 60 years of age. With the increasing longevity of unicompartmental knee replacements, patients who have advanced medial compartment damage with major areas of bone exposure will likely experience symptoms after HTO and are better candidates for partial replacement. Individuals who undergo a unicompartmental

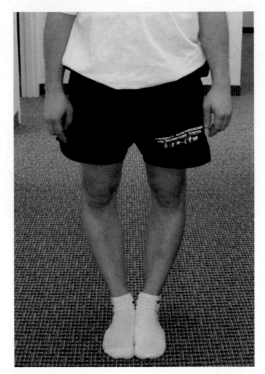

FIGURE 31–1. Bilateral varus malalignment in a 40-year-old man who presented with bilateral medial joint pain after 1 to 2 hours of ambulation.

replacement may participate in recreational activities similar to those who undergo HTO. Osteotomy is performed in patients 55 years of age and younger who are athletically active, have remaining medial tibiofemoral cartilage (although thinned), and wish to maintain reasonable athletic pursuits such as tennis and skiing. These patients have early medial compartment symptoms; however, the joint damage is not advanced to a bone-on-bone state that would warrant unicompartmental replacement. Careful patient selection is the key issue, and the surgeon should not overstate or guarantee results of an HTO because the arthritis will eventually progress. In short, the goal of an HTO is to buy time in younger-aged patients (hopefully 10–15 yr) prior to joint replacement. If there is any question that the arthritis of the medial tibiofemoral compartment is advanced to where the HTO will not last 10 years, it is preferable in patients 50 years of age or older to perform a partial replacement. This is particularly true for sedentary patients in whom the goals of ambulating activities are achieved with partial joint replacement, avoiding the more prolonged postoperative recovery from an HTO.

There exists a group of varus-angulated knees with associated symptomatic ligament deficiencies requiring reconstruction. These ligament deficiencies most commonly involve the anterior cruciate ligament (ACL) and posterolateral structures (fibular collateral ligament [FCL], popliteus muscle-tendon-ligament unit [PMTL], and posterolateral capsule). In these knees (double and triple varus), a normal axial alignment must be achieved before proceeding with ligament reconstructive procedures.

Lower limb varus malalignment in these knees is not overcorrected to valgus when there is no damage to the articular cartilage in the medial tibiofemoral compartment. The goal in these knees is to correct the varus to a neutral alignment and then proceed in a staged manner (if required) with a cruciate

---

Critical Points INDICATIONS

- Varus osseous malalignment: weight-bearing line < 50% of tibial width.
- Mild to moderate symptomatic arthrosis medial tibiofemoral compartment.
- Articular cartilage retained in medial tibiofemoral compartment.
- To achieve normal limb alignment before
  - Medial meniscus transplant.
  - Articular cartilage restorative procedures.
  - Cruciate ligament or posterolateral reconstruction in double and triple varus knees.
- Patients ≤ 50 yr of age, athletically active, wish to maintain reasonable athletic pursuits.

and posterolateral reconstruction as required. Correction of the varus alignment decreases the risks of failure of the ligament reconstructive procedures.[96,98,99,101]

CONTRAINDICATIONS

One commonly debated issue regarding contraindications to osteotomy is the extent of damage to the medial tibiofemoral compartment. In general, HTO is avoided in knees in which there is more than a 15- × 15-mm area of exposed bone on both the tibial and the femoral surfaces. There are knees in younger patients in which the area of exposed bone may be greater and partial replacement is not an option. However, as a general rule, the remaining articular cartilage should be present over the majority of the medial joint surfaces.

Major concavity of the medial tibial plateau with loss of bone stock is a contraindication to HTO. On standing 45° posteroanterior (PA) radiographs,[121] knees that demonstrate no remaining articular cartilage space to the medial compartment are not candidates. An arthroscopic procedure just before HTO helps to assess the amount of remaining articular cartilage and remove symptomatic meniscus fragments and other tissues.

Additional contraindications are a limitation of knee flexion (>10°), lateral tibial subluxation (>10 mm), prior lateral meniscectomy, or lateral tibiofemoral joint damage.

An absolute contraindication for a medial opening wedge osteotomy is the use of nicotine products in any form. The

- Medial tibiofemoral compartment bone exposure over an area greater than 15 x 15 mm on femur and tibia.
- Major concavity medial tibial plateau, loss of bone stock.
- No joint space in medial compartment on standing 45° posteroanterior radiographs.
- Patients 50–60 yr of age with advanced medial compartment damage (candidates for unicompartmental knee replacement).
- Patient > 60 yr of age (candidates for partial or total joint replacement).
- >10° limitation of knee flexion.
- >10 mm of lateral tibial subluxation.
- Prior total lateral meniscectomy, lateral tibiofemoral cartilage damage.
- Use of products containing nicotine.
- Obesity (body mass index > 30).
- Increased slope to affected medal tibial plateau, teeter-totter knee.
- Marked symptomatic and advanced patellofemoral arthrosis.
- Prior joint infection, diabetes, rheumatoid arthritis, autoimmune diseases, malnutrition states.

complication of a nonunion is not worth the risk, and a minimum of 8 to 12 weeks' abstinence before surgery is required. The patient is warned that there may still be an increased risk of osteotomy healing.

A relative contraindication is a body weight over 200 pounds (91 kg) (Fig. 31-2). Although there may be some patients in

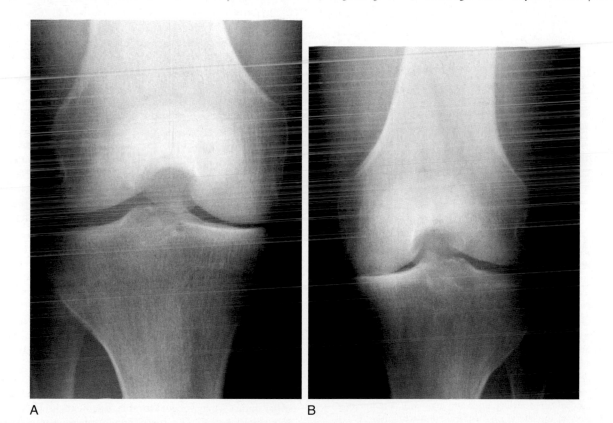

A   B

FIGURE 31–2. Anteroposterior (AP) radiographs of the right (**A**) and the left (**B**) knees in a 45-year-old retired professional football player. The patient's weight was 260 pounds. His chief complaint was bilateral medial joint pain with walking. The patient was advised to lose a significant amount of weight to decrease body size. In the authors' opinion, high tibial osteotomy (HTO) is contraindicated in this case owing to the advanced medial compartment arthritis. Many athletes of large stature with varus malalignment undergo medial meniscectomy, continue athletic participation, and rather promptly lose the remaining cartilage in the medial tibiofemoral joint. An early HTO after weight loss could have been of benefit, but at this point, too much deterioration has occurred.

whom HTO is indicated who weigh up to 225 pounds (102 kg), this operation is avoided in patients with a higher body weight because the beneficial effect of unloading the medial compartment will not be achieved.[28]

A relative contraindication is increased medial slope to the affected medial tibial plateau in the coronal plane due to advanced medial plateau concavity.[27] This finding indicates that it will not be possible to significantly unload the medial compartment with HTO, and the joint will remain with all of the weight-bearing confined to the medial compartment. This problem can be tested prior to surgery with varus-valgus stability tests at 30° knee flexion. In these knees with advanced medial arthritis, there is no neutral point in which there is simultaneous contact of the medial and lateral compartments. The tibia behaves like a teeter-totter, with contact alternating between the medial and the lateral compartment and obvious separation of the noncontacted compartment.

The issue of concurrent patellofemoral arthritis has been addressed by prior studies.[28,83,123] In general, the symptomatic state should be addressed and the patient warned preoperatively that patellofemoral symptoms might continue or progress. Marked patellofemoral symptoms would contraindicate an HTO.[123] The finding of asymptomatic articular cartilage changes to the patellofemoral joint is not a contraindication to HTO, because clinicians have noted that the end result in terms of longevity of the HTO depends on the symptomatic medial tibiofemoral compartment.[28,68,93]

Medical contraindications to HTO include diabetes, rheumatoid arthritis, autoimmune diseases, and malnutrition states.

LOWER LIMB ALIGNMENT: PRIMARY, DOUBLE, AND TRIPLE VARUS KNEES

An added complexity in the varus-angulated knee with medial compartment arthritis is the presence of ACL deficiency. An associated deficiency of the posterolateral structures may add to the varus angulation and clinical symptoms. Patients who have these combined abnormalities often experience pain, swelling, giving-way, and functional limitations that may result

---

Critical Points LOWER LIMB ALIGNMENT: PRIMARY, DOUBLE, AND TRIPLE VARUS KNEES

Primary varus: amount of varus angulation due to:
1. Physiologic tibiofemoral angulation and osteocartilagenous (narrowing) of the medial tibiofemoral compartment.

Double varus: amount of varus angulation due to:
1. Tibiofemoral osteocartilagenous and geometric alignment.
2. Separation of the lateral tibiofemoral compartment from moderate deficiency of the posterolateral structures (>5 mm increased lateral joint opening, 10° increased external tibial rotation).

Triple varus: amount of varus angulation due to:
1. Tibiofemoral osteocartilagenous and geometric alignment.
2. Separation of the lateral tibiofemoral compartment.
3. Varus recurvatum in extension, severe deficiency of posterolateral ligamentous structures.

Restraints resisting lateral tibiofemoral compartment separation under dynamic weight-bearing conditions: quadriceps, biceps femoris, gastrocnemius, iliotibial band.

---

in a disabling condition. In these complex knees, multiple abnormalities exist to the lower limb and knee joint that must be correctly diagnosed to outline a rational treatment program. These include the anatomic tibiofemoral osseous coronal and sagittal alignment, abnormal knee motion limits, abnormal knee positions (subluxations of the medial and lateral tibiofemoral compartments), and the corresponding specific deficiencies of the ligament structures (single and combined).

The terms *primary varus*, *double varus*, and *triple varus* knee were devised to classify varus-aligned knees with associated ligament deficiencies (Table 31–1).[93] This classification system is based on the underlying tibiofemoral osseous alignment and the additional effect of separation of the lateral tibiofemoral compartment (due to deficiency of the posterolateral structures) on the overall varus lower limb alignment, as calculated from the WBL.

In patients with a varus-angulated knee, a bilateral physiologic varus tibiofemoral alignment is usually present. In others, a normal tibiofemoral alignment may convert to a varus malalignment after medial meniscectomy. With loss of the medial meniscus and resultant articular cartilage deterioration, narrowing of the medial tibiofemoral compartment occurs along with an increase in varus lower limb alignment. For example, a patient with a physiologic varus alignment of 3° (mechanical axis) with an additional loss of 3 mm of the medial articular cartilage would develop an overall 6° varus tibiofemoral alignment.

The term *primary varus* refers to the physiologic tibiofemoral osseous angulation and any further increase in angulation owing to altered geometry (narrowing) of the medial osteocartilagenous tibiofemoral joint (Fig. 31–3). The tibiofemoral WBL shifts into the medial tibiofemoral compartment as the narrowing progresses and the lateral compartment is unloaded. Three degrees of varus angulation approximately doubles medial compartment pressures.[36,46]

As the WBL shifts into the medial compartment, there are increased tensile forces in the posterolateral soft tissues, including the iliotibial tract and ligament structures. There is corresponding separation of the lateral tibiofemoral compartment during standing, walking, and running activities (lateral condylar lift-off).[75,125] This is called a *double varus knee* because the lower limb varus malalignment results from two factors: the tibiofemoral osseous and geometric alignment and separation of the lateral tibiofemoral compartment from deficiency of the posterolateral structures.

A combination of active and passive restraints resists separation of the lateral tibiofemoral compartment under dynamic loading conditions.[45,86] The quadriceps, biceps femoris, and gastrocnemius muscles and iliotibial band act in a dynamic manner to resist adduction moments at the knee joint during gait and, with weight-bearing loads, resist lateral tibiofemoral separation. If these muscle forces do not provide a functional restraint to excessive lateral tensile forces, separation of the lateral tibiofemoral joint occurs.

The FCL normally allows a few millimeters of separation of the tibiofemoral compartment, and pathologic stretching (interstitial injury) may occur to this ligament in chronic varus-angulated knees. Under these circumstances, a transfer of all of the weight-bearing loads to the medial compartment occurs, which can be especially deleterious if damaged articular cartilage or prior meniscectomy is present.

The patient symptoms commonly increase with pain in both the medial compartment and the lateral aspect of the knee joint

TABLE 31–1   Causes of Varus Angulation in the Anterior Cruciate Ligament–Deficient Knee

Tibiofemoral Alignment or Geometry	Knee Motion Limits	Knee Joint Position	Ligament Deficiency	Comments
Primary varus Physiologic tibiofemoral varus alignment Narrowing or loss of medial joint cartilage	NA ↑ Varus or adduction rotation	NA ↓ Separation of medial tibiofemoral compartment	NA Pseudolaxity or slackness of medial ligament structures	Medial displacement of weight-bearing tibiofemoral line. Effect on varus alignment is more pronounced when preexisting physiologic varus alignment is present.
Double varus Added deficiency of FCL, posterolateral soft tissue structures	↑↑Varus or adduction rotation Often coupled with lateral tibial translation and secondary support, intercondylar eminence against lateral femoral condyle	Separation of lateral tibiofemoral joint on standing Varus thrust on walking due to lateral condylar lift-off Increased tension in FCL, posterolateral soft tissues	FCL, lateral capsule, iliotibial band (femorotibial portion) Amount of joint opening depends on slackness of lateral soft tissue restraints. Absence of ACL secondary restraint to varus angulation	Weight-bearing tibiofemoral line shifts far enough medially to produce separation of the lateral tibiofemoral joint during walking, sports activities. Under states of maximal muscle contraction (quadriceps, biceps femoris), sufficient compressive forces may exist to prevent lateral condylar lift-off.
Triple varus Added deficiency all PL structures (FCL, PMTL, PL capsule)	↑↑↑Varus or adduction rotation Varus recurvatum in extension • Increased external tibial rotation • Increased hyperextension • Increased external tibial rotation in flexion	↑Separation of lateral compartment plus varus recurvatum may occur on standing, walking. Varus recurvatum thrust if quadriceps and ankle plantar flexors do not prevent knee hyperextension. Posterior subluxation of lateral plateau with external tibial rotation	As above, plus PMTL, PL capsule, Knee hyperextension increases with associated damage to ACL, PCL (partial to complete)	Gait training is required to teach patient not to walk with varus recurvatum thrust, maintaining 5° of knee flexion on initial weight-bearing. Knee hyperextension with physiologic slackness to ACL and PCL may be present without actual injury to cruciates allowing varus recurvatum.

ACL, anterior cruciate ligament; FCL, fibular collateral ligament; NA, not available; PCL, posterior cruciate ligament; PL, posterolateral; PMTL, popliteal muscle-tendon-ligament unit.
From Noyes, F. R.; Simon, R.: The role of high tibial osteotomy in the anterior cruciate ligament–deficient knee with varus alignment. In DeLee, J. C.; Drez, D. (eds.): *Orthopaedic Sports Medicine Principles and Practice*. Philadelphia: W. B. Saunders, 1994; pp. 1401–1443.

owing to excessive medial compressive and lateral soft tissue tensile forces, respectively.

In the triple varus knee, injury to the FCL and posterolateral structures produces a varus recurvatum position of the limb.[54] The *triple varus knee* results from three causes: tibiofemoral varus osseous malalignment, increased lateral tibiofemoral compartment separation due to marked insufficiency of the FCL and PMTL, and varus recurvatum in extension. The varus recurvatum occurs because of abnormal external tibial rotation and knee hyperextension reflecting deficiency of the posterolateral structures and possibly the ACL. Owing to the increase in lateral compartment opening, the WBL shifts farther medially, as shown in Figure 31–3.

HTO is indicated in patients with varus malalignment who demonstrate a varus thrust on walking. An ACL reconstruction in these knees would not address the instability and would be expected to fail if the varus osseous malalignment was not corrected owing to the abnormal lateral tibiofemoral joint opening. A varus recurvatum or back-knee instability indicates a triple varus knee in which the posterolateral structures require reconstruction along with the ACL.

Eckhoff and coworkers[36] reported important three-dimensional measurements in 90 individuals (180 limbs) and showed that there is considerable variation in coronal alignment between subjects and between right-left lower limbs (Fig. 31–4).

One qualification to the data is that the hip-knee-ankle computed tomography (CT) measurements were obtained under non–weight-bearing conditions.

Given the variation in lower limb alignment in individuals, a frequent question is what is the effect of correcting one limb to neutral or a valgus overcorrection on overall gait and the (unoperated) opposite limb, particularly when a marked varus alignment is present bilaterally. In the authors' experience, the opposite extremity does not require operative correction, except in a small percentage of patients who have marked bilateral varus alignment, usually medial tibiofemoral pain in the opposite extremity, and subsequently undergo HTO.

GAIT ANALYSIS

Although a high adduction moment may be anticipated as a result of varus malalignment, the moments and loads on the knee joint cannot be reliably predicted from the static measurement of lower limb alignment on radiographs.[109] Many factors in patients with ACL deficiency, varus malalignment, and posterolateral deficiency can be assessed by gait analysis. Abnormal limb alignment, either varus or valgus in the coronal plane or hyperextension in the sagittal plane, produces substantial alterations in the moments and forces about the knee joint

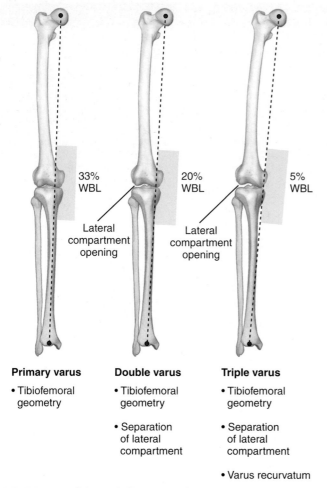

FIGURE 31–3. Schematic illustration of primary, double, and triple varus knee angulation. WBL, weight-bearing line.

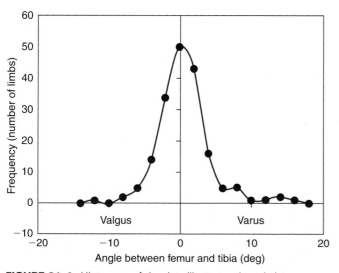

FIGURE 31–4. Histogram of the data illustrates the relative deviation of limb alignment from a straight line in the normal population of 180 limbs. Of the 90 individuals, 37 had bilateral valgus, 22 had bilateral varus, 31 had varus alignment of one limb and valgus of the other limb or varus or valgus alignment of one limb and neutral alignment of the other limb. *(Reprinted with permission from Eckhoff, D. G.; Bach, J. M.; Spitzer, V. M.; et al.: Three-dimensional mechanics, kinematics, and morphology of the knee viewed in virtual reality. J Bone Joint Surg Am 87:71–80, 2005.)*

Critical Points GAIT ANALYSIS

Moments and loads on knee joint cannot be reliably predicted from static measurement of lower limb alignment on radiographs.

Abnormally high knee adduction moments increase the risk for progression of medial tibiofemoral arthrosis. Success of HTO is related to lowering abnormal moments to normal or below-normal values.

Authors' Study Conclusions

• Majority of ACL-deficient varus-angulated knees have abnormally high adduction moments on walking.

• One third normal or low adduction moments, normal to low medial tibiofemoral compartment loads. Gait characteristics/adaptations lowered medial tibiofemoral loads despite varus angulation.

• Significant correlation high adduction moments and high medial tibiofemoral compartment loads, high lateral soft tissue forces.

• In knees with high lateral ligament tensile forces, separation of the lateral tibiofemoral joint may occur with "condylar lift-off" during weight-bearing.

Large tensile loads on posterolateral tissues cause stretching, deficiency (double and triple varus knees), failure of posterolateral reconstructive procedures.

ACL, anterior cruciate ligament; HTO, high tibial osteotomy.

(Fig. 31–5).[109] The analysis of external moments about the knee during gait allows the clinician to understand the effect of the altered gait dynamics on the knee joint. Abnormally high knee adduction moments increase the risk for progression of medial tibiofemoral arthritis owing to excessive loading.[118] The success of HTO has been related to lowering these moments to below-normal values.[118,137] In addition, gait analysis allows calculation of abnormally high tensile forces in the lateral soft tissue restraints that increase the risk of elongating these tissues from lateral condylar lift-off with activity. Abnormal tensile loads on posterolateral soft tissues preclude successful FCL and PMTL reconstruction. Markholf and associates[76] reported that lateral tibiofemoral compartment loading lateral condylar lift-off had a marked effect on providing joint stability.

Many studies have documented that the external moments about the knee joint and the corresponding tibiofemoral compartment loads are markedly influenced by individual gait characteristics and adaptations that occur after injury.[5,8–11,16,23,62,85,118,137] ACL deficiency may produce marked abnormalities in moments about the knee joint in the sagittal plane, which is further affected by lower limb varus malalignment. Patients with ACL deficiency may show a decrease in the magnitude of the external flexion moment (quadriceps-reduced gait) or an increase in the external extension moment (hamstrings-protective muscle force).[6,7] These effects are discussed in Chapter 6, Human Movement and Anterior Cruciate Ligament Function: Anterior Cruciate Ligament Deficiency and Gait Mechanics. The alignment of the foot markedly influences the knee adduction moment. Patients with toe-in, or less than normal external axial rotation of the foot during stance phase, tend to have a higher knee adduction moment as the WBL passes farther medial to the knee joint.[4]

Gait analyses were conducted in a study at the authors' institution[109] involving 32 patients with ACL deficiency and varus angulation. A force plate and an optoelectronic system were used to measure forces and moments of the lower limb and knee joint. Knee joint loads and ligament tensile forces were calculated using a previously described mathematical model.[125] Sixty-two percent of the patients had an abnormally high

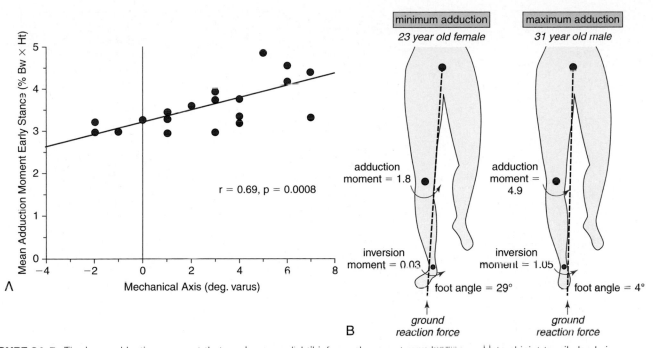

FIGURE 31–5. The knee adduction moment that produces medial tibiofemoral compartment loading and lateral joint tensile loads is dependent on both the mechanical axis (**A**) and patient gait characteristics such as the rotation of the lower limb and the foot angle at stance phase (**B**). (A and B, Reprinted with permission from Andrews, M.; Noyes, F. R.; Hewett, T. F.; Andriacchi, T. P.: Lower limb alignment and foot angle are related to stance phase knee adduction in normal subjects: a critical analysis of the reliability of gait analysis data. J Orthop Res 14:289–295, 1996.)

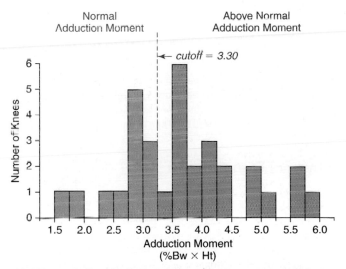

FIGURE 31–6. The distribution of the adduction moments during walking in the anterior cruciate ligament (ACL)–deficient knees. The cutoff value (3.30) (% body weight [BW] x height) represents the control mean minus 1 standard deviation. (Reprinted with permission from Noyes, F. R.; Schipplein, O. D.; Andriacchi, T. P.; et al.: The anterior cruciate ligament–deficient knee with varus alignment. An analysis of gait adaptations and dynamic joint loadings. Am J Sports Med 20:707–716, 1992.)

magnitude of the moment, tending to adduct the affected knee (Fig. 31–6). The calculated medial tibiofemoral loads were excessively high in 66% of the patients ($P < .01$). Forty-seven percent of the patients had predicted abnormally high lateral ligament tensile forces ($P < .05$). The adduction moment showed a statistically significant ($P < .05$) correlation to

predicted high medial tibiofemoral compartment loads and high lateral ligament tensile forces ($P < .01$). A shift had occurred in the center of maximal joint pressure to the medial tibiofemoral compartment, with a corresponding increase in the lateral ligament tensile forces to achieve frontal plane stability (Figs. 31–7 and 31–8). If muscle forces are not sufficient to maintain lateral tibiofemoral compressive loads, tensile forces develop in the lateral ligament tissues. The data indicate that, in knees with high lateral ligament tensile forces, separation of the lateral tibiofemoral joint occurs with "condylar lift-off" during weight-bearing.

The magnitude of the flexion moment (which is related to quadriceps muscle force) was significantly lower in 47% of the patients ($P < .05$), and the extension moment (related to hamstring muscle force) was significantly higher in 50% ($P < .05$). These findings indicated that a gait adaptation occurred that diminished quadriceps muscle activity and enhanced hamstring muscle activity hypothesized to provide anteroposterior stability of the knee joint.[16]

Equally important in the results was the finding that approximately one third of the patients had normal or low adduction moments and corresponding normal to low medial tibiofemoral compartment loads. These patients had gait characteristics or adaptations that lowered medial tibiofemoral loads despite the varus lower limb alignment. Gait analysis allowed identification of patients with a potentially better overall prognosis; the adduction moment and medial tibiofemoral loads were not excessively high, and a HTO would result in a substantial lowering of the loads placed on the medial tibiofemoral joint.

The authors[99] studied patients with varus-angulated knees with insufficient posterolateral structures in whom prior posterolateral reconstructive procedures failed and an HTO was

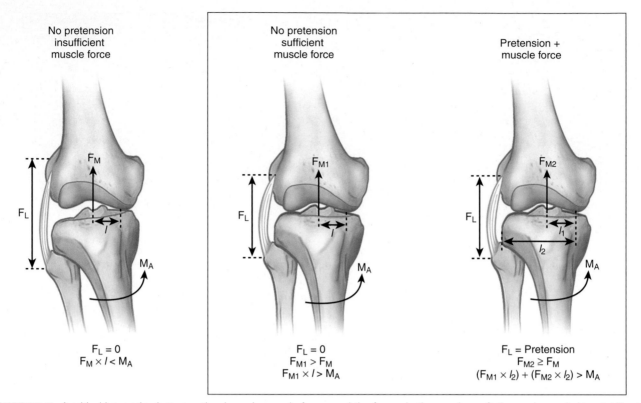

FIGURE 31–7. A critical interaction between the dynamic muscle forces and the forces in the passive soft tissues is needed to stabilize the knee joint during walking. The knee joint remains closed laterally if either pretension in the lateral soft tissues or increased muscle force resulting from antagonistic muscle groups is present. Distances l and $l_1 = 20$ mm; $l_2 = 60$ mm. F_l, soft tissue force; F_m, F_{m1}, F_{m2}, muscle forces; M_A, adducting moment.

required before further soft tissue reconstructive procedures could be done. One explanation for these clinical findings is that these knees had a varus or hyperextension thrust during the stance phase of gait, which placed undue tensile forces on the deficient posterolateral structures (Fig. 31–9). Untreated varus malalignment has also been identified as a predisposing cause of failure of ACL reconstructions[98,101] and posterior cruciate ligament (PCL) reconstructions[96] as well.

CLINICAL EVALUATION

Subjective and Functional Outcome

Patients complete questionnaires and are interviewed for the assessment of symptoms, functional limitations, sports and occupational activity levels, and their perception of the overall knee condition according to the Cincinnati Knee Rating System (see Chapter 44, The Cincinnati Knee Rating System).[13]

Symptoms of pain, swelling, and giving-way are well-recognized consequences of ACL-deficiency.[108] However, in the knee with combined varus malalignment and ACL deficiency, several different knee subluxations may produce symptoms of instability. These include anterior subluxation of the tibia, separation of the lateral tibiofemoral compartment on walking (varus thrust), posterior subluxation of the lateral tibial plateau (with knee flexion and external tibial rotation), and excessive hyperextension or varus recurvatum with a back-knee or feeling of the

knee joint going into hyperextension. By history and asking the patient to demonstrate the knee instability, the surgeon must carefully determine the subluxations present.

Physical Examination

A complaint of medial joint line pain may or may not correlate with the degree of medial compartment articular cartilage damage.[50,58] In the early stages, the patient usually complains of medial pain that occurs with sports activities, but not with daily activities. When pain occurs with daily activities, it is highly likely that extensive damage exists to the joint articular cartilage. Loss of the medial meniscus is the major risk factor for the progression of arthritis in the medial compartment.[37]

The physical examination of the knee joint to detect all of the abnormalities in the varus-angulated knee is comprehensive (Table 31–2) and includes assessment of (1) the patellofemoral joint, especially possible extensor mechanism malalignment due to increased external tibial rotation and posterolateral tibial subluxation; (2) medial tibiofemoral crepitus on varus loading, indicative of articular cartilage damage even if not visible on radiographs; (3) pain and inflammation of the lateral soft tissues due to tensile overloading; (4) gait abnormalities (excessive hyperextension or varus thrust) during walking and jogging[104]; and (5) abnormal knee motion limits and subluxations compared with the contralateral knee.[106]

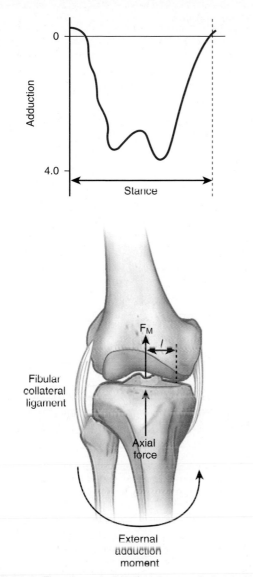

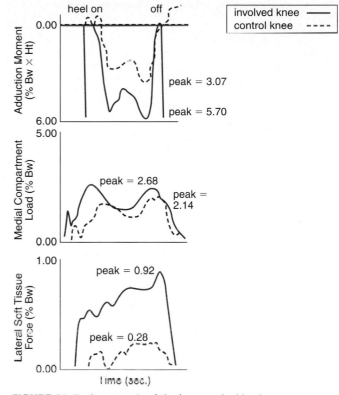

FIGURE 31-8. The external adducting moment is resisted by the minimum sagittal plane muscle force (F$_m$) and axial load acting over l. Pretension in the lateral soft tissues would maintain equilibrium if the muscle force were insufficient.

FIGURE 31-9. An example of the increased adduction moment, medial compartment load, and lateral soft tissue force in an involved knee compared with a control knee. *(Reprinted with permission from Noyes, F. R.; Schipplein, O. D.; Andriacchi, T. P.; et al.: The anterior cruciate ligament–deficient knee with varus alignment. An analysis of gait adaptations and dynamic joint loadings. Am J Sports Med 20:707–716, 1992.)*

Diagnostic Clinical Tests

The medial posterior tibiofemoral step-off on the posterior drawer test is done at 90° of flexion (Fig. 31–10). This test is performed first to identify that the tibia is not posteriorly subluxated, indicating a partial or complete PCL tear. A KT-2000 arthrometer test may be done at 20° of flexion (134 N force) to quantify total anteroposterior (AP) displacement. The Lachman test is performed at 20° of knee flexion. The pivot shift test is done and the result recorded on a scale of 0 to 3, with a grade of 0 indicating no pivot shift; grade 1, a slip or glide; grade 2, a jerk with gross subluxation or clunk; and grade 3, gross subluxation with impingement of the posterior aspect of the lateral side of the tibial plateau against the femoral condyle.

FCL insufficiency is determined by the varus stress test at 0° and 30° of knee flexion (see Fig. 31–10). The surgeon estimates the amount of joint opening (in millimeters) between the initial closed contact position of each tibiofemoral compartment, performed in a constrained manner avoiding internal or external tibial rotation,

and the maximal opened position. The result is recorded according to the increase in the tibiofemoral compartment of the affected knee compared with that of the opposite normal knee. This comparison is crucial, and it is important to avoid measuring only the degrees of varus or valgus rotation in the involved knee.

An increase in medial joint opening may occur compared with the opposite knee that represents a pseudolaxity, because the increase is actually due to medial tibiofemoral joint narrowing. When the test is conducted under a varus stress, the medial joint opening returns the limb to a more normal alignment, and there is no true medial ligamentous damage. The true amount of medial and lateral tibiofemoral compartment opening is later confirmed during the arthroscopic examination with gap tests. The primary and secondary restraints that resist lateral joint opening have been described previously.[45] The abnormal medial joint opening depends on the knee flexion angle at which the test is conducted and the integrity of the secondary restraints.

Tibiofemoral Rotation Test

The tibiofemoral rotation test was first described by the senior author[103] and is used to estimate the amount of posterior tibial subluxation (see Fig. 31–10). The test is conducted in the following manner: (1) the tibia is positioned at 30° of knee flexion, in neutral rotation, (2) the position of the anterior aspect of the medial and lateral tibial plateaus are determined in reference to the femoral condyles by palpation, (3) the tibia is externally rotated to its maximum position, (4) the positions of the

Assessment of symptoms and functional limitations with activity: Cincinnati Knee Rating System

Physical Examination

- Knee flexion and extension
- Joint effusion
- Patellofemoral: extensor mechanism malalignment
- Tibiofemoral crepitus, joint line pain, compression pain, inflammation
- Gait abnormalities
- Abnormal knee motion limits and subluxations

Diagnostic Clinical Tests

- Posterior drawer, 90° knee flexion
- KT-2000, 20° knee flexion, 189 N force
- Pivot shift, Lachman
- Lateral and medial tibiofemoral joint opening 0°, 25° knee flexion
- Varus recurvatum: supine

Tibiofemoral Rotation (Dial Test)

- 30° and 90° knee flexion
- An increase in external tibial rotation represents either a posterior subluxation of the lateral tibial plateau (injury to the posterolateral structures) or an anterior subluxation of the medial tibial plateau (injury to the medial collateral ligament and posteromedial structures).
- Supine position preferred. Difficult to palpate the medial and lateral tibiofemoral position in the prone position.

Radiographic Assessment

- Double-stance, hip-knee-ankle to measure mechanical axis, weight-bearing line, lateral compartment separation
- Lateral, 30° knee flexion (patellar height measurement)
- Posteroanterior, weight-bearing, 45° knee flexion
- Patellofemoral axial
- Lateral stress, neutral tibial rotation, tibia unconstrained, 67 N varus force

TABLE 31–2	**Diagnosis of Abnormalities**
Abnormality	**Diagnostic Test**
Tibiofemoral alignment	Full-length standing radiograph: double support (closure of lateral tibiofemoral joint required).
Narrowing of medial tibiofemoral joint	Change in millimeters from opposite side on weight-bearing 45° posterior on stress radiograph.
FCL insufficiency	Increase in lateral joint opening at 30° of flexion.
FCL, PMTL, PL capsule insufficiency	Further increase in lateral joint opening at 30° of flexion.
	Increase in external tibial rotation at 30° of flexion.
	Varus recurvatum in extension.
Lateral tibiofemoral joint separation	Standing radiograph shows increased joint width compared with opposite side.
	Amount of increase on stress radiograph compared with opposite side.
Varus recurvatum	Defined by degrees of hyperextension and varus angulation.
	Elicited on supine varus recurvatum test.
	Standing tests with patient assuming maximal knee hyperextension position provides greatest subluxation.
	Estimate degrees of increase in varus and hyperextension.

FCL, fibular collateral ligament; PL, posterolateral; PMTL, popliteal muscle-tendon-ligament unit.
From Noyes, F. R.; Simon, R.: The role of high tibial osteotomy in the anterior cruciate ligament–deficient knee with varus alignment. In DeLee, J. C.; Drez, D. (eds.): *Orthopaedic Sports Medicine Principles and Practice.* Philadelphia: W. B. Saunders, 1994; pp. 1401–1443.

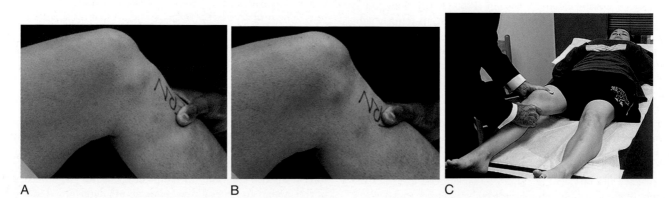

FIGURE 31–10. Manual knee tests. **A** and **B,** Posterior drawer test at 90° knee flexion. **C,** Lachman test.

Continued

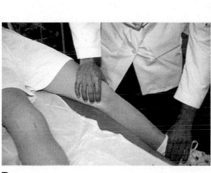

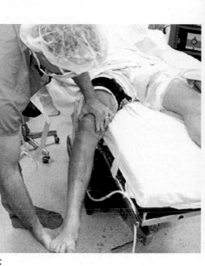

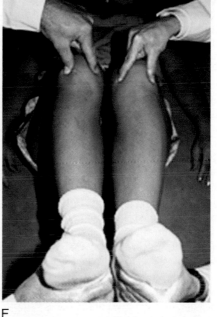

D   E   F

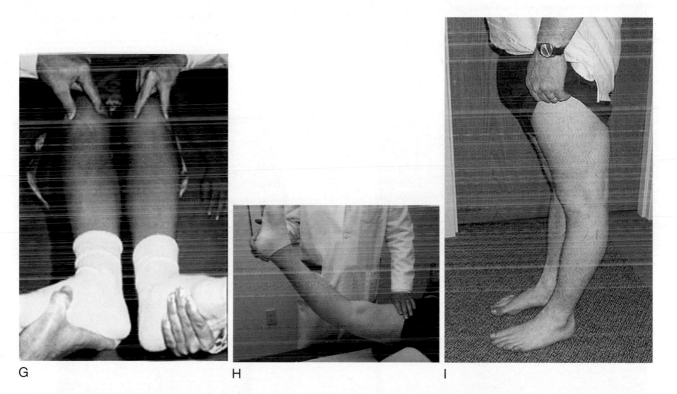

G   H   I

FIGURE 31–10—cont'd D, Valgus manual test for medial joint opening. **E,** Varus manual test for lateral joint opening. Dial test at 90° of knee flexion in neutral tibial rotation (**F**) and maximum external tibial rotation (**G**). Varus recurvatum in the supine (**H**) and the standing (**I**) positions.

medial and lateral tibial plateaus are palpated to determine an abnormal posterior subluxation of the lateral compartment or anterior subluxation of the medial compartment, (5) the examiner observes the location of the tibial tubercle to determine any increase in external tibial rotation compared with the opposite normal knee, and (6) the test is repeated at 90° of knee flexion and may also be conducted by starting at the neutral tibial rotation position and progressing to internal tibial rotation.

If an increase in external tibial rotation is present, it represents either a posterior subluxation of the lateral tibial plateau (indicating injury to the FCL and PMTL) or an anterior subluxation of the medial tibial plateau (indicating injury to the superficial medial collateral ligament [SMCL] and posteromedial structures). In some knees, both anteromedial and posterolateral subluxations are present.

The tibiofemoral rotation test involves close observation of the location of the internal and external tibial rotation axis and comparison of the location of this axis to that in the normal knee. With posterior subluxation of the lateral tibial plateau during external tibial rotation, the examiner may detect a shift in the axis of tibial rotation to the medial tibiofemoral compartment. Alternatively, with an anterior subluxation of the medial tibial plateau, the center of tibial rotation shifts to the lateral tibiofemoral compartment as the maximal external tibial rotation position is reached.

The advantages of the tibiofemoral rotation test over the traditional posterolateral drawer test[55] are (1) the knee may be positioned at varying flexion positions (30° and 90°); (2) the tibia is less constrained because the foot is not held fixed to the examining table; and (3) the axis of tibial rotation can be observed as the tibia is rotated externally and internally. More information is gained when the tibiofemoral rotation tests are performed with the patient in a supine position. In the prone position, it is difficult to palpate the medial and lateral tibiofemoral position required to diagnose the abnormal compartment subluxations. The only indication for the prone dial test is a PCL-deficient knee in which the tibia can be gently displaced to a reduced anterior position during the rotation tests. In the supine position, the tibia can also be displaced anteriorly to prevent posterior subluxation, which makes the interpretation of the dial test more difficult.

A varus recurvatum test in both the supine and the standing positions and the reversed pivot shift test are included in the assessment of posterolateral tibial subluxation. These represent qualitative tests; however, and are difficult to measure in objective terms. Still, they provide useful information regarding the magnitude of the overall subluxation of the knee joint when two or more abnormal motion limits are present.

Radiographic Assessment

Radiographic assessment of lower limb alignment is based on full-length radiographs of the extremity with the patient in the standing position.[35] Separation of the lateral tibiofemoral compartment may occur, preventing a correct assessment of true tibiofemoral osseous alignment. Double-stance, full-length AP radiographs showing both lower extremities from the femoral heads to the ankle joints are obtained. The knee is flexed 3° to 5° to avoid a hyperextension position. If separation of the lateral tibiofemoral joint is observed, it is necessary to subtract the lateral compartment opening so that the true tibiofemoral osseous alignment is determined and a valgus overcorrection at surgery is avoided, as is discussed under Preoperative Planning.

The clinician should assess for a possible teeter-totter effect, in which simultaneous contact of the medial and lateral tibiofemoral compartments is not possible owing to advanced changes of tibial obliquity and bone loss in the medial tibiofemoral joint.

Additional radiographs taken during the initial examination include a lateral at 30° knee flexion, weight-bearing PA at 45° knee flexion, and patellofemoral axial views. Telos medial or lateral stress radiographs may also be required of both knees (Fig. 31–11).

The height of both patellas is measured on lateral radiographs (Fig. 31–12) to determine whether an abnormal patella

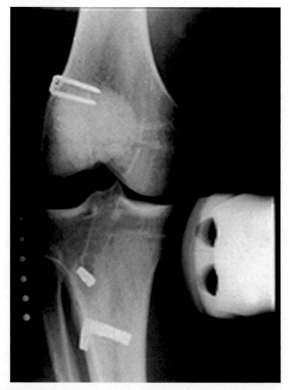

FIGURE 31–11. Lateral stress radiographs used to quantify the increase in lateral tibiofemoral joint opening between knees. Approximately 67 N of varus force is applied and a comparison is made of the millimeters of lateral tibiofemoral compartment opening between the knees.

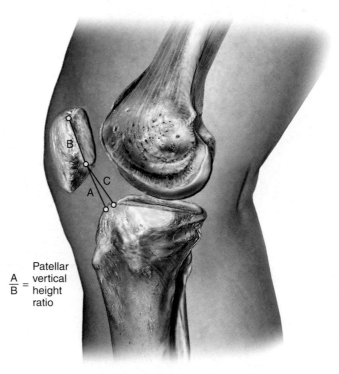

$$\frac{A}{B} = \text{Patellar vertical height ratio}$$

FIGURE 31–12. Method used to determine patellar vertical height ratio on a lateral radiograph. The numerator, *line segment A*, is the distance between the most ventral (anterosuperior) rim of the tibial plateau and the lowest end of the patellar articular surface. The denominator, *line segment B*, is the maximum length of the patellar articular surface. An alternative numerator, *line segment C*, locates the tibial reference point on the middle of the tibial plateau. The patellar vertical-height ratio equals A/B or C/B.

infera or alta position exists that may be a factor in selecting an opening or closing wedge osteotomy, which would further decrease or elevate the patella position.[111,112]

The clinical algorithm for the preoperative clinical and radiographic assessment to determine candidates for either a medial opening wedge or a lateral closing wedge osteotomy is shown in Figure 31–13.

PREOPERATIVE PLANNING

Calculations to Determine Angular Correction

The preoperative calculations for HTO involve precise measurements to determine the amount of angular correction

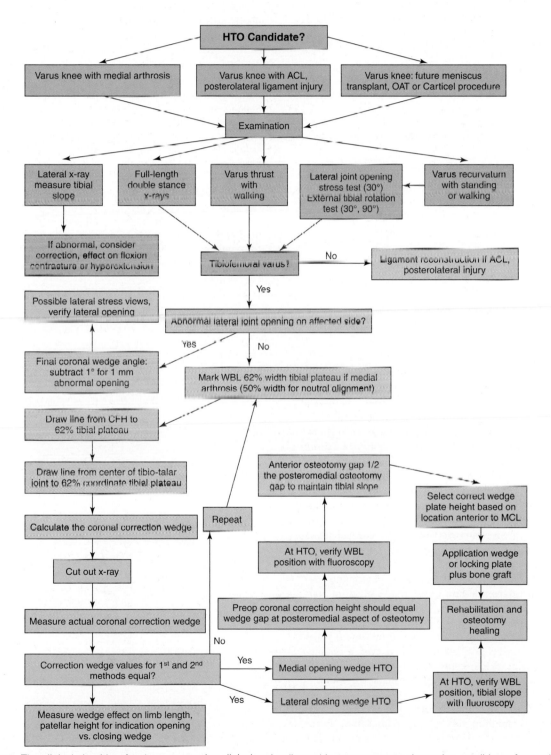

FIGURE 31–13. The clinical algorithm for the preoperative clinical and radiographic assessment to determine candidates for medial opening wedge or lateral closing wedge osteotomy.

Critical Points PREOPERATIVE PLANNING

- Determine angular correction to achieve redistribution of tibiofemoral forces without altering tibial slope.
- Take into account abnormal lateral tibiofemoral separation from deficient posterolateral structures.
- Measure weight-bearing line on bilateral standing hip-knee-ankle radiographs.
  - ○ Weight-bearing line is dependent on femoral and tibial lengths and angular deformity.
- Measure tibial slope on lateral radiographs.
- Increasing tibial slope increases anterior tibial translation; potentially, tensile loads on the ACL.
- Decreasing tibial slope increases posterior tibial translation; potentially, tensile loads on PCL.
- Do not alter normal tibial slope unless it is markedly abnormal.
  - ○ Tibial slope >2 standard deviations above normal.
- Do not alter a normal tibial slope in ACL-deficient or PCL-deficient knees.
- Maintain normal tibial slope: anterior gap at medial opening wedge should be half the posteromedial gap. Every millimeter of anterior gap change = 2° change in tibial slope.

Timing of HTO in Knees with Ligament Deficiencies

Primary Varus Knees
- Cruciate reconstruction with HTO or later (no abnormal lateral joint opening present).

Double Varus Knees
- HTO first.
- Posterolateral structures may shorten with valgus alignment.
- Perform cruciate, posterolateral reconstructions later if required.

Triple Varus Knees
- HTO first, cruciate and posterolateral reconstruction later.

Opening Wedge Advantages
- Avoids lateral dissection, fibular osteotomy.
- Large correction > 12°, avoids tibial shortening.
- Distal advancement or reconstruction of the MCL in chronic MCL ruptures.
- In subsequent posterolateral reconstructions, avoids proximal fibular osteotomy, allows FCL grafts to be fixated securely to proximal fibula.

Closing Wedge Advantages
- Faster healing.
- Earlier resumption of weight-bearing.
- Superior strength initial osteotomy fixation.
- Decreased risk early loss of correction, nonunion.
- More difficult to achieve correction at surgery.
- Large closing wedge may elevate patellar height and decrease lower limb length; reverse applies with opening wedge.

Opening Wedge HTO: Maintenance of Tibial Slope
- Opening wedge angle is dependent on the angle of coronal valgus correction and the angle of obliquity of the anteromedial tibial cortex.
- Every millimeter of alteration in gap height results in a change of 2° in tibial slope.

ACL, anterior cruciate ligament; HTO, high tibial osteotomy; MCL, medial collateral ligament; PCL, posterior cruciate ligament.

---

desired to redistribute tibiofemoral forces while not altering tibial slope and tibiofemoral joint obliquity in the frontal plane.[35,107] The normal tibiofemoral coronal alignment is shown in Figure 31–14. In varus angulated knees, there is a slight increase in obliquity due to medial tibiofemoral joint arthrosis principally involving the medial condyle. An opening wedge femoral osteotomy restores the joint obliquity. The more difficult issue related to joint obliquity involves correcting a valgus malalignment in which a change in joint obliquity is common. An opening wedge osteotomy corrects the joint obliquity, whereas a closing wedge tibial osteotomy increases joint obliquity and therefore is contraindicated.

An undercorrection or overcorrection in the coronal plane may result if the surgeon fails to recognize the effect of lateral tibiofemoral separation on increasing varus angulation that results from slack or deficient lateral soft tissues. Inaccurate calculations may also arise from failure to use the WBL from double-stance, full-length, standing radiographs of both lower extremities to determine the angular deformity. A single-stance radiograph of the affected limb will show the maximum varus angulation due to lateral condylar lift-off. However, a double-stance radiograph helps to close the lateral tibiofemoral compartment so the true osseous alignment is calculated, which is required for surgical correction.

Sabharwal and Zhao[124] compared lower limb coronal alignment on full-length, standing radiographs with supine intraoperative hip-knee-ankle fluoroscopy measurements in 102 limbs. There was a statistically significant mean difference between the two techniques (mean, 13.4 mm deviation in the

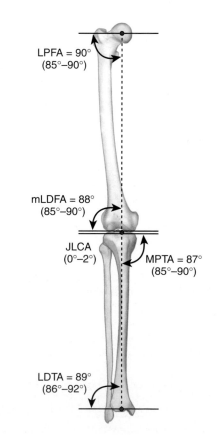

FIGURE 31–14. The normal tibiofemoral coronal alignment.

WBL, measured from the center of the joint). This difference in the two techniques is of concern in the preoperative planning and the final intraoperative osteotomy correction in the coronal plane. The reader should note that there was no description of accounting for the effect of abnormal lateral joint opening on the standing radiographs that would account for errors on full-length, standing radiograph preoperative measurements, as previously discussed. Further, at surgery there was no description of the fluoroscopy technique. The surgeon must verify medial and lateral tibiofemoral joint contact to account for possible opening of the medial or lateral tibiofemoral joint during the WBL measurement. The fluoroscopy technique involves the surgeon placing an axial load against the foot to overcome medial or lateral joint opening, which is verified by the fluoroscopic image. The lower extremity should be held in 10° of knee flexion and approximately 10° to 15° of external rotation (hip to ankle axial alignment simulating the foot progression angle). The limb alignment rod at the knee joint can be observed to move medial to lateral with internal to external limb rotation, which is another source of error in measuring the WBL intersection at the tibia. This is because the alignment rod is placed anterior to the true center of axial rotation at the ankle joint, and therefore, lower limb rotation induces this error. One advantage of the computerized navigation technique is that the WBL is centered through the hip-knee-ankle joints whereas an alignment rod or cord used at surgery is placed anterior to these respective joints.

An example of the potential effect of the failure to account for increased lateral joint opening is shown in Figure 31–15. The case represents a 38-year-old man whose full-length, standing radiograph shows a varus angular deformity (mechanical axis) of 7° and a 4-mm increase in lateral joint opening. The width of the tibial plateau is 81 mm. The equation to determine the angular deformity resulting from the lateral tibiofemoral separation distance is

$$\alpha = 76.4S/TW$$

S, lateral joint opening space; TW, tibial width.

Therefore, in this patient, the calculated amount of varus angular deformity caused by the lateral joint opening increase of 4 mm is

$$76.4(4mm)/81mm = 3.7°, \text{ or approximately } 1°/min$$
increased lateral joint separation

Failure to account for the lateral joint opening would result in approximately 4° of valgus overcorrection after HTO, assuming closure of the lateral tibiofemoral joint (Fig. 31–16). A WBL crossing the knee lateral to the 75% coordinate has the potential for a lift-off of the medial femoral condyle. Unicondylar weight-bearing resulting from distraction of the medial compartment is undesirable and could result in subsequent arthritis of the lateral compartment, medial collateral ligament (MCL) laxity, and a progressive valgus deformity (Fig. 31–17). The WBL-tibial intersection depends on the coronal mechanical axis angle and the femoral and tibial lengths of the patient; the senior author's published study[35] showed the WBL axis to be more accurate than the anatomic axis for osteotomy correction.

Two methods are used to determine the correction wedge on preoperative radiographs.[35] First, the centers of the femoral head and tibiotalar joint (center of the talus) are marked on the full-length radiograph (Fig. 31–18). The desired correction in the WBL coordinate of the tibial plateau is identified and marked. This is usually placed at 62% of the tibial width (just at the down slope of the lateral tibial spine), which allows the WBL to pass through the lateral tibiofemoral compartment, providing a 2° to 3° angular valgus overcorrection. The 62% WBL coordinate is used if there is medial tibiofemoral articular cartilage damage and the intention is to transfer major loads to

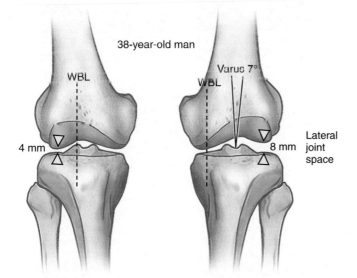

FIGURE 31–15. Sketch of a standing AP roentgenogram. The lateral joint space is 8 mm on the left side and 4 mm on the right side. The calculated angular deformity resulting from the 4-mm joint opening is 3.7° of the total 7° of deformity. WBL, weight-bearing line.

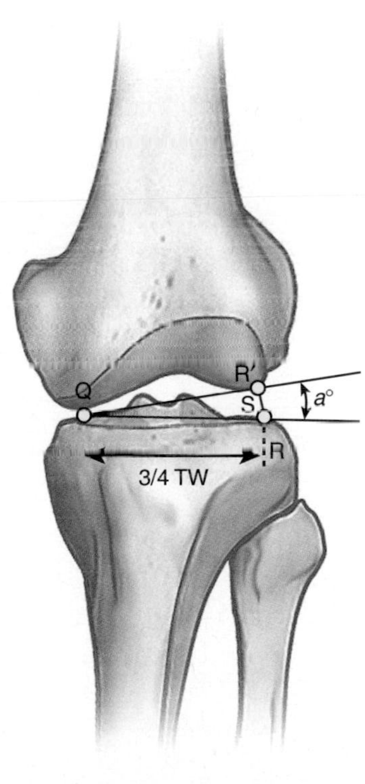

FIGURE 31–16. The effect of abnormal lateral joint opening on varus angular deformity. With a varus moment applied through a fulcrum, or center of rotation (Q), lateral joint space opening (S) occurs in the presence of slack lateral soft tissues resulting in an additional α° of varus angular deformity.

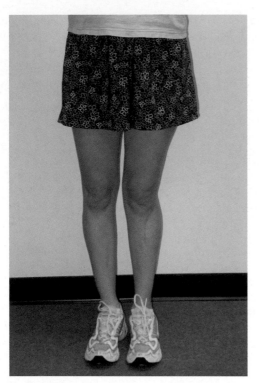

FIGURE 31–17. A 32-year-old woman with abnormal lateral joint opening underwent HTO elsewhere. The preoperative planning failed to account for the abnormal lateral joint opening, which resulted in a severe valgus overcorrection and need for revision osteotomy.

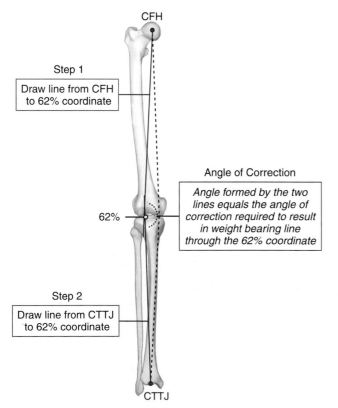

FIGURE 31–18. Graphic depiction of the method used to calculate the correction angle of an HTO using a full-length AP radiograph of the lower extremity. The lines from the centers of the femoral head (CFH) and tibiotalar joint (CTTJ) converge in this example at the 62% coordinate.

the lateral compartment. A 50% WBL coordinate is chosen if there is no medial tibiofemoral joint damage and the surgeon wishes to correct to a neutral axial alignment (e.g., prior to posterolateral reconstruction). One line is drawn from the center of the femoral head to the selected percent WBL intersection at the tibia, and a second line is drawn from the center of the tibiotalar joint to the same tibial coordinate position. The angle formed by the two lines intersecting at the tibia represents the angular correction required to realign the WBL through this coordinate. An alternative method was published[35] in which the previously discussed femoral and tibial axis lines intersect at the hinge point of the tibial osteotomy. This technique ends up with a similar measurement for the angular correction. However, the surgeon does not have the measured WBL tibial intersection required for intraoperative fluoroscopy verification.

The second method of determining the correction wedge involves cutting the full-length, standing radiograph horizontally through the line of the superior osteotomy cut (Fig. 31–19). A vertical cut of the lower tibial segment (opening or closing wedge) is made to converge with the first cut. The distal portion of the radiograph is aligned until the center of the femoral head, the selected WBL coordinate point on the tibial plateau, and the center of the tibiotalar joint are all colinear. With the radiograph taped in this position, the angle of the wedge formed by the overlap of the two radiographic segments

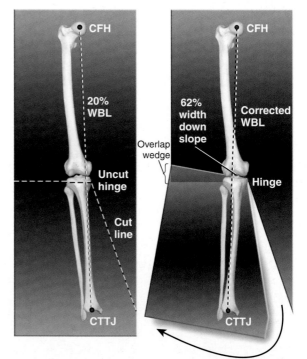

FIGURE 31–19. Graphic depiction of an alternative method used to calculate the correction angle of an HTO using a full-length AP radiograph of the lower extremity. The roentgenograph is cut to allow the center of the femoral head (CFH), the 62% coordinate, and the center of the tibiotalar joint (CTTJ) to become colinear. The angle of the resulting wedge of roentgenograph overlap equals the desired angle of correction. The example is provided for a closing wedge osteotomy. The same technique is used for an opening wedge osteotomy in which the medial tibial opening wedge is made to obtain the desired correction.

is measured and compared with the value obtained using the first method. The mechanical axis is measured to determine the angular correction. If there is a discrepancy between the two correction wedge angles, the procedures should be repeated.

Calculations to Determine Tibial Slope and Clinical Indications to Change Tibial Slope

Lateral radiographs are examined and measurements made of the tibial slope. Abnormal posterior sloping of the tibia in the sagittal plane may occur after tibial osteotomy, tibial fractures, growth abnormalities, or rarely, as a congenital occurrence.

Several methods have been reported to measure the medial and lateral tibial slope based on lateral tibial radiographs (Table 31–3).[17,20,24,25,41,63,79,82,146] Each method results in different slope values for the same tibia (Fig. 31–20), and all studies show high standard deviations and ranges, indicating that tibial slope may show variation among individual patients. Brazier and colleagues[20] measured 83 lateral knee radiographs and concluded that the methods of slope measurement of proximal tibial anatomic axis (PTAA) and posterior tibial cortex were more reliable than other methods. Genin and coworkers[41] and Julliard and associates[63] recommended using the tibial mechanical axis to represent the true tibial slope. The PTAA is the authors' preferred method for HTO, and the anterior tibial cortex measurement is used when cutting the proximal tibia during total knee arthroplasty (TKA).

Most authors have measured the medial tibial slope; only a few have measured and provided data on the lateral tibial slope.[79,146] The lateral tibial slope is less angled than the medial

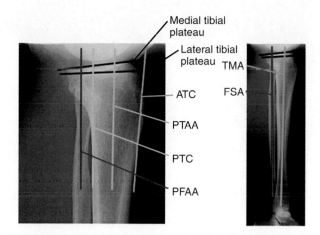

FIGURE 31–20. Some reported radiographic techniques to measure the tibial slope. The values obtained depend on the anatomic site selected on the tibia. Selected literature references for reported values are shown in Table 31–3. ATC, anterior tibial cortex; FSA, fibular shaft axis; PFAA, proximal fibular anatomic axis; PTAA, proximal tibial anatomic axis; PTC, posterior tibial cortex; TMA, tibial mechanical axis. *(Reprinted with permission from Noyes, F. R.; Goebel, S. X.; West, J.: Opening wedge tibial osteotomy: the 3-triangle method to correct axial alignment and tibial slope. Am J Sports Med 33:378–387, 2005.)*

tibial slope. Few investigators have distinguished between the tibial plateau osseous slope and the change that would occur in slope if the articular cartilage and meniscus were added to the calculations. The osseous tibial slope is most commonly noted in the literature and is measured from sagittal radiographs. The true tibial slope, which includes the articular cartilage and meniscus, was noted to be 6° less than the osseous tibial slope, according to Jenny and colleagues.[60]

TABLE 31–3	Literature Review of Medial and Lateral Tibial Plateau Slope Measurements						
		Medial Slope		**Lateral Slope**		
Reference	**Gender**	**Mean ± SD**	**Range**	**Mean ± SD**	**Range**	**Measurement Method**
Ching-Chuan et al., 1994[24]	M	10 ± 3	0–17	NA	NA	PTAA
	F	10 ± 4	0–20	NA	NA	
Matsuda et al., 1999[79]	B	10.7 ± 2.4	5–15.5	7.2 ± 3.8	0–14.5	PTAA
Billings et al., 2000[17]	B	8.7 ± 4.31	NA	NA	NA	TSA
Genin et al., 1993[41]	B	7.03 ± 3.17	–1–+18	NA	NA	Mechanical axis*
		7.9 ± 3.2	–1–+18	NA	NA	ATC
Chiu et al., 2000[25]	B	14.7 ± 3.7	5–22	NA	NA	ATC
		11.5 ± 3.6	2–18.5	NA	NA	TSA
Brazier et al., 1996[20]	B	11.41 ± 3.61	3.47–20.29	NA	NA	ATC
		9.16 ± 3.37	2.54–17.91	NA	NA	PTAA
		10.39 ± 3.72	2.82–19.29	NA	NA	TSA
		6.96 ± 3.28	0–15.44	NA	NA	PTC
		9.54 ± 3.62	0–17.34	NA	NA	PFAA
		8.23 ± 3.51	1.59–16.59	NA	NA	FSA
Julliard et al., 1993[63]	B	7.03 ± 3.17	–2–+19	NA	NA	Mechanical axis*
Yoshioka et al., 1989[146]	M	7 ± 2.2	NA	8 ± 3.7	NA	Mechanical axis*
	F	7 ± 3	NA	7 ± 3.9	NA	Mechanical axis*
Meister et al., 1998[82]	ACL	9.7 ± 1.8	NA	NA	NA	PTAA
	PF	9.9 ± 2.1	NA	NA	NA	PTAA

*Mechanical axis: measurement from center of ankle to center of knee (distal femur) in full extension.

ACL, anterior cruciate ligament; ATC, anterior tibial cortex; FSA, fibula shaft axis; NA, not available; PF, patellofemoral; PFAA, proximal fibular anatomic axis; PTAA, proximal tibial anatomic axis; PTC, posterior tibial cortex; SD, standard deviation; TSA, tibial shaft axis.

From Noyes, F. R.; Goebel, S. X.; West, J.: Opening wedge tibial osteotomy: the 3-triangle method to correct axial alignment and tibial slope. *Am J Sports Med* 33:378–387, 2005.

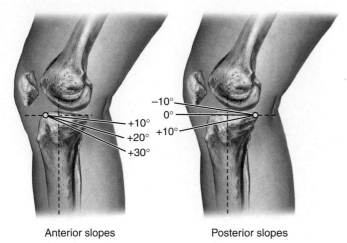

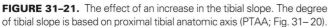

FIGURE 31–21. The effect of an increase in the tibial slope. The degree of tibial slope is based on proximal tibial anatomic axis (PTAA; Fig. 31– 20).

Increasing the tibial slope increases anterior tibial translation and, potentially, tensile loads on the ACL or an ACL reconstruction (Fig. 31–21).[30] Conversely, decreasing the tibial slope theoretically would increase tensile loads on the PCL and shift the tibia to a more anterior position. Giffin and coworkers[44] reported in cadaveric knees that an increase of 5° in the tibial slope produced an anterior shift in the resting position of the tibia (maximum, 3.6 ± 1.4 mm at full extension). However, under a 200-N axial load, there was only a 2-mm anterior shift in the tibiofemoral contact position (30° and 90°) and no increase in ACL forces. The authors concluded that small changes in tibial slope under simulated weight-bearing conditions would have little effect on tibiofemoral position. However, they postulated that larger changes in tibial slope, such as 10°, would cause a greater anterior shift in the tibia resting and loaded positions that might require correction by biplanar osteotomy in knees with ACL injury undergoing HTO.

In a second study conducted by Giffin and associates,[43] a 5-mm anterior opening wedge osteotomy in PCL-sectioned cadaveric knees was performed and an anterior shift in the tibia resting position of approximately 4 mm was measured. The beneficial effect of an increase in tibial slope in a PCL-deficient knee should be viewed in terms of functional loading conditions, and it is questionable whether the resting no-load position data are applicable to in vivo loading conditions. In this study, under a combined 134-N tibial translation load and 200-N axial compressive load, there was no statistical difference in the amount of posterior tibial subluxation between the PCL-deficient and the PCL-deficient-osteotomy knees. The data show that the tibia reached a similar abnormal posterior tibial position (mean 90° AP translation: intact knee 10 mm; PCL-deficient, 20.6 mm; PCL-deficient-osteotomy, 20.3 mm). The authors concluded that "increasing the tibial slope would improve stability in the PCL-deficient knee"; however, this would be true only for conditions of no posterior tibial loading not expected in functional activities. The data in this study may be viewed from an opposite standpoint to indicate that PCL graft reconstruction is warranted in symptomatic knees, because the opening wedge osteotomy is not effective in preventing posterior tibial subluxation under posterior tibial loading conditions.

In cadaveric knees, Agneskirchner and colleagues[2] studied the effect of an opening wedge osteotomy combined with a flexion osteotomy (to change the tibial slope) on tibiofemoral contact pressures and the resultant tibiofemoral position. The study reported that the flexion osteotomy shifted the tibiofemoral contact to a more anterior position (15° flexion osteotomy, ~5 mm, 30° knee flexion), which "neutralized" the effect of sectioning the PCL and reduced pressures of the posterior half of the tibial plateau. The authors suggested in varus-angulated, PCL-deficient knees, with associated posterolateral knee ligament injury and knee hyperextension, that an associated change in tibial slope would have a beneficial effect. Only quadriceps-induced leg extension loading was used, without weight-bearing loads or posterior translational loads to determine the resultant tibiofemoral position under more physiologic loading conditions. The quadriceps loading (to resist the applied external flexion moment) changed with the quadriceps extension force, nearly doubling with the flexion osteotomy (without osteotomy, ~550 N, with 15° flexion; with osteotomy, ~1100 N quadriceps applied load). The increased quadriceps loading in fact increased joint contact pressures.

In contrast to the study just discussed, Rodner and coworkers[120] reported in cadaveric knees that an increase in tibial slope in the ACL-deficient knee at the time of a HTO has the potential to redistribute tibiofemoral contact pressures to a more posterior position on the tibial plateau. From a theoretical standpoint, a redistribution of pressures posterior on the tibial plateau would be detrimental to the long-term success of an HTO in ACL-deficient knees with meniscectomy and posterior tibial plateau articular damage. The cadaver knee studies involved uniaxial loading knee joint loads instead of the quadriceps loading in the study by Agneskirchner and colleagues,[2] thereby demonstrating the marked effect that in vitro experimental loading conditions have on joint contact pressures and study conclusions.

Brandon and associates[19] measured the tibial slope in 100 ACL-deficient patients and 100 controls and reported that female and male patients had similar tibial slope measurements. ACL-deficient female and male patients had increases in tibial slope (mean values increased 3.6° and 2.4°, respectively), and the high-grade pivot-shift patient group had an increase in tibial slope (mean value increased ~2°). The measurements show high standard deviations (~35% of the mean values), and it is probable that the few degrees difference between patient groups is not clinically significant or would result in increased ACL load and anterior tibial displacement.

Dejour and colleagues[32] evaluated chronic ACL-deficient knees with monopodal lateral weight-bearing films (knee flexed 20° to 30° with the quadriceps contracted) and compared the anterior tibial translation with the tibial slope. The tibial slope was defined as the angle between the medial tibial plateau and the long axis of the tibia, which had an average value of 6°. The anterior tibial translation was defined as the distance between a parallel line at the posterior medial tibial plateau and a posterior point on the medial femoral condyle. The authors reported a statistically significant relationship between the standing anterior tibial translation and the tibial slope in both normal and chronic ACL-deficient knees. The regression line showed a 6-mm increase in anterior tibial translation for every 10° increase in tibial slope. However, it should be noted that a wide variation was present in the data between knees. For example, in chronic ACL-deficient knees with a tibial slope of 10°, anterior tibial translation varied from approximately –2° to 12°.

Griffin and Shannon[42] recently summarized the clinical role of HTO with knee ligament instability, showing the benefit of an anterior opening wedge HTO for severe recurvatum and correcting an abnormal increased tibial slope in select patients who had failed multiple ligament reconstructions.

Marti and coworkers[77] recommended that knees with ACL insufficiency and associated medial arthritis with a tibial slope of 10° or more undergo correction at the time of a varus-producing osteotomy. However, no clinical data were provided to demonstrate whether a change in slope decreased instability symptoms. Other authors[33] discussed increases in ACL tensile loads when tibial slope exceeded 10° and postulated the need for correction, again without clinical data.

Griffin and Shannon[42] noted that the anterior tibial subluxation with ACL insufficiency results in a "copula" owing to increased damage of the medial plateau; however, the effect of a medial meniscectomy on producing the same effect should be considered.

The authors of this chapter agree with recommendations to correct tibial slope when a distinct abnormality is present (Figs. 31–22 and 31–23). The published literature does not provide objective data regarding the degrees of abnormal increase or decrease in tibial slope when corrective osteotomy is indicated when there is an associated ACL or PCL insufficiency.

It is probable that a change in AP shear forces, cruciate tensile loads, and tibiofemoral contact under dynamic conditions would not have clinical significance after a 5° change in the tibial slope when the preoperative tibial slope is in the normal range. Therefore, changing the tibial slope to alter the tibiofemoral contact position by a few millimeters to produce an anterior or posterior shift in tibia position (to an area of less cartilage damage) has the theoretical benefits, but has not been proved in clinical studies to be adopted as a treatment recommendation.

There are patients who have a distinctly abnormal tibial slope from a prior osteotomy or tibial fracture or a growth abnormality in which correction of the tibial slope is required prior to cruciate ligament surgery or other conditions discussed. Occasionally, ACL revision patients have an abnormally increased slope that should be corrected prior to repeat ACL surgery. Patients with a severe varus recurvatum require measurement of tibial slope and may fail posterolateral ligament surgery if the normal posterior tibial slope is reversed. Empirically, a tibial slope greater than 2 standard deviations above normal (e.g., a tibial slope of ≥15°) may be considered for correction. In these knees, at the time of HTO, it is possible to decrease the tibial slope to normal or below normal in ACL-deficient knees, or to increase the slope in PCL-deficient knees, to alter loads on the respective cruciate ligament and possibly change the abnormal "resting" tibiofemoral weight-bearing position.

A normal tibial slope should not be increased in ACL-deficient knees or decreased in PCL-deficient knees undergoing a varus-producing opening wedge osteotomy. The rule is described elsewhere in this chapter (Opening Wedge Osteotomy: Preservation of Tibial Slope) that the anterior gap at the medial opening wedge should be one half of the posteromedial gap to maintain a normal tibial slope.[105] For every 1 mm of anterior gap change, an approximately 2° change in tibial slope would be produced. This is based on the angle of the

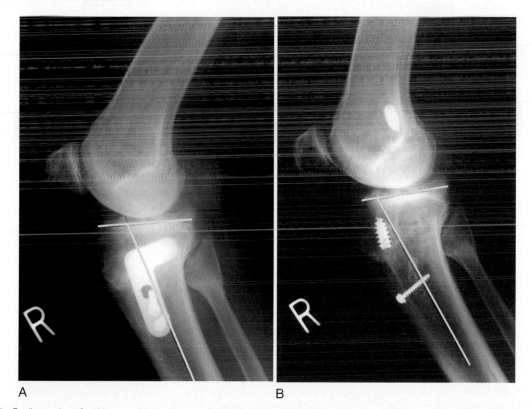

A   B

FIGURE 31–22. Radiographs of a 52-year-old physician referred for treatment after a closing wedge osteotomy (**A**) and subsequent ACL bone–patellar tendon–bone autograft (**B**) that failed. It would have been desirable to correct the abnormal tibial slope, which may have been a factor in the ACL graft failure.

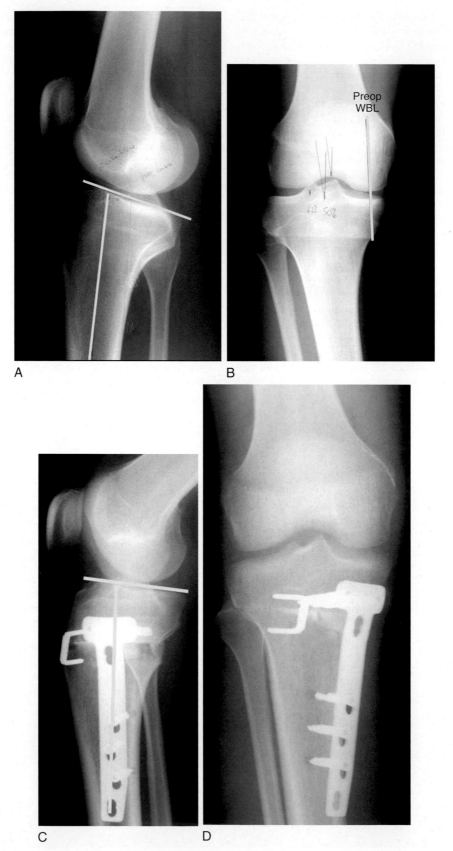

FIGURE 31–23. A and **B,** Preoperative radiographs of a 24-year-old man with bilateral severe varus angulation with medial joint line pain. **C** and **D,** Postoperative radiographs after a biplanar opening wedge osteotomy that was done to correct the abnormal tibial slope. An iliac crest bone graft and locking plate with screws were used in the procedure.

anteromedial tibial cortex, tibial width, and the AP distance where the gap measurement is made (see Table 31–5). It is common in opening wedge osteotomies to incorrectly produce a symmetrical anterior and posterior gap at the osteotomy site, which results in a considerable increase in the tibial slope, potentially leading to a decrease in knee extension and an increase in ACL tensile loads. For example, a change in the tibial slope by 10° would result if an anterior gap measurement error of only 5 mm occurred. The final tibial slope is verified at surgery by lateral fluoroscopic views.

If the surgeon elects to decrease the tibial slope, a staple may be placed at the tibial tubercle while the osteotomy is carefully closed anteriorly to the desired amount. In the senior author's experience, biplanar corrections require the use of a more secure locking plate design to maintain the correction, because it is necessary to section most of the lateral tibial cortex hinge to close the anterior osteotomy gap (Fig. 31–24). Caution is required when closing the anterior osteotomy gap to apply only gentle hyperextension pressure on the tibia. If any resistance is obtained, it is necessary to further weaken the posterolateral tibial cortex (guide pin penetration) to prevent a lateral tibial plateau fracture just anterior to the remaining posterolateral cortex.

Song and associates[127] reported that the normal tibial slope would be maintained if the gap or millimeters of opening along the anteromedial cortex of the anterior plate was two thirds the gap at the location of the posterior plate. The reader should note that the authors are referring to the location of two plates placed along the anteromedial tibial cortex and not the most posterior and anterior gap of the tibial opening wedge discussed in the Noyes and colleagues' study[105] (anterior gap 50% of posterior gap). The data of the Noyes and colleagues' study,[105]

shown in part in Tables 31–6 and 31–7, allows the gap to be computed along the entire anteromedial cortex. The Song and associates' study[127] does not specify where the two plates are placed, and the data in Table 31–7 are more precise to show the actual gap distance where one or two plates would be placed. Further, if the two thirds gap rule of Song and associates were mistakenly applied to the true anterior and posterior gaps along the opening wedge, an increase in tibial slope would occur.

Hohmann and coworkers[51] retrospectively reviewed the radiographs of 67 patients who had a closing wedge HTO and reported a mean decrease of 4.9° in the tibial slope. They suggested that this occurred because of the triangular geometry of the tibia, with more bone removed than required from the anterolateral portion of the lateral tibia.

Timing of Procedures

The timing of HTO and ligament reconstructive procedures is based on several factors (Table 31–4 and Fig. 31–25). In primary varus knees that do not demonstrate abnormal lateral joint opening and external tibial rotation, the HTO and cruciate reconstruction may be performed at the same setting.[93] In double and triple varus knees, the ligament reconstructive procedures are performed after the HTO to reduce the risk of complications.[100] Prolonged rehabilitation and an increased risk of knee arthrofibrosis and motion problems have been described after HTO and ligament reconstructive procedures are performed simultaneously.[18,69,133]

The authors prefer to perform the HTO first and, after adequate healing of the osteotomy, the required ligament reconstructive procedures. In ACL-deficient double varus knees, an

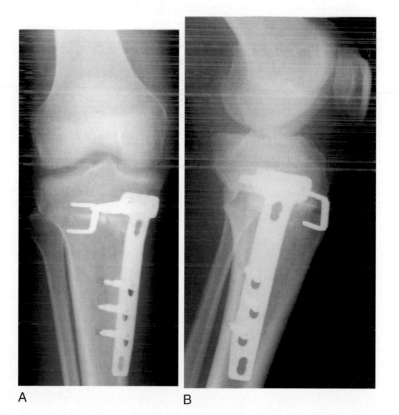

A   B

FIGURE 31–24. A and **B,** A biplanar correction of both the coronal and the sagittal alignment requires the use of a secure locking plate to maintain the correction, because it is necessary to remove more of the lateral tibial cortex hinge in order to close the anterior osteotomy gap.

TABLE 31–4 Indications and Timing of Knee Ligament Reconstructive Procedures

Ligament Deficiency	Surgical Procedure	Timing Related to HTO	Indications/Comments
ACL	Autograft*: 1. Central third B-PT-B 2. Semitendinosus gracilis four-band 3. Quadriceps tendon–patellar bone Allograft: 1. B-PT-B 2. Achillles tendon 3. Others†	Preferably after HTO. With HTO only in primary varus knees that do not have abnormal lateral joint opening.	Any patient who had instability before HTO and who should not risk a further trial of function and possible reinjury. Consider when secondary ligamentous restraints are lost (pivot-shift 3 + impingement, >10 mm increased anterior displacement of the involved knee) and there is associated medial or FCL, PL deficiency. When meniscus repair is performed. Athletically active patient desiring best knee possible for return to sports.
FCL, PMTL (PL structures partial injury, increase 5 mm lateral joint opening, 5°–10° external rotation)	Usually not required after HTO. Confirm negative gap test for abnormal lateral joint opening if ACL reconstruction required (primary vs. double varus knee).	Avoid FCL reconstruction.	Expect adaptive shortening of FCL, lateral tissues in majority after valgus producing osteotomy. At HTO, avoid disrupting proximal tibiofibular joint, which would allow proximal migration and laxity of PL structures.
FCL, PMTL, PL capsule complete deficiency	1. Proximal advancement PL structures (interstitial stretching). 2. FCL, PMTL anatomic reconstruction with autograft or allograft.	Staged procedure: HTO first, followed by combined ACL, FCL/PMTL anatomic reconstruction.	Usually have increased lateral joint opening of 8 mm at the intercondylar notch (≥12 mm at periphery), increased external tibial rotation of 15°, varus recurvatum, requiring PL reconstruction. PL and ACL reconstructions always performed together.

*Ipsilateral or contralateral autogenous grafts preferred over allografts.
†Authors prefer allografts with bone in comparison to anterior tibialis.
ACL, anterior cruciate ligament; B-PT-B, bone–patellar tendon–bone; FCL, fibular collateral ligament; HTO, high tibial osteotomy; PL, posterolateral; PMTL, popliteal muscle-tendon-ligament unit.

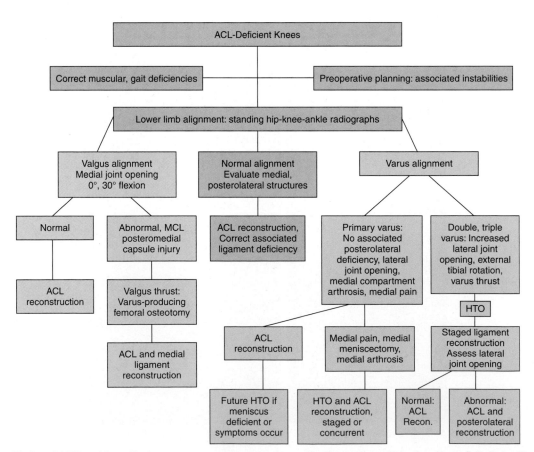

FIGURE 31–25. Timing of HTO and knee ligament reconstructive procedures. *(Reprinted with permission from Noyes, F. R.; Barber-Westin, S. D.: Revision anterior cruciate surgery with use of bone–patellar tendon–bone autogenous grafts. J Bone Joint Surg Am 83:1131–1143, 2001.)*

increase in the lateral tibiofemoral joint gap test contraindicates ACL reconstruction. HTO is effective in decreasing abnormal loads in the lateral and posterolateral tissues, allowing physiologic remodeling and shortening to occur, particularly when the deficiency of the posterolateral structures is only moderate (5–8 mm increased lateral joint opening, 10° increased external tibial rotation).[93,100] In a study conducted by the authors,[93] described later in this chapter (Authors' Clinical Studies), 22 of 41 double varus knees (54%) had abnormally increased lateral joint opening on varus stress testing before osteotomy. Of these, only 5 (12%) had this abnormal joint opening at follow-up. A FCL and posterolateral reconstruction was avoided in these patients. In this same study, a subgroup of 11 patients (27%) did not require ACL reconstruction, because instability symptoms did not exist after the HTO.[93]

In triple varus knees, the ACL and posterolateral structures are reconstructed after the HTO to allow all ligament structures to function together to resist anterior subluxation, abnormal lateral tibiofemoral joint opening, and varus recurvatum. These represent major surgical procedures that are always staged and not combined with the HTO.

Cruciate Graft Options

A four-strand semitendinosus-gracilis (STG) autograft may be harvested from the involved side with little morbidity. Most patients undergoing HTO will not be involved in strenuous athletics, and a STG autograft provides suitable stability for light recreational activities. In revision knees, an STG graft may be used if there are no enlarged femoral or tibial tunnels.

A bone–patellar tendon–bone (B-PT-B) autograft is preferred if there is gross anterior subluxation (grade III pivot shift). In knees undergoing revision ACL reconstruction in which the ipsilateral patellar tendon was previously harvested, the contralateral B-PT-B graft or the ipsilateral quadriceps tendon–patellar bone (QT-PB) graft is a preferred substitute.[94,98] However, care must be taken when harvesting these autografts from the same knee at the time of the osteotomy. The opposite knee may be used for graft harvest.

The use of allografts for ACL reconstruction is controversial owing to the higher graft stretch-out and failure rates compared with B-PT-B autografts, as discussed in detail in Chapter 7, ACL Primary and Revision Reconstruction: Diagnosis, Operative Techniques, and Clinical Outcomes.[90–92,101] If an allograft is required, the B-PT-B has an advantage of more secure bone fixation.

Graft preferences for PCL reconstruction are a two-strand QT-PB autograft or allografts, further described in Chapter 21, Posterior Cruciate Ligament: Diagnosis, Operative Techniques, and Clinical Outcomes.[95,97] The options for surgical restoration of deficient posterolateral structures are described in Chapter 22, Posterolateral Ligament Structures: Diagnosis, Operative Techniques, and Clinical Outcomes.

Opening versus Closing Wedge Osteotomy

The two most common operative techniques for correcting a varus deformity are the opening and the closing wedge tibial osteotomies. An opening wedge avoids the lateral dissection and fibular osteotomy. Knees that require a large angular correction of greater than 12° are candidates for the opening wedge procedure, because it avoids excessive tibial shortening.

Opening wedge osteotomy is advantageous in knees that have chronic medial ligamentous deficiency (MCL, posteromedial capsule), in which a distal advancement or reconstruction of the MCL is required. Knees with rupture of the posterolateral structures requiring posterolateral reconstruction are candidates for opening wedge osteotomy in order to avoid a proximal fibular osteotomy, because a FCL graft will be anchored to the proximal fibula. Opening wedge osteotomy is advantageous in cases of patella alta or decreased lower limb length that would be made worse by a closing wedge osteotomy. A patella infera is a contraindication for an opening wedge osteotomy. A significant patella alta is a relative contraindication for a closing wedge osteotomy.

The major disadvantage of an opening wedge osteotomy is that an appropriate structural corticancellous autograft or allograft is required to restore the anteromedial and posteromedial cortex, add fixation strength, and promote osseous union. Autogenous bone grafting of the open defect aids in achieving stability at the osteotomy site and promoting prompt union with reduced risk of varus collapse due to a delayed union. The potential for many weeks of crutch protection and added disuse effects of the lower limb is lessened by the autogenous grafting. The limited invasive procedure to obtain the outer iliac crest cortical cancellous autograft is discussed in detail in this chapter (Operative Technique: Opening Wedge Tibial Osteotomy).

Several opening wedge plate designs are available. The authors prefer a tibial plate with locking screws to achieve secure osseous fixation.[129] The reader is referred to the appropriate literature by the respective manufacturer, because each locking plate design is different and the recommended technique must be followed. There are rules that must be followed to avoid changing the tibial slope with the use of any fixation plate. A greater chance of increasing the posterior tibial slope exists if an opening wedge buttress plate is placed in an anterior position.[21] With attention to this problem at surgery, the normal tibial slope in the sagittal plane can be preserved with any of the available plate designs.[105]

A disadvantage of an opening wedge osteotomy is that transection of the superficial distal attachment of the MCL is required. In an opening wedge osteotomy of 5 mm, the MCL fibers may be incompletely transected at several different levels (pie-crust approach) to lengthen the ligament. However, osteotomies entailing a correction greater than 5 mm require distal MCL sectioning, careful reflection from the osteotomy site, and reattachment.

The closing wedge osteotomy has the advantage of faster healing and early resumption of weight-bearing because contact of two large cancellous surfaces of the proximal tibia is achieved. The initial interval fixation of the osteotomy is more secure than an opening wedge procedure, and there is less chance for a change in osteotomy position and loss of correction. It is more difficult (compared with the opening wedge technique) to achieve or change the desired amount of bone resection to obtain accurate angular alignment correction at surgery.

The closing wedge osteotomy involves more soft tissue dissection. Osteotomy of the fibula is preferred at the proximal fibular neck region. The lateral dissection must be meticulous to avoid the peroneal nerve. It is more tedious to resect more bone and alter the lower limb valgus correction should it be necessary to achieve additional angular correction. The triangular bone wedge is removed and saved should it be necessary to reinsert bone if an overcorrection is identified at surgery.

Brouwer and associates[22] conducted a prospective clinical trial in 92 patients randomized to either an opening wedge (Puddu plate) or a closing wedge osteotomy. At 1 year postoperatively, a valgus alignment (defined as 0°–6° valgus) was noted in 79% of the closing wedge osteotomies compared with 56% of the closing wedge osteotomies. The authors concluded that the Puddu plate had insufficient strength to maintain the operative correction. The investigation had several flaws because it involved four surgeons and hip-knee-ankle radiographs were not obtained in the initial postoperative period. The number of opening wedge osteotomies that received autogenous bone grafting was not provided. The results emphasize the importance of determining that the appropriate valgus correction is achieved at surgery and maintained in the early postoperative period until union has occurred. The failure to achieve the desired valgus alignment would be expected to decrease long-term success rates. Full-standing weight-bearing hip-knee-ankle radiographs may be obtained by 3 to 4 weeks postoperative after either opening or closing wedge osteotomy to verify that correction has been achieved. In a small percentage of cases in which the correction is found not to be ideal on early postoperative radiographs, a revision angular correction may then be performed.

The use of an external fixator has been advocated with tibial osteotomy, with the advantage of allowing adjustments in lower limb alignment that is helpful in difficult or biplanar corrections.[130,139] A disadvantage of an external fixator is the risk of pin tract infection[74,130,139] and the 12-week period of time that the fixator is typically used. The use of an external fixator is ideal when both coronal lower limb alignment and tibial rotation need to be corrected.

Opening Wedge Osteotomy: Preservation of Tibial Slope

On cross-section, the proximal anteromedial tibial cortex has an oblique or triangular shape, whereas the lateral tibial cortex is more perpendicular at the posterior margin of the tibia. Because of this relationship, a medial opening wedge osteotomy that has an anterior tibial tubercle width equal to the width at the posteromedial margin would increase tibial slope, decrease knee extension, and possibly increase ACL tensile loads. A lateral closing wedge osteotomy with an equal anterior-to-posterior width or gap along the lateral tibial cortex tends to decrease the tibial slope by a few degrees, as is described next.

A study was conducted using three-dimensional analysis of the proximal tibia to determine how the angle of the opening wedge along the anteromedial tibial cortex influences the tibial slope (sagittal plane) and valgus correction (coronal plane) when performing a medial opening wedge osteotomy.[105]

The data in this study on the obliquity of the anteromedial cortex of the proximal tibia relative to the posterior tibial cortex (Fig. 31–26) are presented from 35 magnetic resonance imaging (MRI) films in healthy young individuals (mean age, 32.7 yr).[105] Serial CT images of a cadaveric tibia were made in 1.25-mm slices and digitized using a computer-aided design package to create a solid model of the proximal tibia.

A medial opening wedge osteotomy was created along the AP axis to include a hinge axis on the lateral margin of the tibia. The open wedge osteotomy was just proximal to the tibial tubercle, ending 20 mm below the cortical margin of the lateral tibial plateau. The distal portion of the tibia was rotated on the virtual model about the hinge axis through the lateral point of the

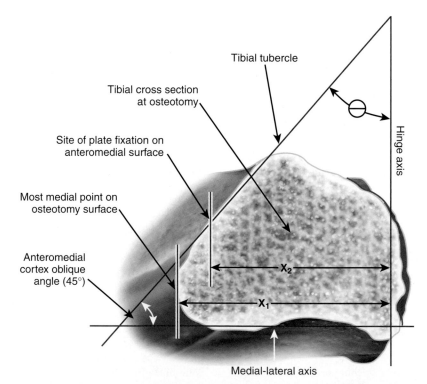

FIGURE 31–26. An axial cut of the proximal tibia at the diaphyseal-metaphyseal junction. The angle formed by the intersection of the mediolateral axis along the posterior tibia and the axis along the anteromedial tibial cortex is called the *anteromedial cortex oblique angle* (θ). This angle measures approximately 45° to the coronal plane.

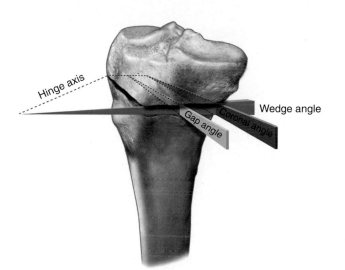

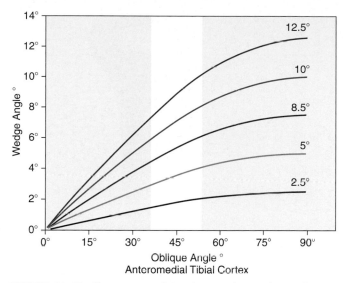

FIGURE 31–27. The distal portion of the tibia was rotated about an AP axis, which ran through the hinge point of the osteotomy to maintain the posterior tibial slope. A solid model of a high tibial osteotomy plate was placed at a series of positions around the medial aspect of the tibia, just anterior to the medial collateral ligament. The anteromedial cortex wedge angle is that angle formed along the oblique anteromedial tibial cortex during a prescribed opening wedge osteotomy (coronal plane). The gap angle is formed by planes that are perpendicular to the wedge angle along the anteromedial tibial surface.

FIGURE 31–28. The anteromedial cortex opening wedge angle depends on the oblique angle of the tibial cortex with respect to the hinge axis. Each line represents the desired calculated degrees of correction for the opening wedge osteotomy in the true coronal (90°) plane. *(Reprinted with permission from Noyes, F. R.; Goebel, S. X.; West, J.: Opening wedge tibial osteotomy: the 3-triangle method to correct axial alignment and tibial slope. Am J Sports Med 33:378–387, 2005.)*

osteotomy, maintaining the anatomic tibial slope (sagittal plane). Measurements of the width of the wedge angle and gap angle (Fig. 31-27) along the anteromedial tibial cortex were made from the resulting computerized model. Standard algebraic calculations were made using the law of triangles to determine the effect of different degrees of opening wedge osteotomy on coronal (valgus) and sagittal (tibial slope) alignment.

The MRI measurement of the anteromedial tibial cortex oblique angle at the site of the opening wedge osteotomy was $45° \pm 6°$ (range, 34°–56°). The opening wedge angle, along the anteromedial tibial cortex to maintain the tibial slope, was found to be dependent on the angle of coronal valgus correction (HTO coronal angle) and the angle of obliquity of the anteromedial tibial cortex. In Figure 31–28, the results are shown for the calculation of the opening wedge angle (along the anteromedial tibial cortex) for five different osteotomy corrections in the coronal valgus plane (2.5°–12.5°).

The gap angle is perpendicular to the anteromedial oblique surface of the tibia with a vertex on the hinge axis posterior to the tibia. This is shown in Figure 31–29, in which the gap angle in degrees is shown for five different osteotomy corrections as a function of the obliquity of the anteromedial tibial cortex.

As an example, a 10° coronal valgus correction (assuming a normal 45° obliquity of the anteromedial tibial cortex) would result in a 7° gap angle at the osteotomy site. An error in the anteromedial tibial cortex opening wedge angle would result in an error in the tibial slope. An example of this is shown in Figure 31–30, which represents the desired wedge angle for a 10° coronal correction. An equal anterior and posterior opening or gap at the osteotomy site would result in an increased tibial slope and loss of normal knee extension.

These variables are shown in Table 31–5. For example, an error of 5 mm in the Y_2 gap (Fig. 31–31) at the tibial tubercle,

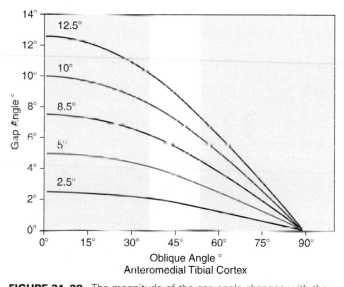

FIGURE 31–29. The magnitude of the gap angle changes with the obliquity of the anteromedial tibial cortex angle. Each line represents the calculated degrees of correction for the opening wedge osteotomy in the coronal plane. *(Reprinted with permission from Noyes, F. R.; Goebel, S. X.; West, J.: Opening wedge tibial osteotomy: the 3-triangle method to correct axial alignment and tibial slope. Am J Sports Med 33:378–387, 2005.)*

assuming the length of the anteromedial cortex (L) is 45 mm, would result in an unexpected change in the tibial slope of 10°. As a general rule in this example, every millimeter of alteration in the gap height induces a change of 2° in the tibial slope.

The opening wedge angle can be set at surgery by measuring and altering the vertical gap (width) at two points along the osteotomy site, Y_1 and Y_2 (Fig. 31–32). This has importance in determining that the correct wedge angle is obtained prior to internal fixation at the osteotomy site. The site at which the

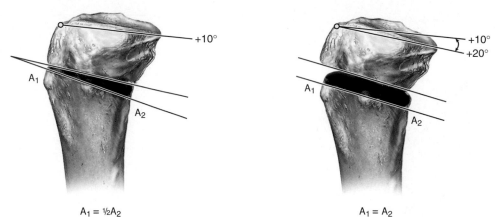

A₁ = ½A₂
Correct wedge opening

A₁ = A₂
Incorrect wedge opening

FIGURE 31–30. Left, Appropriate choice of the wedge angle to maintain the sagittal tibial slope. **Right,** Inappropriate wedge angle results in increased tibial slope.

TABLE 31–5   Errors in the Tibial Slope Caused by Errors in Vertical Gap Height (Y₂)*

Error at Y_2 (mm)	Length of Anteromedial Cortex (mm)							
	25	30	35	40	45	50	55	60
1	4.0	3.2	2.7	2.3	2.0	1.8	1.6	1.5
2	8.1	6.5	5.4	4.6	4.0	3.6	3.2	2.9
3	12.0	9.6	8.1	6.9	6.1	5.4	4.9	4.4
4	15.8	12.8	10.7	9.2	8.1	7.2	6.5	5.9
5	19.5	15.8	13.3	11.4	10.0	8.9	8.1	7.3
6	23.0	18.8	15.8	13.6	12.0	10.7	9.6	8.8
7	26.3	21.6	18.3	15.8	13.9	12.4	11.2	10.2
8	29.5	24.4	20.7	17.9	15.8	14.4	12.8	11.6
9	32.5	27.0	23.0	20.0	17.7	15.8	14.3	13.0
10	35.3	29.5	25.2	22.0	19.5	17.4	15.8	14.4

*Results are given in degrees.

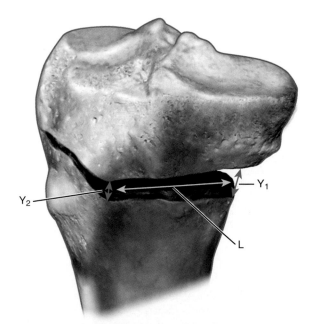

FIGURE 31–31. The opening wedge angle along the anteromedial tibial cortex can be calculated using the three linear measurements along the osteotomy opening wedge. Y₁, gap anterior to Y₂; Y₂, posterior gap; L, length between Y₁ and Y₂.

vertical gap measurement is taken depends on the coronal distance from the hinge axis, obliquity of the anteromedial tibial cortex, and the distance along the osteotomy site on the anteromedial surface (Tables 31–6 and 31–7).

In Table 31–6, the millimeters of opening at the osteotomy site are based on the width of the tibia and the angle of correction. In Table 31–7, an average 45° oblique angle of the anteromedial cortex and a tibial width of 60 mm are assumed. This allows the surgeon to calculate at the time of surgery the desired gap height at two points along the osteotomy to maintain the tibial slope.

For example, the measurement of the posterior tibial width is made at the osteotomy site (X_1). The opening height at the most posteromedial point (Y_1) and the distance between the two measurement points (Y_1–Y_2) are used in Table 31–7 to determine the second opening height at a defined distance (L) along the osteotomy site to maintain tibial slope.

If the tibial plate is placed just anterior to the superficial MCL on the anteromedial tibial cortex, approximately 20 mm anterior to the most posteromedial point of the osteotomy, the osteotomy gap at this site can be determined. In Table 31–7, with a 10-mm posteromedial opening (Y_1), the correct width at the tibial plate would be 7.6 mm (tibial width, 60 mm).

For a 12-mm posteromedial opening, the correct width of the gap at the tibial plate would be 9.2 mm. A wider gap at the

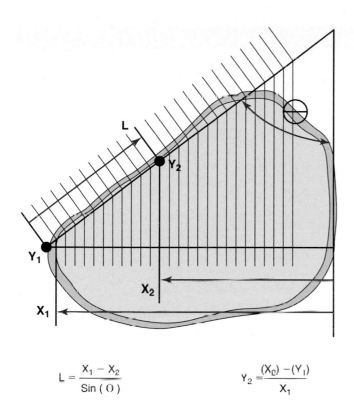

$$L = \frac{X_1 - X_2}{Sin\ (\ O\ )} \qquad Y_2 = \frac{(X_2) - (Y_1)}{X_1}$$

FIGURE 31-32. Vertical gap measurements of the opening wedge osteotomy are a function of distance from the hinge axis of the lateral tibial cortex for the opening wedge (X_1, X_2), oblique angle of the anteromedial tibial cortex (θ), and distance along the osteotomy site (L). *(Reprinted with permission from Noyes, F. R.; Goebel, S. X.; West, J.: Opening wedge tibial osteotomy: the 3-triangle method to correct axial alignment and tibial slope. Am J Sports Med 33:378, 387, 2005.)*

tibial plate would result in excessive valgus alignment and altered tibial slope. The change in the oblique angle of the anteromedial cortex, within the standard deviations reported, would have only a small and negligible effect on the width measurements of the opening wedge (see Table 31–7). To maintain the proper anterior and posterior gaps at the osteotomy site, appropriate distraction instruments at surgery are required to maintain the desired coronal and sagittal angular correction.

Final Recommendations to Obtain Correct Coronal and Slope Alignment

1. Determine the coronal valgus angular correction in degrees based on preoperative full-standing radiographs for the desired placement of the WBL at the tibial plateau and measure the tibial slope based on a lateral radiograph.
2. Determine the millimeters of opening at the posteromedial osteotomy site at surgery (Y_1 gap) using the width of the tibia (X_1 distance) for the coronal valgus correction based on the law of triangles (first triangle; see Table 31–6).
3. Determine the proper gap width of the osteotomy opening wedge along the anteromedial cortex to maintain tibial slope and the proper width beneath the tibial plate based on its location along the anteromedial cortex (see Table 31–7). The opening wedge gap will always be 3 to 4 mm less where the plate is located. If the tibial slope is to be increased or decreased, the effect on the degrees of tibial slope is shown in Table 31–5.
4. Confirm final coronal and sagittal angular correction based on intraoperative fluoroscopy and early postoperative full-standing and lateral radiographs.

INTRAOPERATIVE EVALUATION

An operative "time-out" and identification of the operative limb by the surgeon and patient is performed as described in Chapter 7. All knee ligament subluxation tests should be performed after the induction of anesthesia in both the injured and the contralateral limbs. The amount of increased anterior tibial translation, posterior tibial translation, lateral joint opening, and external tibial rotation should be documented, as previously described.

A thorough arthroscopic examination should be conducted, documenting articular cartilage surface abnormalities[110] and the condition of the menisci. The gap test is done during the arthroscopic examination.[100] The knee is flexed to 30° and a varus load of approximately 89 N is applied. A calibrated nerve hook is used to measure the amount of lateral tibiofemoral compartment opening (Fig. 31–33). Knees that have 12 mm or more of joint opening at the periphery of the lateral tibiofemoral compartment will usually require a staged posterolateral reconstructive procedure.

A medial gap test is performed with a valgus load to measure the opening of the medial tibiofemoral compartment. There may be an

TABLE 31-6	Opening at the Osteotomy Site (mm) Based on the Width of the Tibia and the Angle of Correction								
	Degree of Angular Correction								
TW*	**5**	**6**	**7**	**8**	**9**	**10**	**11**	**12**	**13**
50	4.37	5.25	6.15	7.00	8.00	8.80	9.70	10.85	11.55
55	4.81	5.78	6.77	7.70	8.80	9.68	10.67	11.94	12.71
60	5.25	6.30	7.38	8.40	9.60	10.56	11.64	13.02	13.86
65	5.69	6.83	8.00	9.10	10.40	11.44	12.61	14.11	15.02
70	6.12	7.35	8.61	9.80	11.20	12.32	13.58	15.19	16.17
75	6.56	7.88	9.23	10.50	12.00	13.20	14.55	16.28	17.33
80	7.00	8.40	9.84	11.20	12.80	14.08	15.52	17.36	18.48
85	7.44	8.93	10.46	11.90	13.60	14.96	16.49	18.45	19.64
90	7.87	9.45	11.07	12.60	14.40	15.84	17.46	19.53	20.79
95	8.31	9.98	11.69	13.30	15.20	16.72	18.43	20.62	21.95
100	8.75	10.50	12.30	14.00	16.00	17.60	19.40	21.70	23.10

*TW, coronal tibial width at osteotomy site.

TABLE 31–7   Opening Wedge Height of Y₂ Gap Based on Tibial Width (X₁)*

Opening at Osteotomy (Y₁) (mm)	L (mm)	Tibial Width at Osteotomy (X₁), mm				
		50	55	60	65	70
8	0	8.0	8.0	8.0	8.0	8.0
	20	5.7	5.9	6.1	6.3	6.4
	25	5.2	5.4	5.6	5.8	6.0
	30	4.6	4.9	5.2	5.4	5.6
	35	4.0	4.4	4.7	5.0	5.2
	40	3.5	3.9	4.2	4.5	4.8
	45	2.9	3.4	3.8	4.1	4.4
10	0	10.0	10.0	10.0	10.0	10.0
	20	7.2	7.4	7.6	7.8	8.0
	25	6.5	6.8	7.1	7.3	7.5
	30	5.8	6.1	6.5	6.7	7.0
	35	5.1	5.5	5.9	6.2	6.5
	40	4.3	4.9	5.3	5.6	6.0
	45	3.6	4.2	4.7	5.1	5.5
12	0	12.0	12.0	12.0	12.0	12.0
	20	8.6	8.9	9.2	9.4	9.6
	25	7.8	8.1	8.5	8.7	9.0
	30	6.9	7.4	7.8	8.1	8.4
	35	6.1	6.6	7.1	7.4	7.8
	40	5.2	5.8	6.3	6.8	7.2
	45	4.4	5.1	5.6	6.1	6.5

*By measuring the width of the tibia, the opening wedge height at the most medial point (Y₁), and the distance between vertical measurement points (L), the vertical height at the second measurement point (Y₂) at which the plate implant can be found on the table. Calculations based on a 45° angle of the anteromedial tibial cortex at the osteotomy site.

Critical Points INTRAOPERATIVE EVALUATION

Repeat all knee ligament subluxation tests under anesthesia, both injured and contralateral limb.

Rate All Articular Cartilage Surfaces for Abnormalities and Millimeters of Involvement

- Normal
- Grade 1, softening
- Grade 2A, fissuring and fragmentation < half the depth of the articular surface
- Grade 2B, fissuring and fragmentation > half the depth of the articular surface
- Grade 3, subchondral bone exposed

Gap Test during Arthroscopy

- Knee 30° flexion
- Varus load, valgus load
- Measure millimeters lateral and medial tibiofemoral compartment opening with calibrated nerve hook

increased medial opening due to medial joint damage and loss of cartilage and flattening of the femoral and tibial condyles. In rare cases, there is increased opening due to a chronic MCL rupture. In most knees with varus malalignment, adaptive shortening of the medial ligamentous tissues occurs and MCL advancement and posteromedial plication procedures are not indicated.

OPERATIVE TECHNIQUE: OPENING WEDGE TIBIAL OSTEOTOMY

Step 1: Initial Operating Room Preparation

Preoperative calculations are made as previously described. The entire lower extremity is prepared and draped free with the tourniquet placed high on the proximal thigh to assist visual observation of lower limb alignment. If an autogenous iliac crest autograft is to be performed (authors' choice), the ipsilateral anterior iliac crest is prepared and draped for the limited iliac crest bone harvest of the outer cortex. The patient is positioned to allow fluoroscopic views of the hip-knee-ankle WBL to verify the angular correction at surgery, and lateral views are obtained for tibial slope analysis.

Step 2: Knee Arthroscopy

Arthroscopy is performed at the time of the HTO to evaluate articular surfaces of the medial and lateral tibiofemoral compartments and patellofemoral joint to confirm that the patient is an appropriate candidate for the osteotomy. ACL-deficient knees may have associated meniscus tears that require repair[122] or partial removal. Appropriate débridement of tissues, inflamed synovium, and notch osteophytes limiting knee extension is performed. In particular, a secondary weight-bearing area is established in varus-angulated knees in which the lateral tibial spine produces a bone erosion over the inner margin of the lateral femoral condyle. The femoral condylar bone erosion may be débrided to remove the painful weight-bearing site.

Step 3: Anterior Iliac Crest Bone Graft Harvest

A 4-cm incision is made over the anterior iliac crest and deepened to the periosteum (Fig. 31–34), which is sharply incised and reflected medially only to the inner cortex. Laterally, meticulous subperiosteal dissection is carried along the outer table of the pelvis, avoiding the lateral muscles. The graft size is defined on the outer cortex using electrocautery. In most patients, the graft will be 40 mm in length, 10 mm in width, and 30 mm in depth. However, in smaller

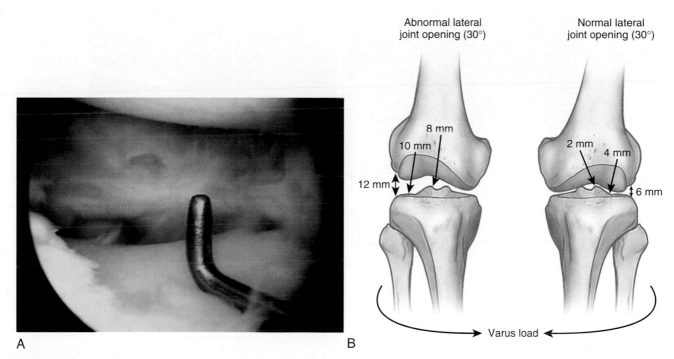

FIGURE 31–33. A and **B,** Arthroscopic gap test for determining the amount of lateral joint opening.

Critical Points OPERATIVE TECHNIQUE OPENING WEDGE OSTEOTOMY

- Arthroscopy prior to HTO to assess all knee compartments, confirm HTO indicated, treat meniscus tears and notch osteophytes blocking knee extension.
- Anterior iliac crest meticulous dissection, remove outer cortex, do not disturb inner cortex or muscle attachments.
  ○ Harvest graft 40 mm in length, 10 mm in width, 30 mm in depth to produce three triangular bone grafts.
- HTO incision: 5 cm vertical medial tibia midway between tibial tubercle and posteromedial tibial cortex, starting 1 cm inferior to joint line.
- Partially detach gracilis and semitendinosus tendons at their tibial insertion, retract posteriorly exposing SMCL and posterior border of the tibia.
- Sharp periosteal incision anterior and posteromedial tibial border of the SMCL, meticulous subperiosteal dissection beneath the SMCL fibers. Protect inferior medial geniculate artery beneath the SMCL.
- Posterior tibial subperiosteal dissection to protect neurovascular structures. Wide dissection not necessary. Surgeon's headlight always used.
- Small osteotomies ≤ 5 mm, "pie-crust" procedure using multiple transverse incisions may effectively lengthen SMCL.
- Osteotomies > 5 mm, transect distal SMCL attachment, carefully elevated to the tibial border, protected and reattached after osteotomy.
- Keith needle placed anteriorly and posteriorly at the joint space to verify the tibial slope and medial sagittal osteotomy plane.
- Anterior and posterior guide pins placed at slight obliquity to tibial shaft (~15°), verify position with fluoroscopy, mark osteotomy line along the anteromedial cortex.

- Ensure guide pins are at least 20 mm distal to the lateral joint line to prevent lateral tibial plateau fracture.
- Begin osteotomy with oscillating saw for medial and anterior cortices. Follow by nonflexible thin ¾-inch osteotome placed anterior, directly above the guide pin, verified by fluoroscopy.
- Use ½-inch osteotomy for posterior cortex, with osteotome edge visualized and palpated posterior to the tibia as the osteotomy is advanced.
- Carry osteotomy to within 10 mm of the posterolateral cortex, confirm by fluoroscopy.
- Place thin spreader bars across osteotomy. Initial distraction requires several minutes to prevent fracture of the lateral cortex; if major resistance, place holes in lateral cortex with guide pin.
- Anterior gap of osteotomy should be half that of the posterior gap to maintain tibial slope. Maintain osteotomy gap; use anterior tibial staple, if necessary, and posterior wedge; confirm alignment by fluoroscopy.
- Apply and fixate locking plate with fluoroscopy verification, confirm final coronal and sagittal (slope) alignment.
- Suture SMCL fibers distally and secure to either plate screws or suture anchors to maintain tension. Reapproximate pes anserine tendons and sartorius fascia.
- Knees with chronic SMCL deficiency require distal advancement if the ligament appears normal without scar replacement.
- Semitendinosus augmentation of SMCL required in knees with scar replacement.
- When the SMCL is advanced distally or reconstructed, incise, reset, and repair medial meniscus attachments.

HTO, high tibial osteotomy; SMCL, superficial medial collateral ligament.

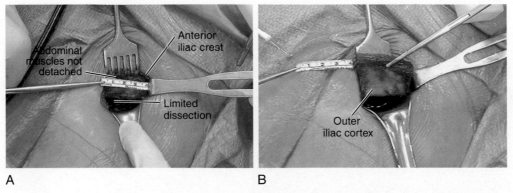

FIGURE 31–34. A, A 4-cm incision over the anterior iliac crest is made to harvest the iliac crest bone graft. The graft is composed of the anterior crest and outer iliac cortex; the inner table is not removed. **B,** The usual iliac crest bone graft dimensions are 40 mm in length, 10 to 12 mm in width, and 30 mm in depth. (*A* and *B, Reprinted with permission from Noyes, F. R.; Mayfield, W.; Barber-Westin, S. D.; et al.: Opening wedge high tibial osteotomy: an operative technique and rehabilitation program to decrease complications and promote early union and function. Am J Sports Med 34:1262–1273, 2006.*)

patients, the graft may be smaller in width and approximately 8 mm in depth. Patients undergoing large osteotomies may require a longer graft of approximately 45 mm to 50 mm.

The inner iliac cortex is not dissected, the muscle attachments are not disturbed, which reduces postoperative pain, and a spacer of the iliac crest defect is not required. Additional cancellous bone is removed from the inner graft site. A drain is not required at the iliac crest harvest site. The wound is closed in layers with deep sutures to close the dead space. The graft is later fashioned into three carefully sized triangles: one triangle is placed posterior to the tibial plate to close the gap at the posterior tibial cortex, one triangle is placed in the midportion of the osteotomy deep to the plate, and one smaller-width triangle

is placed in the gap in the anterior tibial cortex. In large osteotomy corrections (>10-mm gap), autogenous bone is always used and any remaining defect filled with corticocancellous freeze-dried tibial or iliac crest allografts.

Step 4: Initial Anteromedial Tibial Approach

The operative technique is shown in Figure 31–35. A 5-cm vertical skin incision is made medially midway between the tibial tubercle and the posteromedial tibial cortex, starting 1 cm inferior to the joint line. A vertical incision is preferred over an

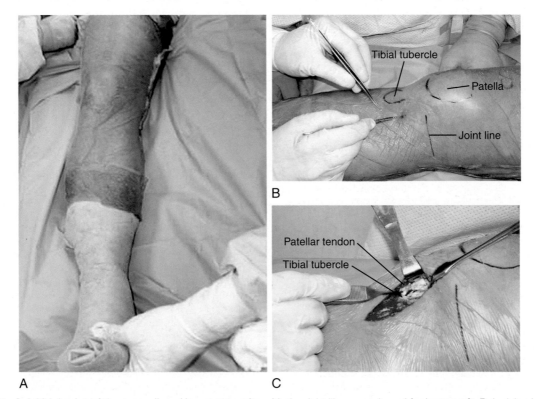

FIGURE 31–35. A, Initial draping of the varus-aligned lower extremity with the right iliac crest draped for bone graft. **B,** Incision location, anterior third of the medial tibia. **C,** Initial exposure beneath the patella tendon under retraction.

Continued

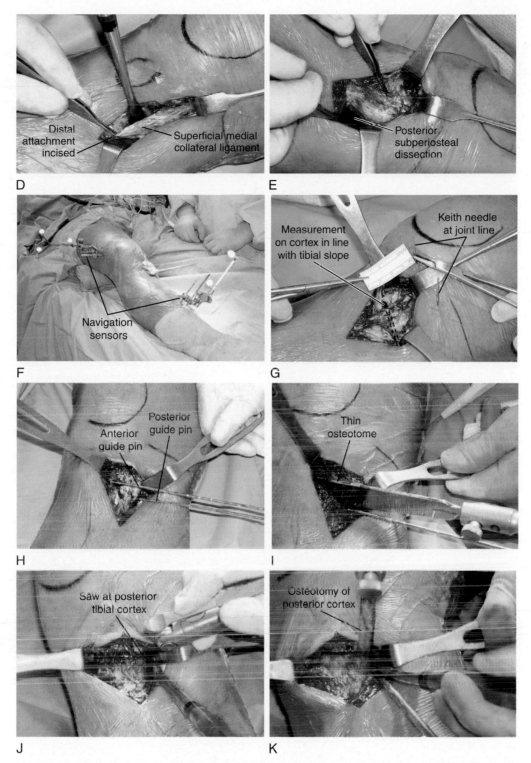

FIGURE 31–35—cont'd   **D,** Initial subperiosteal dissection of the superficial medial collateral ligament (SMCL). The distal attachment has been incised. **E,** Posterior subperiosteal exposure to protect the neurovascular structures. **F,** Placement of the navigation femoral and tibial markers. **G,** A Keith needle placed at the anterior, and later the posterior, aspect of the joint line is used to outline the planned osteotomy. **H,** Two guide pins are placed under fluoroscopic control. **I,** A thin osteotomy blade is placed under fluoroscopic control. Different width blades are used to complete the osteotomy within 8 mm of the lateral cortex. **J,** Initial posterior cortex osteotomy using a thin power saw under direct visualization. **K,** Completion of the posterior cortex osteotomy to within 8 mm of the posterolateral cortex.

Continued

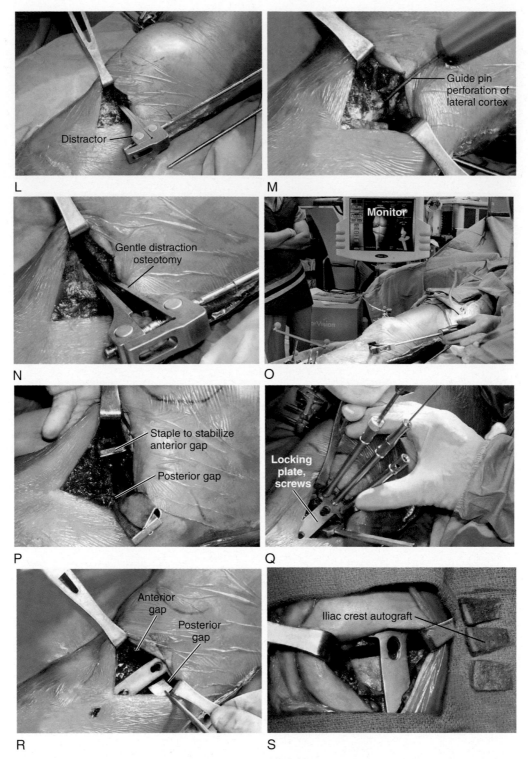

FIGURE 31–35—cont'd   L, Initial gentle dislocation of the osteotomy. **M,** Guide pin perforation of the dense posterolateral tibial cortex to weaken the bone owing to failure of the osteotomy gap to increase under gentle dislocation. **N,** Further dislocation of the osteotomy site. **O,** Use of computerized navigation to monitor valgus alignment. **P,** Staple is placed anterior to the tibial gap to control tibial slope. **Q,** Initial fixation of the osteotomy, maintaining the measured osteotomy correction. **R,** Confirmation of the anterior and posterior osteotomy gap measurement. **S,** Bicortical iliac crest autografts.

Continued

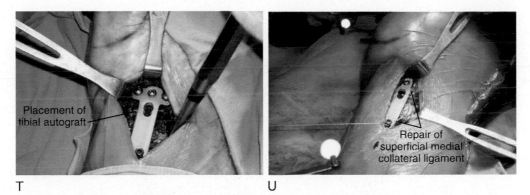

FIGURE 31–35—cont'd. **T,** Placement of the anterior, central and posterior iliac crest autografts. **U,** Fixation of the anterior border of the SMCL to the tibial plate.

oblique or transverse incision because vertical incisions are subsequently used in knees progressing to partial or complete TKA. The sartorius fascia is incised in line with its fibers, proximal to the gracilis tendon, exposing the distal SMCL attachment.

The gracilis and semitendinosus tendons are partially detached at their tibial insertion in an L-shaped manner and retracted posteriorly to further expose the SMCL and posterior border of the tibia. The SMCL is transected at its most distal tibial attachment. Anteriorly, the retropatellar bursa is entered by incising the medial patellar retinaculum, allowing the patellar tendon to be lifted to expose the anterior tibia.

A sharp periosteal incision is made at the posteromedial tibial border, just posterior to the SMCL, to allow the distal SMCL to be dissected subperiosteally in a proximal direction and to allow meticulous posterior tibial subperiosteal dissection by a Cobb elevator. Care is taken to identify the inferior medial geniculate artery, which lies just beneath the SMCL. Only sufficient posterior tibial subperiosteal dissection is used to protect the neurovascular structures; wide dissection is not necessary. A malleable retractor is placed in the subperiosteal posterior tibial space.

Step 5: Proximal Osteotomy and Placement of Tibial Guide Pins

The patellar tendon and retropatellar bursa are exposed medially. The superior attachment of the tendon is recessed 5 mm using a scalpel to provide adequate exposure for the osteotomy. Retractors are placed anteriorly and posteriorly to complete the exposure. A Keith needle is placed in the anteromedial joint just above the tibia, and the distance is marked on the desired point of the osteotomy along the anteromedial cortex. A second Keith needle is placed at the posteromedial tibial joint space, and the same millimeters are marked to provide a measurement of the tibial slope. The two marks are connected to provide the osteotomy line perpendicular to the tibial slope.

A commercial guide system (Arthrex Opening Wedge Osteotomy System, Arthrex Inc., Naples, FL) may be used to facilitate guide wire placement (Fig. 31–36). A 2-mm guide pin is placed at the posteromedial cortex at the marked line and advanced across the tibia at an oblique angle. The anterior and posterior guide pins are placed at 15° of obliquity to the tibial shaft and verified by intraoperative fluoroscopy. An alternative technique is to place the site of the osteotomy directly above

the posterior guide pin, maintaining the oblique angle of the pin across the osteotomy site without using the osteotomy guide system.

To prevent a fracture extending into the joint at the lateral tibial plateau, it is important for the guide pins to be at least 20 mm distal to the lateral joint line. An error that may occur is to have too much obliquity to the guide pin.

At this point, it is imperative to ensure that the medial osteotomy line (from anterior to posterior) is in line with the tibial slope based on the radiographs and prior anteromedial cortex joint line measurements by the Keith needles. A measurement of the perpendicular cut from the joint line confirms the distance of each guide pin from the articular surface of the tibia. The length of the posterior pin (medial to lateral cortex) is measured and used following the law of triangles[105] to determine tibial width and the millimeters of osteotomy opening to obtain the desired angular correction (see Table 31–6).

The osteotomy is initially performed using an oscillating saw for the medial and anterior cortices, followed by a nonflexible, thin ¾-inch and ½-inch osteotome, placed in the same orientation and anterior to the guide pin and verified by fluoroscopy. The lateral cortex is osteotomized to Gerdy's tubercle, leaving the posterolateral tibial cortex hinge. A ½-inch osteotome is used for the posterior cortex, with the osteotome exposed 2 to 3 mm and viewed posterior to the tibia as the osteotome is advanced. The osteotomy is carried to within 10 mm of the posterolateral cortex. It is imperative that the lateral cortex not be fractured because this would produce loss of the lateral cortex buttress and potential collapse and loss of the angular correction. If a fracture of the lateral cortex does occur, with gross instability to the osteotomy site, the lateral tibial cortex may be secured with a two-hole small plate through a limited lateral incision to achieve stability.

Step 6: Opening Wedge Technique and Measurement of Gaps to Confirm Tibial Slope

Commercially available calibrated opening wedges are gently inserted into the osteotomy site to achieve the desired angular correction with the opening medial gap hinging on the intact posterolateral cortex (Fig. 31–37). This step requires several minutes to prevent fracture of the lateral tibial pillar. The spreader bars are inserted entirely across the osteotomy site to prevent a

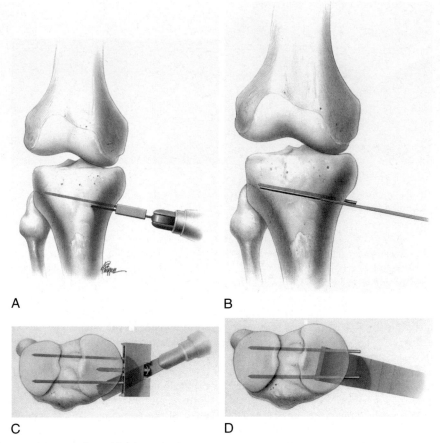

FIGURE 31–36. A–D, Correct placement for guide pin and subsequent osteotomy with a thin osteotome. The lateral cortex is preserved. *(A–D, Reprinted with permission from Noyes, F. R.; Barber-Westin, S. D.; Roberts, C. S.: High tibial osteotomy in knees with associated chronic ligament deficiencies. In Jackson RW [ed.]: Master Techniques in Orthopaedic Surgery, Reconstructive Knee Surgery. Philadelphia: Lippincott Williams & Wilkins, 2003; pp. 229–260.)*

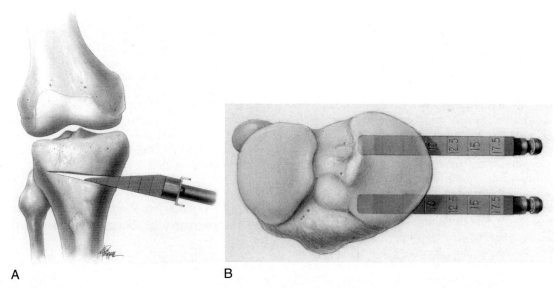

FIGURE 31–37. A and **B,** The use of a commercial (Arthrex Opening Wedge Osteotomy System, Arthrex, Inc., Naples, FL) osteotomy wedge to gradually open the osteotomy site. *(Reprinted with permission from Noyes, F. R.; Barber-Westin, S. D.; Roberts, C. S.: High tibial osteotomy in knees with associated chronic ligament deficiencies. In Jackson RW [ed.]: Master Techniques in Orthopaedic Surgery, Reconstructive Knee Surgery. Philadelphia: Lippincott Williams & Wilkins, 2003; pp. 229–260.)*

fracture extending into the lateral tibial plateau. If there is a rigid nonyielding response to the spreader bars, the lateral cortex is weakened with three to four guide pin perforations.

The anterior gap of the osteotomy site should be one half of the posterior gap, following rules previously described to maintain the tibial slope.[105] The width of the tibial plate along the anteromedial cortex and just anterior to the SMCL is measured and is always less than the millimeters at the posterior medial gap owing to the angular inclination of the anteromedial tibial cortex.

In select cases as previously described, the tibial slope may be purposefully increased in PCL-deficient knees, decreased in ACL-deficient knees, or altered with abnormal knee hyperextension or flexion contracture. The method to complete the desired change in tibial slope and corresponding width of the anterior and posterior osteotomy sites has been presented in an earlier section of this chapter. A locking plate design is always used in single and biplanar corrections.

Step 7: Intraoperative Verification of Desired Limb Alignment Correction

In addition to preoperative measurements of axial alignment (obtained from double-stance hip-knee-ankle radiographs) and calculations to correct for increased lateral joint opening as previously described, the surgeon must verify intraoperatively that the desired limb alignment has been achieved. After the selected wedge correction (which is maintained using one of the commercial wedge-shaped instruments), a small pad is positioned behind the knee to avoid hyperextension and the knee is placed in 5° flexion. With the lower limb lying on the table, the surgeon gently determines that there is closure of both the medial and the lateral tibiofemoral compartments viewed by fluoroscopy. An axial load is placed across the bottom of the foot to compress the knee joint in order to maintain the correct axial alignment. The lower limb is positioned in 12° to 15° of external rotation to simulate the normal lower limb position during gait. A rigid rod is placed at the center of the hip to the center of the ankle, verified by fluoroscopy, and the WBL at the tibia is determined. Adjustment in the millimeters of gap at the osteotomy site is made to obtain the preoperatively selected WBL. The procedure is repeated after internal plate fixation to verify the final alignment correction. The fluoroscopic technique for lower limb positioning to obtain accurate WBL measurements and verify the operative correction does take time and may require repeated steps. The lateral fluoroscopic view determines the final position of the tibial slope. The role of computer navigation is discussed later in this chapter (Role of Computerized Navigation for HTO).

Obtaining an alignment correction in which the WBL is transferred to the lateral tibiofemoral compartment within the desired 50% to 62% range is the key to achieving short- and long-term decreases in pain in the medial tibiofemoral compartment. The surgeon cannot simply rely on the preoperative calculations because the intraoperative hip-knee-ankle fluoroscopic measurements may indicate that the desired correction of the tibial WBL has not been achieved. This problem was demonstrated in a report by Marti and coworkers,[77] who described the accuracy of obtaining the desired alignment correction using preoperative and postoperative double-stance radiographs after opening wedge osteotomy in 32 knees. In their series, only 50% of the limbs demonstrated the desired correction on postoperative radiographs (±5° of calculated correction). An undercorrection was found in

31% and an overcorrection in 19%. The authors did not report on the use of intraoperative fluoroscopy to verify the lower limb correction. Many authors have described problems in obtaining the desired angular correction at surgery, with a substantial percentage of limbs remaining in varus or overcorrected into excessive valgus. The development of computerized navigation techniques to increase the accuracy of obtaining the desired tibial WBL and slope correction is, in the authors' opinion, distinctly advantageous. Both fluoroscopy and computerized navigation techniques require defining accurate anatomic landmarks and precision to obtain accurate measurements.

Step 8: Placement of Bone Graft and Internal Fixation

An appropriate plate is selected and secured. The senior author uses only a locking plate design. If the surgeon elects to use allograft bone, added fixation is required for a longer period of time and a locking plate with screws is strongly recommended to prevent varus collapse at the osteotomy site. Various commercial locking plates and screw systems are available that provide added stability at the operative site.

The senior author recommends structural corticocancellous wedge bone grafts (autograft or allograft) and believes that synthetic grafts or cancellous grafts require further clinical evaluation before being accepted into practice. The clinical studies using these grafts have shown an unacceptable nonunion rate, as is discussed later in this chapter. The author prefers autograft iliac crest grafts or freeze-dried tibia or iliac crest corticocancellous allografts supplemented with a platelet gel.[29]

The three corticocancellous bone graft triangular segments are fashioned based on direct measurements of the anterior and posterior widths at the osteotomy site. The three grafts are impacted tightly into the posterior, middle, and anterior portions of the osteotomy site to obliterate the space and provide added stability, particularly in the sagittal plane. Fluoroscopy is used to confirm the final alignment and tibial slope.

The SMCL fibers are sutured distally and secured either to the plate screws or to suture anchors to maintain tension. The pes anserine tendons and sartorius fascia are reapproximated. A Hemovac drain is rarely required. The tourniquet is deflated and hemostasis obtained. The wound is closed in layers in the usual manner. The lower limb is wrapped with cotton, and additional padding is placed posteriorly and over the peroneal nerve. A commercial ice delivery system with the bladder incorporated a few cotton layers from the wound is always used. A postoperative hinged brace and bilateral ankle-foot compression boots are applied.

The neurovascular status is immediately checked in the operating room and over the initial postoperative period. The importance of limb elevation for the 1st postoperative week and use of a venous compressive system is emphasized. Close observation for lower limb soft tissue swelling is mandatory. There is a high suspicion for a venous thrombosis, and therefore, aspirin is prescribed. There is also a low threshold for venous ultrasound of both lower extremities, which is obtained in the majority of patients in the first 3 to 7 postoperative days.

Management of the SMCL

There are three surgical approaches for management of the SMCL. In a small opening wedge osteotomy of 5 to 7 mm, a "pie-crusting" procedure using multiple transverse incisions at different places may effectively lengthen the SMCL. In larger opening wedge osteotomies, it is necessary to transect the distal attachment and perform a distal elevation of the attachment in a subperiosteal plane. This allows for the SMCL to be reattached distally after the opening wedge osteotomy with the posteromedial portion of the SMCL bridging the osteotomy site. Transecting the SMCL at the most distal attachment site preserves its length, allows excellent exposure and bone grafting, and allows the tibial fixation plate to be placed in a correct midline position. The tibial slope is not altered, and function of the SMCL is retained.

A third approach is used when distal advancement of the SMCL is required as a reconstructive procedure owing to SMCL insufficiency and abnormal medial joint opening. At the conclusion of the osteotomy and plate fixation, the SMCL is dissected to the medial joint, including the deep medial fibers. A posterior incision is made at the junction of the SMCL and posteromedial capsule (posterior oblique ligament). The anterior incision extends only to the joint and preserves the attachment of the medial patellofemoral ligament. The medial meniscus position is carefully examined when a distal advancement of the SMCL is performed. It may be necessary to incise the medial meniscus capsular attachment and then resuture the attachment to preserve the correct anatomic location of the meniscus when the SMCL is advanced.

The SMCL should appear relatively normal without scar replacement, because advancement of only scar tissue would not provide medial stability. In select cases, an STG augmentation of the SMCL may be necessary. The tendon is detached proximally and passed through a small drill hole at the femoral attachment anterior and posterior to the SMCL femoral attachment. The anterior and posterior tendon arms are sutured to the anterior and posterior fibers of the SMCL after the osteotomy is completed. The distal attachment of the tendons is not disturbed. Added tibial fixation at the distal tendons into the bone at the distal tibia may be required.

The need to surgically reconstruct the SMCL is infrequent; however, the surgical techniques presented allow for restoration of function when required. At the conclusion of the SMCL reconstruction, plication of the posteromedial capsule anteriorly to the SMCL is performed to remove any abnormal capsular laxity with the knee at full extension. Overtightening of the SMCL and posteromedial capsules is avoided. The repair allows for full knee extension and a normal range of flexion. The technique is described in further detail in Chapter 24, Medial and Posteromedial Ligament Injuries: Diagnosis, Operative Techniques, and Clinical Outcomes.

OPERATIVE TECHNIQUE: CLOSING WEDGE TIBIAL OSTEOTOMY

Step 1: Initial Operating Room Preparation and Arthroscopy

The entire lower extremity is prepared and draped free with the tourniquet placed high on the proximal thigh to assist visual observation of lower limb alignment. The patient is positioned to allow fluoroscopic views of the hip-knee-ankle WBL in order to verify the angular correction at surgery, and arthroscopy is performed as already described.

Critical Points OPERATIVE TECHNIQUE CLOSING WEDGE OSTEOTOMY

- Arthroscopy first to assess all compartments, confirm HTO indicated, treat meniscus tears and notch osteophytes blocking knee extension.
- Identify anteromedial bare area of fibula when initiating limited subperiosteal exposure of the fibular neck. Be aware of anatomic variability of the superficial peroneal nerve.
- Subperiosteal dissection on tibia begun just distal to Gerdy's tubercle. Clean dissection, relatively bloodless field without damage to muscle tissue.
- Complete dissection posteriorly across width of tibia, extend proximally and distally in posterior tibial subperiosteal plane as required.
- Proximal fibular osteotomy through fibular neck region recommended.
- Fibular bone section removed is 2–3 mm less than the computed tibial wedge to allow compaction at the osteotomy site. Avoid bone step-off adjacent to peroneal nerve.
- Pass a smooth guide pin transversely at the proximal tibia to the medial cortex, 25 mm distal to joint line. Use fluoroscopy to ensure proper placement. Measure tibial width, compute desired bone width to obtain WBL correction. Place second guide pin distal to first guide pin.
- Leave at least 25 mm of proximal tibia to avoid tibial plateau fracture.
- Make initial osteotomy cuts with a micro-oscillating saw to cut only outer cortex. Complete osteotomy with thin osteotomes.
- Place a malleable retractor in the subperiosteal plane posteriorly to protect the neurovascular structures with knee flexed 10°.

- Surgeon seated with a headlamp. Osteotomy plane is maintained in a triangular manner. The midpoint of the tibia width is half of the lateral wedge.
- Posteromedial cortex preserved to provide stability and prevent medial or lateral tibial translation or varus recurrence.
- Close osteotomy gap with gentle valgus force applied over a few minutes to gradually deform remaining medial cortex.
- Sagittal plane of osteotomy should be perpendicular to the long axis of the tibia. Equal width of cortex removed both anteriorly and posteriorly to preserve normal posterior tibial slope.
- Under fluoroscopy, position alignment guide rod over center of femoral head and center of tibiotalar joint to determine corrected WBL intersection at tibial plateau. Axially load the lower limb at the foot to maintain closure of medial and lateral tibiofemoral compartments at 5° flexion to avoid hyperextension.
- Further bone may be resected if necessary to adjust WBL.
- Internal fixation: L-shaped plate, two 6.5-mm cancellous screws in proximal tibia, two or three cortical screws distal to osteotomy.
- Tourniquet released, hemostasis obtained.
- Reattach fascia of the anterior compartment musculature to anterolateral aspect of the tibial border with absorbable sutures.
- Generous cotton Ace compression bandage, multiple layers. Commercial ice delivery system and bilateral venous foot pumps applied.
- Close observation limb swelling, maintain frequent limb elevation, ultrasound within 1st postoperative week in majority of patients.

HTO, high tibial osteotomy; WBL, weight-bearing line.

Step 2: Initial Anterolateral Tibial Approach

A sterile tourniquet is inflated, and an oblique incision is made 1 cm distal to the head of the fibula in a line directed to the center of the tibial tubercle (Fig. 31–38). The subcutaneous tissues are incised down to the fascia of the anterolateral tibial musculature. A fascial incision is made from the lateral aspect of the tibial tubercle sloping up proximally to the distal aspect of Gerdy's tubercle and is extended posteriorly and laterally to the anterior bare area of the fibula. The anterior bare area of the fibula is an important and safe anatomic landmark. The FCL and peroneal nerve are safely avoided when one identifies this area, which is used to initiate the limited subperiosteal exposure of the fibular neck for the fibular osteotomy.

Subperiosteal dissection on the tibia is initiated just distal to Gerdy's tubercle, using a scalpel followed by a Cobb elevator. The dissection is continued just lateral to the patellar tendon and should be done cleanly, with a relatively bloodless field and without damage to muscle tissue. The retinaculum adjacent to the patellar tendon is incised and the retropatellar space entered. The patellar tendon is retracted anteriorly.

The dissection is continued posteriorly on the tibia. It is important to remain in a subperiosteal plane because of the proximity of neurovascular structures. The safe zone is just distal to Gerdy's tubercle to avoid the peroneal nerve. Posteriorly, the dissection is completed across the width of the tibia in one location and is then carefully extended proximally and distally in this safe posterior tibial subperiosteal plane.

Step 3: Fibular Osteotomy

There are three options for the fibula when performing an HTO: proximal slide, proximal fibular osteotomy, and distal fibular osteotomy. A proximal slide (disruption of the tibiofibular joint) is strongly contraindicated because this shortens the FCL and posterolateral structures and may lead to a severe posterolateral instability in an already unstable knee.

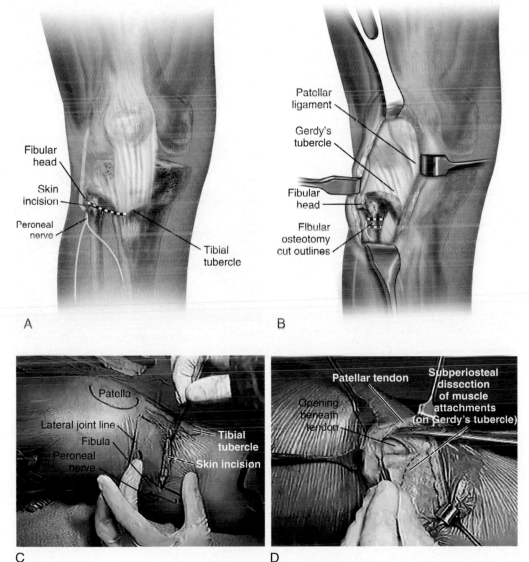

FIGURE 31–38 Closing wedge osteotomy technique. **A,** Skin incision. **B,** Exposure for the lateral tibial and fibular osteotomy. **C,** Landmarks for the skin incision. **D,** Subperiosteal dissection of the muscles to expose the lateral tibia and proximal fibula.

Continued

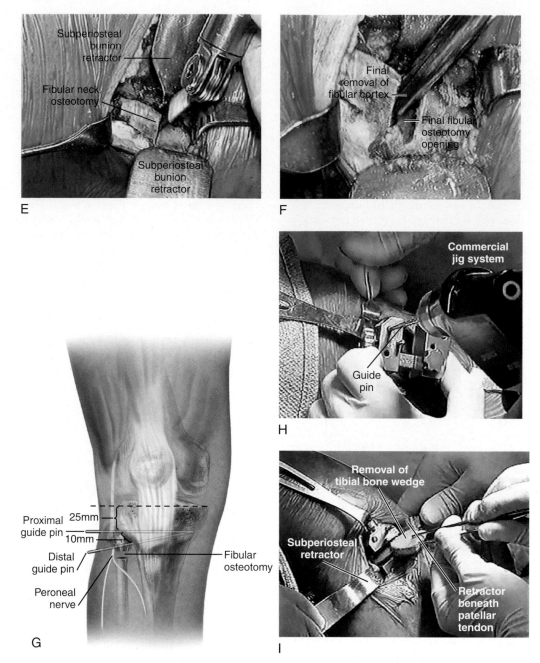

FIGURE 31–38—cont'd. E, Osteotomy of the fibula at the head-neck junction. **F,** Removal of the fibular bone. **G,** Placement of two guide pins at predetermined measured angles and depth for correction. **H,** Alternative use of a commercial guide system for guide pin placement. **I,** Removal of the bone wedge.

Continued

The preferred procedure is a proximal fibular osteotomy through the fibular neck region (see Fig. 31–38). Meticulous surgical technique with protection and palpation of the peroneal nerve is essential. The peroneal nerve is always identified and partially dissected. In order to protect the fibers of the peroneal nerve, the lateral and posterior periosteal sleeve is carefully preserved and not retracted under tension. If there is any question as to the position of the nerve or chance of nerve damage, exposure of the entire nerve is indicated with direct visualization and protection.

The fibular bone section removed is 2 to 3 mm less than the computed tibial wedge to allow compaction at the fibular osteotomy site. Excellent bony apposition is achieved when the osteotomy is closed,

and it is not necessary to add internal fixation. Careful inspection of the fibular osteotomy is done to remove any rough osteotomy edges that would be adjacent to the peroneal nerve.

An alternative choice for a fibular osteotomy is at the junction of the middle and distal thirds of the fibula through a 3-cm posterolateral incision. The peroneal muscles are retracted anteriorly and two bunion retractors can be used for exposure after subperiosteal exposure. A lateral section of the fibula is removed. The medial cortex of the proximal fibula is osteotomized at one site and allowed to slide to maintain bone contact and promote union. A bone graft from the tibial site is added. With this technique, it is not necessary to add internal fixation.

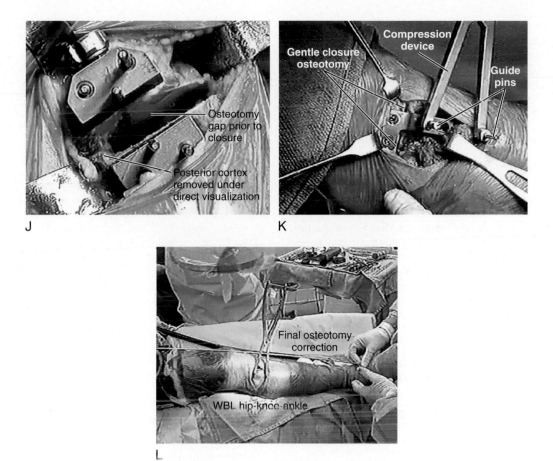

FIGURE 31–38—cont'd. **J,** Lateral gap is equal except for the anterior triangular portion where the gap narrows to prevent alteration of the tibial slope. **K,** Gentle closure of the osteotomy to protect the medial cortex. **L,** Determination of the WBL correction by fluoroscopy and computerized navigation, which is recommended.

The surgeon should be well aware of the anatomic variability of the superficial peroneal nerve (SPN) in the middle third of the leg. Barrett and colleagues[11] reported on this factor in 35 nonpaired and 40 paired cadaver lower extremities. The SPN was identified in the lateral compartment adjacent to the fascial septum in 72%, in the anterior compartment in 23%, or with a branch in both the anterior and the lateral compartments in 5% of the specimens. Ducic and coworkers,[34] in a study of 111 cadaver and clinical specimens, described a similar variability of the location of the SPN in the middle third of the leg. The SPN traveled to the lateral compartment in 70% of the specimens or split with branches in both the lateral and the anterior compartments in 16%. In 6% of the specimens, the SPN was found within the intermuscular septum, and in 8%, traveled only within the anterior compartment.

Step 4: Proximal Osteotomy: Removal of Tibial Wedge

The proximal tibial closing wedge osteotomy technique may be performed using commercially available calibrated osteotomy guide systems, or the bone cuts may be determined using a free-hand method. A smooth guide pin is placed transversely at the proximal tibia to the medial cortex, 25 mm distal to the joint line with the use of fluoroscopy to ensure proper placement. It is critical to leave at least 25 mm of proximal tibia to avoid a tibial plateau fracture. The transverse length of the guide pin determines proximal tibia width.

After the preoperative measurements and based on tibial width (see Table 31–6), the entry point of the second guide pin distally is marked with proper positioning of the guide pins confirmed with fluoroscopy. These guide pins determine the osteotomy triangular bone wedge that is removed to achieve the desired correction. It is important to determine whether the lateral cortex is entirely perpendicular at the osteotomy site. In some knees, there will be a slight triangular anterior slope where it is necessary to downsize the osteotomy gap anteriorly in order not to decrease the tibial slope. The width of the tibia anteriorly is measured and the anterior gap determined (see Table 31–6).

The initial osteotomy cuts are made using a micro-oscillating saw. Initially, only the outer cortex is cut and then the osteotomy is completed with thin osteotomies. An oscillating saw in the cancellous bone may wander and potentially change the correction angle.

A malleable retractor is placed in the subperiosteal plane posteriorly to protect the neurovascular structures at all times with the knee flexed 10°. The lateral half of the wedge is removed as a single piece. Portions of this bone wedge may rarely need to be replaced if an inadvertent overcorrection is obtained at surgery. The remaining triangular wedge of bone is removed under direct visualization.

The surgeon is seated, and a headlamp is always used to view the depth of the osteotomy. The osteotomy plane is maintained in a triangular plane, noting that at the midpoint of the tibia, the tibial width is one half that at the lateral cortex.

The 7 to 10 mm of the wedge adjacent to the posteromedial cortex is left intact to provide stability and prevent medial or lateral tibial translation or varus angulation postoperatively. The posterior tibial cortex of the wedge is removed under direct visualization. The patellar tendon is carefully protected.

Two to three perforations of the posteromedial cortex with a guidewire are often required before the osteotomy gap can be closed with a gentle valgus force that is applied over a few minutes to gradually deform the remaining medial cortex. An option is to use a commercially available compression device to close the osteotomy. Apposition of the bony surfaces of the tibia and fibula should be visualized and inspected.

It is important that the HTO does not increase or decrease the normal posterior tibial slope. The sagittal plane of the osteotomy should be perpendicular to the long axis of the tibia with the width of posterolateral cortex removed based on the coronal angular corrections required (see Table 31–6). In select cases, a biplanar osteotomy for correction of an abnormal tibial slope may be required, as already described. An opening or closing gap in the sagittal plane is performed to the necessary degrees of slope correction.

Step 5: Fluoroscopic Verification of the WBL for Corrected Alignment

Using fluoroscopy, an alignment guide rod (rigid 3–4 mm rod, 1 m in length) is positioned over the center of the femoral head and the center of the tibiotalar joint to determine the corrected WBL intersection at the tibial plateau. A large single staple may be placed across the lateral tibial osteotomy site for provisional fixation. During fluoroscopy, the lower limb is axially loaded at the foot to maintain closure of both the medial and the lateral tibiofemoral compartments at 5° to 10° flexion to avoid hyperextension. It is important to view by fluoroscopy that there is no abnormal opening of the medial or lateral compartment. The knee is taken through a gentle varus-valgus loading to palpate the respective compartments and confirm closure of both because significant errors in the final axial alignment occur if great care is not taken at this junction. A second source of error in the WBL tibial intersection occurs if the lower limb is positioned incorrectly with excessive hip internal or external rotation. The lower limb and foot are positioned with a normal 12° to 15° of external rotation, representing the normal gait foot progression alignment. The alignment guide rod represents a new WBL, which should agree with preoperative calculations. As discussed next, computerized navigation techniques have a distinct advantage in the authors' opinion in improving the accuracy of the WBL determination and final lower limb alignment during the operative procedure. If necessary, further bone may be removed or added to the osteotomy to adjust the WBL.

Internal fixation of the osteotomy is achieved using an L-shaped plate. Two 6.5-mm cancellous screws are placed in the proximal tibia and three cortical screws are placed distal to the osteotomy (Fig. 31–39). Rarely, a 6.5-mm cancellous screw is placed in a lag fashion across the osteotomy site into the

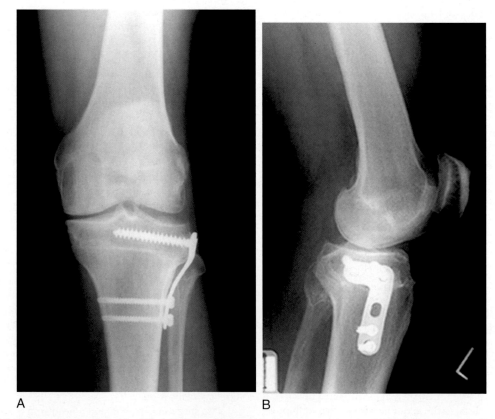

A   B

FIGURE 31–39. AP (**A**) and lateral radiographs (**B**) show the postoperative appearance after proximal tibial osteotomy, fibular osteotomy, and internal fixation. (A and B, *Reprinted with permission from Noyes, F. R.; Barber-Westin, S. D.; Hewett, T. E.: High tibial osteotomy and ligament reconstruction for varus angulated anterior cruciate ligament–deficient knees. Am J Sports Med 28:282–296, 2000.*)

medial aspect of the proximal tibial bone for additional fixation. Newer locking plates and screws provide the advantage of more secure fixation. The final WBL is determined after fixation.

The tourniquet is released and hemostasis obtained. The fascia of the anterior compartment musculature is reattached to the anterolateral aspect of the tibial border with absorbable sutures. It is important to reattach the muscles with adequate suture fixation because muscle tension postoperatively may disrupt the muscle attachment site. A drain is not used.

The lower limb is wrapped with cotton and additional padding is placed posteriorly and over the peroneal nerve, followed by an Ace bandage, postoperative hinged brace, and bilateral ankle-foot compression boots. A commercial ice delivery system with the bladder incorporated over the initial cotton wrapping, a few layers from the wound, is always used. The neurovascular status is checked immediately in the operating room and carefully monitored in the initial postoperative period. A calf or foot compression system is used for the first 24 hours to promote venous blood flow. Aspirin is prescribed and, rarely in high-risk patients, low-molecular-weight heparin (LMWH) or warfarin sodium (Coumadin; Bristol-Myers Squibb Co., Plainsboro, NJ). Early rehabilitation emphasizes early quadriceps isometrics, range of knee motion, ankle pumping, and ambulation (see Chapter 33, Rehabilitation after Tibial and Femoral Osteotomy). The surgeon should have a high suspicion for venous thrombosis and a low threshold for ordering ultrasound evaluation in the postoperative period, which is obtained in the majority of patients in the first few days after surgery.

With the meticulous dissection technique described, a postoperative compartment syndrome should be an exceedingly rare occurrence, if at all. The operative limb is always elevated for the 1st postoperative week, except for periods of ambulation with crutches. The maximum swelling of limb tissues after HTO is usually present 48 to 96 hours postoperatively. The postoperative rehabilitation program is discussed in Chapter 33, Rehabilitation after Tibial and Femoral Osteotomy.

ROLE OF COMPUTERIZED NAVIGATION FOR HTO

For surgeons who are trained on computerized navigation for total knee joint replacement, the addition of the same techniques for HTO offers, in the authors' opinion, a distinct advantage in determining the final WBL and overall limb alignment. The

---

Critical Points ROLE OF COMPUTERIZED NAVIGATION FOR HIGH TIBIAL OSTEOTOMY

- Offers distinct advantage in determining final overall limb alignment.
- Hold lower limb with the knee in 5° flexion to measure WBL, degrees of valgus overcorrection.
- Full standing radiographic measurements may have errors induced in the coronal plane (affecting WBL measurements) owing to the rotation of the lower limb during the radiographic procedure.
- Computerized technique valuable during plate fixation, limb alignment can be checked as often as necessary and is simpler than repeat hip-knee-ankle WBL fluoroscopy.

WBL, weight-bearing line.

---

registration process is easier with fewer points required than for total knee replacement (Fig. 31–40A). The software allows for the preoperative and postoperative varus-valgus position and WBL to be determined (see Fig. 31–40B). We recommend that the lower limb be held with the knee in 5° flexion for the measurement of the WBL and degrees of valgus overcorrection. This compares with the full-standing, hip-knee-ankle radiographs in 5° flexion to avoid a hyperextension position in which different WBL measurements would be erroneously obtained. The operating room setup combining the computerized navigation system with fluoroscopy is shown in Figure 31–40C.

Keppler and associates[64] reported on the use of a computer-aided surgical navigation system of opening wedge tibial osteotomy in a plastic bone model and cadaveric lower limbs. These authors found high consistency between operators in registering anatomic landmarks and concluded that improved accuracy and reliability of correcting the mechanical axis would be the benefits of this approach. A number of studies have shown that full-standing radiographic measurements may have errors induced in the coronal plane (affecting WBL measurements) owing to the rotation of the lower limb during the radiographic procedure.[61,84,143] Song and associates[127] reported that a navigation-assisted opening wedge HTO procedure improved the surgeon's ability to obtain a more accurate postoperative alignment correction.

Clinical studies are still required to determine in a large patient series the increased accuracy obtained with computerized navigation techniques. However, in the authors' experience, the following points are important. It is still necessary to determine the tibial slope (using the Keith needle technique previously described in the Operative Techniques sections) for each knee, although an arbitrary tibial slope may be selected for the navigation technique (see Fig. 31–40D). The navigation of the actual osteotomy cut can be performed as easily as with the placement of guide pins and fluoroscopy. In essence, fluoroscopy is still required on pin placement and to determine the depth of the osteotomes during surgery to maintain integrity of the opposite cortex. Increased accuracy of determining the final WBL, compared with hip-knee-ankle fluoroscopy, is expected because the variable of internal-external limb rotation and its effect on the WBL is nearly eliminated (see Fig. 31–40E). A major error in determining the WBL intersection at the tibia occurs with the standard hip-knee-flexion fluoroscopy method because the measurement line or rigid rod is placed on the limb, but does not correspond to the central measurement line established in the hip-knee-ankle joints based on the navigation registration techniques. This means that with the external rod or line positioned at the hip joint, internal or external rotation at the hip joint with the distal rod at the ankle will result in a potential error of the WBL tibial intersection in a lateral-to-medial direction. The WBL intersection by the computerized method intersects the centers of the hip-knee-ankle, eliminating this major problem. The authors have also found the computerized technique valuable during plate fixation, because the limb alignment can be easily checked as often as necessary and is simpler than repeat hip-knee-ankle WBL fluoroscopy.

OPENING WEDGE FEMORAL OSTEOTOMY

A femoral closing or opening wedge osteotomy is an accepted treatment for the correction of an abnormal valgus lower limb

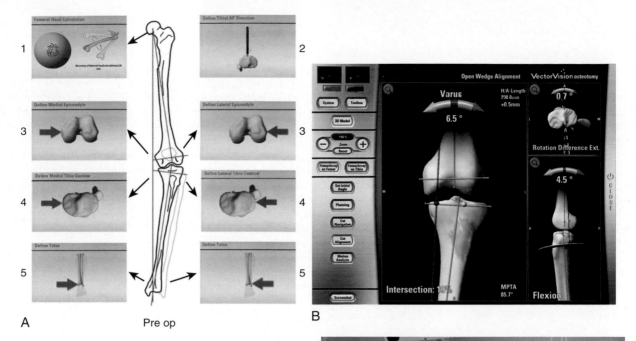

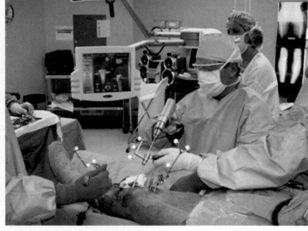

A   Pre op

B

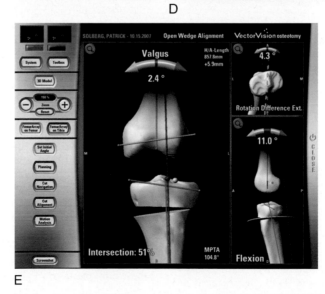

C

D

E

FIGURE 31–40. A, The registration points for the computerized navigation procedure (BrainLAB, Feldkirchen, Germany). **B,** Preoperative measurement shows the angular malalignment of 6.5° varus and a 19% WBL intersection. **C,** Operating room setup. The fluoroscopy and computer navigation instruments are on the operative side. The surgeon is able to perform the medial opening wedge procedure from the medial aspect, usually in a seated position. The photographs show the ability of the surgeon to determine the lower limb alignment from the foot of the table. **D,** Demonstration of the navigation instrumentation that may be used to determine the osteotomy plane (see text). **E,** Final operative correction obtained, with a 2.4° valgus alignment and a 51% WBL intersection.

Critical Points OPENING WEDGE FEMORAL OSTEOTOMY

- Indications, contraindications for surgical treatment are similar to those for an HTO except that the osteotomy is designed to decrease weight-bearing forces on the lateral tibiofemoral compartment.
- Goal is to correct abnormal abduction moment at the knee joint, but not to produce an abnormal adduction moment that would overload the medial compartment.
- Contraindications: absence of remaining lateral tibiofemoral articular cartilage and lateral joint tibial concavity, advanced lateral joint arthritis.
- It is important to determine that there is no abnormal opening of the medial joint space, which must be accounted for in the preoperative correction measurements.
- Target zone is a WBL at the 42%–45% intersection, equal to a 1°–2° varus lower limb alignment, respectively.
- Cosmetic skin incision of limited length, with upper locking screws placed through small 3- to 4-mm skin incisions.
- Guide pins placed in the line of the osteotomy 15 mm proximal to the femoral trochlea region, slight oblique fashion to end at the proximal metaphyseal junction.
- Gradual distraction, leaves 8 mm of the medial femoral cortex intact.
- Maintain equal anterior and posterior osteotomy gap in order to not change the tibiofemoral slope.
- Use autogenous bone graft, locking plate, and screws.

HTO, high tibial osteotomy; WBL, weight-bearing line.

alignment. Details of the operative indications and procedures are covered in Chapter 32, Valgus Malalignment: Diagnosis, Osteotomy Techniques, and Clinical Outcomes, and are therefore only summarized here.

The indications and contraindications for surgical treatment are similar to those for an HTO except that the osteotomy is designed to decrease weight-bearing forces on the lateral tibiofemoral compartment. The most common presentation is a younger patient who has undergone lateral meniscectomy and shows progressive valgus alignment and narrowing of the lateral tibiofemoral compartment and has lateral joint symptoms. The procedure is often performed prior to a lateral meniscus transplantation or other articular cartilage restorative procedures to the lateral compartment. Similar to a corrective procedure for varus malalignment already discussed, the goal of the procedure is to buy time. It is important not to correct the lower limb to an excessive varus alignment, as is discussed next. If there has been a prior medial meniscectomy or if medial tibiofemoral joint damage is present, a relative contraindication to the varus-producing femoral osteotomy may exist or the correction should obtain only a neutral alignment. The goal is to correct an abnormal abduction moment at the knee joint, but not to produce an abnormal adduction moment that would overload the medial compartment (see Fig. 31–5).

Contraindications to a varus-producing osteotomy are similar to those previously discussed for HTO and include the absence of remaining lateral tibiofemoral articular cartilage and lateral joint tibial concavity, indicating advanced lateral joint arthritis.

The clinical evaluation includes an analysis of the patient's gait and observation for a valgus thrust. There is usually lateral joint line tenderness to examination and mild lateral joint crepitus with a valgus loading of the joint during flexion and extension. This maneuver is frequently painful and reproduces the patient's symptoms. It is important to examine specifically for

associate patellofemoral arthritis and articular cartilage damage to the lateral patella facet and trochlea. The valgus lower limb alignment increases the lateral deviation of the patella, producing increased lateral patellofemoral joint loading. Accordingly, symptoms related to the patellofemoral joint may be permanent and should be considered in determining whether the patient is a suitable candidate for the femoral osteotomy.

The radiographic assessment for lower limb alignment has already been presented, including obtaining weight-bearing 45° PA views, axial patellofemoral views, lateral view for tibial slope, and a full-standing radiograph for measurement of the hip-knee-ankle mechanical alignment and WBL. It is important to determine that there is no abnormal opening of the medial joint space that must be accounted for in the preoperative correction measurements. In Figure 31–14, the normal tibiofemoral coronal alignment is shown. In valgus-angulated knees, there is frequently a coronal obliquity to the joint line due to the lateral joint damage primarily affecting the lateral femoral condyle. Owing to this obliquity, an opening wedge tibia osteotomy is contraindicated because this would increase the joint obliquity. An opening or closing wedge femoral osteotomy would correct the joint obliquity. Even though there are reports in the literature on opening wedge tibial osteotomy, the authors have observed clinical cases in which the increased joint obliquity leads to abnormal loading of the lateral tibial tubercle and lateral femoral condyle with subsequent loss of articular cartilage and arthritis. References of publications of closing wedge femoral osteotomy are provided for the reader[12,30,48,81]; this section deals primarily with the surgical technique for an opening wedge femoral osteotomy.

The preoperative planning for the opening wedge osteotomy follows the same rules as previously presented and the measurement techniques are the same except that a final WBL intersection at the tibia is just medial to the 50% tibial width. The target zone is a WBL at the 42% to 45% intersection, which is equivalent to a 1° to 2° varus lower limb alignment, respectively. A WBL more medial to this point would induce a varus overcorrection. The degrees of correction and the corresponding osteotomy opening gap in millimeters (rule of triangles; see Table 31–7) is usually in the 5- to 8-mm range owing to the narrow width of the femur at the osteotomy site. This means that a few millimeters of error would have a major effect in producing an undercorrection or overcorrection. For this reason, the careful and accurate fluoroscopic measurements of surgery of the desired correction and new WBL tibial intersection are important and the added role of computerized navigation to verify the lower limb alignment is encouraged.

The operative steps the senior author follows in performing the opening wedge femoral osteotomy are detailed in Figure 31–41. Important steps in the operative procedure include a cosmetically placed skin incision of limited length, with upper locking screws placed through small 3- to 4-mm skin incisions. The surgeon sits adjacent to the lateral aspect of the lower limb with a headlight for visualization beneath the raised skin flaps. The guide pins are placed in the line of the osteotomy 15 mm proximal to the femoral trochlea region and in a slightly oblique fashion to end at the proximal metaphyseal junction. The osteotomy involves a gradual distraction process that leaves 8 mm of the medial femoral cortex intact. If the medial femoral cortex is thick and dense, it may be necessary to weaken the cortex with two to three small drill holes. It is important to maintain an equal anterior and posterior osteotomy gap in order to not change the tibiofemoral slope. An autogenous limited iliac crest bone harvest (technique already discussed, Operative Technique. Opening Wedge Tibial Osteotomy) is performed and the width of the outer iliac crest that is harvested matches the opening osteotomy gap. Clinical data are insufficient to recommend allografts over autografts for femoral osteotomy, and the authors prefer an autograft for prompt healing and faster resumption of full weight-bearing activities. An autograft approach in combination with a locking plate and screw design provides for secure femoral fixation, avoiding the serious risks of delayed or nonunion and loss of the lower limb angular correction, which should be a rarity.

The rehabilitation program is the same as for an HTO; and radiographs are obtained postoperatively to measure the operative correction obtained and the progression of osteotomy healing. It is usual for partial weight-bearing at 4 weeks and full weight-bearing at 7 to 8 weeks after surgery.

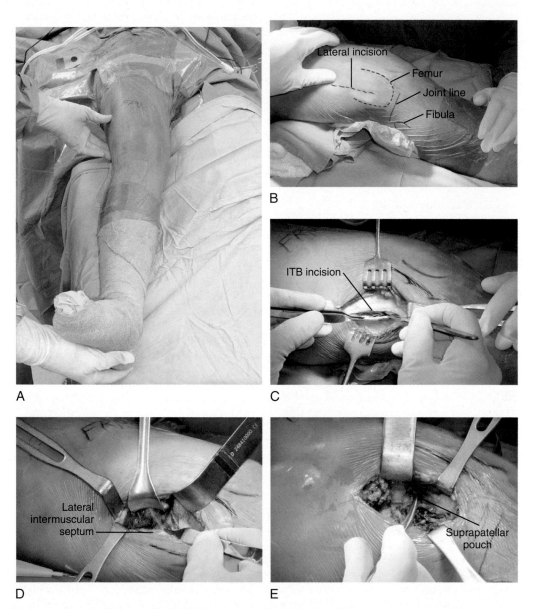

FIGURE 31–41. Demonstration of opening wedge femoral osteotomy for correction of lower limb valgus malalignment. **A,** Surgical setup with high thigh tourniquet and the complete lower extremity draped, including the ipsilateral iliac crest (not shown) for bone graft procedure. **B,** Initial limited incision at the distal lateral thigh just above the joint line. The surgeon is seated with a headlamp for adequate visualization. A small posterior thigh roll is placed to prevent the popliteal neurovascular structures from being displaced anteriorly toward the operative site. **C,** Incision into the posterior third of the iliotibial band that extends in a proximal subcutaneous plane. **D,** A careful dissection of the vastus lateralis insertion at the lateral intermuscular septum is shown with identification of perforating small arteries and veins for control of hemostasis and prevention of hematoma. **E,** An S retractor is placed underneath the vastus lateralis and the proximal joint suprapatellar pouch is identified, which is not opened.

Continued

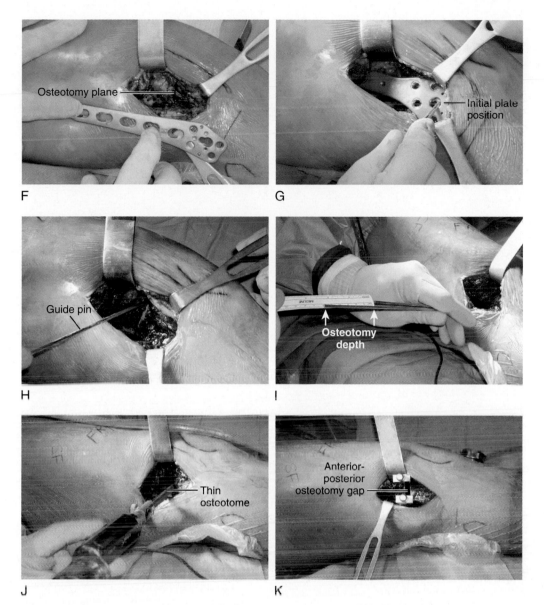

FIGURE 31–41—cont'd.   F, The approximate location of the femoral osteotomy site is identified by fluoroscopy and the locking plate is selected. **G,** Proximal to distal positioning of the locking plate in reference to the distal femoral condyle and osteotomy site. **H,** The anterior guide pin is placed in slight oblique line, 15 mm proximal to femoral trochlea, which can be palpated and verified by fluoroscopy. The guide pin is placed to intersect the proximal medial metaphyseal flare, which is left intact and provides for medial stabilization. Note that there has been no subperiosteal dissection even though the anterior and posterior cortex is visualized for later osteotomy. **I,** The posterior guide pin is placed perpendicular to the femoral shaft and the depth of the planned osteotomy site is measured off a free guide pin. **J,** The initial osteotomy of the lateral cortex is started with a power saw and thin blade followed by a hand-held thin osteotomy blade, which provides better control as the osteotomy progresses. A malleable retractor may be placed posterior to the posterior cortex to protect the neurovascular structures. **K,** The osteotomy site has been gently distracted by thin spreader bars (not shown) and two wedges placed to maintain the opening gap. The medial metaphyseal cortex has been preserved, as confirmed by fluoroscopy.

Continued

AUTHORS' CLINICAL STUDIES

Closing Wedge Osteotomy in ACL-Deficient Varus-Angulated Knees

A study was conducted that reported the results of 41 patients (100% follow-up) who were followed an average of 58 months after closing wedge osteotomy (range, 23–86 mo).[93] These patients also had ACL deficiency, of which 30 were treated with a reconstruction.

Significant improvements were found for all symptoms; the most noteworthy finding was the decrease in pain (Fig. 31–42). Preoperatively, 41% of the patients had moderate to severe pain with activities of daily living whereas only 10% had this level of pain at follow-up. The decrease in pain could have occurred as a result of patient counseling on activity modification and owing to the fact that none of the patients returned to strenuous sports involving jumping, pivoting, and cutting.

Before surgery, 22 patients were participating in some form of sports activities with pain or functional limitations. At

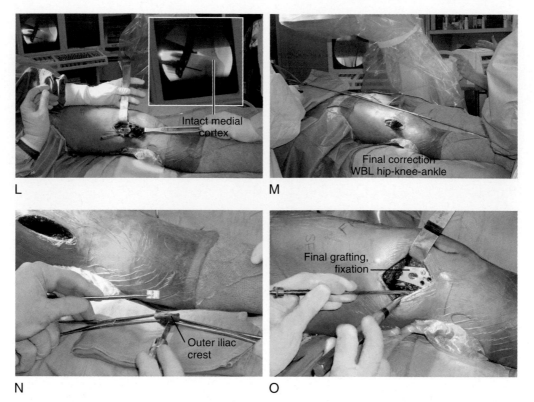

FIGURE 31-41—cont'd. **L,** A rigid rod is placed to establish the new WBL tibial intersection and verify the lower limb alignment. The surgeon provides axial compression at the foot to maintain closure of both the medial and the lateral tibiofemoral joints. An inadvertent joint opening of a few millimeters would result in an inaccurate alignment measurement. **M,** The locking plate is fixed under fluoroscopic control. The monitor shows the osteotomy opening wedge and preservation of the medial metaphyseal cortex. **N,** The iliac crest autograft is sectioned into anterior, middle, and posterior triangles and subsequently gently wedged into the osteotomy opening gap. **O,** The final appearance of the osteotomy with the bone graft in place.

follow-up, 24 patients (59%) had returned to sports with no symptoms; however, the majority were participating in biking or swimming only.

A separate analysis was conducted on a subgroup of 15 patients who had subchondral bone exposed in the medial

Critical Points AUTHORS' CLINICAL STUDIES: CLOSING WEDGE OSTEOTOMY IN ACL-DEFICIENT VARUS-ANGULATED KNEES

- 41 patients, 100% follow-up 2–7 yr postoperative.
- Statistically significant improvements pain, swelling, function.
- 59% returned low-impact sports activities.
- 88% satisfied.
- 22 knees had increased lateral tibiofemoral joint opening preoperatively (double varus knees), which resolved in 17 (77%) without a posterolateral reconstructive procedure.
- 27% did not require subsequent ACL reconstruction.
- Determine each patient's desired level of activity and instability symptoms. ACL reconstruction not required in all.
- Goal of HTO is return to daily activities, not athletics in most patients.
- Goal of HTO in patients with recent onset of pain and no advanced joint damage may be return to athletics or strenuous work activities. ACL reconstruction frequently required in these patients.

ACL, anterior cruciate ligament; HTO, high tibial osteotomy.

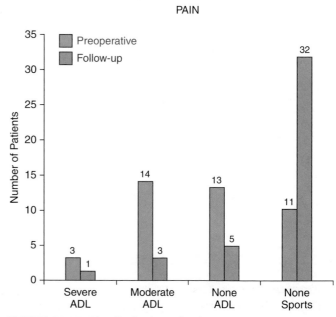

FIGURE 31-42. The distributions of patient responses to the pain scale are shown preoperatively and at follow-up. The improvement was statistically significant ($P < .05$). *(Reprinted with permission from Noyes, F. R.; Barber, S. D.; Simon, R.: High tibial osteotomy and ligament reconstruction in varus angulated, anterior cruciate ligament–deficient knees. A two- to seven-year follow-up study. Am J Sports Med 21:2–12, 1993.)*

tibiofemoral compartment. These patients were followed a mean of 67 months (range, 36–89 mo) postoperatively. A statistically significant improvement was noted in the mean overall rating score at follow-up ($P < .01$). Nine patients returned to light sports activities, whereas the other 6 did not participate, thus following medical advice.

The radiographic evaluation performed in the early postoperative period showed that 37 of 41 patients (90%) were surgically corrected with a WBL between 50% and 80%. Three patients drifted back into varus and 1 had settled into valgus. At the final follow-up examination, 25 patients (61%) still demonstrated optimal correction (mean WBL, 60%; range, 46%–79%). However, 11 patients (27%) were in varus (mean WBL, 37%; range, 25%–44%) and 5 (12%) had an increased valgus position (mean WBL, 90%; range, 81%–108%). These findings indicated that progression of the medial arthritis in the varus-angulated knee continues and long-term correction was not achieved in 1 out of 4 patients. Even in the knees that returned to a varus angulation, there was short-term relief of pain symptoms; however, the long-term function in these patients is expected to decline.

A statistically significant improvement was found between the preoperative and the follow-up overall rating scores (scale, 0–100 points, $P < .01$). The mean increase between evaluations was 14 points (range, –8–38 points).

An interesting finding was that whereas 22 knees (54%) had abnormally increased lateral joint opening on varus stress testing preoperatively, only 5 (12%) had this abnormal joint opening at follow-up. The valgus-producing osteotomy appeared to have unloaded the FCL and posterolateral ligament tissues, allowing physiologic remodeling and shortening to occur. Therefore, no associated posterolateral reconstruction was required during the subsequent ACL reconstruction. This clinical finding appears to support the recommendation to first perform the HTO in double varus knees, and then assess knee stability and symptoms to determine the requirement for future ligament reconstruction.

There was no evidence of infection, peroneal nerve palsy, or tibial nonunion. One patient had a gentle manipulation under anesthesia 24 weeks after the HTO and full motion was successfully regained.

Three patients required a repeat osteotomy owing to complications. One patient settled into a valgus position 16 months postoperatively. One patient required an open reduction and internal fixation 4 weeks postoperatively owing to a loss of fixation at the osteotomy site. A falling injury 3 weeks postoperative caused a 4-mm collapse at the osteotomy site in another patient who underwent an opening wedge osteotomy. In all 3 patients, follow-up examinations performed 2 to 3 years after the revision procedures demonstrated WBLs and mechanical axes within the optimal range.

One patient had a nonunion at the distal fibula osteotomy site; the tibial osteotomy site healed in a satisfactory manner. The fibula nonunion site was resected 12 months postoperatively and symptoms resolved.

Patients who had the ACL reconstruction typically had giving-way symptoms with daily or light sports activities. Because many patients modify their sports activities after surgery, it is not always necessary to perform an ACL reconstruction. Eleven knees in this study that were ACL deficient did not require ACL reconstruction. Patients should be individually profiled regarding the level of activity they wish to resume and an ACL reconstruction done if symptoms warrant the procedure.

Two distinct groups of young, active patients exist in whom the goals of HTO may differ. One group has significant medial tibiofemoral arthritis and pain and swelling with daily activities. The goal of HTO for these patients is to diminish these symptoms, not to return to athletics. These patients are counseled regarding the extent of the disease process and the goal of the HTO, which is to buy time until total joint replacement is required.

The second group of patients does not have advanced joint arthritis; their pain symptoms are of relatively recent onset and occur with sports or manual labor activities. These individuals desire HTO to continue some form of athletics, or they may have a strenuous occupation. These patients also usually require an ACL reconstruction because they have higher activity demands and frequently have experienced a giving-way injury. However, data are not available that accurately predict whether or not athletics are advisable after successful HTO. Large in vivo joint loading occurs with athletics, and patients who resume these activities do so at their own risk of further joint damage.

The Treatment of Double and Triple Varus Knees: Closing Wedge Osteotomy, ACL Reconstruction, and Posterolateral Reconstruction

A second prospective investigation followed 41 knees (23 double, 18 triple varus) for a mean of 4.5 years (range, 2–12 yr after HTO.[100] Prior to referral, 19 ACL reconstructions that had failed had been done in 15 patients. Many of these ACL failures were attributed to an associated posterolateral deficiency that was not corrected at the time of the initial ACL reconstruction. Thirty patients (73%) had a partial or total medial meniscectomy before the HTO.

In 17 patients (12 double, 5 triple varus), gait analysis testing was conducted preoperatively and a mean of 2 years after HTO. The GaitLink system (Computerized Functional Testing Corporation, Chicago, IL) included a two-camera, video-based optoelectronic digitizer for measuring motion, and a multicomponent force plate (Bertec, Columbus, OH) for measuring ground reaction force, which was camouflaged under a 10-m walkway. A control population of 28 age- and sex-matched normal subjects was used for comparisons. All moments were normalized to the product of body weight multiplied by height (BW × HT) and were expressed as a percentage of that product.

Thirty knees had abnormal articular cartilage lesions. Twenty-six (63%) had abnormal lesions in the medial compartment.

In 21 (91%) of the double varus knees, the ACL was reconstructed a mean of 9 months after the HTO, and in 2 knees, the HTO and ACL reconstruction were done simultaneously.

In 13 (72%) of the triple varus knees, the ACL was reconstructed a mean of 8 months after the HTO. One patient had the HTO and ACL reconstruction done simultaneously. Four patients had the ACL reconstruction done before the HTO in an attempt to avoid HTO.

All triple varus knees had a posterolateral reconstruction; 12 (67%) had a proximal advancement of the posterolateral complex with the ACL reconstruction and 6 had an FCL femoral-fibular graft procedure. The knees that had the proximal advancement procedure had a definitive, although lax, FCL of normal width and integrity and intact popliteal muscle-tendon and fibular attachments, previously described as an indication for this procedure. The knees that had the FCL reconstruction had extensive damage to posterolateral tissues.

At follow-up, statistically significant improvements were found for pain, swelling, and giving-way (Fig. 31–43; $P < .001$). Before the HTO, 18 patients (44%) had severe to moderate pain with activities of daily living, whereas at follow-up, only 7 (17%) had such pain. Overall, 29 patients (71%) improved their pain score and 28 (68%) improved their swelling and scores. Giving-way was eliminated in 85%.

Twenty-seven patients (66%) were able to return to mostly low-impact athletics without symptoms. One patient rated the overall knee condition as normal; 14 as very good; 14 as good; 10 as fair; and 2 as poor.

Statistically significant improvements were found in the mean overall rating score from preoperative to follow-up (63 ± 11 points and 82 ± 14 points, respectively; $P = .0001$). The average increase was 20 ± 10 points (range, 2–39 points).

At follow-up, 19 knees (42%) had functional ACL reconstructions, 11 knees (24%) had partial function, and 15 knees (33%) failed. Ten of the 15 knees that failed represented ACL revision cases. A statistically significant difference was found in the failure rate for ACL revision cases compared with primary reconstruction cases (67% and 33%, respectively; $P = .03$).

Preoperatively, all of the triple varus knees had varus recurvatum, increases in lateral joint opening (mean, 8 mm; range, 3–15 mm), and increases in external tibial rotation (mean, 9°; range, 3°–15°). At follow-up, 13 knees were rated as functional, 4 as partially functional, and 1 as failed.

Preoperatively, all patients with double varus knees had abnormal increases in lateral joint opening (mean, 4 mm; range 2–10 mm). At follow-up, no patient had more than 2 mm of increase in lateral joint opening and none had an increase in external tibial rotation. All were rated as functional in lateral joint opening and external tibial rotation.

There was no significant difference in the mean preoperative adduction moment between the double varus and the triple varus knees (4.1% ± 0.3% and 4.2% ± 0.3%, respectively). The preoperative mean adduction moment of the study group was 35% higher ($P < .001$) than the control group value; 10 of the 17 patients (59%) had values that were greater than 1 standard deviation above control values (Fig. 31–44). The study group also had a 22% higher calculated medial compartment load and a 40% higher lateral ligament tensile force compared with the control group (Table 31–8; $P < .01$). Above-normal medial compartment loads were predicted preoperatively in 71% of the involved knees, and above-normal lateral soft tissue forces during walking were predicted in 43% of the involved knees.

Postoperatively, the adduction moment and lateral ligament tensile force decreased to significantly lower than control values.

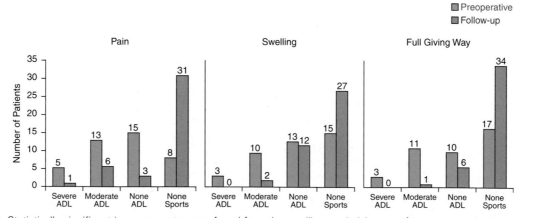

FIGURE 31–43. Statistically significant improvements were found for pain, swelling, and giving-way from preoperative to follow-up ($P < .01$). ADL, activities of daily living. *(Reprinted with permission from Noyes, F. R.; Barber-Westin, S. D.; Hewett, T. E.: High tibial osteotomy and ligament reconstruction for varus angulated anterior cruciate ligament–deficient knees. Am J Sports Med 28:282–296, 2000.)*

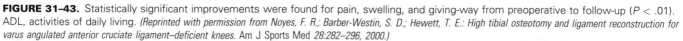

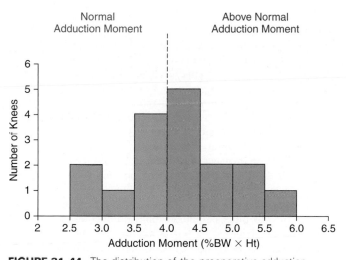

FIGURE 31–44. The distribution of the preoperative adduction moments of the 17 patients tested. The mean adduction moment for the study group was 35% higher than that for the control group (*P* < .001). *(Reprinted with permission from Noyes, F. R.; Barber-Westin, S. D.; Hewett, T. E.: High tibial osteotomy and ligament reconstruction for varus angulated anterior cruciate ligament–deficient knees. Am J Sports Med 28:282–296, 2000.)*

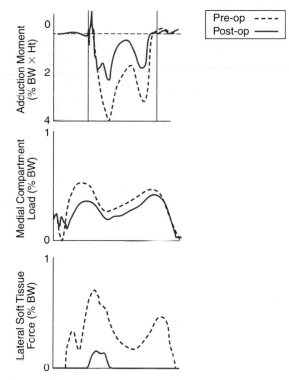

FIGURE 31–45. The preoperative and postoperative adduction moment, medial compartment load, and lateral ligament tensile forces for the 17 patients tested. Postoperatively, the adduction moment and lateral ligament tensile force decreased to significantly lower than control values. The medial compartment load decreased to values equal to those of controls. % BW, percentage of body weight; Ht, height. *(Reprinted with permission from Noyes, F. R.; Barber-Westin, S. D.; Hewett, T. E.: High tibial osteotomy and ligament reconstruction for varus angulated anterior cruciate ligament–deficient knees. Am J Sports Med 28:282–296, 2000.)*

The medial compartment load decreased to values equal to those of controls (Fig. 31–45).

There was no evidence of infection, peroneal nerve palsy, patella infera, or knee motion limitations at follow-up. No patient required additional treatment intervention for losses of knee flexion or extension.

Preoperatively, the mean WBL was 22% (range, 3%–49%) and the mean mechanical axis was –6.2° (range, –12° to –1°). At surgery, all knees were corrected to a WBL of 62%. In 2 knees, a valgus overcorrection occurred; these were subsequently revised.

At follow-up, 33 knees (80%) were in an acceptable position (mean WBL, 61%; range, 50%–75%), 7 knees were in varus, and 1 knee was in valgus (WBL, 81%).

Two knees required revision of the HTO. In both, the optimal correction in the 62% WBL range was obtained at surgery; however, excessive valgus (WBL, 86%) occurred with full weight-bearing. A revision opening wedge osteotomy was done 2 months

postoperative in 1 knee and 6 months postoperative in the other. At follow-up, 1 knee had maintained the optimal WBL position, but the other had reassumed a varus position (WBL, 40%).

One knee had a loss of internal fixation of the osteotomy at the 4th postoperative week that was corrected. The HTO

TABLE 31–8 Gait Analysis Data: Measured and Predicted Peak Values (Mean ± SD)

Variable	Control Group (*N* = 28)	Study Group Preoperative (*N* = 17)	Study Group Postoperative (*N* = 17)	Change (%)
Measured moment*				
Flexion	2.3 ± 0.8	2.2 ± 1.7	2.4 ± 1.3	+9
Extension	2.4 ± 0.7	1.5 ± 1.4	1.4 ± 1.1	–7
Adduction	3.1 ± 0.7	4.2 ± 0.8[†]	2.6 ± 0.6[†]	–38[‡]
Predicted tibiofemoral loads[§]				
Medial	2.3 ± 0.3	2.8 ± 0.3[†]	2.2 ± 0.5	–21[‡]
Lateral	0.9 ± 0.3	1.1 ± 0.3	1.0 ± 0.4	–9
Predicted ligament tensile force[§]				
Lateral	0.5 ± 0.2	0.7 ± 0.2[‖]	0.3 ± 0.2[‖]	–57[‡]

*Percentage of body weight times height.
[†]Significantly different from control subjects (*P* < .01).
[‡]Significantly different from preoperative and postoperative values (*P* < .01).
[§]Percentage of body weight.
[‖]Significantly different from control subjects (*P* < .001).

healed without difficulty. Two patients required resection of a distal fibular painful nonunion osteotomy site 12 and 26 months postoperatively.

Opening Wedge Osteotomy: An Operative Technique and Rehabilitation Program to Decrease Complications and Promote Early Union and Function

A prospective study was conducted of 59 consecutive patients who had a medial opening wedge proximal tibial osteotomy.[107] All but 4 patients were followed for at least 6 months postoperative, the minimum follow-up time period required for this study. The 55 patients were followed a mean of 20 months postoperatively (range, 6–60 mo).

The hypothesis was that a technique for opening wedge osteotomy that incorporated an autogenous iliac crest bone graft would prevent delayed or nonunion and allow early rehabilitation, weight-bearing, and return in function. A second hypothesis was that a methodology for calculating the desired correction of valgus alignment would prevent undesired alterations in tibial slope.

Independent physicians examined radiographs pre- and postoperatively for tibial slope and patellar height and postoperatively for bony union. Postoperative radiographs were taken at 4 and 8 weeks postoperative, and then as required until bone consolidation was evident. *Delayed union* was defined as lack of bridging callous and presence of radiolucent areas within the opening wedge defect past a period of 3 months postoperatively.

In 6 knees, a concurrent operative procedure was performed and included ACL primary reconstruction in 2 knees, ACL revision reconstruction in 1 knee, ACL and MCL reconstructions in 1 knee, and an osteochondral autograft transfer procedure on the medial femoral condyle in 2 knees.

Critical Points AUTHORS' CLINICAL STUDIES: OPENING WEDGE OSTEOTOMY: AN OPERATIVE TECHNIQUE AND REHABILITATION PROGRAM TO DECREASE COMPLICATIONS AND PROMOTE EARLY UNION AND FUNCTION

- 55 patients reviewed mean 20 mo (range, 6–60) postoperative.
- Independent physicians examined preoperative and postoperative radiographs for tibial slope, patellar height, bone consolidation.
- Concurrent ACL reconstruction in 4 knees.
- Staged ACL and posterolateral reconstruction in 3 knees, staged ACL, PCL, and posterolateral reconstruction in 1 knee, staged PCL reconstruction in 2 knees, staged medial meniscus allograft in 3 knees.
- Delayed union in 3 patients (5%), healed by 6–10 mo postoperative.
- Early postoperative loss of fixation 1 patient (noncompliant with weight-bearing rules), HTO revised.
- No patellar infera, change in tibia slope, infection, arthrofibrosis, DVT, vascular injury, fracture, problems at iliac crest harvest site.
- Full weight-bearing achieved mean 8 wk (range, 4–11 wk) postoperative.

ACL, anterior cruciate ligament; DVT, deep vein thrombosis; HTO, high tibial osteotomy; PCL, posterior cruciate ligament.

In 9 knees, staged procedures were performed an average of 8 months (range, 3–19 mo) after the osteotomy. These included knee ligament reconstructions of both the ACL and the posterolateral structures in 3 knees; combined ACL, posterolateral, and PCL reconstruction in 1 knee; PCL reconstruction in 2 knees; and medial meniscus allografts in 3 knees. All 9 knees achieved bony union at the osteotomy site and were full weight-bearing before undergoing the staged procedures. No complications related to the HTO occurred in these 9 knees.

Healing and union at the osteotomy site were radiographically evident an average of 3 months postoperatively in 52 patients (95%). A delay in union (with no loss of fixation or correction) occurred in 3 patients (5%). The size of the opening wedge osteotomy in these 3 patients ranged from 11.0 to 16 mm. In 2 of these patients, a bone stimulator was applied, and union was achieved by 6 to 8 months postoperatively. The other patient achieved union without intervention by 10 months.

An early postoperative loss of fixation occurred in 1 patient who admitted to full weight-bearing immediately after surgery. The osteotomy was successfully revised 10 days postoperatively and proceeded uneventfully to union. There were no instances of shortening of the patellar tendon related to a patella infera syndrome.

There was no significant difference between the mean preoperative (9° ± 4°; range, 2°–16°) and postoperative (10° ± 3°; range, 3°–21°) tibial slope measurements. One patient with a PCL-deficient knee had an intentional increase in posterior slope.

There were no deep infections, loss of knee motion requiring intervention, deep vein thrombosis, nerve or arterial injury, fracture, or complications related to bone grafting.

Full weight-bearing was achieved a mean of 8 weeks (range, 4–11 wk) postoperatively.

The dissection was limited to include only 10 mm of the superior iliac crest. The iliac crest harvest procedure can be painful with trunk flexion activities for up to 4 weeks postoperatively, and patients are advised accordingly. The standard cortical iliac crest graft harvested was 40 mm in length, 12 mm in width, and 30 mm in depth, although larger osteotomies required a longer graft of approximately 45 mm. The width of the osteotomies varied from 5 to 15 mm, with 35% of the procedures being 10 mm or more.

The argument may be made that autogenous bone grafting is required only for large osteotomies, such as those over 10 mm, but in fact, no well-designed clinical studies have been published to date that provide evidence for such recommendations. When an opening wedge osteotomy proceeds to a delayed union or nonunion, there is usually a loss of correction and a prolonged course of restricted weight-bearing, potential muscle disuse, and need for further surgical intervention. In these knees, failure to arrive at the desired goal of the osteotomy ensues, and therefore, specific steps are taken to avoid this sequela in all patients regardless of the size of correction required.

The iliac crest graft harvest adds operative time and most likely increases the risk of complications at a second operative site. In this study, no patient complained of pain at the iliac crest harvest site with activities at follow-up. Two patients had a small hematoma at the iliac crest harvest site, which resolved uneventfully. Still, patients should be advised of the expected postoperative pain and increased risk of complications.

Many commercial allograft wedges are available for opening wedge osteotomies. Allograft bone may have a marked delay in incorporation and healing at the osteotomy site. There may be a higher risk of delayed union, prolonged need for crutch protection, delay in allowing weight-bearing, and disuse effects with both allografts and other substitute materials. A high rate of complications was reported in a series in which tricalcium phosphate was used to fill the wedge defect in 20 knees.[116] Nonunions occurred in 35%, loss of correction in 15%, infections in 10%, and material failure in 30%. No problems with union have been reported in several studies of opening wedge osteotomy when an iliac crest bone autograft was used.[29,78,114,115,138,145]

The following operative principles are promoted to prevent fracture: ensure that a proximal lateral tibial plateau width of at least 20 mm exists, avoid too much obliquity at the osteotomy site, and perforate to within 10 mm of the lateral cortex with the osteotome. Forceful completion of the osteotomy should be avoided. Several surgeon-controlled factors can help minimize the risk of inadequate or loss of correction (Table 31–9). Meticulous preoperative planning is imperative. Intraoperatively, the mechanical axis must be accurately verified. Because the size of the osteotomy is not set prior to fixation, opening wedge osteotomy affords the surgeon ample opportunity to adjust the angular correction and aids in producing the desired alignment. The alignment postoperative should be verified by the 4th postoperative week under partial weight-bearing conditions.

RESULTS FROM OTHER CLINICAL STUDIES

Survival Rates: Closing Wedge Osteotomies

The survival rates reported after HTO are shown in Table 31–10.* Whereas conversion to TKA was uniformly used as an endpoint for survival of HTO, some investigators also incorporated as additional endpoints a low overall Hospital for Special Surgery (HSS) knee rating score, patient dissatisfaction, or the presence of pain in patients who declined TKA.

One study provided a 20-year survival rate of 85.1% on 257 patients after closing wedge osteotomy. Flecher and colleagues[39] found the following factors to be statistically significant in determining the long-term outcome: age at surgery less than 50 years ($P = .01$), body mass index less than 25 ($P = .02$), preoperative Ahlback radiographic grade 1 ($P = .01$), and a postoperative valgus angle of greater than 6° ($P = .02$).

A high long-term survival rate for closing wedge osteotomies was also reported by Koshino and coworkers[68] who followed 75 knees from 15 to 28 years postoperatively. At the final follow-up examination, 93.2% of the patients had not converted to TKA or unicompartmental knee arthroplasty or complained of moderate or severe knee pain. The authors attributed the success of the procedure to the achievement of 10° of anatomic valgus, avoidance of a flexion contracture, and the incorporation of a patellofemoral decompressive procedure in patients with preexisting patellofemoral degeneration.

Other closing wedge osteotomy studies show more modest survival rates 10 and 15 years postoperatively. The 10-year survival rates range from 51% to 78%, with an average rate of 64% when the reports from Koshino and coworkers[68] and

---

*See references 1, 17, 28, 39, 49, 53, 57, 68, 88, 128, 130, 139.

TABLE 31–9   Technical Pearls to Avoid Complications for Opening Wedge High Tibial Osteotomy

1. Perform meticulous subperiosteal dissection to protect SMCL, posterior neurovascular structures.
2. Verify osteotomy starting point medial cortex, use anterior and posterior Keith needles to verify tibial slope.
3. Placement of guide pin and osteotomy too proximal can lead to lateral tibial plateau fracture.
4. Maintain approximately 15° pin angulation to medial tibial site, avoid large obliquity to osteotomy.
5. Measurement pitfalls: anterior tibial gap should be half of posteromedial gap. Downsize plate from posteromedial gap measurement because plate is 15–20 mm from posteromedial corner. Verify coronal, sagittal alignment with fluoroscopy or computerized navigation at surgery, 5° knee flexion, medial and lateral tibiofemoral compartments closed and in contact.
6. Secure fixation SMCL repair to avoid valgus instability.
7. Implement immediate knee motion, patellar mobilization, quadriceps function to avoid patella infera.
8. Maintain lateral cortex hinge by leaving 10 mm laterally, gentle distraction opening wedge.
9. Autograft iliac crest bone graft promotes prompt union, early return to function.
10. Allograft bone grafts: expect delay in union, longer period of crutch protection, delayed weight-bearing.
11. Postoperatively maintain close follow-up, prevent swelling, elevate limb, use TED hose, perform hourly ankle pumps, check for DVT, routine ultrasound.

DVT, deep vein thrombosis; SMCL, superficial medial collateral ligament.

Critical Points RESULTS FROM OTHER CLINICAL STUDIES

Survival Rates Endpoints
- Conversion TKA
- Low HSS score
- Patient dissatisfaction

Survival Rates

Closing Wedge Osteotomy
- 15 yr postoperative: 39%–93.2%
- 10 yr postoperative: 51%–96.2%
- No clear association between survival rates and any factor other than alignment achieved postoperatively

Opening Wedge Osteotomy
- 10 yr postoperative: 63%–85% (only two studies)[49,139]
- 5 yr postoperative: 84%–94%

Effectiveness HTO on Pain Relief
- Correlates with length of follow-up
- Two studies reported pain relief with ADL in 80% at 10 yr postoperative[1,119]

Effectiveness of HTO on Relieving Functional Limitations with ADL
- One study reported 94% of 75 knees could walk more than 1 km without pain 15–28 yr postoperative[68]
- One study found that 57% of 62 knees could walk more than 1 hr 6–14 yr postoperative[117]

ADL, activities of daily living; HSS, Hospital for Special Surgery rating system; HTO, high tibial osteotomy; TKA, total knee arthroscopy.

Flecher and colleagues[39] are excluded.[1,17,28,88,128] The investigations of Naudie and associates[88] and Billings and colleagues[17] had the lowest 10-year survival rates of 51% and 53%, respectively. Naudie and associates[88] reported that the probability of survival increased in patients who were younger than 50 years

TABLE 31-10 Survival Rates after High Tibial Osteotomy (HTO)

Reference	Type of Osteotomy	N, Patient Age (range)	Endpoints for Survival Analysis	Survival Rates			Correlations with Survival Rate
				5 Yr Postoperative (%)	10 Yr Postoperative (%)	15 Yr Postoperative (%)	
Flecher et al., 2006[39]	Closing wedge	257 42 yr (15–76 yr)	1. TKA 2. UKA 3. PFA 4. Débridement 5. Tibial tubercle medialization	94.8	92.8	89.7	Age at surgery, body mass index, preoperative Ahlback grade, overcorrection
Huang et al., 2005[53]	Closing wedge	93 57 yr (38–73 yr)	1. TKA 2. Patient dissatisfaction	94.6	87	75.2	Preoperative tibiofemoral alignment (9° varus)
Koshino et al., 2004[68]	Closing wedge	75 59 yr (46–73 yr)	1. TKA or unicompartmental arthroplasty 2. Moderate pain at final follow-up > 15 yr postoperative	97.8	96.2	93.2	None
Sterett & Steadman, 2004[130]	Opening wedge	38 51 yr (34–79 yr)	1. TKA 2. Revision HTO	84	NA	NA	None
Aglietti et al., 2003[1]	Closing wedge	91 58 yr (36–69 yr)	1. TKA 2. HSS score < 70 points	96	78	57	Alignment at healing, muscle strength, male gender
Sprenger & Doersbacher, 2003[128]	Closing wedge	76 69 yr (47–81 yr)	1. TKA 2. HSS score < 70 points 3. Patient dissatisfaction	86	74	56	Alignment at 1 yr postoperative
Weale et al., 2001[139]	Opening wedge	76 54 yr (36–70 yr)	1. TKA 2. Waiting for TKA 3. Postoperative sepsis precluded revision	88.8	63	NA	None
Hernigou & Ma, 2001[49]	Opening wedge	215 61 yr (48–72 yr)	1. TKA	94	85	68	None
Billings et al., 2000[17]	Closing wedge	64 49 yr (23–69 yr)	1. TKA	85	53	NA	None
Naudie et al., 1999[88]	Closing wedge	106 55 yr (16–76 yr)	1. TKA	73	51	39	Body weight, delayed or nonunion, age, preoperative flex
Coventry et al., 1993[28]	Closing wedge	87 63 yr (41–79 yr)	1. TKA 2. Moderate or severe pain in patients who declined TKA	87%	66%	NA	Body weight, alignment at 1 yr postoperative
Insall et al., 1984[57]	Closing wedge	95 60 yr (30–83 yr)	Survival rate not calculated, but 23% revised to TKA				HSS excellent/good results: 2 yr–97% 5 yr–85% 9 yr–37% Alignment did not correlate with results; passage of time determined result

HSS, Hospital for Special Surgery rating system; NA, not available; PFA, patellofemoral arthroplasty; TKA, total knee arthroplasty; UKA, unicompartmental knee arthroplasty.

of age at the time of the HTO and who had preoperative knee flexion greater than 120°. Billings and colleagues[17] failed to find a statistically significant association between survival rates and patient age, amount of valgus correction achieved, or postoperative complications. More recent studies from Sprenger and Doerzbacher[128] and Aglietti and associates[1] reported more favorable results at 10 years postoperative, with survival rates of 74% and 78%, respectively.

Fifteen-year survival rates of closing wedge osteotomy, provided to date by only a few authors, range from 39% to 57%.[1,53,88,128] Aglietti and associates[1] reported that male gender and preoperative quadriceps strength correlated with a long-term survival rate of 57%. Sprenger and Doerzbacher[128] determined that the survivability of HTO (56% at 15 yr) was related to the achievement of 8° to 16° valgus measured 1 year postoperatively. Naudie and associates[88] reported the probability of survival decreased in patients older than 50 years of age or in whom a previous arthroscopic débridement, presence of a lateral tibial thrust, preoperative knee flexion less than 120°, or delayed union or nonunion postoperatively was present. Huang and coworkers[53] identified only preoperative varus malalignment as predictive of survivability of HTO. Knees with 9° or less of varus had a 10-year survival rate of 93%, whereas those with

more than 9° varus had a 10-year survival rate of only 56% using conversion to TKA as the endpoint.

Survival Rates: Opening Wedge Osteotomies

Fewer data are available regarding survival rates after opening wedge osteotomy. Three studies reported 84%,[130] 89%,[139] and 94%[49] survival rates at 5 years postoperatively. At 10 years, survival rates are available only from two investigations: 63% in Weale and colleagues's series of 73 cases[139] and 85% from Hernigou and Ma's series of 203 knees.[49] Weale and colleagues[139] hypothesized that progression of arthritis in the medial compartment correlated with HTO failure. Hernigou and Ma[49] did not comment on factors that could have affected the survival rates in their investigation. These authors provided the only 15-year survival rate published at the time of writing of opening wedge osteotomy of 68%.

The ability of HTO to alleviate pain has been demonstrated in many studies[1,67,72,114,117,119]; however, the longevity of pain relief correlates with the length of follow-up achieved postoperatively (Table 31–11). Unfortunately, several investigators did

TABLE 31–11   Subjective Results of Isolated HTO

Reference	Type of HTO	Population Data	Pain	Activities of Daily Living	Sports Activities	Patients Satisfied with Results (%)
Sterett & Steadman, 2004[130]	Opening wedge	N = 38 F/U 24–62 mo Mean age 51 yr (range, 34–79 yr)	NA	Lysholm Preoperative mean 43.5 F/U mean 78 WOMAC Preoperative mean 45.8 F/U mean 16.2	Tegner F/U mean 5.0	NA
Amendola et al., 2004[3]	Opening wedge	N = 74 F/U 10–33 mo Mean age 41 yr (range, 14–74 yr)	NA	NA	NA	90
Koshino et al., 2004[68]	Closing wedge	N = 75 F/U 15–28 yr Mean age 60 yr (range, 46–73 yr)	NA	F/U 94% walk > 1 km HSS overall rating Excellent 65%, Good 25% Fair 9% American Knee Society Preoperative mean 37 F/U mean 87	NA	NA
Aglietti et al., 2003[1]	Closing wedge	N = 91 F/U 10–21 yr Mean age 58 yr (range, 36–69 yr)	F/U 79% no or only mild pain	HSS overall score (N = 61) Excellent 31% Good 16% Fair 14% Poor 39% Unlimited walking ability in 43%	NA	NA
Pfahler et al., 2003[117]	Closing wedge	N = 62 F/U 6–14 yr Mean age 54 yr (range, 20–67 yr)	Visual analog Preoperative mean 6.5 F/U mean 3	F/U 57% walk > 1 hr HSS score Preoperative mean 60 F/U mean 87	NA	90
Koshino et al., 2003[67]	Opening wedge	N = 21 F/U 38–114 mo Mean age 66 yr (range, 55–79)	All had relief of pain American Knee Society Preoperative mean 22.9 F/U mean 47.4	89% unlimited walking distance postoperative American Knee Society walking score Preoperative mean 19 F/U mean 46.7 Total function Preoperative mean 48.1 F/U mean 93.1	NA	NA

TABLE 31–11 Subjective Results of Isolated HTO—Cont'd

Reference	Type of HTO	Population Data	Pain	Activities of Daily Living	Sports Activities	Patients Satisfied with Results (%)
Marti et al., 2001[78]	Opening wedge	N = 36 F/U 5–21 yr Mean age 43 yr (range, 17–76)	NA	HSS score Preoperative mean 61.6 F/U mean 95.8 Lysholm F/U. Excellent 26% Good 62% Fair/poor 12%	NA	NA
Billings et al., 2000[17]	Closing wedge	N = 64 F/U 5–13 yr Mean age 49 yr (range, 23–69)	NA	HSS Preoperative mean 71 F/U mean 94	NA	NA
Magyar et al., 1999[72]	Opening wedge	N = 25 F/U 2 yr Mean age 55 yr (range, 36–68 yr)	Visual analog Mean 0 points at 6 wk postoperative	HSS Preoperative mean 69 F/U mean 94	NA	NA
Rinonapoli et al., 1998[119]	Closing wedge	N = 102 F/U 10–21 yr Mean age 61 yr (range, 39–77 yr)	F/U 55% none at rest or on walking	HSS Preoperative mean 55 F/U mean 70 Unlimited walking at F/U 25%	NA	NA
Nagel et al., 1996[86a]	Closing wedge	N = 34 men F/U 2–14 yr Mean age 49 yr (range, 28–60 yr)	Mild 26% Moderate 6%	79% stand 4 hr or more 91% walk at least 1 mile	59% playing sports Tegner: Preoperative mean 6.5 Postoperative mean 5.9	82
Pace et al., 1994[114]	Opening wedge	N = 15 F/U mean 34 mo Age < 50 yr	HSS Pain Preoperative mean 21 F/U mean 37	HSS overall score Preoperative mean 70 F/U mean 93	NA	NA

F/U, follow-up; HSS, Hospital for Special Surgery; HTO, high tibial osteotomy; NA, not available; WOMAC, Western Ontario and McMaster Universities Osteoarthritis Index.

not separately assess pain when determining clinical outcome but provided only final rating scores from knee rating systems such as the Lysholm, HSS, Western Ontario and McMaster Universities Osteoarthritis Index (WOMAC), and the American Knee Society.[3,17,67,78,129,130]

Aglietti and associates[1] followed 61 patients clinically from 10 to 21 years postoperative and reported that 79% had no or only mild knee pain. In a small series of 18 patients, Koshino and colleagues[67] reported that all had relief of pain on follow-up evaluations ranging from 38 to 114 months postoperatively. Only 9 patients had more than 7 years of follow-up in that investigation. Rinonapoli and coworkers[119] followed 60 knees from 10 to 21 years postoperative and reported that pain at rest was absent in 55%, mild in 18%, moderate in 22%, and severe in 5%. Pain on walking was absent or mild in 55%, moderate in 27%, and severe in 18%.

Satisfactory pain relief has been reported in most studies involving patients who had an HTO and ACL reconstruction either concomitant or staged (Table 31–12). Williams and associates[141] followed 25 ACL-deficient varus-angulated knees from 24 to 106 months postoperatively. Thirteen of these knees were treated with a combined HTO and ACL reconstruction, and 12 had an HTO alone. At follow-up, 84% had no pain with vigorous activity. Dejour and coworkers[31] performed a combined HTO and ACL patellar tendon autograft reconstruction in 44 knees. At follow-up, which ranged from 1 to 11 years postoperatively, 66% had no pain or pain only after vigorous activity.

Functional limitations with daily activities such as walking and stair climbing are typically reported in the majority of patients before HTO. In addition, few patients are able to participate in even light sports activities without experiencing noteworthy symptoms. After surgery, the ability to walk an unlimited distance or more than 1 km is an important measure of daily function. Koshino and coworkers[68] reported that 94% of 75 knees could walk more than 1 km without pain at 15 to 28 years postoperative after a closing wedge HTO. A more modest finding was reported by Pfahler and associates,[117] who found that 57% of 62 knees followed 6 to 14 years postoperatively could walk for more than 1 hour.

Koshino and colleagues[67] described a small series of 21 patients who received an opening wedge osteotomy followed 38 to 114 months postoperatively. At the most recent follow-up examination, 89% reported the ability to walk an unlimited distance without limitations. The American Knee Society walking score improved from a preoperative mean of 19 ± 5.4 points to 46.7 ± 7.3 points at follow-up ($P < .0001$). However, a long-term investigation of closing wedge osteotomy from Rinonapoli and coworkers[119] found that only 25% of 102 knees had unlimited walking ability 10 to 21 years postoperatively.

Few authors have reported on the sports activities resumed after HTO; the majority of reports in which these data are provided involve combined HTO and ACL reconstruction (see Table 31–12).

TABLE 31–12　Subjective Results of HTO and ACL Reconstruction

Reference	Type of Osteotomy (N, ACL Reconstruction	Population Data	Pain	ACL	Sports Activities	Patients Satisfied with Results
Bonin et al, 2004[17a]	Closing wedge (25) Opening wedge (5) PT autograft with HTO in all	N = 30 F/U 6–16 yr Mean age 30 yr (range, 18–41 yr)	NA	IKDC subjective F/U mean 78.5	F/U 47% Intense 36% Light	NA
Williams et al, 2003[141]	Closing wedge ACL reconstructed with HTO (13): PT autograft (2) STG autograft (2) PT allograft (9) ACL untreated (12)	N = 25 F/U 24–106 mo Mean age 35 yr	F/U 84% no pain with vigorous activity	HSS overall rating Preoperative mean 81 F/U mean 97 Lysholm Preoperative mean 47 F/U mean 81	F/U 16% strenuous 76% recreational	76% very 16% reasonably
Noyes et al, 2000[100]	Closing wedge ACL reconstructed with HTO (4), before the HTO (34): PT allograft (21) PT autograft (20) PL procedures done in 18 triple varus knees.	N = 41 23 double varus, 18 triple varus F/U 2–12 yr Mean age 29 yr (range, 16–47 yr)	F/U 71% improved pain scores 76% no pain light sports, 7% no pain with ADL, 17% pain with ADL	F/U 93% no problems with walking, 88% no problems with squatting	F/U 66% light sports with no problems	37% rated knee very good, 34% good, 29% fair/poor
Latterman & Jakob, 1996[69]	Closing wedge (17) Opening wedge (10) ACL PT autograft with HTO (8), ACL PT autograft after HTO (8), ACL tear untreated (11)	N = 27 F/U 1.5–11 yr Mean age 37 yr (range, 24–56 yr)	F/U 30% pain at rest 70% pain with moderate sports	NA	NA	93%
Stutz et al, 1996[133]	Closing wedge ACL PT with HTO (14) ACL PT/LAD with HTO (13)	N = 27 F/U 39–166 mo Mean age 36 yr (range, 15–55)	IKDC symptom rating F/U A, B: 52% C, D: 48%	IKDC subjective rating F/U A, B: 67% C, D: 33%	F/U 2 strenuous 7 moderate 9 light	NA
Dejour et al, 1994[30,31]	Closing wedge ACL PT autograft with HTO in all	N = 44 F/U 1–11 yr Mean age 29 yr (range, 18–42 yr)	F/U 12 no pain 17 pain only after vigorous activity	NA	F/U 2% strenuous 60% recreational	50% very satisfied 41% satisfied
Noyes et al, 1993[93]	Closing wedge ACL EA with HTO (14), ACL PT allograft reconstruction after HTO (16), ACL tear untreated (11)	N = 41 F/U 23–86 mo Mean age 32 yr (range, 16–47 yr)	F/U 78% no pain with sports, 12% no pain with ADL, 10% pain with ADL	F/U 93% no problems with walking, 90% no problems with stairs	F/U 59% light sports with no symptoms	88%

ACL, anterior cruciate ligament; ADL, activities of daily living; EA, extra-articular; F/U, follow-up; HSS, Hospital for Special Surgery; HTO, high tibial osteotomy; IKDC, International Knee Documentations Committee; LAD, ligament augmentation device; NA, not available; PL, poster-lateral; PT, patellar tendon; STG, semitendinosus-gracilis.

PREVENTION AND MANAGEMENT OF COMPLICATIONS

Bony Instability, "Teeter Effect"

Kettlekamp and colleagues[65] described the teeter effect in 1975 as a contraindication to proximal tibial osteotomy. Excessive bone loss and concavity on the medial tibial plateau prohibits simultaneous weight-bearing on both plateaus after HTO and results in an unstable knee in the coronal plane. A teeter effect occurs because tibiofemoral contact shifts, or teeters, from one plateau to the other depending on the relationship of the center of gravity to the center of the knee.

Osteotomy is contraindicated when bone loss makes simultaneous contact of both plateaus impossible. Preoperative radiographic evaluation of the bone loss on the tibial plateaus should be performed, specifically evaluating the slope of the plateaus to determine whether loading of both compartments will occur after HTO.

It has been suggested, but not experimentally confirmed, that if the combined cartilaginous and bony loss on the medial side is greater than 1 cm, it would be impossible to achieve loading of both the compartments after HTO. During surgery, the WBL should be evaluated under image intensification with both compartments loaded to confirm that simultaneous medial and lateral tibiofemoral contact is present.

Inadequate or Loss of Axial Correction

Inadequate or overcorrection of lower limb alignment has been reported after HTO by many authors. In the series reported by Matthews and coworkers,[80] 7 of 40 patients (18%) had a partial or complete recurrence of varus deformity up to 14 years postoperatively. Hernigou and associates[50] reported that persistent varus occurred in 10 of 93 knees immediately after closing wedge osteotomy. In that investigation, 71 of 76 knees showed some degree of recurrent varus deformity 10 to 13 years postoperatively. Magyar and colleagues[73] described a loss of correction after closing wedge osteotomy, with 9 of 16 knees collapsing into valgus by 1 year postoperatively despite normal alignment achieved immediately postoperatively.

Marti and coworkers[77] followed 32 knees that had an opening wedge osteotomy with bone grafting. At follow-up, 24 to 62 months postoperative, 31% demonstrated a recurrence of the varus deformity and 19% were in excessive valgus. Stuart and associates[132] evaluated standing tibiofemoral angles, which decreased from a mean of 9.3° of varus to 7.8° of valgus at final follow-up. Using the Kaplan-Meier survival analysis method, the authors predicted that varus alignment was likely to occur in 18% of knees, lateral compartment arthritis was likely to progress in 60%, and medial and lateral compartment arthritis was likely to progress in 83% by 9 years after surgery.

In a biomechanical study, Stoffel and coworkers[131] showed that an intact lateral tibial hinge cortex largely determined the stability after opening wedge HTO. When the lateral cortex was disrupted, a locking plate and screw design showed superior stability in both compression and torsion compared with the Puddu plate.

Loss of the axial alignment obtained at the time of surgery may be attributed to several factors. These include lack of internal fixation or the use of inadequate internal fixation with collapse of the distal fragments settling into the cancellous bone

---

Critical Points PREVENTION AND MANAGEMENT OF COMPLICATIONS

Bony Instability, Teeter Effect
- Preoperative radiographs determine bone loss, slope.
- Intraoperatively, use fluoroscopy with both compartments loaded to confirm simultaneous medial and lateral tibiofemoral contact.

Inadequate or Loss of Axial Correction
- Caused by inadequate internal fixation, progressive loss of articular cartilage medial compartment, stretching or deficiency of posterolateral soft tissues.
- Preoperative: correct calculation mechanical axis and weight-bearing line.
- Intraoperative: confirm adequate correction with fluoroscopy, computerized navigation.

Delayed Union or Nonunion

Closing Wedge
- Perform osteotomy proximal to tibial tubercle to increase amount of cancellous bone surface contact.

Opening Wedge
- Use autogenous iliac crest bone graft, locking plate, and screw fixation.
- Have various plate designs available at surgery.
- Toe-touch weight-bearing 4 wk.

Tibial Plateau Fracture
- Ensure proximal lateral tibial plateau width ≥ 20 mm.
- Avoid forceful closure of osteotomy.

Arterial Injury
- Recognize anterior tibial artery, popliteal artery at risk during surgical dissection owing to anatomic position.
- Flex the knee, gently retract popliteal structures.

Peroneal Nerve Injury, Palsy
- Caused by cast or bandage applied too tightly after surgery, double padding over peroneal nerve.
- Use internal fixation to avoid cast.
- Avoid injury to nerve during surgery.
- Avoid dome osteotomy below the tibial tubercle.

Arthrofibrosis, Patella Infera

Detection
- Bilateral lateral radiographs preoperatively and postoperatively to measure patellar vertical height.
- Inability of patient to perform strong quadriceps contraction.
- Decreased patellar mobility and tension in patellar tendon.
- Distal malposition of involved patella compared with opposite side.

Minimize Risk
- Immediate rehabilitation: straight leg raises, isometrics, electrical muscle stimulation, patellar mobilization.
- Early recognition and treatment of limitation of knee motion.

Iliac Crest Harvest Site Pain
- Limit dissection to only 10 mm of superior iliac crest.
- Meticulous subperiosteal exposure of outer iliac crest.
- Do not violate muscle plane or inner iliac cortex.
- Keep muscle attachments intact.

of the plateau. Late drifting into a varus position may be due to a progressive loss of the medial osteochondral cartilage complex or to stretching of the posterolateral structures. Coventry[26] reported no loss of surgical correction obtained immediately postoperatively. He attributed the success of the procedure to stability of the closing wedge, the hinge effect of the medial periosteum and cortex, internal fixation, and avoidance of a shift of the fragments.

Careful preoperative planning is required to avoid inadequate correction, which begins with the calculation of the mechanical or anatomic axis using full-length, standing radiographs. Stress radiographs may be used to evaluate medial osteocartilagenous complex loss and lateral joint opening.[35] Calculations to determine the amount of bone to be resected should be performed well before the osteotomy.

During surgery, confirmation of adequate correction that was determined by preoperative measurements is done using fluoroscopy. The knee will be placed in an overall excessive valgus position if the amount of lateral opening is not evaluated and if too much bone is resected. Even though an ideal position may be verified at surgery, a change in alignment may be detected when postoperative standing radiographs are obtained. The alignment should be verified by the 4th postoperative week under partial weight-bearing conditions.

Delayed Union or Nonunion

Delayed union or nonunion has been reported after HTO. In the series described by Jackson and Waugh,[59] 19 of 226 (8%) patients had a delayed union; 14 of these were immobilized for more than 12 weeks before union was achieved, and the remaining 5 required bone grafting.

Warden and colleagues[138] reported a low incidence of delayed union (6.6%) and nonunion (1.8%) in 188 opening wedge osteotomies in which an iliac crest bone autograft was used in the majority of knees. There was a trend toward an increased incidence of delayed union or nonunion when a coral wedge was used either alone or in conjunction with the autogenous graft (15%; 5 of 33 knees) compared with when an iliac crest graft was used alone (6%; 8 of 128 knees). No problems with union were reported by Marti and associates,[78] Pace and coworkers,[114] or Patond and Lokhande[115] after opening wedge osteotomy and iliac crest bone autograft procedures. Lobenhoffer and Agneskirchner[71] found that 6% of 101 knees that had an opening wedge HTO with a variety of bone graft substitutes and fixation with an Arthrex plate progressed to a nonunion.

The incidence of healing problems can be reduced drastically by following several technical suggestions for closing wedge osteotomies. First, the osteotomy should be performed proximal to the tibial tubercle because this will increase the amount of cancellous bone surface contact, which will enhance healing and inherent stability. The two surfaces should be cut in a manner that maximizes the amount of surface area that will be in opposition. In opening wedge osteotomies, a stable construct created by the use of an iliac crest autogenous bone graft (in the anterior, middle, and posterior portions of the osteotomy) and appropriate plate fixation with protection of the lateral tibial buttress (cortex) will sustain postoperative compressive and torsional loads. The argument may be made that autogenous bone grafting is required only for large osteotomies or that allograft or synthetic bone substitutes can take the place of an autograft

with no increase in delayed healing or loss of osteotomy correction. In fact, no well-designed clinical studies with a sufficient number of patients have been published to date that provide evidence for such recommendations. Dallari and colleagues[29] showed that the addition of platelet gel or platelet gel combined with bone marrow stromal cells substantially increased the rate of bone healing in a small group of opening wedge osteotomies. In summary, the efficacy of allograft or other bone substitute materials for opening wedge osteotomy has not been adequately determined, even though the introduction of commercially available triangular-shaped corticocancellous allografts (along with rigid plate designs) has led to their increased usage.

Many investigators have demonstrated that external fixators may accomplish adequate union and correction, such as the series reported by Sterett and Steadman[130] in which only 1 of 33 patients had a loss of correction early postoperatively. However, pin tract infections were reported in 45% by these authors, which was similar to the pin tract infection rate reported by Weale and colleagues[139] of 38% (28 of 73 knees) and Magyar and coworkers[74] of 51% (157 of 308 cases).

Plates with different designs should be available during surgery. A locking osteotomy plate and screws with an autogenous bone graft and an intact lateral pillar provides prompt union without loss of correction. Plate designs that incorporate locking screws provide added stability and are necessary in cases of any violation of the lateral tibial cortex to maintain stability under axial compressive or torsional loads. An alternative fixation method for a lateral tibial cortex fracture at osteotomy is to add a lateral two-hole plate through a separate incision; however, angulated locking screws from a medial plate may also be used.

The rehabilitation program allows toe-touch weight-bearing during the first 4 weeks and then allows progression over the next 4 weeks to full weight-bearing based on radiographic signs of osteotomy healing. A delayed union can be treated, if the overall alignment is acceptable, by electrical stimulation.

Tibial Plateau Fracture

The reported prevalence of fracture after closing wedge osteotomy ranges from 1% to 20%.[50,80] This complication appears uncommon after opening wedge osteotomy, although Amendola and associates[3] reported 7 of 37 patients (19%) in their initial series of opening wedge osteotomies had intra-articular fractures that extended into the lateral compartment. The fractures were believed to be caused by a combination of a vertical osteotomy site (closer to the lateral tibial plateau joint line than to the lateral cortex) and use of thick osteotomes. After adjusting the obliquity of the osteotomy and switching to thin, flexible osteotomes, the authors did not experience any more cases of fracture.

Important operative techniques to prevent tibial plateau fracture exist. Fracture of the tibial plateau can be avoided by meticulously following the previously described operative technique. The proximal osteotomy should remain parallel to the joint surface. It is important to keep the proximal tibial portion 20 to 25 mm thick to avoid fracture and to avoid creating a thin medial tibial portion after osteotomy. The cortex on the applicable side of the wedge may be penetrated by multiple drill holes, and forceful closure of the wedge should be avoided. If a tibial plateau fracture does occur, anatomic reduction and internal fixation of the plateau fragments should be performed.

Arterial Injury

Vascular complications are exceedingly rare, with case reports of single episodes of anterior tibial artery injury during surgery. Bauer and colleagues[15] reported on 1 case in 60 in which the anterior tibial artery was severed during the resection of the fibular head. Recognition of the anatomic relationship of the vessels to the surgical dissection is imperative. The anterior tibial artery is at risk because it pierces the proximal interosseous membrane. Injury to this artery may result in an anterior compartment syndrome, which must be recognized and dealt with promptly. The popliteal artery is at risk during posterior dissection and osteotomy of the posterior tibial cortex. By flexing the knee and gently retracting the popliteal structures, the risk of injury to these structures will be significantly reduced.

Peroneal Nerve Injury or Palsy

Jackson and Waugh[59] reported 27 of 226 cases (12%) of partial or complete injury to the peroneal nerve during osteotomy. Because there was a higher incidence of injury during curved osteotomies located below the tibial tuberosity, the authors concluded that osteotomy in this location was too dangerous. A 7% incidence of peroneal nerve injury was reported by Sundaram and coworkers,[134] and a 6% incidence was described by Harris and Kostuik.[47] Slawski and associates[126] reported a 4.3% incidence of peroneal neurapraxias in 225 pediatric tibial osteotomies.

Flierl and colleagues[40] compared the incidence of neurologic complications after opening wedge osteotomy with a technique using a conventional oscillating saw with a technique that created multiple drill holes and osteoclasis. After the conventional method, acute transient peroneal nerve palsy developed in 15.7% of 89 patients, with persistent deficits found in 12.4% 6 months postoperatively. In the osteoclasis group, 14% had acute transient events, and 4.7% reported permanent weakness. Other than the report by Flierl and colleagues,[40] nerve injury after opening wedge HTO appears to be extremely rare.

Peroneal nerve palsy may result from several causes—the most common is a cast or bandage applied too tightly after surgery. The use of internal fixation alleviates the need for casting. The nerve may also be directly injured during surgery.

Osteotomy of the fibula is performed at different sites by different authors depending on the operative technique. A risk of injuring the peroneal nerve exists if the osteotomy is performed in the proximal third of the fibula.[66] In addition, osteotomy in the middle portion of the fibula may injure the peroneal nerve innervation to the extensor hallicus longus. The rate of injury has been reported to be extremely high (25%) after dome osteotomy below the tibial tubercle.[59]

Arthrofibrosis and Patella Infera

Many early HTO studies cited unacceptably high rates of arthrofibrosis and patella infera after postoperative immobilization. Windsor and colleagues[142] reported that 80% of 45 knees had patella infera after closing wedge HTO and postulated that postoperative plaster immobilization allowed the decreased quadriceps muscle forces and shortening of the patellar tendon. Westrich and coworkers[140] demonstrated the beneficial effects of early motion after closing wedge osteotomy: 16 of 34 knees (47%) treated with cast immobilization developed patella infera

compared with 3 of 35 (8%) that received immediate postoperative motion.

A decrease in the patellar height ratio as measured by the Blackburn-Peel ratio is expected after opening wedge osteotomy.[21] Wright and associates[144] reported that all 28 patients in their series of medial opening wedge osteotomies had a decrease in patellar height, but no significant change in patellar ligament length (as measured by the Insall-Salvati ratio[56]). The authors explained that because the osteotomy increased the distance between the tibial tubercle and the tibial articular surface, the patella migrated distally.

Similar findings in decreased patellar height following opening wedge osteotomy have been reported by others.[21,49,87,89,135] Patella infera correlated with the magnitude of angular correction after HTO in two series.[135,144] For example, Wright and associates[144] evaluated patellar height and ligament length in 28 patients and found a relationship between the amount of infera and the degree of angular correction.

Postoperatively, lateral radiographs are taken to detect any decrease in the patellar vertical height ratio; these are repeated often for any patient who shows early signs of developmental patella infera (inability to perform a strong quadriceps contraction after surgery, decreased patellar mobility, decreased palpable tension in the patellar tendon with failure of the patella to displace proximally on quadriceps contraction, or distal malposition of the involved patella compared with the opposite side). Rigid internal fixation should also help to reduce the occurrence of arthrofibrosis and a resultant patella infera.

In the authors' opening wedge osteotomy study, the patellar height was not significantly affected by the magnitude of angular correction owing mostly to the desire not to change the tibial slope and ensuring that the anterior gap at the osteotomy site was less than one half of the posterior gap. In addition, no patient had a limitation in knee motion that required treatment intervention such as manipulation or arthroscopic release of adhesions.

An immediate knee motion program and exercise protocol of straight leg raises, multiangle isometrics, and electrical muscle stimulation are advocated to decrease the incidence of quadriceps weakness and knee motion limitation after HTO. In addition, a phased treatment program is begun for limitations of motion early in the postoperative course when restriction of either extension or flexion is noted.[102] This program is discussed in Chapter 33, Rehabilitation after Tibial and Femoral Osteotomy.

Iliac Crest Harvest Site Pain

Most, if not all, of the complications described in the literature related to iliac crest bone graft harvest may be avoided by the surgical technique described in this chapter. For example, the dissection is limited to include only 10 mm of the superior iliac crest. A meticulous subperiosteal exposure of the outer iliac crest is performed without violating the inner muscle attachments. The inner iliac cortex is never dissected, and the muscle attachments are kept intact. This minimally invasive harvest technique avoids the frequency of complications reported by larger exposures such as those used for spine fusions.

The standard cortical iliac crest graft harvested is 40 mm in length, 12 mm in width, and 30 mm in depth, although larger osteotomies require a longer graft of approximately 45 mm.

The iliac crest harvest procedure may be painful with trunk flexion activities for up to 4 weeks postoperatively, and patients are advised accordingly. Even though there were no complications in the authors' series, added time is required for the operative procedure and a complication is always possible, which must be weighed against the benefits of the rapid healing provided by autogenous bone at the osteotomy site.

Deep Vein Thrombosis

The incidence of deep vein thrombosis (DVT) has not been adequately studied after HTO. Turner and colleagues[136] demonstrated a 41% rate of DVT using venography after HTO in 84 patients; only 15% were clinically diagnosed. Only calf clots were diagnosed clinically; there were 3 proximal and 12 mixed clots diagnosed only with venogram. Leclerc and coworkers[70] performed a randomized, prospective trial comparing LMWH with placebo after 129 HTO. The incidence of DVT was 17% in the LMWH group versus 58% in placebo. Nineteen percent of the placebo group had femoral vein clots compared with none in the treatment group. Thus, it appears that the incidence of DVT after HTO is similar to that in other large reconstructive knee procedures such as TKA.

ILLUSTRATIVE CASES

Case 1 Treatment of Varus Angulation and Severe Articular Cartilage Damage to the Medial Femoral Condyle in a Patient Younger than 20 Years of Age.
A 19-year old male presented with a complaint of pain to the medial aspect of his left knee with activities of daily living. He had a 4-year history of osteochondritis dissecans that had been treated elsewhere with internal fixation of the fragment that failed to heal. A subsequent arthroscopic débridement of the medial femoral condylar fragment was performed. Full-length, standing radiographs revealed a mechanical axis of 5° varus and a WBI of 29% of the tibial width (Fig. 31–46A). All ligamentous structures were intact. Medial tibiofemoral compartment narrowing of 50% was evident on PA 45° weight-bearing radiographs.

HTO was indicated to unload the damaged medial tibiofemoral compartment. The arthroscopic examination showed a 20- x 20-mm area of subchondral bone exposure on the medial femoral condyle (see Fig. 31–46B). A biopsy was obtained for a staged autologous chondrocyte implantation, which was done 5 months later. The full-length, standing radiograph showed correction to 62% WBL (see Fig. 31–46C). At the most recent follow-up evaluation, 3 years postoperative, the patient reported marked improvement in all symptoms with the ability to perform light recreational sports without problems. He rated his overall knee condition as nearly normal. The overall alignment was neutral.

Authors' Comment: There is the expectation that a repeat cartilage restorative procedure will be required in this patient. The importance of measuring the correction obtained at surgery with full-length, standing radiographs and close follow-up of the patient to determine maintenance of the valgus overcorrection is stressed. Future MRI including articular cartilage sequences will be obtained.

Case 2 Treatment Options in a Varus-Angulated, ACL-Deficient, Medial Meniscectomized Knee.
A 33-year old woman presented with moderate to severe medial joint pain and giving-way with daily activities. She had a prior medial meniscectomy 15 years ago and a failed ACL allograft reconstruction 8 years ago. The examination showed a positive pivot shift and 15 mm of increased AP tibial displacement on KT-2000 testing. There was no increase in external tibial rotation, lateral joint opening, or posterior tibial translation. Full-length, standing radiographs revealed a WBL of 20% of the tibial width (Fig. 31–47A) and early narrowing of the medial tibiofemoral compartment.

Arthroscopy demonstrated subchondral bone exposure on the medial femoral condyle and tibial plateau and an absent medial meniscus (see Fig. 31–47B). The lateral tibiofemoral compartment and lateral meniscus were normal. The lateral gap test showed 10 mm of opening under varus loading at 30° of knee flexion.

A closing wedge osteotomy was performed, followed 5 months later with a medial meniscus transplant and osteochondral autograft transfer for the medial femoral condylar defect.

Seven months after the HTO, a revision ACL B-PT-B autograft reconstruction was performed owing to continued instability symptoms. The lateral tibiofemoral compartment gap test was only slightly increased, and therefore, no posterolateral reconstruction was required.

The most recent follow-up examination, 6.7 years after the osteotomy, showed a WBL of 56% (see Fig. 31–47C), no further loss of medial tibiofemoral compartment joint space, and no symptoms with low-impact activities. The patient had negative pivot shift and Lachman tests.

Authors' Comment: In this case, either an opening or a closing wedge osteotomy was indicated. The standing radiograph suggested increased lateral tibiofemoral joint opening (double varus knee), which was confirmed at arthroscopy, contraindicating a concurrent ACL reconstruction. The subsequent ACL revision used a B-PT-B autograft to provide a potentially higher chance of success than that obtained with an allograft (authors' opinion). The vertical femoral tunnel was bypassed with an outside-in reorientation of the femoral tunnel (see Fig. 31–47D and E). A bone graft of prior tunnels was not required. A tibial graft suture and post is always performed in revision knees for added graft fixation strength.

Case 3 Treatment of a Varus-Angulated, PCL-Deficient Knee in a High School–aged Athlete.
A 17-year-old male high school athlete sustained a contact injury during football. A complete PCL rupture was verified by physical examination and arthroscopy performed elsewhere. He was referred to our center 3 months later for treatment. He complained of giving-way sensations with running and cutting activities and mild aching to the medial aspect of his knee with these activities. The preoperative radiographic evaluation demonstrated a WBL of 21% tibial width (Fig. 31–48A) and 10 mm of increased posterior tibial translation (see Fig. 31–48B). All other ligamentous structures were normal on examination. The patient's goal was to play collegiate football and have the "best knee possible."

The patient was treated with an opening wedge osteotomy followed 3 months later with a two-strand QT-PB autogenous

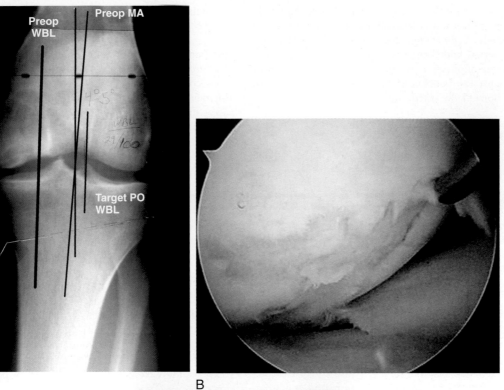

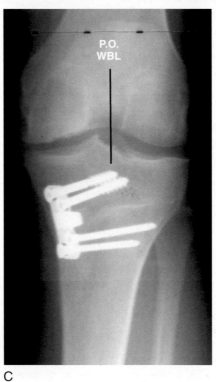

FIGURE 31–46. Case 1.

PCL reconstruction with a tibial inlay approach. All articular cartilage surfaces were normal and both menisci were intact. At 3 years postoperative, the patient had a full range of knee motion and no posterior drawer on physical examination (negative medial tibiofemoral step-off).

Full-length, standing radiographs demonstrated a WBL of 50% (see Fig. 31–48C and D). The posterior stress radiograph showed 3 mm of increased posterior tibial translation (see Fig. 31–48E). He had no symptoms with strenuous athletics and rated the overall condition of his knee as normal.

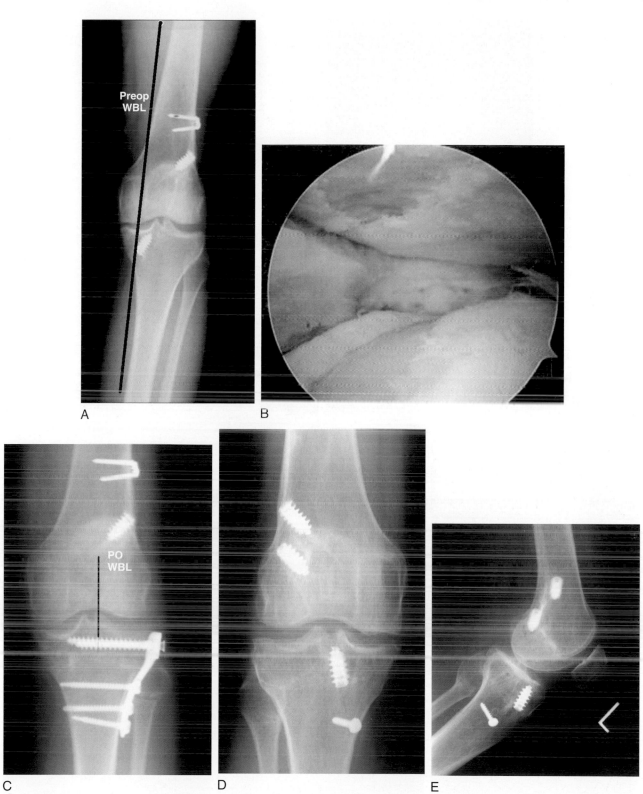

FIGURE 31–47. Case 2.

Authors' Comment: The most controversial aspect of this case was defining the necessity for a corrective osteotomy prior to the PCL reconstruction. Most varus-aligned knees with an intact medial meniscus and ACL or PCL rupture do not require a staged osteotomy. Concurrent medial meniscus loss with early articular cartilage damage would be the usual indication for corrective osteotomy. However, in this knee, the varus angulation (20% WBL) was judged to be so advanced that operative correction was deemed necessary. In addition, early medial tibiofemoral compartment aching symptoms with activity were present. A second option would be to perform the PCL reconstruction and then follow the patient to define the subsequent need for an HTO.

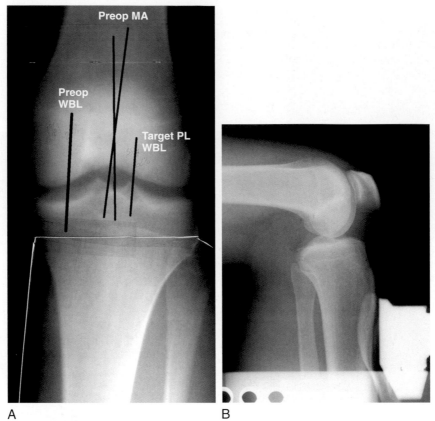

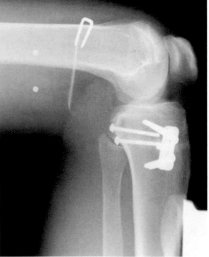

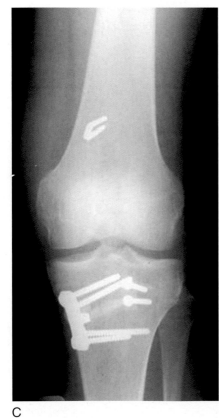

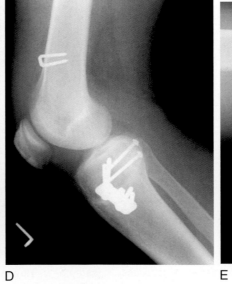

FIGURE 31–48. Case 3.

Case 4 Treatment of Bilateral Varus Malalignment in a Middle-aged Patient.

A 40-year-old woman presented with bilateral varus malalignment and complaints of medial compartment pain with daily activities of many years' duration that had increased in severity over the last 2 years. She expressed a lifelong difficulty with the visual appearance of her lower extremities. Initial evaluation showed an obvious varus malalignment (Fig. 31–49A). Full-length, standing radiographs showed a WBL of 20% (right) and 13% (left) of the lower extremities. All ligaments were intact and no other abnormality was found.

Opening wedge osteotomies with autogenous iliac crest bone grafting were performed 3 months apart (see Fig. 31–49B). The correction was made to a neutral alignment, avoiding an overcorrection. The medial tibiofemoral compartment showed early articular cartilage fibrillation, but no major damage. The postoperative correction is shown in Figure 31–49C.

The most recent evaluation, conducted 4 years postoperative, showed resolution of medial compartment symptoms in both knees. The patient rated both of her knees as normal and stated she was able to wear shorts without feeling embarrassed for the first time.

Authors' Comment: Clinical data on the natural history of severe varus malalignment (WBL <30%) over a patient's lifetime are insufficient. Clinicians have noted the frequent occurrence of medial joint pain in patients in their 40s and 50s, and degenerative medial meniscus tears are common. HTO is not a cosmetically indicated procedure and this patient did have an early onset of medial joint arthritis symptoms, which responded to the corrective procedure.

Case 5 Treatment of Varus-Angulated, ACL-Deficient Knee: Simultaneous Osteotomy and ACL Reconstruction.

A 43-year-old athletically active man presented 9 months after a knee injury sustained while playing basketball. The patient had been diagnosed with an ACL rupture and varus osseous malalignment. He wished to resume sports activities, including basketball and coaching soccer. The patient was referred for surgical management. The initial examination revealed a positive pivot shift, 10 mm of increased AP tibial translation on KT-2000 testing, and a WBL of 18% on full-length, standing radiographs (Fig. 31–50A). All other ligament tests were normal.

The patient elected for a simultaneous opening wedge osteotomy and ACL reconstruction, which was done with a four-strand STG autograft using a two-incision technique. The menisci were intact, and fissuring and fragmentation (classified as 2B damage) were noted in the medial tibiofemoral compartment and on the undersurface of the patella.

Intraoperative fluoroscopy during the osteotomy verified an adequate correction of the varus malalignment. The guide pin was placed to allow maximum width to the lateral plateau to avoid fracture (see Fig. 31–50B). The technique of using thin spreader blades was performed to gradually spread the osteotomy site, which was maintained by a calibrated wedge (see Fig. 31–50C). Placement of the osteotomy plate just prior to iliac crest bone grafting is shown in Figure 31–50D. The HTO healed rapidly with the incorporation of the autogenous bone graft.

At the most recent follow-up, 2.5 years postoperatively, the patient had no symptoms with sports activities. Full-length, standing radiographs demonstrated a WBL of 52% (see Fig. 31–50E),

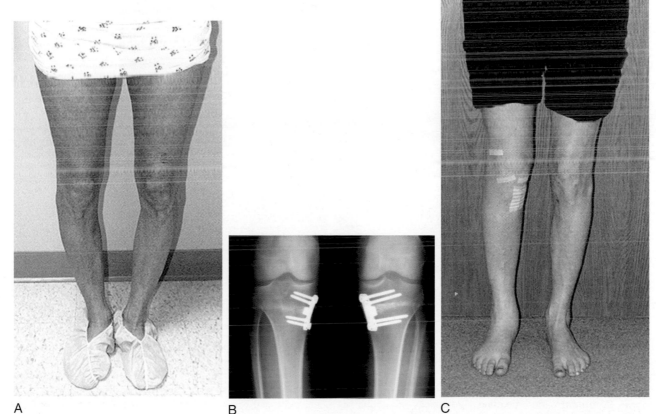

A B C

FIGURE 31–49. Case 4.

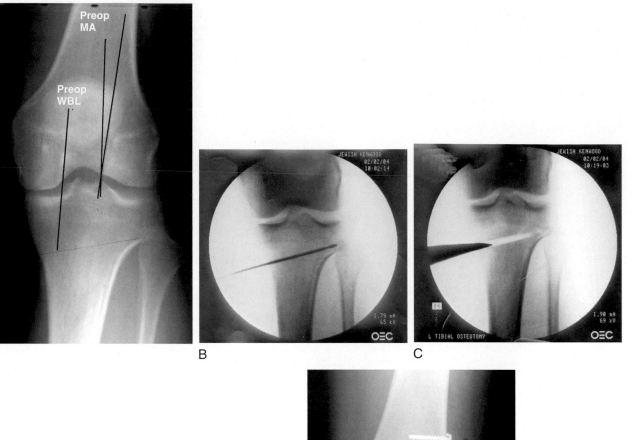

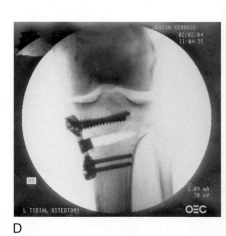

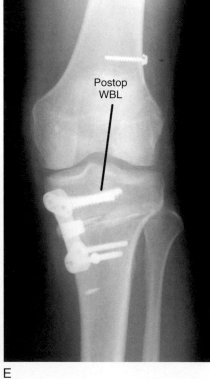

FIGURE 31–50. Case 5.

and KT-2000 examination revealed 4 mm of increased AP tibial translation (25° of flexion, 134 N). He rated the overall condition of his knee as very good.

Authors' Comment: The operative fluoroscopy photographs show proper placement of the guide pin and distraction of the opening wedge, which was done gradually to preserve the lateral

tibial cortex. Loss of the lateral tibial cortical buttress produces an unstable osteotomy that requires additional fixation such as a locking plate. The four-strand STG graft was anatomically placed at insertion sites using an outside-in technique to achieve a coronal graft with maximum femoral and tibial tunnel lengths. The STG graft fixation was achieved using both a suture post and absorbable interference screws.

Case 6 Treatment of Excessive Valgus Lower Limb Malalignment after Closing Wedge Osteotomy.

A 26-year-old woman presented 9 months after a left lateral closing HTO performed for medial joint line pain and early medial tibiofemoral damage. The patient was unable to participate in any athletic activities, had developed hip pain over the past 3 to 4 months, and complained of increasing diffuse knee pain located primarily in the lateral aspect of the knee during standing and walking. She was aware of the abnormal lower limb alignment and highly concerned with the cosmetic appearance (Fig. 31–51A).

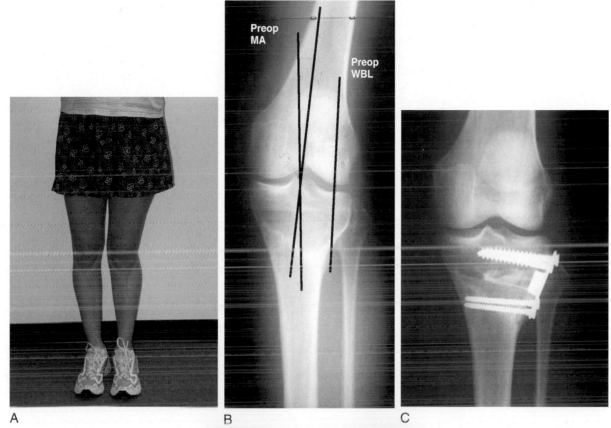

A

B

C

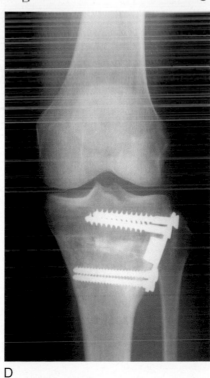

D

FIGURE 31–51. Case 6.

On physical examination, the patient ambulated with a marked valgus angulation and valgus thrust. The lower extremity neurovascular examination was normal, and the range of knee motion was 0° to 155°. There was pain on palpation over the lateral joint line. There was no increase in anterior or posterior tibial translation. The patient had 15° of increased external tibial rotation at 30° of flexion, but only 5° of increased external tibial rotation at 90° of flexion. Varus stress radiographs showed 10 mm of increased lateral joint opening. Full-length, standing radiographs revealed a healed lateral closing wedge HTO. The coronal joint line was sloped laterally and the WBL was 80% (see Fig. 31–51B).

Two major problems were identified in this patient. First, a valgus overcorrection was noted, which occurs when the WBL is greater than 70% of the tibial width. A WBL of 62% normally represents an approximate 2° to 3° overcorrection. The overcorrection of the HTO in this patient was 6° mechanical axis (80% WBL), which resulted in a cosmetically unacceptable appearance. This amount of overcorrection frequently results in arthritis of the lateral tibiofemoral compartment. To avoid this error, the degrees of correction of the WBL must be measured on full-length, standing double-stance radiographs as described in this chapter. Single-stance radiographs allow abnormal lateral joint opening to occur, which must then be subtracted in the calculation for the true degrees of tibial correction required. In addition, the lower limb alignment must be verified at surgery and early postoperatively.

If an abnormal valgus alignment is detected, it can be easily corrected within the first 4 weeks postoperatively by readjusting the osteotomy gap. In this patient, osseous healing had already occurred and the revision procedure was therefore more difficult.

The second problem was that a fibular osteotomy (at either the fibular neck or the distal one third region) had not been performed. The proximal tibiofibular joint was disrupted, which allowed the fibula to slide proximally. The abnormal fibular position produced laxity of the FCL and other posterolateral structures that attached to the proximal fibula. The operative plan was to restore the normal tibiofibular relationship to retension the posterolateral structures. The patient was warned that if the tibiofibular joint was destroyed, a tibiofibular fusion would be required, placing the fibula into a normal tibial relationship to restore the proper length-tension relationship of the native or reconstructed posterolateral structures.

The patient was treated with a revision opening wedge osteotomy. At surgery, the proximal tibiofibular joint and attached ligaments were carefully dissected after the common peroneal nerve was identified and protected. An opening wedge osteotomy was performed, preserving the medial tibial buttress. Careful distraction of the osteotomy with spacer plates that spanned the length of the osteotomy was performed to prevent fracture of the tibial plateau, which was osteopenic from the prior surgery. The fibula was gradually relocated to a normal position relative to the tibia. In other revision cases, the author has used two proximal tibiofibular 4.0 cancellous screws to provide temporary stabilization of the joint; however, this was not required. An autogenous iliac crest bone graft was used and healing successfully occurred.

Immediately postoperative, radiographs demonstrated correction of the abnormal valgus alignment and a normal tibiofibular position (see Fig. 31–51C). The position was maintained at the most recent evaluation, 16 months postoperative (see Fig. 31–51D). There was no increase in lateral joint opening or external tibial rotation with functional posterolateral ligament structures.

Case 7 Treatment of Failed Internal Fixation after Opening Wedge Osteotomy.

A 41-year-old man presented complaining of pain to the medial aspect of his right knee joint. He had previously undergone a partial medial meniscectomy, chondroplasty, and microfracture of the medial femoral condyle. The patient was employed as an automobile mechanic and had discomfort with squatting and kneeling.

On physical examination, the patient had an obvious varus malalignment and walked with a mild varus thrust. He had mild lateral joint line pain, moderate patellofemoral crepitus, and moderate patellar pain on compression. The ligament examination was normal. Radiographs demonstrated a WBL of 20% (Fig. 31–52A) and preserved medial tibiofemoral joint space. MRI revealed a posterior horn medial meniscus tear and articular cartilage damage to the trochlea.

The patient underwent an opening wedge osteotomy with autogenous iliac crest bone graft and internal fixation with a Puddu plate. A 62% WBL was confirmed intraoperatively.

The initial postoperative course was normal with initial radiographs showing correction of the malalignment. However, at 5 months postoperative, the patient complained of a new onset of pain in the region of the anteromedial tibial osteotomy. Radiographs demonstrated nonunion of the osteotomy site and two broken distal screws with loss of the valgus alignment correction (see Fig. 31–52B and C). The patient underwent a revision osteotomy with a locking plate (see Fig. 31–52D and E), which successfully corrected the malalignment. The tibial slope was maintained and the mechanical axis postoperatively was 2° valgus. The osteotomy healed without problems.

Authors' Comment: This case demonstrates the potential inherent weakness of the Puddu plate. If there is any delay in healing after opening wedge osteotomy, even with autogenous bone grafting, early failure can be expected and revision indicated. A locking plate, which became available during the treatment of this patient, provides a more stable construct and is now preferred by the authors.

Case 8 Treatment of a Varus-Angulated Knee after Failed Multiple Ligament Procedures.

A 27-year-old man presented after a knee dislocation from an industrial accident, which had been treated with an ACL STG reconstruction and MCL primary repair. The patient complained of medial tibiofemoral compartment pain and instability with daily activities.

On physical examination, the patient demonstrated varus malalignment and a varus thrust on ambulation. There was a mild effusion and a normal range of motion. A positive pivot shift was elicited, indicating failure of the ACL reconstruction. In addition, an increase of 8 mm in lateral tibiofemoral opening was noted. Radiographs revealed a WBL of 20% and mild medial tibiofemoral joint space narrowing (Fig. 31–53A). Posterior stress radiographs demonstrated 7 mm of increased posterior tibial translation compared with the contralateral limb, indicating partial PCL deficiency.

The patient was treated with an opening wedge osteotomy with an autogenous iliac crest bone graft and a locking plate for secure fixation; fluoroscopy confirmed correction of the WBL at 62% (see Fig. 31–53B–D). Six months later, a revision ACL reconstruction was performed using the contralateral patellar tendon autograft. The lateral tibiofemoral gap at surgery was 5 mm, and therefore, no posterolateral reconstruction was required.

Authors' Comment: With large angular corrections, the authors prefer to stage osteotomy and ACL revision reconstructive

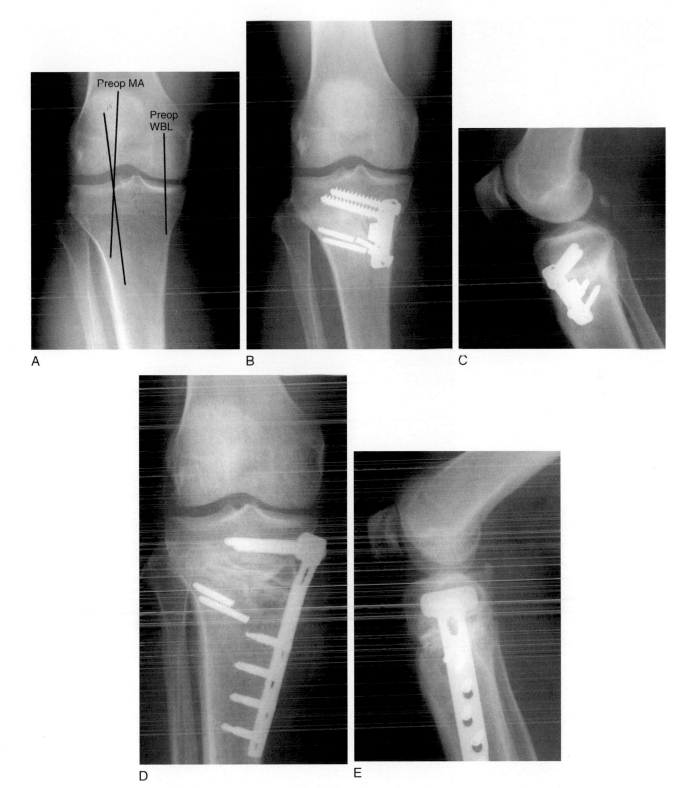

FIGURE 31-52. Case 7.

procedures. Staging the procedures ensures that the osteotomy correction will be maintained postoperatively and reduces the risk of complications, especially arthrofibrosis. In addition, adaptive shortening of the FCL and posterolateral structures occurred, avoiding a posterolateral reconstructive procedure.

Case 9 Treatment of Severe Bilateral Varus Malalignment. A 44-year-old male teacher presented with complaints of bilateral medial compartment pain of 16 months' duration. He had pain at rest, with walking tolerance of only 1 minute. He had undergone multiple cortisone injections of both

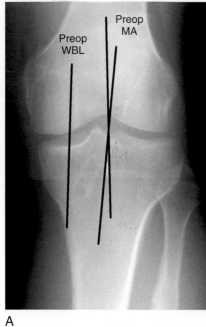

A

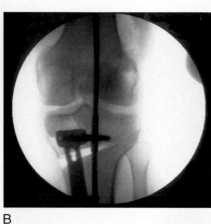

B

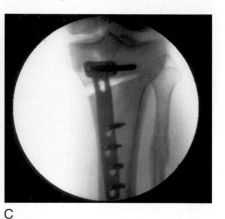

C

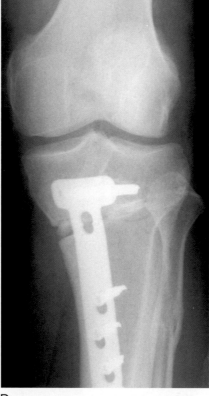

D

FIGURE 31–53. Case 8.

knees and had also tried an unloading brace on the left knee, which made the pain worse. Physical examination revealed a full range of motion in both knees, severe bilateral medial joint line pain, no patellofemoral symptoms, intact ligaments, and a bilateral varus thrust on ambulation. Radiographs demonstrated severe medial tibiofemoral compartment narrowing in both the right (Fig. 31–54A) and the left (see Fig. 31–54B) knees. Marked varus malalignment was present bilaterally.

Although another surgeon recommended HTO, the patient was advised that the loss of joint space was too severe for an HTO to be effective. The patient underwent bilateral unicompartmental knee replacement, first in the left knee (see Fig. 31–54C)

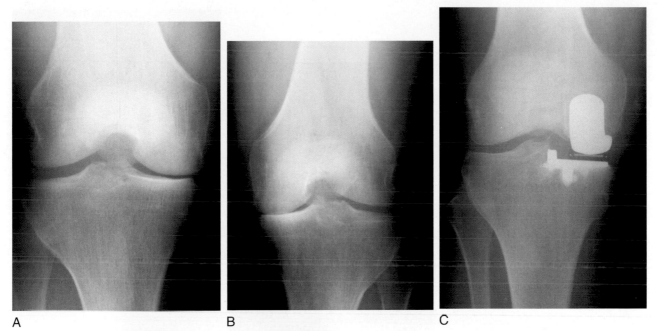

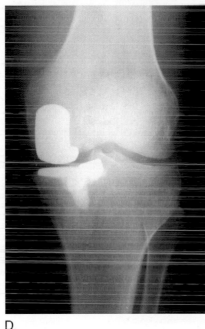

FIGURE 31–54. Case 9.

and then 3 months later in the right knee (see Fig. 31–54D). The patient recovered uneventfully from both procedures.

Case 10 Treatment of a Valgus-Angulated Knee after Lateral Meniscus Transplantation.
An elite female gymnast initially presented to the authors' center at age 16 with complaints of aching pain in the posterior and lateral aspect of her left knee. She denied any specific episode of trauma. Arthroscopy and partial lateral meniscectomy were performed. The patient continued with high-level training for Olympic gymnastics competition, and subsequently, her symptoms of pain and swelling became worse, requiring repeat arthroscopy. Grade III changes were noted on the weight-bearing surface of the lateral femoral condyle (Fig. 31–55A).

Two years later, physical examination demonstrated a mild increase in the valgus alignment (58%). Standing radiographs, at 30° of knee flexion, demonstrated narrowing of approximately 50% joint width. The patient had tenderness to the lateral tibiofemoral compartment and mild swelling in the joint. She elected to have a lateral meniscus transplant and osteochondral autograft transfer procedure.

The patient did well for 7 years after the lateral meniscus transplant and osteochondral plug procedure. She returned with chief complaints of pain, catching, and swelling in the knee. Over the course of treatment, it had been noted that the patient had a progression of symptoms in the lateral compartment as well as an increase in valgus malalignment. Physical examination revealed obvious valgus alignment present of the left lower

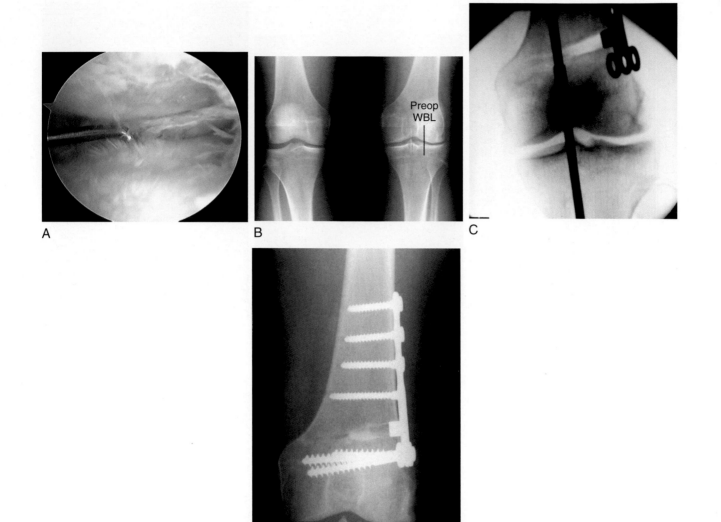

FIGURE 31–55. Case 10.

extremity, full range of motion, no joint effusion, no ligamentous instability, and no crepitus to the lateral compartment. Standing 45° PA radiographs demonstrated 50% narrowing of the lateral compartment. Full-length, standing radiographs demonstrated a 5° valgus mechanical axis and a 65% WBL (see Fig. 31–55B).

The patient underwent an opening wedge femoral osteotomy with an autogenous iliac crest graft (see Fig. 31–55C), which obtained a correction to a 45% WBL. Postoperative radiographs show the correction of the valgus alignment and healing of the osteotomy site (see Fig. 31–55D).

Case 11 Treatment of Valgus Malalignment in a Young Patient with Pain with Activities of Daily Living.

A 20-year-old female presented with a chief complaint of lateral knee pain with activities of daily living and anterior knee pain when ascending stairs. She had a total lateral meniscectomy 5 years previously. Prior arthroscopy demonstrated moderate articular cartilage damage to the lateral tibiofemoral joint. She had given up running and squatting activities as a result of the pain in her knee.

Physical examination demonstrated a mild effusion, a standing valgus position of the lower extremity, and a valgus thrust on walking. The patient had normal ligamentous stability. Standing 45° PA radiographs demonstrated 50% joint narrowing. Full-length, standing views showed a WBL of 71% and a mechanical axis of 4° valgus (Fig. 31–56A).

The patient underwent an opening wedge femoral osteotomy for correction of the valgus malalignment. A locking plate with screws was used with an iliac crest autogenous bone graft (see Fig. 31–56B). Postoperative radiographs show a correction to 45% WBL (see Fig. 31–56C and D).

Case 12 Revision Opening Wedge Femoral Osteotomy.

A 33-year-old woman presented to the authors' center with a chief complaint of pain to the lateral aspect of the knee joint. She had undergone a lateral meniscectomy 15 years previously and had noted increasing joint pain over the past 2 years.

Full-length, standing radiographs demonstrated a valgus malalignment to the left leg (Fig. 31–57A). Standing 45° PA radiographs revealed 50% narrowing of the lateral tibiofemoral compartment. The recommendation was an opening wedge femoral osteotomy with autogenous bone grafting, followed by a staged meniscus transplant.

The patient underwent an opening wedge femoral osteotomy with allograft bone at another center that was closer to her home. In addition, the patient had a staged lateral meniscus transplantation that failed within a few months postoperatively.

The patient returned to our center 7 months after the opening wedge femoral osteotomy and lateral meniscus transplant with pain and delayed union of the osteotomy site (see Fig. 31–57B). Physical examination confirmed lateral joint line tenderness and varus malalignment of the lower extremity without ligament deficiency. A revision opening wedge femoral osteotomy was performed (see Fig. 31–57C) using an autogenous bone graft, which obtained correction to a 45% WBL.

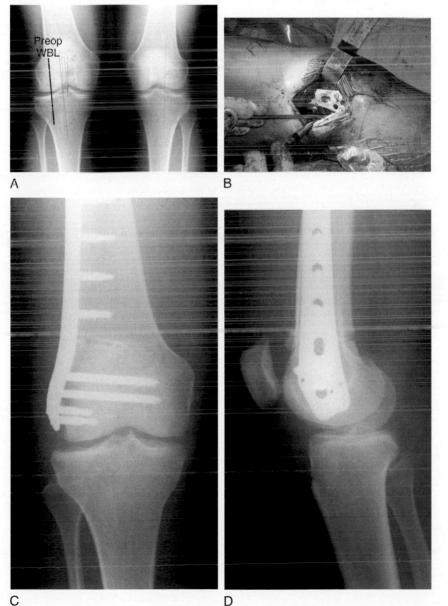

FIGURE 31–56. Case 11.

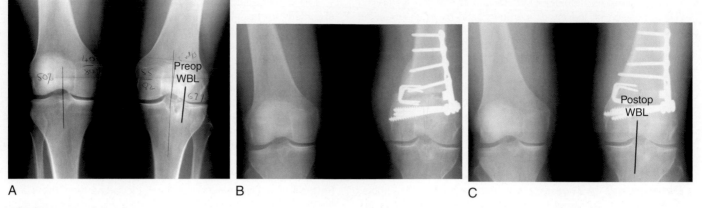

FIGURE 31–57. Case 12.

REFERENCES

1. Aglietti, P.; Buzzi, R.; Vena, L. M.; et al.: High tibial osteotomy for medial gonarthrosis. A 10- to 21-year study. *Am J Knee Surg* 16:21–26, 2003.
2. Agneskirchner, J. D.; Hurschler, C.; Stukenborg-Colsman, C.; et al.: Effect of high tibial flexion osteotomy on cartilage pressure and joint kinematics: a biomechanical study in human cadaveric knees. Winner of the AGA-DonJoy Award 2004. *Arch Orthop Trauma Surg* 124:575–584, 2004.
3. Amendola, A.; Fowler, P. J.; Litchfield, R.; et al.: Opening wedge high tibial osteotomy using a novel technique: early results and complications. *J Knee Surg* 17:164–169, 2004.
4. Andrews, M.; Noyes, F. R.; Hewett, T. E.; Andriacchi, T. P.: Lower limb alignment and foot angle are related to stance phase knee adduction in normal subjects: a critical analysis of the reliability of gait analysis data. *J Orthop Res* 14:289–295, 1996.
5. Andriacchi, T. P.: Biomechanics and gait analysis in total knee replacement. *Orthop Rev* 17:470–474, 1988.
6. Andriacchi, T. P.: Dynamics of pathological motion: applied to the anterior cruciate–deficient knee. *J Biomech* 23(suppl 1):99–105, 1990.
7. Andriacchi, T. P.: Functional analysis of pre- and post-knee surgery: total knee arthroplasty and ACL reconstruction. *J Biomech Eng* 115:575–581, 1993.
8. Andriacchi, T. P.; Andersson, G. B. J.; Fermier, R. W.; et al.: Study of lower-limb mechanics during stair-climbing. *J Bone Joint Surg Am* 62:749–757, 1980.
9. Andriacchi, T. P.; Hampton, S. J.; Schultz, A. B.; Galante, J. O.: Three-dimensional coordinate data processing in human motion analysis. *J Biomech Eng* 101:279–283, 1979.
10. Andriacchi, T. P.; Ogle, J. A.; Galante, J. O.: Walking speeds as a basis for normal and abnormal gait measurements. *J Biomech* 10:261–268, 1977.
11. Andriacchi, T. P.; Schipplein, O. D.; Galante, J. O.: Dynamic analysis of medial compartment loading in assessment of high tibial osteotomy. *Trans Orthop Res Soc* 10:281, 1985.
12. Backstein, D.; Morag, G.; Hanna, S.; et al.: Long-term follow-up of distal femoral varus osteotomy of the knee. *J Arthroplasty* 22(4 suppl 1):2–6, 2007.
13. Barber-Westin, S. D.; Noyes, F. R.; McCloskey, J. W.: Rigorous statistical reliability, validity, and responsiveness testing of the Cincinnati Knee Rating System in 350 subjects with uninjured, injured, or anterior cruciate ligament-reconstructed knees. *Am J Sports Med* 27:402–416, 1999.
14. Barrett, S. L.; Dellon, A. L.; Rosson, G. D.; Walters, L.: Superficial peroneal nerve (superficial fibularis nerve): the clinical implications of anatomic variability. *J Foot Ankle Surg* 45:174–176, 2006.
15. Bauer, G. C.; Insall, J.; Koshino, T.: Tibial osteotomy in gonarthrosis (osteo-arthritis of the knee). *J Bone Joint Surg Am* 51:1545–1563, 1969.
16. Berchuck, M.; Andriacchi, T. P.; Bach, B. R.; Reider, B.: Gait adaptations by patients who have a deficient anterior cruciate ligament. *J Bone Joint Surg Am* 72:871–877, 1990.
17. Billings, A.; Scott, D. F.; Camargo, M. P.; Hofmann, A. A.: High tibial osteotomy with a calibrated osteotomy guide, rigid internal fixation, and early motion. Long-term follow-up. *J Bone Joint Surg Am* 82:70–79, 2000.
17a. Bonin, N.; Ait Si Selmi, T.; Donell, S. T.; et al.: Anterior cruciate reconstruction combined with valgus upper tibial osteotomy: 12 years follow-up. *Knee* 11:431–437, 2004.
18. Boss, A.; Stutz, G.; Oursin, C.; Gachter, A.: Anterior cruciate ligament reconstruction combined with valgus tibial osteotomy (combined procedure). *Knee Surg Sports Traumatol Arthrosc* 3:187–191, 1995.
19. Brandon, M. L.; Haynes, P. T.; Bonamo, J. R.; et al.: The association between posterior-inferior tibial slope and anterior cruciate ligament insufficiency. *Arthroscopy* 22:894–899, 2006.
20. Brazier, J.; Migaud, H.; Gougeon, F.; et al.: [Evaluation of tibial slope radiographic methods. Analysis of 83 healthy knees]. *Rev Chir Orthop* 82:7–13, 1996.
21. Brouwer, R. W.; Bierma-Zeinstra, S. M.; van Koeveringe, A. J.; Verhaar, J. A.: Patellar height and the inclination of the tibial plateau after high tibial osteotomy. The open versus the closed-wedge technique. *J Bone Joint Surg Br* 87:1227–1232, 2005.
22. Brouwer, R. W.; Bierma-Zeinstra, S. M.; van Raaij, T. M.; Verhaar, J. A.: Osteotomy for medial compartment arthritis of the knee using a closing wedge or an opening wedge controlled by a Puddu plate. A one-year randomised, controlled study. *J Bone Joint Surg Br* 88:1454–1459, 2006.
23. Chao, E. Y.; Laughman, R. K.; Schneider, E.; Stauffer, R. N.: Normative data of knee joint motion and ground reaction forces in adult level walking. *J Biomech* 16:219–233, 1983.
24. Ching-Chuan, J.; Yip, K. M.; Liu, T. K.: Posterior slope angle of the medial tibial plateau. *J Formos Med Assoc* 93:509–512, 1994.
25. Chiu, K. Y.; Zhang, S. D.; Zhang, G. H.: Posterior slope of tibial plateau in Chinese. *J Arthroplasty* 15:224–227, 2000.
26. Coventry, M. B.: Upper tibial osteotomy for gonarthrosis. The evolution of the operation in the last 18 years and long term results. *Orthop Clin North Am* 10:191–210, 1979.
27. Coventry, M. B.; Bowman, P. W.: Long-term results of upper tibial osteotomy for degenerative arthritis of the knee. *Acta Orthop Belg* 48:139–156, 1982.
28. Coventry, M. B.; Ilstrup, D. M.; Wallrichs, S. L.: Proximal tibial osteotomy. A critical long-term study of eighty-seven cases. *J Bone Joint Surgery Am* 75:196–201, 1993.
29. Dallari, D.; Savarino, L.; Stagni, C.; et al.: Enhanced tibial osteotomy healing with use of bone grafts supplemented with platelet gel or platelet gel and bone marrow stromal cells. *J Bone Joint Surg Am* 89:2413–2420, 2007.
30. Dejour, H.; Bonnin, M.: Tibial translation after anterior cruciate ligament rupture. Two radiological tests compared. *J Bone Joint Surg Br* 76:745–749, 1994.
31. Dejour, H.; Neyret, P.; Boileau, P.; Donell, S. T.: Anterior cruciate reconstruction combined with valgus tibial osteotomy. *Clin Orthop* 299:220–228, 1994.

32. Dejour, H.; Neyret, P.; Bonnin, M.: Monopodal weight-bearing radiography of the chronically unstable knee. In Jakob, R. P.; Staubli, H.-U. (eds.): *The Knee and the Cruciate Ligaments*. London: Springer-Verlag, 1992; pp. 568–576.

33. Dejour, H.; Walch, G.; Neyret, P.; Adeleine, P.: La dysplasie de la trochlee femorale. *Rev Chir Orthop* 76:45, 1990.

34. Ducic, I.; Dellon, A. L.; Graw, K. S.: The clinical importance of variations in the surgical anatomy of the superficial peroneal nerve in the mid-third of the lateral leg. *Ann Plast Surg* 56:635–638, 2006.

35. Dugdale, T. W.; Noyes, F. R.; Styer, D.: Preoperative planning for high tibial osteotomy: the effect of lateral tibiofemoral separation and tibiofemoral length. *Clin Orthop Relat Res* 274:248–264, 1992.

36. Eckhoff, D. G.; Bach, J. M.; Spitzer, V. M.; et al.: Three-dimensional mechanics, kinematics, and morphology of the knee viewed in virtual reality. *J Bone Joint Surg Am* 87:71–80, 2005.

37. Fairbank, F. J.: Knee joint changes after meniscectomy. *J Bone Joint Surg Br* 30:664–670, 1948.

38. Finkelstein, J. A.; Gross, A. E.; Davis, A.: Varus osteotomy of the distal part of the femur. A survivorship analysis. *J Bone Joint Surg Am* 78:1348–1352, 1996.

39. Flecher, X.; Parratte, S.; Aubaniac, J. M.; Argenson, J. N.: A 12- to 28-year follow-up study of closing wedge high tibial osteotomy. *Clin Orthop Relat Res* 452:91–96, 2006.

40. Flierl, S.; Sabo, D.; Hornig, K.; Perlick, L.: Open wedge high tibial osteotomy using fractioned drill osteotomy: a surgical modification that lowers the complication rate. *Knee Surg Sports Traumatol Arthrosc* 4:149–153, 1996.

41. Genin, P.; Weill, G.; Julliard, R.: [The tibial slope. Proposal for a measurement method]. *J Radiol* 74:27–33, 1993.

42. Giffin, J. R.; Shannon, F. J.: The role of the high tibial osteotomy in the unstable knee. *Sports Med Arthrosc* 15:23–31, 2007.

43. Giffin, J. R.; Stabile, K. J.; Zantop, T.; et al.: Importance of tibial slope for stability of the posterior cruciate ligament deficient knee. *Am J Sports Med* 35:1443–1449, 2007.

44. Giffin, J. R.; Vogrin, T. M.; Zantop, T.; et al.: Effects of increasing tibial slope on the biomechanics of the knee. *Am J Sports Med* 32:376–382, 2004.

45. Grood, E. S.; Noyes, F. R.; Butler, D. L.; Suntay, W. J.: Ligamentous and capsular restraints preventing straight medial and lateral laxity in intact human cadaver knees. *J Bone Joint Surg Am* 63:1257–1269, 1981.

46. Guettier, J. H.; Glisson, R. R.; Stubbs, A. J.; et al.: The triad of varus malalignment, meniscectomy, and chondral damage: a biomechanical explanation for joint degeneration based on pressure and force distribution within the medial knee compartment. In: *Meeting of the American Orthopaedic Society of Sports Medicine*. Edited, Orlando, FL, 2002.

47. Harris, W. R.; Kostuik, J. P.: High tibial osteotomy for osteoarthritis of the knee. *J Bone Joint Surg Am* 52:330–336, 1970.

48. Healy, W. L.; Anglen, J. O.; Wasilewski, S. A.; Krackow, K. A.: Distal femoral varus osteotomy. *J Bone Joint Surg Am* 70:102–109, 1988.

49. Hernigou, P.; Ma, W.: Open wedge tibial osteotomy with acrylic bone cement as bone substitute. *Knee* 8:103–110, 2001.

50. Hernigou, P.; Medevielle, D.; Debeyre, J.; Goutallier, D.: Proximal tibial osteotomy for osteoarthritis with varus deformity. A ten- to thirteen-year follow-up study. *J Bone Joint Surg Am* 69:332–354, 1987.

51. Hohmann, E.; Bryant, A.; Imhoff, A. B.: The effect of closed wedge high tibial osteotomy on tibial slope: a radiographic study. *Knee Surg Sports Traumatol Arthrosc* 14:454–459, 2006.

52. Holden, D. L.; James, S. L.; Larson, R. L.; Slocum, D. B.: Proximal tibial osteotomy in patients who are fifty years old or less. A long-term follow-up study. *J Bone Joint Surg Am* 70:977–982, 1988.

53. Huang, T. L.; Tseng, K. F.; Chen, W. M.; et al.: Preoperative tibiofemoral angle predicts survival of proximal tibia osteotomy. *Clin Orthop Relat Res* 432:188–195, 2005.

54. Hughston, J. C.; Jacobson, K. E.: Chronic posterolateral rotatory instability of the knee. *J Bone Joint Surg Am* 67:351–359, 1985.

55. Hughston, J. C.; Norwood, L. A., Jr.: The posterolateral drawer test and external rotational recurvatum test for posterolateral rotatory instability of the knee. *Clin Orthop Relat Res* 147:82–87, 1980.

56. Insall, J.; Salvati, E.: Patella position in the normal knee joint. *Radiology* 101:101–104, 1971.

57. Insall, J. N.; Joseph, D. M.; Msika, C.: High tibial osteotomy for varus gonarthrosis. A long-term follow-up study. *J Bone Joint Surg Am* 66:1040–1048, 1984.

58. Ivarsson, I.; Myrnerts, R.; Gillquist, J.: High tibial osteotomy for medial osteoarthritis of the knee. A 5- to 7- and 11- to 13-year follow-up. *J Bone Joint Surg Br* 72:238–244, 1990.

59. Jackson, J. P.; Waugh, W.: The technique and complications of upper tibial osteotomy. A review of 226 operations. *J Bone Joint Surg Br* 56:236–245, 1974.

60. Jenny, J. Y.; Rapp, E.; Kehr, P.: [Proximal tibial meniscal slope: a comparison with the bone slope]. *Rev Chir Orthop Reparatrice Appar Mot* 84:435–438, 1997.

61. Jiang, C. C.; Insall, J. N.: Effect of rotation on the axial alignment of the femur. Pitfalls in the use of femoral intramedullary guides in total knee arthroplasty. *Clin Orthop Relat Res* 248:50–56, 1989.

62. Johnson, F.; Leitl, S.; Waugh, W.: The distribution of load across the knee. A comparison of static and dynamic measurements. *J Bone Joint Surg Br* 62:346–349, 1980.

63. Julliard, R.; Genin, P.; Weil, G.; Palmkrantz, P.: [The median functional slope of the tibia. Principle. Technique of measurement. Value. Interest]. *Rev Chir Orthop Reparatrice Appar Mot* 79:625–634, 1993.

64. Keppler, P.; Gebhard, F.; Grutzner, P. A.; et al.: Computer aided high tibial open wedge osteotomy. *Injury* 35(suppl 1):S–A68–S–A78, 2004.

65. Kettelkamp, D. B.; Leach, R. E.; Nasca, R.: Pitfalls of proximal tibial osteotomy. *Clin Orthop Relat Res* 106:232–241, 1975.

66. Kirgis, A.; Albrecht, S.: Palsy of the deep peroneal nerve after proximal tibial osteotomy. An anatomical study. *J Bone Joint Surg Am* 74:1180–1185, 1992.

67. Koshino, T.; Murase, T.; Saito, T.: Medial opening-wedge high tibial osteotomy with use of porous hydroxyapatite to treat medial compartment osteoarthritis of the knee. *J Bone Joint Surg Am* 85:78–85, 2003.

68. Koshino, T.; Yoshida, T.; Ara, Y.; et al.: Fifteen to twenty-eight years' follow-up results of high tibial valgus osteotomy for osteoarthritic knee. *Knee* 11:439–444, 2004.

69. Lattermann, C.; Jakob, R. P.: High tibial osteotomy alone or combined with ligament reconstruction in anterior cruciate ligament-deficient knees. *Knee Surgery Sports Traumatol Arthrosc* 4:32–38, 1996.

70. Leclerc, J. R.; Geerts, W. H.; Desjardins, L.; et al.: Prevention of deep vein thrombosis after major knee surgery—a randomized, double-blind trial comparing a low molecular weight heparin fragment (enoxaparin) to placebo. *Thromb Haemost* 67:417–423, 1992.

71. Lobenhoffer, P.; Agneskirchner, J. D.: Improvements in surgical technique of valgus high tibial osteotomy. *Knee Surg Sports Traumatol Arthrosc* 11:132–138, 2003.

72. Magyar, G.; Ahl, T. L.; Vibe, P.; et al.: Open-wedge osteotomy by hemicallotasis or the closed-wedge technique for osteoarthritis of the knee. A randomised study of 50 operations. *J Bone Joint Surg Br* 81:444–448, 1999.

73. Magyar, G.; Toksvig-Larsen, S.; Lindstrand, A.: Changes in osseous correction after proximal tibial osteotomy: radiostereometry of closed- and open-wedge osteotomy in 33 patients. *Acta Orthop Scand* 70:473–477, 1999.

74. Magyar, G.; Toksvig-Larsen, S.; Lindstrand, A.: Hemicallotasis open-wedge osteotomy for osteoarthritis of the knee. Complications in 308 operations. *J Bone Joint Surg Br* 81:449–451, 1999.

75. Markolf, K. L.; Bargar, W. L.; Shoemaker, S. C.; Amstutz, H. C.: The role of joint load in knee stability. *J Bone Joint Surg Am* 63:570–585, 1981.

76. Markolf, K. L.; Kochan, A.; Amstutz, H. C.: Measurement of knee stiffness and laxity in patients with documented absence of the anterior cruciate ligament. *J Bone Joint Surg Am* 66:242–253, 1984.

77. Marti, C. B.; Gautier, E.; Wachtl, S. W.; Jakob, R. P.: Accuracy of frontal and sagittal plane correction in open-wedge high tibial osteotomy. *Arthroscopy* 20:366–372, 2004.

78. Marti, R. K.; Verhagen, R. A.; Kerkhoffs, G. M.; Moojen, T. M.: Proximal tibial varus osteotomy. Indications, technique, and five- to twenty-one–year results. *J Bone Joint Surg Am* 83:164–170, 2001.

79. Matsuda, S.; Miura, H.; Nagamine, R.; et al.: Posterior tibial slope in the normal and varus knee. *Am J Knee Surg* 12:165–168, 1999.

80. Matthews, L. S.; Goldstein, S. A.; Malvita, T. A.; et al.: Proximal tibial osteotomy. Factors that influence the duration of satisfactory function. *Clin Orthop Relat Res* 229:193–200, 1988.

81. McDermott, A. G.; Finklestein, J. A.; Farine, I.; et al.: Distal femoral varus osteotomy for valgus deformity of the knee. *J Bone Joint Surg Am* 70:110–116, 1988.

82. Meister, K.; Talley, M. C.; Horodyski, M. B.; et al.: Caudal slope of the tibia and its relationship to noncontact injuries to the ACL. *Am J Knee Surg* 11:217–219, 1998.

83. Miller, B. S.; Joseph, T. A.; Barry, E. M.; et al.: Patient satisfaction after medial opening high tibial osteotomy and microfracture. *J Knee Surg* 20:129–133, 2007.

84. Moreland, J. R.; Bassett, L. W.; Hanker, G. J.: Radiographic analysis of the axial alignment of the lower extremity. *J Bone Joint Surg Am* 69:745–749, 1987.

85. Morrison, J. B.: Function of the knee joint in various activities. *Biomed Eng* 4:573–580, 1969.

86. Muller, W.: Kinematics of the cruciate ligaments. In Feagin, J. (ed.): *The Cruciate Ligaments. Diagnosis and Treatment of Ligamentous Injuries About the Knee.* New York: Churchill Livingstone, 1988; pp. 217–233.

86a. Nagel, A.; Insall, J. N.; Scuderi, G. R.: Proximal tibial osteotomy. A subjective outcome study. *J Bone Joint Surg Am* 78:1353–1358, 1996.

87. Nakamura, E.; Mizuta, H.; Kudo, S.; et al.: Open-wedge osteotomy of the proximal tibia with hemicallotasis. *J Bone Joint Surg Br* 83:1111–1115, 2001.

88. Naudie, D.; Bourne, R. B.; Rorabeck, C. H.; Bourne, T. J.: Survivorship of the high tibial valgus osteotomy. A 10- to 22-year follow-up study. *Clin Orthop Relat Res* 367:18–27, 1999.

89. Naudie, D. D.; Amendola, A.; Fowler, P. J.: Opening wedge high tibial osteotomy for symptomatic hyperextension-varus thrust. *Am J Sports Med* 32:60–70, 2004.

90. Noyes, F. R.; Barber, S. D.: Allograft reconstruction of the anterior and posterior cruciate ligaments: report of ten-year experience and results. *Instr Course Lect* 42:381–396, 1993.

91. Noyes, F. R.; Barber, S. D.: The effect of a ligament-augmentation device on allograft reconstructions for chronic ruptures of the anterior cruciate ligament. *J Bone Joint Surg Am* 74:960–973, 1992.

92. Noyes, F. R.; Barber, S. D.: The effect of an extra-articular procedure on allograft reconstructions for chronic ruptures of the anterior cruciate ligament. *J Bone Joint Surg Am* 73:882–892, 1991.

93. Noyes, F. R.; Barber, S. D.; Simon, R.: High tibial osteotomy and ligament reconstruction in varus angulated, anterior cruciate ligament–deficient knees. A two- to seven-year follow-up study. *Am J Sports Med* 21:2–12, 1993.

94. Noyes, F. R.; Barber-Westin, S. D.: Anterior cruciate ligament revision reconstruction: results using a quadriceps tendon–patellar bone autograft. *Am J Sports Med* 34:553–564, 2006.

95. Noyes, F. R.; Barber-Westin, S. D.: Two-strand posterior cruciate ligament reconstruction with a quadriceps tendon–patellar bone autograft: Technical considerations and clinical results. *Inst Course Lect* 55:509–528, 2006.

96. Noyes, F. R.; Barber-Westin, S. D.: Posterior cruciate ligament revision reconstruction, part 1: causes of surgical failure in 52 consecutive operations. *Am J Sports Med* 33:646–654, 2005.

97. Noyes, F. R.; Barber-Westin, S. D.: Posterior cruciate ligament revision reconstruction, part 2: results of revision using a 2-strand quadriceps tendon–patellar bone autograft. *Am J Sports Med* 33:655–665, 2005.

98. Noyes, F. R.; Barber-Westin, S. D.: Revision anterior cruciate surgery with use of bone–patellar tendon–bone autogenous grafts. *J Bone Joint Surg Am* 83:1131–1143, 2001.

99. Noyes, F. R.; Barber-Westin, S. D.; Albright, J. C.: An analysis of the causes of failure in 57 consecutive posterolateral operative procedures. *Am J Sports Med* 34:1419–1430, 2006.

100. Noyes, F. R.; Barber-Westin, S. D.; Hewett, T. E.: High tibial osteotomy and ligament reconstruction for varus angulated anterior cruciate ligament–deficient knees. *Am J Sports Med* 28:282–296, 2000.

101. Noyes, F. R.; Barber-Westin, S. D.; Roberts, C. S.: Use of allografts after failed treatment of rupture of the anterior cruciate ligament. *J Bone Joint Surg Am* 76:1019–1031, 1994.

102. Noyes, F. R.; Berrios-Torres, S.; Barber-Westin, S. D.; Heckmann, T. P.: Prevention of permanent arthrofibrosis after anterior cruciate ligament reconstruction alone or combined with associated procedures: a prospective study in 443 knees. *Knee Surg Sports Traumatol Arthrosc* 8:196–206, 2000.

103. Noyes, F. R.; Cummings, J. F.; Grood, E. S.; et al.: The diagnosis of knee motion limits, subluxations, and ligament injury. *Am J Sports Med* 19:163–171, 1991.

104. Noyes, F. R.; Dunworth, L. A.; Andriacchi, T. P.; et al.: Knee hyperextension gait abnormalities in unstable knees. Recognition and preoperative gait retraining. *Am J Sports Med* 24:35–45, 1996.

105. Noyes, F. R.; Goebel, S. X.; West, J.: Opening wedge tibial osteotomy: the 3-triangle method to correct axial alignment and tibial slope. *Am J Sports Med* 33:378–387, 2005.

106. Noyes, F. R.; Grood, E. S.; Torzilli, P. A.: Current concepts review. The definitions of terms for motion and position of the knee and injuries of the ligaments. *J Bone Joint Surg Am* 71:465–472, 1989.

107. Noyes, F. R.; Mayfield, W.; Barber-Westin, S. D.; et al.: Opening wedge high tibial osteotomy: an operative technique and rehabilitation program to decrease complications and promote early union and function. *Am J Sports Med* 34:1262–1273, 2006.

108. Noyes, F. R.; Mooar, P. A.; Matthews, D. S.; Butler, D. L.: The symptomatic anterior cruciate–deficient knee. Part I: the long-term functional disability in athletically active individuals. *J Bone Joint Surg Am* 65:154–162, 1983.

109. Noyes, F. R.; Schipplein, O. D.; Andriacchi, T. P.; et al.: The anterior cruciate ligament–deficient knee with varus alignment. An analysis of gait adaptations and dynamic joint loadings. *Am J Sports Med* 20:707–716, 1992.

110. Noyes, F. R.; Stabler, C. L.: A system for grading articular cartilage lesions at arthroscopy. *Am J Sports Med* 17:505–513, 1989.

111. Noyes, F. R.; Wojtys, E. M.: The early recognition, diagnosis and treatment of the patella infera syndrome. In Tullos, H. S. (ed.): *Instructional Course Lectures.* Rosemont, IL: AAOS, 1991; pp. 233–247.

112. Noyes, F. R.; Wojtys, E. M.; Marshall, M. T.: The early diagnosis and treatment of developmental patella infera syndrome. *Clin Orthop* 265:241–252, 1991.

113. Odenbring, S.; Tjornstrand, B.; Egund, N.; et al.: Function after tibial osteotomy for medial gonarthrosis below aged 50 years. *Acta Orthop Scand* 60:527–531, 1989.

114. Pace, T. B.; Hofmann, A. A.; Kane, K. R.: Medial-opening high-tibial osteotomy combined with Magnuson intra-articular débridement for traumatic gonarthrosis. *J Orthop Tech* 2:21–28, 1994.

115. Patond, K. R.; Lokhande, A. V.: Medial open wedge high tibial osteotomy in medial compartment osteoarthrosis of the knee. *Natl Med J India* 6:105–108, 1993.

116. Patt, T. W.; Kleinhout, M. Y.; Albers, R. G.; van der Vis, H. M.: Paper #142 Early complications after high tibial osteotomy—a comparison of two techniques (open vs. closed wedge). *Arthroscopy* 19:74, 2003.

117. Pfahler, M.; Lutz, C.; Anetzberger, H.; et al.: Long-term results of high tibial osteotomy for medial osteoarthritis of the knee. *Acta Chir Belg* 103:603–606, 2003.

118. Prodromos, C. C.; Andriacchi, T. P.; Galante, J. O.: A relationship between gait and clinical changes following high tibial osteotomy. *J Bone Joint Surg Am* 67:1188–1194, 1985.

119. Rinonapoli, E.; Mancini, G. B.; Corvaglia, A.; Musiello, S.: Tibial osteotomy for varus gonarthrosis. A 10- to 21-year follow-up study. *Clin Orthop Relat Res* 353:185–193, 1998.

120. Rodner, C. M.; Adams, D. J.; Diaz-Doran, V.; et al.: Medial opening wedge tibial osteotomy and the sagittal plane: the effect of increasing tibial slope on tibiofemoral contact pressure. *Am J Sports Med* 34:1431–1441, 2006.

121. Rosenberg, T. D.; Paulos, L. E.; Parker, R. D.; et al.: The forty-five-degree posteroanterior flexion weight-bearing radiograph of the knee. *J Bone Joint Surg Am* 70:1479–1483, 1988.

122. Rubman, M. H.; Noyes, F. R.; Barber-Westin, S. D.: Technical considerations in the management of complex meniscus tears. *Clin Sports Med* 15:511–530, 1996.

123. Rudan, J. F.; Simurda, M. A.: High tibial osteotomy. A prospective clinical and roentgenographic review. *Clin Orthop Relat Res* 255:251–256, 1990.

124. Sabharwal, S.; Zhao, C.: Assessment of lower limb alignment: supine fluoroscopy compared with a standing full-length radiograph. *J Bone Joint Surg Am* 90:43–51, 2008.

125. Schipplein, O. D.; Andriacchi, T. P.: Interaction between active and passive knee stabilizers during level walking. *J Orthop Res* 9:113–119, 1991.

126. Slawski, D. P.; Schoenecker, P. L.; Rich, M. M.: Peroneal nerve injury as a complication of pediatric tibial osteotomies: a review of 255 osteotomies. *J Pediatr Orthop* 14:166–172, 1994.

127. Song, E. K.; Seon, J. K.; Park, S. J.: How to avoid unintended increase of posterior slope in navigation-assisted open-wedge high tibial osteotomy. *Orthopedics* 30(10 suppl):S127–S131, 2007.

128. Sprenger, T. R.; Doerzbacher, J. F.: Tibial osteotomy for the treatment of varus gonarthrosis. Survival and failure analysis to twenty-two years. *J Bone Joint Surg Am* 85:469–474, 2003.

129. Staubli, A. E.; De Simoni, C.; Babst, R.; Lobenhoffer, P.: TomoFix: a new LCP-concept for open wedge osteotomy of the medial proximal tibia—early results in 92 cases. *Injury* 34(suppl 2):B55–B62, 2003.

130. Sterett, W. I.; Steadman, J. R.: Chondral resurfacing and high tibial osteotomy in the varus knee. *Am J Sports Med* 32:1243–1249, 2004.

131. Stoffel, K.; Stachowiak, G.; Kuster, M.: Open wedge high tibial osteotomy: biomechanical investigation of the modified Arthrex Osteotomy Plate (Puddu Plate) and the TomoFix Plate. *Clin Biomech (Bristol, Avon)* 19:944–950, 2004.

132. Stuart, M. J.; Grace, J. N.; Ilstrup, D. M.; et al.: Late recurrence of varus deformity after proximal tibial osteotomy. *Clin Orthop Relat Res* 260:61–65, 1990.

133. Stutz, G.; Boss, A.; Gachter, A.: Comparison of augmented and non-augmented anterior cruciate ligament reconstruction combined with high tibial osteotomy. *Knee Surg Sports Traumatol Arthrosc* 4:143–148, 1996.

134. Sundaram, N. A.; Hallett, J. P.; Sullivan, M. F.: Dome osteotomy of the tibia for osteoarthritis of the knee. *J Bone Joint Surg Br* 68:782–786, 1986.

135. Tigani, D.; Ferrari, D.; Trentani, P.; et al.: Patellar height after high tibial osteotomy. *Int Orthop* 24:331–334, 2001.

136. Turner, R. S.; Griffiths, H.; Heatley, F. W.: The incidence of deep-vein thrombosis after upper tibial osteotomy. A venographic study. *J Bone Joint Surg Br* 75:942–944, 1993.

137. Wang, J. W.; Kuo, K. N.; Andriacchi, T. P.; Galante, J. O.: The influence of walking mechanics and time on the results of proximal tibial osteotomy. *J Bone Joint Surg Am* 72:905–909, 1990.

138. Warden, S. J.; Morris, H. G.; Crossley, K. M.; et al.: Delayed- and non-union following opening wedge high tibial osteotomy: surgeons' results from 182 completed cases. *Knee Surg Sports Traumatol Arthrosc* 13:34–37, 2005.

139. Weale, A. E.; Lee, A. S.; MacEachern, A. G.: High tibial osteotomy using a dynamic axial external fixator. *Clin Orthop Relat Res* 382:154–167, 2001.

140. Westrich, G. H.; Peters, L. E.; Haas, S. B.; et al.: Patella height after high tibial osteotomy with internal fixation and early motion. *Clin Orthop Relat Res* 354:169–174, 1998.

141. Williams, R. J.; Kelly, B. T.; Wickiewicz, T.; et al.: The short-term outcome of surgical treatment for painful varus arthritis in association with chronic ACL deficiency. *Am J Knee Surg* 16:9–16, 2003.

142. Windsor, R. E.; Insall, J. N.; Vince, K. G.: Technical considerations of total knee arthroplasty after proximal tibial osteotomy. *J Bone Joint Surg Am* 70:547–555, 1988.

143. Wright, J. G.; Treble, N.; Feinstein, A. R.: Measurement of lower limb alignment using long radiographs. *J Bone Joint Surg Br* 73:721–723, 1991.

144. Wright, J. M.; Heavrin, B.; Begg, M.; et al.: Observations on patellar height following opening wedge proximal tibial osteotomy. *Am J Knee Surg* 14:163–173, 2001.

145. Yacobucci, G. N.; Cocking, M. R.: Union of medial opening-wedge high tibial osteotomy using a corticocancellous proximal tibial wedge allograft. *Am J Sports Med* 36:713–719, 2008.

146. Yoshioka, Y.; Siu, D. W.; Scudamore, R. A.; Cooke, T. D.: Tibial anatomy and functional axes. *J Orthop Res* 7:132–137, 1989.

Chapter 32

Valgus Malalignment: Diagnosis, Osteotomy Techniques, and Clinical Outcomes

Simon Görtz, MD ■ *William D. Bugbee*, MD

INTRODUCTION

Originally described in the German literature in the 19th century, multiple reports on knee osteotomy have appeared in the English literature over the last 50 years, most of which have detailed the proximal tibial valgus osteotomy for varus arthrosis. The popularity of these procedures decreased in the latter part of the century as confidence in the durability and outcomes of total knee replacement (TKR) improved. However, interest in osteotomy has recently undergone resurgence with the advent of biologic treatments for cartilage deterioration and loss of meniscal tissue and function.

Fewer reports have been published regarding osteotomy for valgus knee arthrosis, probably owing to the lower incidence of valgus deformity of the knee. Valgus malalignment may be either a cause or a consequence of lateral unicompartmental gonarthritis in young, active adults. Osteotomy is a biologic treatment alternative for unicompartmental disease in patients in whom TKR is undesirable owing to age, life expectancy, or activity level that would be considered inappropriate for prosthetic replacement. In this patient population, distal femoral osteotomy (DFO) can be an appropriate joint-preserving solution that relies on the redistribution of forces in the knee joint away from a mechanically overloaded, and thus symptomatic, lateral tibiofemoral compartment. Opening wedge techniques generally allow a more physiologic approach and precise correction and have gained popularity lately to adequately address cases of dysplastic lateral femoral condyles in valgus knees as well as medial tibial plateau defects in varus gonarthrosis.

INDICATIONS

Despite less predictable pain relief and relatively inferior long-term results compared with total knee arthrosis (TKA), joint-preserving osteotomy is an appealing, yet reluctant, choice for high-demand patients with increased life expectancy and reservations about prosthetic replacement. The traditional indication for DFO is the correction of valgus limb malalignment in a knee with symptomatic lateral compartment osteoarthritis or post-traumatic arthrosis. The procedure has also gained significance as part of a joint-preserving treatment for less advanced cartilage or meniscal disease of the lateral compartment. At the authors' institution, osteotomy has also been used increasingly to unload and optimize the biologic environment of a compartment undergoing osteochondral or meniscal transplantation. Therefore,

---

Critical Points INDICATIONS FOR DFO

- Valgus limb malalignment in a knee with symptomatic lateral compartment arthrosis in young, active patients.
- Joint preservation in less advanced cartilage or meniscal disease of the lateral compartment.
- Ancillary procedure to osteochondral repair or meniscal transplantation procedures.

two distinct groups of patients with valgus limb malalignment may benefit from the procedure.

Primary osteotomy to correct malalignment will alleviate symptoms by reducing stresses on the articular cartilage and the underlying subchondral bone. Secondary osteotomy, adjunct to resurfacing procedures addressing osteoarticular lesions resulting from a pathologic biomechanical environment, putatively protects the resultant repair tissue by correcting the underlying condition that contributed to the original lesion.

The ideal patient for DFO has an extended life expectancy, isolated lateral compartment symptoms, knee flexion greater than 90°, less than 15° of flexion contracture, no ligamentous instability, normal body mass index, and reasonable expectations. Although some have considered men to be better candidates for osteotomy than women, the authors have not found a correlation with gender and outcome. Rather, other criteria such as age, motivation, and fitness have been found to be far more critical. Other considerations when indicating DFO include age, activity level, and magnitude of deformity.

Because of the generally good clinical results and survivorship of TKR, the threshold for considering osteotomy over arthroplasty is typically patients aged 65 and younger. Older, physically active patients may be candidates for DFO if they are expected to return to an activity level that would be inappropriate for TKR. Young, active patients (<50 yr of age) are better candidates for joint-preserving osteotomy owing to the absence of implant-related activity restrictions, despite the relatively inferior long-term results compared with TKA. In these individuals, the osteotomy should be considered a temporizing procedure amenable to possible future conversion to TKA. The 50- to 65-year-old group presents a unique challenge in determining whether osteotomy is the most appropriate treatment choice. Finally, young patients (<40 yr of age) with even small amounts of valgus limb malalignment should be carefully evaluated for osteotomy when there is symptomatic loss of lateral compartment chondral or meniscal tissue. In this setting, it may be reasonable to consider (though not proven) that the osteotomy may delay the progression to more advanced arthrosis. When cartilage or meniscal restoration is performed in the lateral compartment, the adjunctive use of DFO may help protect the reconstruction as well.

CONTRAINDICATIONS

Absolute contraindications to DFO include the presence of symptomatic medial compartment arthrosis, inflammatory arthrosis including advanced crystal-induced arthropathy, and metabolic bone disorders that would significantly interfere with osseous healing of the osteotomy. Conversely, neuromuscular disorders

are not a contraindication, because the osteotomy may be a more reasonable and durable operation than TKA in this setting.

Relative contraindications include severe angular deformity (consideration in these cases should be given to a double osteotomy of the distal femur and proximal tibia), limited knee range of motion (>15° flexion contracture or <90° of flexion), poor motivation, or poor rehabilitation potential. Rehabilitation issues would include the inability to follow postoperative weight-bearing restrictions and the use of drugs or substances such as nicotine that may interfere with bone healing. The extent of lateral joint arthrosis (as defined by amount of cartilage loss on femoral and tibial surfaces) has, to our knowledge, not been shown to have a demonstrable effect on outcome. Therefore, we do not use the amount of radiographic or clinical joint space loss as a criterion or contraindication. The presence of patellofemoral arthrosis as a relative contraindication is controversial. Some studies have shown that arthrosis of the patellofemoral joint has no bearing on the outcome, whereas others have even shown improvement in patellofemoral symptoms with DFO.[11]

CLINICAL BIOMECHANICS

The *weight-bearing line* (WBL) of the lower extremity is defined as the line drawn from the center of the femoral head through the center of the ankle mortise. Based on where this line crosses the knee joint, overall limb alignment is considered varus (medial to the center of the knee), valgus (lateral to the center of the knee), or neutral relative to the center of the knee. Based on morphologic studies of normal subjects with neutral overall alignment, Hsu and coworkers[8] determined that 75% of weight-bearing forces are transmitted through the medial compartment of the knee in a one-legged simulated weight-bearing stance. Other studies have determined that 60% of the load is passed through the medial compartment during weight-bearing.[1,11] Alterations in the overall alignment will change these forces and create an unfavorable mechanical environment, potentially leading to injury and degeneration of the over stressed compartment that may be stopped or slowed by timely correction of the malalignment.[13]

With a valgus deformity, the mechanical axis passes through (or lateral to) the lateral compartment of the knee, thus overburdening that compartment and leading to pain and development of arthritis. Additional pathologic features of the valgus knee include progressive posterolateral soft-tissue contractures including the iliotibial band, popliteus, lateral collateral ligament, posterolateral capsule, lateral head of the gastrocnemius, lateral intermuscular septum, and long head of the biceps. In addition, these contractures may lead to attenuation of the medial collateral ligament and medial capsular laxity.

Osseous deformities should be understood in the context of "normal" anatomy and "physiologic" valgus. Kapandji[9] illustrated that the average distal femoral angle is 7% to 9% of valgus, and the average proximal tibial angle is 0% to 3% of varus, producing the overall tibiofemoral angle of 5% to 7% of valgus, which, after accounting for hip offset, leads to a mechanical limb axis through the center of the knee. Osseous deformities in the valgus knee are usually limited to the lateral femoral condyle, which is typically hypoplastic, thus leading to excessive distal femoral valgus. Conversely, the lateral tibial plateau is usually well preserved, except in the case of fracture.

The important distinction is that for the majority of valgus knees, the deformity lies in the distal femur and not in the tibia. In some cases, this excessive distal femoral valgus may be minimal, but in other more severe cases, the distal femoral angle can approach 15% to 20% of valgus. Whereas the exact prevalence of valgus deformity of the knee is unknown, it is generally considered less common than varus deformity about the knee. Cooke and associates[3] examined full-length radiographs of 167 white patients with osteoarthritis. Valgus alignment was seen in 24% and varus in 76%. In addition, valgus deformity has been noted to be more common in females, patients with inflammatory arthritis, post-traumatic arthritis, and those with metabolic abnormalities such as rickets or renal osteodystrophy.

The rationale of the DFO is to correct the excessive tibiofemoral valgus by shifting the mechanical axis line from the lateral compartment to a more median or even medial position. Historically, this correction has been performed both above and below the level of the joint line. Initial reports of correction of painful valgus deformity described a proximal tibial varus-producing osteotomy. However, Coventry[4] recommended that deformity of greater than 12% of tibiofemoral valgus should be corrected above the joint line in order to avoid excessive joint line obliquity, which leads to increased shear stresses across the joint, ligamentous and capsular attenuation, and subsequent joint subluxation. A general rule is that the osteotomy should be performed at the site of the primary deformity, which in most patients with valgus deformity lies in the distal femur.

CLINICAL EVALUATION

History and Physical Examination

Patients who are candidates for DFO are rare, but when they present, the deformity is quite evident. Symptoms are localized to the lateral compartment, and patients complain of difficulty ascending and descending stairs, often with a feeling of giving-way. On physical examination, range of motion should be at least 90° and any flexion contracture less than 15°. The knee should be ligamentously stable and the medial and patellofemoral compartments should have minimal or no articular cartilage damage. Ambulation demonstrates genu valgum with an occasional abduction-type lurch and a stiff-knee gait, attempting to avoid the worn cartilage in the posterior aspect of the knee, which makes contact in flexion.

Radiographic Evaluation

All patients who are candidates for DFO obtain full-length, standing anteroposterior (AP) radiographs of bilateral lower extremities. In addition, standing AP views of both knees,

Critical Points RADIOGRAPHIC EVALUATION

- Full-length, standing anteroposterior (AP) radiographs of bilateral lower extremities.
- Standing AP views of bilateral knees.
- Standing posteroanterior (PA) view in 45° of flexion (Rosenberg).
- Lateral flexion view of the knee.
- Patellofemoral (Merchant) view.
- Reestablish the mechanical axis to fall through the center or just medial to center of the knee.
- Correct distal femoral angle to between 0% and 4% of valgus, depending on the patient's circumstance and proximal tibial anatomy.
- Millimeter value of the linear correction at the osteotomy site is roughly equivalent to the degree correction of axial alignment.
- Stage osteotomy to be the last of the concomitant procedures performed.

standing posteroanterior (PA) views in 45° of flexion (Rosenberg), lateral flexion views of the knee, and patellofemoral (Merchant) views are obtained. The long-alignment films help determine the overall mechanical axis of the limb and whether the lateral compartment is experiencing overload due to overall genu valgum. The standing AP and Rosenberg views of the knee allow determination of the amount of joint space narrowing in the anterior and posterior portions of the lateral compartment, respectively. The lateral and patellofemoral views are helpful for determining the condition of the patellofemoral joint. If there is any concern, stress radiographs may be obtained to test for ligamentous stability and joint subluxation.

PREOPERATIVE PLANNING

The radiographic studies are essential in the preoperative planning of the intended corrections. These are determined by calculating the tibiofemoral angle and the proximal tibial and distal femoral angles (Fig. 32–1). The goal is to shift the mechanical axis so that it falls through the center or just medial to the center of the knee. Overcorrection of the deformity, as for example in high tibial osteotomy (HTO), will place extreme loads through the medial compartment. The authors recommend instead aiming for the 0% to 4% of valgus that the literature suggests as acceptable. When performing an osteotomy as an ancillary procedure to cartilage repair in young patients, the goal of correction is to restore the WBL through the center of the knee, because overcorrection may be detrimental to long-term joint health. When used to treat cases of arthritis, in which undercorrection can lead to poor outcome, the minimum correction should result in neutral alignment with the maximum correction resulting in the WBL falling through the medial tibial spine. These corrections result in various degrees of tibiofemoral valgus alignment depending on other parameters such as hip offset. This is most easily determined preoperatively using tracing paper cutouts of the proposed osteotomy on standing long-alignment films.

The millimeter value of the linear correction at the osteotomy site is roughly equivalent to the degree of correction of axial alignment (e.g., a 10-mm opening will usually result in 10% of correction). In general, the distal femoral angle is corrected to between 0% and 4% depending on the patient's circumstance and proximal tibial anatomy.

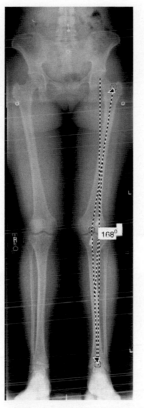

FIGURE 32–1. Preoperative weight-bearing long-leg anteroposterior (AP) radiographs show valgus alignment of the left lower extremity in a 45-year old woman with left lateral knee pain.

The use of arthroscopy preceding the osteotomy to indicate or predict outcome has not been well defined. Currently, no substantial scientific evidence exists that findings at arthroscopy predict the outcome of DFO, and therefore, these data should not be used in isolation, but rather used with careful correlation with clinical and radiographic evaluation. When considering realigning osteotomy as an adjunct procedure to an osteochondral graft of the ipsilateral lateral femoral condyle, staging the procedure is advised so as not to jeopardize the microvascularity of the recipient bone bed.

OPERATIVE TECHNIQUE

The patient is placed supine on a radiolucent operating table that will allow fluoroscopic imaging of the entire lower extremity from the hip to the ankle. The authors' anesthesia preference for surgery is a regional anesthetic that will provide 1 to 2 days of postoperative pain control. If the osteotomy is to be combined with arthroscopy or an allografting procedure (e.g., lateral tibial plateau allograft), the osteotomy is generally the last procedure performed.

The operated limb including the ipsilateral hip is prepared free, and a small bump is placed under the hip to align the extremity in the coronal plane. For reasons described previously, a lateral opening wedge osteotomy fixed with an osteotomy plate and filled with either allograft or iliac crest bone graft is preferred. A sterile tourniquet is placed, but used only if necessary. An 8- to 10-cm incision is made over the lateral aspect of the distal femur. The iliotibial band is incised in line with the

Critical Points SURGICAL TECHNIQUE

- Establish starting point under fluoroscopy, approximately 3 cm above the lateral femoral epicondyle.
- Angle guide pin medial and distal to exit the cortex at the level of the medial epicondyle.
- Palpate the superior trochlea to ensure guide pin position proximally and avoid violating the patellofemoral joint.
- Second guide pin should completely overlap the first guide pin on AP view.
- Confirm symmetry and perpendicularity of the osteotomy on multiple fluoroscopic views before making bone cuts.
- Start osteotomy with an oscillating 1-inch saw using both pins as a guide.
- Complete osteotomy with wide osteotomes, preserving the medial cortex as a hinge.
- Insert the distraction device and distract osteotomy slowly.
- Assess weight-bearing line on fluoroscopy by stretching a radioopaque cord from the center of the femoral head to the center of the ankle.
- Secure the osteotomy plate with three unicortical cancellous screws distally and three bicortical cortical screws proximally.
- Bone graft can utilize autograft or allograft bone products or a combination thereof.

incision, and the vastus lateralis is dissected posteriorly off the lateral intermuscular septum to expose the femoral shaft and the metaphyseal flare (Fig. 32–2). The joint can be entered, if necessary.

Using fluoroscopy, the starting point for the osteotomy is located, which is approximately 3 cm above the lateral femoral epicondyle. The guide pin is angled medially and distally so that it exits the cortex at the level of the medial epicondyle (Fig. 32–3). The goal is to create the osteotomy in the metaphyseal bone, which has excellent healing potential without violating the patellofemoral joint. The superiormost aspect of the trochlea should be palpated to ensure that the guide pin is not too distal. If this is the case, the superior aspect of the joint will be violated during the osteotomy. In these instances, the guide pin should be removed and placed more proximally.

It is important to consider the angle of the osteotomy not only on the AP view but also in the lateral plane. In order to

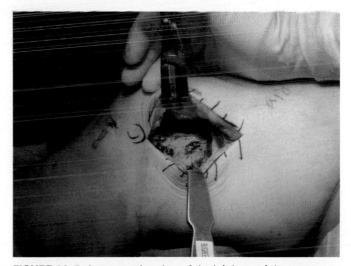

FIGURE 32–2. Intraoperative view of the left knee of the same patient shows exposure of the femoral shaft and the metaphyseal flare.

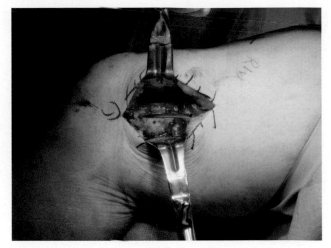

FIGURE 32–3. Intraoperative view of guide pin placement.

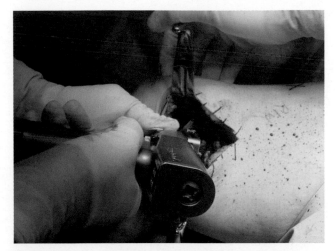

FIGURE 32–5. The osteotomy is begun with the oscillating saw.

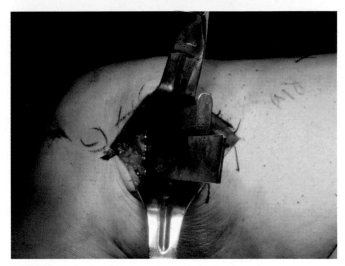

FIGURE 32–6. Osteotomes are used to complete the osteotomy.

preserve the sagittal plane alignment of the femur, the osteotomy should be performed perpendicular to the axis of the femur in the lateral plane. Any deviation will create either excessive flexion or extension of the femur, depending on the angle of the osteotomy. This may be desirable, for example, if the patient has a fixed flexion contracture at the knee and the goal is to create a mild hyperextension of the distal femur to counter the contracture. In general, however, the authors' preference is to create a symmetrical osteotomy perpendicular to the axis of the femur in the lateral plane.

Once the first guide pin is accurately placed, a second guide pin should be placed either directly anterior or directly posterior to that pin in the same plane, so that both pins completely overlap on an AP view of the distal femur. This ensures that an osteotomy created parallel to the plane of both guide pins will be perpendicular to the long axis of the femur in the lateral plane. After the guide pins have been placed in the appropriate position on the AP view (Fig. 32–4), the osteotomy may then be performed using both pins as a guide. An oscillating saw with a 1-inch saw blade is used to start the osteotomy, either just above or just below the guide pins, to create the proper plane (Fig. 32–5). Once this has been done, wide osteotomes are used to complete the osteotomy (Fig. 32–6). The goal is not to create a complete fracture, but

instead to keep the medial cortex intact to act as a hinge. Occasionally, the medial cortex is perforated to allow for opening of the osteotomy, which may be done with a small K-wire.

Once the majority of the cortex has been freed, the distraction device is placed in the osteotomy site (Fig. 32–7) and slowly distracted (Fig. 32–8). The goal is for the mechanical axis to pass through the medial tibial spine. The amount of distraction required to attain this goal correlates with the amount of correction attained. For small osteotomies, this is usually 5 to 8 mm, and for large osteotomies, 10 to 15 mm. Once the desired amount of correction is obtained, fluoroscopy is used to evaluate the WBL. An electrocautery cord is stretched from the center of the femoral head to the center of the ankle and the overall mechanical axis is assessed (Fig. 32–9). Undercorrection is associated with a higher rate of failure, whereas overcorrection places extreme loads on the medial side. If the mechanical axis is over- or undercorrected, it can be adjusted at this time using the distraction device. Once the correction is believed to be appropriate, a plate is used to secure the osteotomy (Fig. 32–10). The plate is fixed using three unicortical cancellous screws distally and three bicortical cortical screws proximally (Figs. 32–11 to 32–13). Depending on the patient, either autologous iliac crest bone graft and/or allograft bone is used (Fig. 32–14). For younger, female patients and those concerned with cosmesis, allograft is preferred, but both

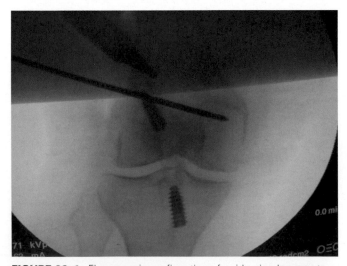

FIGURE 32–4. Fluoroscopic confirmation of guide pin placement, with retained interference screws from prior anterior cruciate ligament reconstruction.

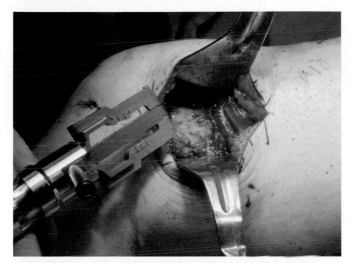

FIGURE 32–7. The distraction device is introduced into the osteotomy.

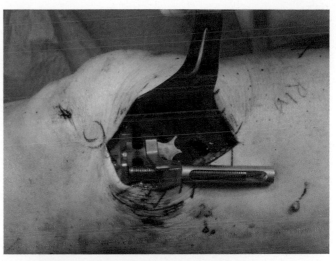

FIGURE 32–10. The osteotomy is secured with an osteotomy plate.

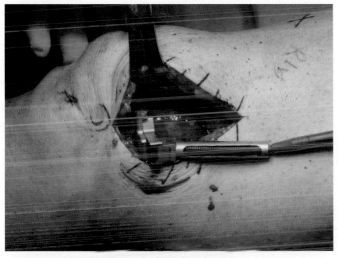

FIGURE 32–8. The osteotomy is distracted.

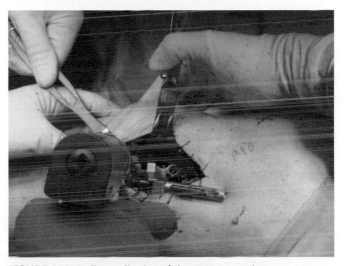

FIGURE 32–11. Screw fixation of the osteotomy plate.

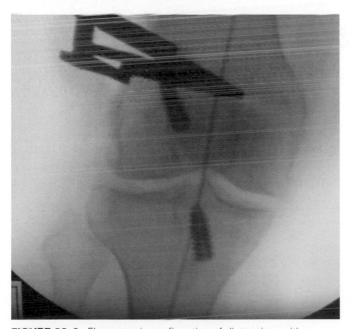

FIGURE 32–9. Fluoroscopic confirmation of distraction, with radiopaque cord indicating the approximate weight-bearing line.

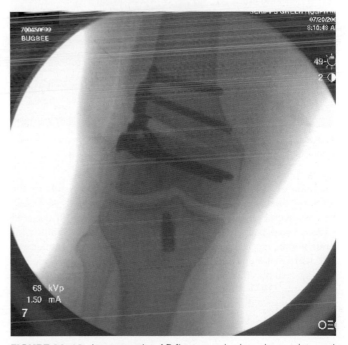

FIGURE 32–12. Intraoperative AP fluoroscopic view shows plate and screw fixation of the osteotomy.

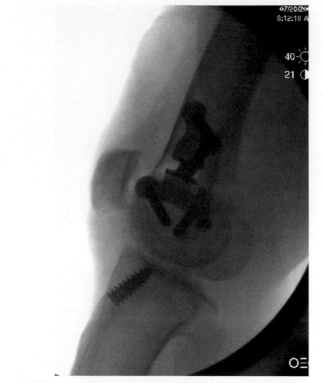

FIGURE 32–13. Intraoperative lateral fluoroscopic view shows plate and screw fixation of the osteotomy.

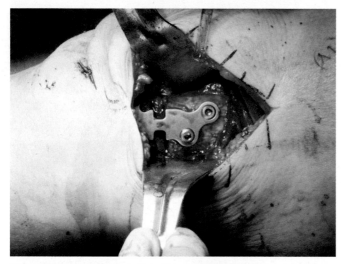

FIGURE 32–14. Intraoperative view of fixed osteotomy plate after placement of the autologous bone graft and bone matrix.

methods of bone grafting have been equally successful. In the authors' clinical experience since 2005 (encompassing 44 cases), no instance of delayed union or nonunion occurred. Of these 44 cases, 13 were performed using only autograft, 7 received only allograft, and 23 received a combination of both. This was supplemented with demineralized bone matrix (DBM) in 21 cases, and platelet-rich plasma (PRP) in 4 cases. One osteotomy was secured using only DBM putty. Although studies to date show no clear superiority of either method, our experience suggests that more rapid healing occurs when autograft is used in some fashion, but patient characteristics and the size of correction also play an important role in the healing process of opening wedge osteotomies.

Postoperatively, the patient is placed in a knee immobilizer overnight for pain control. If osteochondral allografting has also been performed concomitantly, a range of motion brace is placed on postoperative day 1. Patients are started on range of motion exercises immediately, and isometric strengthening is initiated when pain and swelling subside. Patients are kept touch-down weight-bearing for 8 to 12 weeks or until radiographic evidence of healing is confirmed. At 4 weeks, patients are started on a low-resistance exercise bike; resistance training is initiated when the osteotomy is healed (Fig. 32–15). Regular activities are usually resumed at approximately 6 months postoperatively, with continued improvement up to a year.

AUTHORS' CLINICAL OUTCOMES

Thirty-eight distal femoral osteotomies have been performed in 37 individuals. Of these, 17 were done in association with a cartilage (osteochondral allograft) transplant or lateral meniscus

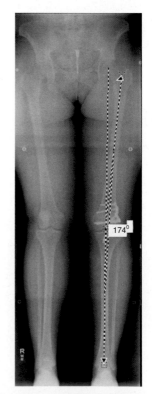

FIGURE 32–15. Postoperative weight-bearing long-leg AP radiographs shows physiologic valgus and normal alignment of the left lower extremity.

transplant, and the remaining 21 were performed for lateral compartment arthrosis with associated mild to severe genu valgum. Thirty-seven of 38 were opening wedge osteotomies. Four knees (11%) have been converted to TKR or partial knee replacement. One patient developed a delayed union, and 3 underwent hardware removal. Overall survivorship of the osteotomy at follow-up at a mean of 4 years (range, 1–9 yr) is 89%.

CLINICAL OUTCOMES FROM OTHER AUTHORS

Compared with HTO, very few reports have been published in the orthopaedic literature on the results of distal femoral varus-producing osteotomy for painful lateral compartment gonarthrosis. The first study for lateral compartment gonarthrosis was published by Coventry in 1987,[4] who described the results of 31 knees that underwent a varus-producing proximal tibial osteotomy. In this report, 77% of cases were considered successful. Failures occurred in patients with a large valgus deformity or in whom the results of the surgery produced a tilt of the articular surface greater than 10%. For these patients, Coventry[4] recommended a distal femoral varus-producing osteotomy.

The first report of varus-producing DFO was by Healy and colleagues in 1988.[7] The series included 23 patients (average age, 56 yr) with painful valgus deformity of the knee with lateral joint space narrowing. Diagnoses included osteoarthritis in 15, post-traumatic osteoarthritis in 3, rheumatoid arthritis in 3, and renal osteodystrophy in 2. The technique used in this series included a medial closing wedge osteotomy in all patients, fixed with a blade plate. Results an average of 4 years postoperatively were good or excellent in 83% (19 of 23). In the osteoarthritis subgroup, 93% had good or excellent outcomes. The authors of this study concluded that 86% of the patients were satisfied with their outcome; however, they did not recommend the procedure in patients with rheumatoid arthritis or decreased range of motion.

McDermott and coworkers[10] reported their experience with distal femoral varus-producing osteotomy in 24 patients with painful valgus deformity of the knee. The average age at the time of operation was 53 years. The goal of the procedure was to obtain a final tibiofemoral angle of 0°. A medial closing wedge osteotomy technique was used, fixed with a blade plate in all patients. At follow-up 4 years postoperatively, 22 patients (92%) had a successful result and were satisfied. The greatest improvement was in the category of pain. There was 1 fixation failure, and 1 patient developed medial compartment gonarthrosis and converted to TKR.

Edgerton and associates[5] followed 24 knees for 5 to 11 years (average, 8.3 yr) after DFO for painful valgus deformity of the knee. At follow-up, 71% of patients had good or excellent results, with no differences in those followed for longer periods. Complications occurred in 63% of the cases, including nonunion (25%), and loss of correction (21%). Both of these complications were associated exclusively with staple fixation, which the authors subsequently abandoned. Thirteen percent of the cases converted to TKR. The authors concluded that with current indications and techniques, a DFO is effective in up to 80% at long-term evaluation if the fixation is rigid, the correction is adequate, and the procedure is done relatively early in the course of the disease.

Finkelstein and colleagues[6] reported on 21 knees that underwent DFO for painful valgus deformity and were followed long term (mean, 133 mo; range, 97–240 mo) or until failure. A medial-based closing wedge osteotomy fixed with a blade plate was performed. The study reported that 13 osteotomies survived, 7 failed, and 1 patient died. The probability of survival at 10 years was 64%. The authors concluded that this is an effective procedure for relieving pain in patients with symptomatic valgus deformity of the knee.

Wang and Hsu[14] reported on 30 knees in 30 patients that were managed with distal femoral varus osteotomy (DFVO) for the treatment of noninflammatory lateral compartment arthritis of the knee associated with a valgus deformity. Twelve knees had isolated lateral compartment arthritis, 10 had mild to moderate degenerative changes in the other two compartments, and 8 knees had severe patellofemoral arthritis in addition to lateral compartment disease. The osteotomy site was fixed with a 90° blade plate. At an average follow-up of 99 months, 25 patients (83%) had a satisfactory result and 2 had a fair result according to the Hospital for Special Surgery rating system. The remaining 3 patients converted to a TKR. With conversion to TKR as the endpoint, the cumulative 10-year survival rate for all patients was 87% (95% confidence interval [CI], 69%–100%). Improvement in patellar tracking, which persisted at the time of the latest follow-up, was observed in 7 of 8 knees with associated severe patellofemoral arthritis. The authors concluded that DFVO with blade plate fixation is a reliable procedure for the treatment of lateral compartment osteoarthritis of the valgus knee and that the result of the osteotomy does not appear to be affected by the presence of severe patellofemoral arthritis.

Backstein and coworkers[2] reported on 40 DFOs followed a mean of 123 months. At the most recent follow-up, 24 knees (60%) had good or excellent results, 3 (7.5%) had fair results, and 3 (7.5%) had poor results. Four in the fair or poor categories were awaiting TKR and 8 (20%) had been converted to TKR. The mean Knee Society objective score improved from 18 points (range, 0–74) to 87.2 points (range, 50–100). The mean Knee Society function score improved from 54 points (range, 0–100) to 85.6 points (range, 40–100). The 10-year survival rate of the DFO was 82% (95% CI, 75%–89%) and the 15-year survival rate was 45% (95% CI, 33%–57%).

COMPLICATIONS

The complications reported for DFO are similar to those reported for HTO. It should be noted that this is mostly empirical because reports on the results of opening wedge distal femoral osteotomy in the literature are limited. Usual concerns include loss of fixation, nonunion, loss of correction, and conversion to arthroplasty. With the opening wedge technique, the authors have experienced since 2002 one distal femoral nonunion in an arthritis patient that required conversion to TKA. No loss of fixation has resulted using this technique and hardware, and thus no loss of correction has been noted on serial radiographs. Joint stiffness after osteotomy has not been an issue with rigid fixation and early mobilization, although some patients do have preexisting flexion contractures that may persist for many months. As with HTO, particular attention to avoiding flexion or extension of the osteotomy site is critical to avoid an asymmetrical opening wedge.

One concern after DFO is the potential difficulty in performing a subsequent knee replacement, if necessary. Nelson and associates[12] retrospectively evaluated the results of TKR performed after varus osteotomy of the distal part of the femur. The study group included nine patients (11 knees) with an average age of 44 years. The mean interval from osteotomy to TKR was 14 years, and the average time to follow-up after TKR was 5 years. The Knee Society score increased from 35 points before TKR to 84 points after TKR. Of note, a constrained prosthesis was required in 5 of the 11 knees. Two knees reported excellent results, 5 had a good result, and 4 had a fair result. The authors concluded that whereas TKR is effective for pain relief and improvement of function after DFO, it is technically more challenging and the results are inferior when compared with the results of primary arthroplasty performed without prior osteotomy of the knee.

In contrast to the previous report, Finklestein and colleagues[6] reported on seven knees that converted to TKR after DFVO. The authors believed that at the time of conversion, there was little or no scarring and no difficulty with exposure. Similarly, there was no difficulty gaining correct femoral alignment. The authors believed that in some patients in whom there is difficulty with soft-tissue balancing and patellar tracking because of severe valgus deformity, a varus osteotomy of the distal part of the femur could make a future TKR technically easier. It should be noted that these studies involved conversion of closing wedge osteotomies rather than of opening wedge osteotomies. This scarce and somewhat conflicting data reflect the limited experience with conversion of lateral opening wedge osteotomies to TKR.

SUMMARY

The treatment of symptomatic lateral compartment gonarthrosis with a varus-producing DFO has proved to be a successful procedure at the authors' institution. The indications for this procedure have been expanded to include unloading of an allograft performed for lateral compartment disease and genu valgum. Failure of fixation or healing of the osteotomy has not been a serious problem, with sound union usually achieved at 6 to 8 weeks. The pain relief from osteotomy can be dramatic, but usually is inferior to relief from knee arthroplasty. However, the authors believe that this is an excellent biologic solution that preserves the native joint and is an excellent surgical option for younger patients who are too active to be considered for prosthetic joint replacement. The opening wedge technique is technically less demanding than previously described techniques and may be more easily converted to TKR should this be necessary in the future.

ACKNOWLEDGMENTS

The authors would like to thank Judy Blake and Allison De Young for their assistance in preparation of this chapter.

REFERENCES

1. Andriacchi, T. P.: Dynamics of knee malalignment. *Orthop Clin North Am* 25:395–403, 1994.
2. Backstein, D.; Morag, G.; Hanna, S.; et al.: Long-term follow-up of distal femoral varus osteotomy of the knee. *J Arthroplasty* 22(4 suppl 1):2–6, 2007.
3. Cooke, T. D.; Li, J.; Scudamore, R. A.: Radiographic assessment of bony contributions to knee deformity. *Orthop Clin North Am* 25:387–393, 1994.
4. Coventry, M. B.: Proximal tibial varus osteotomy for osteoarthritis of the lateral compartment of the knee. *J Bone Joint Surg Am* 69:32–38, 1987.
5. Edgerton, B. C.; Mariani, E. M.; Morrey, B. F.: Distal femoral varus osteotomy for painful genu valgum. A five- to 11-year follow-up study. *Clin Orthop Relat Res* 288:263–269, 1993.
6. Finkelstein, J. A.; Gross, A. E.; Davis, A.: Varus osteotomy of the distal part of the femur. A survivorship analysis. *J Bone Joint Surg Am* 78:1348–1352, 1996.
7. Healy, W. L.; Anglen, J. O.; Wasilewski, S. A.; Krackow, K. A.: Distal femoral varus osteotomy. *J Bone Joint Surg Am* 70:102–109, 1988.
8. Hsu, R. W.; Himeno, S.; Coventry, M. B.; Chao, E. Y.: Normal axial alignment of the lower extremity and load-bearing distribution at the knee. *Clin Orthop Relat Res* 255:215–227, 1990.
9. Kapandji, A.: The Physiology of the Joints. II. The Lower Extremity. Philadelphia: Churchill Livingstone, 1988; p. 68.
10. McDermott, A. G.; Finklestein, J. A.; Farine, I.; et al.: Distal femoral varus osteotomy for valgus deformity of the knee. *J Bone Joint Surg Am* 70:110–116, 1988.
11. Morrey, B. F.; Edgerton, B. C.: Distal femoral osteotomy for lateral gonarthrosis. *Instr Course Lect* 41:77–85, 1992.
12. Nelson, C. L.; Saleh, K. J.; Kassim, R. A.; et al.: Total knee arthroplasty after varus osteotomy of the distal part of the femur. *J Bone Joint Surg Am* 85:1062–1065, 2003.
13. Phillips, M. J.; Krackow, K. A.: High tibial osteotomy and distal femoral osteotomy for valgus or varus deformity around the knee. *Instr Course Lect* 47:429–436, 1998.
14. Wang, J. W.; Hsu, C. C.: Distal femoral varus osteotomy for osteoarthritis of the knee. *J Bone Joint Surg Am* 87:127–133, 2005.

Rehabilitation after Tibial and Femoral Osteotomy

Frank R. Noyes, MD ■ Timothy P. Heckmann, PT, ATC ■ Sue D. Barber-Westin, BS

CLINICAL CONCEPTS

The protocol described in this chapter was designed for opening wedge high tibial osteotomy (HTO) and distal femoral osteotomy (DFO) in which an autogenous iliac crest bone graft is used along with internal fixation with a locking plate and screw. The operative techniques, detailed in Chapter 31, Primary, Double, and Triple Varus Knee Syndromes: Diagnosis, Osteotomy Techniques, and Clinical Outcomes, prevent delayed union or nonunion and collapse at the osteotomy site and allow a rehabilitation program of immediate knee motion and early weight-bearing, preventing the complications of arthrofibrosis and patella infera.[1-5] As discussed in Chapter 31, allograft instead of an iliac crest autograft is frequently used for open wedge osteotomy. In these knees, a more cautious approach is required for resuming weight-bearing because healing is delayed approximately twofold. Full weight-bearing is not allowed until the surgeon advises based on radiographic evidence of healing. In addition, the physical therapist is informed whether a locking plate and screw fixation was used because this provides more rigid fixation. If a smaller non–locking plate and screw was used, protection from weight-bearing is required until osteotomy healing is advanced. In rare cases in which the opening wedge has been compromised at the lateral tibial cortex, inducing a fracture, no weight-bearing is allowed until complete healing of the osteotomy is verified.

Patients receive instructions before surgery regarding the postoperative protocol so they have a thorough understanding of what is expected after the procedure. The supervised rehabilitation program is supplemented with home exercises that are performed daily. The therapist routinely examines the patient in the clinic postoperatively in order to progress the patient through the protocol in a safe and effective manner. Therapeutic procedures and modalities are used as required to achieve a successful outcome.

The overall goals of the osteotomy and rehabilitation are to control joint pain, swelling, and hemarthrosis; regain normal knee flexion and extension; resume a normal gait pattern and neuromuscular stability for ambulation; regain lower extremity

---

Critical Points CLINICAL CONCEPTS

- Protocol designed for opening wedge high tibial osteotomy and distal femoral osteotomy
  - Autogenous iliac crest bone graft, internal fixation with locking plate and screw.
  - Allograft bone graft, delayed weight-bearing until radiographic evidence healing.
- Immediate knee motion, early weight-bearing prevent arthrofibrosis and patella infera.
- Preoperative patient education essential.
- Program is supervised, patient performs exercises at home daily.

Goals

- Control joint pain, swelling, hemarthrosis.
- Regain normal knee flexion and extension.
- Resume normal gait pattern and neuromuscular stability for ambulation.
- Regain lower extremity muscle strength, proprioception, balance, coordination.
- Achieve optimal functional outcome based on orthopaedic and patient goals.

Prophylaxis for Deep Vein Thrombosis

- Intermittent compression foot boots in both extremities.
- Immediate knee motion exercises.
- Antiembolism stockings.
- Ankle pumps performed hourly.
- Aspirin.

muscle strength, proprioception, balance, and coordination for desired activities; and achieve the optimal functional outcome based on orthopaedic and patient goals.

Immediately after surgery, the lower limb is wrapped with cotton with additional padding placed posteriorly, followed by a double compression and cotton bandage, postoperative hinged brace, and bilateral ankle-foot compression boots. A commercial ice delivery system is used with the bladder incorporated over the initial cotton wrapping, a few layers from the wound. The neurovascular status is checked immediately in the operating room and carefully monitored in the initial postoperative period. A calf or foot compression system is used for the first 24 hours to promote venous blood flow. Aspirin is prescribed and, rarely in high-risk patients, low-molecular-weight heparin (LMWH) or warfarinsodium (Coumadin; Bristol-Myers Squibb Co., Plainsboro, NJ). During the 1st postoperative week, patients are ambulatory for short periods of time, but are instructed to elevate their limb, remain home, and not resume usual activities.

Prophylaxis for deep venous thrombosis (DVT) includes intermittent compression foot boots in both extremities, immediate knee motion exercises, antiembolism stockings, ankle pumps performed hourly, and aspirin (600 mg/day for 10 days). Doppler ultrasound is obtained if a patient demonstrates abnormal calf tenderness, a positive Homans sign, or increased edema.

Important postoperative signs to monitor include (Table 33–1):

■ Loss of correction, reoccurrence of varus or valgus malalignment.
■ Delayed union or nonunion.
■ Swelling of the knee joint or soft tissues.
■ Abnormal pain response, increased pain with weight-bearing.
■ Abnormal gait pattern.
■ Insufficient flexion or extension, limited patellar mobility.
■ Weakness (strength/control) of the lower extremity.
■ Insufficient lower extremity flexibility.
■ Peroneal nerve palsy.
■ DVT (calf pain, Homans', tibial edema).

TABLE 33–1 Postoperative Signs and Symptoms Requiring Prompt Treatment

Postoperative Sign, Symptom	Treatment Recommendations
Failure to meet knee extension and flexion goals (see text)	Overpressure program, early gentle manipulation under anesthesia if 0°–135° not met by 6 wk postoperatively.
Decreased patellar mobility (indicative of early arthrofibrosis)	Aggressive knee flexion, extension overpressure program, or gentle manipulation under anesthesia to regain full knee ROM and normal patellar mobility.
Decrease in voluntary quadriceps contraction and muscle tone, advancing muscle atrophy	Aggressive quadriceps muscle–strengthening program, EMS.
Persistent joint effusion, joint inflammation	Aspiration, rule out infection, close physician observation.
Loss of angular correction	Immediate referral to physician for revision.
DVT: abnormal calf tenderness, a positive Homans sign, or increased edema	Immediate ultrasound evaluation.

DVT, deep venous thrombosis; EMS, electrical muscle stimulation; ROM, range of motion.

POSTOPERATIVE REHABILITATION PROTOCOL

Modalities

The postoperative rehabilitation protocol after tibial and femoral osteotomy is summarized in Table 33–2. In the immediate postoperative period, knee pain and effusion must be controlled to avoid quadriceps muscle inhibition or shutdown.

Critical Points POSTOPERATIVE REHABILITATION PROTOCOL

Modalities
• Electrogalvanic stimulation or high-voltage electrical muscle stimulation.
• Biofeedback therapy.
• Cryotherapy.

Postoperative Bracing and Weight-Bearing
• Long-leg brace 8–12 wk.
• Unloading brace if required.
• Immediate toe-touch weight-bearing.
• 25% weight-bearing 4 wk, based on x-ray.
• Full weight-bearing 8–10 wk.

Range of Knee Motion
• Regain 0°–90° within first 2 wk. If unsuccessful, placed into overpressure program.
• Goals knee flexion: 110° by 3–4 wk, 130° by 5–6 wk, 135° by 7–8 wk.

Patellar Mobilization
• Patellar glide performed in all four planes beginning 1st postoperative day with sustained pressure applied to the appropriate patellar border for at least 10 sec.
• Done for 8 wk postoperative.

Flexibility
• Hamstring, gastrocnemius-soleus begun 1st day after surgery.
• Quadriceps, iliotibial band begun 9th postoperative wk.

Strengthening
• Quadriceps isometrics, straight leg raises hip flexion plane 1st day after surgery.
• Straight leg plus exercise.
• Toe-raises 3rd–4th wk as tolerated.
• Closed kinetic chain 5th–6th wk.
• 7–8 wk: lateral step-ups, hip machine.

Balance, Proprioceptive, and Perturbation Training
• Cup-walking when partial weight-bearing.
• Weight-shifting when full weight-bearing.
• Double-, single-leg balance exercises.
• Perturbation training.
• Walking half foam rolls.
• Balance board.

Conditioning and Return to Activities
• Upper body cycle as soon as tolerated.
• Stationary bicycling, water-walking 5–6 wk.
• Cross-country ski, elliptical, and stair-climbing machines 9–12 wk.
• Return to only light, low-impact activities recommended.

TABLE 33–2   Rehabilitation after High Tibial or Femoral Osteotomy

	Postoperative Weeks					Postoperative Months		
	1–2	3–4	5–6	7–8	9–12	4	5	6
Brace								
Long-leg postoperative	X	X	X	X	X			
Unloading						(X)*	(X)*	(X)*
Range of motion minimum goals								
0°–110°	X							
0°–130°		X						
0°–135°			X					
Weight-bearing								
None to toe-touch	X	X						
25%–50% body weight			X					
Full (fracture site healed)				X	(X)*			
Patella mobilization	X	X	X	X				
Modalities								
EMS	X	X	X	X				
Pain/edema management (cryotherapy)	X	X	X	X	X	X	X	X
Stretching								
Hamstring, gastrocnemius-soleus, iliotibial band, quadriceps	X	X	X	X	X	X	X	X
Strengthening								
Quadriceps isometrics, straight leg raises, active knee extension	X	X	X	X	X			
Closed chain: gait retraining, toe-raises, wall-sits, mini-squats		(X)*	X	X	X	X		
Knee flexion hamstring curls (90°)				X	X	X	X	X
Knee extension quads (90°–30°)				X	X	X	X	X
Hip abduction adduction, multi-hip				X	X	X	X	X
Leg press (70°-10°)			X	X	X	X	X	X
Balance/proprioceptive training								
Weight-shifting, minitrampoline, BAPS, BBS, plyometrics				X	X	X	X	X
Conditioning								
UBC		X	X	X				
Bike (stationary)				X	X	X	X	X
Aquatic program			X	X	X	X	X	X
Swimming (kicking)					X	X	X	X
Walking					X	X	X	X
Stair-climbing machine					X	X	X	X
Ski machine					X	X	X	X
Recreational activities								X

*(X), see text—based on patient symptoms, function, resumption of weight-bearing, fracture site healing.
BAPS, Biomechanical Ankle Platform System (Camp, Jackson, MI); BBS, Biodex Balance System (Biodex Medical Systems, Inc., Shirley, NY); UBC. upper body cycle (Biodex Medical Systems, Inc., Shirley, NY).

Electrogalvanic stimulation or high-voltage electrical muscle stimulation (EMS) may be used to augment ice, compression, and elevation to control swelling. The treatment duration is approximately 30 minutes and the intensity is set to patient tolerance.

Once the joint effusion is controlled, functional EMS is begun for muscle reeducation and facilitation of an adequate quadriceps contraction. One electrode is placed over the vastus medialis obliquus and the second electrode is placed on the central to lateral aspect of the upper third of the quadriceps muscle belly. The patient is instructed to actively contract the quadriceps muscle simultaneously with the machine's stimulation. The treatment duration is 20 minutes. A portable EMS machine for use at home may be required in individuals whose muscle rating is poor. EMS is continued until the muscle grade is rated as good.

Biofeedback therapy is an important adjunct to facilitate an adequate quadriceps muscle contraction early postoperatively. The surface electrode is placed over the selected muscle component to provide feedback to the patient and the clinician regarding the quality of active or voluntary quadriceps contraction. Biofeedback is also useful in enhancing hamstring relaxation if the patient experiences difficulty achieving full knee extension secondary to knee pain or muscle spasm. The electrode is placed over the belly of the hamstring muscle while the patient performs range of motion exercises.

Cryotherapy is begun immediately after surgery. The standard method is an ice bag or commercial cold pack. However, patients prefer motorized cooler units because they maintain a constant temperature and circulation of ice water, which provides excellent pain control. Gravity flow units are also effective;

however, temperature maintenance is more difficult with these devices than with the motorized cooler units. Cryotherapy is used from three times a day to every waking hour for 20 minutes at a time depending upon the extent of pain and swelling. In some cases, the treatment time is extended owing to the thickness of the buffer that exists between the skin and the device. Cryotherapy is typically done after exercise or when required for pain and swelling control and is maintained throughout the entire postoperative rehabilitation protocol.

Postoperative Bracing and Weight-Bearing

A long-leg postoperative brace is worn for the first 8 to 12 weeks postoperatively. Patients then discontinue use of the brace, but if they continue to experience pain, Visco heel pads are used to unload the affected compartment. A lateral wedge is used for patients who underwent HTO, whereas a medial wedge is used for those who had a DFO. If pain remains, an unloading brace, used initially in a neutral position and then adjusted based on patient response, is recommended (Fig. 33–1).

Initially, patients are allowed only toe-touch weight-bearing. They are encouraged during this time period to lightly touch the ground with the toes of the operated limb while standing, with the visual image of stepping on a sponge, as frequently as possible during the day. At 4 weeks postoperative, double-stance, full-length antero-posterior radiographs are taken to determine osteotomy healing. Patients are then allowed to bear 25% of their body weight if the radiographs demonstrate adequate healing and maintenance of the osteotomy position and fixation implant (Fig. 33–2). A normal gait pattern is advocated that encourages normal knee flexion throughout the gait cycle. This technique allows for normal patterning of heel-

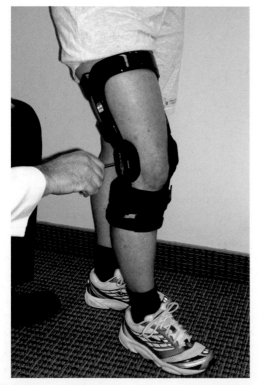

FIGURE 33–1. An unloading brace may be used and adjusted based on patient pain response.

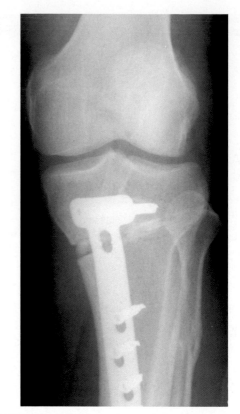

FIGURE 33–2. Postoperative anteroposterior radiograph after opening wedge tibial osteotomy with an iliac crest autograft and locking plate–screw fixation shows beginning healing and maintenance of the fixation position, although full activities are possible only with complete filling-in of the osteotomy gap.

to-toe ambulation, quadriceps contraction during midstance, and hip and knee flexion during the gait cycle. Average healing of the fracture site occurs at approximately 8 to 10 weeks postoperatively. In patients in whom allograft bone is used to fill the osteotomy gap, an additional delay in full weight-bearing may be required for up to 12 weeks postoperatively to allow for bony consolidation.

Range of Knee Motion

The postoperative goals for knee flexion and extension are shown in Table 33–3. Patients are encouraged to regain 0° to 90° within the first 2 weeks. Patients perform passive and active range of motion exercises in a seated position for 10 minutes a session, approximately three to four times per day.

Patients that have difficulty regaining at least 0° by the 2nd week are placed into an overpressure program using a propped foot/ankle position (Fig. 33–3). This position is maintained for 10 minutes and repeated four to six times per day. A 10-pound weight may be added to the distal thigh and knee to provide overpressure to stretch the posterior capsule. If this method is not successful in achieving full extension, or if the clinician notes a firm end feel, an extension board or additional weight of 15 to 20 pounds may be used up to six times a day.

Knee flexion is gradually increased to 110° by the 3rd to 4th postoperative week, 130° by the 5th to 6th week, and 135° by the 7th to 8th week. Methods to assist in achieving flexion greater than 90° include chair-rolling, wall-slides, knee flexion devices, and passive quadriceps stretching exercises (Fig. 33–4).

TABLE 33–3   Range of Motion, Flexibility, and Modality Usage after Osteotomy

Time Postoperative, Frequency	Extension-Flexion Limits	Patellar Mobilization	Flexibility (5 reps x 20 sec)	Electrical Muscle Stimulation (20 min)	Cryotherapy (20 min)
1–2 wk 3–4 x/day, 10-min sessions	0°–90°	Medial-lateral Superior-inferior	Hamstring, gastrocnemius-soleus	Yes	Yes
3–4 wk 3–4 x/day, 10-min sessions	0°–110°	Medial-lateral Superior-inferior	Hamstring, gastrocnemius-soleus	Yes	Yes
5–6 wk 3 x/day, 10-min sessions	0°–130°	Medial-lateral Superior-inferior	Hamstring, gastrocnemius-soleus	Yes	Yes
7–8 wk 2 x/day, 10-min sessions	0°–135°	(If required)	Hamstring, gastrocnemius-soleus	Yes	Yes
9–52 wk 2 x/day, 10-min sessions	(Should be full)		Hamstring, gastrocnemius-soleus, quadriceps, iliotibial band		Yes

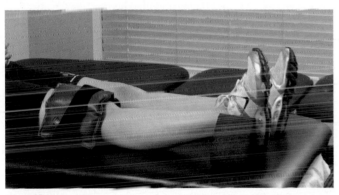

FIGURE 33–3. Overpressure extension exercise.

Patellar Mobilization

The resumption of normal patellar mobility is critical to regain a normal range of knee motion. The loss of patellar mobility is often associated with arthrofibrosis and, in extreme cases, the development of patella infera. Patellar glides are performed in all four planes (superior, inferior, medial, and lateral) beginning the 1st postoperative day with sustained pressure applied to the appropriate patellar border for at least 10 seconds (Fig. 33–5). This exercise is done for 5 minutes before range of motion exercises. Caution is warranted if an extensor lag is detected because this may be associated with poor superior migration of the patella, indicating the need for additional emphasis on this exercise. Patellar mobilization is performed for approximately 8 weeks postoperatively.

Flexibility

Hamstring and gastrocnemius-soleus flexibility exercises are begun the 1st day after surgery. A sustained static stretch is held for 30 seconds and repeated five times. Common methods for stretching these muscle groups include the modified hurdler

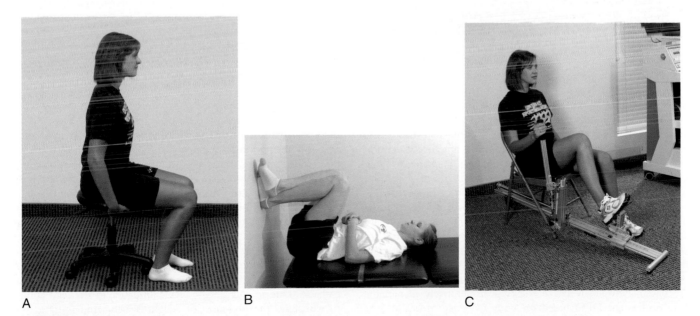

A   B   C

FIGURE 33–4. Flexion overpressure exercise options include rolling stool (**A**), wall-slides (**B**), and commercial devices (**C**).

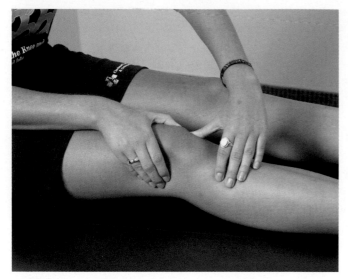

FIGURE 33–5. Patellar mobilization.

stretch and the towel pull. These exercises help control pain due to the reflex response created in the hamstrings when the knee is maintained in the flexed position. As well, the towel-pulling exercise can help lessen discomfort in the calf, Achilles tendon, and ankle. Quadriceps and iliotibial band flexibility exercises are begun at the 9th postoperative week.

Strengthening

The strengthening program is begun on the 1st postoperative day (Table 33–4). Isometric quadriceps contractions are done hourly using the repetition rules of 10-second holds, 10 repetitions, 10 times per day. The patient is taught to monitor the contractions by visual or manual means, comparing the quality with those achieved by the contralateral limb. The superior migration of the patella is observed and should be approximately 1 cm during contractions, with inferior migration also seen during the initial relaxation of the contraction. The knee is held in a slightly flexed position during isometric contractions. Biofeedback may be used to reinforce an adequate quadriceps contraction.

Open kinetic chain extension exercises are incorporated within the first few weeks to further develop quadriceps muscle strength. Caution is warranted owing to the potential problems these exercises may create for the patellofemoral joint. Resisted knee extension is begun with Velcro ankle weights from 90° to 30°. The terminal phase of extension is avoided owing to the high forces placed on the patellofemoral joint. The patellofemoral joint must be monitored for changes in pain, swelling, and crepitus to avoid a patellar conversion in which painful patellofemoral crepitus develops with articular cartilage damage.

Straight leg raises are begun the 1st postoperative day in the hip flexion plane (supine position) only. These exercises are advanced to include the hip extension plane during the 3rd week. Patients who underwent HTO begin straight leg raises in the abduction/adduction planes between 4 and 6 weeks postoperatively based on x-ray evidence of healing. These exercises are begun between 6 and 8 weeks postoperatively in patients who underwent DFO based on x-ray evidence of healing. As these exercises become easy to perform, ankle weights are added

to progress muscle strengthening. Initially, 1 to 2 pounds of weight are used, and eventually, up to 10 pounds is added as long as this is not more than 10% of the patient's body weight. Initially, weight is applied above the patella to control forces to the healing fracture. The use of rubber tubing to provide increased resistance may also be of benefit starting at the 7th to 8th postoperative week.

Another common exercise effective in helping with quadriceps reeducation is the straight leg plus raise (Fig. 33–6). The quadriceps is contracted, the leg is lifted approximately 6 inches off the table or chair, held in the lifted position for 15 seconds, and then lowered and relaxed for 45 seconds. This 1-minute cycle is maintained and progressed in ratios (1:3, 1:2, and eventually, 1:1), and then progressed from 5 to 10 repetitions, with additional ankle weight added to increase the difficulty of the exercise.

Toe-raises are begun during the 3rd to 4th week as tolerated. Closed kinetic chain exercises may be initiated during the 5th to 6th week. Mini-squats from 0° to 45° are begun when tolerated by the patient. Initially, the patient's body weight is used as resistance, and gradually, TheraBand or surgical tubing is added for resistance (Fig. 33–7). Quick, smooth, rhythmic squats are performed to a high-set/high-repetition cadence to promote muscle fatigue. Wall-sitting exercises are also begun during this time period. The goal of wall-sitting is to improve quadriceps contraction by performing the exercise to muscle exhaustion. If anterior knee pain is experienced, either the knee flexion angle of the sit or the toe-out/toe-in angle is altered. The exercise may also be modified by the patient squeezing a ball between the distal thighs, holding dumbbell weights, or shifting the body weight over the involved side to stimulate a single-leg contraction. This exercise is promoted as an excellent one to perform at home four to six times a day to achieve quadriceps fatigue in a knee flexion angle that does not induce anterior knee pain. Leg press exercises in the range of 70° to 10° are begun during this time period as well.

Lateral step-ups are initiated when the patient has achieved full weight-bearing, at approximately 7 to 8 weeks. The height of the step is gradually increased based on patient tolerance. Strengthening is also initiated during this time for hip abductors, adductors, flexors, and extensors by using either a multi-hip or cable system machine, or a hip abductor/adductor machine. Hamstring curls on a weight machine are begun at 9 to 12 weeks postoperative.

Balance, Proprioceptive, and Perturbation Training

Cup-walking is an exercise that promotes symmetry between the surgical and the uninvolved limbs. This exercise helps develop hip and knee flexion and quadriceps control during midstance of gait to prevent knee hyperextension (see Chapter 34, Correction of Hyperextension Gait Abnormalities: Preoperative and Postoperative Techniques). In addition, cup-walking controls hip and pelvic motion during midstance, gastrocnemius-soleus activity during push-off, and excessive hip hiking (Fig. 33–8). This exercise may be initiated during the partial weight-bearing phase.

Balance and proprioceptive training are initiated when the patient has resumed full weight-bearing. Initially, the patient stands and shifts the body weight from side-to-side and front-to-back. This activity encourages confidence in the leg's ability to withstand the pressures of weight-bearing and initiates the stimulus to knee joint position sense.

TABLE 33–4   Muscle Strengthening Exercises after Osteotomy

Time Postoperative, Frequency	Quadriceps Isometrics (Active)	Straight Leg Raises	Knee Extension (Active-Assisted) 90°–30°	Toe-Raises	Wall-Sits (To Fatigue)	Mini-Squats	Lateral Step-ups (5- to 10-cm Block)	Hamstring Curls (0°–90°)	Multi-Hip (Flex, Ext, Abd, Add)	Leg Press (70°–10°)
1–2 wk 3 x/day 15 min	1 set x 10 reps (every hr)	Flex, 3 sets x 10 reps	3 sets x 10 reps							
3–4 wk 2–3 x/day 20 min	Multiangle 0°, 60° 1 set x 10 reps each	Flex, ext, 3 sets x 10 reps	3 sets x 10 reps	3 sets x 10 reps						
5–6 wk 2 x/day 20 min	Multiangle 30°, 60°, 90° 2 sets x 10 reps	Add ankle weight ≤ 10% of body weight, 3 sets x 10 reps	Active 3 sets x 10 reps	3 sets x 10 reps	3 sets to fatigue	3 sets to fatigue				3 sets x 10 reps
7–8 wk 2 x/day 20 min		Add abd, add, 3 sets x 10 reps Add rubber tubing, 3 sets x 30 reps	Active 3 sets x 10 reps	3 sets x 10 reps	3 sets to fatigue	3 sets to fatigue Add rubber tubing, 0°–30°	3 sets x 10 reps		3 sets x 10 reps	3 sets x 10 reps
9–12 wk 2 x/day 20 min		3 sets x 10 reps Rubber tubing, 3 sets x 30 reps	With resistance, 3 sets x 10 reps	3 sets x 10 reps	3 sets to fatigue	Add rubber tubing, 0°–40°, 3 sets x 20 reps	3 sets x 10 reps	Active, 3 sets x 10 reps	3 sets x 10 reps	3 sets x 10 reps
13–26 wk 2 x/day 20 min		Rubber tubing, high speed, 3 sets x 30 reps	With resistance, 3 sets x 10 reps			3 sets x 20 reps		Active, 3 sets x 10 reps	3 sets x 10 reps	3 sets x 10 reps

abd, abduction; add, adduction; ext, extension; flex, flexion.

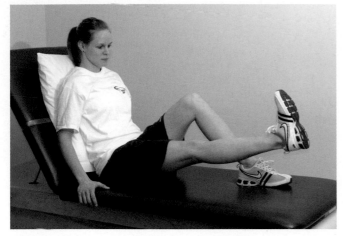

FIGURE 33–6. The straight leg raise plus exercise.

Double- and single-leg balance exercises in the stance position are also beneficial. During the single-leg exercise, the foot is pointed straight ahead, the knee flexed 20° to 30°, the arms extended outward to horizontal, and the torso positioned upright with the shoulders above the hips and the hips above the ankles. The patient is encouraged to remain in this position until balance is disturbed. A minitrampoline or unstable platform may be used to make this exercise more difficult. Patients may assume the single-leg stance position and throw or catch a weighted ball against an inverted minitrampoline until fatigue occurs.

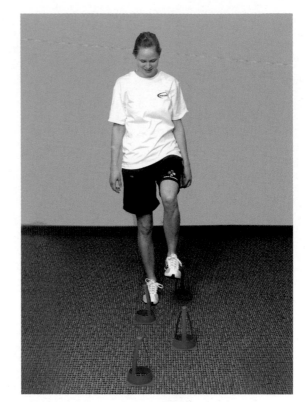

FIGURE 33–8. Cup- (or cone-) walking.

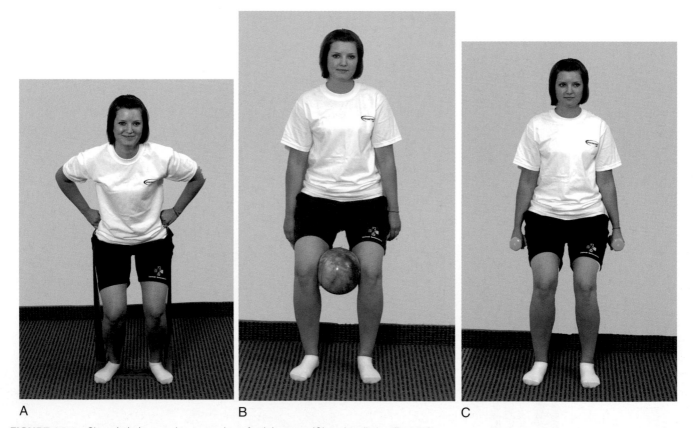

A   B   C

FIGURE 33–7. Closed chain exercise examples of mini-squats (**A**) and wall-sits (**B** and **C**).

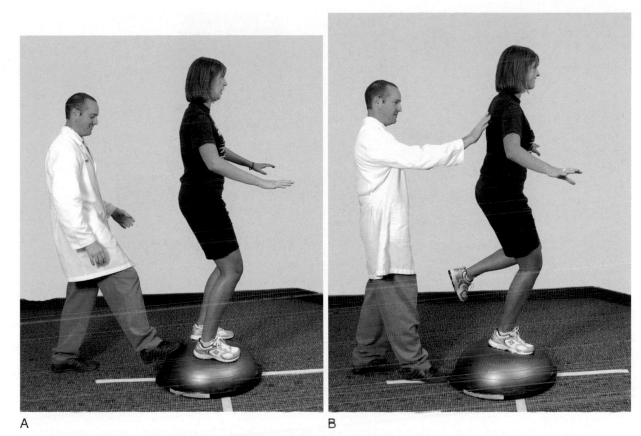

A   B

FIGURE 33–9. A and B, Perturbation-training techniques.

Perturbation-training techniques are also performed during balance exercises. The therapist stands behind the patient and disrupts her or his body posture and position periodically to enhance dynamic knee stability (Fig. 33–9). The techniques involve either direct contact with the patient or disruption of the platform the patient is standing on, and the patient is then instructed to correct the unbalanced position.

Half foam rolls are also used in this time period as part of the gait-retraining and balance program (Fig. 33–10A). This technique helps the patient develop balance and dynamic muscular control required to maintain an upright position and be able to walk from one end of the roll to the other. Use of a balance board or other unstable platform in double-leg and single-leg stance is another effective measure (see Fig. 33–10B). Developing a center of balance, limb symmetry, quadriceps control in midstance, and postural positioning are benefits obtained from this type of training.

Conditioning and Return to Activities

Depending on accessibility, a cardiovascular program with an upper body cycle may be initiated as soon as tolerated by the patient (Table 33–5). The surgical limb should be elevated to minimize lower extremity swelling. Stationary bicycling is begun during the 5th to 6th postoperative weeks. Water-walking is also begun during this time period.

Cross-country ski, elliptical, and stair-climbing machines are permitted 9 to 12 weeks postoperatively. Protection against high stresses to the patellofemoral joint is required. The seat height of the bicycle is adjusted to its highest level based on patient body size, and a low resistance level is recommended. Stair-climbing machines are adjusted to produce a short step with low resistance. An aquatic program that includes lap work using freestyle or flutter kicking, water-walking, and water aerobics is encouraged if the patient has access to a pool. In order to improve cardiovascular endurance, the program should be done at least three times per week for 20 to 30 minutes, with the exercise performed to at least 60% to 85% of maximal heart rate.

The majority of patients who undergo HTO or DFO are advised to return to only light, low-impact activities to maintain an active and healthy lifestyle and weight control. Patients who express the desire to return to higher-impact sports activities are advised of the risk of further cartilage deterioration if damage was noted during the operation. Because the usual goal of osteotomy is to buy time before the necessity for a partial or total joint replacement, participation in high-loading activities is discouraged.

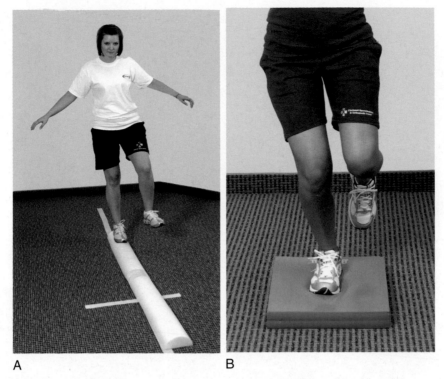

A   B

FIGURE 33–10. Balance training techniques include walking on half foam roll (**A**) and single-leg stance on an unstable surface (**B**).

TABLE 33–5   Aerobic Conditioning Exercises after Osteotomy

Time Postoperative, Frequency	Upper Body Cycle	Bicycle (Stationary)	Water-Walking	Swimming	Walking	Stair-Climbing Machine (Low Resistance, Low Stroke)	Ski Machine (Short Stride, Level, Low Resistance)
3–4 wk 1–2 x/day	10 min						
5–6 wk 2 x/day	10 min	10 min	10 min				
7–8 wk 1–2 x/day	15 min	15 min	15 min				
9–12 wk 1 x/day (select one activity per session)		15–20 min	15–20 min	15–20 min	15–20 min	15–20 min	15–20 min
13–26 wk 3 x/wk (select one activity per session)		20 min	20 min	20 min	20 min	20 min	20 min

REFERENCES

1. Noyes, F. R.; Mayfield, W.; Barber-Westin, S. D.; et al.: Opening wedge high tibial osteotomy: an operative technique and rehabilitation program to decrease complications and promote early union and function. *Am J Sports Med* 34:1262–1273, 2006.
2. Noyes, F. R.; Wojtys, E. M.; Marshall, M. T.: The early diagnosis and treatment of developmental patella infera syndrome. *Clin Orthop* 265:241–252, 1991.
3. Noyes, F. R.; Barber, S. D.; Simon, R.: High tibial osteotomy and ligament reconstruction in varus angulated, anterior cruciate ligament-deficient knees. A two to seven year follow-up study. *Am J Sports Med* 21:2–12, 1993.
4. Noyes, F. R.; Barber-Westin, S. D.; Hewett, T. E.: High tibial osteotomy and ligament reconstruction for varus angulated anterior cruciate ligament deficient knees. *Am J Sports Med* 28:282–296, 2000.
5. Noyes, F. R.; Berrios-Torres, S.; Barber-Westin, S. D.; Heckmann, T. P.: Prevention of permanent arthrofibrosis after anterior cruciate ligament reconstruction alone or combined with associated procedures: A prospective study in 443 knees. *Knee Surg Sports Traumat Arthrosc* 8:196–206, 2000.

Chapter 34

Correction of Hyperextension Gait Abnormalities: Preoperative and Postoperative Techniques

Timothy P. Heckmann, PT, ATC ■ *Frank R. Noyes*, MD ■ *Sue D. Barber-Westin*, BS

INTRODUCTION AND DIAGNOSIS

It is well appreciated that patients with chronic insufficiency of the lateral and posterolateral structures of the knee may develop a gait abnormality characterized by excessive knee hyperextension during the stance phase (initial contact or heel-strike, loading response, midstance, and toe-off) of the gait cycle (Fig. 34–1). The primary lateral and posterolateral structures of the knee joint are the fibular collateral ligament (FCL) and popliteus muscle-tendon ligament unit (PMTL), including the popliteofibular ligament (PFL) and the posterolateral capsule (PLC). These structures function together to resist lateral tibiofemoral compartment opening, posterior subluxation of the lateral tibial plateau with tibial rotation, knee hyperextension, and varus recurvatum (see Chapter 20, Function of the Posterior Cruciate Ligament and Posterolateral Ligament Structures).[8,9,12,13,19,26] Posterolateral injuries are frequently accompanied by a rupture to the anterior cruciate ligament (ACL) and, in some cases, a rupture to the posterior cruciate ligament (PCL).[5,7,11] In addition, many knees with insufficiency to the posterolateral structures also have varus osseous malalignment. The comprehensive physical examination and radiographic evaluation required to determine all of the abnormalities that exist in these complex knee joint injuries are detailed in Chapter 21, Posterior Cruciate Ligament: Diagnosis, Operative Techniques, and Clinical Outcomes, and 31, Primary, Double, and Triple Varus Knee Syndromes: Diagnosis, Osteotomy Techniques, and Clinical Outcomes.

The gait abnormality described in this chapter is easily identifiable in the clinic if the examiner devotes a small amount of time to observation during the initial patient presentation. An abnormal knee hyperextension gait pattern involves increased extension (>0°) in the sagittal plane and, frequently, associated varus malalignment in the coronal plane (varus recurvatum). The varus recurvatum position of the knee will be markedly worse if there is associated osseous tibiofemoral varus malalignment. The *triple varus knee*, described in detail in Chapter 31,

Critical Points INTRODUCTION AND DIAGNOSIS

- Patients with chronic insufficiency of the lateral and posterolateral structures may develop a gait abnormality characterized by excessive knee hyperextension during the stance phase of the gait cycle.
- Gait abnormality is easily identifiable in the clinic: increased extension (>0°) in the sagittal plane, associated varus recurvatum.
- Patients with knee hyperextension gait problems present with varying amounts of altered gait mechanics, symptoms, and functional limitations.
- Degree of the gait abnormality during the stance phase depends on the magnitude of associated ligamentous deficiencies, quadriceps muscle atrophy, and symptomatic patellofemoral arthrosis.
- Complaints of either partial or full giving-way during routine daily activities are frequent.
- Pain is in medial compartment, posterolateral tissues.
- Increased risk of failure of cruciate and posterolateral reconstructions exists if the gait abnormality is not corrected before surgery.

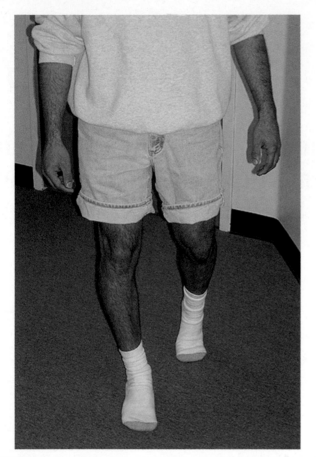

FIGURE 34–1. A lower limb varus deformity and hyperextension gait abnormality are evident in this 32-year-old man with chronic deficiency of the posterolateral structures and varus malalignment.

Primary, Double, and Triple Varus Knee Syndromes: Diagnosis, Osteotomy Techniques, and Clinical Outcomes, refers to varus alignment caused by three factors: tibiofemoral varus osseous malalignment, increased lateral tibiofemoral compartment separation due to marked insufficiency of the FCL and PMTL, and varus recurvatum in extension. An abnormal increase in hyperextension usually indicates damage to not only the posterolateral structures but the ACL as well.

Some knees with uninjured but physiologically slack posterolateral structures demonstrate a passive varus recurvatum and excessive knee hyperextension. After a knee injury or muscle atrophy of any cause, the patient may demonstrate a hyperextension gait pattern due to muscle weakness. Other patients with symptomatic patellofemoral arthrosis develop a hyperextension gait pattern to avoid knee flexion that loads the patellofemoral joint and causes anterior knee pain. These patients are the most difficult to manage, because the knee arthrosis symptoms require treatment to relieve the painful state in addition to correcting quadriceps weakness and the knee hyperextension gait pattern.

In the authors' experience, patients with knee hyperextension gait problems present with varying amounts of altered gait mechanics, symptoms, and functional limitations. Some may demonstrate a markedly abnormal gait that is severely disabling and limits ambulation, requiring crutch or cane support. Others may have a less noticeable alteration, with the abnormal knee hyperextension occurring only after excessive walking (or other weight-bearing activities) and muscle fatigue. The degree of

the gait abnormality during the stance phase depends on the magnitude of associated ligamentous deficiencies, quadriceps muscle atrophy, and symptomatic patellofemoral arthrosis.

Subjective complaints of knee instability of either partial or full giving-way during routine daily activities often accompany the knee hyperextension gait abnormality. Pain is frequently located in the medial tibiofemoral compartment, which is caused by increased compressive forces owing to the varus malalignment. Pain in the posterolateral tissues also occurs from increased soft tissue tensile forces. In addition to the pain and instability caused by this gait pattern, there is an increased risk of failure of posterolateral reconstructions if the gait abnormality is not corrected before surgery. This is due to the excessively high tensile forces from high knee extension and adduction moments that are expected to be resumed during weight-bearing activities after surgery.[16] In addition, patients with associated ACL or PCL deficiency may have an increased risk of failure of cruciate ligament reconstructions if the hyperextension pattern is not corrected before surgery.[14,15] Therefore, gait retraining and avoidance of the gait hyperextension pattern are paramount for both resolution of patient symptoms and reduction of the risk of failure of soft tissue ligament reconstructive procedures.

Many investigators have described a quadriceps-avoidance abnormal gait pattern in patients with ACL ruptures.[1,2,6,18,20,27] An investigation at the authors' center[18] documented diminished quadriceps activity and enhanced hamstring muscle activity in one half of 32 ACL-deficient varus-angulated knees. Whereas the increased hamstring muscle force could be assumed to be beneficial because it provides a protective mechanism in decreasing anterior tibial translation, the increased muscle force creates high axial compressive forces and, therefore, increases medial and lateral joint compartment (calculated) loads. These loads could be deleterious to the joint over the long term, especially in knees with associated varus osseous malalignment. The abnormal gait characteristics of the ACL-deficient knee are discussed in detail in Chapter 6, Human Movements and ACL Function: ACL-Deficiency and Gait Mechanics.

A hyperextension gait abnormality pattern is also found in patients who have suffered a stroke or traumatic brain injury, cerebral palsy, and poliomyelitis.[10] In these instances, the disorder may occur owing to many factors including quadriceps weakness, ankle plantar flexion spasticity, heel cord contracture, and gastrocnemius-soleus weakness. The concern is that the abnormal knee hyperextension may cause stretching of the posterior ligamentous and capsular structures from the increased external extensor torque that is placed across the knee during stance. It is not the purpose of this chapter to discuss the treatment of this problem in patients with neurologic pathology. Rather, this chapter focuses on the treatment of this gait disorder in patients with chronic insufficiency of the posterolateral structures, with or without cruciate ligament ruptures or varus malalignment.

ABNORMAL KNEE HYPEREXTENSION PATTERNS

The normal pattern of knee motion that occurs during the gait cycle is shown in Figure 34–2. A detailed description of normal human gait mechanics is beyond the scope of this chapter and has been presented by many authors.[3,4,21,24,25] The loss of the normal knee flexion and extension patterns throughout the stance phase noted in patients with hyperextension gait abnormalities has important functional implications. During the loading response, normal amounts of knee flexion are required for the knee joint to absorb shock. A limb that is instead hyperextended transfers body weight directly from the femur to the tibia, resulting in abnormally high compressive forces. The usual muscle energy absorption and cushioning effect a flexed knee provides is lost.[22,23] The thrusting hyperextension motion at the knee is associated with an abnormally high adduction moment, which tends to increase medial tibiofemoral compartment compressive forces and lateral distraction forces. The increased compressive forces manifest as pain in the medial tibiofemoral compartment and posterolateral soft tissues.

The authors have reported two distinct knee hyperextension gait patterns. In *pattern I*, the abnormal hyperextension occurs during two periods of the stance phase, heel-strike and terminal extension (Fig. 34–3), with knee flexion noted during the loading response. Exceedingly high knee extension moments are present, along with an abnormal reversal of hip extension and ankle dorsiflexion. *Pattern II* is characterized by a prolonged knee hyperextension pattern from heel-strike throughout

midstance (Fig. 34–4). In these patients, the knee flexion moment is markedly below normal, with its effects incurred primarily at the knee with only a slight delay in ankle dorsiflexion.

The authors' clinical observations[17] on the various types of abnormal knee motions and thrusts in the sagittal, coronal, and transverse rotational planes that occur during the stance phase of gait are summarized in Table 34–1. Any abnormality in tibiofemoral alignment (varus-valgus osseous malalignment or anterior-posterior tibial slope) may affect knee-thrusting motions in the sagittal or coronal plane. The most common of these is a varus-thrusting gait abnormality, caused by a varus tibiofemoral osseous malalignment. The thrusting motion occurs with the knee near full extension immediately after heel-strike, during the loading response. There may be an associated external or internal rotational subluxation with the varus thrust, depending on the presence of associated deficiency to the posterolateral structures. A less common abnormality, a valgus-thrusting gait, is usually associated with valgus lower limb malalignment. This disorder is typically accompanied by external rotation of the tibia. Knees with these osseous malalignments and associated knee ligament deficiencies require surgical correction of the malalignment by osteotomy prior to ligament reconstructive procedures.

GAIT-RETRAINING PROGRAM FOR ABNORMAL KNEE HYPEREXTENSION

A gait-retraining program has been successfully used at the authors' center[17] for knee hyperextension abnormalities since the mid-1980s. The program requires two to four initial clinical sessions (held preferably every other week) with an experienced physical therapist to instruct the patient on the abnormal gait mechanics that occur and the adaptations required to restore a normal gait pattern (Table 34–2). The patient is instructed to practice at home for at least 2 to 4 hours daily. In addition, the patient undergoes muscle strengthening and neuromuscular coordination training as part of the comprehensive rehabilitation process. In order to have a successful outcome, the patient must be compliant with the time commitment and constant motivation required of this program. A family member is also taught the

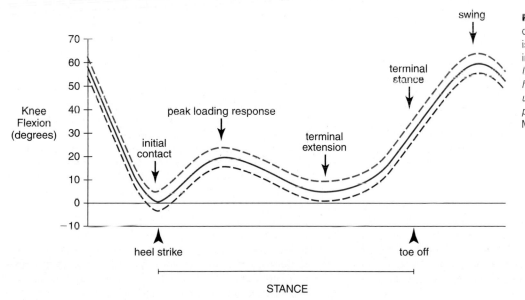

FIGURE 34–2. Knee motion (in degrees) during a normal gait cycle is shown. Phases of stance gait are indicated. (*From Noyes, F. R.; Dunworth, L. A.; Andriacchi, T. P.; et al.: Knee hyperextension gait abnormalities in unstable knees. Recognition and preoperative gait retraining. Am J Sports Med 24:35–45, 1996.*)

PATTERN I

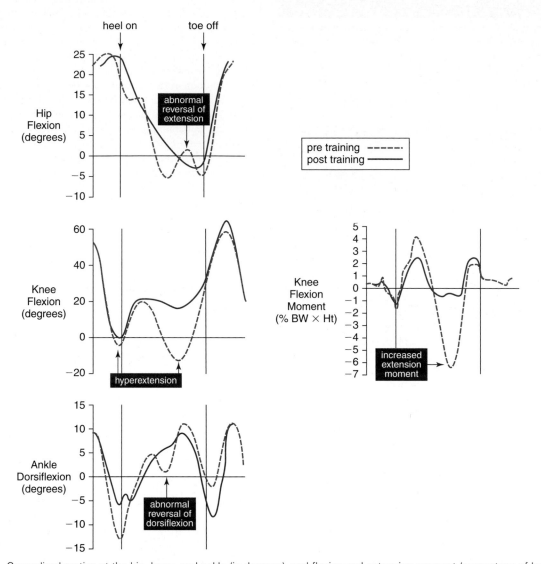

FIGURE 34–3. Generalized motion at the hip, knee, and ankle (in degrees), and flexion and extension moment (percentage of body weight x height) for patients showing pattern I, knee hyperextension at heel-strike and midstance only. *(From Noyes, F. R.; Dunworth, L. A.; Andriacchi, T. P.; et al.: Knee hyperextension gait abnormalities in unstable knees. Recognition and preoperative gait retraining. Am J Sports Med 24:35–45, 1996.)*

same instructions so that she or he can observe and assist with the patient's retraining at home. It is also helpful to video the patient's abnormal and corrected gait to aid the educational process.

The initial focus of the retraining process is placed on the hyperextension of the knee in order for the patient to understand that this is the primary abnormality that requires modification (Fig. 34–5). The patient is instructed to maintain 5° of flexion with every step. This requires walking in a very slow and deliberate manner. A visual aid to provide to the patient is the mental image of a woman walking in high heels, which produces 5° to 8° of knee flexion. In addition, a 1- to 2-inch elevated heel may be used to help maintain flexion throughout stance phase. The clinician should be aware that problems might occur during gait retraining when the patient practices the flexed knee stance. While the flexed knee gait is advantageous in contributing to quadriceps strengthening, it may aggravate preexisting patellofemoral pain, which must be treated promptly.

The second step of the training process involves educating the patient on the abnormal ankle and foot motions that occur concurrently with knee hyperextension. The patient practices elevating the heel and pushing off with the forefoot and toes in the midstance phase to avoid knee hyperextension. The patient must limit excessive ankle plantar flexion and assume early ankle dorsiflexion to maintain forward progression of the tibia and flexion of the knee joint. It is helpful to have the patient notice and feel the pressure against the forefoot during the end of stance phase. With the first and second steps, the patient is taught to say "knee-foot" with each stance cycle as a reminder of the normal gait pattern.

When the patient is not practicing the "knee-foot" adaptation, he or she will revert to the abnormal knee hyperextension pattern. However, within 2 to 4 weeks, it is surprising to note that the gait pattern returns to normal and the patient is no longer required to perform a conscious reminder of the gait adaptation. In short, the gait pattern becomes routine.

PATTERN II

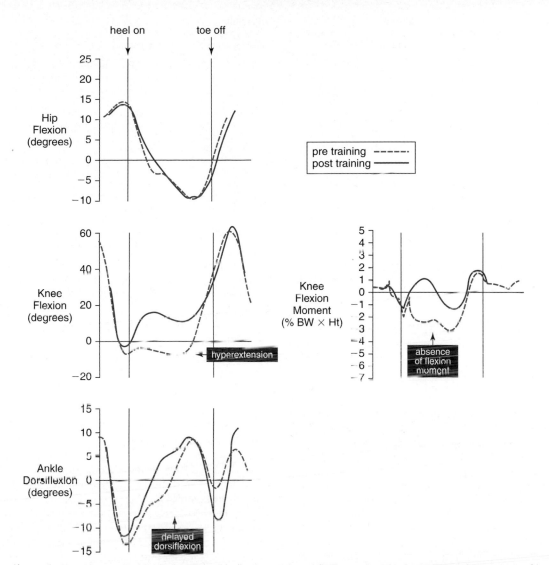

FIGURE 34–4. Generalized motion at the hip, knee, and ankle (in degrees), and flexion and extension moment (percentage of body weight x height) for patients showing pattern II, hyperextension of the knee throughout the stance phase. *(From Noyes, F. R.; Dunworth, L. A.; Andriacchi, T. P.; et al.; Knee hyperextension gait abnormalities in unstable knees. Recognition and preoperative gait retraining. Am J Sports Med 24:35–45, 1996.)*

The third step analyzes the hip and body trunk position (see Table 34–2). The fourth and final step of the retraining program determines whether an abnormal lower limb alignment (varus or valgus thrust) or an external or internal rotational knee subluxation occurs during stance. This is important because a primary cause of a patient's abnormal knee hyperextension may be instability of the knee with flexion, so that coronal plane or rotational transverse plane subluxations occur. In these patients, a functional knee brace and additional gait retraining may be required.

In some cases, a heel wedge may be used to place the knee in slight flexion in order to minimize the midstance hyperextension that can occur with poor quadriceps control. A significant varus or valgus malalignment may require use of an unloading brace or a lateral or medial heel wedge.

There are primarily two different types of unloading braces: single-hinged and bilateral-hinged. Single-hinged braces are able to create a pulling mechanism through the affected compartment, thereby creating the unloading (e.g., when the brace has a medial hinge, the medial compartment is unloaded). With a double upright-hinged system, the brace will typically have a pushing mechanism of unloading (e.g., when attempting to unload the medial compartment, the lateral hinge mechanism will be adjusted to push through the lateral to the medial joint). In custom unloading braces, a fixed amount of unloading can also be built into the brace. The potential added advantage of double upright-unloading braces is the ability to compensate for cruciate and/or collateral ligament insufficiency. If a brace or heel wedge is used, the patient is reminded to actively practice the gait-retraining techniques and not to solely use the brace/wedge as a passive limit to hyperextension. These devices also assist in decreasing the medial or lateral pain complaints that can accompany either joint instability or arthrosis.

Voluntary muscle control is critical to help minimize hyperextension gait mechanisms related to diminished quadriceps

TABLE 34–1 Abnormal Knee Motion Patterns and Subluxations during Stance Phase

Stance Phase Event	Abnormal Knee Position	Motion Limit Increased	Phase of Stance	Possible Additional Subluxations	Comments
Hyperextension motion (thrust)	Hyperextension (pattern I)	Extension	Initial contact, terminal extension phases	Varus–external tibial rotation (recurvatum)	Sudden knee hyperextension-flexion-hyperextension even during stance. Markedly abnormal gait, retraining difficult.
Hyperextension motion (thrust)	Hyperextension (pattern II)	Extension	Entire stance phase	Varus–external tibial rotation (recurvatum)	No back-and-forth motion during stance. Gait retraining less difficult.
Varus thrust	Tibial adduction (lateral joint opening)	Adduction	Initial contact and loading response phase	Tibiofemoral compartment rotational subluxation*	Usually occurs at loading response. Gait retraining not possible. External tibial rotation may decrease thrusting; internal rotation increases thrusting. Increased external tibial rotation (lateral-posterolateral injury, medial-posteromedial injury, or both). Increased internal tibial rotation is rare, usually anterior cruciate ligament plus lateral ligament injury.
Valgus thrust	Tibial abduction (medial joint opening)	Abduction	Initial contact and loading response phase	Tibiofemoral compartment rotational subluxation*	Increased external tibial rotation (medial-posteromedial ligament injury) with anterior subluxation of medial plateau. Increased external tibial rotation with lateral-posterolateral injury with posterior subluxation of the medial plateau.

*Rotational subluxations may also occur in the absence of a varus or valgus thrust.

From Noyes, F. R.; Dunworth, L. A.; Andriacchi, T. P.; et al.: Knee hyperextension gait abnormalities in unstable knees. Recognition and preoperative gait retraining. *Am J Sports Med* 24:35–45, 1996.

Critical Points GAIT-RETRAINING PROGRAM FOR ABNORMAL KNEE HYPEREXTENSION

- Program requires two to four sessions (held preferably every other week) with an experienced physical therapist to instruct the patient on the abnormal gait mechanics that occur and the adaptations required to restore a normal gait pattern.
- Patient practices at home for at least 2 to 4 hr daily.
- Muscle strengthening and neuromuscular coordination training are also performed.
- Initial focus is on the knee hyperextension. Patient is instructed to maintain 5° of flexion with every step, walking in a very slow and deliberate manner.
- Patient is educated on the abnormal ankle and foot motions that occur concurrently with knee hyperextension. Patient practices elevating the heel and pushing off with the forefoot and toes in the midstance phase to avoid knee hyperextension.
- Hip and body trunk position are analyzed.
- Clinician determines whether an abnormal lower limb alignment (varus or valgus thrust) or an external or internal rotational knee subluxation occurs during stance. Functional knee brace and additional gait retraining may be required.
- Heel wedge may be used to place the knee in slight flexion.
- Unloading brace or a lateral or medial heel wedge is used for significant varus or valgus malalignment.
- Exercises are done to target specific muscles used during gait: toe-raises for gastrocnemius-soleus complex, straight leg plus raise and wall-sits for quadriceps.
- Balance and proprioception: weight-shifting, tandem balance, single-leg balance (stable and unstable), rocker board (front-to-back and side-to-side), cup-walking, resisted gait activity with a heavy elastic band.
- Two to 3 months may be required to complete the training to the point at which a normal gait pattern becomes routine on a subconscious level.

function. Normal gait requires adequate push-off from the gastrocnemius-soleus complex, sufficient quadriceps contraction in midstance, hip and knee flexion during swing, and an upright posture. Defects in any of these mechanisms will permit gait alterations and, when completed with sufficient frequency, become the default gait pattern for the patient. Gait is a learned activity and eventually becomes habitual. Therefore, gait retraining should include exercises to target the specific muscles used during gait, pre-gait activities to methodically force the patient to think about using these muscles functionally, and then the act to practice the new gait pattern so it eventually becomes the learned default pattern to avoid the hyperextension gait mechanism. It should be noted that it is not always necessary to correct a marked varus or valgus thrust due to an associated tibiofemoral osseous malalignment. In these knees, the associated high adduction or abduction moment is rarely counterbalanced, even with an unloader brace or heel wedges. In some knees with varus malalignment, there is an associated internal tibial torsion and toe-in gait. The patient may voluntarily decrease the varus thrust by purposely walking with a toe-out gait; however, when the patient is not practicing, the toe-in gait resumes. The same situation applies to a valgus knee alignment with a pronated toe-out gait. The gait retraining, therefore, is primarily to address knee hyperextension in which most patients will achieve a beneficial response to the program.

The following sections represent examples of how exercises may be coupled with other activities to assist with gait retraining. An important component of gait retraining is to target exercises for the specific muscles required during the gait cycle. For the gastrocnemius-soleus complex, the patient is instructed on the toe-raise exercise. This exercise can be progressed to move from using double stance to eccentric/negative repetitions (up with two legs/down with a single leg) and eventually to single-ankle plantar flexion

TABLE 34–2   Gait-Retraining Program for Abnormal Knee Stance Hyperextension

Anatomic Part	Retraining Program
Trunk–upper body	1. Maintain erect position, avoid forward loading position, which shifts body weight anteriorly to knee joint during stance phase. 2. Avoid excessive medial-lateral sway during stance phase, which induces varus-valgus moments about the knee and hip.
Hip	1. Avoid excessive hip flexion during stance phase, which encourages knee hyperextension and fatigues hip extensors. 2. For valgus lower limb alignment, avoid excessive internal femoral rotation. Encourage external femoral rotation and walking on lateral foot border. Avoid knock-knee position (important for valgus thrusts). 3. For varus lower limb alignment, avoid external femoral rotation. Encourage internal femoral rotation, knock-knee position.
Knee	1. Avoid any knee hyperextension throughout stance phase by always maintaining a knee flexion position. 2. Practice knee flexion-extension control walking in a slow manner; often begin with crutches. Initially use an excessive knee flexion position. 3. Gradually resume a more normal walking speed, after flexion-extension control and a more normal gait pattern are resumed. 4. Look for increase in patellofemoral pain. 5. Look for varus or valgus thrust with knee flexion position. 6. Look for external or internal rotational tibiofemoral subluxations when flexion position resumed.
Ankle	1. Avoid excessive plantar flexion. Maintain dorsiflexion using soleus muscle to induce early heel rise (rocker action) to encourage forward tibial progression and knee flexion. 2. Initially use excessive dorsiflexion and walking aids (elevated heel) to increase early heel-off in stance phase.
Foot	1. Encourage push-off against forefoot and toes along with early heel-off in stance phase to assist knee flexion during stance phase. 2. With associated varus alignment, encourage toe-out position. For valgus alignment, encourage toe-in position.

From Noyes, F. R.; Dunworth, L. A.; Andriacchi, T. P.; et al.: Knee hyperextension gait abnormalities in unstable knees. Recognition and preoperative gait retraining, *Am J Sports Med* 24:35–45, 1996.

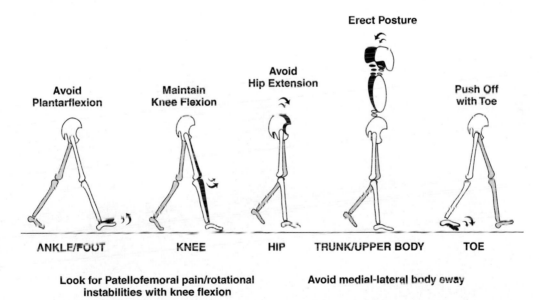

FIGURE 34–5. Graphic representation of gait abnormalities observed in patients before retraining. *Filled gray anatomic structures represent the correct, retrained positions at the trunk, upper body, hip, knee, foot, ankle, and toes. (From Noyes, F. R.; Dunworth, L. A.; Andriacchi, T. P.; et al.: Knee hyperextension gait abnormalities in unstable knees. Recognition and preoperative gait retraining. Am J Sports Med 24:35–45, 1996.).*

lifting. Other options are to move from the floor to the edge of a step or to add additional weight for increasing the workload. The exercise can also be combined with traditional step-up exercises.

Quadriceps control is critical for normal gait and represents the muscle group that demands the most attention. Common exercises shown to be effective in helping with quadriceps reeducation include the straight leg plus raise (Fig. 34–6), performed with the patient in the seated position. The quadriceps is contracted, the leg is lifted approximately 6 inches off the table or chair, held in the lifted position for 15 seconds, and then lowered and relaxed for 45 seconds. This 1-minute cycle is maintained and progressed in ratios (1:3, 1:2, and eventually, 1:1), and then progressed from 5 to 10 repetitions, with additional ankle weight added to increase the difficulty of the exercise.

Isometric wall-sits are an excellent method of facilitating quadriceps activation. The desired angle of knee flexion is typically between 45° and 70°. Patients with patellofemoral joint changes may need to maintain the angle of flexion between 30°

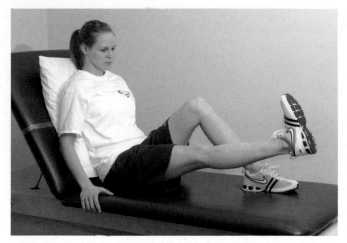

FIGURE 34–6. The straight leg plus raise exercise.

and 45° in order to decrease patellofemoral pain. Patients who do not have joint damage or pain may perform this exercise in deeper degrees of knee flexion to allow for an increase in quadriceps muscle fiber recruitment. Having the patient keep weight pressures through the heels will also decrease the potential for patellar pain complaints. This exercise is similar to a stationary leg press and is performed as two repetitions, four times a day to a maximum fatigue, experiencing a quadriceps burning sensation. The patient tries each exercise and attempts to reach a 3-minute-total duration for each wall-sit repetition.

Active isometric hip adduction during the wall-sit by compressing a ball between the knees may assist vastus medialis obliquus recruitment. In addition to obtaining adequate quadriceps control, it is important to improve hip abduction control. A heavy elastic exercise band may be placed proximal to the knee (avoiding patellar pressure) and "clamshells" are performed in either the long-sitting (hook) (Fig. 34–7A and B) or the side-lying (see Fig. 34–7C and D) position. Three to five sets of 10 repetitions are performed. Adjustments to either knee flexion or hip flexion angles can make the exercise easier or more difficult depending on what is necessary to challenge the gluteal musculature.

Balance and proprioception are important components of a gait-retraining program. The patient must be able to maintain single-stance control, as well as move the opposite leg through swing and be ready for the transition into the next stride. Standard progression of balance activities is typically sufficient to allow for return of a normal gait. A sample of these activities includes the following: weight-shifting, tandem balance, single-leg balance (stable and unstable), rocker board (front-to-back and side-to-side), and Biodex Stabilometer (Biodex Medical Systems, Shirley, NY) for postural stability (random control and maze control). Focus of balance control is part of both the clinical treatment and the home exercise programs.

In order to create a functional gait-retraining program, a blending of the individual exercise programs must progress to include specific gait activities. Patients must overcome a variety of contributing factors including apprehension, muscle weakness, lack of range of motion, compensation, and pain. These factors must be resolved in order for the patient to restore a

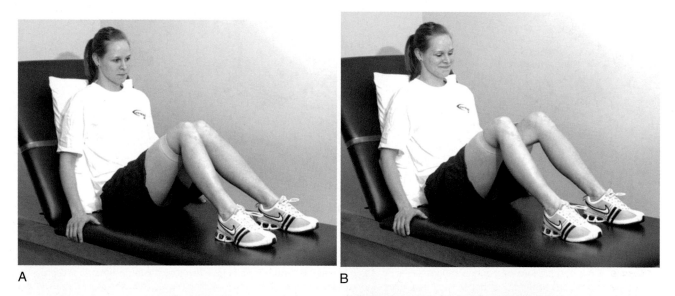

A   B   C   D

FIGURE 34–7. The clamshell exercise is performed in either the long sitting (**A** and **B**) or the side-lying (**C** and **D**) position.

normal gait cycle. Each of the following factors contributes to a symmetrical gait pattern: adequate push-off, midstance quadriceps control, hip and knee flexion, and maintenance of an upright posture. Two common gait activities can be used quite successfully to assist both in the early time period after injury or surgery and in later time periods. Initially, an activity known as *cup-walking* is used to encourage the patient to break down the actual gait cycle into more manageable tasks. Cups are set up in two staggered rows with symmetrical stride lengths (Fig. 34–8). The patient is asked to walk or march over the cups, emphasizing each of the earlier four mentioned tasks. This activity allows the clinician to observe the gait cycle to determine where emphasis needs to be placed. Common compensatory mechanisms that patients exhibit include circumduction of the lower extremity, inadequate push-off, midstance hyperextension, lack of coordinated hip and knee flexion, positive Trendelenburg sign, and forward-flexed trunk. The clinician must be able to identify the deficiency in order to teach the patient and her or his support system how to observe the deficiency and to perform the corrective strategy. The normal automatic nature of gait now becomes a "thinking" activity for the patient. The patient is asked to exaggerate the gait cycle by stepping over the cups. This methodical approach allows the patient to apply a part of the gait cycle to the entire, normal gait pattern. Gait-retraining activities such as this must be repeated thousands of cycles over time in order to create a "new default" gait pattern.

As time progresses from the injury or surgery, another gait activity may be used that requires the patient to wear a heavy elastic band around the distal thighs (~2 finger widths above the patella) and then produce a marching pattern to provide a resisted-gait cycle. With a central line on the floor, the patient, while marching, must maintain right foot-strike on the right side of the line and left foot-strike on the left side of the line (Fig. 34–9). This movement into swing ensures that adequate hip flexion and hip abduction musculature is used during the gait cycle. In addition, the stance limb requires adequate push-off of the gastrocnemius as well as a voluntary quadriceps contraction to prevent a hyperextension episode. This resisted-gait activity can be completed in forward, backward, and lateral directions. Each direction allows the clinician to emphasize what muscle groups are used to allow for adequate voluntary muscle control. Again, these activities require voluntary thought processes to focus on recruiting the quadriceps to avoid the hyperextension mechanism from occurring.

In the authors' experience, after approximately two to four sessions, the patient will understand the abnormal mechanics and recognize when the hyperextension patterns occur. As already discussed, mental reminders, such as "knee bent, toe push-off," are helpful in this stage. After approximately 4 weeks of training, the patient should convert to a more normal gait pattern. However, it may require 2 to 3 months to complete the training process to the point at which a normal gait pattern becomes routine on a subconscious level and the patient does not resume the hyperextension gait pattern when walking quickly.

CLINICAL INVESTIGATION

Methods and Materials

The authors' gait-retraining program[17] was studied in 5 patients with symptomatic knee hyperextension and deficiency of the posterolateral structures. Computerized gait analysis testing was conducted before and after the retraining program using a two-camera video-based optoelectronic digitizer for measuring motion and a multicomponent force plate for measuring ground reaction force. The force plate was camouflaged under a 10-m walkway. Patients were asked to walk at three speeds (normal, fast, slow), and measurements were obtained over these ranges to enable comparison of similar walking speeds. Data from complete cycles of stance and swing phase were obtained.

Kinematic data in the sagittal plane and kinetic data in the sagittal, coronal, and transverse planes of the hip, knee, and ankle were evaluated. Peak values during the stance phase were recorded for each patient. Using a previously described mathematical model,[3,24] joint reaction loads, lateral soft tissue forces, and muscle forces were calculated. The patient data were compared with those obtained from a control group of 11 subjects matched for age and walking speed. All moments, which were expressed as external moments, were normalized to body weight and height.

Analysis of Gait Mechanics before Retraining

Statistically significant differences were found between the pretrained patients and the control subjects in the mean values for knee hyperextension during heel-strike and terminal extension (Table 34–3 and Fig. 34-10), with the patients demonstrating a range of 5.4° to 18.4° less flexion ($P < .05$). The patients had a significantly higher mean knee midstance extension moment (127%; $P < .01$), knee adduction moment (28%; $P < .05$)

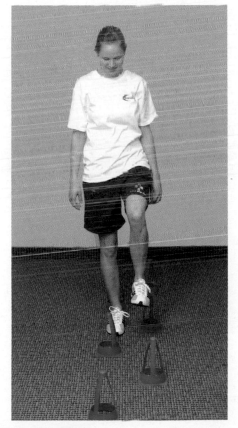

FIGURE 34–8. Cup-walking.

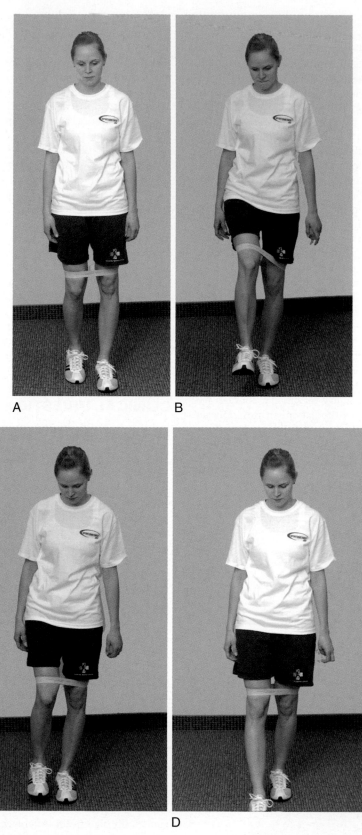

FIGURE 34–9. A–D, Elastic band gait retraining.

Critical Points CLINICAL INVESTIGATION

Gait-retraining program studied in five patients with symptomatic knee hyperextension and deficiency of the posterolateral structure.

Computerized gait analysis testing conducted before and after retraining using a two-camera video-based optoelectronic digitizer for measuring motion and a multicomponent force plate for measuring ground reaction force.

Patient data compared with control group of 11 subjects matched for age and walking speed.

Significant differences between pretrained patients and controls. Patients had

- Less knee hyperextension during heel-strike and terminal extension.
- Greater knee midstance extension moments, knee adduction moments, calculated medial tibiofemoral compartment loads.

After retraining, patients demonstrated

- Significant increases in knee flexion during heel-strike, terminal extension, and toe-off.
- Significant decreases in the knee extension moment at heel-strike and terminal extension.
- Significant decrease in mean adduction moment to a normal value.
- Decrease in hip abduction moment at heel-strike.
- Decrease in hip adduction moment during midstance.
- Decrease in ankle plantar flexion motion.

Four out of five patients successfully resolved or markedly reduced hyperextension at the knee and abnormal motion patterns at the hip and ankle.

Four out of five patients improved from experiencing moderate pain and instability with daily activities before retraining to walking several hours per day without appreciable symptoms.

and calculated medial tibiofemoral compartment loads (43%; $P < .001$) than the controls. The two knee hyperextension patterns previously discussed were identified: 3 patients demonstrated pattern I and 2 patients, pattern II.

Analysis of Gait Mechanics after Retraining

After the program of gait retraining, the patients demonstrated a statistically significant increase in the degrees of knee flexion during heel-strike, terminal extension, and toe-off (mean, 10°). At terminal extension, an average increase of 18° of flexion was measured compared with the pretraining value ($P < .01$). There were significant decreases in the knee extension moment at heel-strike (23%) and terminal extension (80%). The mean adduction moment decreased to a normal value, and a significant reduction (30%) occurred in the predicted medial tibiofemoral load ($P < .05$).

There was a 36% decrease in the hip abduction moment at heel strike ($P < .01$) and an 18% decrease in hip adduction moment during midstance after gait retraining ($P < .01$). The ankle plantar flexion motion decreased by 7° ($P < .01$), which was associated with an 8% decrease in the ankle dorsiflexion moment.

Four of the 5 patients successfully resolved or markedly reduced hyperextension at the knee and abnormal motion patterns at the hip and ankle. These individuals converted the knee flexion-extension moment to a normal biphasic pattern. One patient failed to complete the program and demonstrated continued gait abnormalities.

Effect of Retraining on Patient Symptoms

The patient symptoms before and after gait retraining were evaluated with the symptom rating scale of the Cincinnati Knee Rating System (see Chapter 44, The Cincinnati Knee Rating System). A statistically significant improvement occurred in the pain scale (0-10 points) from a mean of 1.6 ± 0.9 points before training to 4.8 ± 2.3 points after training ($P < .05$) and in the partial giving-way scale from a mean of 2.4 ± 0.9 points before training to 5.2 ± 2.3 points after training ($P < .05$). Four

TABLE 34–3   Measured and Calculated Peak Values for Control and Involved Limbs

Variable	Control Group	Study Group Pretraining	Study Group Post-Training
Knee motion (°)			
Heel-strike	1.3 ± 1.6	−5.6 ± 2.8*	−0.2 ± 2.6[†]
Peak loading response	14.9 ± 5.0	6.2 ± 10.9[‡]	16.4 ± 4.2
Terminal extension	6.6 ± 4.0	−7.3 ± 4.4*	11.1 ± 5.8[†]
Toe-off	35.0 ± 7.0	36.1 ± 5.3	41.8 ± 5.9[§]
Ankle plantar flexion motion (°)	11.4 ± 6.0	16.1 ± 8.5	9.4 ± 1.5
Hip moments (% BW x Ht)			
Abduction	1.2 ± 0.9	1.1 ± 0.4	0.7 ± 0.4[†]
Adduction	5.1 ± 0.9	6.0 ± 1.0	4.9 ± 1.4[†]
Knee moments (% BW x Ht)			
Heel-strike extension	2.4 ± 0.5	2.6 ± 0.7	2.0 ± 0.5[§]
Peak midstance extension	1.5 ± 1.0	3.4 ± 2.0[‡]	0.7 ± 0.7[§]
Adduction	3.6 ± 0.5	4.6 ± 1.4[‡]	3.6 ± 0.7
Ankle dorsiflexion moment (% BW x Ht)	9.0 ± 0.5	9.1 ± 0.9	8.4 ± 0.9
Predicted forces (BW)			
Flexor muscle group	1.5 ± 0.3	2.2 ± 0.7[‡]	1.3 ± 0.4[§]
Extensor muscle group	1.0 ± 0.4	1.1 ± 0.5	0.9 ± 0.4
Medial tibiofemoral load	2.1 ± 0.2	3.0 ± 0.4*	2.1 ± 0.5[§]

*$P < .01$ for pretraining versus control.
[†]$P < .01$ for post-training versus pretraining.
[‡]$P < .05$ for pretraining versus control.
[§]$P < .05$ for post-training versus pretraining.
BW, body weight; Ht, body height.

FIGURE 34–10. An analysis of the pre- and post-training knee flexion angles and how the amount of flexion relates to the ground reaction force. Hyperextension tends to place the ground reaction force anterior to the knee, requiring that the posterior structures rather than the quadriceps muscle balance the ground reaction force. *(From Noyes, F. R.; Dunworth, L. A.; Andriacchi, T. P.; et al.: Knee hyperextension gait abnormalities in unstable knees. Recognition and preoperative gait retraining. Am J Sports Med 24:35–45, 1996.)*

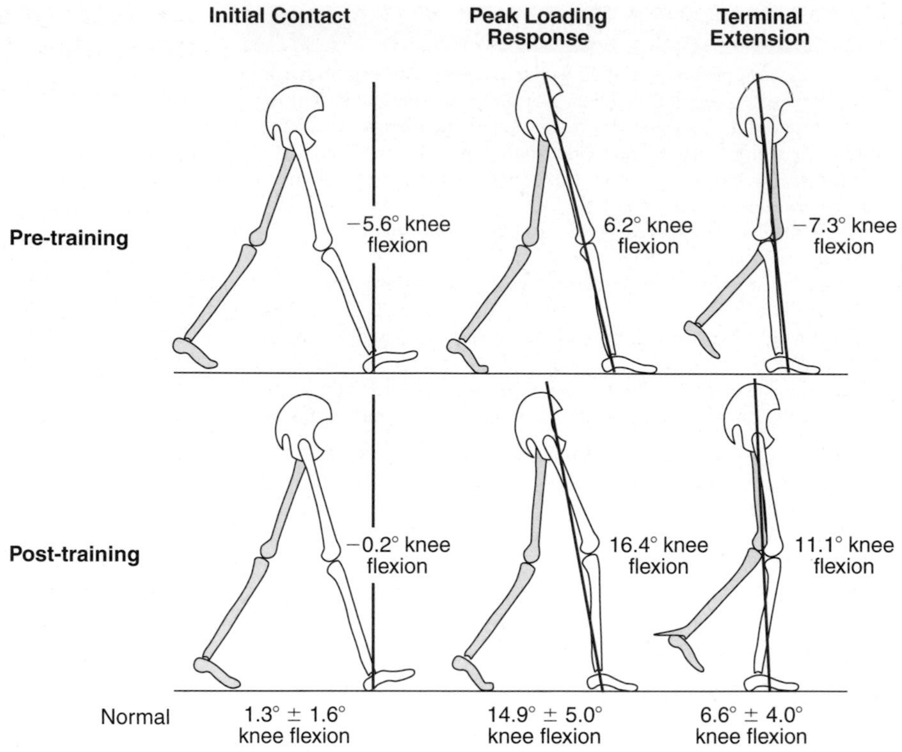

Initial Contact   Peak Loading Response   Terminal Extension

Pre-training   −5.6° knee flexion   6.2° knee flexion   −7.3° knee flexion

Post-training   −0.2° knee flexion   16.4° knee flexion   11.1° knee flexion

Normal   1.3° ± 1.6° knee flexion   14.9° ± 5.0° knee flexion   6.6° ± 4.0° knee flexion

of the 5 patients improved from experiencing moderate pain and instability with daily activities before retraining to walking several hours per day without appreciable symptoms. Because of this improvement, 2 patients did not require ligament reconstructive surgery after retraining.

SUMMARY

In patients with chronic deficiency of the posterolateral structures, the use of gait analysis techniques and retraining can successfully change the kinetics and kinematics of the hip, knee, and ankle to more normal levels. The abnormal knee hyperextension can be significantly reduced, along with adduction and extension moments about the knee and medial tibiofemoral compartment loads. Hip abduction and adduction moments may be restored to normal levels. In addition, ankle plantar flexion and its counterbalancing dorsiflexion moment can be decreased. Gait retraining is indicated in knees with a hyperextension gait abnormality prior to any ligament reconstructive procedure and may, in some cases, eliminate the requirement for such soft tissue operations. If the gait abnormality is not corrected, cruciate and posterolateral ligament reconstructions may fail from the high tensile forces placed on the grafts postoperatively as the patient resumes weight-bearing activities. These same principles apply to other patients with knee hyperextension gait patterns such as those that occur with quadriceps muscle weakness from a variety of knee injuries and early symptomatic patellofemoral arthrosis.

ILLUSTRATIVE CASES

Case 1. A 32-year-old physical therapist with chronic ACL deficiency of the left knee had given up strenuous athletics in order to avoid ACL reconstruction. She had no pain, swelling, or giving-way for several years. The patient participated in a light recreational volleyball game and experienced a partial giving-way episode. She presented with increasing medial joint line pain and a feeling of knee instability and believed she required ACL reconstruction. The patient had a bilateral standing physiologic varus recurvatum and walked with marked varus recurvatum thrust to the left lower extremity (Fig. 34–11). She was unaware that her gait pattern had changed. and the obvious hyperextension thrust became readily apparent to her after it was revealed under examination. The patient underwent the gait-retraining program and adapted to a normal gait pattern. Within 3 weeks, her medial joint pain and instability symptoms resolved. She returned to her preinjury compensated status and had no further symptoms to warrant ACL reconstruction. Because she was a physical therapist and could understand the retraining program, she had a fast response.

Case 2. A 38-year-old woman presented 1 year after a motor vehicle accident with a diagnosis of a PCL rupture. She experienced frequent instability and shifting episodes and severe medial joint line pain. Physical examination revealed marked quadriceps atrophy, 12 mm of increased posterior tibial translation, 10 mm of increased lateral joint opening, 15° of increased

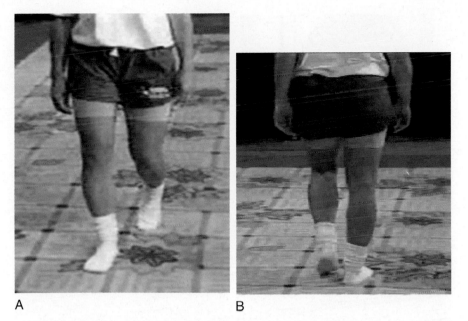

A   B

FIGURE 34–11. Patient with bilateral standing physiologic varus recurvatum who walked with marked varus recurvatum thrust to the left lower extremity.

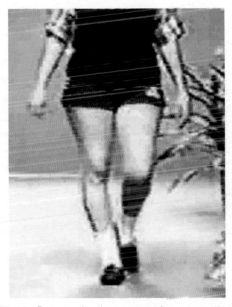

FIGURE 34–12. Patient who demonstrated a severe varus recurvatum with every step.

external tibial rotation, and a varus alignment. On standing alignment, the patient showed a varus position, but did not demonstrate a varus recurvatum. However, on walking with increased forces, a severe varus recurvatum occurred with every step (Fig. 34–12). The patient first underwent gait retraining to correct the varus thrust and rehabilitation for quadriceps muscle strengthening for 3 months. Then, an opening wedge osteotomy was performed to correct the varus osseous malalignment, followed 6 months later with a PCL and posterolateral reconstruction.

Case 3. A 24-year-old woman presented 2 years after a motor vehicle accident with a severe gait abnormality and limp on the left lower extremity (Fig. 34–13). She had pain throughout the knee joint. Physical examination revealed complete deficiency of the PCL and posterolateral structures. The patient had seen three other orthopaedic surgeons who were all reluctant to perform surgery owing to the severe gait abnormality and lower extremity muscle atrophy. She required 6 months of gait retraining. Although she was never fully able to control her knee stability, she did experience marked improvement and could consciously control the severe varus recurvatum.

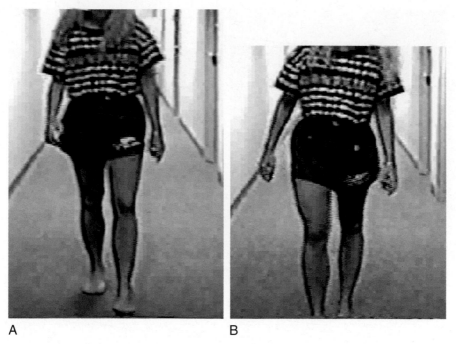

A   B

FIGURE 34–13. Patient who presented 2 years after a motor vehicle accident with a severe gait abnormality and limp on the left lower extremity.

REFERENCES

1. Andriacchi, T. P.: Dynamics of pathological motion: applied to the anterior cruciate–deficient knee. *J Biomech* 23(suppl 1):99–105, 1990.
2. Andriacchi, T. P.; Birac, D.: Functional testing in the anterior cruciate ligament–deficient knee. *Clin Orthop Relat Res* 288:40–47, 1993.
3. Andriacchi, T. P.; Hampton, S. J.; Schultz, A. B.; Galante, J. O.: Three-dimensional coordinate data processing in human motion analysis. *J Biomech Eng* 101:279–283, 1979.
4. Andriacchi, T. P.; Ogle, J. A.; Galante, J. O.: Walking speeds as a basis for normal and abnormal gait measurements. *J Biomech* 10:261–268, 1977.
5. Baker, C. L., Jr.; Norwood, L. A.; Hughston, J. C.: Acute posterolateral rotatory instability of the knee. *J Bone Joint Surg Am* 65:614–618, 1983.
6. Berchuck, M.; Andriacchi, T. P.; Bach, B. R.; Reider, B.: Gait adaptations by patients who have a deficient anterior cruciate ligament. *J Bone Joint Surg Am* 72:871–877, 1990.
7. DeLee, J. C.; Riley, M. B.; Rockwood, C. A., Jr.: Acute posterolateral rotatory instability of the knee. *Am J Sports Med* 11:199–207, 1983.
8. Gollehon, D. L.; Torzilli, P. A.; Warren, R. F.: The role of the posterolateral and cruciate ligaments in the stability of the human knee. A biomechanical study. *J Bone Joint Surg Am* 69:233–242, 1987.
9. Grood, E. S.; Noyes, F. R.; Butler, D. L.; Suntay, W. J.: Ligamentous and capsular restraints preventing straight medial and lateral laxity in intact human cadaver knees. *J Bone Joint Surg Am* 63:1257–1269, 1981.
10. Kerrigan, D. C.; Deming, L. C.; Holden, M. K.: Knee recurvatum in gait: a study of associated knee biomechanics. *Arch Phys Med Rehabil* 77:645–650, 1996.
11. LaPrade, R. F.; Terry, G. C.: Injuries to the posterolateral aspect of the knee. Association of anatomic injury patterns with clinical instability. *Am J Sports Med* 25:433–438, 1997.
12. Nielsen, S.; Ovesen, J.; Rasmussen, O.: The posterior cruciate ligament and rotatory knee instability. An experimental study. *Arch Orthop Trauma Surg* 104:53–56, 1985.
13. Nielsen, S.; Rasmussen, O.; Ovesen, J.; Andersen, K.: Rotatory instability of cadaver knees after transection of collateral ligaments and capsule. *Arch Orthop Trauma Surg* 103:165–169, 1984.
14. Noyes, F. R.; Barber-Westin, S. D.: Posterior cruciate ligament revision reconstruction, part 1: causes of surgical failure in 52 consecutive operations. *Am J Sports Med* 33:646–654, 2005.
15. Noyes, F. R.; Barber-Westin, S. D.: Revision anterior cruciate surgery with use of bone–patellar tendon–bone autogenous grafts. *J Bone Joint Surg Am* 83:1131–1143, 2001.
16. Noyes, F. R.; Barber-Westin, S. D.; Albright, J. C.: An analysis of the causes of failure in 57 consecutive posterolateral operative procedures. *Am J Sports Med* 34:1419–1430, 2006.
17. Noyes, F. R.; Dunworth, L. A.; Andriacchi, T. P.; et al.: Knee hyperextension gait abnormalities in unstable knees. Recognition and preoperative gait retraining. *Am J Sports Med* 24:35–45, 1996.
18. Noyes, F. R.; Schipplein, O. D.; Andriacchi, T. P.; et al.: The anterior cruciate ligament–deficient knee with varus alignment. An analysis of gait adaptations and dynamic joint loadings. *Am J Sports Med* 20:707–716, 1992.
19. Pasque, C.; Noyes, F. R.; Gibbons, M.; et al.: The role of the popliteofibular ligament and the tendon of popliteus in providing stability in the human knee. *J Bone Joint Surg Br* 85:292–298, 2003.
20. Patel, R. R.; Hurwitz, D. E.; Bush-Joseph, C. A.; et al.: Comparison of clinical and dynamic knee function in patients with anterior cruciate ligament deficiency. *Am J Sports Med* 31:68–74, 2003.
21. Perry, J. (ed.): *Gait Analysis: Normal and Pathological Function.* Thorofare, NJ, Slack, 1992; pp. 49–281.
22. Perry, J.; Antonelli, D.; Ford, W.: Analysis of knee joint forces during flexed-knee stance. *J Bone Joint Surg Am* 57:961–967, 1975.
23. Saunders, J.; Inman, V.; Eberhart, H.: The major determinants in normal and pathological gait. *J Bone Joint Surg Am* 35:543–558, 1953.
24. Schipplein, O. D.; Andriacchi, T. P.: Interaction between active and passive knee stabilizers during level walking. *J Orthop Res* 9:113–119, 1991.
25. Simon, S. R.: Gait—normal and abnormal. In Insall, J.; Scott, W. N. (eds.): *Surgery of the Knee.* Philadelphia: Churchill Livingstone, 2001; pp. 232–254.
26. Veltri, D. M.; Deng, X. H.; Torzilli, P. A.; et al.: The role of the cruciate and posterolateral ligaments in stability of the knee. A biomechanical study. *Am J Sports Med* 23:436–443, 1995.
27. Wexler, G.; Hurwitz, D. E.; Bush-Joseph, C. A.; et al.: Functional gait adaptations in patients with anterior cruciate ligament deficiency over time. *Clin Orthop Relat Res* 348:166–175, 1998.

Articular Cartilage Procedures and Rehabilitation of the Arthritic Knee

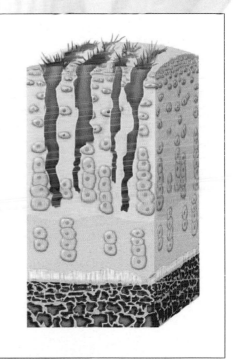

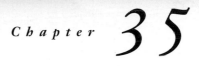

Chapter **35**

Autologous Chondrocyte Implantation

Lars Peterson, MD, PhD

INTRODUCTION

The ancient Greeks acknowledged ulcerated cartilage as troublesome to treat, with little to no natural healing capacity. Articular cartilage lesions have for a long time been undiagnosed and their severity underestimated. The increased surgical approach to ligament injuries, along with the introduction of arthroscopy and magnetic resonance imaging (MRI), has increased the diagnostic possibilities for articular cartilage lesions and activated the search for an improved treatment. Articular cartilage lesions are much more common than earlier recognized.

Anterior cruciate ligament (ACL) and meniscus injuries are often combined with articular cartilage injuries, in which the cartilage injury is the most serious and most difficult to treat in the end. Noyes and coworkers[18,19] and Shelbourne and associates[24] found that acute and chronic ACL injuries were associated with articular cartilage injuries in 40% to 70% of knees. There are reports that in cases of meniscus injury, 40% to 50% of patients also have cartilage damage.[25] Hjelle and colleagues[11] reported on 1000 consecutive patients with symptoms requiring arthroscopy. Chondral or osteochondral lesions of any type were found in 61% of the patients. Curl and coworkers[5] found that in 31,516 patients who underwent arthroscopy,

63% had a cartilage lesion and 19% had an Outerbridge grade IV cartilage lesion. Bone bruises have been reported in acute knee injuries[12] and in combination with ACL injuries in 80%.[17] The damage to the trabecular bone may heal, but the overlying cartilage may degrade over time.

Since the early 1980s different treatments for full-thickness cartilage lesions have been developed that show promise. Some treatments have been discarded whereas others have been further developed. However, no "gold standard" is currently established and injuries to articular cartilage are still difficult to treat. Without proper management, articular cartilage injuries may degrade through enzymatic and mechanical breakdown into post-traumatic osteoarthritis.

Autologous chondrocyte implantation (ACI) has been in clinical practice since 1987, with over 25,000 patients treated worldwide. ACI was approved by the U.S. Food and Drug Administration in 1997.

INDICATIONS

ACI is indicated for full-thickness cartilage lesions or osteochondral lesions, including osteochondritis dissecans (OCD) in the knee (International Cartilage Repair Society [ICRS]

Critical Points INDICATIONS

- Full-thickness chondral or osteochondral lesion.
- Symptomatic.
- Size between 2 and 16 cm².
- Bone-to-bone conditions can be tried as a salvage procedure.

---

or Outerbridge classification grade III or IV). The size of the lesion should be between 2 and 16 cm², but larger lesions and multiple lesions can be treated in the same joint. The lesions should be situated on either the patella, the femur, or the tibia, and the opposing articular surface should be undamaged or have only superficial cartilage damage. Bone-to-bone conditions between the tibia and the femur or between the trochlea and the patella can be tried as a salvage procedure in young patients. The age recommendation is between 15 and 55 years, but there is no definite limit. Ligamentous instability, varus or valgus deformities, patella malalignment or instability, meniscus deficiency, and bone pathology or defect are not contraindications, but these must be addressed in the treatment.

The recognition of serious articular cartilage injuries, including bipolar lesions in young and middle-aged individuals, has along with increased experience widened the indications for ACI (Fig. 35–1).

CONTRAINDICATIONS

ACI is contraindicated in the treatment for general osteoarthritis, rheumatoid arthritis, or other systemic diseases affecting the joints. The effect of high body mass index on the outcome after surgery has not been studied, but overweight or obesity should be considered a relative contraindication. It is likely that smoking affects the cell proliferation and tissue maturation after ACI in a negative way, but because it is not known to what extent, smoking is not an absolute contraindication.

CLINICAL EVALUATION

History

The patient often presents with a history of trauma, repeated trauma, or microtrauma. Typical symptoms are pain on weight-bearing, catching, locking, crepitus, and pain and swelling after activity. The onset may be acute, but in many patients, especially those with patellar lesions, the onset of symptoms is gradual and no specific trauma has been involved or recognized.

Physical Examination

When planning the treatment, a thorough physical examination—including tests for instability; varus or valgus deformity;

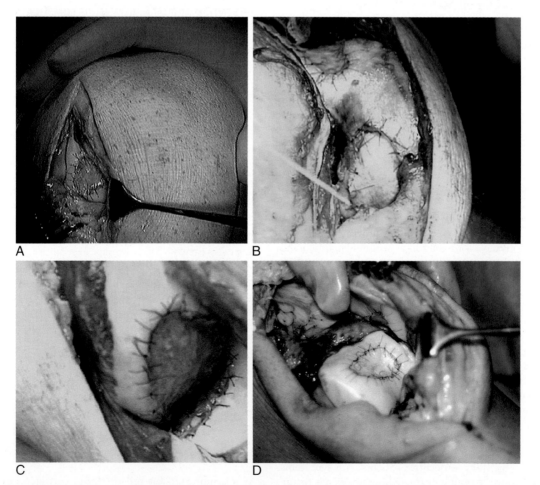

FIGURE 35–1. The original indication for autologous chondrocyte implantation (ACI) was a single contained lesion on the femoral condyle (**A**), but with increased experience, lesions to other locations as well as multiple lesions (**B**) have been included. **C** and **D**, Kissing lesions can be tried as a salvage procedure.

patellar malalignment, instability or maltracking; and other background factors that may require surgical correction—is mandatory. To create an optimal environment for the short- and long-term survival of the repair tissue, the background factors must be corrected for a successful outcome.

Diagnostic Tests

To further investigate the pathology including background factors, x-rays, MRI, and computed tomography (CT) with and without contrast medium are useful tools. Standing x-rays with the knees in extension and in 45° of flexion, and standing hip-knee-ankle x-rays are valuable for evaluating the joint space, the subchondral bone, and varus or valgus deformity. MRI with or without gadolinium can be helpful to diagnose the articular cartilage injury, the condition of other soft tissues such as the ligaments and menisci, and the pathology of the subchondral bone in further detail. CT with or without contrast injection is helpful to evaluate patellofemoral pathology, especially in combination with comparison between quadriceps muscle relaxation and contraction with the knee in extension.

PREOPERATIVE PLANNING

ACI is a staged procedure with an initial arthroscopic evaluation and harvest of cartilage. The cultivation of chondrocytes takes a minimum of 2 weeks. However, the cells may be frozen after 1 week of culturing and thawed at a later stage for continued culturing without decreased viability. The second stage is the implantation of chondrocytes, which is performed through an arthrotomy.

Correcting background factors must be planned in advance. The procedure can be performed either at the same time as the arthroscopic evaluation (e.g., ACL reconstruction) or prior to, concomitant with, or after the ACI and must be decided on a case-by-case basis. For the tibiofemoral compartment, procedures such as varus or valgus osteotomy, meniscus transplantation, bone grafting (e.g., for OCD), or knee ligament reconstruction must be planned. For the patellofemoral joint, patella realignment or unloading or stabilizing the medial patellofemoral ligament procedures must be considered. In principal, two consecutive arthrotomies should be avoided if possible.

INTRAOPERATIVE EVALUATION

During the first-stage arthroscopy, knee stability is reassessed under anesthesia. The lesion is examined to decide whether it meets the indications for ACI. The lesion should be surrounded by healthy cartilage (but uncontainment is not a contraindication) and the opposing articular surface should be undamaged or have only minor superficial cartilage injury (Fig. 35–2). All intra-articular structures should be examined. The location, size, and depth should be noted using, for instance, the ICRS Knee Evaluation Package. Slices of cartilage with subchondral bone are harvested with a curet. The recommended harvest sites are the medial and lateral proximal rim of the femoral trochlea and the lateral aspect of the intercondylar notch in the knee joint. In more than 1400 patients who have had cartilage removed from the proximal medial trochlea for cell culturing, no complications or late symptoms have occurred from the donor site area. An optimal harvesting of cartilage is of great

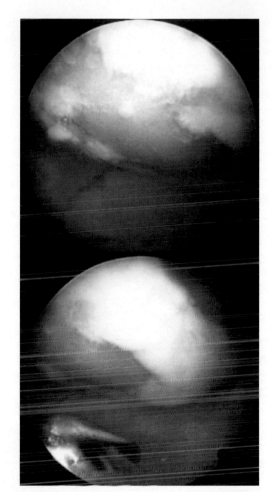

FIGURE 35–2. Arthroscopic evaluation of a lesion indicated for ACI.

importance for the success of the cell culturing. Optimal cell quality is necessary for a successful result of this procedure and should be performed according to good laboratory practice or national regulations if present.

Other pathology within the knee should also be noted. If present, loose bodies are removed before the cartilage harvest. Meniscal tears are treated after the cartilage biopsy has been harvested. Always consider the possibility of meniscus repair, especially in young patients.

OPERATIVE TECHNIQUE

Either general or spinal anesthesia is used, and a tourniquet-controlled blood field is optional. A central straight skin incision is used. If previous incisions are present, these are used if

---

Critical Points OPERATIVE TECHNIQUE

- Radical excision of all damaged cartilage.
- Careful débridement, avoid bleeding.
- Template for correct size and form.
- Periosteum as thin as possible.
- Sizing of periosteum.
- Anchor, suture, glue for watertight integrity.
- Correct instability.
- Unload when needed.

possible to avoid further scar formation. The cartilage injury is approached through either a medial or a lateral arthrotomy depending on the location of the lesion and concomitant procedures, and the arthrotomy is adjusted for adequate access to the lesion. When the lesion is difficult to reach, the patella may have to be dislocated. In posterior femoral and tibial lesions, the anterior meniscus attachment has to be released or the medial or lateral collateral ligament femoral insertion detached with a bone block. The injured area is excised with vertical edges including all damaged cartilage and débrided without causing any bleeding from the subchondral bone. This avoids possible contamination with fibroblasts and undifferentiated stem cells from the bone marrow. Intralesional osteophytes may be present as a result of an intrinsic healing attempt or a previous microfracture or drilling procedure. Smaller osteophytes are carefully tapped down to the level of the subchondral bone plate, whereas larger and prominent osteophytes may be carefully curetted down to the bone plate. Surprisingly, there is very little bleeding from the curettage. If bleeding is present, use an epinephrine sponge or a drop of fibrin glue to stop the bleeding. Avoid electrocautery to prevent any necrosis in the bone.

The length and width of the defect is measured, and a template of the lesion is made with sterile paper or aluminum foil. Through a separate incision on the upper medial tibia, below the pes anserinus and the medial collateral ligament insertion, the periosteum is dissected free from overlying fascia, fat, fibrous tissue, and crossing vessels. A periosteal flap of the correct size and form is excised using a template, but because of shrinkage and room for suturing, the flap is oversized with 1 to 2 mm in the periphery. The flap with intact cambium layer is gently dissected from the cortical bone with a periosteal elevator. The periosteal flap should be as thin as possible and transparent, which will give more volume in the defect, allowing diffusion of synovial fluid and the cells to spread and expand and produce hyaline matrix. A thin flap also reduces the risk of periosteal complications. With increased age and inactivity, the periosteum atrophies and can become so thin that it is impossible to harvest. In smokers and obese patients, the quality of the periosteum is also decreased. The periosteum is thicker and more fibrous on the medial and lateral femoral condyle, proximal to the articular surface, and covered with a rich vascular network with risk for bleeding. This can lead to postoperative hematoma with swelling, adhesions, and arthrofibrosis. Therefore, the distal shaft of the femur is a better option as a second region for periosteal flap harvesting.

The flap is sutured to the cartilage rim of the defect at the level of the surrounding cartilage and the periosteum-cartilage border is sealed with fibrin glue. A gentle saline injection under the flap reveals any leakage along the cartilage rim, which must be sealed. After aspiration of the saline, the cultured chondrocytes are injected underneath the periosteal cover and the injection site is sutured and sealed (Fig. 35–3). The arthrotomy is closed in separate layers. Bandaging including the foot, lower leg, and knee is applied.

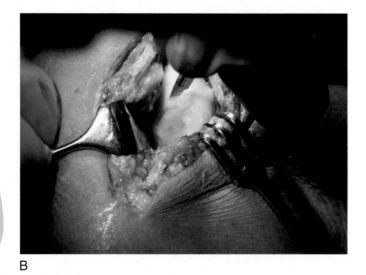

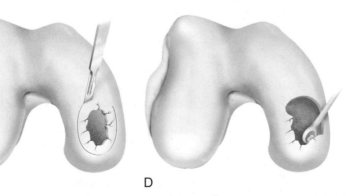

A   B

C   D

FIGURE 35–3. A lesion (**A**) is radically excised (**B** and **C**) and débrided (**D**) and made ready for transplantation (**E**).

Continued

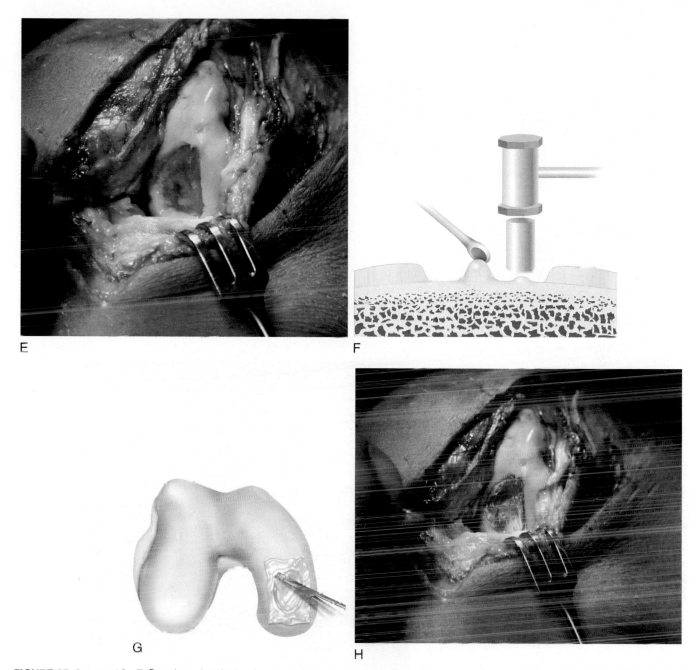

FIGURE 35–3—cont'd. F, Prominent intralesional osteophytes are curetted and smaller ones can be tapped down. A template of the lesion is made (**G** and **H**) and used when excising the periosteal flap (**I**).

Continued

Concomitant Stabilizing Procedures

For an optimal environment for the repair tissue, any instability must be corrected. In the tibiofemoral joint, an ACL or posterior cruciate ligament reconstruction or a medial or lateral collateral ligament shortening may be prepared before ACI. These procedures are usually done concomitantly with ACI. The aim is to avoid a second arthrotomy when staging. When performed concomitantly with ACI, a ligament reconstruction or shortening is done after the cartilage lesion is débrided and covered with periosteum but before the chondrocytes are injected.

Patellofemoral lesions are often related to an unstable patella, and the patella must thus be stabilized for good healing. Stabilizing procedures may include anteromedialization of the tibial tuberosity and sometimes slight distalization owing to patella alta, lateral release, proximal medial soft tissue (medial patellofemoral ligament and vastus medialis obliquus) shortening, and trochlear groove plasty[21] (if the patella is dysplastic) (Fig. 35–4).

Patellofemoral (trochlear) lesions are often related to patellar instability. If a 6-month training program does not restore functional stability, the background factors present must be corrected. These factors are increased Q-angle (>15°–20°), patella alta, ligament instability (medial patellofemoral ligament

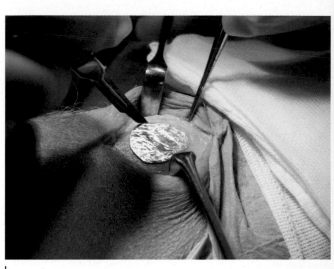

I

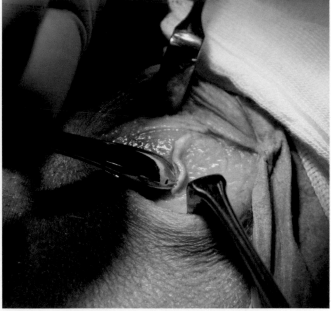

J

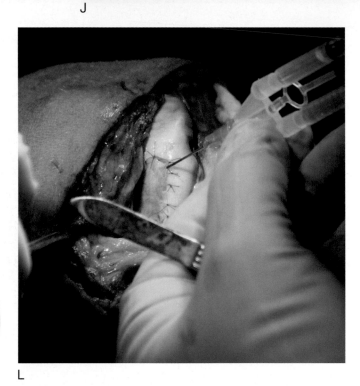

K

L

FIGURE 35–3—cont'd. The periosteal flap is gently elevated (**J**), placed on the defect with the cambium layer facing the bone, and anchored to the cartilage (**K**). After suturing is completed, the intervals are sealed with fibrin glue (**L**),

Continued

[MPFL]), muscular imbalance (musculus vastus medialis obliquus [VMO] weakness) and trochlear dysplasia (flat, convex, and extended in a proximal direction or a flat articulating lateral trochlea) (Fig. 35–5).

Tibial tuberosity transfer is used to correct the Q-angle by approximately 8 to 12 mm of medialization. Tibial tuberosity ventralization unloads the patella-trochlear joint (used in bipolar and large, uncontained lesions). To distalize a patella alta, the tibial tuberosity is moved distally 3 to 5 mm to secure so that the apex of the patellae will articulate on the trochlea. This can be achieved by a tibial tuberosity oblique osteotomy. Stabilizing and unloading procedures may include anteromedialization when needed.

The trochlea groove plasty is performed to establish the skeletal stability of the patella in the trochlea groove in the first 0° to 30° of flexion when the patella is skeletally unstable. Release the synovial membrane from the proximal attachment to the trochlear articular cartilage with a knife. Dissect the membrane free from the femur. Take a curved osteotome and remove the cartilage and bone starting in the center, aiming to the top of the intercondylar notch. Extend 8 to 10 mm distal to the horizontal

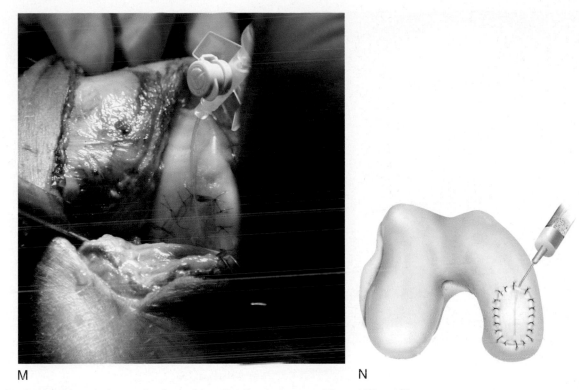

FIGURE 35-3—cont'd. and after testing for leakage, the chondrocytes are injected (**M** and **N**).

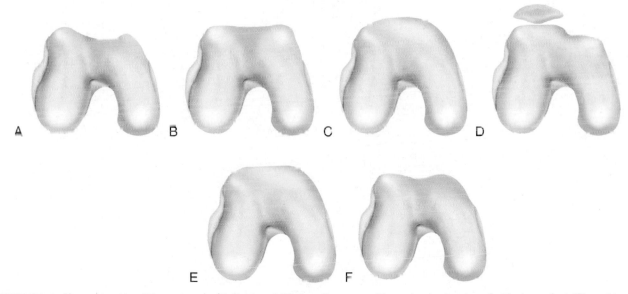

FIGURE 35-4. Normal trochlea (**A**) compared with flat type I (**B**), type II convex with proximal extension of articular surface (**C**), and type III flat articulating lateral trochlea (**D**). The aim (**E**) and goal (**F**) of the trochlea groove plasty of a flat trochlea.

of the trochlear articular cartilage and widen the groove 15 mm medial and lateral to the center, for a total of approximately 30 mm. If the cortical femoral bone is flat or convex, continue the removal of the bone proximally. Reattach the synovial membrane to the articular cartilage using mattress sutures starting in the synovial edge, cutting through the edge surface 5 to 6 mm into the cartilage. Then, proceed transversely and return the suture through the articular cartilage and the synovial membrane. Adapt the synovial membrane to the cut edge of the articular surface. A maximum of three to five sutures should be used. Inject a layer

of fibrin glue under the membrane and compress with a dry sponge for 60 to 120 seconds. Check the sliding of the patella in the new groove and adjust the edges when necessary. This technique preserves the congruity between the trochlea and the patella during the remaining flexion. The author does not address the patella dysplastic forms at any time (Fig. 35-6).

When a stabilization procedure is required, a midline incision is used, starting 3 cm proximal to the base of the patella and ending 4 to 5 cm distal to the patellar tendon insertion. Dissect medially and laterally and perform a lateral release and a medial

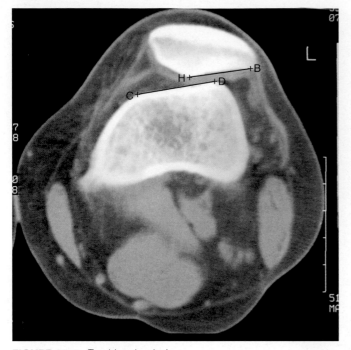

FIGURE 35–5. Trochlea dysplasia.

arthrotomy 3 to 5 mm medial to patella in the VMO tendon. Divide the VMO proximal from the rectus femoris 1 to 2 cm proximal to the base of the patella. Distally, open the infrapatellar bursa medially and laterally. Predrill the tibial tuberosity for later fixation and perform the necessary osteotomy. Perform the ACI on the patella and/or trochlea defects and inject the cells. Fix the tibial tuberosity with one or two screws. Roughen the bone between the VMO and MPFL insertions and the articular cartilage. Suture the VMO and MPFL medial end to the roughened bony surface of the patella. Implicate the lateral flap by suturing it to the VMO tendon. Complete the closure distally. Round the sharp edges of the tibial tuberosity medially and distally. Leave an extra-articular drainage for 12 to 24 hours lateral to the tibial tuberosity. After each step of the procedure, check the range of motion (ROM) and the adequate correction of the Q-angle. Use a brace to limit the ROM to 0° to 60° for the first 3 weeks and then from 0° to 90° or 110° the following 3 weeks.

Concomitant Unloading Procedures

Pathologic mechanics affecting the joint reduce the chances of a successful repair. Correcting varus or valgus malalignment with a high tibial or distal femoral osteotomy may be done before or after ACI. The correction is done to unload the repair tissue,

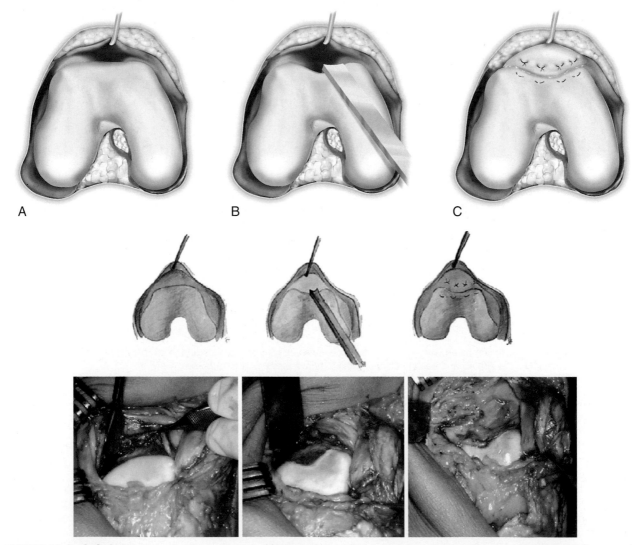

FIGURE 35–6. A–C, A dysplastic trochlea is treated with removal of cartilage and bone, and then the synovial membrane is sutured to the cartilage edge.

especially in large, uncontained, or kissing lesions, and the correctional angle is recommended to be 2° to 3°.

In trochlear and patellar lesions without malalignment, unloading with ventralization of the tibial tuberosity is performed in large, uncontained, or kissing lesions. A brace limiting ROM is used after unloading procedures.

Meniscus Transplantation

Meniscus transplantation should be considered after previous total or subtotal meniscectomy. The author recommends a staged procedure, with meniscus transplantation performed 9 to 12 months after ACI.

Concomitant Bone Grafting

When treating osteochondral lesions with bone defects and pathologic bone deeper than 6 to 7 mm, ACI is not enough and staged or concomitant autologous bone grafting is required. A staged procedure is preferable when both bone grafting and high tibial osteotomy are required. This can then be done concomitantly with the cartilage harvesting. Start by abrading away the sclerotic bottom of the defect and all pathologic bone down to spongy bone and undercut the subchondral bone plate. Use a 2-mm burr and drill holes into the spongy bone. Débride the cartilage to healthy cartilage with vertical edges. Then, harvest the cancellous bone used for grafting the bony defect. If the bony defect is small, use bone from the tibia or femoral condyle; if the defect is larger, harvest the bone from the iliac crest. Pack the bone from the bottom up and contour the bone graft just

below the subchondral bone plate. Harvest a periosteal flap to cover the bone graft at the level of the subchondral bone plate, the cambium layer facing the joint. Anchor the graft with horizontal sutures into the cartilage and inject fibrin glue under the flap for fixation to the bone graft. Use a dry sponge to compress the area for 2 to 3 minutes. This will avoid bleeding into the cartilage defect. When required, use bone sutures through small 1.2-mm drill holes or resorbable microanchors (Mitec). Harvest another periosteal flap and suture to the cartilage edges, with the cambium layer facing the defect. Use fibrin glue to seal off the intervals between the sutures. Test the watertightness with a gentle saline injection. If there is no leakage, aspirate the saline and inject the chondrocytes. Close the last opening and seal with fibrin glue (Fig. 35–7).

Postoperative Treatment

Analgesics are given to reduce pain and allow early motion and quadriceps activation. Prophylactic antibiotic and antithrombotic treatment is important.

REHABILITATION

Six to 8 hours after surgery, the patient begins passive motion training using a continuous passive motion machine in a pain-free ROM, usually 0° to 30° or 40°. The day after surgery, quadriceps activation, active ROM training, and gait training are the important parts of the rehabilitation, in addition to controlling swelling.

To avoid overloading, but still stimulate the chondrocytes and increase the exchange of fluids and nutrients in the

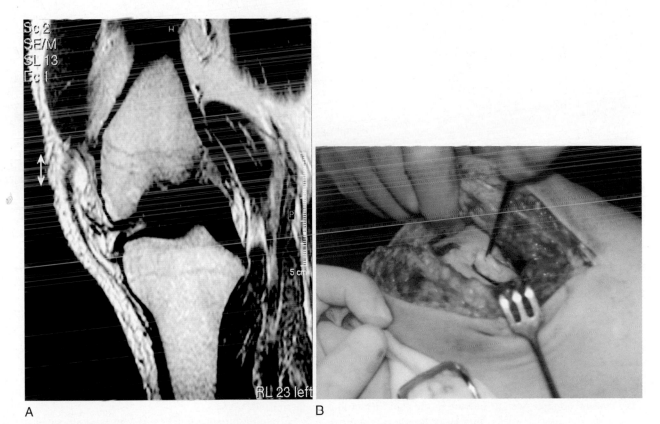

A   B

FIGURE 35–7. A, Magnetic resonance imaging (MRI) of a deep osteochondritis dissecans. The loose fragment is removed (**B**), and the damaged cartilage and fibrous and sclerotic bottom are débrided (**C**).

Continued

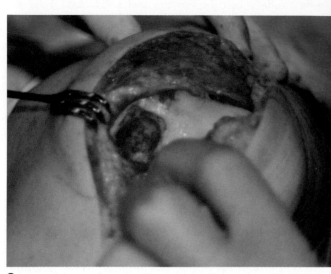

C

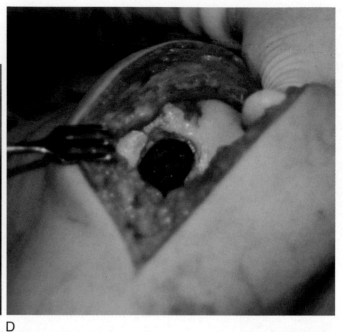

D

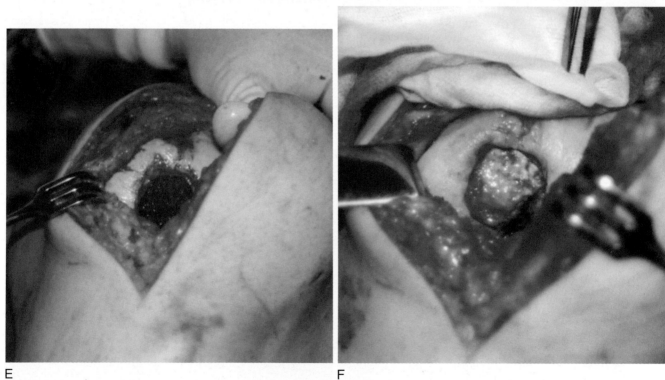

E

F

FIGURE 35–7—cont'd. D, The sclerotic bottom is abraded to a bleeding spongy surface, and drill holes are burred into the subchondral bone. The bone defect is packed with bone graft (**E**), and a periosteal flap is placed on top of the bone graft (**F**), glued to the bone graft and sutured to the cartilage.

Continued

cartilage, weight-bearing on the operated leg is kept partial for the first weeks. The amount of weight allowed depends on the size, location, and number of transplanted defects and possible concomitant procedures. After ACI to a small, contained lesion on the femoral condyle, weight-bearing to the pain threshold is allowed for the first 6 weeks. For large lesions or multiple lesions with concomitant procedures, weight-bearing is limited

to 30 to 40 pounds for 6 to 8 weeks, and is then gradually increased up to full after the following 6 to 8 weeks. For patellar and trochlear contained lesions, weight-bearing to the pain threshold for the first 6 weeks is used, but stair climbing is not permitted.

Training on a stationary bike can be done when the wound is healed and knee flexion permits; low resistance is used.

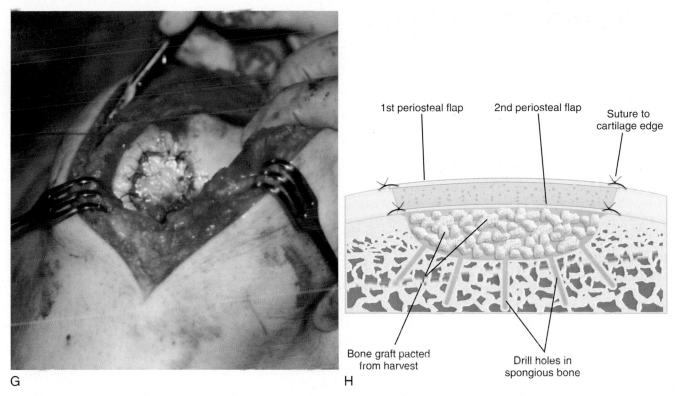

G   H

FIGURE 35-7—cont'd. G, Another periosteal flap is sutured to the cartilage rim. **H**, Schematic drawing of the bone graft and ACI.

Encourage bicycling during the entire rehabilitation program. Training in water may be initiated when the wound is healed. Gradually increased functional and proprioceptive training is important during the entire course of rehabilitation.

When full weight-bearing is achieved, increase distances of walking. If possible, use skating, inline skating, or cross-country skiing on even surfaces as intermediate training before returning to running. Running should be postponed at least 6 to 9 months for small, contained, shouldered femoral condyle defects and begun on an individual basis. For larger or unshouldered femoral condyle defects or defects on patella, trochlea, tibia, or bipolar defects, running should be postponed longer, possibly for up to 12 to 18 months after ACI.

Return to professional athletic training and competition should be judged on an individual basis, including assessment of ROM, muscle strength and endurance, and arthroscopic evaluation and probing/indentation test of the repair area (Fig. 35-8).

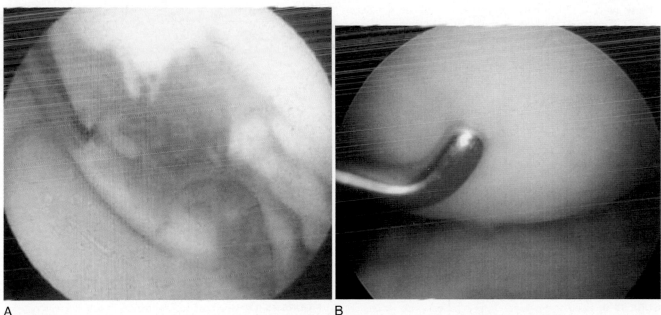

A   B

FIGURE 35-8. Arthroscopic evaluation before (**A**) and after (**B**) osteochondritis dissecans on the medial femoral condyle treated with ACI.

AUTHOR'S EVIDENCE-BASED CLINICAL OUTCOMES

Subjective

A clinical evaluation at an intermediate to long-term follow-up of the first 101 patients showed that overall, 77% were considered a good or excellent result.[22] The patients were divided into groups according to the location and type of the lesion as well as concomitant ACL reconstruction. In the isolated femoral condyle group, 92% were clinically graded as good or excellent; in the OCD group, 89% were in this category; and in the femoral condyle with ACL reconstruction, 75% were in this category. Patients with multiple lesions had a 67% good or excellent rate. The patellar lesions were often treated with concomitant transfer of the tibial tubercle, medial patellofemoral ligament and VMO shortening, and trochlea groove plasty. At follow-up, 65% had a good or excellent result[22] compared with 28% in the initial follow-up study.[2]

An early consecutive cohort of 61 patients were followed for a mean of 7.4 years (range, 5–11 years).[20] At the 2-year follow-up, 50 patients had a good or excellent clinical result; at the 5-to 11-year follow-up, 51 patients were considered good or excellent.

In a study published in 2003,[23] 58 patients with OCD were treated with ACI and followed an average of 5.6 years. The average age was 26.4 years, and the average defect size was 5.7 cm², with a maximum defect of 12 cm². Forty-eight patients had had a mean of 2.1 previous operations because of the injury. The modified Cincinnati clinical rating score was 2.0 points preoperatively and 9.8 points at follow-up. The overall clinical grading was excellent in 53%, good in 38%, fair in 7%, and poor in 2%. Self-assessed improvement was 93%.[23] (Figs. 35–9 to 35–12). At the ICRS meeting in Toronto in 2002,[3] results were presented for patients treated with ACI for cartilage lesions on tibia and trochlea as well as tibiofemoral kissing lesions and multiple lesions (Fig. 35–13).

Objective

Different objective tools have been used to evaluate the repair after ACI of chondral and osteochondral lesions including arthroscopic macroscopic assessment and indentation tests as well as repair tissue biopsy for histology and histochemistry. In the first 101 patients, 37 biopsies from the repair tissue were assessed for

collagen type II.[22] There was correlation between hyaline-like repair tissue and good or excellent clinical outcomes.

In the 61-patient cohort, biopsies from the repair tissue were obtained in 12 patients.[20] Eight of the biopsies were characterized as hyaline-like by Safranin O staining and homogeneous appearance under polarized light. Eight hyaline-like and 3 fibrous biopsies stained positive to aggrecan and cartilage oligomeric matrix protein. Hyaline-like biopsies stained positive

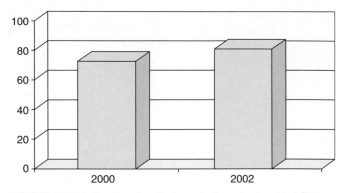

FIGURE 35–10. Good or excellent results in patients with ACI to femoral condyle lesions and concomitant anterior cruciate ligament reconstruction in studies published in 2000 ($n = 16$)[22] and 2002 ($n = 11$).[20]

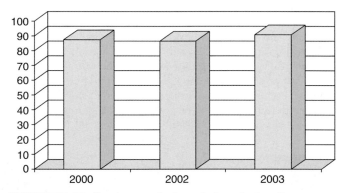

FIGURE 35–11. Good or excellent results in patients with osteochondritis dissecans (OCD) in studies published in 2000 ($n = 18$),[22] 2002 ($n = 14$),[20] and 2003 ($n = 58$).[23]

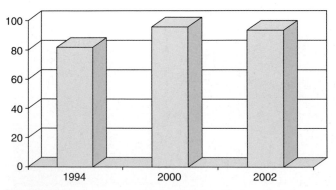

FIGURE 35–9. Good or excellent results in patients with lesions on the femoral condyle in studies published in 1994 ($n = 17$),[2] 2000 ($n = 25$),[22] and 2002 ($n = 18$).[20]

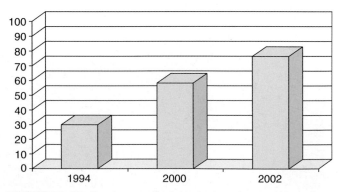

FIGURE 35–12. Good or excellent results in patients with patella lesions in studies published in 1994 ($n = 7$),[2] 2000 ($n = 19$), and 2002 ($n = 17$).[20]

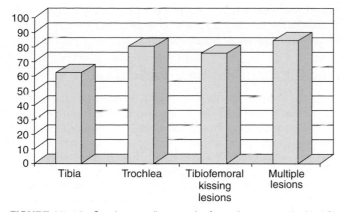

FIGURE 35–13. Good or excellent results for patients treated with ACI to the tibia ($n = 8$; mean size, 4.5 cm^2) and trochlea ($n = 15$; mean size, 5.2 cm^2) as well as tibiofemoral kissing lesion ($n = 14$, mean size, 11.8 cm^2) and multiple lesions ($n = 43$; mean size, 10.8 cm^2). *(From Brittberg, M.; Peterson, L.; Björnum, S.; Lindahl, A.: Multiple lesions in the knee treated with autologous chondrocyte implantation. Read at the meeting of the International Cartilage Repair Society, June 14-16, 2002, Toronto, Canada.)*

for collagen type II and fibrous biopsies stained positive for collagen type I. All histologic evaluations were performed by independent scientists.[20]

An arthroscopic indentation probe was used to measure the stiffness of the repair tissue in 11 of the 61 patients at a mean of 54.3 months (range, 33-84 mo).[20] The mean stiffness of repair tissue characterized as hyaline-like by histologic evaluation was 3.0 ± 1.1 N, compared with 1.5 ± 0.35 N of fibrous repair tissue. Good and excellent clinical results correlated with hyaline-like repair tissue, whereas fair or poor clinical results correlated with fibrous repair tissue.[20]

Vasara and associates[26] arthroscopically measured the stiffness of the repair tissue 8 to 18 months after ACI using an indentation probe, and compared it with the stiffness of normal surrounding cartilage. The mean stiffness of the repair tissue was 2.04 ± 0.83 N, and the mean stiffness of the surrounding cartilage was 3.58 ± 1.04 N. Non-OCD repair tissue was stiffer (2.37 ± 0.72 N) than the repair tissue of OCD defects (1.45 ± 0.46 N).[26]

Functional

In the study of the first 101 consecutive patients with chondral or osteochondral lesions of the knee treated with ACI, the activity levels of the patients were evaluated.[22] According to the Tegner/Wallgren score, the patients were able to resume an active lifestyle that included sports with high demands on the knee (e.g., soccer). The modified Cincinnati score was an average 9 out of 10, indicating the patients returned to high-level sports.[22]

In one study, 45 soccer players treated with ACI were followed for a mean of 40 months.[16] Eighty-three percent of the young players below 26 years of age, high–skill-level players, and players operated within 12 months after trauma returned to preinjury levels. The time to return from surgery to soccer was 12 to 18 months.[16]

Twenty adolescent athletes were followed for a mean of 47 months after ACI.[15] At follow-up, the 0 to 10 Tegner activity score had increased from 4 to 8 points, and 96% of patients

had returned to impact sports, 60% at the same or higher level than before the injury. Treatment with ACI within 12 months from injury lead to 100% return to preinjury sport, whereas 42% of the chronic cases returned to preinjury sport.[15]

Complications

In the first 23 patients, 4 graft failures occurred, whereas in the following 78 patients, only 3 grafts failed. Arthroscopically verified periosteal overgrowth was found in 26 patients; however, only 7 were symptomatic and these resolved after débridement.[22]

OUTCOMES FROM OTHER AUTHORS

Gillogly[6-8] evaluated 112 patients 2 to 5 years after ACI. The locations of the lesions were diverse and included 15 lesions on the patella, 27 on the trochlea, and multiple lesions in 22. When using the clinician evaluation portion of the modified Cincinnati scale, 93% were considered good or excellent. Using the patient evaluation portion, 89% considered themselves good or excellent.

Minas[14] reported on 130 patients treated with ACI in the patellofemoral joint with a follow-up of 2 to 9 years. In a patient satisfaction survey, 80% rated themselves as good or excellent.

Bentley and colleagues[1] compared ACI and mosaicplasty in a randomized, prospective study of 100 consecutive patients (58 ACI and 42 mosaicplasty) with a follow-up mean of 19 months. Functional assessment using the modified Cincinnati and Stanmore rating systems as well as clinical assessment showed good or excellent results in 88% after ACI and 69% after mosaicplasty. Arthroscopic assessment 1 year after treatment showed good or excellent repair in 82% after ACI and 34% after mosaicplasty.

In another study, Knutsen and coworkers[13] reported on 80 patients with single symptomatic cartilage defects on the femoral condyle treated with either ACI ($N = 40$) or microfracture ($N = 40$). Ten patients in each group were treated at four different hospitals. At the 2-year follow-up, both groups had significant clinical improvement. However, according to the Short-Form 36-item questionnaire (SF-36) physical component score, the improvement in the patients treated with microfracture was significantly better than in the ACI group. Three failures were reported, 2 in the ACI group and 1 in the microfracture group. Biopsies from the repair tissue were taken arthroscopically in 67 patients. In the ACI group, 72% of the biopsies showed hyaline-like tissue and 25% showed a mix of hyaline and fibrocartilage. Only 3% showed fibrocartilage. In the biopsies from the microfracture group, 40% were identified as hyaline-like, 29% were a mix of hyaline and fibrocartilage, and 31% contained fibrocartilage.[13]

Henderson and associates[9,10] evaluated 53 patients (72 lesions) with MRI 3 months, 12 months, and 2 years after ACI. The 3-month MRI demonstrated a filling of the defect of at least 50% in 75.3% of the lesions, 46.3% had a near-normal signal, 68.1% had mild or no effusion, and 66.7% had mild or no underlying bone marrow edema. At 12 months, 94.2% had at least 50% defect fill with 86.9% demonstrating a near-normal signal. By 2 years, 97% had at least 50% defect fill and 97% had a near-normal signal. The values for mild or no effusion and mild or no bone marrow edema increased to 91.3% and

88.4%, respectively, at 12 months and 95.6% and 92.6%, respectively, at 2 years. A clinical evaluation of the patients and results from second-look arthroscopy and repair tissue biopsy correlated well with the 12-month MRI.[9,10]

Brown and colleagues[4] evaluated 180 MRIs of 112 patients treated with cartilage resurfacing techniques, including microfracture (MRI done a mean of 15 mo) and ACI (MRI done a mean of 13 mo). Lesions treated with ACI showed better filling of the defect, but graft hypertrophy was present in 63%. The repair tissue after microfracture was depressed compared with the native cartilage and had a propensity for bone development and loss of adjacent cartilage.[4]

PREVENTION AND MANAGEMENT OF COMPLICATIONS

General Complications

Four serious general complications have occurred, involving one deep infection and three deep vein thrombosis in 1400 patients treated since 1987.

Local Complications: Arthrofibrosis

The complication of arthrofibrosis with decreased ROM is, in the author's experience, a rare event. This usually occurs owing to bleeding from concomitant procedures such as ACL reconstruction, osteotomy, or intra-articular harvesting of periosteal flaps from the femoral condyles. Arthrofibrosis and decreased ROM can be prevented by careful hemostasis and intra-articular drainage without suction or extra-articular drainage with suction. Postoperative pain control, continuous passive motion, early motion, and muscle activation are mandatory. Early and regular follow-up is necessary to ensure a return of motion, muscle activity, and progressive increase of weight-bearing.

Local Complications: Periosteal

Superficial fibrillation of the periosteal surface that causes crepitus has occurred (Fig. 35–14). Periosteal hypertrophy overlapping the surrounding normal cartilage may cause symptoms of clicking, catching, or crepitus (Fig. 35–15). This complication may appear between 3 and 9 months postoperatively and, in most patients, disappears spontaneously during continued rehabilitation. When this problem interferes with the rehabilitation, it is first handled with change and modification of the rehabilitation program and then with gentle arthroscopic resection. The frequency of periosteal complications was initially reported to be about 25%. By improved surgical technique and adapted rehabilitation, the incidence of this problem has been reduced to 5% to 8%. Other authors have reported frequencies between 5% and 65%.

Periosteal delamination has occurred in a few cases (Fig. 35–16). The delamination can be marginal, partial, or total. In a marginal delamination, the periosteal flap is avulsed from the surrounding cartilage up to 10 mm and should be excised or gently débrided. In a partial delamination, the periosteal flap is partly separated from the underlying repair tissue and can be removed by shaving or excising the superficial periosteal delamination. A total periosteal delamination can either be detached or appear as a loose body. It should be removed from the joint or the transplanted area. Usually, the repair tissue will continue filling the defect and motion will stimulate it to produce a new sliding surface. During the 6 to 8 weeks after periosteum removal, ROM training and bicycling with low resistance should be performed, but no running is

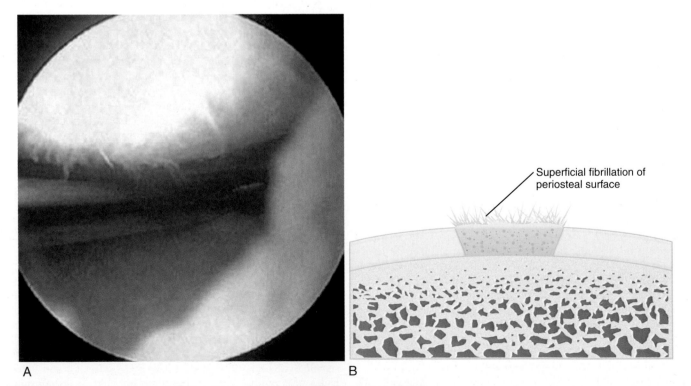

Superficial fibrillation of periosteal surface

A   B

FIGURE 35–14. Arthroscopic view (**A**) and schematic drawing (**B**) of periosteal fibrillation.

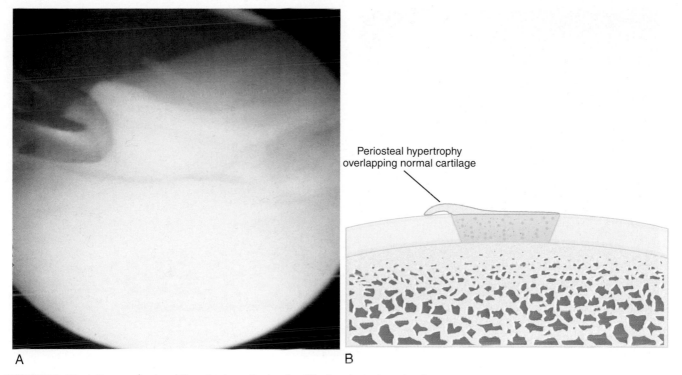

FIGURE 35-15. Arthroscopic view (**A**) and schematic drawing (**B**) of periosteal overlapping

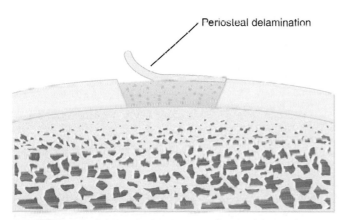

FIGURE 35-16. Schematic drawing of periosteal delamination

permitted. Periosteal complications are benign and, when adequately addressed, will have no impact on the end result.

Local Complications: Graft Delamination

Separation and delamination of the total repair tissue down to the subchondral bone is a rare complication (Fig. 35–17). In a marginal graft delamination of less than 10 mm, the area is débrided and left alone. If any bone is visible, the bone is microfractured to create a fibrous repair filling, which will stabilize the area. In a partial graft delamination, the defect is excised and new cartilage is harvested for retransplantation of chondrocytes. In smaller defects up to 1.5 cm², osteochondral cylinders or

microfracture may be first options. In a total graft delamination, it either is detached in a small area or appears as a loose body. A loose body is removed and a delaminated graft excised. New cartilage is harvested for reoperation with ACI. Good results can be achieved after a second ACI procedure.

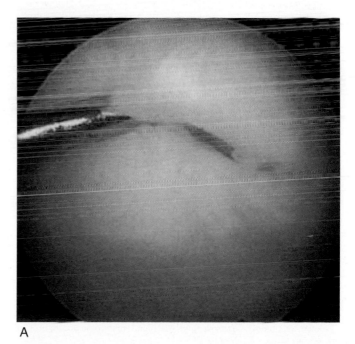

FIGURE 35-17. A, Arthroscopic view of marginal graft delamination.
Continued

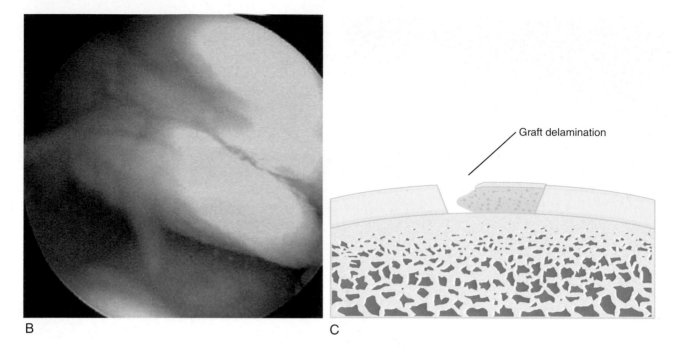

FIGURE 35–17—cont'd. B, In a total graft delamination, the graft can become a loose body. **C**, Schematic drawing of partial graft delamination.

REFERENCES

1. Bentley, G.; Biant, L. C.; Carrington, R. W.; et al.: A prospective, randomized comparison of autologous chondrocyte implantation versus mosaicplasty for osteochondral defects in the knee. *J Bone Joint Surg Br* 85:223–230, 2003.
2. Brittberg, M.; Lindahl, A.; Nilsson, A.; et al.: Treatment of deep cartilage defects in the knee with autologous chondrocyte transplantation. *N Engl J Med* 331:889–895, 1994.
3. Brittberg, M.; Peterson, L.; Björnum, S.; Lindahl, A.: Multiple lesions in the knee treated with autologous chondrocyte implantation. Read at the meeting of the International Cartilage Repair Society, June 14-18, 2002, Toronto, Canada.
4. Brown, W. E.; Potter, H. G.; Marx, R. G.; et al.: Magnetic resonance imaging appearance of cartilage repair in the knee. *Clin Orthop Relat Res* 422:214–223, 2004.
5. Curl, W. W.; Krome, J.; Gordon, E. S.; et al.: Cartilage injuries: a review of 31,516 knee arthroscopies. *Arthroscopy* 13:456–460, 1997.
6. Gillogly, S. D.: Clinical results of autologous chondrocyte implantation for large full-thickness chondral defects of the knee: 5-year experience with 112 consecutive patients. Read at the annual meeting of the American Society for Sports Medicine, June 2001, Keystone, CO.
7. Gillogly, S. D.: Autologous chondrocyte implantation: complex defects and concomitant procedures. *Oper Tech Sports Med* 10:120–128, 2002.
8. Gillogly, S. D.: Treatment of large full-thickness chondral defects of the knee with autologous chondrocyte implantation. *Arthroscopy* 19 (suppl 1):147–153, 2003.
9. Henderson, I. J.; Tuy, B.; Connell, D.; et al.: Prospective clinical study of autologous chondrocyte implantation and correlation with MRI at 3 and 12 months. *J Bone Joint Surg Br* 85:1060–1066, 2003.
10. Henderson, I. J.; Tuy, B.; Connell, D.; et al.: Autologous chondrocyte implantation for treatment of focal chondral defects of the knee—a clinical, arthroscopic, MRI and histologic evaluation at 2 years. *Knee* 12:209–216, 2005.
11. Hjelle, K.; Solheim, E.; Strand, T.; et al.: Articular cartilage defects in 1000 knee arthroscopies. *Arthroscopy* 18:730–734, 2002.
12. Johnson, D. L.; Urban, W. P., Jr.; Caborn, D. N.; et al.: Articular cartilage changes seen with magnetic resonance imaging–detected bone bruises associated with acute anterior cruciate ligament rupture. *Am J Sports Med* 26:409–414, 1998.
13. Knutsen, G.; Engebretsen, L.; Ludvigsen, T. C.; et al.: Autologous chondrocyte implantation compared with microfracture in the knee. A randomized trial. *J Bone Joint Surg Am* 86:455–464, 2004.
14. Minas, T.: A surgical algorithm for the management of patellofemoral disease. Read at the meeting Advanced Concepts in ACI, November 2007, Philadelphia, PA.
15. Mithöfer, K.; Minas, T.; Peterson, L.; et al.: Functional outcome of knee articular cartilage repair in adolescent athletes. *Am J Sports Med* 33:1147–1153, 2005.
16. Mithöfer, K.; Peterson, L.; Mandelbaum, B. R.; Minas, T.: Articular cartilage repair in soccer players with autologous chondrocyte transplantation: functional outcome and return to competition. *Am J Sports Med* 33:1639–1646, 2005.
17. Noyes, F. R.; Barber-Westin, S. D.; Butler, D. L.; Wilkins, R. M.: The role of allografts in repair and reconstruction of knee joint ligaments and menisci. In Cannon, W. D., Jr. (ed.): Instructional Course Lectures, Vol. 47. Rosemont, IL: American Academy of Orthopaedic Surgeons, 1998; pp. 379–396.
18. Noyes, F. R.; Bassett, R. W.; Grood, E. S.; Butler, D. L.: Arthroscopy in acute traumatic hemarthrosis of the knee: incidence of anterior cruciate tears and other injuries. *J Bone Joint Surg Am* 62:687–695, 1980.
19. Noyes, F. R.; Mooar, P. A.; Matthews, D. S.; Butler, D. L.: The symptomatic anterior cruciate–deficient knee: part I. The long-term functional disability in athletically active individuals. *J Bone Joint Surg Am* 65:154–162, 1983.
20. Peterson, L.; Brittberg, M.; Kiviranta, I.; et al.: Autologous chondrocyte transplantation: biomechanics and long-term durability. *Am J Sports Med* 30:2–12, 2002.
21. Peterson, L.; Karlsson, J.; Brittberg, M.: Patellar instability with recurrent dislocation due to patellofemoral dysplasia. Results after surgical treatment. *Bull Hosp Jt Dis Orthop Inst* 48:130–139, 1988.
22. Peterson, L.; Minas, T.; Brittberg, M.; et al.: Two- to 9-year outcome after autologous chondrocyte transplantation of the knee. *Clin Orthop Relat Res* 374:212–234, 2000.
23. Peterson, L.; Minas, T.; Brittberg, M.; Lindahl, A.: Treatment of osteochondritis dissecans of the knee with autologous chondrocyte

transplantation: results at two to ten years. *J Bone Joint Surg Am* 85 (suppl 2):17–25, 2003.

24. Shelbourne, K. D.; Jari, S.; Gray, T.: Outcome of untreated traumatic articular cartilage defects of the knee. *J Bone Joint Surg Am* 85(suppl 2):8–16, 2003.

25. Schimmer, R. C.; Brülhart, K. B.; Duff, C.; Glinz, W.: Arthroscopic partial meniscectomy: a 12-year follow-up and two-step evaluation of the long-term course. *Arthroscopy* 14:136–142, 1998.

26. Vasara, A. I.; Nieminen, M. T.; Jurvelin, J. S.; et al.: Indentation stiffness of repair tissue after autologous chondrocyte transplantation. *Clin Orthop Relat Res* 433:233–242, 2005.

Chapter 36

Osteochondral Grafts: Diagnosis, Operative Techniques, and Clinical Outcomes

Simon Görtz, MD ■ *William D. Bugbee*, MD

INTRODUCTION

Hyaline articular cartilage is an avascular and insensate tissue that allows low-friction transmission of physiologic loads in diarthrodial joints. Its functional structure ideally is maintained in homeostasis over the lifetime of an individual, but remains incapable of mounting an effective repair response when injured in the skeletally mature adult.[10,35] The treatment threshold for surgical intervention is not unequivocal, but patients with symptomatic lesions are generally considered candidates for cartilage restoration procedures.[3]

The use of osteochondral grafts of autologous or allogeneic origin is well supported on a basic science level and has a long successful clinical history as a means of biologic resurfacing.[9,16] Both modalities rely on transplanting mature hyaline cartilage containing viable chondrocytes attached to subchondral bone to restore the architecture and characteristics of native tissue in acquired osteoarticular defects. By transplanting structurally complete osteochondral units with an intact tidemark, the fixation issue is mostly relegated to that of osseous ingrowth.[31] Whereas both graft sources represent a common cartilage organ transplantation paradigm and are complementary, each has its unique, reciprocal challenges with regard to tissue availability and safety that must be weighed, managed, and communicated whenever the use of osteochondral grafts is being considered.

INDICATIONS

Autografts

In the authors' hands, autologous grafts are best used to address relatively small, yet symptomatic, focal articular lesions of the femoral condyles, especially if these present with associated subchondral abnormalities such as a bone cyst or an intralesional osteophyte. Autologous plugs are also a potential salvage option as in situ fixation for a delaminating osteochondritis dissecans (OCD) lesion (International Cartilage Repair Society [ICRS] grade II–IV, see Chapter 47, Articular Cartilage Rating Systems).[19,41]

Advantages of autologous grafts are immediate availability, relatively low cost, and their nonantigenic and osteogenic behavior that routinely lead to reliable osteointegration.[11] The possibility of arthroscopic delivery of these smaller grafts is appealing, albeit technically challenging.

One obvious disadvantage of autologous graft sources is that the maximum graft surface area is self-limited by donor volume or lack thereof, for small and at most medium-sized lesions. This is especially true in the previously injured and/or operated knee, in which suitability regarding tissue quality and overall joint topography has to be critically assessed. In addition, donor-site morbidity can significantly add to the disease burden during intra-articular transfer.[9]

Allografts

Osteochondral allografts are ideally suited to treat medium to large chondral and osteochondral lesions.[24] In particular, osteochondral allografting may be considered the current "gold standard" treatment for high-grade (ICRS grade III–IV) OCD about the knee. Other specific conditions amenable to allografting include osteonecrosis and post-traumatic defects, such as after periarticular fractures. Further indications for allografting of the knee include treatment of patellofemoral chondrosis or arthrosis and highly select cases of multifocal or bipolar post-traumatic or degenerative lesions. In a case in which meniscus replacement is also necessary, a composite tibial plateau with attached meniscus can be transplanted. Allografts are also increasingly employed in the salvage of knees that have failed other cartilage resurfacing procedures. Primary treatment may be considered in large chondral defects, whose size presents a relative contraindication for other treatments and for which the surgeon believes other procedures may be inadequate.

Osteochondral allografting is the only treatment option that restores mature orthotopic hyaline cartilage and reproduces the site-appropriate anatomy of the native joint both macroscopically and microscopically, without the risk of inducing donor-site morbidity.[23] Osteochondral allografts are versatile addressing even very large, complex, or multiple lesions in topographically challenging environments, especially if they involve an osseous component.

Obvious drawbacks to the allograft paradigm are the relative scarcity of donor tissue, financial and logistical issues of graft procurement, and residual risk of infection, a discussion that is an essential part of the informed consent process.[24] Although rare allograft-associated bacterial infections have been reported,[49] there are no available published data quantifying this risk or that of viral transmission. Patients are counseled that the risk for disease transmission from a fresh osteochondral allograft is comparable with that associated with banked blood transfusion. In a 30-year experience at the authors' institution, using over 500 fresh allografts, no cases of transmission of disease from donor to recipient have been documented.

Fresh, cold-stored osteochondral allografts have shown to maintain viable chondrocytes and mechanical properties of the matrix many years after transplantation.[4,14–16,30,38,52] These findings have generally supported the use of tissue for small osteochondral allografts in the setting of reconstruction of chondral and osteochondral defects. Chondrocyte viability and structural integrity of the matrix are preserved during hypothermal storage in nutritive culture medium containing human serum, with cell density, viability, and metabolic activity remaining essentially unchanged from baseline for as many as 14 days before deteriorating significantly after 28 days while the hyaline matrix remains relatively intact.[6,45,47,50,53] The clinical consequences of these storage-induced graft changes have yet to be determined, but 28 days is generally considered the threshold of graft utility in present clinical practice.

CONTRAINDICATIONS

Persisting impairments to the mechanical or biologic milieu of the knee joint are considered contraindications to osteochondral grafting procedures. These include uncorrected ligamentous instability, meniscal deficiency, or axial malalignment of the lower extremity, as well as the presence of inflammatory or crystal-induced arthropathy or any unexplained global synovitis of the knee.

Autologous plugs are not advised in lesions presenting with a lack of containment or substantial subchondral bone loss, which might lead to loss of fixation and graft failure. Whereas "kissing" lesions are also widely considered unsuitable for autologous grafting, bipolar and multicompartmental allografting has been modestly successful in the younger individual. However, advanced multicompartmental arthrosis is a relative contraindication to the allografting procedure, and neither osteochondral grafting technique should be considered an alternative to prosthetic arthroplasty in an individual with symptoms and acceptable age and activity level for prosthetic replacement.

CLINICAL EVALUATION

A careful and focused history and physical examination are essential to determine candidacy for any cartilage restoration procedure. Because articular cartilage itself is insensate, it is important to identify contributory pain generators and to distinguish them from mechanical symptoms. Tools such as the ICRS Cartilage Injury Evaluation Package, which incorporates several validated outcome measures, can be helpful in systematically documenting the anatomic condition and functional envelope of the knee and in establishing a baseline for therapy.[1]

The clinician should elucidate the location and quality of pain, onset (acute vs. chronic) and duration of symptoms, alleviating and exacerbating events or measures, prior treatment and surgical history (if any), as well as activity at the time of injury and expected future level of occupational and recreational performance. Significant medical factors potentially relating to knee pathology should be sought such as prior trauma, collagen-vascular/inflammatory disorders, or corticosteroid use.

It should be noted that the time since the initial cartilage injury and pending disability compensation claims are universally recognized as inversely related to outcome. The onset and character of symptoms are worth noting in an effort to distinguish pain at rest (indicative of an underlying, more advanced degenerative process) from activity-related pain or mechanical symptoms such as catching or locking that suggest meniscal injury, loose bodies, or cartilage flaps associated with acute injury or early degenerative disease.

The physical examination should begin with a visual inspection of the patient's gait and limb alignment. With the patient placed supine, the examiner can commence with a closer inspection of the knee joint and comparison with the uninjured side, focusing on the area of the chief complaint. Range of motion (ROM) and ligamentous stability should be noted using standard maneuvers. Presence of effusion should be noted, and the patellofemoral joint should be assessed for alignment, baja or alta position, mobility, grind, tracking, tilt, and signs of apprehension. It is particularly useful to palpate the femoral condyles and other accessible articular surfaces, because focal tenderness at the site of cartilage lesions is an important physical finding. Symptomatic trochlear or patellar lesions can be stressed with a bounce test or by applying prepatellar pressure during the grind test, whereas condylar lesions will often become painful when loaded with a valgus or varus stress test or during a McMurray maneuver. Accordingly, joint line pain and other complaints due to meniscal or synovial symptoms or originating from extra-articular structures such as bursae or the iliotibial band should be distinguished from chondral pathology. A diagnostic injection of an anesthetic agent can help differentiate the intra-articular pain component that might be amenable to surgical intervention from extra-articular stimuli.

Patients who are considered for an osteochondral grafting procedure should optimally be fully imaged, including a complete radiologic series and magnetic resonance imaging (MRI) studies with cartilage-specific sequencing, if available. Depending on the type and location of cartilage injury being suspected, this should include at least standing anteroposterior (AP) weight-bearing and flexed knee lateral radiographs. Many chondral lesions and their subchondral sequelae are detectable on the AP views (Fig. 36–1), which also give an indication of possible secondary changes such as joint space narrowing and osteophytes. Imaging both knees side-by-side allows for a built-in comparison view. Of note, OCD presents with bilateral lesions in about a third of cases that are often easily detected on an x-ray in their typical location on the lateral aspect of the medial femoral condyle toward the intercondylar notch. The lateral flexed view is an important supplementary tool to help assess lesion size, triangulate locations, and identify patient morphology such as patella alta or baja and trochlear groove topography. Additional views that can be obtained include standing posteroanterior 45° flexed knee (Rosenberg) views and supine flexed knee (Merchant) views. The Rosenberg view brings the posterior condyles into view, which helps assess the posterior joint space during loading. Merchant views are standard for the evaluation of the patellofemoral articulation. Long-leg (hip to ankle) standing AP weight-bearing films should be obtained if axial alignment is deemed contributory to the patient's symptomatology and are essential for preoperative planning if a realignment procedure is being considered.

MRI remains an invaluable tool for assessing the status of the articular cartilage and associated structures of the knee[46]

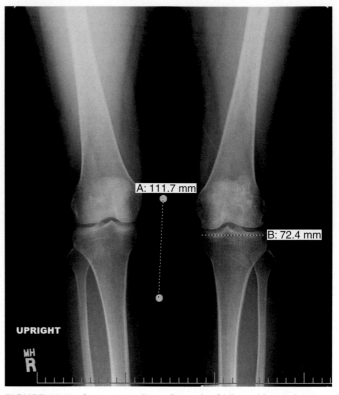

FIGURE 36–1. Anteroposterior radiograph of bilateral knees in a 44-year-old patient with osteonecrotic changes to her left lateral femoral condyle, displaying a tibial measurement and a radiographic magnification marker for allograft sizing.

(Fig. 36–2). While T_2-weighted relaxation time maps are currently recognized as the gold standard for imaging the ultrastructure of the articular cartilage, a standard fat-saturated T_2-weighted fast-spin-echo sequence usually conveys sufficient detail on cartilage morphology to guide surgical decision-making and preoperative planning. T_1-weighted sequences are generally better suited to assess involvement of the subchondral bone and menisci.

Early degenerative ICRS grade I or II changes (softening, fibrillation) and associated surface irregularities often present as subtle alterations in contour morphology and thickness on MRI. Decreases in thickness can indicate cartilage volume loss, whereas increases in thickness can signal intrasubstance collagen degeneration and free water accumulation. Advanced degenerative grade III or IV lesions are usually more overt on MRI, manifesting as poorly marginated substance defects often associated with corresponding signal-intensive subchondral edema or cysts, apposing joint surface changes, localized synovitis, or general joint effusion. In contrast, acute, traumatic defects routinely present as focal chondral or osteochondral lesions with distinct margins, often with underlying bone signal changes.

PREOPERATIVE PLANNING

If the patient has had prior surgery, the corresponding operative reports and arthroscopic photographs (if available) are usually helpful not only in assessing the index lesion but also in gauging the overall disease burden and suitability for autologous graft harvest, if applicable. Obviously, results of any modalities and

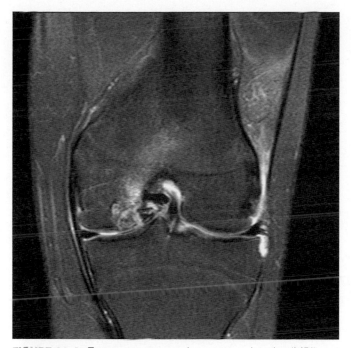

FIGURE 36–2. T_2 sequence magnetic resonance imaging (MRI) of the left knee of an 18-year-old female demonstrates an osteochondritis dissecans lesion in typical location on the lateral aspect of the left medial femoral condyle.

examinations described previously will also factor into the decision and any surgical planning.

Common to all fresh allografting procedures is matching the donor with the recipient. It should be noted that in current practice, small-fragment fresh osteochondral allografts are not human leukocyte antigen- (HLA-) or blood type–matched between donor and recipient and that no immunosuppression is used. The allografts are matched to recipients on size alone. In the knee, an AP radiograph with a magnification marker is

---

Critical Points GENERAL SURGICAL PRINCIPLES OF ALLOGRAFTING

1. Careful consideration of patient and surgeon goals.
2. Assessment of biologic and mechanical environment of joint.
3. Adequate confirmation of inclusion criteria for fresh osteochondral allografting.
4. Careful informed consent process, including risks of infection.
5. Confirm graft recipient match, in both size and side.
6. Review other graft characteristics, including donor age, history, and length of graft storage time since harvest.
7. Inspect graft material before making incision.
8. Be prepared to fashion graft and recipient site with a freehand technique, if necessary.
9. Utilize fluoroscopy to confirm the clinical perspective, especially in tibia and patella allografts.
10. Minimize the osseous portion of the allograft to 3–6 mm except in tibial plateau grafts, for which minimal graft thickness should be 10 mm.
11. Always remove all soft tissue and perform pressurized lavage of osseous graft portion prior to insertion.
12. Avoid excessively impacting the graft during insertion.
13. Ensure adequate fixation; utilize adjunctive fixation where necessary.

---

used (see Fig. 36–1), and a measurement of the mediolateral dimension of the tibia, just below the joint surface, is made and corrected for magnification of the radiograph. This corrected measurement is used, and the tissue bank makes a direct measurement on the donor tibial plateau. Alternatively, a measurement of the affected condyle can be performed.[28] A match is considered acceptable at ± 2 mm; however, it should be noted that there is a significant variability in anatomy, which is not reflected in size measurements. In particular, in treating OCD, the pathologic condyle is typically larger, wider, and flatter; therefore, a larger donor generally should be used.

Lastly, when considering realigning osteotomy on the same articulating side of an osteochondral graft, staging the procedure is advised in order not to jeopardize the microvascularity of the recipient bone bed.

INTRAOPERATIVE PLANNING

The patient is positioned in a supine fashion to allow for full flexion of the knee. A tourniquet is recommended to assist with intraoperative visualization. A leg or foot holder can help to position and maintain the leg between 70° and 100° of flexion during open procedures.

Autografting

Historically, the intercondylar notch and lateral trochlea were presumed to be non–load bearing and thus recommended as donor sites for autologous osteochondral grafting. More recent reports have demonstrated that these areas do bear significant weight, which can theoretically contribute to increased donor-site morbidity. The lateral trochlea appears to be the most involved in loading, followed by the intercondylar notch and the distal medial trochlea.[2] Because the lateral trochlea is wider than the medial side, the medial trochlea may best be suited for smaller donor plugs (<5 mm).[20] Larger plugs can be taken from the lateral trochlea, starting proximal to the sulcus terminalis, where the lowest contact pressures of the lateral trochlea were measured. Owing to its load-bearing demands, the lateral trochlea appears to have the thicker articular cartilage, making it the favorite graft source of most surgeons. Plugs taken from the far medial and lateral margins of the femoral trochlea, just proximal to the sulcus terminalis, also appear to provide the most accurate reconstruction of the surface anatomy of central lesions in the weight-bearing portion of either femoral condyle.[7]

Smaller grafts (4 or 6 mm) from the lateral intercondylar notch can also provide precise matches to similar lesions; however, significant inaccuracies are noted when the lateral intercondylar notch grafts are increased in size (8 mm). Whereas all traditional donor sites have less cartilage thickness than common recipient sites, this discrepancy is most profound between the lateral intercondylar notch and the weight-bearing portion of the femoral condyles.[48] In addition, the concave central intercondylar notch grafts do not match the topography of the convex femoral condyles,[2] and their harvest jeopardizes the integrity of the trochlear subchondral bone, which might be responsible for the increased incidence of anterior knee pain in some studies.

In general, matching articular geometry becomes more difficult and the potential for donor-site morbidity increases with larger dowels.

Allografting

Usually, patients have undergone prior surgery or are at least fully imaged; otherwise, a diagnostic arthroscopy is performed prior to the allografting procedure to confirm the extent of the lesion and, thus, adequacy of the available graft. It is the surgeon's responsibility to inspect the graft and to confirm the adequacy of the size match and quality of the tissue prior to surgery.

OPERATIVE TECHNIQUE

Autografting

The technique can be performed through a standard arthrotomy or miniarthrotomy or arthroscopically. Even in arthroscopic approaches, graft harvest from the trochlea almost always necessitates a mini-incision, and the surgeon should be prepared for conversion to a standard arthrotomy because certain locations (e.g., the posterior femoral condyle) may be difficult to access with less invasive approaches and perpendicularity in graft harvest and placement might be difficult to achieve.

After the entire knee joint has been inspected and tissue adequacy of the potential donor sites validated, the lesion to treat is accessed, probed, and measured and a corresponding graft match is established. In current practice, available donor plug sizes vary from 4 to 10 mm depending on the technique and instrumentation system used and on the size of the chondral lesion treated. For reasons outlined previously, the authors advocate medium-sized trochlear plugs, optimally harvested through the same ipsilateral incision. The procedure should begin with the graft harvest to ensure availability of a suitable graft before creating a recipient tunnel or to at least have a fallback option available, such as bone void filler.

Proprietary instrument systems generally use a hollow-core instrument for the graft harvest. An appropriately sized T-handled recipient harvester is tapped perpendicular to the articular surface of the far ipsilateral margin of the trochlea, just proximal to the sulcus terminalis. The depth should be a minimum of 8 mm or more, depending on subchondral involvement of the lesion to treat. It is paramount to check the perpendicularity of the harvesting device from several angles after introduction and before advancing it farther. Once tapped, the harvester chisel is then removed by rotating the driver to amputate the graft. The functional length of the graft is measured, and efforts should be made to fashion the recipient socket so that it provides a secure press-fit circumferentially and has enough depth to accommodate the plug easily lengthwise.

Biomechanical studies have confirmed that optimally sized, level-seated plugs face nearly normal joint contact pressures in situ.[34] Results also show that slightly countersunk grafts and angled grafts with the highest edge placed flush to neighboring cartilage demonstrate fairly normal contact pressures. Conversely, elevated angled grafts increase contact pressures as much as 40%, making them biomechanically disadvantageous.[33] The general consensus is that it is more favorable to leave a graft slightly countersunk than elevated with respect to the neighboring cartilage.[42] The authors thus advise slightly lengthening the recipient tunnel to avoid leaving the graft proud or subjecting it to undue insertion forces in an effort to bury an oversized graft.

Depending on the instrument systems, the recipient socket can be prepared using either a core or a drill. The traditional osteochondral autograft system employs a tubular coring device. Using the same technique described previously with a slightly smaller circumference T-handled harvester and maintaining strict perpendicularity, the recipient socket is created. Again, it is advisable to not oversize the recipient tunnel; rather, it should be of equal or greater depth than the donor plug's length. Drilling the recipient site might produce a more precise socket depth. In either event, the recipient socket should be measured for accuracy. The bony portion of the plug can be rasped down to the desired depth measurement, if necessary. After the donor graft's length is verified, it is then transplanted into the recipient site using the donor insertion guide, which dilates the cartilage layer with its beveled edge creating a tight press-fit. The last 1 mm of impaction should be performed by lightly tapping a bone tamp over the cartilaginous cap. The bone tamp should be oversized or placed offset to avoid countersinking a slightly shorter graft.

If required, the process can be repeated until a reasonable tissue fill is achieved in the lesion, but careful spacing of the plugs is essential. A 2-mm bone bridge between recipient sockets is recommended to help achieve and maintain a secure press-fit. The resulting margins on the articular surface should fill with fibrocartilage. To avoid premature amputation of the graft, the osseous portions should not intersect with one another. This can be most problematic with longer grafts obtained in areas of the knee where there is high curvature, such as the posterior femoral condyle. Finally, to prevent recipient tunnel wall fracture, each plug transfer should be completed prior to proceeding with additional recipient sockets.

The surgeon may choose to retrofill the created defects to minimize donor-site morbidity. Using the plugs removed from the recipient sockets carries the risk of displacement owing to their undersized nature relative to the donor voids. However, osteobiologic plugs that correspond to the diameters of commercial coring devices are available for this purpose and are optional. After the graft process, surface congruity is confirmed, and the joint is put through an ROM to ensure graft stability and lack of impingement. The knee is closed in a standard fashion over a drain after irrigation of the joint and inspection for loose bodies.

Allografting

The technique of fresh osteochondral allografting generally relies on an open arthrotomy of variable size, depending on the position and dimension of the lesion. For most femoral condyle lesions, eversion of the patella is not necessary. A standard midline incision is made from the center of the patella to the tip of the tibial tubercle and elevated subcutaneously. Depending on the location of the lesion (either medial or lateral), the joint is entered by incising the fat pad, taking care not to disrupt the anterior horn of the meniscus or to damage the articular surface. In some cases in which the lesion is posterior or very large, the ipsilateral meniscus must be detached and reflected. Generally, this can be done safely, leaving a small cuff of tissue adjacent to the anterior insertion of the meniscus for reattachment during closure. Once the joint capsule and synovium have been incised and retractors carefully placed, the knee is brought to a degree of flexion that presents the lesion into the arthrotomy site. The lesion is then inspected and palpated with a probe to determine the extent, stable margins, and maximum size.

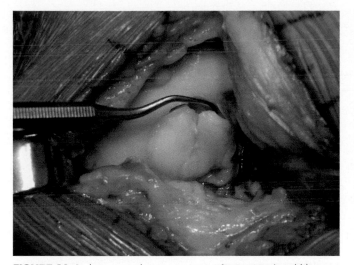

FIGURE 36–3. Intraoperative appearance of an osteochondritis dissecans lesion in typical location on the left medial femoral condyle of an 18-year-old female.

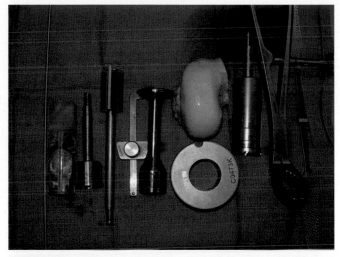

FIGURE 36–4. Common proprietary instrumentation used for dowel allograft preparation.

The two commonly used techniques for the preparation and implantation of osteochondral allografts include the press-fit plug technique and the shell-graft technique. Each technique has advantages and disadvantages. The press-fit plug technique is similar in principle to the autologous osteochondral transfer systems described previously. This technique is optimal for contained condylar lesions between 15 and 35 mm in diameter (Fig. 36–3). Fixation is generally not required owing to the stability achieved with the press fit, unless the lesion falls into the intercondylar notch. Disadvantages include the fact that very posterior femoral and trochlear lesions are not conducive to the use of a circular coring system and may be more amenable to shell allografts. In addition, the more ovoid a lesion in shape, the greater amount of normal cartilage that needs to be sacrificed at the recipient site in order to accommodate the circular donor plug. Shell grafts are technically more difficult to perform and typically require fixation. However, depending on the technique employed, less native host cartilage may need to be sacrificed.

Dowel Allograft

As with autologous dowels, several proprietary instrumentation systems are currently available (Fig. 36–4) for the preparation and implantation of press-fit dowel allografts up to 35 mm in diameter, and surgical techniques are similar.

After a size determination is made, a guidewire is driven into the center of the lesion, perpendicular to the curvature of the articular surface. The size of the graft is then determined using sizing dowels, remembering that overlapping dowels (in a "master card" or "snowman" configuration) can possibly deliver the best area fit. The remaining articular cartilage is scored to subchondral bone, and a core reamer is used to remove the articular cartilage remnants and at least 3 to 4 mm of subchondral bone (Fig. 36–5). Because it merely serves as an osteoconductive scaffold for healing to the host by creeping substitution, which is a rate-limited process, the portion of transplanted bone should be minimized wherever possible, without compromising stability of the graft as warranted by the clinical situation (Fig. 36–6). This will also minimize the potential antigenic burden of

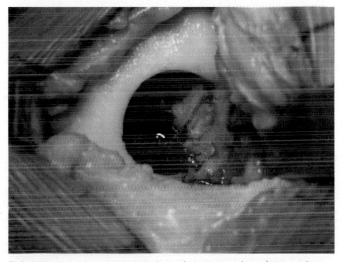

FIGURE 36–5. Intraoperative view after preparation of the graft bed via core reaming of the osteochondral defect and débridement down to bleeding bone.

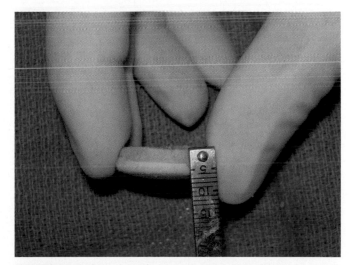

FIGURE 36–6. Side view of prepared dowel allograft prior to implantation displays the thickness of the articular cartilage in relationship to the subchondral bone portion.

marrow elements possibly remaining in the transplanted spongiosa.[18] In deeper lesions, fibrous and sclerotic bone is removed to a healthy, bleeding osseous base that does not exceed 10 mm in depth. Lesions below this depth should be curetted manually, and packed morselized autologous bone graft should be used to fill any deeper or more extensive osseous defects. Circumferential depth measurements are made of the prepared recipient site after the guide pin has been removed.

The graft is then placed into a graft holder or held manually with bone-holding forceps. The correspondent anatomic location is identified on the graft, and after a circular saw guide has been placed in the position, again perpendicular to the articular surface, an appropriate-sized tube saw is used to core out the graft. Prior to removing the graft from the condyle, identifying marks are made to ensure proper orientation. Once the dowel is removed, the recipient's depth measurements are transferred to the graft. This graft is then cut with an oscillating saw and trimmed with a rasp to the precise thickness in all four quadrants. The deep edges of the bone plug can be further chamfered with a rongeur and bone rasp to ease insertion.

The graft is then irrigated copiously with a high-pressure lavage (Fig. 36–7) to remove all marrow elements possible, and the recipient site is dilated using a slightly oversized tamp. This may ease the insertion of the graft to prevent excessive impact loading of the articular surface when the graft is inserted, while compacting the subchondral bone to prevent subsidence of the graft. At this time, any remaining osseous defects are bone-grafted to a level base. The allograft is then inserted by hand in the appropriate rotation and is gently tamped into place until it is flush, again minimizing mechanical insult to the articular surface of both the graft and the surrounding native tissue. Alternatively, the graft can be seated by gently ranging the knee, using the apposing joint surface as a fulcrum.

After the graft is seated, additional fixation with absorbable polydioxanone pins may be added if necessary, particularly if the graft is large or has an exposed edge within the notch (Fig. 36–8). The knee is then brought through a complete ROM in order to confirm that the graft is stable and that there is no catching or soft-tissue obstruction noted. The wound is then copiously irrigated, and routine closure is performed.

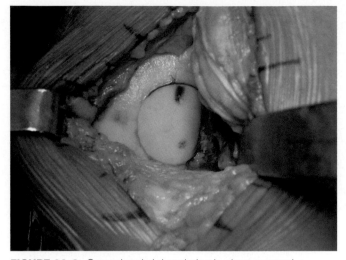

FIGURE 36–8. Osteochondral dowel plug in place, secured by several absorbable polydioxanone pins. Note the flush fit with the surrounding joint surface and the ink marks ensuring orthotopic orientation of the graft.

Shell Allograft

The defect is identified through the previously described arthrotomy, and the dimensions of the lesion are marked with a surgical pen. Minimizing the sacrifice of normal cartilage, a geometric shape is created that is amenable to handcrafting a shell graft (Figs. 36–9 and 36–10). A No. 15 scalpel blade is used to demarcate the lesion, and sharp ring curets are used to remove all tissue inside this mark. Using motorized burrs and sharp curettes, the lesion is débrided down to a depth of 4 to 5 mm (Fig. 36–11). The shape is transferred to the graft, which is molded in a freehand fashion (Fig. 36–12), initially slightly oversizing the graft and carefully removing excess bone and cartilage from the template as necessary through multiple trial fittings. If there is deeper bone loss in the defect, more bone can be left on the graft and the defect can be grafted with cancellous bone prior to graft insertion. The graft and host bed are then copiously irrigated and the graft placed flush with the articular surface.

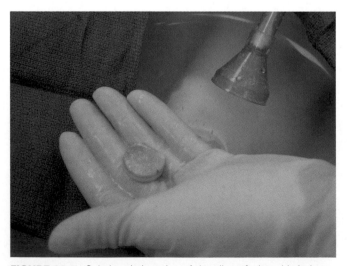

FIGURE 36–7. Subchondral portion of the allograft dowel is being thoroughly pulse-lavaged to remove potentially antigenic marrow elements and debris.

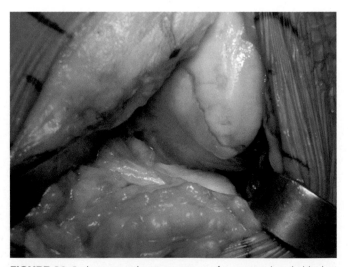

FIGURE 36–9. Intraoperative appearance of an osteochondral lesion secondary to osteonecrosis of the left lateral femoral condyle in a 44-year-old woman.

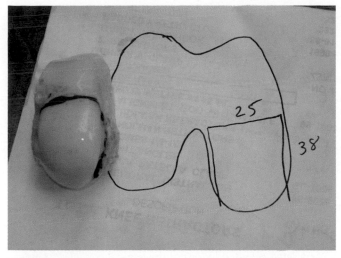

FIGURE 36–10. Left lateral femoral condyle allograft illustrates the templating for a shell allograft. Note the ink marks on the native cartilage and measurement transferred to a corresponding map.

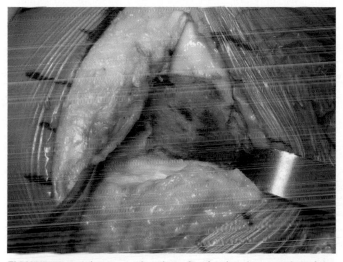

FIGURE 36–11. Intraoperative view after freehand preparation of the graft bed in preparation for a shell allograft.

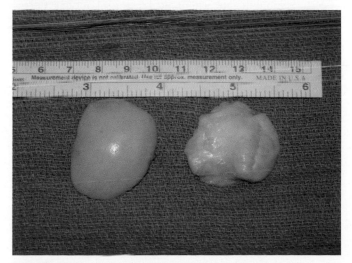

FIGURE 36–12. Comparison of the removed collapsed native condyle on the *right* and the shell allograft on the *left*.

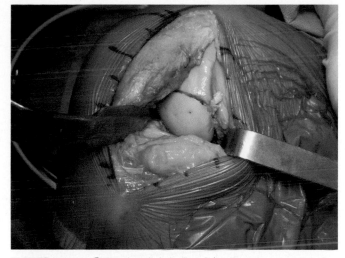

FIGURE 36–13. Osteochondral shell graft in place shows restoration of the condylar topography and weight-bearing portion of the articular cartilage in the lateral femoral condyle.

The need for fixation is based on the degree of inherent stability. Bioabsorbable pins, as described previously, are typically used when fixation is required (Fig. 36–13), but countersunk compression screws may be used as an alternative, optimally avoiding the weight-bearing portion. After cycling the knee through a full ROM and irrigating the joint, standard closure is performed.

Postoperative Management

The use of continuous passive motion during early postoperative management is optional. Patients generally are allowed full ROM, unless the graft involves the patellofemoral joint or there are other additional reconstructive procedures, such as meniscal repair, anterior cruciate ligament (ACL) reconstruction, or osteotomy that would alter the rehabilitation plan. Typically, braces are not used postoperatively except for patellofemoral grafts where flexion is limited to less than 45° for the first 4 to 6 weeks or in cases of bipolar tibial femoral grafts where an unloader or ROM brace is used to prevent excessive stress on the grafted compartment.

Patients are begun on early ROM exercises and quadriceps strengthening (such as straight leg raises) and are maintained in a toe-touch–only weight-bearing status for a period of at least 8 weeks, and often 12 weeks, depending on the size and containment of the graft, type of fixation, and ultimately, radiographic evidence of incorporation. At 4 weeks, patients are allowed closed chain exercises such as cycling. Progressive weight-bearing as tolerated is usually allowed at 3 months, and if functional rehabilitation is complete, the patient is allowed to return to recreation and sports at approximately 6 months. Patients are generally cautioned about excessive impact loading of the allograft, particularly in the 1st year. As with any cartilage replacement procedure, long-term outcomes in osteochondral allografting are directly and inversely related to the time to treatment and overall burden of disease in the afflicted joint. In a young patient with a focal lesion (traumatic or OCD), it is not unrealistic to expect this person to go back to normal impact-loading activities after 12 months and to return to preinjury function, whereas the goals in a salvage situation are usually to delay or even eliminate the need for prosthetic replacement by reducing pain and allowing a return to functional activities of daily living as well as low-impact recreational activities.

AUTHORS' CLINICAL OUTCOMES

The authors believe that osteochondral allografting is an excellent treatment option for advanced OCD lesions. The authors previously published the results of 66 knees in 64 patients with OCD of the femoral condyle, treated with fresh osteochondral allografts, implanted within 5 days of graft recovery.[17] Patients were evaluated pre- and postoperatively using an 18-point modified D'Aubigne and Postel scale, which measures function, ROM, and absence of pain, allotting 1 to 6 points each, for a maximum of 18 points (Table 36-1).

There were 45 males and 19 females, with a mean age of 28.6 years (range, 15–54 yr). All lesions were ICRS grade III–IV OCD; 40 involved the medial femoral condyle, and 25 the lateral femoral condyle. All patients had undergone an average of 1.6 previous operations. The average allograft size was 7.5 cm². The mean follow-up was 7.7 years (range, 2–22 yr); 1 patient was lost to follow-up. Overall, 47 of 65 knees (72%) were rated good or excellent, scoring 15 points or above on the 18-point scale. Seven (11%) were rated fair, and 1 (2%) was rated poor. The average clinical score improved from 12.9 points preoperatively to 16.1 points postoperatively (P < .01). Preoperative, immediate postoperative, and most recent follow-up AP and lateral radiographs were available for 32 of 66 knees, with a mean follow-up of 3.1 years. In these, evidence of graft union, collapse, resorption, and the presence of degenerative changes were recorded by a musculoskeletal radiologist.

TABLE 36–1   18-Point Scale

	CRITERIA	
Points	**PAIN**	
1	Severe	Not relieved by rest and analgesics
2	Severe	Relieved by rest and analgesics
3	Moderate	Regular analgesics needed
4	Mild	Occasional analgesics needed
5	Minimum	Occasional ache
6	None	
Points	**FUNCTION**	
1	Bedridden or household walker with two canes or crutches	
2	Time and distance outside limited; walks with external aids	
3	Walks < 0.8 km with external aids; stair climbing limited	
4	Walks > 0.8 km with external aids; stair climbing not limited	
5	No external aids; limps	
6	Unlimited walking without a limp	
Points	**RANGE OF MOTION**	
1	<60° of flexion	
2	15°–90° of flexion	
3	0°–90° of flexion	
4	>90° of flexion; ≤15° contracture	
5	>90° of flexion without contracture	
6	≥130° of flexion without contracture	

Twenty-four of the grafts (75%) demonstrated healing, and 26 (81%) were intact. Subchondral cysts were present in 5 (16%) in knees. Sclerosis was found in 6 (19%) cases. Ten patients had reoperations on the allograft, with a mean time to reoperation of 56 months, including 3 patients who went on to arthroplasty. Subjective knee function improved from a mean of 3.4 points to 8.4 points (P <.01) on a 10-point scale for the 59 patients who completed questionnaires. With greater than 70% good or excellent results, fresh osteochondral allograft transplantation has proved to be a successful surgical treatment for OCD of the femoral condyle in multiply operated knees. In the authors' experience, results are even more favorable for osteochondral allografts as a primary treatment measure in native OCD lesions.

Whereas OCD remains a perfect indication for osteochondral allografting, focal lesions of diverse etiologies are amenable to this application, and the results were presented of 43 knees with isolated chondral lesions of the femoral condyle.[25] Clinical evaluation was performed with the modified D'Aubigne and Postel (18-point) scale. Subjective outcome measures included a patient questionnaire evaluating pain, function, and satisfaction. The study population included 23 males and 20 females, with a mean age of 35 years. Twenty-nine lesions involved the medial femoral condyle, 13 the lateral femoral condyle, and 1 both condyles. All patients had undergone an average of 1.9 previous operations (range, 1–5 operations) before allograft transplantation. The mean allograft area was 5.88 cm². Of these knees, 38 (88%) were considered successful (score, ≥15 on the 18-point modified D'Aubigne and Postel scale) a mean of 54 months postoperatively. The average score improved from 11.5 points to 16.7 points (P <.05). Fifteen patients had further surgery on the knee, not all related to the allograft: 10 arthroscopies, 3 revision allografts, 1 ACL reconstruction, and 1 osteotomy. Twenty-one of 43 patients completed questionnaires, of which 90% were satisfied and 90% reported less pain and improved function. In conclusion, fresh osteochondral allografting was successful in 88% of patients and resulted in significant improvement in function and pain with high patient satisfaction. Osteochondral allografting is a reasonable option for patients with cartilage lesions of the femoral condyle, especially in a salvage situation after prior failure of other cartilage procedures.

Osteonecrosis of the knee is a serious potential complication of corticosteroid therapy with limited treatment options. Osteochondral allografting is a salvage alternative in patients who are of an age and activity level not ideally suited for arthroplasty. The authors[26] reported the clinical outcomes of fresh osteochondral allografting in individuals with steroid-induced modified Association Research Circulation Osseous (ARCO) stage 3/4 osteonecrosis of the femoral condyles. Clinical evaluation was performed using the modified D'Aubigne and Postel (18-point) scale. Subjective outcome measures included a patient questionnaire evaluating pain, function, and satisfaction. Of 24 patients who underwent osteochondral allografting for osteonecrosis between 1984 and 2005, 17 (12 females and 5 males) fulfilled inclusion criteria with minimum 2-year follow-up (mean follow-up, 65 mo; range, 24–236 mo). The 17 patients had a mean age of 28.8 years (range, 16–68 yr). Five had bilateral surgery, for a total of 22 knees. Of these knees, 16 had unicondylar lesions (12 lateral, 4 medial) and 6 had bicompartmental involvement. Fifty-six percent of knees had previous surgery (average, 1.5; range, 1–5 surgeries). The mean graft surface area was 11.0 cm² (range, 5.3–19.0 cm²). Twelve of 22 (54.5%) required additional bone grafting. Seventeen of 22 (77%) were considered successful (score, ≥ 15 points). The mean score improved from 11.1 points to 15.9 points ($P < .0001$). Two patients had further surgery: 1 underwent arthroscopic débridement and another underwent total knee arthroplasty 76 months after the index surgery. Fourteen patients completed questionnaires; all reported statistically significant higher ($P < .0001$) pain relief, improved function, and overall satisfaction with their outcome. Fresh osteochondral allografting was successful in 77% of these relatively young patients and resulted in significant improvement in function and pain with high patient satisfaction, leading us to consider osteochondral allografting as a reasonable salvage option for patients with avascular necrosis of the knee joint.

Treatment options also remain limited in younger, active individuals with impeding knee arthrosis. The authors[44] reported the results of osteochondral allografting in 37 knees with multifocal chondral lesions and arthritic changes. All patients demonstrated radiographic evidence of arthrosis. Assessment was performed with the modified D'Aubigne and Postel (18-point) scale and International Knee Documentations Committee (IKDC) score. Radiographs were evaluated by modified Fairbanks/Ahlbäck criteria. Again, subjective outcome measures included a patient questionnaire evaluating pain, function, and satisfaction. The 37 patients (25 males, 12 females) had a mean age of 42 years (range, 15–67 yr) and an activity level not ideally suited for arthroplasty. The mean follow-up was 36 months (range, 24–84 mo). Three patients were lost to follow-up. Nineteen of the allografts were unipolar, 10 involved bipolar/kissing lesions, and 5 multiple surfaces. The mean allograft area was 10.5 cm². Twenty-six of 34 (76%) were considered successful (score, ≥ 15 points) and 8 (24%) were unsuccessful (3 converted to total knee arthroplasty, 2 underwent repeat allografting, 3 declined further surgery but were considered failures owing to fair/poor postoperative scores). The average 18-point scores improved from 11.5 points to 16.2 points, whereas IKDC scores improved from 33.0 points to 61.7 points ($P < .01$).

Nineteen of 31 preoperative radiographs (61%) were grade 3 (>50% joint space narrowing) and 12 of 31 (39%) were grade 1 to 2 (<50% narrowing). Postoperatively, 13 of 31 radiographs (42%) were grade 3 and 18 of 31 (58%) were grade 1 to 2. Eighteen of 34 patients (53%) were extremely satisfied, 15 (44%) were satisfied, 1 (3%) was somewhat satisfied, and 0 were dissatisfied. Overall, clinical success of fresh allografting for knee arthrosis was 76%. Objective and subjective improvements were statistically significant. Success may be challenged with longer follow-up. Treatment options for knee arthritis in the young, active patient are currently extremely limited, and fresh osteochondral allografting is an emergent bio-orthologic alternative in this growing and challenging segment of the population.

CLINICAL OUTCOMES FROM OTHER AUTHORS

Autografts

Hangody and Fules[27] reported their 10-year clinical experience with autologous osteochondral mosaicplasty (Table 36–2). These investigators performed 831 mosaicplasties, involving 597 femoral condyles, 118 patellofemoral (patella and/or trochlea) joints, 76 talar domes, 25 tibial condyles, 6 capitulum humeri, 6 femoral heads, and 3 humeral heads. Concomitant

TABLE 36–2   Selected Outcomes of Osteochondral Autografting in the Knee

Reference	Site of Lesion	Knees (Number)	Follow-up (yr)	Outcome (%)
Hangody & Fules[27]	Femur	597	1–10	92 G/E
Hangody & Fules[27]	PFJ	118	1–10	87 G/E
Hangody & Fules[27]	Tibia	25	1–10	79 G/E
Marcacci et al.[37]	Femur	37	2.0	78 G/E
Marcacci et al.[36]	Femur	30	7.0	77 G/E
Jakob et al.[29]	Femur	52	3.1	92 I
Chow et al.[12]	Femur	30	3.8	83 G/E
Outerbridge et al.[43]	Femur	18	7.6	81 H
Karataglis et al.[32]	Femur & PFJ	37	3.1	87 H

G/E, good/excellent; H, high functional level; I, improved knee function; PFJ, patellofemoral joint.

surgery (ACL reconstruction, realignment procedures, and meniscal surgeries) was performed in 85% of the patients. Good to excellent results were reported in 92% of the patients who had femoral condyle grafts, 87% of those who had tibial grafts, and 79% of those who had patella grafts. Long-term donor-site morbidity was found in 3% of the patients.

Marcacci and coworkers[37] reported on 37 athletes younger than 50 years of age with at least a 2-year follow-up. In this study, 23 of 37 patients (62%) underwent an associated procedure with arthroscopic mosaicplasty of the femoral condyle. The data revealed that 78% of the patients had good to excellent results. Twenty-seven patients returned to sports at the same level, 5 patients returned at a lower level, and 5 were unable to return to sports. Medial femoral condyle lesions statistically did not fare as well as lateral condyle lesions. Donor site morbidity was not an identifiable problem in this case series.

The same group prospectively evaluated 30 patients with full-thickness chondral lesions (<2.5 cm²) of the knee treated with arthroscopic autologous osteochondral transplantation.[36] The ICRS objective evaluation showed 76.7% of patients had good or excellent results at 7-year follow-up, and IKDC subjective score significantly improved from preoperative (34.8 points) to 7-year follow-up (71.8 points). The Tegner score showed a significant improvement after the surgery at 2- and 7-year follow-up (from 2.9 points to 6.2 and 5.6 points, respectively); however, sports participation declined from 2- to 7-year follow-up. MRI evaluation showed good integration of the graft in the host bone and complete maintenance of the grafted cartilage in more than 60% of cases.

In a study by Jakob and associates,[29] 92% of patients (48 of 52) demonstrated improved knee function at the latest follow-up (average, 37 mo) from open knee mosaicplasty. In 30 of 52 patients (58%), a concomitant procedure was performed. Four patients required reoperation because of graft failure.

With a mean follow-up of 45.1 months, Chow and colleagues[12] reported on 30 patients who had undergone arthroscopic autologous osteochondral transplantation to the femoral condyle. Good to excellent results were reported in 83% (25 of 30) of patients. Lysholm scores increased from an average of 43.6 points preoperatively to a mean of 87.5 points postoperatively. Two patients (7%) had poor results and later underwent total knee arthroplasty.

Outerbridge and coworkers[43] followed 18 knees for an average of 7.6 years after osteochondral autografting of the femoral condyle using the ipsilateral lateral patellar facet as the donor graft. These investigators reported an increase in Cincinnati knee scores from an average preoperative score of 37 points to an average final follow-up score of 85 points. Eighty-one percent (13 of 16) of the patients returned to a high functional level. Twelve percent (2 of 16) experienced moderate patellofemoral joint symptoms. Nevertheless, all patients were satisfied with the procedure results and, given the choice, would have the same surgery done again for an identical lesion on the contralateral knee.

Karataglis and associates[32] reported on their mid- and long-term functional outcomes of 36 patients (37 knees) who underwent the osteochondral autograft transplantation technique with an average follow-up of 36.9 months. The lesions were located on the femoral condyle in 26 cases, on the trochlea in 7 cases, and on the patella in 4 cases. Thirty-two out of 37 patients (86.5%) reported significant improvement of their preoperative symptoms. All but 5 patients returned to previous daily and work activities. Eighteen patients returned to sports. Nine patients required second-look arthroscopies because of swelling, pain, or clicking. In 2 of those cases, the grafts were found to be loose and required revision. Symptoms improved significantly in 4 out of those 9 patients after repeat arthroscopy. Donor-site morbidity was not seen in this series.

Allografts

Garrett[21] reported on the experience with fresh osteochondral allografts used as both a press-fit plug and a large shell graft in the treatment of 17 patients with OCD, all of whom had undergone previous surgery (Table 36–3). Sixteen patients (94%) reported relief of symptoms at 2- to 9-year follow-up. This work is remarkable for the first reported use of dowel grafts in the literature.

Chu and colleagues[13] reported on 55 consecutive knees undergoing osteochondral allografting for diagnoses such as traumatic chondral injury, avascular necrosis, OCD, and patellofemoral disease. The mean age was 35.6 years, with follow-up averaging 75 months (range, 11–147 mo). Of the 55 knees, 43 were unipolar replacements and 12 were bipolar resurfacing replacements. On the 18-point scale, 45 of 55 of these knees (76%) were rated good to excellent, and 3 as fair. Of note, 36 of the 43 knees (84%) that underwent unipolar femoral grafts were rated good to excellent compared with only 6 of the 12 knees (50%) with bipolar grafts.

McDermott and coworkers[40] reported on 100 patients treated with fresh osteochondral grafts implanted within 24 hours of recovery. Fifty patients had a unifocal traumatic defect of the tibial plateau or femoral condyle, 38 of which (76%) were considered successful at an average follow-up of 3.8 years. Patients with osteoarthritis and osteonecrosis had poorer results.

Ghazavi and associates[22] reported on 126 knees in 123 patients with an average follow-up of 7.5 years. One hundred and five of 123 patients (85%) were rated as successful, and the remaining 18 failed. Advanced age (>50 yr), bipolar defects, malalignment, and Workers' Compensation cases were considered main factors related to failure.

Beaver and colleagues[8] performed a survivorship study on 92 knees allografted for post-traumatic cartilage lesions with failure defined as the need for a revision operation or the persistence of symptoms. There was a 75% success rate at 5 years, 64% at 10 years, and 63% at 14 years. Advanced age (>60 yr) and bipolar defects were again identified as factors for failure.

Aubin and coworkers[5] later followed 60 patients, 41 of whom (68%) had undergone simultaneous realignment osteotomy and 10 (15%) concomitant meniscal transplantation. Kaplan-Meier survivorship analysis showed 51 grafts (85%) survived at 10 years and 44 (74%) at 15 years.

McCulloch and associates[39] presented the results of 25 consecutive patients who underwent prolonged fresh osteochondral allograft transplantation for defects in the femoral condyle. The average patient age was 35 years (range, 17–49 yr). The average length of follow-up was 35 months (range, 24–67 mo). Statistically significant improvements ($P < .05$) were reported for the Lysholm (39 points to 67 points), IKDC scores (29 points to 58 points), all five components of the Knee Injury and Osteoarthritis Outcome Score (KOOS) and the Short Form-12 physical component score (36 points to 40 points). Overall, patients reported 84% satisfaction (range, 25%–100%) with their results and believed that the knee functioned at 79% of their unaffected knee (range, 35%–100%). Radiographically, 22 of the grafts (88%) were incorporated into host bone.

Williams and colleagues[51] prospectively followed 19 patients with symptomatic chondral and osteochondral lesions of the knee who were treated with fresh osteochondral allografts, with a mean preimplantation storage time of 30 days (range, 17–42 days). The mean age at the time of surgery was 34 years. The mean lesion size was 602 mm². MRI was used to evaluate the morphologic characteristics of the implanted grafts. The mean duration of clinical follow-up was 48 months (range, 21–68 mo). The mean score

---

TABLE 36–3   Selected Outcomes: Osteochondral Allografting in the Knee

Reference	Site of Lesion	Diagnosis/Indication	Patients (N)	Mean Follow-Up (yr)	Successful Outcome (%)
Chu et al.[13]	Knee	Multiple	55	6.2	84 G/E
Görtz et al.[25]	Femur	Multiple	43	4.5	88 G/E
McCulloch et al.[39]	Knee	Multiple	25	3.9	84 SCS
Williams et al.[51]	Knee	Multiple	19	4.0	100 SVS
McDermott et al.[40]	Knee	Trauma	50	3.8	76 SCS
Ghazavi et al.[22]	Knee	Trauma	126	7.5	85 SVS
Beaver et al.[8]	Knee	Trauma	92	14.0	63 SVS
Aubin et al.[5]	Femur	Trauma	60	10.0	85 SVS
Garrett[21]	Femur	OCD	17	2.9	94 G/E
Emmerson et al.[17]	Femur	OCD	69	5.2	80 G/E
Görtz et al.[26]	Knee	Osteonecrosis	21	5.3	88 G/E
Park et al.[44]	Knee	Osteoarthrosis	37	5.3	76 G/E

G/E, good/excellent; OCD, osteochondritis dissecans; SCS, successful; SVS, survivorship.

(and standard deviation) on the Activities of Daily Living Scale increased from a baseline of 56 ± 24 points to 70 ± 22 points at the time of the final follow-up ($P < .05$). The mean Short Form-36 (SF-36) score increased from a baseline of 51 ± 23 points to 66 ± 24 points at the time of final follow-up ($P < .005$). At a mean follow-up interval of 25 months, cartilage-sensitive MRI demonstrated that the normal articular cartilage thickness was preserved in 18 implanted grafts, and allograft cartilage signal properties were isointense relative to normal articular cartilage in 8 of the 18 grafts. Osseous trabecular incorporation of the allograft was complete or partial in 14 patients and poor in 4 patients. Complete or partial trabecular incorporation positively correlated with SF-36 scores at the time of follow-up ($R = 0.487; P < .05$).

COMPLICATIONS

The unique issue regarding possible postoperative complications with fresh allografts relates to transmission of disease from the graft. Infection after the implantation of a fresh osteochondral allograft is rare, but its consequences can be devastating. Generally, all grafts are currently harvested and tested in accordance with American Association of Tissue Banks standards. However, allograft-associated bacterial infections have been reported. Death in the immediate postoperative period has even occurred as the result of implantation of a contaminated fresh osteochondral graft. As with most procedures, infection may become apparent between days to weeks after surgery. Deep infection needs to be distinguished from a superficial infection with the use of physical examination findings and joint aspiration. Deep infection involving the allograft should be addressed immediately with removal of the allograft because of the risk that the fresh tissue is the source of the infection or a nidus for a recurrence. Patients need to be informed of this risk preoperatively and again counseled to look for signs of infection prior to and after discharge from the hospital.

Failure of the allograft procedure can occur owing to non-union or late fragmentation and graft collapse. Disease progression (arthritis) may also lead to inferior clinical outcome. Whereas healing of the graft-host interface reliably occurs, particularly with smaller grafts, the degree of revascularization appears to be variable. Fragmentation and collapse typically occur in areas of unvascularized allograft bone. Patients typically present with new-onset pain or mechanical symptoms. Radiographs may show joint space narrowing, cysts, or sclerotic regions. MRI can help rule out contributory concomitant joint pathology in the differential diagnosis of postoperative symptoms. In the event of mechanical allograft failure, MRI will often show areas of graft collapse. However, care must be taken in the interpretation of MRI because even normal, well-functioning grafts demonstrate signal abnormalities. Depending on the status of the knee joint, the treatment options include observation, removal of the fragmented portion of the graft, repeat allografting, or conversion to arthroplasty.

ACKNOWLEDGMENT

The authors would like to thank Judy Blake for her assistance in preparation of this chapter.

REFERENCES

1. http://www.cartilage.org/_files/contentmanagement/ICRS_evaluation.pdf (accessed October 1, 2007).
2. Ahmad, C. S.; Cohen, Z. A.; Levine, W. N.; et al.: Biomechanical and topographic considerations for autologous osteochondral grafting in the knee. *Am J Sports Med* 29:201–206, 2001.
3. Alford, J. W.; Cole, B. J.: Cartilage restoration, part 1: basic science, historical perspective, patient evaluation, and treatment options. *Am J Sports Med* 33:295–306, 2005.
4. Allen, R. T.; Robertson, C. M.; Pennock, A. T.; et al.: Analysis of stored osteochondral allografts at the time of surgical implantation. *Am J Sports Med* 33:1479–1484, 2005.
5. Aubin, P. P.; Cheah, H. K.; Davis, A. M.; Gross, A. E.: Long-term follow-up of fresh femoral osteochondral allografts for posttraumatic knee defects. *Clin Orthop Relat Res* 391(suppl):S318–S327, 2001.
6. Ball, S. T.; Amiel, D.; Williams, S. K.; et al.: The effects of storage on fresh human osteochondral allografts. *Clin Orthop Relat Res* 418:246–252, 2004.
7. Bartz, R. L.; Kamaric, E.; Noble, P. C.; et al.: Topographic matching of selected donor and recipient sites for osteochondral autografting of the articular surface of the femoral condyles. *Am J Sports Med* 29:207–212, 2001.
8. Beaver, R. J.; Mahomed, M.; Backstein, D.; et al.: Fresh osteochondral allografts for post-traumatic defects in the knee. A survivorship analysis. *J Bone Joint Surg Br* 74:105–110, 1992.
9. Bobic, V.: [Autologous osteo-chondral grafts in the management of articular cartilage lesions]. *Orthopade* 28:19–25, 1999.
10. Buckwalter, J. A.: Articular cartilage. *Instr Course Lect* 32:349–370, 1983.
11. Burchardt, H.: The biology of bone graft repair. *Clin Orthop Relat Res* 174:28–42, 1983.
12. Chow, J. C.; Hantes, M. E.; Houle, J. B.; Zalavras, C. G.: Arthroscopic autogenous osteochondral transplantation for treating knee cartilage defects: a 2- to 5-year follow-up study. *Arthroscopy* 20:681–690, 2004.
13. Chu, C. R.; Convery, F. R.; Akeson, W. H.; et al.: Articular cartilage transplantation. Clinical results in the knee. *Clin Orthop Relat Res* 360:159–168, 1999.
14. Convery, F. R.; Akeson, W. H.; Amiel, D.; et al.: Long-term survival of chondrocytes in an osteochondral articular cartilage allograft. A case report. *J Bone Joint Surg Am* 78:1082–1088, 1996.
15. Czitrom, A. A.; Keating, S.; Gross, A. E.: The viability of articular cartilage in fresh osteochondral allografts after clinical transplantation. *J Bone Joint Surg Am* 72:574–581, 1990.
16. Czitrom, A. A.; Langer, F.; McKee, N.; Gross, A. E.: Bone and cartilage allotransplantation. A review of 14 years of research and clinical studies. *Clin Orthop Relat Res* 208:141–145, 1986.
17. Emmerson, B. C.; Gortz, S.; Jamali, A. A.; et al.: Fresh osteochondral allografting in the treatment of osteochondritis dissecans of the femoral condyle. *Am J Sports Med* 35:907–914, 2007.
18. Enneking, W. F.; Campanacci, D. A.: Retrieved human allografts: a clinicopathological study. *J Bone Joint Surg Am* 83:971–986, 2001.
19. Fonseca, F.; Balaco, I.: Fixation with autogenous osteochondral grafts for the treatment of osteochondritis dissecans (stages III and IV). *Int Orthop* 33:139–144, 2007.
20. Garretson, R. B., 3rd; Katolik, L. I.; Verma, N.; et al.: Contact pressure at osteochondral donor sites in the patellofemoral joint. *Am J Sports Med* 32:967–974, 2004.
21. Garrett, J. C.: Treatment of osteochondral defects of the distal femur with fresh osteochondral allografts: a preliminary report. *Arthroscopy* 2:222–226, 1986.
22. Ghazavi, M. T.; Pritzker, K. P.; Davis, A. M.; Gross, A. E.: Fresh osteochondral allografts for post-traumatic osteochondral defects of the knee. *J Bone Joint Surg Br* 79:1008–1013, 1997.
23. Gortz, S.; Bugbee, W. D.: Allografts in articular cartilage repair. *J Bone Joint Surg Am* 88:1374–1384, 2006.
24. Gortz, S.; Bugbee, W. D.: Fresh osteochondral allografts: graft processing and clinical applications. *J Knee Surg* 19:231–240, 2006.

25. Görtz, S.; Ho, A.; Bugbee, W.: Fresh osteochondral allograft transplantation for cartilage lesions in the knee. *Trans Am Acad Orthop Surg* 73:151, 2006.

26. Görtz, S.; Khadavi, B.; Jamali, A.; Bugbee, W.: Fresh osteochondral allografting for steroid-induced osteonecrosis of the femoral condyles. *Knee Surg Sports Traumatol Arthrosc* 16(suppl 1):S3–23, 2008.

27. Hangody, L.; Fules, P.: Autologous osteochondral mosaicplasty for the treatment of full-thickness defects of weight-bearing joints: ten years of experimental and clinical experience. *J Bone Joint Surg Am* 85(suppl 2):25–32, 2003.

28. Highgenboten, C. L.; Jackson, A.; Trudelle-Jackson, E.; Meske, N. B.: Cross-validation of height and gender estimations of femoral condyle width in osteochondral allografts. *Clin Orthop Relat Res* 298:246–249, 1994.

29. Jakob, R. P.; Franz, T.; Gautier, E.; Mainil-Varlet, P.: Autologous osteochondral grafting in the knee: indication, results, and reflections. *Clin Orthop Relat Res* 401:170–184, 2002.

30. Jamali, A. A.; Hatcher, S. L.; You, Z.: Donor cell survival in a fresh osteochondral allograft at twenty-nine years. A case report. *J Bone Joint Surg Am* 89:166–169, 2007.

31. Kandel, R. A.; Gross, A. E.; Ganel, A.; et al.: Histopathology of failed osteoarticular shell allografts. *Clin Orthop Relat Res* 197:103–110, 1985.

32. Karataglis, D.; Green, M. A.; Learmonth, D. J.: Autologous osteochondral transplantation for the treatment of chondral defects of the knee. *Knee* 13:32–35, 2006.

33. Koh, J. L.; Kowalski, A.; Lautenschlager, E.: The effect of angled osteochondral grafting on contact pressure: a biomechanical study. *Am J Sports Med* 34:116–119, 2006.

34. Koh, J. L.; Wirsing, K.; Lautenschlager, E.; Zhang, L. O.: The effect of graft height mismatch on contact pressure following osteochondral grafting: a biomechanical study. *Am J Sports Med* 32:317–320, 2004.

35. Mankin, H. J.: The response of articular cartilage to mechanical injury. *J Bone Joint Surg Am* 64:460–466, 1982.

36. Marcacci, M.; Kon, E.; Delcogliano, M.; et al.: Arthroscopic autologous osteochondral grafting for cartilage defects of the knee: prospective study results at a minimum 7-year follow-up. *Am J Sports Med* 35:2014–2021, 2007.

37. Marcacci, M.; Kon, E.; Zaffagnini, S.; et al.: Multiple osteochondral arthroscopic grafting (mosaicplasty) for cartilage defects of the knee: prospective study results at 2-year follow-up. *Arthroscopy* 21:462–470, 2005.

38. Maury, A. C.; Safir, O.; Heras, F. L.; et al.: Twenty-five-year chondrocyte viability in fresh osteochondral allograft. A case report. *J Bone Joint Surg Am* 89:159–165, 2007.

39. McCulloch, P. C.; Kang, R. W.; Sobhy, M. H.; et al.: Prospective evaluation of prolonged fresh osteochondral allograft transplantation of the femoral condyle: minimum 2-year follow-up. *Am J Sports Med* 35:411–420, 2007.

40. McDermott, A. G.; Langer, F.; Pritzker, K. P.; Gross, A. E.: Fresh small-fragment osteochondral allografts. Long-term follow-up study on first 100 cases. *Clin Orthop Relat Res* 197:96–102, 1985.

41. Miniaci, A.; Tytherleigh-Strong, G.: Fixation of unstable osteochondritis dissecans lesions of the knee using arthroscopic autogenous osteochondral grafting (mosaicplasty). *Arthroscopy* 23:845–851, 2007.

42. Nakagawa, Y.; Suzuki, T.; Kuroki, H.; et al.: The effect of surface incongruity of grafted plugs in osteochondral grafting: a report of five cases. *Knee Surg Sports Traumatol Arthrosc* 15:591–596, 2007.

43. Outerbridge, H. K.; Outerbridge, R. E.; Smith, D. E.: Osteochondral defects in the knee. A treatment using lateral patella autografts. *Clin Orthop Relat Res* 377:145–151, 2000.

44. Park, D.; Chung, C.; Bugbee, W.: Fresh osteochondral allografts for younger, active individuals with osteoarthrosis of the knee. *Trans Int Cart Rep Soc* 5:10, 2006.

45. Pennock, A. T.; Wagner, F.; Robertson, C. M.; et al.: Prolonged storage of osteochondral allografts: does the addition of fetal bovine serum improve chondrocyte viability? *J Knee Surg* 19:265–272, 2006.

46. Potter, H. G.; Foo, L. F.: Magnetic resonance imaging of articular cartilage: trauma, degeneration, and repair. *Am J Sports Med* 34:661–677, 2006.

47. Robertson, C. M.; Allen, R. T.; Pennock, A. T.; et al.: Up-regulation of apoptotic and matrix-related gene expression during fresh osteochondral allograft storage. *Clin Orthop Relat Res* 442:260–266, 2006.

48. Thaunat, M.; Couchon, S.; Lunn, J.; et al.: Cartilage thickness matching of selected donor and recipient sites for osteochondral autografting of the medial femoral condyle. *Knee Surg Sports Traumatol Arthrosc* 15:381–386, 2007.

49. Vangsness, C. T., Jr.; Garcia, I. A.; Mills, C. R.; et al.: Allograft transplantation in the knee: tissue regulation, procurement, processing, and sterilization. *Am J Sports Med* 31:474–481, 2003.

50. Williams, R. J., 3rd; Dreese, J. C.; Chen, C. T.: Chondrocyte survival and material properties of hypothermically stored cartilage: an evaluation of tissue used for osteochondral allograft transplantation. *Am J Sports Med* 32:132–139, 2004.

51. Williams, R. J., 3rd; Ranawat, A. S.; Potter, H. G.; et al.: Fresh stored allografts for the treatment of osteochondral defects of the knee. *J Bone Joint Surg Am* 89:718–726, 2007.

52. Williams, S. K.; Amiel, D.; Ball, S. T.: Analysis of cartilage tissue on a cellular level in fresh osteochondral allograft retrievals. *Am J Sports Med* 35:2022–2032, 2007.

53. Williams, S. K.; Amiel, D.; Ball, S. T.; et al.: Prolonged storage effects on the articular cartilage of fresh human osteochondral allografts. *J Bone Joint Surg Am* 85:2111–2120, 2003.

Rehabilitation after Articular Cartilage Procedures

Kevin E. Wilk, DPT, PT ■ *Michael M. Reinold*, PT, DPT, ATC, CSCS

INTRODUCTION

Articular cartilage defects of the knee appear to be an increasing cause of pain and functional disability in orthopaedics and sports medicine. This pathology creates a significant challenge to the health care team, especially the physician who must decide on the appropriate treatment plan. The avascular nature of articular cartilage predisposes the individual to progressive symptoms and degeneration owing to the extremely slow and frequent inability to heal. Nonoperative rehabilitation and palliative care are frequently unsuccessful, and further treatment is required to alleviate symptoms. This presents a significant challenge for patients, particularly young and more active individuals. Traditional methods of treating these lesions have led to unfavorable results, stimulating the need for newer surgical procedures designed to facilitate the repair or transplantation of autogenous cartilage tissue. Postoperative rehabilitation programs vary greatly between patients and are individualized based on specifics of the lesion (size, depth, location, containment, quality of tissue), patient (age, activities, goals, quality of tissue, lower extremity alignment, body mass index (BMI), general health, and nutrition), and surgery (exact procedure, tissue involvement, and concomitant surgeries). Thus, the development of an appropriate rehabilitation program is challenging and must be highly individualized to ensure successful outcomes. These programs are designed according to the knowledge of basic science, anatomy, and biomechanics of articular cartilage as well as the biologic course of healing after surgery. The goal is to restore full function in each patient as quickly as possible without overloading the healing articular cartilage. In this chapter, the essential principles of rehabilitation after articular cartilage repair procedures are discussed as well as specific rehabilitation guidelines for débridement, abrasion chondroplasty, microfracture, osteochondral autograft transplantation (OATS), and autologous chondrocyte implantation (ACI).

PRINCIPLES OF ARTICULAR CARTILAGE REHABILITATION

Several principles exist that must be considered when designing a rehabilitation program after articular cartilage repair procedures (Table 37–1). These key principles have been designed based upon the authors' understanding of the basic science and mechanics of articular cartilage. These principles include individualization, creating a healing environment, understanding the biomechanics of the knee, reducing pain and effusion, restoring soft tissue balance, restoring muscle function, restoring proprioception and

Critical Points PRINCIPLES OF ARTICULAR CARTILAGE REHABILITATION

Individualization

- Develop the program based on specifics regarding the patient (demands of activities of daily living, work, and/or sport activities, body mass index), lesion (location, size), and operative procedure.
- Age, obesity, poor nutrition, history of repetitive impact loading may result in osteoarthritic changes.
- Younger patients with isolated defects and relatively healthy surrounding articular cartilage will progress more rapidly than older individuals with degenerative changes.

Create a Healing Environment

- Biologic phases of maturation have been identified.
- Controlled weight-bearing and range of motion are essential to facilitate healing and prevent degeneration: stimulate matrix production, improve the tissue's mechanical properties, nourish the articular cartilage.
- Use pool and force platforms in early phases.

Biomechanics of the Knee

- Articulation between the femoral condyle and the tibial plateau is constant throughout knee range of motion.
- Area of contact between the patella and the trochlea gradually increases as the knee is flexed.
- Rate of weight-bearing, passive range of motion, and exercise progression is based on the exact location of the lesion.
- Exercises are altered based on the biomechanics of the knee to avoid excessive compressive or shearing forces.
- Open kinetic chain exercises are performed from 90° to 40° of flexion.
- Closed kinetic chain exercises are performed initially from 0° to 30° and then progressed to 0° to 60°.

Reduce Pain and Effusion

- Look for a progressive decrease in volitional quadriceps activity with knee pain, distention.
- Any increase in intra-articular joint temperature stimulates proteoglytic enzyme activity, detrimental to articular cartilage.

- Reduction in knee pain and swelling is crucial to minimize reflexive inhibition and restore normal quadriceps activity.

Restore Soft Tissue Balance

- Avoid arthrofibrosis by restoring full passive knee extension, patellar mobility, and soft tissue flexibility of the knee and entire lower extremity.
- Achieve at least 0° of extension within the first few days after surgery.

Restore Muscle Function

- Use electrical muscle stimulation and biofeedback with exercises to facilitate active contraction of the quadriceps musculature.
- Machine weights and closed kinetic chain exercises are included as the patient progresses. Emphasize total leg strength rather than concentrating solely on the quadriceps.
- Train core, hip, and ankle.

Enhance Proprioception and Neuromuscular Control

- Proprioceptive and neuromuscular control drills of both lower extremities are included to restore dynamic stabilization of the knee.

Control the Application of Loads

- Gradually increase the amount of stress applied to the injured knee as the patient returns to functional activities.
- Monitor pain and effusion.
- Consider orthotics, insoles, and bracing to alter the applied loads on the articular cartilage during functional activities.

Team Communication

- Communication between surgeon, physical therapist, and patient before and after surgery is essential.

Rehabilitation Philosophy

- All members of the health care team should convey the same rehabilitation message.
- Slower is better for healing and maturation of articular cartilage.
- Medical team is more interested in long-term results rather than outcome 6 mo after surgery.

TABLE 37–1   Key Principles to Consider when Designing Rehabilitation Programs after Articular Cartilage Repair Procedures

1. Individualize the program.
2. Create a healing environment.
3. Avoid overloading healing tissue.
4. Understand the arthrokinematics of the knee.
5. Understand the biomechanics of exercises.
6. Reduce pain and effusion.
7. Restore soft tissue balance.
8. Restore muscle function.
9. Enhance proprioception and neuromuscular control.
10. Control the application of loads.
11. Promote team communication.
12. Rehabilitation philosophical approach:
    - Gradual progressive loading.
    - "Slower functional progression is better."
    - Think long-term functional results.

neuromuscular control, controlling the application of loads, and team communication. Each of these principles is briefly described as they relate to the rehabilitation program after articular cartilage repair procedures.

Individualization

One of the most important principles involving rehabilitation after articular cartilage repair procedures is the need for an individualized approach for each patient. Several variables must be considered when developing a unique rehabilitation progression for each patient. These include specifics regarding the patient, lesion, and surgery (Table 37–2).

The quality of each individual's articular cartilage is the result of several factors including age, BMI, general health, nutrition, history of previous injuries, and genetics. The composition of articular cartilage undergoes a gradual degeneration over time that results in a breakdown of tissue matrix and a reduction in the load-bearing capacity of the cartilage.[8] The specific factors that contribute to this deterioration remain controversial, but it appears that age, obesity, poor nutrition, and a history of repetitive impact loading (through work or sport activities) may result in osteoarthritic changes.[8] Thus, younger patients with isolated defects and relatively healthy surrounding articular cartilage will progress more rapidly than older individuals with more degenerative changes and less dense cartilage structure.

TABLE 37–2 Specific Variables that Must be Considered when Designing Postoperative Rehabilitation Protocols after Articular Cartilage Procedures

Lesion specifics	Location of lesion
	Size of lesion
	Depth of lesion
	Containment of lesion
	Quality of surrounding tissue
Patient specifics	Age
	Body mass index
	General health
	Nutrition
	Quality of articular cartilage
	Previous activity level
	Specific goals
	Motivation level
Surgical specifics	Surgical procedure
	Tissue involvement
	Concomitant procedures

Furthermore, the patient's motivation and previous activity levels must be considered when determining the rehabilitation approach to ensure that the goals of each patient are addressed. The rehabilitation program should be individualized to the specific demands of each patient's activities of daily living, work, and/or sport activities.

Several variables must be considered in regard to the lesion that may have a dramatic effect on the rehabilitation process. Most important are the exact location and size of the lesion. Lesions on a weight-bearing surface of a femoral condyle must avoid deleterious compressive forces and will require a different rehabilitation approach than those located within the trochlea or undersurface of the patella, where shear forces should be avoided. Furthermore, the size, depth, and containment of each lesion must be considered. Lesions that are large or deep or that have poor containment with healthy surrounding articular cartilage may require a slightly slower rehabilitation progression to ensure that the repair tissue or graft has an adequate amount of time to heal. In addition, the patient's lower extremity alignment must be carefully considered. A patient's knee in a genu varum alignment with a medial compartment lesion may also require a high tibial osteotomy or an osteoarthritis unloader brace.

BMI is another factor to consider. Mithoefer and coworkers[30] reported a correlation between BMI and outcomes after microfracture, because the greater the BMI, the more likely the clinical outcome would be less favorable.

Lastly, the specifics of each surgical procedure will vary the rehabilitation process. Arthroscopic procedures such as chondroplasty or microfracture may progress at a different pace than those with larger incisions and greater tissue involvement, such as OATS or ACI, which require a slower rehabilitation process to protect the healing structures. Each specific surgical procedure has different biologic healing responses postoperatively, which are discussed in detail later in this chapter. Furthermore, any concomitant procedures to address alignment, stability, or meniscal function may also alter the rehabilitation program because of the need to protect other healing tissues. The importance of communication between the surgical team and the rehabilitation team cannot be overemphasized. Appropriate information regarding the specifics of each surgical procedure must be shared to ensure the highest quality of care for each individual.

Create a Healing Environment

The next principle of articular cartilage rehabilitation involves creating an environment that facilitates the healing process while avoiding potentially deleterious forces to the repair site. This involves a thorough knowledge of the physiologic repair process after surgery. Through animal studies, as well as closely monitoring the maturation of repair tissue in human patients via arthroscopic examination, the biologic phases of maturation have been identified after several articular cartilage repair procedures.[4,5,16,36,38] Knowledge of the healing and maturation process after these procedures will ensure that the repair tissue is gradually loaded and that excessive forces are not introduced too early in the healing process. These are discussed in detail in regard to each specific surgical procedure.

Two of the most important modes of rehabilitation of articular cartilage procedures are weight-bearing restrictions and range of motion (ROM) limitations. Unloading and immobilization have been shown to be deleterious to healing articular cartilage, resulting in proteoglycan loss and gradual weakening.[2,17,50] Therefore, controlled weight-bearing and ROM are essential to facilitate healing and prevent degeneration. This gradual progression has been shown to stimulate matrix production and improve the tissue's mechanical properties.[6,7,51]

Controlled compression and decompression forces observed during weight-bearing may nourish the articular cartilage and provide the necessary signals to the repair tissue to produce a matrix that will match the environmental forces.[2,17,50] A progression of partial weight-bearing with crutches is used to gradually increase the amount of load applied to the weight-bearing surfaces of the joint. The use of a pool or aquatic therapy may also be beneficial to initiate gait training and lower extremity weight-bearing exercises. The buoyancy of the water has been shown to decrease the amount of weight-bearing forces to approximately 25% of the individual's body weight when submerged to the level of the axilla and 50% of the individual's body weight when submerged to the level of the waist.[20] Commercially available devices to unload the patient's body weight during treadmill ambulation may also be useful.

A force platform is another useful tool during the early phases of rehabilitation when weight-bearing is limited. This can be used to monitor the percentage of weight-bearing on each extremity during closed kinetic chain (CKC) exercises such as weight-shifts, mini-squats, and leg press (Fig. 37–1).

The pool and force platforms may be used during early phases of rehabilitation to perform limited weight-bearing activities designed to facilitate a normal gait pattern and enhance strength, proprioception, and balance. The goal of these techniques is to initiate weight-bearing activities during the early protective phases of rehabilitation, rather than remain strictly non–weight-bearing and immobilized. The authors' opinion is that beginning controlled weight-bearing activities is a critical component to the overall successful outcome of the procedure. Although the return to functional activities will differ for each patient, early initiation of controlled exercise enables the individual to return to functional activities sooner than those who are immobilized and non–weight-bearing. This may have a positive effect on patient satisfaction.

Passive range of motion (PROM) activities, such as continuous passive motion (CPM) machines or manual PROM, performed by a rehabilitation specialist are also begun immediately after surgery in a limited ROM to nourish the healing articular cartilage and prevent the formation of adhesions. Motion exercises may assist in creating a smooth low-frictional surface by sliding against the joint's articular surface and may be an essential component in

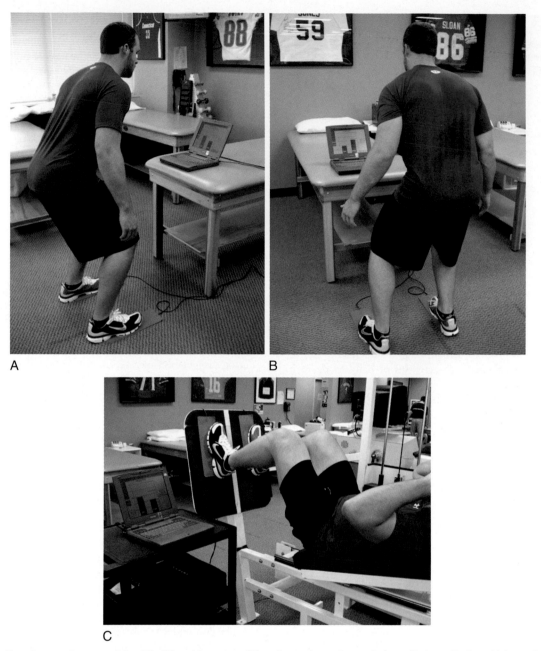

FIGURE 37–1. Exercises such as a weight-shift (**A**) and leg press (**B**) performed on a force platform (Balance Trainer, Unicam Corporation, Ramsey, NJ) that can measure the amount of weight distribution between each extremity (**C**).

cartilage repair.[44,45] The authors' opinion is that PROM is a safe and effective exercise to perform immediately postoperatively, with minimal disadvantageous shear or compressive forces, if done with patient relaxation. This ensures that muscular contraction does not create deleterious compressive or shearing forces. Furthermore, the use of CPM has been shown to enhance cartilage healing and long-term outcomes after articular cartilage procedures.[41,42] In a study comparing the outcomes of patients after microfracture procedures, Rodrigo and associates[41] reported an 85% satisfactory outcome in patients who used a CPM machine for 6 to 8 hours per day for 8 weeks as compared with a 55% satisfactory outcome in patients who did not use a CPM machine. PROM may also be performed on an isokinetic device (Biodex Corporation, Shirley, NY) in the passive mode or with a bike with adjustable pedals that can alter the available ROM (Unicam

Corporation, Ramsey, NJ) (Fig. 37–2). The authors advocate low-intensity (light-resistance) bicycling for long duration to stimulate articular cartilage regeneration.

Biomechanics of the Knee

The next rehabilitation principle involves the biomechanics of the tibiofemoral and patellofemoral joints during normal joint articulation. Articulation between the femoral condyle and the tibial plateau is constant throughout knee ROM. The anterior surface of each femoral condyle is in articulation with the middle aspect of the tibial plateau near full knee extension. With weight-bearing, as the knee moves into greater degrees of knee flexion, the femoral condyles progressively roll posteriorly and slide anteriorly causing the articulation to shift posteriorly on the femoral condyle and tibial plateaus.[24,28]

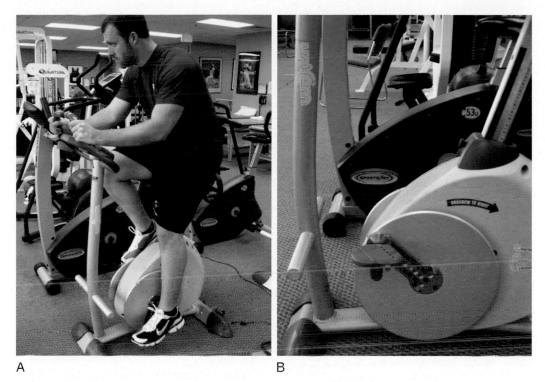

A   B

FIGURE 37–2. Bicycle riding on a Unicam machine (**A**) that can adjust the pedal axis (**B**) to alter the range of motion performed.

The articulation between the inferior margin of the patella and the trochlea begins at approximately 10° to 20° of knee flexion depending on the size of the patella and the length of the patella tendon.[23] As the knee proceeds into greater degrees of flexion, the contact area of the patellofemoral joint moves proximally along the patella. At 30°, the area of patellofemoral contact (inferior facets) is approximately 2 cm².[23] The area of contact gradually increases as the knee is flexed. At 60° of knee flexion, the middle facets of the patella articulate with the trochlea. At 90° of knee flexion, the contact area increases up to 6 cm² and the superior facets articulate.[23]

Using this knowledge of joint arthrokinematics, the rate of weight-bearing, PROM, and exercise progression may be based on the exact location of the lesion (Fig. 37–3).[3,12,14,15] For example, a patient with a lesion on the anterior aspect of the femoral condyle may perform exercises into deeper degrees of knee flexion without causing articulation at the repair site. Conversely, lesions on the posterior condyle may require the avoidance of exercise in deep knee flexion owing to the rolling and sliding component of the articulation during deeper knee flexion. Furthermore, the rehabilitation program for lesions on a non–weight-bearing surface, such as the trochlea, may include immediate partial weight-bearing with a brace locked in full knee extension without causing excessive compression on the repair site.

Rehabilitation exercises are altered based on the biomechanics of the knee to avoid excessive compressive or shearing forces. Whereas the exact ROM in which articulation of the lesion occurs is the most important factor to consider when designing the rehabilitation program, the amount of compressive and shear forces observed at the joint also vary throughout the ROM. Open kinetic chain (OKC) exercises, such as knee extension, are commonly performed from 90° to 40° of knee flexion. This ROM provides the lowest amount of patellofemoral joint reaction forces while exhibiting the greatest amount of patellofemoral contact area,[22,23,49] thus distributing the force along a greater surface area. CKC exercises such as the leg press, vertical squats, lateral step-ups, and wall-squats are performed initially from 0° to 30° and then progressed to 0° to 60° where tibiofemoral and patellofemoral joint reaction forces are lowered.[22,23,49] Clinically, these exercises are begun using a leg press machine rather than the vertical mini-squat owing to the ability to control the amount of weight applied to the lower extremities in the horizontal position in comparison with the vertical squat. As the repair site heals and symptoms subside, the ROM in which exercises are performed is progressed to allow greater muscle strengthening in a larger arc of motion. Exercises are progressed based on the patient's symptoms and the clinical assessment of swelling and crepitation.

Reduce Pain and Effusion

Numerous authors have studied the effect of pain and joint effusion on muscle inhibition. A progressive decrease in volitional quadriceps activity has been noted as the knee exhibits increased pain and distention.[48,52] Therefore, the reduction in knee joint pain and swelling is crucial to minimize this reflexive inhibition and restore normal quadriceps activity. Furthermore, any increase in intra-articular joint temperature has been shown to stimulate proteoglytic enzyme activity, which has a detrimental effect on articular cartilage.[21,34]

Treatment options for swelling reduction include cryotherapy, elevation, high-voltage stimulation, and joint compression through the use of a knee sleeve or compression wrap (Fig. 37–4). Patients presenting with chronic joint effusion may also benefit from a knee sleeve or compression wrap to apply constant pressure while performing everyday activities in an attempt to minimize the development of further effusion (Fig. 37–5).

Pain can be reduced passively through the use of cryotherapy, transcutaneous electrical nerve stimulation, and analgesic medication. Immediately after injury or surgery, the use of a commercial cold wrap can be extremely beneficial. PROM may also provide neuromodulation of pain during acute or exacerbated conditions.[43]

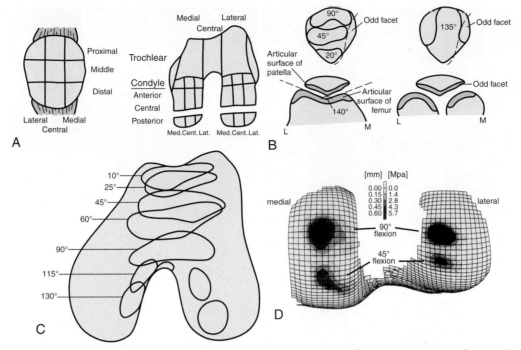

FIGURE 37–3. **A**, The lesion location diagram from the International Knee Documentation Committee evaluation form used to document the location of articular cartilage lesions on the patella, trochlea, and femoral condyles. This form may be used to correlate with the exact location of lesion articulation with the patella (**B**), trochlea (**C**), and femoral condyles (**D**). The diagrams represent the point of articulation of the patellofemoral and tibiofemoral joints at various degrees of knee range of motion. Surface displacements (mm) and surface stresses (MPa) at 45° and 90° of knee flexion are depicted on **D**. *(**A**, Reprinted with permission from the International Knee Documentation Committee; **B** and **C**, Reprinted with permission from McConnell, J.; Fulkerson, J.: The knee: patellofemoral and soft tissue injuries. In Zachazewski, J. E.; Magee, D. J.; Quillen, W. S. [eds.]: Athletic Injuries and Rehabilitation. Philadelphia: W. B. Saunders, 1996; pp. 693–729; **D**, Reprinted with permission from Blankevoort, L.; Kuiper, J. H.; Huiskes, R.; Grootenboer, H. J.: Articular contact in a three-dimensional model of the knee. J Biomech 24:1019–1031, 1991.)*

Restore Soft Tissue Balance

One of the most important aspects of articular cartilage rehabilitation involves the avoidance of arthrofibrosis, particularly with the OATS and ACI procedures, owing to the large open incision and extensive soft tissue trauma. This is achieved through the restoration of full passive knee extension, patellar mobility, and soft tissue flexibility of the knee and entire lower extremity. The inability to fully extend the knee results in abnormal joint arthrokinematics and subsequent increases in patellofemoral and tibiofemoral joint

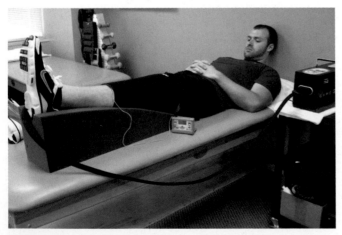

FIGURE 37–4. Cryotherapy and intermittent compression applied through a commercial cold device (Gameready, Coolsystems Corporation, Berkeley, CA) with elevation and high-voltage electrical stimulation (300PV, Empi Corporation, St. Paul, MN) for swelling control.

contact pressure, increased strain on the quadriceps muscle, and muscular fatigue.[35] Therefore, a drop-lock postoperative knee brace locked into 0° of extension is used during ambulation, and PROM out of the brace is performed immediately after surgery.

The goal is to achieve at least 0° of knee extension within the first few days after surgery. Specific exercises include manual PROM exercises performed by the rehabilitation specialist, supine hamstring stretches with a wedge under the heel, and gastrocnemius stretching with a towel. Overpressure of 6 to 12 pounds may be used for a low-load long-duration stretch as needed to achieve full extension (Fig. 37–6). Patients are instructed to perform low, long-duration stretches for 10 to 12 minutes several times each day (usually five to six times per day). Modalities such as moist heat and ultrasound may also be applied to facilitate greater ROM improvements before and/or during these stretching techniques.[25,40]

The loss of patellar mobility after surgery may be due to various reasons including excessive scar tissue adhesions from the incision anteriorly as well as along the medial and lateral gutters. The loss of patellar mobility may result in ROM complications and difficulty in recruiting a quadriceps contraction. Patellar mobilizations in the medial-lateral and superior-inferior directions are performed by the rehabilitation specialist and independently by the patient during his or her home exercise program.

Soft tissue flexibility and pliability are also important for the entire lower extremity. Soft tissue mobilization and scar management are performed to prevent the development of adhesions around the anterior, medial, and lateral aspects of the knee. In addition, flexibility exercises are performed for the entire lower

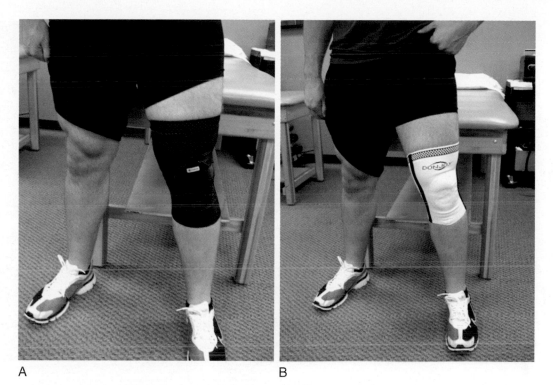

A   B

FIGURE 37–5. A, Knee compression sleeve (Bauerfeind Corp, Atlanta, GA) **B**, Compression sleeve (DJ Orthopaedics, Carlsbad, CA).

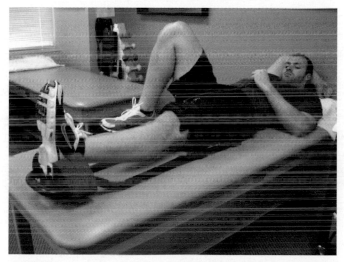

FIGURE 37–6. Low load long duration stretching into knee extension using 8 to 10 pounds of overpressure. A wedge is applied under the heel to facilitate full extension (ERMI device, Get Motion Corporation, Atlanta, GA).

extremity including the hamstrings, hip, and calf musculature. As ROM improves and the lesion begins to heal, quadriceps stretching may be performed as tolerated by the patient.

Restore Muscle Function

The next principle involves restoring muscle function of the lower extremity. As previously stated, inhibition of the quadriceps muscle is a common clinical enigma in the presence of pain and effusion during the acute phases of rehabilitation. Electrical muscle stimulation (EMS) and biofeedback are often incorporated with therapeutic exercises to facilitate the active contraction of the quadriceps musculature (Fig. 37–7A)

EMS and biofeedback on the quadriceps musculature appear to facilitate the return of muscle activation and may be valuable additions to therapeutic exercises.[9,46] Clinically, EMS is begun immediately after surgery while the patient performs isometric and isotonic exercises such as quadriceps sets, straight leg raises, hip adduction and abduction, and knee extensions (see Fig. 37–7B). EMS is used before biofeedback when the patient presents acutely with the inability to activate the quadriceps musculature. EMS is useful to attempt to recruit a maximum amount of muscle fibers during active contraction and may be used throughout the rehabilitation process. Once independent muscle activation is present, biofeedback may also be incorporated to facilitate further neuromuscular activation of the quadriceps. The patient must concentrate on neuromuscular control to independently activate the quadriceps during rehabilitation. The quadriceps and the hip/core muscles are emphasized to assist in dissipating ground reaction forces.

Exercises that strengthen the entire lower extremity, such as machine weights and CKC exercises, may be included as the patient progresses to more advanced phases of rehabilitation. It is important that total leg strength be emphasized rather than concentrating solely on the quadriceps. Furthermore, the importance of incorporating core stability exercises cannot be overlooked. Training of the core, hip, and ankle located proximally and distally along the kinetic chain is emphasized to assist in controlling the production and dissipation of forces in the knee. In addition, the hip and ankle assist in controlling abduction and adduction moments at the knee joint.

Enhance Proprioception and Neuromuscular Control

Proprioceptive and neuromuscular control drills of the lower extremities should be included to restore dynamic stabilization of the knee joint postoperatively. Proprioceptive deficits have been noted in the injured and postoperative knee.[10,39] Specific

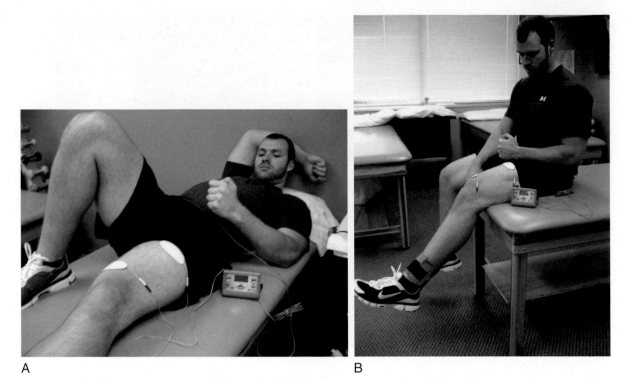

A   B

FIGURE 37–7. Neuromuscular electrical stimulation (300PV, Empi Corporation, St. Paul, MN) applied to the quadriceps muscle (**A**) during exercises such as knee extension (**B**).

drills initially include weight-shifting side-to-side, weight-shifting diagonally, mini-squats, and mini-squats on an unstable surface such as a tilt board (Fig. 37–8). Perturbations can be added to challenge the neuromuscular system as well as additional exercises including lunges, step-ups, and balance onto unstable surfaces (Figs. 37–9 and 37–10).

Control the Application of Loads

The next principle of rehabilitation involves gradually increasing the amount of stress applied to the injured knee as the patient returns to functional activities. The rehabilitation process involves a progressive application of therapeutic exercises designed to

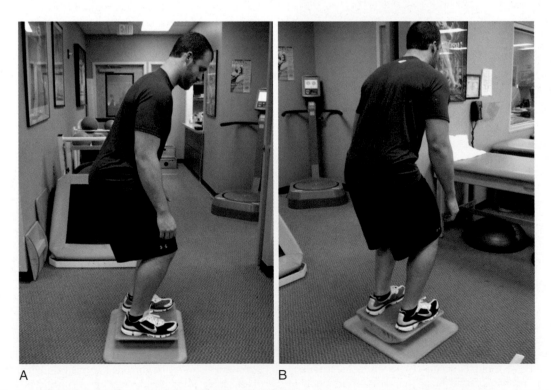

A   B

FIGURE 37–8. **A** and **B**, Mini-squats on an unstable surface such as a tiltboard. The patient is instructed to squat while preventing movement of the board.

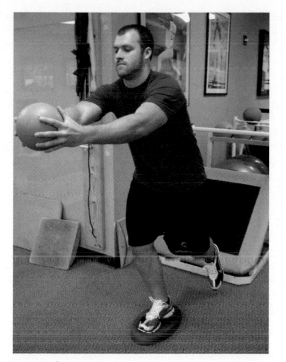

FIGURE 37-9. Single-leg balance on an unstable surface such as foam. The patient may use a weighted ball while performing reciprocal movement patterns with the uninvolved upper and lower extremities to alter the center of gravity throughout the exercise.

gradually increase function in the postoperative knee. This progression is used to provide a healthy stimulus for healing tissues while ensuring that forces are gradually applied without causing damage. Common clinical signs that a patient may be progressing too quickly and overloading the healing tissue are joint line

pain and effusion. This should be monitored throughout the rehabilitation process.

In addition, patients may benefit from the use of orthotics, insoles, and bracing to alter the applied loads on the articular cartilage during functional activities. These devices are used to avoid excessive forces by unloading the area of the knee where the lesion is located. Unloading braces are often used for patients with subtle uncorrected abnormal alignments (genu varum) or large or uncontained lesions or who had concomitant osteotomies and meniscal allografts (Fig. 37-11).

Team Communication

The next principle of rehabilitation involves communication between the surgeon, the physical therapist, and the patient. Communication between the surgeon and the rehabilitation team is essential to determine the accurate rate of progression based on the location and size of the lesion, tissue quality, and concomitant surgical procedures. As well, communication between the medical team and the patient is essential to provide the patient with education regarding the avoidance of deleterious forces as well as improving compliance with precautions. Frequently, a preoperative physical therapy evaluation may be useful to mentally and physically prepare the patient for the articular cartilage procedure and postoperative rehabilitation.

Rehabilitation Philosophy

It is important that all members of the health care team (e.g., physician, physical therapist, athletic trainer, nurses) convey the same rehabilitation message. The authors advocate gradual progressive loading of healing articular cartilage. The purpose of this concept is to recondition the articular cartilage. Another message is "slower

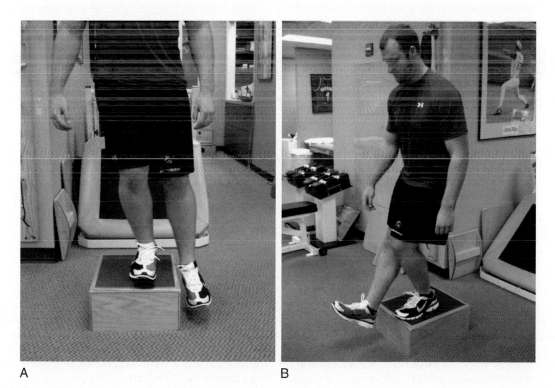

A   B

FIGURE 37-10. A and B, Lateral step up exercises performed while standing on an unstable surface such as a piece of foam. This exercise requires eccentric control of the lower extremity to perform the step-up exercise as well as to balance throughout the movement.

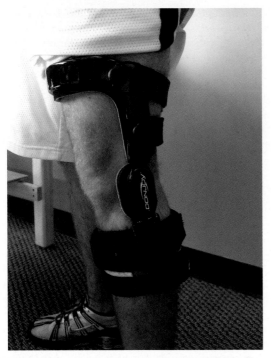

FIGURE 37–11. An osteoarthritis unloading brace (OA Defiance, Don Joy Corporation, Vista, CA) using a four-point leverage system to unload the medial compartment of the knee by providing a mild valgus stress to the knee.

is better." It takes a long period of time for articular cartilage to heal, mature, and return to weight-bearing activities. One last philosophical point is "faster is not better, even if you feel pain-free." Patients are instructed that the medical team is more interested in long-term results than outcome 6 months after surgery.

REHABILITATION AFTER ARTICULAR CARTILAGE REPAIR PROCEDURES

The rehabilitation progression is designed based on the four biologic phases of cartilage maturation: proliferation, transitional, remodeling, and maturation.[4,5,11,16,19,33,36,38] The length of each phase will vary depending on the lesion, patient's age and general health, and surgical specifics discussed previously; however, the concepts of each phase are consistent. The following sections overview the generalized rehabilitation process during each of the four phases.

Phase I: Early Protection Phase

The first phase of cartilage healing is the *proliferation phase*, which typically involves the first 4 to 6 postoperative weeks. During this phase, the initial healing process begins. It is imperative to decrease swelling, gradually restore PROM, and enhance volitional control of the quadriceps during this period of rehabilitation.

Controlled active ROM and PROM and a gradual weight-bearing progression are critical components to the rehabilitation process. As previously discussed, PROM and controlled partial weight-bearing will help promote the nurturing of the cartilage

through diffusion of synovial fluid as well as provide the proper stimulus for the cells to produce specific matrix markers. Individuals begin with partial weight-bearing activities using crutches. Progressive loading exercises using the pool and force platforms are gradually implemented to increase the amount of load applied to the weight-bearing surfaces of the joint. The use of a pool or aquatic therapy may be beneficial to begin gait training and lower extremity exercises once the incisions are well healed.

PROM activities, such as manual PROM performed by a rehabilitation specialist and CPM machines, are also begun immediately after surgery to nourish the healing articular cartilage and prevent the formation of adhesions. The use of a CPM typically begins 6 to 8 hours after surgery and is performed for at least 2 to 3 weeks, with recommended use up to 6 to 8 weeks. It is recommended that the CPM be used throughout the day for up to 6 to 8 hours. The patient is instructed to also perform active-assisted ROM frequently throughout the day. Patella mobilization, soft tissue mobilization, and soft tissue flexibility exercises are also performed to minimize scar tissue formation and avoid loss of motion. Low-intensity stationary cycling may be implemented in this phase.

Early strengthening exercises are performed to restore volitional quadriceps control and neuromuscular control through the use of concomitant EMS. Exercises performed during this phase are limited based on the specific weight-bearing status of each patient and typically include quadriceps sets, straight leg raises, and early baseline proprioception exercises such as weight-shifting.

Phase II: Transition Phase

The second phase is the *transitional phase*, which typically includes postoperative weeks 4 through 12. The repair tissue at this point is gaining strength, which will allow for the progression of rehabilitation exercises. During this phase, the patient progresses from partial to full weight-bearing, while full ROM and soft tissue flexibility are achieved. Continued maturation of the repair tissue is fostered through higher-level functional and ROM exercises. It is during this phase that patients typically resume most normal activities of daily living. The rehabilitation program will gradually progress strengthening activities to include machine weights and CKC exercises, such as leg press, front lunges, wall-slides, and lateral step-ups, as the patient's weight-bearing status returns to normal.

At this time, the rehabilitation process involves the progressive application of therapeutic exercises designed to gradually increase function in the postoperative knee. The progression of weight-bearing activities and restoration of ROM, as previously discussed, involves the gradual advancement of activities to ensure that complications do not arise while facilitating healing. A principle of gradual progressive loading is implemented during this phase. Once weight-bearing is initiated, the clinician may consider an osteoarthritis unloader brace. Common complications include motion restrictions and scar tissue formation. Furthermore, an overaggressive approach early within the rehabilitation program may result in increased pain, inflammation, or effusion as well as graft damage. This simple concept may be applied to the progression of strengthening exercises, proprioception training, neuromuscular control drills, and functional drills. For example, exercises such as weight-shifts and lunges are progressed from straight-plane anterior-posterior or medial-lateral directions to involve multiplane and rotational movements. Exercises using two legs, such as leg press and balance activities, are progressed to single-leg exercises. Thus, the progression through the postoperative rehabilitation program involves a gradual progression of applied and functional stresses. This progression is used to provide a healthy stimulus for healing tissues while ensuring that forces are gradually applied without causing damage.

Phase III: Remodeling Phase

The third phase, known as the *remodeling phase*, generally occurs from 3 to 6 months postoperatively. During this phase, there is a continuous remodeling of tissue into a more organized structure. The tissue continues to increase in strength and durability. As the tissue becomes more firm and integrated, more functional training activities may be performed. At this point, the patient typically notes improvement of symptoms and has normal ROM. The patient is encouraged to continue with her or his rehabilitation program independently to maximize strength and flexibility. Low- to moderate-impact activities such as bicycle riding, golfing, and recreational walking may often be gradually incorporated. The senior author's experience has shown that during this phase when overzealous patients are "feeling good," they may overexert their program, which may compromise the repair site.

Phase IV: Maturation Phase

The final phase is known as the *maturation phase*, which typically begins in a range of 4 to 6 months and can last up to 15 to 18 months. This depends on the type of surgery, size, and location of the lesion. During this phase, the repair tissue reaches its full maturation. The duration of this phase varies based on several factors such as lesion size and location and the specific surgical procedure performed. The patient will gradually return to full premorbid activities as tolerated. Impact-loading activities are gradually introduced. Although such procedures as OATS and ACI are designed to restore function rather than to facilitate return to high impact athletic activities, a return to athletic activities is determined based on the unique presentation of each patient. A return to competitive athletics has been documented after microfracture,[44] OATS,[19] and ACI[27,28] procedures.

SPECIFIC POSTOPERATIVE GUIDELINES

Débridement and Chondroplasty

Rehabilitation after an arthroscopic débridement or chondroplasty is fairly simple owing to the nature and goal of the procedure to facilitate tissue healing rather than create repair tissue. Initial weight-bearing is limited for the first 3 to 5 days using axillary crutches, although weight-bearing is permitted as tolerated. PROM exercises are progressed as tolerated immediately with no postoperative limitations in motion. Full passive motion is typically achieved within 2 to 3 weeks. OKC exercises are performed initially, although CKC strengthening exercises and bicycle riding are normally incorporated by the end of the 1st week. The patient is allowed to return to full functional activities and progress to moderate-impact activities, such as light jogging and sports, beginning at week 4. The progression of impact loading may be delayed if significant degenerative changes are present within the knee or if symptoms of pain and/or effusion persist.

Microfracture

Rehabilitation after a microfracture procedure progresses more cautiously than that of a débridement or chondroplasty (Table 37-3). The program is based on size, location, number of areas treated, and concomitant procedures. The early protection phase begins immediately after surgery and lasts until the 4th week postoperatively. During this time, defects begin to fill with a fibrin clot, although no fibrocartilage is present.[11] A period of non–weight-bearing is applied for the first 2 to 6 weeks postoperatively for most lesions. A recent study by Marder and colleagues[27] compared the results of patients with small focal lesions of less than 2.0 cm² using two postoperative rehabilitation programs. Group I used touch-down weight bearing and a CPM machine for 6 to 8 hours a day for 6 weeks. Group II was allowed weight-bearing as tolerated immediately after surgery and used active-assisted heel-slides for ROM (without the use of a CPM). The authors reported significant improvements in both groups and no significant differences in the subjective or objective outcomes between groups a minimum of 2 years postoperatively. Thus, it appears that it may be possible to begin early controlled weight bearing for small, focal lesions without applying deleterious forces to the repair site. Initial controlled touch-down weight-bearing is initiated for lesions that are localized and smaller than 2.0 cm² in patients with good tissue quality. For patients with patellofemoral lesions, immediate weight-bearing is performed owing to the lack of lesion articulation during weight-bearing; however, a drop-locked knee brace is worn to avoid deleterious sheer forces to the healing repair site.

Owing to the arthroscopic nature of the procedure, PROM is performed immediately without restrictions. Full PROM of at least 0° to 125° is achieved between weeks 3 and 4, often with little difficulty.

The transition phase begins at week 4 and progresses to week 8. During this phase, the patient may progress to full weight bearing and more functional CKC exercises. At 6 weeks postoperatively, a thin layer of tissue covers the base of the lesion.[13] Although the repair is still incomplete, fibrocartilagenous tissue is present, and by 8 weeks, some tissue with hyaline-like characteristics has been detected.[11] By 12 weeks, the defect is completely filled and the quality of cartilaginous tissue improves significantly.[13]

Weight-bearing is thus progressed to full at week 8 for most lesions when the strength of the repair tissue is increasing. However, the progression to more advanced exercises, including impact loading, is delayed until the end of the remodeling phase when the defect is completely filled. The patient may gradually begin to return to former activities during the maturation phase between months 4 to 6; however, larger lesions may need to delay the progression to high-impact activities for up to 8 months.

Clinical outcome studies indicate that a significant number of patients will be able to return to sports after a microfracture procedure. Mithoefer and coworkers[31] reported on 32 patients who routinely participated in high impact and pivoting sports. At a minimum 2-year follow-up, 66% had good to excellent results and 44% had returned to high-impact sports. However, after initial improvement, scores decreased in 47% of athletes. Return to sports was significantly higher in athletes younger

TABLE 37–3   Rehabilitation after Microfracture Procedure

PHASE I: EARLY PROTECTION PHASE (WEEKS 0–4)

Goals	Protect healing tissue from load and shear forces. Decrease pain and effusion. Restore full passive knee extension. Gradually restore knee flexion. Regain quadriceps control.
Brace	No brace; may use elastic wrap to control swelling.
WB	WB status varies based on lesion location, size. For medium to large femoral condyle lesions (>2.0 cm^2): non-WB for 2 wk, begin toe-touch WB ($\sim$20–30 lb) wk 3; progress to partial WB ($\sim$25% body weight) at wk 4. For small femoral condyle lesions (<2.0 cm^2): immediate toe-touch WB (per physician) ($\sim$20-30 lb) wk 0–2; progress to 50% WB wk 3, 75% WB wk 4. For patellofemoral lesions: immediate toe-touch WB of $\sim$25% body weight with brace locked in full extension; progress to 50% WB at wk 2, 75% WB wk 3 with brace locked in full extension, full WB wk 4.
ROM	Immediate motion exercise day 1. Full passive knee extension immediately. Initiate CPM day 1 for total of 8–12 hr/day (0°–60°; if patellofemoral lesion > 6.0 cm^2, 0°–40°). Progress CPM ROM as tolerated 5°–10°/day. May continue CPM for total of 6–8 hr/day for up to 6 wk. Patellar mobilization (4–6 times/day). Motion exercises throughout the day. Passive knee flexion ROM at least 2–3 times/day. Progress passive knee ROM as tolerated, no restrictions. Minimum ROM goals 0°–90° wk 1; 0°–105° wk 2; 0°–115° wk 3; and 0°–125° wk 4. Stretch hamstrings and calf.
Strengthening program	Ankle pump using rubber tubing. Quadriceps setting. Multiangle isometrics (co-contractions Q/H). Active knee extension 90°–40° for femoral condyle lesions (no resistance), avoid for patellofemoral patients. Straight leg raises (four directions). Stationary bicycle when ROM allows—low resistance. EMS and/or biofeedback during quadriceps exercises. Initiate weight-shifting exercises with knee in extension wk 1–2 for patellofemoral lesions and small femoral condyle lesions, wk 3 for larger femoral condyle lesions. Leg press 0°–60° wk 3 for small femoral condyle lesions and patellofemoral lesions; progress to 0°–90° wk 4 Toe-calf-raises wk 4 for small femoral condyle and patellofemoral lesions. May begin use of pool for gait training and exercises wk 3–4 (when incision is fully healed). May begin stationary bike wk 3–4, low resistance. NO active knee extension exercises for patellofemoral lesions.
Functional activities	Gradual return to daily activities. If symptoms occur, reduce activities to reduce pain and inflammation.
Swelling control	Ice, elevation, compression, and effusion modalities as needed.
Criteria to progress to phase II	Full passive knee extension. Knee flexion to 125°. Minimal pain and swelling. Voluntary quadriceps activity.

PHASE II: TRANSITION PHASE (WEEKS 4–8)

Goals	Gradually improve quadriceps strength/endurance. Gradual increase in functional activities.
WB	Progress as tolerated. Large femoral condyle lesions: 50% WB with crutches 6 wk; 75% WB wk 7, full WB wk 8, discontinue crutches.
ROM	Gradual increase in ROM. Maintain full passive knee extension. Progress knee flexion to ≥135° by wk 8. Continue patellar mobilization and soft tissue mobilization, as needed. Continue stretching program.
Strengthening exercises	Progress CKC exercises. Initiate leg press for large femoral condyle lesions wk 6. Mini-squats 0°–45° wk 7. Toe-calf-raises wk 8 for femoral condyle lesions. Progress balance and proprioception drills. Initiate front lunges, wall-squats, front and lateral step-ups wk 5 for small femoral condyle and patellofemoral lesions, wk 8 for large femoral condyle lesions.

PHASE II: TRANSITION PHASE (WEEKS 4–8)—Cont'd

	For femoral condyle lesions, progress OKC knee extension, 1 lb/wk.
	For patellofemoral lesion, may begin OKC knee extension without resistance in an ROM that does not allow for articulation of the lesion.
	Continue stationary bicycle, low resistance (gradually increase time).
	Continue use of EMS and/or biofeedback as needed.
	Continue use of pool for gait training and exercise.
Functional activities	As pain and swelling (symptoms) diminish, the patient may gradually increase functional activities.
	Gradually increase standing and walking.
Criteria to progress to phase III	Full ROM.
	Acceptable strength level
	• Hamstrings within 20% of contralateral leg.
	• Quadriceps within 30% of contralateral leg.
	Balance testing within 30% of contralateral leg.
	Able to bike for 30 min.

PHASE III: REMODELING PHASE (WEEKS 8–16)

Goals	Improve muscular strength and endurance.
	Increase functional activities.
ROM	Patient should exhibit 125°–135°+ flexion.
Exercise program	Leg press (0°–90°).
	Bilateral squats (0°–60°).
	Unilateral step-ups progressing from 2" to 8".
	Forward lunges.
	Walking program wk 10.
	Progress OKC extension (0°–90°); for patellofemoral lesions, may begin wk 12, perform from 90°–40° or avoid angle where lesion articulates—progress 1 lb every 2 wk beginning wk 20 if no pain or crepitation—must monitor symptoms.
	Continue progressing balance and proprioception.
	Bicycle.
	Stairmaster.
	Swimming.
	Nordic-Trak/elliptical.
Functional activities	As patient improves, increase walking (e.g., distance, cadence, incline)
Maintenance program	Initiate at wk 12–16.
	Bicycle: low resistance, increase time.
	Progressive walking program.
	Pool exercises for entire lower extremity.
	Straight leg raises.
	Leg press.
	Wall-squats.
	Hip abduction/adduction.
	Front lunges.
	Step ups.
	Stretch quadriceps, hamstrings, calf.
Criteria to progress to phase IV	Full non-painful ROM.
	Strength within 80–90% of contralateral extremity.
	Balance and/or stability within 75–80% of contralateral extremity.
	No pain, inflammation, or swelling.

PHASE IV: MATURATION PHASE (WEEKS 16–26)

Goals	Gradual return to full unrestricted functional activities.
Exercises	Continue maintenance program progression 3–4 times/wk.
	Progress resistance as tolerated.
	Emphasis on entire lower extremity strength and flexibility.
	Progress agility and balance drills.
	Impact-loading program should be specialized to patient's demands.
	Progress sport programs depending on patient variables.
Functional activities	Patient may return to various sport activities as progression in rehabilitation and cartilage healing allows. Generally, low-impact sports such as swimming, skating, rollerblading, and cycling are permitted at about 2 mo for small femoral condyle and patellofemoral lesions and at 3 mo for large femoral condyle lesions. Higher-impact sports such as jogging, running, and aerobics may be performed at 4 mo for small lesions or 5 mo for larger lesions. High-impact sports such as tennis, basketball, football and baseball are allowed at 6–8 mo.

CKC, closed kinetic chain; CPM, continuous passive motion; EMS, electrical muscle stimulation; OKC, open kinetic chain; Q/H, quadriceps/hamstring; ROM, range of motion; WB, weight-bearing.

than 40 years of age, patients with a lesion size less than 200 mm^2, those with preoperative symptoms less than 12 months' duration, and patients who had no prior surgical intervention. Mithoefer and associates[29] reported results of microfracture on isolated femoral chondral lesions. They reported that 67% of patients had a good to excellent result; 25%, a fair result; and 8%, a poor result. The investigators were able to obtain follow-up magnetic resonance imaging (MRI) on 50% of the patients. MRI revealed good tissue healing and filling in 54%, moderate tissue filling in 29%, and poor healing result in 17%. Successful outcomes correlated to a low BMI, good healing or lesion filling, and short duration of symptoms. The worst results were seen in patients with a BMI of 30 kg/m. Kreuz and colleagues[26] compared the results of microfracture in patients older than 40 years of age and younger than 40 years of age. The authors reported superior outcomes in patients 40 years or younger. Between 18 and 36 months postoperatively, the investigators found a deterioration in International Cartilage Repair Society (ICRS) scores, which was significantly pronounced in older patients. Furthermore, MRI performed at 36 months after surgery indicated better fill in patients younger than 40 years of age.

OATS

Rehabilitation after OATS procedures requires the avoidance of early deleterious forces to avoid disrupting the healing transplanted bone plugs (Table 37–4). Currently, the pace of the rehabilitation program after OATS procedures is based not only on the size of the lesion but also on the amount of transplanted bone plugs. The program is progressed more cautiously when numerous bone plugs are used owing to the potential for a less congruent surface. The early protection phase lasts until the 8th week postoperatively. During this phase, an initial 44% reduction in the push-in and pull-out strength of the transplanted bone plugs has been observed (at 1 wk postoperatively),[52] emphasizing the need for strict non–weight-bearing postoperatively. Partial weight-bearing is usually initiated 2 to 4 weeks after surgery based on the size of the lesion and the number of transplanted bone plugs. Although the original hyaline cartilage remains intact and viable,[33] the strength of the bone plugs is the limiting factor when designing the postoperative rehabilitation program.

By 4 weeks, the cancellous bone plugs have united,[19] and by 6 weeks, there is full subchondral integration and 29% of grafts show bonding between the articular cartilage of the bone plugs and the surrounding articular cartilage.[33] Although integration has occurred, a 63% decrease in graft stiffness is still observed at 6 weeks postoperative.[33] During this time, weight-bearing is gradually progressed as the strength of the repair increases. At 8 weeks postoperative, fibrocartilage has been observed to grow to the surface and seal the recipient and donor site hyaline cartilage, and weight-bearing is progressed to full. Immediate weight-bearing is initiated for patellofemoral lesions with a drop-lock knee brace and progressed to full without the brace at approximately 6 to 8 weeks postoperative.

ROM during the early protective phase is gradually progressed to ensure that adhesion formation and loss of motion is avoided. Owing to the large incision and invasive nature of the procedure, motion is progressed gradually to minimize effusion formation.

Exercises are progressed from non–weight-bearing, such as quadriceps sets and multiangle straight leg raises, to gentle weight-bearing in a restricted weight tolerance after week 6.

During the transition phase, full ROM and weight-bearing are achieved typically between weeks 8 to 10, although larger lesions may need to further delay the progress to full weight-bearing for up to 12 to 14 weeks. At this point, the strengthening program is progressed to include weight-bearing CKC and machine exercises. Again, during this phase, patients return to low-impact functional activities.

During the remodeling and maturation phases, strength, proprioception, and neuromuscular control are enhanced while impact-loading stresses are gradually applied as tolerated without an increase in symptoms. Patient may return to various sport activities as progression in rehabilitation and cartilage healing allows, although this is more delayed than the previously discussed rehabilitation progressions. Generally, low-impact sports such as golf, swimming, cycling, and walking for exercise are permitted at 4 to 5 months postoperatively. Moderate-impact sports such as tennis and hiking are permitted at 6 to 8 months (depending on size and location of the lesion). The return to high-impact sports is controversial, although some clinicians allow sports such as jogging, running, and aerobics at 8 to 10 months and tennis, basketball, and baseball at 12 to 18 months. There are too few studies to indicate the long-term success in allowing the return to strenuous activities, which may risk deterioration of the reparative cartilage.

Clinical outcome results after mosaicplasty indicate good results. Hangody and Fules[18] followed 831 patients and reported a good to excellent result in 92% of those who exhibited a lesion of the femoral condyle, and the same in 87% with a tibial plateau lesion. Lesions of the patella rendered the lowest outcomes, with only 79% exhibiting a good to excellent result. Furthermore, the authors reported a 3% rate of donor site morbidity. Lastly, 36 patients exhibited a painful postoperative hemarthroses. Bartha and coworkers[1] reported on 89 patients who underwent second-look arthroscopy, 77% of whom exhibited congruent surfaces and healing of the lesion.

ACI

The rehabilitation program after ACI is vital to the success and long-term outcomes of patients (Table 37–5). Early controlled ROM and weight-bearing are necessary to stimulate chondrocyte development, although caution is placed on overaggressive activities that may result in cell damage or graft delamination.

Knowledge of the biologic healing response is vital for the development of appropriate rehabilitation guidelines. Rehabilitation may begin as early as the recovery room in the form of CPM. At this time, the chondrocytes are aligned and attached to the underlying surface.[47] It is imperative that the patient be appropriately positioned to allow for the effect of gravity to evenly distribute the chondrocytes on the base of the defect during these first 4 hours as the cells adhere to the surface. A study by Sohn and associates[47] showed that the defect orientation during these first 4 hours can be an important factor in the uniformity of cell distribution in the ACI procedure. These authors advanced the hypothesis, which has not yet been proved clinically, that the effects of gravity within the first few hours of cell implantation could lead to localization of induced cells in one area of the graft but not in other areas, which may affect healing

TABLE 37–4   Rehabilitation after Osteochondral Autograft Transplantation

PHASE I: EARLY PROTECTION PHASE (WEEKS 0–6)

Goals	Protection of healing tissue from load and shear forces. Decrease pain and effusion. Restoration of full passive knee extension. Gradual improvement of knee flexion. Regain quadriceps control.
Brace	Locked at 0° during WB activities. Sleep in locked brace for 2–4 wk.
WB	WB status varies based on lesion location and size. For femoral condyle lesions: non-WB for 2–4 wk (physician direction); if large lesion (>5 cm²) may need to delay WB up to 4 wk, progress to toe-touch WB (~20–30 lb) wks 3–4 and partial WB (~25–50% body weight) at wk 6. For patellofemoral lesions: immediate toe-touch WB 25% body weight with brace locked in full extension. Progress to 50% WB wk 2–3 in brace and 75% wk 4–5 in brace.
ROM	Immediate motion exercise day 1. Full passive knee extension immediately. Initiate CPM day 1 for total of 8–12 hr/day (0°–60°; if patellofemoral lesion > 6.0 cm², 0°–40°). Progress CPM ROM as tolerated 5°–10°/day. May continue CPM for total of 6–8 hr/day for up to 6 wk. Patellar mobilization (1–6 times/day). Motion exercises throughout the day. Passive knee flexion ROM at least 2–3 times/day. Passive knee ROM as tolerated. For femoral condyle lesions, minimum knee flexion ROM goal is 90° by 1–2 wk; 105° wk 3; 115° wk 4; and 120°–125° by wk 6. For patellofemoral lesions, minimum knee flexion ROM goal is 90° by wk 2–3; 105° by 3–4 wk; and 120° by wk 6. Stretch hamstrings and calf.
Strengthening program	Ankle pump using rubber tubing. Quadriceps setting. Multiangle isometrics (co-contractions Q/H). Straight leg raises (four directions). Active knee extension 90°–40° for femoral condyle lesions if not articulation wk 4 (no resistance). EMS and/or biofeedback during quadriceps exercises. Stationary bicycle when ROM allows—low resistance. Isometric leg press at wk 4 (multiangle). May begin use of pool for gait training and exercises wk 6. Initiate weight-shifting exercises with knee in extension wk 3–4 for patellofemoral lesions. NO active knee extension exercises for patellofemoral lesions. NO CKC exercises for femoral condyle lesions.
Functional activities	Gradual return to daily activities. If symptoms occur, reduce activities to reduce pain and inflammation. Extended standing should be avoided.
Swelling control	Ice, elevation, compression, and edema modalities as needed to decrease swelling.
Criteria to progress to phase II	Full passive knee extension. Knee flexion to 120°. Minimal pain and swelling.

PHASE II: TRANSITION PHASE (WEEKS 6–12)

Goals	Gradually increase ROM and WB to full. Gradually improve quadriceps strength/endurance. Gradual increase in functional activities.
Brace	Discontinue brace at 6 wk, consider unloading brace for femoral condyle lesions.
WB	Progress WB as tolerated. For femoral condyle lesions: 75% body weight with crutches at 6–7 wk, and progress to full WB at 8–10 wk, may need to delay full WB up to 14 wk if large lesion, discontinue crutches at 8–10 wk. For patellofemoral lesions, progress to full WB and discharge crutches at 6–8 wk.
ROM	Gradual increase in ROM. Maintain full passive knee extension. Progress knee flexion to 125°–135° by wk 8–10. Continue patellar mobilization and soft tissue mobilization, as needed. Continue stretching program.
Strengthening exercises	Initiate weight-shifts wk 6–8 for femoral condyle lesions. Initiate mini-squats 0°–45° wk 6–8 for patellofemoral lesions. CKC exercises (leg press) wk 8–10 for femoral condyle lesions: mini-squats 0°–45°, front lunges, step-ups, wall-squats; may need to delay CKC up to 14 wk if large lesions. Leg press wk 8–10 (0°–90° for femoral condyle, 0°–60° for patellofemoral, progressing to 0°–90° as tolerated). Toe-calf-raises wk 10–12.

Continued

	PHASE II: TRANSITION PHASE (WEEKS 6–12)—Cont'd
	Progress active knee extension: begin resistance with femoral condyle lesions progressing 1 lb every 10–14 days; for patellofemoral lesions, begin with 0°–30° at wk 12 and progress to deeper angles as tolerated.
	Stationary bicycle (gradually increase time).
	Balance and proprioception drills.
	Continue use of electrical stimulation and biofeedback as needed.
	Continue use of pool for gait training and exercise.
Functional activities	As pain and swelling (symptoms) diminish, the patient may gradually increase functional activities. Gradually increase standing and walking.
Criteria to progress to phase III	Full ROM. Acceptable strength level: • Hamstrings within 20% of contralateral leg. • Quadriceps within 30% of contralateral leg. Balance testing within 30% of contralateral leg. Able to bike for 30 min.

	PHASE III: REMODELING PHASE (WEEKS 12–26)
Goals	Improve muscular strength and endurance. Increase functional activities.
ROM	Patient should exhibit 125°–135° flexion—no restrictions.
Exercise program	Continue progressing exercises. Leg press 0°–90°. Bilateral squats (0°–60°). Unilateral step-ups progressing from 2" to 8". Forward lunges. Begin walking program on treadmill. OKC knee extension (0°–90°) as tolerated, do not progress to heavy resistance with patellofemoral lesions—must monitor symptoms of pain and crepitation. Bicycle. Stairmaster. Swimming. Nordic-Trak/elliptical.
Functional activities	As patient improves, increase walking (e.g., distance, cadence, incline)
Maintenance program	Initiate at wk 16–20. Bicycle—low resistance. Progressive walking program. Pool exercises for entire lower extremity. Straight leg raises into flexion. Leg press. Wall-squats. Hip abduction/adduction. Front lunges. Stretch quadriceps, hamstrings, gastrocnemius.
Criteria to progress to phase IV	Full nonpainful ROM. Strength within 80%–90% of contralateral extremity. Balance and/or stability within 75%–80% of contralateral extremity. No pain, inflammation, or swelling.

	PHASE IV: MATURATION PHASE (WEEKS 26–52)
Goals	Gradual return to full unrestricted functional activities.
Exercises	Continue maintenance program progression 3–4 times/wk. Progress resistance as tolerated. Emphasis on entire lower extremity strength and flexibility. Progress agility and balance drills. Impact-loading program should be specialized to patient's demands. Progress sport programs depending on patient variables.
Functional activities	Patient may return to various sport activities as progression in rehabilitation and cartilage healing allows. Generally, low-impact sports such as skating, rollerblading, and cycling are permitted at about 6–8 mo. Higher-impact sports such as jogging, running, and aerobics may be performed at 8–10 mo. High-impact sports such as tennis, basketball, and baseball are allowed at 12–18 mo.

CKC, closed kinetic chain; CPM, continuous passive motion; EMS, electrical muscle stimulation; OKC, open kinetic chain; Q/H, quadriceps/hamstring; ROM, range of motion; WB, weight-bearing.

TABLE 37–5 Rehabilitation after Autologous Chondrocyte Implantation

PHASE I: EARLY PROTECTION PHASE (WEEKS 0–6)

Goals	Protect healing tissue from load and shear forces. Decrease pain and effusion. Restoration of full passive knee extension. Gradually improve knee flexion. Regain quadriceps control.
Brace	Locked at 0° during WB activities. Sleep in locked brace for 2–4 wk.
WB	WB status varies based on lesion location and size. For femoral condyle lesions: non-WB for 1–2 wk, may begin toe-touch WB immediately per physician if lesion < 2.0 cm^2; begin toe-touch WB (~20–30 lb) wk 2–3; progress to partial WB (~25% body weight) at wk 4–5. For patellofemoral lesions: immediate toe-touch WB of ~25% body weight with brace locked in full extension; progress to 50% WB at wk 2 and 75% WB wk 3–4 with brace locked in full extension.
ROM	Immediate motion exercise day 1. Full passive knee extension immediately. Initiate CPM day 1 for total of 8–12 hr/day (0°–60°; if patellofemoral lesion > 6.0 cm^2, 0°–40°). Progress CPM ROM as tolerated 5°10°/day. May continue CPM for total of 6–8 hr/day for up to 6 wk. Patellar mobilization (4–6 times/day). Motion exercises throughout the day. Passive knee flexion ROM at least 2–3 times/day. Passive knee ROM as tolerated. For femoral condyle lesions, knee flexion ROM goal is 90° by 1–2 wk; 105° wk 3; 115° wk 4; and 120°–125° by wk 6. For patellofemoral lesions, knee flexion ROM goal is 90° by wk 2–3; 105° by 3–4 wk; and 120° by wk 6. Stretch hamstrings and calf.
Strengthening program	Ankle pump using rubber tubing. Quadriceps setting. Multiangle isometrics (co-contractions Q/H). Active knee extension 90°–40° for femoral condyle lesions (no resistance). Straight leg raises (four directions). Stationary bicycle when ROM allows—low resistance. EMS and/or biofeedback during quadriceps exercises. Isometric leg press at wk 4 (multiangle). May begin use of pool for gait training and exercises wk 4. Initiate weight-shifting exercises with knee in extension wk 2–3 for patellofemoral lesions. NO active knee extension exercises for patellofemoral lesions.
Functional activities	Gradual return to daily activities. If symptoms occur, reduce activities to reduce pain and inflammation. Extended standing should be avoided.
Swelling control	Ice, elevation, compression, and edema modalities as needed to decrease swelling.
Criteria to progress to phase II	Full passive knee extension. Knee flexion to 120°. Minimal pain and swelling. Voluntary quadriceps activity.

PHASE II: TRANSITION PHASE (WEEKS 6–12)

Goals	Gradually increase ROM. Gradually improve quadriceps strength/endurance. Gradual increase in functional activities.
Brace	Discontinue brace at wk 6. Consider unloading knee brace for femoral condyle lesions.
WB	Progress WB as tolerated. For femoral condyle lesions: 50% body weight with crutches at 6 wk; progress to full WB at 8–9 wk, discontinue crutches. For patellofemoral lesions: progress to full WB wk 6–8, discontinue crutches.
ROM	Gradual increase in ROM. Maintain full passive knee extension. Progress knee flexion to 125°–135° by wk 8. Continue patellar mobilization and soft tissue mobilization, as needed. Continue stretching program.
Strengthening exercises	Progress CKC exercises. Initiate weight-shifts wk 6 for femoral condyle lesions. Leg press wk 7–8. Mini-squats 0°–45° wk 8. Toe-calf-raises wk 6 for patellofemoral lesions, wk 8 for femoral condyle lesions. Progress balance and proprioception drills.

Continued

PHASE II: TRANSITION PHASE (WEEKS 6–12)—Cont'd	
	Initiate front lunges, wall-squats, front and lateral step-ups wk 8–10.
	For femoral condyle lesions, progress OKC knee extension, 1 lb/wk.
	For patellofemoral lesion, may begin OKC knee extension without resistance in an ROM that does not allow for articulation of the lesion.
	Stationary bicycle, low resistance (gradually increase time).
	Treadmill walking program wk 10–12.
	Continue use of EMS and/or biofeedback as needed.
	Continue use of pool for gait training and exercise.
Functional activities	As pain and swelling (symptoms) diminish, the patient may gradually increase functional activities. Gradually increase standing and walking.
Criteria to progress to phase III	Full ROM. Acceptable strength level: • Hamstrings within 20% of contralateral leg. • Quadriceps within 30% of contralateral leg. Balance testing within 30% of contralateral leg. Able to walk 1–2 miles or bike for 30 min.

PHASE III: REMODELING PHASE (WEEKS 12–26)	
Goals	Improve muscular strength and endurance. Increase functional activities.
ROM	Patient should exhibit 125°–135° flexion.
Exercise program	Leg press (0°–90°). Bilateral squats (0°–60°). Unilateral step-ups progressing from 2" to 8". Forward lunges. Walking program. Progress OKC extension (0°–90°), for patellofemoral lesions perform from 90°–40° or avoid angle where lesion articulates—progress 1 lb every 2 wk beginning wk 20 if no pain or crepitation—must monitor symptoms. Continue progressing balance and proprioception. Bicycle. Stairmaster. Swimming. Nordic-Trak/elliptical.
Functional activities	As patient improves, increase walking (e.g., distance, cadence, incline)
Maintenance program	Initiate at wk 16–20. Bicycle—low resistance, increase time. Progressive walking program. Pool exercises for entire lower extremity. Straight leg raises. Leg press. Wall-squats. Hip abduction/adduction. Front lunges. Step-ups. Stretch quadriceps, hamstrings, calf.
Criteria to progress to phase IV	Full nonpainful ROM. Strength within 80%–90% of contralateral extremity. Balance and/or stability within 75%–80% of contralateral extremity. No pain, inflammation, or swelling.

PHASE IV: MATURATION PHASE (WEEKS 12–26)	
Goals	Gradual return to full unrestricted functional activities.
Exercises	Continue maintenance program progression 3–4 times/wk. Progress resistance as tolerated. Emphasis on entire lower extremity strength and flexibility. Progress agility and balance drills. Impact-loading program should be specialized to patient's demands. Progress sport programs depending on patient variables.
Functional activities	Patient may return to various sport activities as progression in rehabilitation and cartilage healing allows. Generally, low-impact sports such as swimming, skating, rollerblading, and cycling are permitted at about 6 mo. Higher-impact sports such as jogging, running, and aerobics may be performed at 8–9 mo for small lesions or 9–12 mo for larger lesions. High-impact sports such as tennis, basketball, football and baseball are allowed at 12–18 mo.

CKC, closed kinetic chain; CPM, continuous passive motion; EMS, electrical muscle stimulation; OKC, open kinetic chain; Q/H, quadriceps/hamstring; ROM, range of motion; WB, weight-bearing.

of the defects. This suggests two possibilities. First, that the position of the patient with a patellar defect in the prone position would contraindicate CPM, because it would produce an abnormal gravity effect. Second, that the use of CPM immediately after surgery is warranted to produce a "more even distribution of implanted cells within the defect." At present, no in vivo or clinical studies have been published to support this hypothesis.

Proliferation of the chondrocytes occurs in the first 6 weeks after cell implantation. During the first 24 hours after cell implantation, the cells line the base of the lesion and multiply several times to produce a matrix that will fill the defect with a soft repair tissue up to the level of the periosteal cover.[16,38] At this time, PROM and controlled partial weight-bearing will help to promote cellular nutrition through synovial fluid diffusion as well as provide the proper stimulus for the cells to produce specific matrix markers. During this initial phase, controlled PROM and a gradual weight-bearing progression are two of the most important components of the rehabilitation process.

Immediate toe-touch weight-bearing is performed in knees with smaller lesions, progressing to 25% body weight at weeks 2 to 4, 50% body weight at weeks 5 to 6, and full weight-bearing at week 8. This progression may be delayed approximately 2 weeks, with 2 weeks of non–weight-bearing, if the lesion is large, deep, or uncontained. For lesions within the patella or trochlea, the patient is allowed to bear weight as tolerated immediately after surgery with a brace locked in full extension. ROM is progressed cautiously to avoid swelling similar to the OATS procedure, with at least 90° of flexion at week 1, 105° at weeks 2 to 3, 115° at week 4, and 125° at week 6. Early strength and proprioceptive exercises are performed within the patient's weight-bearing status.

During the transition phase, which includes weeks 7 through 12, the repair tissue is spongy and compressible with little resistance. Upon arthroscopic examination, the tissue may in fact have a wavelike motion when a probe is slid over the tissue.[16,38] During this phase, the patient achieves full ROM and progresses from partial to full weight-bearing. Continued maturation of the repair tissue is fostered through higher level functional and motion exercises. CKC exercises, such as front lunges, step-ups, and wall-squats are performed as well as machine exercises for the entire lower extremity. Again, caution should be placed on exercises that produce sheer forces in patients with patellofemoral lesions.

The remodeling phase occurs from 12 weeks through 32 weeks postoperatively. During this phase, there is a continuous production of matrix with further remodeling into a more organized structural tissue. The tissue at this point has the consistency of soft plastic upon probing.[16,38] As the tissue becomes more firm and integrated, it allows for more functional training activities to be performed as well as elliptical, bicycle, and a gradual walking program.

The final maturation phase can last up to 15 to 18 months depending upon the size and location of the lesion. During this phase, the repair tissue reaches its full maturation. The stiffness of the cartilage resembles that of the surrounding tissue.[16,38] The duration of this phase varies based on several factors such as lesion size and location.

Basic science studies have shown that it may take up to 6 months for the graft site to become firm and at least 9 months to become as durable as the surrounding healthy articular cartilage.[16,38] Thus, low-impact activities (such as golf, swimming, cycling, and walking) are initiated by months 5 to 6 and progressed to moderate-impact activities (such as tennis, hiking, skating) from months 7 to 9 as tolerated. Usually, high-impact activities such as running and skiing are permitted with a gradual return beginning at 11 to 12 months postoperative.

The results of clinical outcomes after ACI are encouraging. Mithoefer and colleagues[32] reported a 72% good to excellent result and return to play in competitive soccer players, with 80% returning back to the same level of play. Peterson and co-workers[37] reported a 90% good to excellent result using ACI on osteochondritis dissecans lesions of the knee in patients with a mean age of 26.4 years (range, 14–52 yr).

CONCLUSION

The rehabilitation process after articular cartilage repair procedures is vital to the long-term success and functional outcome of the patient. The rehabilitation programs discussed are performed based on current understanding of articular cartilage and the natural healing response observed after articular cartilage repair procedures. Rehabilitation is based on several key principles designed to facilitate the repair process by creating a healing environment while avoiding deleterious forces that may overload the healing tissue. It is imperative that these principles be incorporated into the rehabilitation process along with the knowledge of the basic science and maturation process of each specific repair procedure. The medical team should consider the long-term results of the patients and functional outcomes at 1, 2, and 5 years after the surgical procedure. The basic principles outlined in this chapter may be applied and integrated as the understanding and clinical use of the next generation of procedures (such as collagen-covered ACI and matrix-induced ACI) continue to evolve. Long-term clinical studies are needed to determine the effectiveness of the surgical techniques and postoperative rehabilitation programs discussed in this chapter.

REFERENCES

1. Bartha, L.; Vajda, A.; Duska, Z. L.; et al.: Autologous osteochondral mosaicplasty grafting. *J Orthop Sports Phys Ther* 36:739–750, 2006.
2. Behrens, F.; Kraft, E. L.; Oegema, T. R., Jr.: Biochemical changes in articular cartilage after joint immobilization by casting or external fixation. *J Orthop Res* 7:335–343, 1989.
3. Blankevoort, L.; Kuiper, J. H.; Huiskes, R.; Grootenboer, H. J.: Articular contact in a three-dimensional model of the knee. *J Biomech* 24;1019–1031, 1991.
4. Brittberg, M.; Lindahl, A.; Nilsson, A.; et al.: Treatment of deep cartilage defects in the knee with autologous chondrocyte transplantation. *N Engl J Med* 331:889–895, 1994.
5. Brittberg, M.; Nilsson, A.; Lindahl, A.; et al.: Rabbit articular cartilage defects treated with autologous cultured chondrocytes. *Clin Orthop Relat Res* 326:270–283, 1996.
6. Buckwalter, J. A.: Articular cartilage: injuries and potential for healing. *J Orthop Sports Phys Ther* 28:192–202, 1998.
7. Buckwalter, J. A.; Mankin, H. J.: Articular cartilage: tissue design and chondrocyte-matrix interactions. *Instr Course Lect* 47:477–486, 1998.
8. Cohen, N. P.; Foster, R. J.; Mow, V. C.: Composition and dynamics of articular cartilage: structure, function, and maintaining healthy state. *J Orthop Sports Phys Ther* 28:203–215, 1998.

9. Delitto, A.; Rose, S. J.; McKowen, J. M.; et al.: Electrical stimulation versus voluntary exercise in strengthening thigh musculature after anterior cruciate ligament surgery. *Phys Ther* 68:660–663, 1988.

10. Friden, T.; Roberts, D.; Ageberg, E.; et al.: Review of knee proprioception and the relation to extremity function after an anterior cruciate ligament rupture. *J Orthop Sports Phys Ther* 31:567–576, 2001.

11. Frisbie, D. D.; Oxford, J. T.; Southwood, L.; et al.: Early events in cartilage repair after subchondral bone microfracture. *Clin Orthop Relat Res* 407:215–227, 2003.

12. Fujikawa, K.; Seedhom, B. B.; Wright, V.: Biomechanics of the patello-femoral joint. Part I: a study of the contact and the congruity of the patello-femoral compartment and movement of the patella. *Eng Med* 12:3–11, 1983.

13. Gill, T. J.; McCulloch, P. C.; Glasson, S. S.; et al.: Chondral defect repair after the microfracture procedure: a nonhuman primate model. *Am J Sports Med* 33:680–685, 2005.

14. Goodfellow, J.; Hungerford, D. S.; Woods, C.: Patello-femoral joint mechanics and pathology. 2. Chondromalacia patellae. *J Bone Joint Surg Br* 58:291–299, 1976.

15. Goodfellow, J.; Hungerford, D. S.; Zindel, M.: Patello-femoral joint mechanics and pathology. 1. Functional anatomy of the patello-femoral joint. *J Bone Joint Surg Br* 58:287–290, 1976.

16. Grande, D. A.; Pitman, M. I.; Peterson, L.; et al.: The repair of experimentally produced defects in rabbit articular cartilage by autologous chondrocyte transplantation. *J Orthop Res* 7:208–218, 1989.

17. Haapala, J.; Arokoski, J.; Pirttimaki, J.; et al.: Incomplete restoration of immobilization induced softening of young beagle knee articular cartilage after 50-week remobilization. *Int J Sports Med* 21:76–81, 2000.

18. Hangody, L.; Fules, P.: Autologous osteochondral mosaicplasty for the treatment of full-thickness defects of weight-bearing joints: ten years of experimental and clinical experience. *J Bone Joint Surg Am* 85(suppl 2):25–32, 2003.

19. Hangody, L.; Kish, G.; Karpati, Z.: Autogenous osteochondral graft technique for replacing knee cartilage defects in dogs. *Orthop Int* 5:175–181, 1997.

20. Harrison, R. A.; Hillman, M.; Bulstrode, S.: Loading of the limb when walking partially immersed. *Physiotherapy* 78:112–116, 1992.

21. Horvath, S. M.; Hollander, J. L.: Intra-articular temperature as a measure of joint reaction. *J Clin Invest* 28:469–473, 1949.

22. Huberti, H. H.; Hayes, W. C.: Patellofemoral contact pressures. The influence of Q-angle and tendofemoral contact. *J Bone Joint Surg Am* 66:715–724, 1984.

23. Hungerford, D. S.; Barry, M.: Biomechanics of the patellofemoral joint. *Clin Orthop Relat Res* 144:9–15, 1979.

24. Iwaki, H.; Pinskerova, V.; Freeman, M. A.: Tibiofemoral movement 1: the shapes and relative movements of the femur and tibia in the unloaded cadaver knee. *J Bone Joint Surg Br* 82:1189–1195, 2000.

25. Knight, C. A.; Rutledge, C. R.; Cox, M. E.; et al.: Effect of superficial heat, deep heat, and active exercise warm-up on the extensibility of the plantar flexors. *Phys Ther* 81:1206–1214, 2001.

26. Kreuz, P. C.; Erggelet, C.; Steinwachs, M. R.; et al.: Is microfracture of chondral defects in the knee associated with different results in patients aged 40 years or younger? *Arthroscopy* 22:1180–1186, 2006.

27. Marder, R. A.; Hopkins, G., Jr.; Timmerman, L. A.: Arthroscopic microfracture of chondral defects of the knee: a comparison of two postoperative treatments. *Arthroscopy* 21:152–158, 2005.

28. Martelli, S.; Pinskerova, V.: The shapes of the tibial and femoral articular surfaces in relation to tibiofemoral movement. *J Bone Joint Surg Br* 84:607–613, 2002.

29. Mithoefer, K.; Williams, R. J., 3rd; Warren, R. F.; et al.: Chondral resurfacing of articular cartilage defects in the knee with the microfracture technique. Surgical technique. *J Bone Joint Surg Am* 88(suppl 1 pt 2):294–304, 2006.

30. Mithoefer, K.; Williams, R. J., 3rd; Warren, R. F.; et al.: The microfracture technique for the treatment of articular cartilage lesions in the knee. A prospective cohort study. *J Bone Joint Surg Am* 87:1911–1920, 2005.

31. Mithoefer, K.; Williams, R. J., 3rd; Warren, R. F.; et al.: High-impact athletics after knee articular cartilage repair: a prospective evaluation of the microfracture technique. *Am J Sports Med* 34:1413–1418, 2006.

32. Mithofer, K.; Peterson, L.; Mandelbaum, B. R., Minas, T.: Articular cartilage repair in soccer players with autologous chondrocyte transplantation: functional outcome and return to competition. *Am J Sports Med* 33:1639–1646, 2005.

33. Nam, E. K.; Makhsous, M.; Koh, J.; et al.: Biomechanical and histological evaluation of osteochondral transplantation in a rabbit model. *Am J Sports Med* 32:308–316, 2004.

34. Osbahr, D. C.; Cawley, P. W.; Speer, K. P.: The effect of continuous cryotherapy on glenohumeral joint and subacromial space temperatures in the postoperative shoulder. *Arthroscopy* 18:748–754, 2002.

35. Perry, J.; Antonelli, D.; Ford, W.: Analysis of knee joint forces during flexed-knee stance. *J Bone Joint Surg Am* 57A:961–967, 1975.

36. Peterson, L.; Brittberg, M.; Kiviranta, I.; et al.: Autologous chondrocyte transplantation. Biomechanics and long-term durability. *Am J Sports Med* 30:2–12, 2002.

37. Peterson, L.; Minas, T.; Brittberg, M.; Lindahl, A.: Treatment of osteochondritis dissecans of the knee with autologous chondrocyte transplantation. Results at two to ten years. *J Bone Joint Surg* 85(suppl 2):17–24, 2003.

38. Peterson, L.; Minas, T.; Brittberg, M.; et al.: Two- to 9-year outcome after autologous chondrocyte transplantation of the knee. *Clin Orthop Relat Res* 374:212–234, 2000.

39. Roberts, D.; Friden, T.; Stomberg, A.; et al.: Bilateral proprioceptive defects in patients with a unilateral anterior cruciate ligament reconstruction: a comparison between patients and healthy individuals. *J Orthop Res* 18:565–571, 2000.

40. Robertson, V. J.; Ward, A. R.; Jung, P.: The effect of heat on tissue extensibility: a comparison of deep and superficial heating. *Arch Phys Med Rehabil* 86:819–825, 2005.

41. Rodrigo, J. J.; Steadman, J. R.; Silliman, J. F.: Improvement of full-thickness chondral defect healing in the human knee after débridement and microfracture using continuous passive motion. *Am J Knee Surg* 7:109–116, 1994.

42. Salter, R.: The biological concept of continuous passive motion of synovial joints: the first 18 years of basic research and its clinical application. In Ewing, J. (ed.): *Articular Cartilage and Knee Joint Function*. New York: Raven, 1990; pp. 127–139.

43. Salter, R. B.; Hamilton, H. W.; Wedge, J. H.; et al.: Clinical application of basic research on continuous passive motion for disorders and injuries of synovial joints: a preliminary report of a feasibility study. *J Orthop Res* 1:325–342, 1984.

44. Salter, R. B.; Simmonds, D. F.; Malcolm, B. W.; et al.: The biological effect of continuous passive motion on the healing of full-thickness defects in articular cartilage. An experimental investigation in the rabbit. *J Bone Joint Surg Am* 62:1232–1251, 1980.

45. Shimizu, T.; Videman, T.; Shimazaki, K.; Mooney, V.: Experimental study on the repair of full thickness articular cartilage defects: effects of varying periods of continuous passive motion, cage activity, and immobilization. *J Orthop Res* 5:187–197, 1987.

46. Snyder-Mackler, L.; Delitto, A.; Bailey, S. L.; Stralka, S. W.: Strength of the quadriceps femoris muscle and functional recovery after reconstruction of the anterior cruciate ligament. A prospective, randomized clinical trial of electrical stimulation. *J Bone Joint Surg Am* 77:1166–1173, 1995.

47. Sohn, D. H.; Lottman, L. M.; Lum, L. Y.; et al.: Effect of gravity on localization of chondrocytes implanted in cartilage defects. *Clin Orthop Relat Res* 394:254–262, 2002.

48. Spencer, J. D.; Hayes, K. C.; Alexander, I. J.: Knee joint effusion and quadriceps reflex inhibition in man. *Arch Phys Med Rehabil* 65:171–177, 1984.

49. Steinkamp, L. A.; Dillingham, M. F.; Markel, M. D.; et al.: Biomechanical considerations in patellofemoral joint rehabilitation. *Am J Sports Med* 21:438–444, 1993.

50. Vanwanseele, B.; Lucchinetti, E.; Stussi, E.: The effects of immobilization on the characteristics of articular cartilage: current concepts and future directions. *Osteoarthritis Cartilage* 10:408–419, 2002.

51. Waldman, S. D.; Spiteri, C. G.; Grynpas, M. D.; et al.: Effect of biomechanical conditioning on cartilaginous tissue formation in vitro. *J Bone Joint Surg Am* 85(suppl 2):101–105, 2003.

52. Whiteside, R. A.; Bryant, J. T.; Jakob, R. P.; et al.: Short-term load bearing capacity of osteochondral autografts implanted by the mosaicplasty technique: an in vitro porcine model. *J Biomech* 36:1203–1208, 2003.

Chapter 38

Aquatic Therapy for the Arthritic Knee

Lori Thein Brody, PT, PhD, SCS, ATC

INTRODUCTION

Water has been used for healing, spiritual, and religious purposes since at least 2400 BC.[15] Water was used by the people of Asia to combat fevers as early as 1500 BC. Hippocrates (460–375 BC) used water for relief of muscle spasms and joint pain.[23] For many years, water exercise was dismissed as a medical intervention and considered to be purely recreational. The advent of spas in Europe and around the world moved water-based interventions into the leisure and recreation category, making reimbursement for water-based medical interventions difficult.

Despite a history spanning over 4000 years, a resurgence of aquatics as an intervention has occurred in the past quarter century. The Aquatic Section of the American Physical Therapy Association was organized as recently as 1992. Throughout this history, many different terms have been used to describe rehabilitation that takes place in the water. Some of these terms include *hydrotherapy*, *aquatic therapy*, *spa therapy*, *water therapy*, *water gymnastics*, *balneotherapy*, and *pool therapy*. Currently, the term *balneotherapy* is still distinguished from other forms of hydrotherapy. Balneotherapy refers to the use of hot-water or thermal treatments to decrease pain and stiffness and promote muscle relaxation. Balneotherapy often uses minerals, salts, or sulfur treatments, mud packs, and water jets to achieve these goals. *Hydrotherapy* is a general term covering any type of water intervention, which might include balneotherapy or exercise. For the purposes of this chapter, the focus remains on the use of exercise in water for the treatment of knee arthritis. For further information on balneotherapy, the reader is referred to Verhagen and coworkers.[36]

Physical therapy for patients with knee arthritis focuses on decreasing pain while improving mobility, strength, motor control, and function. This is often achieved through stretching, strengthening, and balance exercises. However, many patients are unable to perform these exercises on land owing to pain, comorbidities, or other limitations. These patients often do well in an unweighted environment in which they are able to perform a full range of exercises directed at improved function. Preferably, exercises are not confined to a single environment, but represent a comprehensive program of both land-based and water-based rehabilitation. It is not suggested that aquatic rehabilitation results in superior outcomes compared with land-based rehabilitation. Rather, the pool provides an effective, safe alternative for those who cannot tolerate a comprehensive rehabilitation program on land.

The purpose of this chapter is to discuss the scientific basis for rehabilitative exercise in the water, and then apply this information to the treatment of patients with arthritis of the knee. Understanding the physical properties of water is critical for building a successful rehabilitation program in the water. This understanding is both cognitive and kinesthetic. The reader is encouraged to experiment with these properties in order to fully understand how the body responds differently to exercises in the water compared with those done on land.

SCIENTIFIC BASIS

The scientific foundation for aquatic rehabilitation in patients with arthritic knees is found in two major areas. The first is the basis in aqua physics in which two key forces are critical for treatment planning. The first force is that of buoyancy. Buoyancy is used to unweight an arthritic extremity, normalize gait, and increase pain-free exercise. Buoyancy can also be used as resistance depending upon equipment choices and patient positioning. The second force is that of viscosity. Viscosity is used to provide resistance for strengthening muscles from the core to the foot and to provide postural challenges that improve balance. The second major scientific foundational area is that of clinical research in which aquatic rehabilitation has been shown to increase measures of physical performance and to improve patient outcomes.

Aqua Physics

The principles supporting the use of water in rehabilitation are based in physics. Several physical properties of water are key to understanding how water is a useful exercise mode for patients with arthritis of the knee. Capitalizing on these properties can increase the opportunity for a successful outcome for these patients with complicated problems. Failure to recognize or understand how these principles work in harmony or in opposition can lead to poor outcomes. The key properties include buoyancy, hydrostatic pressure, and viscosity.

Buoyancy

Buoyancy is the upward thrust experienced during immersion that is in direct opposition to gravity. Buoyancy is used to unload the lower extremity from the effects of gravity, making it a useful tool for those with knee arthritis. Archimedes' principle states that an immersed body at rest experiences an upward thrust equal to the weight of the same fluid volume it displaces.[6]

Buoyancy is related to a person's specific gravity (SG), which varies with body composition. Any object with an SG less than 1.0 g/cm^2 will float, whereas any object with an SG greater than 1.0 g/cm^2 will sink. This property forms the basis of underwater weighing to determine body composition. Because lean body mass is heavier than fat mass, those with a high lean body mass tend to sink whereas those with a greater fat mass float. This fact makes it difficult to know precisely how much weight-bearing any given individual is achieving at a given water depth. Harrison and

Bulstrode[20] performed studies on the percentage of weight-bearing during static standing in various water depths ranging from the hips to the neck. The authors found considerable variability in the amount of weight-bearing with immersion at various depths. This variation might have been partly due to using a fixed-depth pool and only nine subjects. However, the disparity may also be the result of differences in body composition and body fat distribution among individual study subjects, suggesting that a weight-bearing prescription is difficult in this medium. A follow-up study by Harrison and associates[21] showed that, compared with static standing, fast walking increased weight-bearing forces up to 76%. Understanding Archimedes' principle highlights the difficulties in assigning a specific percentage of weight-bearing at any given depth: the weight on the limb will vary with body composition and speed of movement.

The moment of buoyancy is also important in exercise prescription. As with moments of gravity on land, the moment of buoyancy increases with increasing lever arm length and nearer the parallel. If the movement is in an upward direction, the same direction as the force of buoyancy, the activity is considered to be *buoyancy assisted*. If the movement is toward the pool bottom in opposition to buoyancy, it is considered to be *buoyancy resisted*. Movements parallel to the bottom that are neither assisted nor resisted by buoyancy are considered *buoyancy-supported* exercises. For example, in a standing position, a straight leg lift forward would be assisted by buoyancy, whereas the return motion back to the neutral position would be buoyancy resisted. In a supine position, hip abduction and adduction would be buoyancy-supported activities. An important application of this information is used in strengthening hip extensor muscles. In a standing position, the motion of hip extension from neutral to 15° extension (the normal range of hip extension) occurs through such a small range of motion (ROM), with a short moment arm, and is buoyancy assisted, making the exercise little more than a gluteal isometric exercise (Fig. 38–1). However, the motion from 90° hip flexion returning to neutral is also hip extension, but is now moving through a larger range with a longer moment arm against the upward force of buoyancy, making this an effective hip extensor muscle–strengthening exercise (Fig. 38–2).

Critical Points AQUA PHYSICS

- Buoyancy can unweight an arthritic joint while permitting rehabilitation activities to continue.
- The precise amount of weight-bearing at any given depth is unknown and is related to the individual's body composition and speed of movement.
- Buoyancy can assist, support, or resist a movement depending upon how the individual is oriented in the water.
- Viscosity can always override buoyancy as resistance if the surface area and speed are great enough.
- Hydrostatic pressure can minimize swelling and edema in the lower limb that can occur with land-based exercise.
- Hydrostatic pressure causes a centralization of peripheral blood flow with subsequent changes in the pulmonary and heart blood volumes.
- Heart rates for exercise while immersed to the neck will be approximately 20 beats/min lower than comparable land-based exercise owing to hydrostatic pressure.

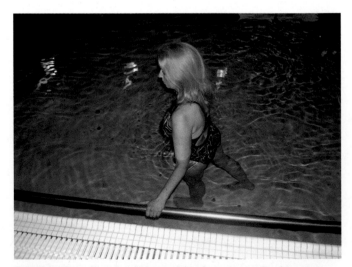

FIGURE 38–1. Standing hip extension from 0° to 15° of extension. This is a buoyancy-assisted exercise with a short moment arm, making it a less effective exercise for gluteal muscle strengthening.

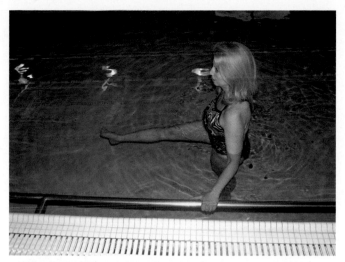

FIGURE 38–2. Hip extension from 90° of flexion to neutral is a buoyancy-resisted exercise with a longer moment arm, making it a more effective gluteal muscle–strengthening exercise.

Hydrostatic Pressure

Pascal's law states that a fluid exerts pressure equally on an object at a given depth.[6] Hydrostatic pressure increases with a greater depth of immersion owing to the weight of the volume of fluid overhead. The increased hydrostatic pressure close to the bottom of the pool assists venous return to the heart and prevents fluid accumulation in the lower extremities. This is useful for patients with knee or ankle arthritis, who tend to experience swelling with exercise. The increased venous return to the heart also affects the cardiorespiratory system. The hydrostatic pressure when the body is immersed to the neck produces an increase in heart volume, intrapulmonary blood volume, right atrial pressure, left ventricular end-diastolic volume, stroke volume, and cardiac output.[2,9] Heart rate is unchanged or decreased compared with similar land-based activities.[2] Peripheral circulation and vital capacity are decreased.[9] This cardiopulmonary response is significant for patients with cardiorespiratory conditions and for those who are trying to achieve training heart rates in deep-water exercise.[19] These changes have been noted in individuals both with and without cardiac disease.[10,11] Aerobic exercise in neck-deep water will result in heart rates that are approximately 17 to 20 beats/min lower than comparable land-based exercise.[3,18,31,34]

Viscosity and Hydrodynamics

The *viscosity* of a fluid is its resistance to adjacent fluid layers sliding freely by one another.[6] Viscosity causes a resistance to flow when a body is moving through the water. As such, viscosity is clinically insignificant when a body is stationary. The viscous quality of water allows it to be used effectively for resistance because of its *hydrodynamic properties*, or fluid mechanics. The key hydrodynamic properties are turbulence and drag.[33] Turbulent flow occurs when the speed of movement of an object (or person or body part) reaches a critical velocity or when the flow of water encounters an object (or person or body part).[4] In turbulent flow, resistance is proportional to the velocity squared, and increasing the speed of movement significantly increases the resistance.[27] Eddies are formed in the wake behind the moving body, creating drag that is greater in

the unstreamlined object than in a streamlined object (Figs. 38–3 and 38–4).

When moving through the water, the body experiences a frontal resistance proportional to the presenting surface area. Resistance can be increased by enlarging the surface area. For example, walking forward or backward will produce greater drag in most people than walking sideways because of the greater surface area. Increasing the surface area or otherwise increasing drag increases the resistance to movement. The clinician has two variables to alter resistance produced by viscosity: the velocity of movement and the surface area or streamlined nature of the object.

Several areas of research provide evidence for these variables. A study by Law and Smidt[25] examined the impact of surface area and velocity on force production. Hydrotone (Hydro-Tone Fitness Systems, Inc., Huntington Beach, CA) bells were used at different speeds and angles to assess the impact on force production. Results showed a 50% increase in force production at fast speeds. Force also increased at fast speeds when the bells were

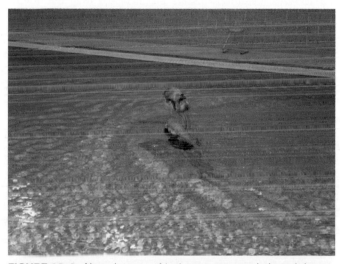

FIGURE 38–3. Note the area of high pressure anteriorly and the area of low pressure evidenced by the eddies formed in the wake.

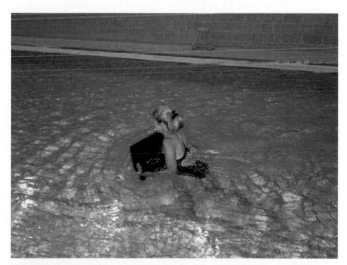

FIGURE 38–4. Adding the plow increases the surface area and creates additional drag.

oriented at 45° compared with 0°. Orientation had no impact on force production when performed at slow speeds. Therefore, both speed and surface area influence force production when using viscosity. Another study using the Hydrotone boots showed increased drag compared with a barefoot condition.[28]

A third study examined electromyographic (EMG) data from the shoulder musculature during arm elevation at three different speeds (30°/sec, 45°/sec, and 90°/sec) on land and in the water.[24] The percentage of maximum voluntary contraction of the deltoid and rotator cuff musculature was consistently higher on land at the slowest speeds, but higher in the water at 90°/sec, highlighting the positive relationship among viscosity, speed, and force generation.

Poyhonen and colleagues[27–29] performed several research studies on the hydrodynamics of knee flexion and extension exercises in water and on land in barefoot and increased surface area conditions. The authors found that increasing the surface area of the lower leg significantly increased the level of water resistance. They also found that the EMG activity of the knee flexors and extensors was similar between barefoot and increased surface area conditions despite the increased drag due to the Hydrotone Boot.

Research in the cardiopulmonary effects of speed on measures of exertion also supports the positive relationship between speed and work in the water. Whitley and Schoene[38] examined walking on land and in the water at four different speeds. Heart rates were significantly higher after water-walking versus treadmill-walking at all four speeds. In addition, heart rates rose significantly with each increasing speed in water-walking, suggesting increasing cardiopulmonary workloads at increasing speeds. Cassady and Nielsen[8] measured oxygen consumption during calisthenic arm and leg exercises at three different speeds on land and in the water. They also found increasing heart rate with increasing speed of exercise in the water. The higher metabolic cost of exercises at a faster speed supports the theory of increased work at faster speeds in the water.

CLINICAL RESEARCH

New clinical research has shown the effectiveness of aquatic rehabilitation for patients with musculoskeletal problems, particularly those with knee arthritis. A study examining outcomes following a water-based program for patients with lower limb osteoarthritis found that group-based water exercise classes over 1 year produced significant reductions in pain and improvements in function.[12] A randomized, controlled trial (RCT) compared the effects of a water-based resistance program with a land-based program on function and strength in patients with osteoarthritis of the hip or knee.[16] The authors found improvements in strength and function in both the land- and the water-based groups as compared with the control group. Compliance rates were 84% for water therapy and 75% for land therapy. In a similar study, Wyatt and coworkers[39] examined changes in function following a land-based or an aquatic exercise program in patients with knee osteoarthritis. Both groups showed significant improvements in measures of ROM, thigh girth, pain scales, and 1-mile walk test. However, the aquatic group had significantly lower pain levels than the land group. Silva and associates[32] followed 64 patients with knee osteoarthritis randomly assigned to a land-based or a hydrotherapy program. Both land and water exercises reduced knee pain and increased function,

but the hydrotherapy group had significantly lower knee pain scores before and after the 50-foot walk test. The results reinforce the notion that patients can improve strength and function effectively in either a land or an aquatic environment. The key is the ability to provide a comprehensive program, whether on land, in the water, or some combination of both.

Recently, Hinman and colleagues[22] performed an RCT randomly assigning 71 participants with hip or knee osteoarthritis to 6 weeks of aquatic physical therapy or no physical therapy. Those in the aquatic physical therapy program had less pain and joint stiffness and greater physical function, quality of life, and hip muscle strength than the control group. Nearly 75% of participants reported improvements in pain and function compared with 17% in the control group. More importantly, 84% of participants continued the aquatic program independently at the conclusion of the study.

Whereas the previous study compared aquatic physical therapy with no physical therapy, Fransen and coworkers[17] compared hydrotherapy with Tai Chi or a control group in an RCT of 152 patients with hip or knee osteoarthritis. Results showed that both hydrotherapy and Tai Chi participants improved in the pain and physical function subscales of the Western Ontario and McMaster Osteoarthritis Index (WOMAC), but only the hydrotherapy group achieved significant improvements in the physical performance measures of the Short Form-12-item questionnaire (SF-12). In addition, compliance with the hydrotherapy classes was higher than that with Tai Chi.

Pools are expensive to maintain and operate. An RCT examined the cost-effectiveness of water-based therapy for lower limb osteoarthritis. A group of 312 patients with hip or knee osteoarthritis was randomized into control and water-exercise groups. The control group received usual care, and the intervention group received aquatic exercise for 1 year with follow-up for an additional 6 months. Results showed a favorable cost-benefit ratio as measured by a reduction in WOMAC pain as the measure of benefit.

An RCT of the effects of a water-based program on balance, fear of falling, and quality of life was performed in community-dwelling older women with osteopenia or osteoporosis.[14] The intervention group received a 10-week water-based and self-management program. The intervention group showed significant improvement over the control group in balance and quality of life, but not in fear of falling.

Although structured aquatic physical therapy for patients with knee arthritis is relatively new, there is evidence supporting the clinical effectiveness and cost-effectiveness of this intervention in this population. A *Cochrane Review* examining the effectiveness of aquatic physical therapy for the treatment of hip and knee osteoarthritis is ongoing.[5]

APPLICATIONS

Although patients with knee arthritis have individualized problems and differing comorbidities, some generalizations about preferred applications in this population can be made based upon the pathology and commonly associated limitations. A thorough examination is the foundation for determining the appropriate exercise intervention. Awareness of the interrelationships among lower extremity joints and the spine can ensure proper positioning and targeting of the tissue of interest. Altering the position of the hip or foot can significantly affect the loads across the knee. The following discussion is meant to provide examples of how the physical properties of water can be exploited to improve function in patients with knee osteoarthritis.

Mobility

Many activities typically performed on land can be modified, adapted, and used in the pool. *Mobility* has both a static and a dynamic component. Functional mobility requires both appropriate soft tissue extensibility, achieved through stretching exercises, and dynamic mobility, achieved through a combination of stretching, strengthening, balance, and neuromuscular retraining.

Soft tissue stretching exercises are readily and easily performed in the pool. Many patients with arthritis have difficulty stretching on land owing to the positions or postures required. For example, some individuals are unable to get up and down off the floor or lack a sufficient supportive surface to perform the exercises appropriately. Some stretches require bending, twisting, or reaching or have weight-bearing components that patients are unable to accomplish on land. For example, hamstring or quadriceps muscle stretches often require balancing on a single leg or getting up and down off the floor. Many of these exercises are easily performed in the pool with stationary or buoyant equipment. The water's warmth and support from buoyancy make it easier and more relaxing to achieve a successful stretch.

As on land, muscles crossing both the hip and the knee or both the knee and the ankle are stretched together. Thus, the position of the adjacent joint becomes important. Because many of the stretches use buoyancy, it is easy to adjust the stretch to decrease stress on the joints and emphasize the soft tissue component.

Key muscles to be stretched in patients with knee arthritis include the gastrocnemius and soleus muscles as well as the quadriceps, hamstring, lateral hip muscles (iliotibial band), and gluteal/buttock muscles (Figs. 38–5 to 38–7). As with stretching exercises on land, the intensity should be subjectively between "low" and "medium" and should be pain-free. The patient should feel stretching in the muscle of interest and not in the joint itself. The patient should be able to hold the stretches for 60 seconds without an increase in pain.[4] Repeat the stretches for two or three repetitions.

Dynamic mobility is easily accomplished in the pool. Dynamic mobility has been advocated as an appropriate means to increase functional mobility, because it requires not only static flexibility

Critical Points MOBILITY

- Stretching is readily performed in the pool because positioning is simple and gravity is minimized.
- Stretching can be performed in functional upright positions using buoyant equipment or stationary features of the pool.
- Static stretching should be combined with dynamic mobility exercises for functional mobility.
- Buoyancy, viscosity, or the water's hydrodynamic principles can be used for strengthening.
- Rapid direction changes can challenge buoyancy and elicit eccentric muscle contractions.
- Utilizing a variety of arm and trunk movements will challenge dynamic balance.
- The water- and land-based programs can be progressed in tandem, with an eye to the long-term medium that will best support a lifetime of exercise.

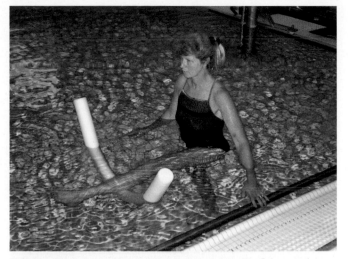

FIGURE 38–5. Hamstring stretching using a noodle. Other stationary equipment in the pool can also be used for stretching.

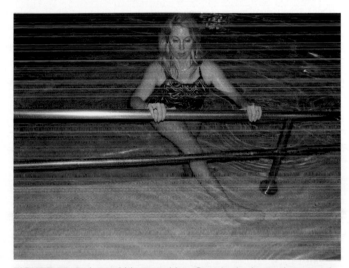

FIGURE 38–6. Lateral hip stretching. Start in the hamstring stretch position, then horizontally adduct approximately 15° and internally rotate.

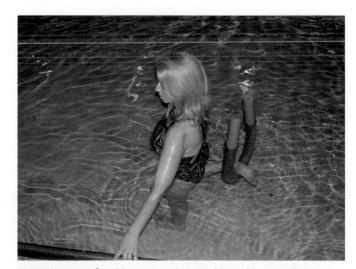

FIGURE 38–7. Quadriceps muscle stretching with a noodle.

but also strength, balance, and neuromotor coordination.[26] Dynamic mobility activities in the pool take place in a gravity-lessened environment, which decreases joint-loading forces. The water's viscosity also slows movement and increases the reaction time for patients with balance difficulties. This property makes the pool a safe environment for such individuals.

Dynamic mobility activities can easily replicate similar activities performed on land. Walking forward with varying speed and step length can be modified to emphasize lower extremity mobility. Cue the patient for increased knee flexion and extension during the swing phase of gait. Ankle or hip mobility can be similarly cued to increase sagittal plane mobility. Backward walking is useful for increasing dynamic knee flexion, because increased knee flexion is required to clear the ground during walking this direction. Frontal plane mobility is emphasized by walking sideways.

Other dynamic mobility activities include marching in place and marching across the pool. Vary the amount of hip and knee flexion based upon patient needs. Marching does not need to proceed in a straight line, but can be on a diagonal to encourage more functional movement patterns. Proprioceptive neuromuscular facilitation (PNF) patterns also encourage functional movement patterns in the lower extremity. Cueing the patient appropriately can emphasize motion at the knee joint when tolerated. For closed chain dynamic mobility, perform squats for hip, knee, and ankle mobility in shallow water or fully flex the hips and knees by flexing and extending these joints at a ladder (Figs. 38–8 and 38–9). These closed chain activities can be progressed by asking the patient to lunge during ambulation (Fig. 38–10).

Dynamic mobility can also be performed non–weight-bearing. Bicycling or running with a belt or a noodle is a good way to perform repeated hip and knee flexion and extension. The range of movement can be modified as needed for any given patient. Similarly, deep-water cross-country skiing requires repeated non–weight-bearing sagittal plane mobility, with greater hip motion and less knee motion. These repeated movements provide lubrication via mobility, but lack the weight-bearing component necessary for articular cartilage lubrication (Table 38–1).[37]

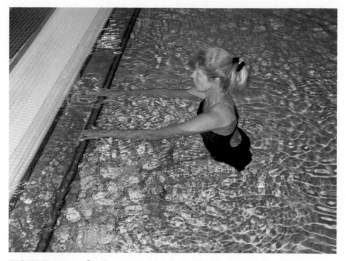

FIGURE 38–9. Shallow water squat to facilitate mobility and functional movement patterns.

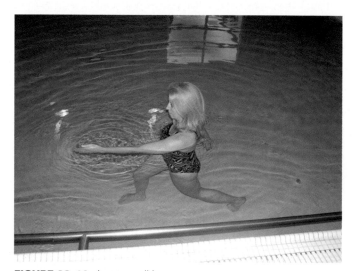

FIGURE 38–10. Lunge walking.

Strength

Clinicians can use buoyancy, viscosity, or hydrodynamics as tools to increase lower extremity and core strength in individuals with arthritis. A variety of activities using all components will produce a well-rounded rehabilitation program. The starting point is established during the patient examination when the strength of surrounding muscles and the irritability of the joint are determined. For example, in a patient with an irritable knee and decreased strength, buoyancy might be used to assist the exercise, whereas in a patient with a less irritable joint and greater strength, buoyancy might be used as resistance. Whether using buoyancy or viscosity, exercises can be performed in either an open chain, a closed chain, or a combination of both.

Exercise Using Buoyancy

For patients needing buoyancy assistance, squats, step-ups, or step-downs in deeper water will provide the necessary assistance in both the eccentric and the concentric phases of the exercise.

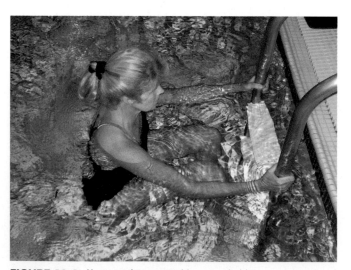

FIGURE 38–8. Knee-to-chest stretching on a ladder.

TABLE 38-1   Exercises for Mobility*

Level 1 Exercise	Level 2 Exercise	Level 3 Exercise	Additional Challenge
Passive knee extension with noodle under midcalf	Noodle under ankle	Foot on rigid object	Provide downward pressure on knee
Passive knee flexion with noodle under midshin	Noodle under ankle	Foot on rigid object	Provide overpressure into flexion
March in place	March across pool	Emphasize gait components such as knee flexion or extension, vary step length	Add stop to provide additional balance challenge
Standing knee flexion/extension with support	Increase range of motion	Add buoyant equipment	Remove support
Bicycle in stable, supported position	Bicycle on noodle or with vest	Increase range of motion, speed	Vary activity to emphasize flexion or extension or both
Squats at railing	Increase depth of squat	Progress to hip and knee flexion on ladder	Bring knees closer to chest as tolerated
Stationary lunges	Increase stride length	Increase depth of lunge	Progress to forward-moving lunges
Hip mobility through single plane with support	Hip flexion/extension, abduction/adduction, figure-eights	Increase range of motion, remove support	Add karioka walking, walking with direction changes and varying step length

*Progress exercises from one level to the next after successful completion of the previous level.

Specially designed boxes can be submerged in water of any depth to find the appropriate amount of assistance/resistance for a given patient. A box submerged in 4 to 4.5 feet of water is a good place to start for the average adult. Remember that the amount of assistance provided by buoyancy will vary with body type. Thus, the exercise prescription must be specific to the individual. As the patient improves, progress the buoyancy-assisted exercises by moving the exercise to more shallow water. This will increase the forces of gravity and lessen the assistance by buoyancy. Exercises can also be progressed to positions such as the lunge position, which is more challenging. Lunges can be performed in place or moving forward, backward, or sideways.

Strengthening exercises can also use buoyancy as resistance. Adding buoyant equipment to the foot or ankle will increase the challenge of these exercises. Straight leg lifts in the sagittal or frontal planes will result in concentric and eccentric contractions of the muscle groups positioned in opposition to buoyancy. For example, lifting the leg forward and back down will result in eccentric and concentric contractions of the hip extensor muscles if sufficient buoyant equipment is used. If the amount of buoyant equipment is inadequate, the muscle contractions become alternating concentric contractions of the hip flexor muscles and hip extensor muscles. Therefore, the relative amounts of muscle strength and buoyant equipment will determine which muscle groups are working and in what type of muscle contraction. These straight leg lifts strengthen the core hip muscles isotonically while challenging the muscles at the knee isometrically. To challenge these muscles directly, perform buoyancy-resisted hamstring curls in a standing position with the hip flexed to 90° (Fig. 38–11). Buoyancy-resisted quadriceps exercises are performed in a standing position with the knee moving from extension to flexion (Fig. 38–12). Realize that while the moving limb is working in an open chain, the opposite limb is working in a closed chain to stabilize the body against the hydrodynamic forces created by the moving limb. This principle is one of the strengths of working in the aquatic medium.

Functional movement patterns can be trained using buoyant equipment. The same PNF patterns used for mobility can be used for strengthening using buoyant equipment. For example, place a Wet Vest strap (Hydro-Fit, Inc., Eugene, OR) around

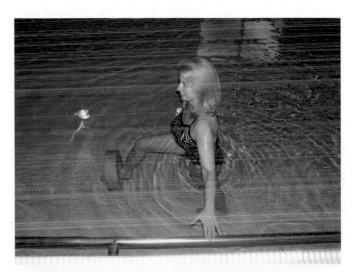

FIGURE 38-11. Hamstring curls with buoyant equipment.

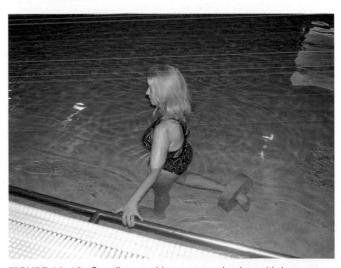

FIGURE 38-12. Standing quadriceps strengthening with buoyant equipment.

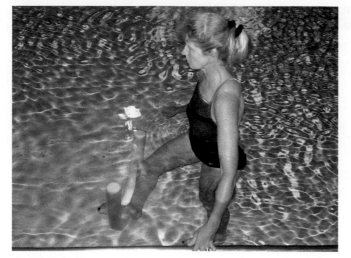

FIGURE 38–13. Noodle leg press.

the ankle and perform PNF diagonals, alphabet writing, or other functional movement patterns with the leg straight. This type of movement provides resistive exercise to muscles throughout the entire leg. Place a noodle under the bottom of a foot and press down as in a leg press for a buoyancy-resisted leg press activity (Fig. 38–13).

Exercise Using Viscosity

Open or closed chain exercises using viscosity provide an opportunity to strengthen lower extremity muscles isotonically. It is important to consider *how* the exercises are performed to ensure that the structures of interest are being challenged. A study of the hydrodynamic responses to single and repeated knee flexion and extension in the water found high levels of antagonist activity with the repeated activity and lower levels with the single-repetition activity.[29] This is an important issue for those wanting to provide both concentric and eccentric muscle contractions during aquatic rehabilitation. Whereas concentric and eccentric contractions of a single muscle group can be achieved using buoyancy-resisted exercise (such as a hamstring curl), this same exercise using viscosity produces reciprocal concentric contractions. A standing hamstring curl with the hip at 90° of flexion will produce reciprocal concentric contractions of the quadriceps and hamstring muscles. However, research by Poyhonen and associates[28] suggested that the muscle activity is influenced by the surface area, speed, and limb orientation. During both the flexion and the extension phases of a knee flexion and extension activity in water, the agonist EMG activity decreased with a concurrent increase in the antagonist EMG during the final portion of the ROM. This finding suggests that the moment of the moving water produces lift that tends to "carry" the limb through the final ROM, requiring antagonist activation to decelerate the limb at end ROM. This is more evident in the extension phase of seated knee extension than in the knee flexion phase owing to the additional lift from buoyancy. Therefore, the quadriceps muscles will be activated through a greater ROM if performed in standing and the hip in neutral than in a seated or standing position with the hip at 90°. Similarly, if the goal is to facilitate hamstring muscle activation and minimize quadriceps muscle activation near full knee extension (as in

anterior cruciate ligament injuries), then the 90° hip flexion position would be preferable.

Progress activities using viscosity as resistance by increasing the speed and/or surface area of the exercise. Flippers or fins are good choices for increasing the surface area. Flippers tend to work best in the sagittal plane, whereas Aquafins (The Hygienic Corporation, Akron, OH) can be placed in any plane, providing resistance in the sagittal plane, frontal plane, or on any diagonal in between. Other resistive equipment, such as a Hydro Boot provides a larger surface area for greater resistance.[29] Leg kicks, knee exercises, or walking activities can be performed with resistive fins around the ankle. Different components of the activity can be emphasized depending upon how the exercise is cued. For example, during backward walking, emphasizing the knee flexion component will challenge the hamstring and gastrocnemius muscles whereas stressing the hip extension component will challenge the hamstring and gluteal muscles. Generate more resistance by positioning the arms with increased surface area. For example, walk forward with the arms held at 90° abduction or increase the challenge by walking forward while simultaneously horizontally adducting the shoulders. Be aware of the additional stress this will place on the shoulders (Table 38–2).

Balance and Stabilization

The hydrodynamic forces of water provide excellent opportunities for activities to challenge the core muscles and balance. A study of balance training on land and in water found both mediums resulted in improvements in the center of pressure variables.[30] No differences were found between the water and the land, suggesting that balance training can be equally effective when performed in water. Exercises can be stationary or moving and can be challenged in a variety of different ways. Whereas strength is important, it is only one component of a program to enhance balance. Muscle activation patterns and knowledge of position in space also contribute to good balance.

Patients can use their arms to create forces that are resisted by their trunk and core muscles. Reciprocal shoulder flexion and extension produce rotational forces that are resisted by the core muscles. Turning the palms to the direction of movement increases surface area and increases the challenge. Likewise, symmetrical, bilateral shoulder internal and external rotation also creates rotational forces resisted by the trunk. Anterior-posterior sway is produced with any bilateral anterior-posterior movement of the arms such as flexion/extension or horizontal abduction/adduction. Increase the challenge of these exercises by increasing the exercise speed or surface area or by decreasing the base of support by bringing the feet closer together. Further increase the challenge by removing the bilateral symmetry. For example, performing shoulder horizontal abduction/adduction with a single arm minimizes the anterior-posterior sway and produces trunk rotation (Fig. 38–14).

Progress the narrow base of support to exercise on a single foot as appropriate. Rotational activities will be difficult on a single foot and may not be appropriate for all patients with complex knee problems. Other sagittal or frontal plane activities may be appropriate on a single leg and also challenge balance. Simple hip flexion/extension or hip abduction/adduction on a single leg will challenge balance if no external support is provided. For patients with chronic knee problems, continuous standing for

TABLE 38–2   Aquatic Strengthening Activities*

Level 1 Exercise	Level 2 Exercise	Level 3 Exercise	Level 4 Exercise	Comments
Standing hip flexion/extension	Add fins or buoyant equipment	Increase speed in controlled fashion	Progress to unsupported will further challenge balance	Buoyant equipment will emphasize hip extensors; fins will equally emphasize flexors and extensors
Standing hip abduction/adduction	Add fins or buoyant equipment	Increase speed in a controlled fashion	Progress to unsupported will further challenge balance	Buoyant equipment will emphasize hip adductors; fins will equally emphasize adductors and abductors
Standing knee flexion/extension	Add fins or buoyant equipment	Increase speed in a controlled fashion	Progress to unsupported will further challenge balance	Buoyant equipment will emphasize knee flexors with hip at 90°, extensors with hip in neutral; fins will equally emphasize flexors and extensors
Wall-sits	Progress to single leg	Add arm and/or contralateral leg movement to perturb	Decrease depth to increase weight-bearing	Buoyant equipment will emphasize knee flexors with hip at 90°, extensors with hip in neutral; fins will equally emphasize flexors and extensors
Squats with arm support	Progress to single leg	Bilateral squat without support	Decrease depth to increase weight-bearing	Can add toe-raise to increase calf muscle work
Lunge	Stationary lunge with support	Stationary lunge without support	Lunge walk across pool	Can be performed in any direction
Noodle depression activities	Noodle leg press	Noodle figure-eights or alphabet writing	Increase depth and/or buoyancy to increase resistance	Remove support to add balance challenge
Stepping activities	Step-ups on box	Decrease depth to increase weight-bearing	Perform in a variety of directions	Decrease depth to increase challenge
Deep water activities	Bicycling, cross-country skiing, running, vertical or supine kicking	Add fins	Increase speed or add interval training	If safety allows, deep water exercises without a flotation support increases the challenge

*Progress to higher levels upon successful completion of prior levels.

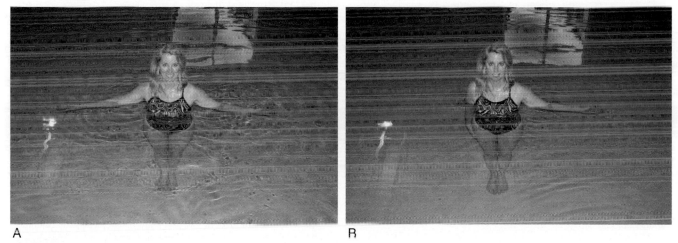

A   B

FIGURE 38–14. **A,** Balance exercise performing shoulder horizontal abduction and adduction bilaterally. This creates anterior-posterior sway. **B,** Same balance exercise with a single arm. This creates transverse plane rotation.

several repetitions on a single leg may be inappropriate. Consider alternating legs every repetition or every few repetitions for these patients.

Other dynamic activities can capitalize on the physical properties of water. Continuous moving in one direction is not particularly challenging to the core muscles, other than the generalized strengthening that occurs with walking against resistance. Once an individual begins moving through the water, the momentum of the water produces lift, carrying the body along through the water. The real challenge to balance occurs with stopping and changing direction once this momentum is achieved. A beginning activity is simply stepping forward onto

one foot and balancing followed by a step backward and balancing again. Increase the challenge by taking three or four steps forward, stop and balance, followed by three or four steps backward, stop and balance. A few steps in one direction is enough to get the water moving along with the patient. Stopping and balancing then changing direction produces significant balance challenges. This same pattern can be repeated moving in different directions. Further increase the challenge of the activity by increasing the speed of walking, decreasing arm assistance by placing the arms across the chest and/or decreasing visual input by closing the eyes. Finally, tip or turn the head to include the vestibular component.

Other balance exercises use movements of the arms or opposite leg while stabilizing on a single leg. A stepping motion with a concurrent pushing and pulling motion with resistive equipment makes an excellent core strengthening and balance exercise. In single-leg stance, pushing a ball down works on stability of the entire lower extremity. To increase the challenge, these exercises can be performed on an unstable base such as Therafoam (The Hygienic Corporation, Akron, OH) submerged in the water (Table 38–3).

Cardiopulmonary

Regular aerobic exercise is an important component of general fitness and weight loss. The American College of Sportsmedicine[1] and the American Heart Association recommend performing moderately intense cardiopulmonary activity 30 minutes a day, 5 days a week, or performing vigorously intense cardiopulmonary activity 20 minutes a day, 3 days a week. These organizations also recommend regular strength-training exercises. For patients with arthritis or complex problems at the knee, many of the traditional cardiopulmonary-training activities are too painful. Most of these activities involve some weight-bearing through the knee. Walking, running, elliptical trainers, stair-steppers, and ski machines all require weight-bearing through the knee. Bicycling places lower weight-bearing loads across the knee than other cardiopulmonary-training activities, but still places large demands on this joint.

The water is an excellent alternative to cardiopulmonary training on land. Patients do not need to be skilled swimmers to achieve a training effect in the pool. Alternative non–weight-bearing activities include deep-water bicycling, cross-country skiing, or deep-water running. Vertical kicking or deep-water aerobics classes also provide a good training stimulus. For some individuals, walking in chest-deep water at a steady pace is sufficient cardiopulmonary training. Circuit-training or interval-training techniques can also be incorporated into the cardiopulmonary program. For those who like to swim, traditional swim strokes can be modified to improve their efficiency. Adding a mask and snorkel decreases the amount of neck and trunk rotation necessary during the crawl stroke and the amount of extension necessary during breaststroke. This may increase the efficiency of the stroke and decrease stresses on the spine, allowing people to swim continuously enough to obtain the desired cardiopulmonary results. Adding flippers increases the torque production of the leg muscles and may decrease loads on the knees due to inefficient kicking techniques. Simple flutter kicking with flippers is a good cardiopulmonary exercise.

Research has shown that subjects exercising in the water can achieve a sufficient training stimulus.[7,13,35] D'Acquisto and colleagues[13] and Campbell and coworkers[7] found that controlling the frequency, intensity, and duration of shallow water exercise resulted in a training response sufficient to meet the American College of Sportsmedicine's guidelines in younger and older women. Takeshima and associates[35] found that exercising three times per week for 12 weeks resulted in an increase in peak volume of oxygen consumption (VO_2). Improvements in muscle strength, power, flexibility, agility, and subcutaneous fat were also found. All of these changes are positive for people who have complex knee problems.

Training parameters in the water are basically the same as those on land. Manipulating the frequency, intensity, and duration to meet the American College of Sportsmedicine's guidelines[1] follows the same thought process as those on land. One important issue is skill level in the water. Unskilled deep-water exercisers report higher rates of perceived exertion and have higher lactate levels than skilled deep-water runners. As patients become skilled and comfortable with the new techniques, the exertion levels and heart rate will decrease. Exercise in deep

TABLE 38–3 Aquatic Balance Activities*				
Level 1 Exercise	**Level 2 Exercise**	**Level 3 Exercise**	**Level 4 Exercise**	**Comments**
Bilateral shoulder flexion/extension	Narrow base of support	Single foot	On unstable surface, such as immersible foam	Close eyes, add head movement to increase balance challenge; can also add gloves to increase resistance, or use single arm to emphasize core
Bilateral horizontal abduction/adduction	Narrow base of support	Single foot	On unstable surface, such as immersible foam	Close eyes, add head movement to increase balance challenge; can also add gloves to increase resistance, or use single arm to emphasize core
Reciprocal shoulder internal/external rotation	Narrow base of support	Single foot	On unstable surface, such as immersible foam	Close eyes, add head movement to increase balance challenge; can also add gloves to increase resistance
Stepping exercises	Step and hold forward and backward, with, then without, arm balance	Three-step stop, with, then without, arm balance	Stepping push-pull with resistive equipment	Close eyes, increase speed; perform in any direction
Single-leg activities, unsupported	Hip flexion/ extension, abduction/ adduction	Standing knee flexion/ extension	Arms across chest	Close eyes, add unstable surface
Hop in place, with stable balance in between	Hop forward/ backward, side-to-side	Hop on diagonal	Arms across chest, close eyes	Perform 2–2, 2–1, 1–2, 1–1 footed with emphasis on stability upon landing

*Progress to higher levels upon successful completion of the previous level.

water will result in a heart rate approximately 20 beats/min lower than comparable land-based exercise owing to the effects of hydrostatic pressure.[34]

TRANSITION TO LAND

Transition to land-based activities should be a part of the patient's treatment program. The balance between land-based and aquatic-based activities will vary from one patient to the next. Several issues must be considered when determining this balance. The patient's tolerance for land-based activities is a key consideration. If the patient is unable to achieve a sufficient training stimulus on land owing to pain, swelling, or other mechanical symptoms, then the majority of the rehabilitation and maintenance program will likely contain an aquatic component. This can be achieved through an independent rehabilitation and exercise program at a local pool or a community aquatic exercise class. In contrast, some people may not tolerate regular aquatic exercise owing to reactions to pool chemicals. These individuals may need more land-based activities or find an alternative pool with fewer chemicals such as a salt-water system pool. Other considerations are pool availability and the patient's preferences.

The transition to land occurs in a manner similar to other transitions in rehabilitation. Frequently, patients begin with programs that are primarily in the water, with the addition of a few land-based exercises that they tolerate and can complement the water activities. As the patient tolerates this program and healing progresses, the land-based component is gradually increased and the aquatic component is maintained or increased in parallel, as the patient tolerates. The long-term progression and outcome depend on the patient's long term goals and whether these are best met with an aquatic program, a land program, or some combination of both. The ultimate goal should be the design of a program that the patient can easily maintain because of its ease, effectiveness, and enjoyment. This requires a partnership and communication between the therapist and the patient.

SUMMARY

The water is an excellent exercise, training, and rehabilitation medium for patients with arthritis. The water's buoyancy unweights painful joints, allowing greater ease of movement and the ability to train and strengthen without high joint compressive forces. The unweighting reduces pain and allows more active participation in the rehabilitation process. The hydrostatic pressure controls lower extremity swelling that may accompany exercise in patients with arthritis. Finally, the water's viscosity provides resistance for strengthening and support against falls due to poor balance. Research into the efficacy of water-based exercise is ongoing. As with all interventions, exercise in the water is not for everyone. However, for those who tolerate or enjoy the water, this environment can provide opportunities to rehabilitate and exercise across the lifespan.

REFERENCES

1. American College of Sportsmedicine: Guidelines for exercise testing and prescription. *Physical Activity and Public Health Guidelines.* 7th ed. Philadelphia: Lippincott Williams & Wilkins, 2006.
2. Arborelius, M.; Balldin, U.; Lilja, B.; Lundgren, C.: Hemodynamic changes in man during immersion with the head above water. *Aerospace Med* 43:592–598, 1972.
3. Avellini, B.; Shapiro, Y.; Pandolf, K.: Cardio-respiratory physical training in water and on land. *Eur J Appl Physiol* 50:255–263, 1983.
4. Bandy, W.; Irion, J.: The effect of time of static stretch on the flexibility of the hamstring muscles. *Phys Ther* 74:845–852, 1994.
5. Bartels, E.; Lund, H.; Hagen, K.; et al.: Aquatic exercise for the treatment of knee and hip osteoarthritis. Review. *Cochrane Database Syst Rev* 4:CD005523, 2005.
6. Beiser, A. (ed.): Basic physical principles and their application. *Physics.* Menlo Park, CA: Benjamin/Cummings, 1978.
7. Campbell, J.; D'Acquisto, L.; D'Acquisto, D.; Cline M. G.: Metabolic and cardiovascular responses to shallow water exercise in young and older women. *Med Sci Sports Exerc* 35:675–681, 2003.
8. Cassady, S.; Nielsen, D.: Cardiorespiratory responses of healthy subjects to calisthenics performed on land versus in the water. *Phys Ther* 72:532–538, 1992.
9. Christie, J.; Sheldahl, L.; Tristani, F.: Cardiovascular regulation during head-out immersion exercise. *J Appl Physiol* 69:657–664, 1990.
10. Cider, A.; Sunnerhagen, K.; Schaufelberger, M.; Andersson, B.: Cardiorespiratory effects of warm water immersion in elderly patients with chronic heart failure. *Clin Physiol Funct Imaging* 25:313–317, 2005.
11. Cider, A.; Svealv, B.; Tang, M.; et al.: Immersion in warm water induces improvement in cardiac function in patients with chronic heart failure. *Eur J Heart Fail* 8:308–313, 2006.
12. Cochrane, T.; Davey, R.; Matthes Edwards, S.: Randomised controlled trial of the cost-effectiveness of water-based therapy for lower limb osteoarthritis. *Health Technol Assess* 9(31):1–114, 2005.
13. D'Acquisto, L.; D'Acquisto, D.; Renne, D.: Metabolic and cardiovascular responses in older women during shallow water exercise. *J Strength Cond Res* 15:12–19, 2001.
14. Devereux, K.; Robertson, D., Briffa, N.: Effects of a water-based program on women 65 years and over: a randomised controlled trial. *Aust J Physiother* 51.102–108, 2005.
15. Finnerty, G.; Corbitt, T. (eds.): *Hydrotherapy.* New York: Frederick Ungar, 1960.
16. Foley, A.; Halbert, J.; Hewitt, T.; Crotty, M.: Does hydrotherapy improve strength and physical function in patients with osteoarthritis; a randomised controlled trial comparing a gym-based and a hydrotherapy-based strengthening program. *Ann Rheum Dis* 62:1162–1167, 2003.
17. Fransen, M.; Nairn, L.; Winstanley, J.; et al.: Physical activity for osteoarthritis management: a randomized controlled clinical trial evaluating hydrotherapy or Tai Chi classes. *Arthritis Rheum* 57:407–414, 2007.
18. Hall, J.; Macdonald, I.; Maddison, P.; O'Hare, J.: Cardiorespiratory responses to underwater treadmill walking in healthy females. *Eur J Appl Physiol Occup Physiol* 77:278–284, 1998.
19. Hall, J.; Skevington, S.; Maddison, P.; Chapman, K.: A randomized and controlled trial of hydrotherapy in rheumatoid arthritis. *Arthritis Care Res* 9:206–215, 1996.
20. Harrison, R.; Bulstrode, S.: Percentage weightbearing during partial immersion in the hydrotherapy pool. *Physiother Pract* 3:60–64, 1987.
21. Harrison, R.; Hillman, M.; Bulstrode, S.: Loading the lower limb when walking partially immersed: implications for clinical practice. *Physiother Pract* 78:164–166, 1992.
22. Hinman, R.; Heywood, S.; Day, A.: Aquatic physical therapy for hip and knee osteoarthritis: results of a single-blind randomized controlled trial. *Phys Ther* 87:32–43, 2007.
23. Irion, J.: Historical overview of aquatic rehabilitation. In Ruoti, R.; Morris, D.; Cole, A. (eds.): *Aquatic Rehabilitation.* Philadelphia: Lippincott, 1997; pp. 3–13.
24. Kelly, B.; Roskin, L.; Kirkendall, D.; Speer, K.: Shoulder muscle activation during aquatic and dry land exercises in nonimpaired subjects. *J Orthop Sports Phys Ther* 30:204–210, 2000.
25. Law, L.; Smidt, G.: Underwater forces produced by the Hydro-Tone bell. *J Orthop Sports Phys Ther* 23:267–271, 1996.

26. Mandelbaum, B.; Silvers, H.; Watanabe, D.: Effectiveness of a neuromuscular training on the incidence of knee injury in female athletes: 2-year follow-up. *Am J Sports Med* 33:1003–1010, 2005.

27. Poyhonen, T.; Keskinen, K.; Hautala, A.; Malkia, E.: Determination of hydrodynamic drag forces and drag coefficients on human leg/foot model during knee exercise. *Clin Biomech* 15:256–260, 2000.

28. Poyhonen, T.; Keskinen, K.; Kyrolainen, H.; et al.: Neuromuscular function during therapeutic knee exercise under water and on dry land. *Arch Phys Med Rehabil* 82:1446–1452, 2001.

29. Poyhonen, T.; Kyrolainen, H.; Keskinen, K.; et al.: Electromyographic and kinematic analysis of therapeutic knee exercises under water. *Clin Biomech* 16:496–504, 2001.

30. Roth, A.; Miller, M.; Ricard, M.; Ritenour, D.: Comparisons of static and dynamic balance following training in aquatic and land environments. *J Sport Rehabil* 15:299–311, 2006.

31. Shono, T.; Fujishima, K.; Hotta, N.; et al.: Physiological responses and RPE during underwater treadmill walking in women of middle and advanced age. *J Physiol Anthropol Appl Human Sci* 19:195–200, 2000.

32. Silva, L.; Valim, V.; Pessanha, A.; et al.: Hydrotherapy versus conventional land-based exercise for the management of patients with osteoarthritis of the knee: a randomized clinical trial. *Phys Ther* 88:12–21, 2008.

33. Skinner, A.; Thomson, A. (eds.): *Duffield's Exercise in Water.* London: Bailliere Tindall, 1983.

34. Svedenhag, J.; Seger, J.: Running on land and in water: comparative exercise physiology. *Med Sci Sports Exerc* 24:1155–1160, 1992.

35. Takeshima, N.; Rogers, M.; Watanabe, E.: Water-based exercise improves health-related aspects of fitness in older women. *Med Sci Sports Exerc* 33:544–551, 2002.

36. Verhagen, A.; Bierma-Zeinstra, S.; Cardoso, J.; et al.: Balneotherapy for rheumatoid arthritis. *Cochrance Database Syst Rev* CD000518:(1), 2003.

37. Walker, J.: Connective tissue plasticity: Issues in histological and light microscopy studies of exercise and aging in articular cartilage. *J Orthop Sports Phys Ther* 14:189–212, 1991.

38. Whitley, J.; Schoene, L.: Comparison of heart rate responses: water walking versus treadmill walking. *Phys Ther* 67:1501–1504, 1987.

39. Wyatt, F.; Milam, S.; Manske, R.; Deere, R.: The effects of aquatic and traditional exercise programs on persons with knee osteoarthritis. *J Strength Cond Res* 15:337–340, 2001.

Patellofemoral Disorders

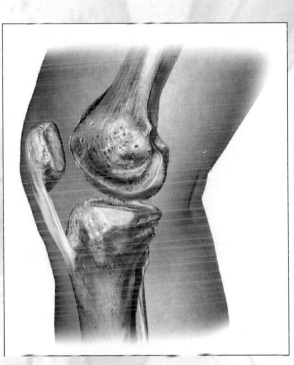

Operative Options for Extensor Mechanism Malalignment and Patellar Dislocation

Frank R. Noyes, MD ■ *Sue D. Barber-Westin*, BS

INDICATIONS

Disorders of the patellofemoral joint are one of the most common causes of anterior knee pain related to inflammation of the parapatellar soft tissues, articular cartilage damage, and instability (subluxation, dislocation). Although the majority of patients respond favorably to conservative measures, surgical treatment is required for recalcitrant cases with distinct anatomic abnormalities that require correction. The key to the indications for surgical treatment is the diagnosis of the specific anatomic defects that cause the patient's symptoms. This underscores the importance of the history and physical examination discussed later in this chapter.

The terminology used to describe patellofemoral disorders in the literature can be confusing. *Patellar malalignment* may be defined as a translational or rotational deviation of the patella relative to any axis. It is caused by an abnormal relationship between the patella, the soft tissues surrounding the patella, and the femoral and tibial osseous structures. The source of such abnormal patellar kinematics may be peripatellar tissue tightness or laxity; osteochondral dysplasias, such as a shallow or convex trochlear groove; bony abnormalities of the patella; rotational malalignment of the femur and tibia proximal and distal to the knee joint; an excessive proximal or distal position of the patella relative to the trochlea (patella alta and patella baja); and inflexibility or weakness of the quadriceps, hamstrings, and iliotibial band (ITB).

Many surgical procedures have been described for realignment of the patellofemoral mechanism including proximal realignment procedures, distal realignment procedures, or a combination of both. Proximal realignment procedures alter the medial-lateral position of the patella through balancing of soft tissue restraints proximal to its inferior pole. Included in this category are lateral retinacular release, medial retinacular capsular and medial patellomeniscal ligament (MPML) plication, vastus medialis obliquus (VMO) advancement, and medial patellofemoral ligament (MPFL) repair or reconstruction. Distal realignment procedures modify the medial-lateral, anterior-posterior, and proximal-distal positions of the patella by transfer of the tibial tubercle. Included in this category are anterior (Maquet[55]), medial (Elmslie-Trillat[93]), and anteromedial (Fulkerson[33]) transfer of the tibial tubercle. Literally hundreds of articles have been written on these operative procedures regarding their indications, technique, and clinical outcome and the reader is referred to recent review articles for further information.[2-4,27,31,32,36,61]

The purpose of this chapter is to provide an algorithm of the surgical treatment of specific patellofemoral disorders. Because this is an evolving surgical field, the authors recognize many approaches and strategies to the treatment of these problems are published in the review articles cited previously. In this chapter, the technique of a proximal and distal patellar realignment, a modification of Elmslie-Trillat procedure, is described. It includes an arthroscopic lateral release if a contracted lateral retinaculum is present, a modified VMO advancement, and a modified medial transfer of the tibial tubercle. The goals of this procedure are to release abnormal lateral tethering tissues when present, provide a balanced medial tissue-ligament complex, and realign the quadriceps–patella–tibial tubercle relationship. The procedure is performed using cosmetically appealing incisions with rapid rehabilitation, immediate knee motion, early weight-bearing, and early return to function.

The second operative procedure described in detail is an MPFL reconstruction using the quadriceps tendon (QT) based on the proximal patella. This procedure is performed through a limited cosmetic incision and avoids harvesting the semitendinosus tendon or bony fixation at the patella or medial femur. This procedure has proved to be useful in revision cases that failed after a prior proximal realignment in which an inadequate

MPFL was not addressed. The operative procedure is combined with a distal realignment when indicated, as is discussed. Other operative procedures the senior author has found useful for correcting patella alta and ITB lengthening are also described. Surgical procedures for rotational malalignment of excessive femoral anteversion and external tibial torsion are discussed in Chapter 40, Patellofemoral Disorders: Correction of Rotational Malalignment of the Lower Extremity, and not repeated here.

The majority of patients with patellofemoral malalignment respond favorably to conservative treatment programs, covered in detail in other publications.[17,18,96] In general, three types of extensor mechanism problems present for treatment. The first group of patients have diffuse anterior knee pain without distinct anatomic abnormalities in alignment, subluxation, or joint damage that can be identified. Commonly, these are younger athletes who are involved in multiple sports, and frequently, the only finding is the presence of tenderness of peripatellar soft tissues and the anterior fat pad tissues. On occasion, a mild joint effusion may be present. Authors have stressed that these symptoms frequently represent an overuse condition from excessive participation in athletics.[45,91] Treatment consists of allowing the soft tissues time to heal and inflammation to recede by modification of athletics, followed by appropriate strengthening and stretching of the muscle groups. Specific factors that may contribute to the symptomatic state include excessive conditioning, type of sport, and duration and frequency of athletic participation. Recurrence of symptoms is not an indication for surgical treatment, because distinct anatomic abnormalities of the extensor mechanism are not present. A cartilage-sensitive magnetic resonance imaging (MRI) may be helpful in recurrent symptomatic knees to determine the status of the patellofemoral joint and the presence of early articular cartilage damage that is aggravated by vigorous athletic activities.

There is a second group of patients with anterior knee pain who are similar in all aspects to the first group described previously, except that mild to moderate abnormalities are detected on the physical examination. For example, there may be a lateral subluxation (lateral glide) up to 50% of the patellar width and a mild to moderate increase in the Q-angle. There may be a physiologic posterolateral ligament laxity allowing increased external tibial rotation during activities (dynamic Q-angle). These patients are also treated conservatively and are not candidates for extensor mechanism realignment surgery.

The third group of patients comprises those who demonstrate definite anatomic signs of an extensor mechanism malalignment who are candidates for surgery. An example is those patients with symptomatic lateral patellofemoral subluxation events that do not respond to conservative treatment and have a deficient MPFL. Included in this group are patients who have had a prior patellofemoral dislocation and remain symptomatic, with either recurrence of lateral patellofemoral subluxation or a repeat dislocation event.

Nonoperative treatment of first-time patella dislocations has a re-dislocation rate that ranges from 14% to 57% in adult populations[15,30,40,50,52,53,92] and from 36% to 71% in pediatric populations.[12,72] Stefancin and Parker[87] conducted a systematic review of 70 articles that focused on the management of traumatic first-time patellar dislocations and concluded that conservative treatment was indicated initially except in specific circumstances. These included the finding of an osteochondral fracture, a substantial disruption of the MPFL, a laterally subluxated patella with normal alignment of the contralateral knee, or after failed conservative treatment or recurrent dislocations.

Patients with an acute lateral first-time dislocation are separated into three categories:

1. Dislocation with underlying anatomic abnormalities such as congenital laxity of the MPFL, increased Q-angle, and trochlear dysplasia, with similar abnormalities present in the opposite extremity. These patients undergo conservative treatment and are candidates for surgery if symptoms occur in the future. These patients require an MPFL reconstruction, because the hyperlaxity indicates deficiency of the medial soft tissue stabilizers. This surgery is not indicated in an acute knee injury situation and may be performed on an elective basis after the patient has recovered muscle function and conditions are more ideal for surgery.

2. Dislocation with or without underlying anatomic abnormalities, as detailed previously, in which there is a major joint hemarthrosis and MRI evidence of a well-defined or probable patellar or femoral osteochondral fracture. These patients require arthroscopic examination, removal of loose bodies, and fixation of a large osteochondral fracture when present (rare).[28] Under ideal circumstances, an MPFL repair is performed and the MRI helps to define the location of the tear. The MPFL may be avulsed at its femoral or patellar attachment, contain an interstitial disruption throughout its substance, or demonstrate a combination of these.[34,67,78] The goal is to restore a functional MPFL to allow immediate knee motion after surgery. The surgeon may elect to perform only the arthroscopic procedure for joint lavage and removal of loose bodies when signs of the acute dislocation (swelling, edema, limitation of joint motion) indicate that only a minimal intervention is required.

3. Dislocation without distinct trochlear or patellar tendon insertion abnormalities in which the primary defect is an acute disruption of the MPFL. In an athletic patient desiring an early return to athletics, an MPFL repair of a well-defined patella or femoral attachment tear may be indicated. Less clear are indications for acute repair of MPFL tears that are interstitial without a patella or femoral attachment tear. These interstitial tears have the ability to heal by conservative treatment and may not require further surgery.[72,85,87]

In a majority of chronic knees with recurrent bilateral patellar subluxation or dislocation, patient education is essential to explain the goals of the operative procedure. Patients are advised that any associated articular cartilage damage will likely cause future symptoms that limit athletic participation, even though the recurrent patellar instability has been successfully treated.

CONTRAINDICATIONS

The primary contraindication for extensor mechanism malalignment surgery is the absence of a distinct anatomic defect, because the goal of surgery is to restore normal anatomy of the extensor mechanism. The presence of chronic recurrent anterior knee pain is not an indication for surgery when the

---

Critical Points CONTRAINDICATIONS

- Primary contraindication surgery: absence of a distinct anatomic defect.
- Excessive hip anteversion or abnormal external tibial torsion.
- Distal realignment contraindicated in skeletally immature patients.
- Patellofemoral arthritis relative contraindication; however, in select knees, a realignment procedure is indicated along with a cartilage restoration procedure.
- Severe lower limb muscle atrophy.
- Obesity.

---

specific etiology of the pain symptoms cannot be determined. This point is worthy of emphasis, because many patients present with anterior knee pain in which the specific diagnosis is not apparent despite a thorough and careful examination and evaluation. It is probable that there are pain generation factors related to early patellofemoral cartilage deterioration that is still early in the disease course. Alternatively, peripatellar and intra-articular soft tissues may be an explainable source of pain.[24,32] A common cause of unexplained pain is a subtle infrapatellar neuroma or neuritis of the sensory nerves about the knee joint, discussed in Chapters 42, Knee Pain of Neural Origin, and 43, Diagnosis and Treatment of Complex Regional Pain Syndrome.

A specific contraindication to extensor mechanism surgery is the presence of excessive hip anteversion or abnormal external tibial torsion as discussed in Chapter 40, Patellofemoral Disorders: Correction of Rotational Malalignment of the Lower Extremity. An MRI or computed tomography (CT) scan for axial rotation of the lower extremity from the hip to the ankle is required. The measurements obtained include femoral anteversion, trochlear groove–tibial tubercle offset, and external tibial torsion as are described. The anterior knee pain is due to excessive lateral patellofemoral forces induced by external tibial torsion or increased femoral anteversion (Fig. 39–1). In these patients, a femoral or tibial derotation osteotomy may be indicated and not a proximal or distal patellofemoral procedure.[58,89]

A distal realignment is contraindicated in the skeletally immature patient. However, a proximal realignment that may include a QT autograft (for deficient, thin MPFL and retinaculum) may be performed because there is no drilling of osseous tunnels. In cases of recurrent dislocation in the skeletally immature patient, even with an abnormal lateral patellar tendon insertion offset (increased Q-angle), the MPFL reconstruction is usually very successful in providing patellar stability. After growth is complete, the need for correction of the lateral patellar tendon attachment may be assessed, which is frequently not required in the authors' experience.

A relative contraindication is the presence of patellofemoral arthritis; however, in select knees, a realignment procedure may be performed with a cartilage restoration procedure.[9,10,38,43,54,64,74,76]

Often, patients with chronic extensor mechanism malalignment disorders have limited their activity, gained excessive body weight, and have articular cartilage damage that limits rehabilitation. These problems cause muscle atrophy of the entire lower extremity. These patients require a comprehensive evaluation and team approach involving nutrition counseling, weight reduction to normal indices, prolonged rehabilitation,

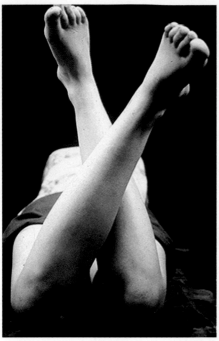

A

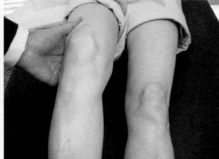

B

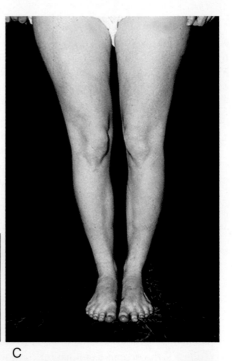

C

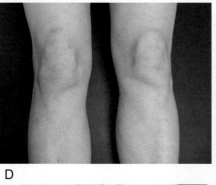

D

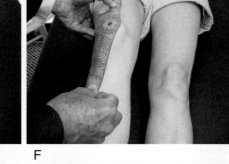

E

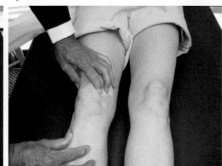

F

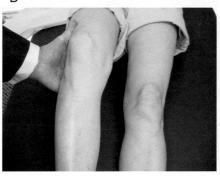

G

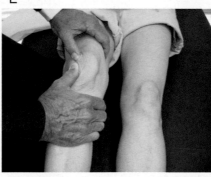

H

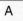

I

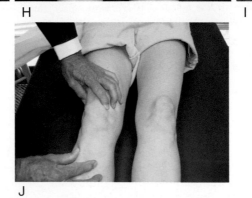

J

FIGURE 39–1. See legend on pg. 999

occupational rating and modification, and management of patellofemoral pain before any consideration of surgery. An abnormal body mass index in a patient with symptomatic patellofemoral cartilage damage contraindicates extensor mechanism surgery.

BIOMECHANICS OF MEDIAL AND LATERAL PATELLOFEMORAL RESTRAINTS

Three factors influence patellar stability: articular geometry, dynamic muscle actions, and passive soft tissue restraints.[2,27] The geometry of the trochlear groove,[2] the height and slope of the lateral femoral condyle, and the angle of knee flexion all affect lateral patellar translation. Amis[2] described objective patellar stability in terms of two factors: the amount of force required to displace the patella a given linear distance from its equilibrium position (translation) and the turning moment required to induce a rotation, such as a lateral tilt. Methods used to determine patellar mobility include manual measurement, instrumented quantitative measurement, and radiographic measurement. Kolowich and coworkers[47] measured patellar glide by dividing the patella into four quadrants and describing medial and lateral mobility as a fraction of patellar width. Normal subjects had less than two quadrants of translation with the knee flexed 30°. Teitge and associates[90] developed a stress radiographic method to measure patellar medial-lateral stability. Knees of normal subjects and symptomatic patients were tested between 30° and 40° of flexion with 71 N of force applied. Wide variation was noted in the normal knees, because lateral displacement ranged from 1 to 32 mm, and medial displacement ranged from 2 to 22 mm. The mean difference in lateral displacement

between right and left knees was 1.3 ± 1.1 mm, and the mean difference in medial displacement was 1.2 ± 1.08 mm. The investigators determined that a difference between knees in lateral displacement of 3.7 mm, or a difference in medial displacement of 3.46 mm, was abnormal.

Hautamaa and colleagues[39] developed an instrumented measurement device to determine patella medial-lateral translation in the coronal plane. In 17 cadaver knees, with the knee flexed 30 ± 5°, 5 pounds of laterally directed force produced an average of 9.3 ± 0.9 mm of lateral translation. Instrumented measurement of medial-lateral patellar translation was also conducted by Fithian and coworkers[29] in normal and symptomatic patients. Right versus left knee comparisons revealed small mean differences in the control subjects for medial and lateral patellar translation (30° flexion, 2.5-lb force, 0.1 ± 1.9 mm and 0.2 ± 1.0 mm, respectively). Significant differences were found between the control and the symptomatic subjects in the mean differences in lateral translation (P < .01), with the patients demonstrating 1.6 ± 2.5 mm difference under a 2.5-pound force at 30° of flexion.

It is well appreciated that the patella is most unstable in the range of 0° to 30° of flexion. When the knee is near full extension, the Q-angle is maximized owing to the external rotation of the tibia. In addition, with the quadriceps muscle relaxed, the patella is not engaged in the trochlear groove and thus is easily mobilized in a medial-lateral direction. As the knee is flexed, patellar stability is increased owing to the combined tensions of the quadriceps muscles and the patellar tendon that pull the patella into the trochlear groove. A shallow or dysplastic trochlear groove allows the patella to displace more easily.[81] A patella alta condition results in a loss of the trochlea geometric restraint until 30° to 40° of flexion when patellotrochlear contact finally occurs.

In regard to passive soft tissue restraints, the MPFL is the primary restraint to lateral patellar translation, providing 53% to 67% restraint up to 30° of flexion.[4,11,16,23,39,73] Desio and associates[23] examined nine cadaver knees (mean age, 57 yr; range, 43–70 yr) at 20° of flexion and reported that the MPFL provided a mean of 60% of the restraining force to lateral patellar translation. The MPML provided a mean of 13% of the restraining force; the lateral retinaculum, 10%; and the medial retinaculum and medial patellotibial ligament, 3% each. Conlan and colleagues[16] reported similar findings from 25 cadaver specimens (Fig. 39–2); the MPFL provided an average of 53% of the total restraining force, followed by the MPML (22% contribution), the medial retinaculum (11% contribution), and the medial patellotibial ligament (5% contribution). Sectioning of the MPFL decreased the restraining force significantly; the average stiffness decreased from 225 N/cm in the intact specimens to 104.6 N/cm (P = .001).

Nomura and coworkers[68] measured the lateral patellar translation in 10 cadaver knees (aged 45–60 yr) with the quadriceps tensed to 10 N and a lateral force of 10 N applied before and

---

Critical Points BIOMECHANICS OF MEDIAL AND LATERAL PATELLOFEMORAL RESTRAINTS

- Factors influencing patellar stability: geometry trochlear groove, dynamic muscle actions, passive soft tissue restraints, angle of knee flexion.
- Methods to measure patellar mobility: manual, instrumented, radiographic.
- Patella most unstable 0°–30° of knee flexion.
- Shallow or dysplastic trochlear groove allows patella to displace more easily.
- Patella alta results in a loss of the trochlea geometric restraint until 30°–40° of flexion.
- MPFL primary restraint to lateral patellar translation, providing 53%–67% restraint ≤30° of flexion.
- Mean failure load MPFL 208 N.

MPFL, medial patellofemoral ligament.

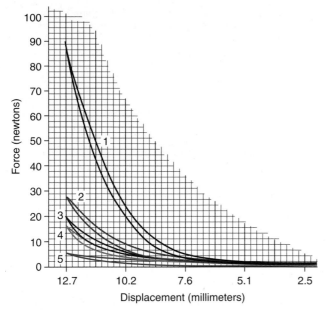

FIGURE 39–2. Superimposed force-displacement curves, recorded during the 16th testing cycle for one specimen. The medial patellofemoral ligament (MPFL) provided 67% of the medial soft tissue restraint to lateral patellar displacement (13% more than average) and the medial patellomeniscal ligament provided 12% (14% less than average). Curve 1 represents the intact ligaments and curves 2, 3, 4, and 5, the MPFL, medial retinaculum, medial patellotibial ligament, and medial patellomeniscal ligament, respectively, after sectioning. *(From Conlon, T.; Garth, W. P., Jr.; Lemons, J. E.: Evaluation of the medial soft-tissue restraints of the extensor mechanism of the knee. J Bone Joint Surg Am 75:682–693, 1993.)*

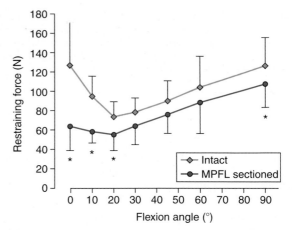

FIGURE 39–3. Graph of patellar lateral displacing force at 10 mm displacement, for the intact knee with 175 N quadriceps tension, and after transection of the MPFL. The drop between the two curves shows that the contribution of the MPFL was greatest in the extended knee. *Significant difference (P value not provided). *(From Amis, A. A.; Firer, P.; Mountney, J.; et al.: Anatomy and biomechanics of the medial patellofemoral ligament. Knee 10:215–220, 2003.)*

Critical Points PREOPERATIVE PLANNING

- Physical examination
  ○ Palpation of parapatellar soft tissues.
  ○ Patellar compression test with knee flexion-extension.
  ○ Patellar subluxation, 0° and 30° flexion, medial-lateral.
  ○ Rule out other sources of pain.
- Lower limb rotational alignment: femoral anteversion, tibial torsion, Q-angle 0° and 30° of flexion.
- CT, MRI: trochlear dysplasia, TT/TG distance, femoral anteversion, tibial torsion.

CT, computed tomography; MRI, magnetic resonance imaging; TT/TG, tibial tubercle/trochlear groove.

---

after sectioning of the MPFL. Isolated sectioning of the MPFL significantly increased the lateral patellar translation from 20° to 90° of flexion ($P < .05$).

Amis and associates[3] reported a mean failure load of the MPFL of 208 N from 10 cadaveric specimens (mean age, 70 yr) and interpreted these findings as "surprisingly strong for such an insubstantial appearance." These investigators also reported that the contribution of the MPFL in restraining lateral patellar translation was greatest with the knee at 0° extension. Significant increases in lateral translation occurred from 0° to 20° after the MPFL was sectioned (P value not provided; Fig. 39–3).

PREOPERATIVE PLANNING

The physical examination is crucial in preoperative planning for patellar realignment surgery. The examination should be performed with the patient in the standing, sitting, and supine positions (see Fig. 39–1D–J). Palpation of parapatellar soft tissues and the fat pad is performed for swelling and elicitation of pain. The examiner should look for evidence of lateralization of the extensor mechanism and tilt. The patellar compression test should be performed with flexion and extension of the knee to evaluate for articular crepitus or pain. Passive patellar tilt and tightness of the lateral retinaculum should be noted. Patellar subluxation tests (patellar glide at 0° and 30° flexion) should be performed in medial and lateral directions, and patellar mobility noted. Other sources of pain such as neuroma, patellar tendinitis, synovial plica, synovitis,

meniscus tears, osteochondritis dissecans, complex regional pain syndrome, and advanced tibiofemoral arthritis should be excluded.

Lower limb rotational alignment, including femoral anteversion and tibial torsion, is measured. The Q-angle is the angle formed between one line connecting the anterior superior iliac spine to the center of the patella and a second line connecting the center of the patella to the tibial tubercle. The Q-angle is measured with the knee in 0° and 30° of flexion. The Q-angle arc is measured at 30° with internal and external tibial rotation. Patients with a physiologic laxity of the posterolateral ligament structures have an increased lateral patellar tendon deviation by virtue of the increased external tibial rotation. The clinical measurement of the Q-angle can be inaccurate for a number of reasons. If the patella is subluxed laterally, the central reference point of measurement is also lateral, with a decrease in the Q-angle measurement unless the patella is carefully positioned within the center of the femoral groove. The Q-angle will vary depending on the amount of knee flexion and foot position; it increases with foot pronation and external tibial rotation. The proximal line to the anterior superior iliac spine is only an approximation.

Conventional radiographic techniques are often inadequate for the assessment of patellofemoral malalignment. The most commonly used Merchant technique requires 30° to 45° of knee flexion. The difficulty with this technique and others is that images are not obtained near full extension where the trochlea is most shallow. As the knee flexes, the trochlear groove deepens and the patella undergoes medialization and becomes more congruent with the femoral sulcus. The extent of trochlear dysplasia and patellar subluxation or tilt may be underestimated on the axial view owing to the amount of flexion required to obtain the image. A lateral radiograph in 30° of flexion may be used to evaluate patellar height, patellar tendon length, and trochlear dysplasia. However, a true lateral radiograph, in which the distal and posterior aspects of the femoral condyles are perfectly superimposed, is required to evaluate trochlear depth, which is measured more accurately on an axial MRI.

CT and MRI have been used to assess lower limb rotational alignment and are important tests for a complete diagnosis of the anatomic abnormalities that may be present. These studies obtain axial images of the patellofemoral joint at or near full extension to evaluate trochlear dysplasia and the tibial tubercle/trochlear groove (TT/TG) distance. Various investigators have studied this distance and found that it is increased in patients with patellofemoral pain and instability.[21,46,82]

Femoral anteversion has been measured by a variety of techniques by many authors. Yoshioka and Cooke[97] measured anteversion from the bone in 32 femora and reported a mean of 13.1° ± 8° (range, −11°–+22°) in both males and females when the distal measurement was the tangent across the femoral condyles, and a mean of 7.4° when measured across the epicondyles. These authors conducted a review of the literature on this measurement and found reported normal values were between 8° and 16° in twelve different investigations. Teitge and associates[90] arbitrarily selected 13° as the goal for correction (see Chapter 40, Patellofemoral Disorders: Correction of Rotational Malalignment of the Lower Extremity).

The technique for measuring tibial torsion by CT has not been standardized and wide variation exists in the literature regarding normal values. Yoshioka and colleagues[98] reported a mean lateral tibial torsion of 21° + 4.9° in males and 27° ± 11.0° in females, a significant difference ($P < .05$). Eckhoff and coworkers[25] reported mean tibial "version" of 37.0° ± 1.7° in control knees and 32.8° ± 1.7° in a group of symptomatic knees. Turner[94] measured a mean of 19° ± 4.8° in a control group compared with a mean of 24.5° ± 6.3° in a group with unstable patella. Sayli and associates[79] reported an average of tibial torsion in females of 31.07° for the right side and 30.02° for the left. For males, the averages were 32.7° and 35.26° for the right and left sides, respectively. Tamari and colleagues[88] conducted a reliability study that examined different methods of measuring tibial torsion. The results showed that clinical methods currently available do not accurately measure true torsion of the femur and tibia. The authors stressed that even so, these methods may be useful for screening and descriptive purposes as indices of true torsion and use of different reference axes could improve their reliability.

MRI has some advantages over CT, including improved ability to image cartilaginous structures, better anatomic approximation of the trochlear articular cartilage groove, and avoidance of radiation exposure. MRI also provides meaningful information about all of the soft tissue structures about the knee joint. The MRI is obtained in standard fashion, with images obtained of the hip parallel to the femoral neck and axial images obtained of the knee and ankle (Fig. 39–4). These individual images are then measured based on the techniques described by Murphy and coworkers[65] and Guenther and associates[37] (Figs. 39–5 and 39–6).

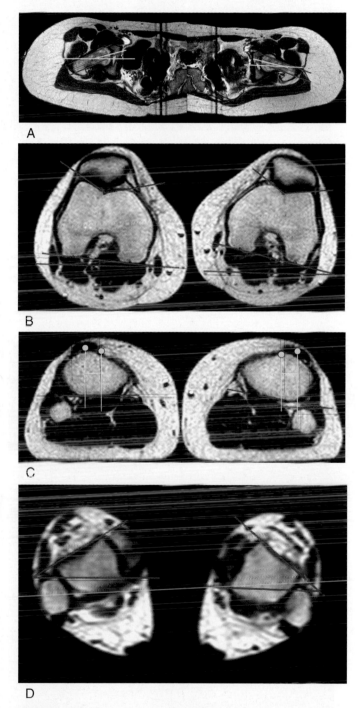

FIGURE 39–4. A–D, An example of a patient's lower limb rotational magnetic resonance imaging (MRI) profile. **A** and **B,** The femoral anteversion for the right knee was 16° on the left and 3° on the right. **B** and **C,** The knee version was 3° on the right and 0° on the left. The tibial tubercle/trochlear groove (TT/TG) was 14 mm on the right and 12 mm on the left. **C** and **D,** External tibial torsion was 30° on the right and 33° on the left. An increased signal alternation is shown for the lateral patellar facet, which is related to the patient's primary abnormality of a bilateral external tibial torsion.

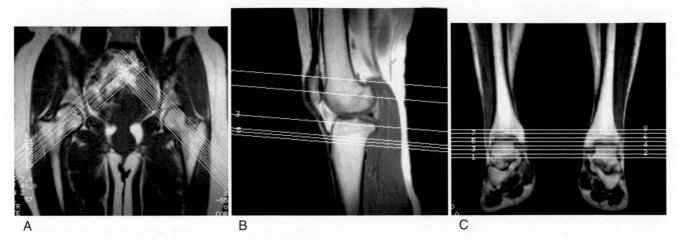

FIGURE 39–5. MRI T$_1$ images are obtained at the hip (**A**), knee (**B**), and ankle (**C**). This allows selection of the proper images for the measurements shown in Figure 39–6. (**A–C**, *From Parikh, S. N.; Noyes, F. R.; Albright, J.: Proximal and distal extensor mechanism realignment: the surgical technique. Tech Knee Surg 5:27–38, 2006.)*

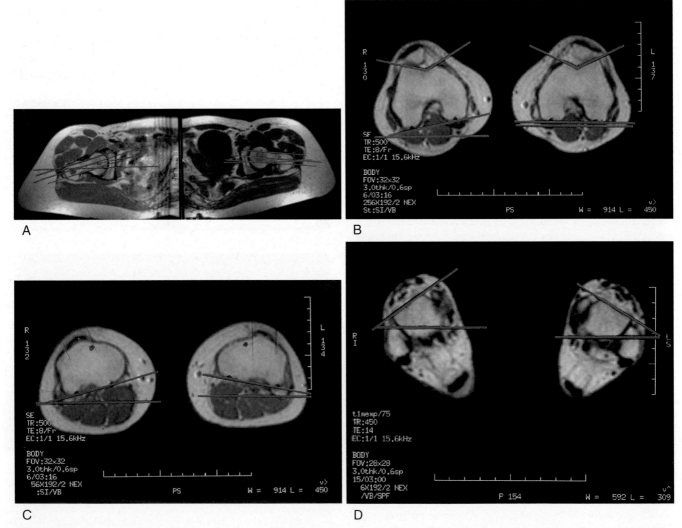

FIGURE 39–6. A, Axial view of the hip is taken through the center of the femoral neck. **B**, The femoral view is taken at the proximal aspect of the femoral trochlea. **C**, The proximal tibia view is taken at the proximal insertion of the patellar tendon on the tubercle. The center of the patellar tendon is taken for the TT/TG ratio. **D**, The axial ankle view is taken at the level of the flat edge of the talar dome (often at the same level and angle as the medial and lateral maleoli). (**A–D**, *From Parikh, S. N.; Noyes, F. R.; Albright, J.: Proximal and distal extensor mechanism realignment: the surgical technique. Tech Knee Surg 5:27–38, 2006.)*

The angle between the femoral neck and the horizontal line is subtracted from the positive angle of the flat portion of the posterior cortex of the distal femur. In rare cases, the rotation of the femoral neck and posterior femoral condyle are in opposite directions, which necessitates addition for the true femoral anteversion. The version of the knee is measured by adding or subtracting the posterior femoral angle (to the horizontal) from the proximal tibial angle (angle between the posterior aspect of the proximal tibia and the horizontal line). The tibial torsion is the difference between the proximal tibia angle and the anterior talus from the horizontal line.

TT/TG is measured using the trochlear groove–patellar tendon insertion distance. TT/TG is measured in millimeters and is the difference from the center of the deepest point of the femoral groove to the center of the patellar tendon attachment to the tibial tubercle. This is done by superimposing the line perpendicular to these points and measuring the distance between the two lines, adjusting for magnification. Dejour and Walch[22] reported a mean TT/TG distance of 12.7 ± 3.4 mm in a group of asymptomatic knees. In a group of knees with patellar instability, the mean TT/TG distance significantly increased to 19.8 ± 1.6 mm ($P < .001$). The authors concluded that the pathologic threshold is 20 mm, which has been agreed upon by others.[89] In some knees with trochlear dysplasia, it is difficult to determine the true center point for the measurement, rendering the TT/TG offset to be inaccurate. In these knees, this measurement cannot be used as an evaluation measurement of the desired operative correction.

The TT/TG plays a role in estimating the amount of correction required at the time of tibial tubercle realignment procedure. Intraoperatively, it is easier to accomplish linear corrections (in millimeters) than to assess angular relationships (in degrees), as in the Q-angle measurement. Importantly, this helps to prevent excessive medial translation of the tibial tubercle. The TT/TG measurement may not reflect the lateral deviation of the patellar tendon attachment with knee flexion and external tibial rotation, and therefore, the MRI measurements must be correlated with the physical examination. The tibial tubercle abnormality may also involve both a lateral translation and an outward (external rotation) orientation.

SURGICAL TECHNIQUES

The operative extremity is signed by the patient and surgeon with nursing personnel present. A time-out is performed with the patient's name, procedure, allergies, preoperative antibiotics, special precautions given and agreed upon by the surgeon, anesthetist, and nursing personnel.

The patient is positioned supine on the operating table. Under anesthesia, the peripatellar retinaculum, patellofemoral crepitation, patellar tilt, passive medial-lateral patellar glide (0°, 30° flexion), and Q-angle are assessed and compared with preoperative measurements. A sterile thigh tourniquet is applied as proximal as possible, so that an intraoperative assessment of the Q-angle can be made. Routine diagnostic arthroscopy is performed, and any intra-articular pathology is evaluated and treated. Particular attention is paid to patellar position, mobility, tracking, and articular surface. Approximately one fourth of the patella should establish trochlear contact at 0° to 5° of knee flexion. The medial and lateral translation of the patella is assessed at 0° and 30° of knee flexion (Fig. 39–7).

This is an important test, because a lateral translation of the patella greater than 50% of its width indicates incompetency of the MPFL. The medial translation of the patella tests for lateral retinacular tightness, and a normal lateral translation of 10 to 12 mm should be obtained with the knee at 30° of flexion. The patella and femoral groove are assessed for articular cartilage pathology or dysplasia. Articular cartilage lesions are evaluated for nature, location, and depth. The finding of loose flaps of articular cartilage requires a careful débridement; otherwise, fibrillated cartilage is left alone because it is possible to produce further damage by the débridement procedure. Radiofrequency cartilage débridement devices are never used, because excessive cartilage damage may occur. Most important at the time of arthroscopy is the critical assessment of whether the realignment procedure will transfer the loading from soft or fragmented articular surface to an intact or less involved cartilage surface. The articular cartilage is graded by the classification system described in Chapter 47, Articular Cartilage Rating Systems.[70]

Lateral Retinacular Release

A lateral retinacular release is performed only if the patellar medial subluxation test is abnormal (the patellar medial subluxation ≤ 5 mm on the manual medial translation test at 30° flexion). The goal is to perform a lateral release only when abnormally tight lateral structures and loss of normal lateral translation are demonstrated under direct visualization at arthroscopy, and not to weaken the vastus lateralis obliquus (VLO). A subcutaneous pouch is created with a scissor from the anterolateral portal over the site of the anticipated lateral release, which keeps the skin from being damaged by the intra-articular procedure. An arthroscopic retinacular release is performed using a commercial radiofrequency wand through the anterolateral portal. The lateral release is performed in two stages, from proximal to distal. The release is initiated from the 9 o'clock position (right knee) and continued distally to 1 cm below the inferior pole of the patella with the knee in full extension. The patellar medial subluxation test is then performed at 30° flexion to check for the adequacy of the release and restoration of a normal manual medial translation test. In a majority of knees, no further release is required. If the release is inadequate, it is extended proximally to a 10 o'clock position. The depth of the release involves division of the retinaculum, with care taken to avoid cutting the VLO insertion. The goal is not to perform a release of lateral soft tissue restraints, which would allow the patellar to be everted or have an abnormal medial translation. In select knees, excessive tightness of the VLO may exist, warranting a Z-plasty lengthening through a limited lateral incision to preserve VLO function. Upon completion of the procedure, complete hemostasis is achieved by coagulation of all sources of bleeding, especially the superior lateral geniculate artery at the superolateral border of the patella.

In addition to determining that there is no abnormal restraint to lateral patellar glide at 20° to 30° of flexion as already described, it is also important at 90° to confirm the absence of tight lateral tissues. This is difficult to do, because lateral patellar tilting cannot be measured at high flexion angles. A measure of excessive lateral tissues can be qualitatively estimated by placing a thin-blade scissor (Metzenbaum) beneath the lateral retinaculum and observing, with knee flexion, if there is a bowstringing effect with excessive tension in the lateral soft

- Operative extremity signed by patient and surgeon with nursing personnel present.
- Patient's name, procedure, allergies, preoperative antibiotics, special precautions given and agreed upon by the surgeon, anesthetist, and nursing personnel.
- Under anesthesia, the peripatellar retinaculum, patellofemoral crepitation, patellar tilt, passive medial-lateral patellar glide (0°, 30° flexion), Q-angle assessed.
- Articular cartilage lesions evaluated, loose flaps débrided.
- Lateral retinacular release
  ○ Performed only if patellar medial subluxation test is abnormal (patellar medial subluxation ≤ 5 mm on the manual medial translation test, knee at 30° flexion).
  ○ Subcutaneous pouch created with a scissor from the anterolateral portal.
  ○ Arthroscopic retinacular release performed with commercial radiofrequency wand through anterolateral portal.
  ○ Initiated from 9 o'clock position (right knee), continued distally to 1 cm below inferior pole of patella with the knee in full extension.
  ○ Patellar medial subluxation test performed at 30° flexion.
  ○ If the release is inadequate, it is extended proximally to a 10 o'clock position.
  ○ Determine that there is no abnormal restraint to lateral patellar glide at 20°–30° of flexion, confirm absence of tight lateral tissues at 90°.
- Proximal realignment
  ○ 3-cm vertical skin incision made along medial aspect of the patella.
  ○ Medial parapatellar incision made through medial retinaculum.
  ○ Superficial and deep retinaculum MPFL incised, 2–3 cm of VMO insertion into patella detached.
  ○ Quality of MPFL and medial retinaculum inspected.
  ○ Extensor mechanism reconstructed with medial plication of VMO and MPFL so that the VMO advancement is in line with its fibers and prior insertion.
  ○ VMO tissue sleeve is translated laterally and imbricated in a vest-over-pants fashion.
  ○ Suture placed at 1 o'clock position (right knee) so that the distal part of the VMO is brought laterally in the line of its attachment to restore normal tension at 30° flexion.
  ○ Suture placed at 2 o'clock position through MPFL and medial patellar insertion.
  ○ Suture placed at 4–5 o'clock position through MPML and medial retinaculum to plicate these structures in line with their normal patellar attachment.
  ○ Final tensioning of sutures 30° knee flexion, patella centered within trochlea.
  ○ Knee is taken through 0°–135° to observe normal tracking of the patella.
- MPFL reconstruction
  ○ See Table 39–1.

- Distal realignment
  ○ 3-cm vertical skin incision placed lateral to tibial tubercle.
  ○ Longitudinal incision made over periosteum, along lateral border of patellar tendon.
  ○ Planned tibial tubercle osteotomy 12–15 mm wide, 8 mm thick, 35 mm in length.
  ○ Hole drilled through tibial cortex, four to five holes drilled on anterolateral tibial cortex.
  ○ Axial 90° cut made just proximal to patellar tendon insertion.
  ○ Drill holes along anterolateral surface of tibia connected using a ½-inch osteotome.
  ○ Osteotome carried through medial cortex directly adjacent to tibial tubercle.
  ○ Bone fragment mobilized and translated medially 8–10 mm.
  ○ Tibial tubercle secured with a 3.2-mm drill bit.
  ○ When a proximal advancement is also performed, medial plication and reconstruction completed.
  ○ Patellar glide, tracking assessed, Q-angle measured at 0° and 30° of flexion.
  ○ Final fixation of tibial tubercle with three 4-mm cancellous screws
- Lateral patellofemoral (iliopatellar tract) reconstruction
  ○ Indicated symptomatic medial patellar subluxation, manual medial glide at 30° of flexion grossly positive.
  ○ Goal is to restore lateral muscle function by reattachment of the VLO if possible and reconstruct lateral soft tissue restraints.
  ○ Dissect VLO attachment to the quadriceps tendon and patella.
  ○ Reattach VLO to lateral border of the quadriceps tendon.
  ○ Dissect distal VLO tendon proximally, reattach VLO as distally as possible to restore normal anatomy.
  ○ Knee flexed 135°.
  ○ Semitendinosus tendon autograft used to reconstruct lateral soft tissue restraints.
  ○ Tendon placed through a lateral patellar tunnel (10 mm), which enters and exits at the one third and two third junction points along the vertical height of the patella.
  ○ Tendon ends sutured, length 25 mm.
  ○ Incision made at junction of iliopatellar tract and iliotibial band.
  ○ Usual site for graft is posterior just above the lateral intermuscular septum and proximal to the lateral epicondyle.
  ○ Drill hole placed, Beath pin used to pass the two ends of the tendon into the tunnel.
  ○ Graft tensioned with knee at 30° of flexion, allow a normal 10–12 mm manual medial glide.
  ○ Soft tissue interference screw used for fixation.
- Patella alta correction
  ○ See Table 39–3.

MPFL, medial patellofemoral ligament; MPML, medial patellomeniscal ligament; VLO, vastus longus obliquus; VMO, vastus medialis obliquus.

tissues. The surgeon should always be able to gently lift and anteriorly displace the lateral soft tissues away from the lateral femoral condyle.

In select cases in which there is extensive contracture of the lateral retinacular tissues and the VLO with associated arthrofibrosis, an open Z-plasty release is indicated as presented in Chapter 41, Prevention and Treatment of Knee Arthrofibrosis.

Proximal Realignment

The patient positioning and arthroscopic examination are performed as already described. The knee is fully flexed prior to inflation of the tourniquet to lengthen the quadriceps muscle. A 3-cm vertical skin incision is made along the medial aspect of the patella. The subcutaneous tissues are undermined sufficiently to create a skin flap that will allow the skin incision to

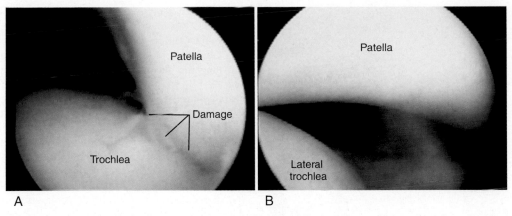

FIGURE 39–7. Arthroscopic medial-lateral translation manual test at 30° of knee flexion shows third quadrant lateral subluxation with cartilage deterioration (**A**) and lateral subluxation viewed through the anterolateral portal (**B**).

be moved in proximal-distal and medial-lateral directions using four vein retractors. This decreases the length of the skin incision and allows for a cosmetic approach. The proximal retraction exposes the distal quadriceps tendon, superomedial border of the patella, and VMO insertion. The distal retraction exposes the medial border of patella, medial retinaculum, and distal retinaculum fibers referred to as the MPML. A medial parapatellar incision is then made through the medial retinaculum, extending from approximately 2 cm proximal to the superomedial aspect of the patella to the medial border of patella and progressing distally to the patella. The superficial and deep retinaculum MPFL is incised, taking care to avoid cutting through the muscle or underlying synovium. The proximal extent of the incision extends in the QT, thus detaching 2 to 3 cm of the VMO insertion into the patella. The free medial edge of the retinaculum is grasped and the underlying synovium is dissected free. This allows the VMO, PMFL, and MPML tissue sleeve and medial retinacular tissues to be mobilized for later tensioning and advancement as required. The joint is not entered and the synovium over the femoral condyle and medial pouch is protected to lessen postoperative scar formation at this location.

The quality of the MPFL and medial retinaculum is inspected and a decision is made whether a MPFL reconstruction is necessary. The medial tissues should be 3 to 4 mm in thickness. A thin, abnormal medial retinaculum and MPFL indicates that an MPFL graft is required, to be described later. The mistake that is made is to accept marginal MPFL tissue, because it is relatively easy at this point to augment the surgery with an MPFL graft. If there is adequate MPFL tissue by visual inspection, proximal realignment is commenced. The closure procedure to be described next is performed if no distal realignment is planned; otherwise, the proximal closure is performed after the distal realignment described.

The extensor mechanism is reconstructed with medial plication of the VMO and MPFL so that the VMO advancement is in line with its fibers and prior insertion. The VMO tissue sleeve is translated laterally and imbricated in a vest-over-pants fashion. Three No.1 nonabsorbable sutures are used. Three Ellis clamps are placed at the VMO center, MPFL, and MPML medial anatomic sites to reestablish a normal tension. The first suture is placed at the 1 o'clock position (right knee) so that the distal part of the VMO is brought laterally in the line of its attachment, overlapping the superior medial border of the patella and QT by 5 to 10 mm to restore normal tension at 30° of flexion. The second suture is placed at the

2 o'clock position through the MPFL and medial patellar insertion. The third suture is placed at the 4 to 5 o'clock position through the MPML and medial retinaculum to plicate these structures in line with their normal patellar attachment. It is important that the final tensioning of the sutures be performed with the knee at 30° flexion with the patella held centered within the trochlea. The mistake is to adjust the tension with the knee at extension. The tightening procedure at 30° flexion allows for a normal slackness of the medial tissues and the MPFL and for a normal medial glide of 10 to 12 mm (~25% of patella width). The mistake is to apply too much tension that limits normal medial translation, which restricts postoperative knee motion and potentially results in medial facet cartilage damage from excessive pressure. The lateral subluxation of the patella is also assessed at 0° to ensure that a normal medial restraint exists, preventing abnormal lateral patellar subluxation at knee extension. The knee is taken through a range of motion of 0° to 135° to observe normal tracking of the patella. If the sutures disrupt, this is an indication that the medial advancement was excessive and the suture placement and tensioning procedure is repeated.

MPFL Reconstruction

MPFL deficiency is diagnosed when the patella translates greater than 50% of its width from the center of the sulcus. Symptomatic patients with chronic dislocations or subluxations will frequently demonstrate patellar translation of 75% to 100% (of its width) under manual pressure at both 0° and 30° of flexion (Fig. 39–8). An MPFL reconstruction is almost always indicated in revision surgery when a prior proximal realignment procedure has failed and a residual lateral patellar subluxation exists. The intraoperative examination includes the lateral subluxation test at 0° and 30° of flexion. The balancing of the medial soft tissue restraints requires that tension be restored at both knee positions to guide the patella into the trochlea and resist lateral patellar subluxation at full extension and with knee flexion. The operative procedure includes a balancing of three structures, namely, the MPFL, VMO, and medial retinacular fibers, including the MPML. Preoperative radiographs and MRI define whether a patella alta or a lateral tibial tendon offset exists, requiring distal correction.

The patient is placed in a supine position on the operating table with the foot of the bed flexed 20° to 30°. A high-thigh tourniquet is placed (sterile or nonsterile) so that the entire

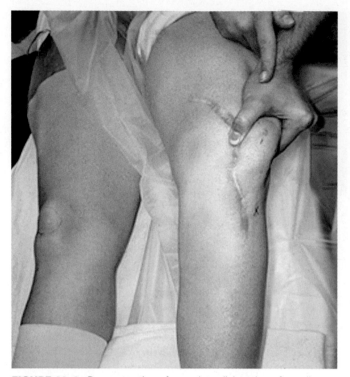

FIGURE 39–8. Demonstration of complete dislocation of patella at the time of surgery after multiple prior operative procedures. A reconstruction of the medial patellofemoral ligament was required. *(From Parikh, S. N.; Noyes, F. R.; Albright, J.: Proximal and distal extensor mechanism realignment: the surgical technique. Tech Knee Surg 5:27–38, 2006.)*

lower extremity is draped and provides an estimate of patellofemoral alignment. A diagnostic arthroscopy is performed as already described and the condition of the patellofemoral articular cartilage documented. Medial-lateral glide tests are performed at 30° flexion to determine the resisting function of the medial and lateral soft tissue restraints. The leg is elevated, exsanguinated, and the tourniquet inflated.

The operative steps of MPFL reconstruction are shown in Figure 39–9 and summarized in Table 39–1. A 5- to 6-cm incision is made at the medial border of the patella and extended 1 to 2 cm proximally (see Fig. 39–9A). A dissection of the skin flaps is carefully performed beneath the fascia layer to preserve the skin blood supply. This allows the incision to be mobilized in a proximal-distal direction, providing a cosmetic incision one half the usual length. The dissection is carried over the medial aspect of the knee and medial epicondyle to the adductor tendon. A head light and careful dissection technique is used at this point to avoid the infrapatellar nerve branches, which can result in injury and a painful neuroma. The medial nerves are highly variable in their course, as shown in Chapter 1, Medial and Anterior Knee Anatomy. The skin flaps are further developed in all directions to be able to reach the proximal aspect of the QT, a distance of 6 to 7 cm from the patellar insertion for the planned turn-down of the medial QT graft.

A medial incision through the medial retinaculum is made 5 mm from the medial border of the patella from the inferior to superior pole. The medial incision is extended distally to the level of the joint. This is an incision similar to that used for a proximal realignment procedure already described, which is performed in conjunction with the MPFL reconstruction.

Using an Army/Navy retractor, the insertion of the VMO into the QT is identified. A ruler is used to measure the MPFL attachment length from the medial border of the patella, past the epicondyle to the adductor tubercle and tendon. This provides the length of the QT graft to be harvested (see Fig. 39–9B). A ruler is used to mark the medial QT to harvest a graft 8 mm wide and usually 60 mm in length. In a smaller knee, the graft is 6 mm in thickness. The full-thickness medial QT graft is harvested 5 mm from the medial border of the VMO to allow for VMO tendon-to-tendon suturing after harvest. The proximal graft never extends into the proximal QT-muscle junction, because this would weaken the attachment. Two full-thickness incisions are made into the medial QT at the marked graft site, avoiding penetration into the capsule. The incision connects to the prior medial patella retinaculum incision. The medial QT graft is transected proximally, preserving its attachment to the superomedial border of the patella (see Fig. 39–9C). The three tendon components of the QT (rectus, confluent VMO-VLO, intermedius) are carefully identified and the proximal end of the graft is sutured with a baseball-type stitch (No. 1 nonabsorbable suture).

With care taken not to transect the graft, subperiosteal dissection of the patella attachment of the graft is performed to a point approximately 30% of the proximal height of the patella at the normal MPFL attachment (see Fig. 39–9D). Later in the procedure, appropriate sutures are placed to secure the proximal patella attachment of the QT graft to adjacent tissues. Preserving the medial synovial pouch and avoiding penetration of the joint, the medial retinaculum is dissected off the capsule past the medial epicondyle to the adductor tendon (see Fig. 39–9E). At the junction immediately anterior to the adductor, distal to the insertion of the VMO, and superficial to the medial epicondyle, a hole is punctured in the retinaculum with a right-angle hemostat (see Fig. 39–9F). The graft is turned 90° and folded over on itself at the proximal medial portion of the patella. The free end of the QT graft is passed beneath the retinaculum, adjacent to the VMO attachment, and through the created retinaculum hole to exit and lay over the adductor tubercle and tendon.

The final proximal realignment tensioning procedure is then performed following the steps previously outlined (and after the distal realignment when added to the overall realignment surgery). With the knee flexed 30° and the patella located within the trochlea, the medial vest-over-pants procedure is performed, including closure of the QT graft harvest site. The entire medial soft tissue and VMO is grasped with an Ellis clamp placed at the 1 o'clock (VMO), 2 o'clock (MPFL), and 4 o'clock (retinaculum, MPTL) areas and gently brought in line of its attachments to determine the amount of plication and overlap for suturing. Three sutures are placed at these respective sites with care taken not to overtension the repair. It is emphasized that there must always be a normal lateral glide of 25% of the width of the patella at 0° and 30° of flexion under manual pressure to avoid limiting normal patellar mobility. The imbrication procedure restores the patella to its reduced position (see Fig. 39–9G).

The final portion of the procedure consists of tensioning the MPFL-QT graft. Two absorbable sutures are passed into the adductor tendon, avoiding penetrating the medial geniculate at the posterior border of the VMO and the medial retinacular nerve (see Chapter 1, Medial and Anterior Knee Anatomy). The sutures are brought up through the free end of the graft that lays on the adductor tendon. No tension is applied to the

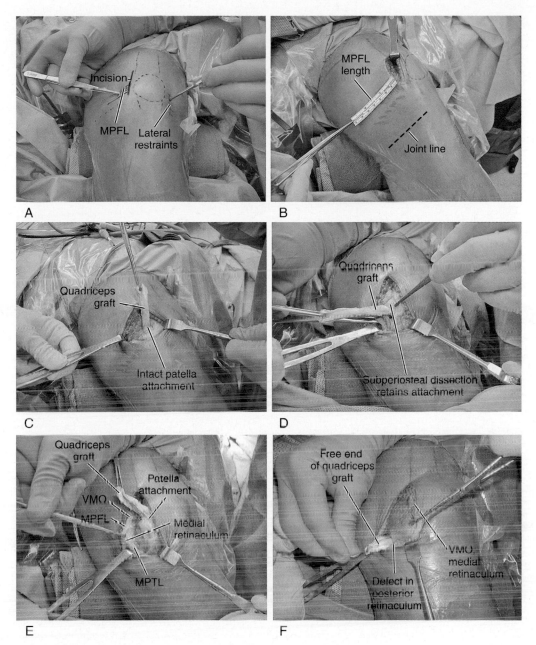

FIGURE 39–9. Medial patellofemoral ligament reconstruction with quadriceps tendon. **A,** After arthroscopic evaluation, the planned surgical incision (*thick black line*) over medial aspect of the widest portion of the patella is shown. **B,** Measurement of length of graft needed (60–70 mm); limited cosmetic incision is shown. **C,** A medial full-thickness quadriceps tendon graft, 60–70 × 8 mm (measured to the superior edge of the patella) is harvested with the patellar attachment retained. Two to 3 mm of remaining quadriceps tendon is left attached to the vastus medialis obliquus (VMO) for later closure. **D,** Completed 70 mm quadriceps tendon graft after dissection from the superior-medial patella down to the normal anatomic attachment site of the medial patellofemoral ligament. **E,** Dissection deep to the medial retinaculum and above the synovial pouch, MPFL, medial patellomeniscal ligament (MPML) and medial patellotibial ligament (MPTL). **F,** Puncture of the medial retinaculum, posterior to the medial femoral epicondyle at the adductor tendon with passage of graft beneath retinaculum. Setting of the normal tension of the medial soft tissues (see text).

(Continued)

graft, which simply lies in its created tunnel underneath the retinaculum and over the adductor tendon, because the tension in the medial soft tissue restraints has already been set by the proximal realignment just described. Three to four absorbable sutures are passed through the medial retinaculum into the graft to complete the procedure. Again, the lateral glide test is performed to make sure the graft is not under any resting tension and that the combined medial soft tissue imbrication and MPFL reconstruction is initially lax and allows the patella to be

displaced 25% of its width, restoring the normal length of the medial soft tissues. After suturing is complete, the knee should be ranged from 0° to 135° restoring normal patellofemoral tracking. An additional two to three sutures are then placed in a figure-eight fashion, reinforcing the fixation of the graft to the medial retinaculum around the rent created for the graft to pass through the retinaculum (see Fig. 39–9H).

The advantage of this procedure is that no bone tunnels are placed into the patella or medial femoral condyle, as described

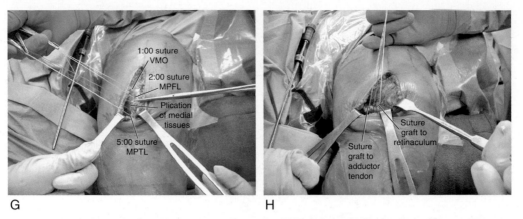

FIGURE 39–9—cont'd. G, Imbrication of the VMO, medial retinaculum, MPFL, and MPTL. **H**, Suturing of the quadriceps graft to the medial retinaculum and adductor tendon. The graft and medial tissues are not overtensioned and should allow a normal lateral translation (glide) of 25% patellar width. *(A–H, From Noyes, F. R.; Albright, J.: Reconstruction of the medial patellofemoral ligament with autologous quadriceps tendon. Arthroscopy 22:904e1–904e7, 2006.)*

TABLE 39–1   Key Points to Successful Medial Patellofemoral Ligament Reconstruction

Preoperative

1. Complete rehabilitation for muscle and motion deficits.
2. Comprehensive evaluation of patellar soft tissue restraints, Q-angle (0° and 30° flexion) and with internal-external rotation, standing rotational alignment, and gait (see text).
3. Complete radiographic and MRI evaluation, femoral anteversion, hip rotation, trochlear dysplasia, trochlear groove, patella height, patella-trochlear contact at 0°, lateral tibial tubercle offset, and external tibial torsion.

Operative Steps

1. Confirm preoperative examination under anesthesia, medial-lateral translation tests, lateral translation > 50% patella width 0° and 30° knee flexion, measure resting Q-angle at 0° and Q translation arc with internal-external tibial rotation at 30°.
2. Arthroscopic procedure defines patellofemoral abnormalities, confirms medial-lateral translation 30°, and need for proximal realignment. Limited arthroscopic lateral release only with contracted lateral tissues and absence of normal medial glide (see text).
3. High thigh tourniquet to view entire lower extremity and patellofemoral tracking.
4. Cosmetic limited medial incision medial to patellar border and 1–2 cm proximal to patella, undermine incision for skin mobilization.
5. Careful subcutaneous dissection medially to adductor magnus tendon avoiding infrapatellar nerves and proximally along medial VMO and quadriceps tendon.
6. Incise medial retinaculum adjacent to patella to the joint line, confirm thin medial tissues, insufficient MPFL requiring graft reconstruction.
7. Harvest full-thickness medial quadriceps graft 60–70 mm long, 6–8 mm wide, and 10 mm deep leaving 5 mm medial VMO tendon for closure and patellar graft insertion intact. Connect medial quadriceps tendon incision to prior medial retinaculum incision.
8. Careful subperiosteal dissection of quadriceps graft attachment proximal and medial aspect of the patella to native MPFL attachment.
9. At the posterior junction of the medial retinaculum, preserve medial synovial pouch, penetrate retinaculum just above adductor tendon, rotate graft 90° at patella. Pass free end of graft beneath retinaculum to exit through retinaculum hole overlying adductor tendon.
10. Perform proximal realignment advancing the entire medial retinaculum sleeve and VMO, carefully setting tension to allow normal 25% patellar width, lateral glide at 30° flexion (see text). Perform knee flexion-extension to observe normal patellofemoral tracking.
11. Quadriceps graft sutured to adductor tendon and overlying retinaculum under minimal graft tension to avoid overconstraining normal lateral patellar glide. Perform medial-lateral glide tests again and full flexion to confirm normal medial restraint and patellar stability restored. Closure of remaining quadriceps tendon incision.
12. Additional sutures to reinforce quadriceps graft at medial patellar attachment may be required

MPFL, medial patellofemoral ligament; MRI, magnetic resonance imaging; VMO, vastus medialis obliquus.

in other MPFL reconstructions. The graft is sutured along the path of the native MPFL by pliable soft tissue fixation, reproducing patella and femoral attachments. It is not necessary to add a harvest of a medial hamstring tendon. The disadvantage of the procedure is related to the medial QT graft harvest, because this adds additional postoperative pain in comparison with a hamstring autograft. In knees with previous dislocations or revision cases, the restoration of the normal proximal VMO tension is performed with closure of the proximal harvest site. It is important that MPFL reconstruction be performed in the majority of knees with a prior dislocation, because it is usual to find a medial retinaculum that is thin with no identifiable MPFL structure. The resultant cosmetic appearance of the incision and restoration of full knee flexion are demonstrated in Figure 39–10.

Distal Realignment

A lateral radiograph is used to confirm that a normal patella tendon length and patella height exist, as presented in Chapter 41, Prevention and Treatment of Knee Arthrofibrosis. A 3-cm vertical skin incision is placed lateral to the tibial tubercle (Fig. 39–11). The subcutaneous tissues are undermined sufficiently to create a skin flap that would allow the skin incision to be moved in all directions and maintain a small cosmetic incision. The patellar tendon insertion is identified and a retractor placed behind it to identify its insertion site on the tibial tubercle. A longitudinal incision is made over the periosteum, along the lateral border of patellar tendon. Subperiosteal dissection is carefully performed to expose the anterolateral aspect of the tibia, reflecting the

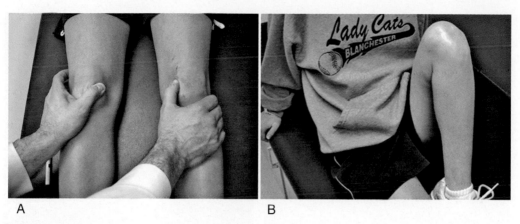

FIGURE 39–10. Three-month postoperative case demonstrates excellent healing and function of reconstructed MPFL in resisting lateral patellar translation (**A**) and full flexion of the knee (**B**). *(A and B, From Noyes, F. R.; Albright, J.: Reconstruction of the medial patellofemoral ligament with autologous quadriceps tendon.* Arthroscopy *22:904e1–904e7, 2006.)*

periosteum and the muscular origin of the anterior compartment. Care is taken in the dissection not to enter into the muscle tissues to decrease postoperative pain and swelling. The planned tibial tubercle osteotomy measures 12 to 15 mm width, 8 mm thick, and 35 mm long. At the distal extent of the osteotomy, a hole is drilled through the tibial cortex, using a 3.2-mm drill bit and drill guide. This is to prevent the osteotomy from extending distally. The drill hole is placed beneath the anterior tibial periosteum, which maintains the normal proximal-to-distal position of the tibial tubercle. Similarly, four to five holes are drilled on the anterolateral tibial cortex, along the line of the planned osteotomy; the angle of the osteotomy is oblique by 15° to 20° from a posterolateral-to-anteromedial direction. An axial 90° cut is made just proximal to the patellar tendon insertion to mark the proximal extent of the osteotomy. This step-cut produces a bony buttress to

prevent proximal migration of the tibial tubercle. The drill holes along the anterolateral surface of the tibia are then connected using a ½-inch osteotome. The osteotome is carried through the medial cortex directly adjacent to the tibial tubercle, while the distal periosteal hinge remains intact. The bone fragment is carefully mobilized and translated medially, according to a predetermined amount based on TT/TG distance correction. This distance is usually 8 to 10 mm. The tibial tubercle is secured with a 3.2-mm drill bit.

The tourniquet is deflated so that there is no pressure on the quadriceps muscle during assessment of quadriceps function. When a proximal advancement is also performed, it is at this point that the medial plication and reconstruction are completed as already described. The ability to glide the patella medially and laterally by one quadrant, with the knee in 30° of flexion, is

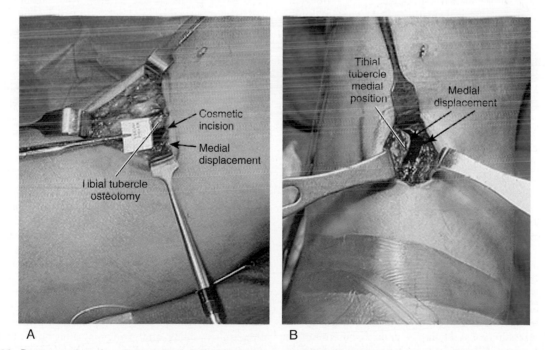

FIGURE 39–11. Demonstration of a proximal-distal realignment when a medial patellofemoral ligament reconstruction is not required. **A**, The medial retinaculum and VMO 2 cm above the patella are advanced in line of their insertions to restore patellar stability. **B**, The millimeters of tibial tubercle medial displacement required are measured at surgery.

(Continued)

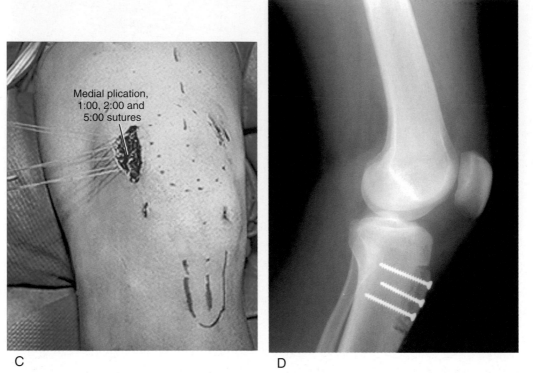

C   D

FIGURE 39–11—cont'd. C, A dovetail tibial tubercle osteotomy has been performed, maintaining the distal and medial soft tissues. **D,** Postoperative radiograph. *(A–C, From Parikh, S. N.; Noyes, F. R.; Albright, J.: Proximal and distal extensor mechanism realignment: the surgical technique. Tech Knee Surg 5:27–38, 2006.)*

verified. The patellofemoral tracking is next assessed by taking the knee through a range of motion. The patella should remain centralized within the femoral sulcus, with no medial or lateral tilt or subluxation in flexion or extension. The Q-angle is assessed using a goniometer, with the knee in 30° of flexion in neutral, internal, and external rotation. The Q-angle should always be positive, even with maximum internal tibial rotation. The correction based on preoperative TT/TG distance and the preoperative measurements is confirmed. A goniometer is placed over the anterior knee region and the Q-angle measurement made at 0° and 30° of flexion with maximum internal and external tibial rotation. These measurements are only approximations and the goal is to restore as closely as possible a normal lateral patellar offset. Once the ideal position is determined, the final fixation of the tibial tubercle is done with three 4-mm cancellous screws. A compression technique with overdrilling the tibial tubercle is performed, and the screw head is countersunk to prevent prominence under the skin. If the bone quality is questionable, cortical screws can be used for bicortical fixation. The screws should be tightened gently to avoid fracturing the bone fragment.

At this point, hemostasis is achieved, followed by the closure of the wound in layers. There is a lateral tibial tubercle defect after the medial displacement that requires a simple shifting of the anterolateral tissues (Fig. 39–12), which closes the defect and prevents a cosmetically unappealing indentation and concavity in this area after healing of the incision. The skin is closed using subcuticular stitches. A Hemovac drain is not routinely used. A double-cotton, double-Ace compression dressing is applied, and the lower extremity is placed in a brace. Cryotherapy is instituted immediately after surgery in the operating room.

Lateral Patellofemoral (Iliopatellar Tract) Reconstruction

The anatomy of the lateral iliopatellar tract is presented in detail in Chapter 1, Medial and Anterior Knee Anatomy. The iliopatellar tract is divided into the superficial oblique retinaculum and a second layer termed the *deep transverse fibers*. The attachment of the VLO to the superolateral aspect of the patellae is shown in Chapter 1, Medial and Anterior Knee Anatomy (see Fig. 1–13).

As previously discussed, a lateral release should be performed only when there is an abnormal contracture of these tissues, with an inability to perform a manual lateral translation (glide) at 30° of flexion. This condition may occur with joint arthrofibrosis or from a developmental standpoint referred to as the *lateral patellar compression syndrome* that may be associated with a bipartite patella. In the 1970s and 1980s, some authors recommended a lateral release that included resection of the VLO attachment for lateral patellar subluxation.[57,59,60] It is now appreciated that the appropriate treatment of a lateral patellar subluxation is restoration of the MPFL, and not by weakening the VLO. There remain descriptions of the lateral release of soft tissues and VLO to the extent that the patella can be everted, which should be avoided.

The syndrome of a medial subluxation after a release of the lateral restraining structures and VLO has been identified by numerous authors.[5,42,44,69,84] Nonweiler and DeLee[69] reported on a series of five patients who presented with medial subluxation, pain, swelling, and giving-way after isolated lateral release. All underwent reconstruction of the lateral retinaculum. An average of 3.3 years postoperatively, four of the five had no symptoms of instability and the patellar stability was similar to that of the contralateral limb. Hughston and Deese[42] described

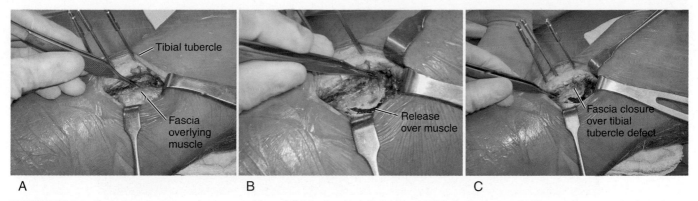

FIGURE 39–12. Technique for cosmetic closure of lateral tibial tubercle defect after medial displacement. **A,** The gap between the lateral soft tissues and the tibial tubercle is shown. **B,** Incision 15 mm lateral to the defect and at the proximal extent of the soft tissue flap. **C,** Rotation of soft tissue flap into defect with closure to the soft tissues along the lateral border of the tibial tubercle. This simple transposition of adjacent soft tissues prevents the lateral indentation commonly visible after tibial tubercle medialization.

a series of 60 knees treated after failure of a lateral release to improve symptoms. Thirty knees had developed medial subluxation of the patella, 17 of whom underwent an isolated lateral release and 13 of whom underwent a concomitant proximal or distal realignment. Twenty-seven of these 30 knees had disabling symptoms postoperatively, and all demonstrated marked quadriceps atrophy and retraction of the VLO. Biedert and Friederich[5] described 41 cases of patients who had pain after a lateral release; 32 had also had medial subluxation of the patella.

Christoforakis and colleagues[11] measured the effects of lateral release on the lateral stability of the patella in cadaveric specimens (aged 65–82 yr). The patella was displaced 10 mm laterally while measuring the required force, with 175 N quadriceps force. Patellar force-displacement behavior was measured from 0° to 60° of knee flexion in intact knees and then after lateral release, which extended from the proximal limit of the lateral retinaculum to Gerdy's tubercle. At 0°, 10°, and 20° of flexion, the mean force required to displace the patella (10 mm laterally) was significantly reduced after lateral release by 16% to 19% ($P = .002–.001$). The investigators concluded that the procedure decreased the lateral stability of the patella in normal elderly knees.

The diagnosis of a symptomatic medial patellar subluxation is not difficult. The patient complains of medial subluxation events that produce a partial giving-way and pain that commonly occurs with normal activities of daily living. The patient can usually distinguish the medial subluxation position of the patella from a lateral subluxation. The manual medial glide at 30° of flexion is usually grossly positive, producing patient apprehension. The defect in the VLO attachment is palpable and the patella can be everted. There is often extensive muscle atrophy, which requires months of physical therapy prior to surgery.

The goal of surgical treatment is to restore lateral muscle function by reattachment of the VLO if possible and to reconstruct the lateral soft tissue restraints. The skin incision for the surgical approach depends on the placement of incisions from prior surgery and either a medial or a lateral parapatellar incision provides exposure. It is necessary to dissect the VLO attachment to the QT and patella. It is usually possible to reattach the VLO to the lateral border of the QT. Often, a layer of scar tissue at the site of the prior release is identified, and it is a simple matter to excise the scar and reattach the VLO. It may also be possible to reattach a portion of the VLO to the superior lateral border of the patella; however, frequently, a contracture and shortening of the VLO has occurred. The distal

VLO tendon is dissected proximally and an attempt is made to reattach the VLO as distally as possible to restore normal anatomy. The knee is flexed to 135° to ensure that the distal attachment of the VLO does not limit flexion or the sutures pull out from a shortened VLO muscle.

The reconstruction of the lateral soft tissue restraints is accomplished with a semitendinosus tendon autograft, which is preferred over an allograft to avoid delayed remodeling (Fig. 39–13). If the semitendinosus tendon is small in diameter, the gracilis tendon is also incorporated into the construct. The tendon is placed through a lateral patellar tunnel, which enters and exits at the one third and two thirds junction points along the vertical height of the patella. The lateral patella tunnel for the graft is approximately 10 mm in length, with a diameter matching that of the tendon. Each end of the tendon is sutured with a baseball-type stitch and the length adjusted so that 25 mm of tendon will pass into the femoral tunnel used for the posterior attachment of the graft. An incision is made at the junction of the iliopatellar tract and the ITB to expose the lateral aspect of the femoral condyle and lateral intramuscular septum. The isometric point for the femoral tunnel on the lateral femoral condyle is identified by using a suture fixed to the lateral patella tunnel site and a guidewire placed at the lateral femur with full extension-flexion produced. The usual site for the graft is posterior just above the lateral intermuscular septum and proximal to the lateral epicondyle. A drill hole is placed at this site and a Beath pin used to pass the two ends of the tendon into the tunnel. A soft tissue interference screw is used for fixation. The tension in the graft prior to fixation is adjusted by placing the knee at 30° of flexion and allowing a normal 10 to 12 mm manual medial glide. The graft should be under no tension in its resting state and under tension only to resist manual medial patellar displacement. It is important not to overtension the graft and produce a lateral soft tissue contracture, which would potentially lead to articular cartilage damage (iatrogenic lateral patellar compression syndrome). Following tensioning, the knee is taken through a full range of motion. The wound closure is routine and a drain is not necessary. The rehabilitation program is the same as that described for an MPFL reconstruction.

Patella Alta Correction

Patella alta represents a congenital abnormality of an increased vertical position of the patella due to an elongated patellar tendon resulting in the patella not engaging within the trochlea

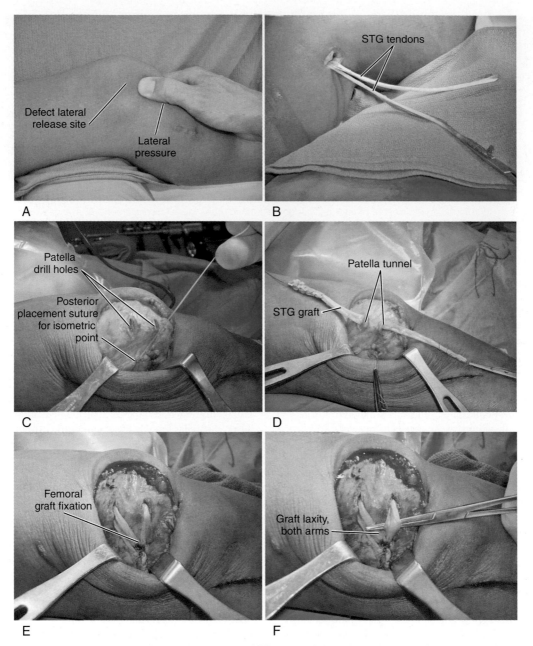

FIGURE 39–13. Surgical demonstration of semitendinosus-gracilis (STG) autograft lateral reconstruction for symptomatic medial subluxation after a prior proximal realignment involving complete release of the lateral soft tissue restraints. **A**, Positive manual medial glide test shows obvious medial subluxation. **B**, Harvest of STG autograft through limited medial incision. **C**, Placement of two drill holes on the lateral border of the patella. A suture is placed to identify the location of the lateral femoral tunnel for the STG graft. The previously transected and scarred lateral retinaculum is not disturbed. In this case, the vastus lateralis obliquus (VLO) insertion is shown to be intact. If it was previously released, it would be dissected and reattached. **D**, Passage of the two arms of the STG graft through the lateral patella tunnel. **E**, Final STG graft fixation. **F**, Demonstration that the graft is under no tension with the patellar at 30° knee flexion; however, the graft is adjusted to resist a 10-mm medial patella glide (see text).

until a midflexion range of motion. Patients typically present with significant complaints related to lateral patellar subluxation or dislocation that can affect all activities of daily living. Ward and coworkers[95] studied patients with patella alta with MRI under partial weight-bearing loads that induced quadriceps tension at various knee flexion angles and reported increased lateral displacement and lateral tilt at 0° degrees of knee flexion only (Fig. 39–14). There was a decrease in patellofemoral joint contact area in subjects with patella alta at all knee flexion angles. The data did not explain the basis for anterior knee pain in

symptomatic patella alta patients, and the authors recommended the need for further studies. In most patients, the patella alta abnormality does not occur in isolation and other abnormalities of the extensor mechanism are usually present. Some patients with patella alta and anterior knee pain and joint swelling have signs of patellofemoral crepitus and arthritis, but do not experience subluxation symptoms.

The major factors for patellar instability include patella alta, MPFL deficiency, trochlear dysplasia, and patellar tendon lateral offset, as already discussed. Associated increased femoral

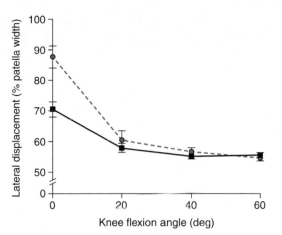

FIGURE 39–14. Lateral patellar displacement as a function of knee flexion angle in controls (*solid line*) and subjects with patella alta (*dotted line*). *Error bars* indicate 1 standard error. The difference between the patella alta group and the control groups at 0° of knee flexion was significant (*P* < .05). *(From Ward, S. R.; Terk, M. R.; Powers, C. M.: Patella alta: association with patellofemoral alignment and changes in contact area during weight bearing. J Bone Joint Surg Am 89:1749–1755, 2007.)*

anteversion and increased external tibial torsion add to the predisposition for lateral patellar instability. The decision to correct an abnormal patellar tendon length to allow the patella to engage within the trochlear would address only one aspect of the problem in cases of lateral patellar subluxation or dislocation. Additional correction of an MPFL deficiency and lateral patellar offset may be required. At surgery, the tibial tubercle is advanced distally to restore a normal patellotrochlear relationship. In this corrected position, the medial-lateral manual translation tests determine the new tension relationship of the MPFL and lateral restraints and the need for rebalancing the tension by surgical correction. The senior author has no experience with correcting trochlear dysplasia and this has not been a part of the operative procedure. Dejour and Walch[22] analyzed the radiographs and CT scans of 143 knees with symptomatic patellar instability and 67 contralateral asymptomatic knees to determine the factors affecting patellar instability. These authors reported that trochlear dysplasia was present in 96% of unstable patella. Although it would be ideal to correct a trochlear dysplasia, the problem remains that the patella is still flattened and dysplastic and it is therefore not possible to restore a normal patellofemoral contact pattern by surgically deepening the trochlear groove. Abnormally high patellofemoral contact pressures would be expected after

trochlearplasty procedures that may lead to short-term cartilage deterioration. Rather, the approach taken is to restore a normal patellotrochlear contact and MPFL function and correct an abnormal lateral patellar offset when present.

There are differences in the methods used for measurement of patellar height regarding the anatomic points selected and the values used for the classification of an alta, normal, or infera position of the patella. Seil and colleagues[80] compared five different patellar height ratio techniques in 21 patients and reported that the classification of alta, normal, and infera depended on the normative data chosen for each technique. The normal values for patellar height, and those selected to determine the presence of patella alta and patella infera, are shown in Table 39–2. Noyes and colleagues[71] conducted a study to determine normal right to left patellar vertical height ratios within the same individual in a group of 51 patients (102 knees). The difference in the vertical height ratio of the patella between these two methods ranged from 0% to 9%, with an average difference of 3%. Large variations existed in the ratios between individual patients (range, 0.75–1.46).

Shabshin and coworkers[83] reported patellar tendon length to patellar length on MRI in 245 patients using the Insall-Salvati method. The results of the measurement are shown in Figure 39–15. The patients were not selected out as to diagnosis and were referred for orthopaedic evaluation for a number of disorders; thus, it is not known how many patients had a clinical diagnosis of a patellar subluxation or dislocation, which is an unaccounted variable in the study. In addition, the measurements were made with the knee in full extension with the possibility of an inaccurate length for the patellar tendon in a resting position.

Biedert and Albrecht[6] described an MRI method to measure the true articular cartilage sagittal patellotrochlear relationship at 0° extension. The ratio of the patella to trochlea cartilage contact was described as a percentage and the mean index was 32% ± 12%. An index value greater than 50% documented a patella infera and less than 12.5% documented a patella alta (Fig. 39–16). This is a useful index in surgical cases of patella alta in terms of determining at surgery the distal displacement of the tibial tubercle required to establish a normal patellotrochlear relationship. The authors believed this index is more accurate than the numerous published indices (e.g., Blackburne and Peel,[7] Linclau,[51] and Caton and colleagues[13]), which rely on the length of the patella articular cartilage to a defined tibial reference point, but do not indicate the final patellofemoral joint position or define an alta or an infera relationship. The main problem with the patellotrochlear index method is the inability to obtain a quadriceps contraction during the MRI to define that

TABLE 39–2   Published Values for Patellar Height: Normal, Alta, Infera

Reference	Technique Source	Normal Mean ± SD (Range)	Alta	Infera
Insall & Salvati, 1971[42a]	Authors' own	1.02 ± 0.13 (0.7 – 1.3)	>1.2	<0.8
Blackburne & Peel, 1977[7]	Authors' own	0.8 ± 0.13 (0.54 – 1.06)	>1.2	<0.5
Caton et al., 1982[13]	Authors' own	<1.2	>1.2	≤0.6
Linclau, 1984[51]	Caton et al.[13]	1.0 ± 0.08 (0.84 – 1.16)	>1.2	<0.8
	Blackburne & Peel[7]	0.8 ± 0.10 (0.61 – 1.01)	>1.0	<0.6
Noyes et al., 1991[71]	Caton et al.[13]	1.04 ± 0.13 (0.75 – 1.36)	NA	≥15%*
	Blackburne & Peel[7]	0.84 ± 0.14 (0.61 – 1.33)	NA	≥14%*
	Insall & Salvati[42a]	1.05 ± 0.11 (0.86 – 1.28)	NA	≥11%*

*Decrease in patellar height between the involved and the contralateral knee.
SD, standard deviation.

FIGURE 39–15. Histogram demonstrates the distribution of the Insall-Salvati Index (ISI) applied to the study population. Note the asymmetrical curve, which is skewed toward the higher ratios. The *solid line* shows the mean (1.05), and the *dotted line* represents the proposed normal range, which is defined by calculating the extreme 2.5% of the ratio at each end of the curve. *(From Shabshin, N.; Schweitzer, M. E.; Morrison, W. B.; Parker, L.: MRI criteria for patella alta and baja. Skeletal Radiol 33:445–450, 2004.)*

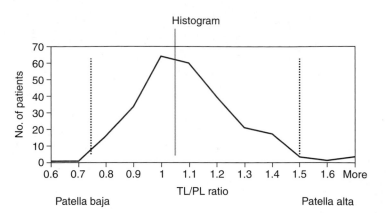

FIGURE 39–16. Left, Method used to determine patellar vertical height ratio on lateral radiograph with a quadriceps contraction to show the maximum elevated position of the patella. The numerator, *line segment A,* is the distance between the most ventral (anterosuperior) rim of the tibial plateau and the lowest end of the patellar articular surface. The denominator, *line segment B,* is the maximum length of the patellar articular surface. An alternative numerator, *line segment C,* locates the tibial reference point on the middle of the tibial plateau. The patellar vertical-height ratio equals A/B or C/B. **Right,** Alternative patellotrochlear ratio measurement. The mean ratio is 32 ± 12%; >50% indicates patellar infera; <12% indicates patella alta.

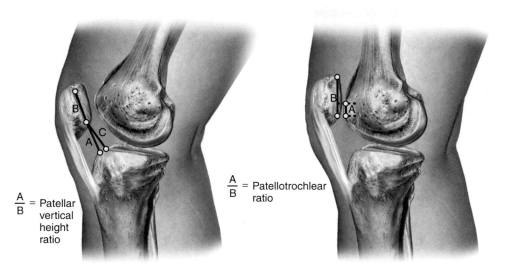

the patella is at a maximum proximal relationship. In the absence of a quadriceps contraction, the patellar may appear to be lower and the maximum patellar height will not be measured.

In Figure 39–17, radiographs of a 16-year-old male who had multiple recurrent lateral patellar dislocations are shown that demonstrate bilateral patella alta. The Linclau ratio was 1.6 and the patellotrochlear index demonstrated no patellar contact at full extension. The corrective bilateral operative procedures had to be delayed 2 years to allow for completion of growth. A distal transfer of the tibial tubercle was performed to restore these two indices to normal values. Lateral radiographs taken at surgery are required to measure that the normal patellar height ratio has been restored and to prevent too distal a transfer and a patella infera condition. A concurrent MPFL reconstruction was also performed.

Neyret and colleagues[66] measured the patellar tendon length on lateral radiographs and MRI in 42 knees with patellar dislocation and 51 control knees and reported that the patellar tendon was 8 mm longer in the former group (mean length, 52 ± 6 mm, and range, 39–61 mm; and 44 ± 7 mm and range, 32–62 mm, respectively; $P < .0001$). The wide range in patellar length shows the marked variation in patellar length from patient to patient even in the dislocation group. The Caton-Deschamps index was abnormal (>1.20) in 48% of the dislocation group and 12% of

controls, and the values for the MRI were 60% and 12%, respectively. There was no difference in the distance of the tendon insertion on the tibia compared with that on the tibial plateau. The authors suggested that when a distal transfer of the patellar tendon in patellar alta cases is performed, a tenodesis of the tendon at the tibial insertion site would restore normal tendon length and decrease side-to-side patellar mobility, given the high percentage of associated trochlear dysplasia. The senior author of this chapter has no experience with this operative technique.

Lancourt and Cristini[49] used the Insall-Salvati method; however, these authors used the patellar tendon length as the denominator and the patellar length as the numerator, which is the reverse of the original description of this method. They reported that the Insall-Salvati index was 1.0 in normal patients, 0.80 in dislocating patella (alta), and 0.86 (infera) in chondromalacia (patella grating, crepitus), with the differences statistically significant ($P < .05$). The authors believed that patella alta results in patellotrochlear incongruity and risk for early patellofemoral arthritis. Marks and Bentley[56] used a similar Insall-Salvati method in 51 patients with patellar chondromalacia graded at arthroscopy and reported no definite relationship to patella alta, suggesting that recurrent dislocation provided a stronger relationship.

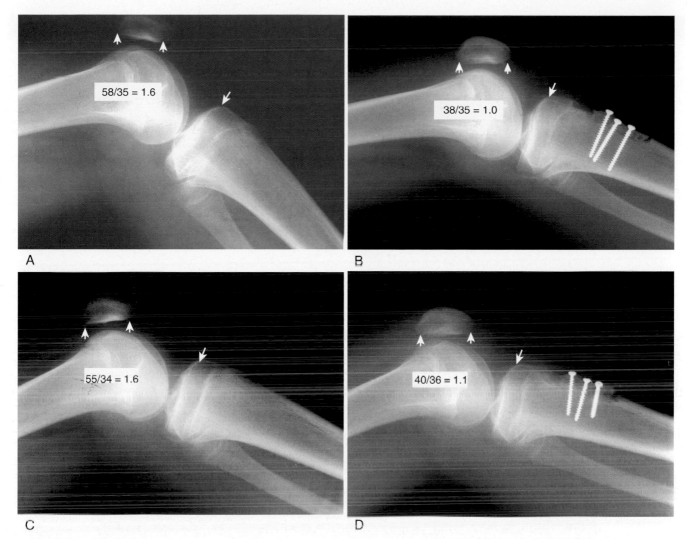

FIGURE 39–17. Demonstration of a symptomatic bilateral patella alta with multiple recurrent dislocations. **A** and **B**, Preoperative and postoperative radiographs of the left knee. **C** and **D**, Preoperative and postoperative radiographs of the right knee. An MPFL reconstruction was performed with a quadriceps tendon (QT) autograft as previously described on both knees. The right knee was initially performed, followed 4 months later by the left knee reconstruction. The patient's growth was complete and the tibial tubercle physes closed. The patient had an uneventful successful recovery without further patellar dislocations.

Al-Sayyad and Cameron[1] reported short-term improvements in patellofemoral scores (1–4 yr postoperatively) in 25 patients with painful patella alta and no history of patellar dislocation who underwent distal transfer of the tibial tubercle. The authors did not provide a system for computing the measurement of the millimeters of distal transfer of the tibial tubercle, except for maintaining a minimum of 13 mm from the inferior patella pole and proximal tibial surface. A patient satisfaction rate of 88% was reported. Patients with a normal-appearing trochlea had higher scores compared with those with trochlea articular cartilage damage. The study reported cartilage lesions typically involved the inferolateral portion of the lateral patella facet, with possible involvement of the lateral region of the trochlea. The authors stressed that patella alta may be a source of anterior knee pain not responsive to nonoperative treatment as well as a leader to the development of patellofemoral arthritis.

The indications for correcting a patella alta are recurrent dislocations and symptomatic anterior knee pain (and an obvious patella alta) that has not responded to conservative treatment.

Commonly, there are associated patellar crepitus and articular cartilage degeneration, and the patient is advised that symptoms of anterior knee pain related to the arthritis will continue. It is thus preferable to correct a symptomatic patellar alta condition early prior to the development of cartilage deterioration. At the time of a proximal or distal realignment, a patella alta results in the distal patella articular cartilage not engaging the trochlea, but lying in a more cephalad position. It is at this point that lateral subluxation or dislocation events occur, particularly with a dysplastic shallow trochlea. In addition to correcting the patella alta, a functional MPFL is required, because there is a loss of the normal geometric restraint provided by the trochlear groove. There are no established clinically proven rules regarding when correction of an abnormal patella height is required or the amount of correction to be obtained at surgery. The goal is to restore a normal patellar height index for the index chosen and to confirm that patellotrochlear contact (~30% of the inferior patellar articular cartilage) has engaged the trochlear at full extension. These rules are empirical; however, they do provide

TABLE 39–3 Operative Steps in the Technique to Correct Patella Alta

1. Determine abnormal patellar height indices in Figure 39–17. Determine millimeters of distal tibial tubercle transfer necessary to restore patellar height indices to normal values.
2. Determine whether any other abnormality is present requiring correction: MPFL, lateral restraints, patellar tendon offset (TT/TG ratio).
3. Supine position operating table, lower limb draped with high thigh tourniquet.
4. Arthroscopic procedure performed, determine articular cartilage condition of patellofemoral joint, patellotrochlear dysplasia. Medial-lateral manual glide at 30° knee flexion to confirm function MPFL, medial and lateral restraints.
5. Skin incision 4 cm just lateral to tibial tubercle, excise lateral and medial patellar tendon retinaculum, preserve blood supply fat pad and patellar tendon. Subperiosteal limited dissection medial and lateral to tibial tubercle 35 mm.
6. Osteotomize tibial tubercle 8 mm depth × 35 mm length × 15 mm wide. Leave the tibia section proximal to the tibial tubercle which is not included in the osteotomy as described for distal realignment technique. Remove anterior tibial cortex just distal to tibial tubercle the calculated distance to allow distal tibial tubercle displacement. Displace the tibial tubercle distally, avoiding recession, and correcting abnormal lateral tibial tubercle offset when present. Temporary fixation by single 2.7-mm drill bit.
7. Lateral radiograph or fluoroscopy at 0° and 30° knee flexion, measure patellar height indices and adjust tibial tubercle position to restore normal index indices. Patella should engage trochlea at 0° knee flexion (~30% patellar cartilage length).
8. Internal fixation tibial tubercle at new distal position, three cancellous 4.0 mm lagged screws or cortical screws as required.
9. Repeat medial-lateral manual translation (glide) tests at 0 and 30° knee flexion. Majority of knees will require MPFL reconstruction (steps already described). Lateral restraints usually do not require tensioning or release.

MPFL, medial patellofemoral ligament; TT/TG, tibial tubercle/trochlear groove.

the surgeon with guidelines to follow during the surgical technique. The operative steps for the correction of a patella alta are shown in Table 39–3.

Iliotibial Band Z-Plasty Release for Contracture

The technique for a Z-plasty release of a tight ITB is demonstrated in Figure 39–18. After conservative modalities have failed, including one or two local cortical steroid injections, ITB stretching exercises over 4 to 6 months, and a return of symptoms, an ITB release may be indicated. The goal of the procedure is to restore the normal length of the ITB and the normal tension in both arms of the released ITB. The alternative technique that has been described is to remove a window of the ITB, which has the disadvantage of essentially removing the function of the ITB. In addition, there may be remaining anterior and posterior portions of the ITB that still require release. The Z-plasty release has the advantage of restoring normal anatomy. It is important to explore the soft tissues beneath the ITB for abnormal bursae tissue and a sensory nerve.

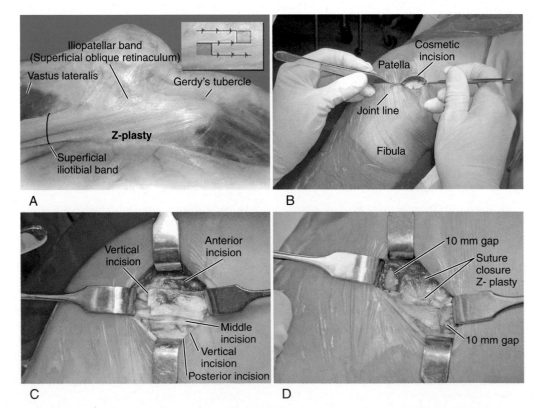

FIGURE 39–18. **A**, The Z-plasty iliotibial band (ITB) procedure for lengthening and preserving function. **B**, Cosmetic incision. **C**, Z-Plasty incision of the ITB. Note three longitudinal incisions and two vertical incisions. **D**, Final appearance of Z-plasty after closure.

POSTOPERATIVE MANAGEMENT

The postoperative rehabilitation protocol is summarized in Table 39–4. This protocol was developed for patients undergoing proximal and distal extensor mechanism realignment procedure, including MPFL reconstruction. Patients are placed into a postoperative long-leg brace for the first 4 weeks. Patellar mobilization in superior-inferior and medial-lateral directions is begun immediately after surgery to prevent parapatellar

Critical Points POSTOPERATIVE MANAGEMENT
• See Table 39–4.
• Postoperative long-leg brace first 4 wk.
• Patellar mobilization begun immediately postoperative.
• 0°–90° 1st wk, full by 8th wk.
• Return to strenuous activities depends on appearance of articular cartilage in the patellofemoral joint

TABLE 39–4 Postoperative Rehabilitation Protocol

	Postoperative			Postoperative Months	
	1-4	5-8	9-12	4-6	7-12
Brace					
Soft postoperative motion	X				
Patellar (optional, symptoms)		X	X	X	X
ROM minimum goals:					
0°–90° (wk 1-2)	X				
0°–110° (wk 3-4)	X				
0°–135°		X			
Weight-bearing:					
25% body weight (wk 1-2)	X				
100% body weight (wk 3-4)	X				
Patella mobilization	X	X			
Modalities					
EMS	X	X			
Biofeedback	X	X			
Pain/edema management (cryotherapy)	X	X			
Stretching					
Hamstring, gastrocnemius-soleus, iliotibial band, quadriceps	X	X	X	X	X
Strengthening					
Quadriceps isometrics, straight leg raises	X	X			
Active knee extension	X	X	X		
Closed-chain; gait retraining, toe raises, wall sits, mini-squats	X	X	X	X	
Knee flexion hamstring curls (90°)	X	X	X	X	X
Knee extension quads (90°–30°)	X	X	X	X	X
Hip abduction-adduction, multi-hip		X	X	X	X
Leg press (70°–10°)		X	X	X	X
Balance/proprioceptive training					
Weight-shifting, minitrampoline, BAPS, KAT, plyometrics	X	X	X	X	X
Conditioning					
UBC	X	X			
Bike (stationary)				X	X
Water-walking		X	X	X	X
Swimming (kicking)			X	X	X
Walking		X	X	X	X
Ski machine		X	X	X	X
Running: straight			X*	X	X
Cutting: lateral carioca, figure eights				X*	X
Full sports				X*	X

*Only for patients with normal articular cartilage in the patellofemoral joint.
BAPS, Biomechanical Ankle Platform System (Camp, Jackson, MI); EMS, electrical muscle stimulation; KAT, Kinesthetic Awareness Trainer (Breg, Inc., Vista, CA); ROM, range of motion; UBC, upper body cycle.

contractures. The goal for the 1st week is to obtain 0° to 90° of motion. Knee flexion is gradually increased to 110° by the 4th week and then full motion of at least 135° is allowed by the 8th week. This limitation of flexion in the first 4 weeks is designed to protect the suture lines and the repair when a proximal realignment procedure is performed. Patients are allowed to bear 25% of their body weight for 2 weeks; full weight-bearing is allowed between the 4th and the 6th week. When a distal realignment osteotomy has not been performed, full weight-bearing after 3 to 4 weeks is allowed based on patient control and muscle strength parameters.

Radiographs are taken the 1st and the 4th postoperative week to ensure adequate position and healing of the osteotomy. Weight-bearing may be delayed if problems are detected in bony healing or in quadriceps control. Flexibility exercises including stretching of hamstrings, gastrocnemius-soleus, quadriceps, and ITB are started in the 1st week. The strengthening program for quadriceps mechanism is begun during the 1st week and gradually progressed. Straight leg raises are allowed after the 3rd week. Open kinetic chain exercises are begun between the 4th and the 6th weeks, because there is usually rapid healing of the osteotomy. In order to initiate a running program, the patient must demonstrate at least 70% of the strength of the noninvolved limb for quadriceps and hamstrings on isometric testing, be at least 3 months postoperative, and have normal articular cartilage surfaces. The return to strenuous activities is markedly dependent on the appearance of the articular cartilage in the patellofemoral joint. Unfortunately, the majority of patients already have deterioration from chronic patellofemoral malalignment. In these patients, the goal of surgery is to return to light, low-impact activities only.

COMPLICATIONS

The common pitfalls related to lateral retinacular release are improper patient selection, incomplete release, excessive or inappropriate release, and inadequate hemostasis. Sectioning of the VLO tendon will cause it to retract, with resultant weakness of quadriceps muscle and patellofemoral imbalance. The ability to evert the patella even at 30°, and certainly at 90°, indicates excessive release of lateral restraints and the VLO tendon insertion, and should be avoided to prevent medial patellar subluxation. A lateral release should also be avoided in a patient with hypermobile patella.

Critical Points COMPLICATIONS

- Lateral retinacular release pitfalls: improper patient selection, incomplete release, excessive or inappropriate release, inadequate hemostasis.
- Proximal realignment: fail if MPFL incompetent, medial plication overtensioned.
- Distal realignment: loss of patellar tendon fixation, delayed union or nonunion of the tibial tubercle, fracture of the bony fragment, inadequate correction, overcorrection with iatrogenic medial subluxation, prominent hardware.
- Other rare complications: infection, compartment syndrome, neurovascular injury, deep venous thrombosis, pulmonary embolism, hemarthrosis, subcutaneous hematoma, arthrofibrosis, patella baja, complex regional pain syndrome.

MPFL, medial patellofemoral ligament.

During the proximal realignment procedure, the three primary sutures should be tied with the knee in 30° of flexion, followed by knee flexion-extension to ensure a full range of motion and normal patellofemoral tracking. The MPFL may be incompetent owing to repeat dislocations or prior surgery. A proximal plication of a thin attenuated MPFL is likely to stretch and fail and should be reconstructed using a QT graft or other tendon graft. Overtensioning of the medial plication or MPFL may produce abnormal patellofemoral contact forces and cartilage deterioration, pain, and limitation of knee flexion.

Potential complications related to distal realignment surgery include loss of patellar tendon fixation, delayed union or nonunion of the tibial tubercle, fracture of the bony fragment, inadequate correction, overcorrection with iatrogenic medial subluxation, and prominent hardware. Rapid healing of the tibial metaphyseal bony fragment is generally achieved owing to the inherent stability of the step-cut osteotomy and intact medial tissues. If the osteotomy is too superficial through the tibial tubercle, resulting in mostly a cortical bony fragment, the potential for delayed union or nonunion is increased. At the distal extent of the osteotomy, a hole is drilled through the tibial cortex to prevent the osteotomy from extending distally. Two to three smaller-diameter screws are used for tibial tubercle fixation to control rotation of the osteotomized bony fragment. These screws often require removal in the future through a minimal approach.

Other postoperative complications should be very rare and include infection, compartment syndrome, neurovascular injury, deep venous thrombosis, pulmonary embolism, hemarthrosis, subcutaneous hematoma, arthrofibrosis, patella baja, and complex regional pain syndrome. The patient should also be informed about the risk of worsening of patellofemoral arthritis symptoms.

CLINICAL STUDIES

MPFL Reconstruction

A summary of the published clinical studies on MPFL graft reconstructions is shown in Table 39–5. A variety of grafts were used, including the gracilis and semitendinosus tendons, the QT, the patellar tendon, the adductor magnus, and artificial ligaments, along with different fixation methods. In the majority of studies, the prevention of recurrent dislocation or subluxation episodes was used as a primary outcome factor, along with rating activities of daily living. Typically, fewer than 5% of patients suffered dislocation or subluxation episodes postoperatively. The most widely used outcome rating instrument was the Kujala score[48] (0–100 points), which was designed to rate patellofemoral disorders by measuring the following factors: limp, support, walking, stairs, squatting, running, jumping, prolonged sitting with knees flexed, pain, swelling, knee subluxation, thigh atrophy, and flexion deficiency. All of the studies reviewed reported statistically significant improvement in this score postoperatively.

Few authors assessed activity levels postoperatively with a validated rating system or determined the effect of articular cartilage damage on outcome. Various techniques were used to ascertain patellar stability, including physical examination and stress radiographs.[19,20,62,63] Because most of the study cohorts were followed short- to mid-term postoperatively (<10 yr), the percentage of patients in whom progression of patellofemoral arthritis occurs after this operation is unknown.

TABLE 39–5   Results of MPFL Reconstruction

Reference	Number of Subjects, Follow-up	Population	Graft, Fixation, Concomitant Procedures	Outcome Measures	Results
Christiansen et al., 2008[13a]	N = 44 Mean, 22 mo (range, 12–32 mo)	Chronic patellar instability, ≥ two prior dislocations, median age 22 yr (range, 12–47 yr), 29 females, 15 males	Gracilis tendon autograft, bioresorbable interference screw femoral condyle, medial tibial tuberosity for significant trochlear dysplasia (N = 12)	Kujala score KOOS scores	64% no pain ADL, 59% no pain sports. Mean Kujala preoperative 46 points, follow-up 84 points. 1 patient dislocation, 3 patients sensation subluxation. Positive apprehension 41%, patellar pain 43%. 1 patella fracture postoperative.
Gomes 2008[35a]	N = 24 Mean, 53 mo (range, 30–71 mo)	N = 12 ST graft N = 12 pedicled adductor magnus graft, mean age 19.3 yr (range, 16–24 yr)	ST free graft, fixation: 2 sutures to lateral retinaculum. Adductor magnus graft: 1 suture to lateral retinaculum, lateral release.	ADL scale	ST group: mean preoperative 50.1 ± 3.73, mean follow-up 72.8 ± 1.7 (NS), no dislocations, 8 patients recreational sports. Adductor magnus group: mean preoperative 50.6 ± 3.8, mean follow-up 72.7 ± 1.27 (NS), 1 patient subluxation, 4 patients recreational sports.
Nomura et al., 2007[68a]	N = 24 knees Mean, 11.9 yr (range, 8.4–17.2 yr)	18 females, 4 males, mean age 22.5 yr (range, 13–48 yr)	Leeds-Keio artificial ligament, staple lateral release 14 knees	Kujala score, Crosby/ Insall score, Kellgren/ Lawrence score x-rays	Mean Kujala preoperative 63.2 points, follow-up 94.2 points (P < .0001), 88% satisfactory clinical results. 2 patients dislocation/subluxation, positive apprehension 5 knees, x-ray slight progression PF arthritis 5 knees, definite progression 2 knees.
Steiner et al., 2006[87a]	N = 34 Mean, 66.5 mo (range, 24–130 mo)	22 females, 12 males, mean age 27 yr. Group A: prior patella dislocations (19) Group B: subjective sensation subluxation (10) Group C: no dislocation or subluxation (5)	Adductor magnus (23), quadriceps tendon (6), patellar tendon (5). Grafts double over patella, sutured to lateral retinaculum, medial retinaculum, quadriceps expansion	Kujala, Lysholm, Tegner	No difference between groups clinical outcomes. Mean Kujala preoperative 53.3 ± 10.2 points, follow-up 90.7 ± 9.0 points (P < .001). Mean Lysholm preoperative 52.4 ± 12.6 points, follow-up 92.1 ± 8.4 (P < .001) points. No dislocations/subluxations.
Mikashima et al., 2006[63]	N = 24 Mean, 41 mo (range, 28–52 mo)	14 females, 10 males, mean age 21.8 yr (range, 13–24 yr)	ST tendon. Group A, ST sutured onto tissue overlying surface of patella. Group B, ST sutured into patellar bone tunnel. MPFL reconstruction combined with distal realignment (Elmslie-Trillat) in knees with > 8° tibial external rotation angle	Kujala score	Mean Kujala preoperative 30.5 ± 6.7 points, mean follow-up 95.2 ± 12.9 points (P not given). 13 sports activities same level, 4 sports reduced level. Patellar fracture 2 patients, positive apprehension test 1 patient. Stress lateral patella shift x-rays: no difference between groups A and B or between all patients and control group.
Nomura & Inoue 2006[67a]	N = 12 Mean, 4.2 yr (range, 3.1–5.6 yr)	All recurrent patellar dislocation, normal Q-angle, 8 females, 4 males, mean age 24.8 yr (range, 13–49 yr)	ST tendon, fixation screw/washer, lateral release 3 knees.	Kujala score Insall grading	Mean Kujala preoperative 56.3 points, follow-up 96 points (P not given). Insall: excellent 8 knees, good 2 knees, fair 2 knees.

Continued

TABLE 39–5 Results of MPFL Reconstruction—Cont'd

Reference	Number of Subjects, Follow-up	Population	Graft, Fixation, Concomitant Procedures	Outcome Measures	Results
Schottle et al., 2005[79a]	N = 15 knees Mean, 47.5 mo (range, 24–70 mo)	All > 1 patellar dislocation, 8 female, 4 male, mean age 30.1 yr (range, 19–36 yr)	ST tendon, fixation absorbable soft tissue interference screw, medialization tibial tuberosity for tibial tuberosity-trochlear groove distance > 15 mm (N = 8)	Kujala score	No dislocation/subluxation events, positive apprehension signs, complications. Mean Kujala preoperative 53.5 points, follow-up 85.7 points ($P < .001$). 86% patients believed knee condition improved. Positive apprehension 4 knees, recurrent instability 2 knees.
Deie et al., 2005[19]	N = 46 knees Mean, 9.5 yr (range, 5–12 yr)	All recurrent patellar dislocation, 34 females, 9 males, mean age 19.2 yr (range, 6–43 yr)	ST tendon left attached distally, fixation sutures either through patellar bone tunnel or onto surface of patella, concurrent lateral release and advancement vastus medialis in 42.	Kujala score	Significant improvement Kujala score ($P < .01$) at 6, 12, 60, 120 mo postoperatively. Positive apprehension in 4 knees, no recurrent instability/dislocation. Stress lateral patella shift x-rays: within normal range postoperatively all patients.
Cossey & Paterson 2005[16a]	N = 21 knees Mean, 23 mo (range, 11–37 mo)	All recurrent patellar dislocation, 11 females, 8 males, mean age 21 yr (range, 18–29 yr)	Strip medial retinacular tissue, lateral release, distal realignment	Lysholm score Tegner score Turba score	Postop Lysholm mean 95.6 points (range, 90–100 points), no recurrent subluxation or dislocation.
Fernandez et al., 2005[27a]	N = 30 knees Mean, 38 mo (range, 12–48 mo)	All recurrent patellar dislocation, 20 females, 8 males, mean age 23 yr (range, 17–28 yr)	ST tendon, lateral release in 2, fixation soft tissue staple, medial transfer tibial tubercle in 2 (Q-angle > 25°)	Larsen and Lauridsen	90% excellent, 7% good, 3% fair. No recurrent subluxation or dislocation.
Mikashima et al., 2004[62]	N = 40 2-yr follow-up	Group E (Elmslie-Trillat realign only): 15 females, 5 males, mean age 26.4 yr (range, 14–45 yr), mean follow-up 41 mo (range, 28–52 mo) Group M (MPFL reconstruction with Elmslie-Trillat realignment): 15 females, 6 males, mean age 26 yr (range, 16–55 yr), mean follow-up 31.7 mo (range, 24–44 mo)	N/A	Kujala score	Group E: mean Kujala preoperative 30.5 points, follow-up 79.6 points. Group M: mean Kujala preoperative 30.1 points, follow-up 89 points. Apprehension sign positive 6 knees in group E, no knees in group M. Lateral stability stress x-rays significantly better in group M than in group E. No complications.
Ellera Gomes et al., 2004[25a]	N = 16 knees 5-yr follow-up	All recurrent patella instability, 11 females, 4 males, mean age 26.7 yr (range, 21–37 yr)	Free ST tendon, suture fixation	Crosby-Insall Aglietti	Crosby-Insall: 11 knees excellent, 4 good, 1 poor Aglietti: 11 excellent, 3 good, 1 fair, 1 poor 8 returned sports, level unknown Apprehension sign positive 1 knee
Deie et al., 2003[20]	N = 6 knees Mean, 7.4 yr (range, 4.8–10 yr)	All recurrent patella instability, 2 girls, 2 boys aged 6–10 yr	ST tendon transfer, fixation sutured to surface of patella	Kujala	Mean Kujala follow-up 96.3 points (range, 89–100 points). No recurrent dislocations. Apprehension sign positive 2 knees in same patient. Lateral and medial stress x-ray ratios abnormal, patella alta 5 knees.
Drez et al., 2001[23a]	N = 14	Majority recurrent patella dislocations, 9 males,	ST tendon (6), STG tendons (5), strip	Kujala Fulkerson	Mean Kujala follow-up 88.6 points (range,

TABLE 39-5   Results of MPFL Reconstruction—Cont'd

Reference	Number of Subjects, Follow-up	Population	Graft, Fixation, Concomitant Procedures	Outcome Measures	Results
	Follow-up, 24–43 mo	5 females, mean age 22 yr (range, 14–52 yr)	ITB (3), fixation suture to periosteum at adductor tubercle and tibial periosteum.	Tegner	57–100 points). 11 patients returned to preinjury activity level (Tegner). Fulkerson: 10 excellent, 4 good, 1 fair. No positive apprehension. Recurrent instability.
Muneta et al., 1999[64a]	N = 6 Follow-up not given	Not described	Gracilis tendon (4), ST tendon (1), ITB allograft (1), fixed spiked staple, sutured surrounding tissue	N/A	"Good stabilization of the patella was achieved in all 6 patients, resulting in improved confidence in higher levels of activity."
Avikainen et al., 1993[3a]	N = 14 Mean, 6.9 yr	Acute or chronic patellar dislocation, 10 females, 4 males, mean age 20 yr (range, 15–27 yr)	Adductor magnus tendon tenodesis	Lysholm	12 patients rated knee as good, 2 as fair. Mean Lysholm follow-up 84 ± 15 points. 1 patient recurrent patellar dislocation.

ADL, activities of daily living; ITB, iliotibial band; KOOS, Knee Injury and Osteoarthritis Outcome Score; MPFL, medial patellofemoral ligament; NS, not significant; PF, patellofemoral, ST, semitendinosus, STG, semitendinosus-gracilis.

Smith and coworkers[86] conducted a systematic review of the existing literature of MPFL reconstruction and found eight studies that met their selection criteria. The authors concluded that the procedure may provide a favorable outcome; however, many methodological problems exist in the published investigations that should be appropriately resolved in future studies. Owing to the heterogeneity of the studies, a formal meta-analysis could not be conducted.

Autologous Chondrocyte Implantation

The initial report of autologous chondrocyte implantation (ACI) used for patellar articular cartilage lesions noted disappointing results,[8] although improvements were noted in two small series of patients[75,77] when the procedure was done with an extensor mechanism realignment. Minas and Bryant[64] reported on 45 patients followed a mean of 46.4 months (range, 2–7 yr) after ACI for lesions in the patellofemoral joint. The lesions were either isolated to the patella or trochlea or combined with condylar defects. Either a concomitant tibial tubercle osteotomy or a high tibial osteotomy was done in 29 of the patients (64%). At follow-up, significant improvements were reported in several subjective scores (Medical Outcomes Study Short-Form 36-item questionnaire [SF-36], Western Ontario and MacMaster Universities [WOMAC], modified Cincinnati activity, all $P < .001$). There were 8 failures caused by a patella or trochlea graft failure. Seventy-one percent of the patients were satisfied with the outcome.

Mandelbaum and associates[54] reported the outcomes of 40 patients (mean age, 37.1 ± 8.5 yr) from 34 centers treated with ACI for isolated trochlear lesions. Before the operation, 48% had undergone a failed microfracture, abrasion arthroplasty, or drilling procedure; 23% had a tibiofemoral osteotomy; and 13% had a lateral release or Fulkerson procedure. At a mean of 59 months (range, 24–84 mo) postoperatively, significant

improvements were noted in scores for pain, swelling, and overall function of the knee. The pain score improved from 2.6 ± 1.7 to 6.2 ± 2.4 points (modified Cincinnati Knee Rating System, scale 0–10 points, $P < .0001$), the swelling score improved from 3.9 ± 2.7 to 6.3 ± 2.7 points ($P < .0001$), and the overall condition score improved from 3.1 ± 1.0 and 6.4 ± 1.7 points ($P < .0001$).

Gobbi and colleagues[35] followed 32 patients who received a "second-generation ACI" Hyalograft-C (Fidia Advanced Biopolymers, Abano Terme, Italy), a tissue-engineered graft composed of autologous chondrocytes grown on a hyaluronan-based three-dimensional scaffold, for isolated defects in the patellofemoral joint. Twenty-two knees had lesions on the patella and 10 on the trochlea. At follow-up, 24 months postoperatively, significant improvement was noted in the mean International Knee Documentation Committee (IKDC) subjective score from 43.2 to 73.6 points ($P < .001$), as well in the objective IKDC rating ($P < .001$). Before the operation, 6 patients were rated on the IKDC objective knee evaluation as nearly normal and the remaining 26, as abnormal or severely abnormal. At follow-up, 29 patients were rated as normal or nearly normal and only 3 as abnormal on this scale. MRI at 24 months postoperatively showed 23 of the grafted defects had greater than 50% fill to complete fill, 25 had a normal or nearly normal signal, and none demonstrated hypertrophy or delamination.

Farr[26] presented the results of a series of 34 knees that received ACI for isolated patella or trochlear lesions. The majority (95%) underwent a staged or concomitant procedure to correct an anatomic disorder, such as anteromedialization (Fulkerson). At follow-up, 2 years postoperatively, a significant improvement was noted in the Cincinnati overall condition rating score ($P < .01$). Nine patients rated their knee condition as excellent, 11 as very good, 11 as good, and 8 as fair or poor. Seven patients required follow-up surgery for mechanical symptoms related to the graft and 5 patients required débridement for arthrofibrosis. There were 3 treatment failures. The author concluded that combining ACI and corrective procedures is worthy of further study.

Henderson and Lavigne[41] compared the results of a group of 22 patients who underwent ACI and concomitant proximal and distal extensor realignment with a group of 22 patients who underwent ACI only, without patellar malalignment. All patients had isolated patellar lesions and were followed from 9 to 55 months postoperatively. There was an even distribution between groups regarding the severity of patellar articular cartilage lesions. At follow-up, significantly higher mean scores were reported in the combined procedure group in the modified Cincinnati overall rating of the knee condition ($P = .001$) score, the SF-36 physical component score ($P < .001$), and IKDC clinical outcome score ($P < .001$). Nine reoperations were required for hypertrophy or extrusion of the graft, but there were no graft failures. The authors postulated that the difference in outcome between the groups may have been from the unloading effect of the realignment (osteotomy), because patellar tracking was normal in all patients postoperatively. The suggestion was made to unload the patellofemoral joint via a realignment procedure when ACI is performed, even in knees with normal patellar tracking.

Peterson and coworkers[74] reported on 17 patients who received ACI for isolated grade III to IV (Outerbridge) patellar lesions. All patients were followed a mean of 7.4 years (range, 5–11 yr) postoperatively and none underwent a concomitant procedure with the ACI. The overall Brittberg clinical score was good or excellent in 65%. Significant improvements were noted in the modified Cincinnati grading of the knee condition score (from 1.6 to 6.8 points), the Lysholm score, and the Brittberg score visual analog score ($P < .001$). There were 4 treatment failures of patients who did not improve in symptoms; however, none of the grafts failed. The authors did not comment on the potential necessity to perform a concomitant proximal-distal realignment with ACI.

Osteochondral Autograft Transfer

Hangody and Fules[38] summarized the results of 831 mosaicplasties, 118 of which were done for lesions located in the patellofemoral joint. The majority of patients (percentage unknown) underwent concomitant patellar realignment procedures. The results were assessed with a variety of scoring systems (modified Hospital for Special Surgery, modified Cincinnati, Lysholm). The clinical scores demonstrated "good-to-excellent" results in 79% of this subset of patients, which were the only data reported. This is the only series published to date to the authors' knowledge on the results of this operation for patellofemoral articular cartilage lesions.

The authors of this chapter have prospectively followed all patients in whom a patellar osteochondral autograft transfer procedure was performed at their center. Between July 1996 and June 2004, a total of 50 osteochondral autograft transfer procedures were done in 43 knees for isolated patellar lesions. Nineteen of these had failed at the time of writing, leaving 31 procedures that have been followed a mean of 62 months (range, 12–121 mo). The 19 procedures that failed occurred in 16 women and 3 men whose mean age at the time of surgery was 36 years (range, 26–50 yr). The average time from surgery to the failure (defined as either revision osteochondral autograft transfer, total knee arthroplasty, patellectomy, patella allograft, or patient designated as requiring any of these procedures) was 36 months (range, 5–120 mo). All but 4 of these patients had sustained an injury to their knee; during daily activities in 6, during work activities in 6, and during sports in 3. An average of 96 months had elapsed (range, 2–324 mo) between the injury or onset of symptoms and the osteochondral autograft transfer procedure.

The 31 patellar osteochondral autograft transfer procedures that had survived at the time of writing were performed in 24 females and 7 males. The mean age at the time of the procedure was 32 years (range, 14–45 yr). Seventeen patients sustained an injury, and 14 patients had a gradual onset of symptoms without an injury. The mean time from the injury or onset of symptoms to the operation was 93 months (range, 6–283 mo). Significant improvements were found in the mean Cincinnati Knee Rating System scores (see Chapter 44, The Cincinnati Knee Rating System) from preoperative to follow-up for pain (2.4 ± 1.2 and 5.2 ± 1.9 points, respectively; $P < .0001$), swelling (3.8 ± 2.1 and 5.5 ± 1.9 points, respectively; $P < .01$), patient perception of the knee condition (2.6 ± 1.2 and 6.1 ± 2.1 points, respectively; $P < .0001$), walking (28 ± 9 and 36 ± 8 points, respectively; $P < .001$), and squatting (10 ± 2 and 16 ± 3 points, respectively; $P = .01$). Two patients rated their knee condition as poor, 3 as fair, 9 as good, 11 as very good, and 1 as normal. Complications included manipulation under anesthesia in 2 patients and reflex sympathetic dystrophy in two patients. The 5 patients who rated their knee condition as fair or poor did not improve in their subjective and functional scores.

The authors of this chapter conclude that current procedures for patellar cartilage lesions provide inconsistent and unpredictable results, representing an unsolved problem and dilemma for the patient and treating surgeon.

ILLUSTRATIVE CASE

Acute Patellar Tendon Rupture. A demonstration of the surgical technique for an acute patellar tendon rupture is shown in Figure 39–19. In Figure 39–19A, the preoperative photograph shows subcutaneous hemorrhage along the anterior aspect of the knee in a patient who sustained a fall and acute rupture of the patellar tendon. The preoperative MRI showed extensive disruption throughout the entire patellar tendon. In Figure 39–19B, the initial exploration shows a "mop-end" appearance to the midsubstance patellar tendon rupture. Figure 39–19C and D shows the method of repair with interrupted baseball locking sutures from the distal tendon to the proximal tendon or through the patellar tunnel based on site of tendon rupture. In this case, a

tendon-to-tendon repair was performed. Two wire sutures are placed through the tibial tubercle and distal one third of patella. One wire suture is placed through the tibial tubercle and distal quadriceps patellar attachment to function as a tension band. The use of wire fixation does involve the need for later removal; however, it provides a firm fixation of low cross-sectional area, which is an advantage over synthetic tape. The length of the repaired patellar tendon is adjusted at surgery and verified by fluoroscopy to be equal to the opposite lateral knee preoperative radiograph. It is important that immediate range of motion from 0° to 90° be initiated within the first 2 weeks after surgery, along with quadriceps muscle exercises to prevent a patella infera.

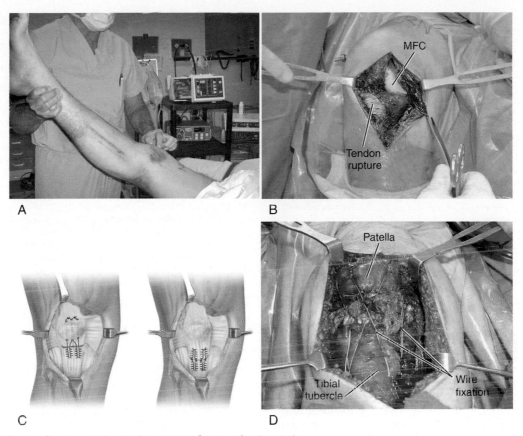

FIGURE 39-19. Repair of acute patellar tendon rupture. See text for description.

The wire fixation allows initial weight-bearing with the knee in extension. A semitendinosus-gracilis graft augmentation was not required in this case, but may be indicated if the patellar tendon is severely disrupted, preventing primary tendon suture. This patient had a successful result and was weaned from crutches at 8 weeks postoperatively, regained a normal range of knee motion, and had a normal patellar height equal to that of the opposite knee. He was cautioned to avoid full weight-bearing on the operative limb in ascending and descending stairs until 20 weeks from surgery, and no sporting activities until 6 months after surgery.

REFERENCES

1. Al-Sayyad, M. J.; Cameron, J. C.: Functional outcome after tibial tubercle transfer for the painful patella alta. *Clin Orthop Relat Res* 396:152–162, 2002.
2. Amis, A. A.: Current concepts on anatomy and biomechanics of patellar stability. *Sports Med Arthrosc* 15:48–56, 2007.
3. Amis, A. A.; Firer, P.; Mountney, J.; et al.: Anatomy and biomechanics of the medial patellofemoral ligament. *Knee* 10:215–220, 2003.
3a. Avikainen, V. J.; Nikku, R. K.; Seppanen-Lehmonen, T. K.: Adductor magnus tenodesis for patellar dislocation. Technique and preliminary results. *Clin Orthop Relat Res* 297:12–16, 1993.
4. Bicos, J.; Fulkerson, J. P.; Amis, A.: Current concepts review: the medial patellofemoral ligament. *Am J Sports Med* 35:484–492, 2007.
5. Biedert, R. M.; Friederich, N. F.: Failed lateral retinacular release: clinical outcome. *J Sports Traumatol* 16:162–173, 1994.
6. Biedert, R. M.; Albrecht, S.: The patellotrochlear index: a new index for assessing patellar height. *Knee Surg Sports Traumatol Arthrosc* 14:707–712, 2006.
7. Blackburne, J.; Peel, T.: A new method for measuring patellar height. *J Bone Joint Surg Br* 58:241–242, 1977.
8. Brittberg, M.; Lindahl, A.; Nilsson, A.; et al.: Treatment of deep cartilage defects in the knee with autologous chondrocyte transplantation. *N Engl J Med* 331:889–895, 1994.
9. Bugbee, W. D.: Fresh osteochondral allografts. *J Knee Surg* 15:191–195, 2002.
10. Bugbee, W. D.; Convery, F. R.: Osteochondral allograft transplantation. *Clin Sports Med* 18:67–75, 1999.
11. Burks, R. T.; Luker, M. G.: Medial patellofemoral ligament reconstruction. *Tech Orthop* 12:185–191, 1997.
12. Cash, J. D.; Hughston, J. C.: Treatment of acute patellar dislocation. *Am J Sports Med* 16:244–249, 1988.
13. Caton, J.; Deschamps, G.; Chambat, P.; et al.: [Patella infera. Apropos of 128 cases]. *Rev Chir Orthop Reparatrice Appar Mot* 68:317–325, 1982.
13a. Christiansen, S. E.; Jacobsen, B. W.; Lund, B.; Lind, M.: Reconstruction of the medial patellofemoral ligament with gracilis tendon autograft in transverse patellar drill holes. *Arthroscopy* 24:82–87, 2008.
14. Christoforakis, J.; Bull, A. M.; Strachan, R. K.; et al.: Effects of lateral retinacular release on the lateral stability of the patella. *Knee Surg Sports Traumatol Arthrosc* 14:273–277, 2006.
15. Cofield, R. H.; Bryan, R. S.: Acute dislocation of the patella: results of conservative treatment. *J Trauma* 17:526–531, 1977.
16. Conlan, T.; Garth, W. P., Jr.; Lemons, J. E.: Evaluation of the medial soft-tissue restraints of the extensor mechanism of the knee. *J Bone Joint Surg Am* 75:682–693, 1993.
16a. Cossey, A. J.; Paterson, R.: A new technique for reconstructing the medial patellofemoral ligament. *Knee* 12:93–98, 2005.
17. Cowan, S. M.; Bennell, K. L.; Crossley, K. M.; et al.: Physical therapy alters recruitment of the vasti in patellofemoral pain syndrome. *Med Sci Sports Exerc* 34:1879–1885, 2002.
18. Crossley, K.; Bennell, K.; Green, S.; et al.: Physical therapy for patellofemoral pain: a randomized, double-blinded, placebo-controlled trial. *Am J Sports Med* 30:857–865, 2002.

19. Deie, M.; Ochi, M.; Sumen, Y.; et al.: A long-term follow-up study after medial patellofemoral ligament reconstruction using the transferred semitendinosus tendon for patellar dislocation. *Knee Surg Sports Traumatol Arthrosc* 13:522–528, 2005.

20. Deie, M.; Ochi, M.; Sumen, Y.; et al.: Reconstruction of the medial patellofemoral ligament for the treatment of habitual or recurrent dislocation of the patella in children. *J Bone Joint Surg Br* 85:887–890, 2003.

21. Dejour, H.; Neyret, P.; Walch, G.: Factors in patellar instability. In Aichroth, P. M.; Cannon, W. D. (eds.): *Knee Surgery. Current Practice.* New York, Raven, 1992; pp. 403–412.

22. Dejour, H.; Walch, G.; Nove-Josserand, L.; Guier, C.: Factors of patellar instability: an anatomic radiographic study. *Knee Surg Sports Traumatol Arthrosc* 2:19–26, 1994.

23. Desio, S. M.; Burks, R. T.; Bachus, K. N.: Soft tissue restraints to lateral patellar translation in the human knee. *Am J Sports Med* 26:59–65, 1998.

23a. Drez, D. Jr.; Edwards, T. B.; Williams, C. S.: Results of medial patellofemoral ligament reconstruction in the treatment of patellar dislocation. *Arthroscopy* 17:298–306, 2001.

24. Dye, S. F.: The pathophysiology of patellofemoral pain: a tissue homeostasis perspective. *Clin Orthop Relat Res* 436:100–110, 2005.

25. Eckhoff, D. G.; Brown, A. W.; Kilcoyne, R. F.; Stamm, E. R.: Knee version associated with anterior knee pain. *Clin Orthop Relat Res* 339:152–155, 1997.

25a. Ellera Gomes, J. L.; Stigler Marczyk, L. R.; Cesar de Cesar, P.; Jungblut, C. F.: Medial patellofemoral ligament reconstruction with semitendinosus autograft for chronic patellar instability: a follow-up study. *Arthroscopy* 20:147–151, 2004.

26. Farr, J.: Autologous chondrocyte implantation improves patellofemoral cartilage treatment outcomes. *Clin Orthop Relat Res* 463:187–194, 2007.

27. Feller, J. A.; Amis, A. A.; Andrish, J. T.; et al.: Surgical biomechanics of the patellofemoral joint. *Arthroscopy* 23:542–553, 2007.

27a. Fernandez, E.; Sala, D.; Castejon, M.: Reconstruction of the medial patellofemoral ligament for patellar instability using a semitendinosus autograft. *Acta Orthop Belg* 71:303–308, 2005.

28. Ferris, B.; Aichroth, P.: The treatment of congenital knee dislocation. A review of nineteen knees. *Clin Orthop Relat Res* 216:135–140, 1987.

29. Fithian, D. C.; Mishra, D. K.; Balen, P. F.; et al.: Instrumented measurement of patellar mobility. *Am J Sports Med* 23:607–615, 1995.

30. Fithian, D. C.; Paxton, E. W.; Stone, M. L.; et al.: Epidemiology and natural history of acute patellar dislocation. *Am J Sports Med* 32:1114–1121, 2004.

31. Froelke, B. M.; Elias, J. J.; Cosgarea, A. J.: Surgical options for treating injuries to the medial patellofemoral ligament. *J Knee Surg* 19:296–306, 2006.

32. Fulkerson, J. P.: Diagnosis and treatment of patients with patellofemoral pain. *Am J Sports Med* 30:447–456, 2002.

33. Fulkerson, J. P.; Becker, G. J.; Meaney, J. A.; et al.: Anteromedial tibial tubercle transfer without bone graft. *Am J Sports Med* 18:490–496; discussion 496–497, 1990.

34. Garth, W. P., Jr.; DiChristina, D. G.; Holt, G.: Delayed proximal repair and distal realignment after patellar dislocation. *Clin Orthop Relat Res* 377:132–144, 2000.

35. Gobbi, A.; Kon, E.; Berruto, M.; et al.: Patellofemoral full-thickness chondral defects treated with Hyalograft-C: a clinical, arthroscopic, and histologic review. *Am J Sports Med* 34:1763–1773, 2006.

35a. Gomes, J. E.: Comparison between a static and a dynamic technique for medial patellofemoral ligament reconstruction. *Arthroscopy* 24:430–435, 2008.

36. Grelsamer, R. P.; Stein, D. A.: Patellofemoral arthritis. *J Bone Joint Surg Am* 88:1849–1860, 2006.

37. Guenther, K. P.; Tomczak, R.; Kessler, S.; et al.: Measurement of femoral anteversion by magnetic resonance imaging—evaluation of a new technique in children and adolescents. *Eur J Radiol* 21: 47–52, 1995.

38. Hangody, L.; Fules, P.: Autologous osteochondral mosaicplasty for the treatment of full-thickness defects of weight-bearing joints: ten years of experimental and clinical experience. *J Bone Joint Surg Am* 85(suppl 2):25–32, 2003.

39. Hautamaa, P. V.; Fithian, D. C.; Kaufman, K. R.; et al.: Medial soft tissue restraints in lateral patellar instability and repair. *Clin Orthop Relat Res* 349:174–182, 1998.

40. Hawkins, R. J.; Bell, R. H.; Anisette, G.: Acute patellar dislocations. The natural history. *Am J Sports Med* 14:117–120, 1986.

41. Henderson, I. J.; Lavigne, P.: Periosteal autologous chondrocyte implantation for patellar chondral defect in patients with normal and abnormal patellar tracking. *Knee* 13:274–279, 2006.

42. Hughston, J. C.; Deese, M.: Medial subluxation of the patella as a complication of lateral retinacular release. *Am J Sports Med* 16:383–388, 1988.

42a. Insall, J.; Salvati, E.: Patella position in the normal knee joint. *Radiology* 101:101–104, 1971.

43. Jamali, A. A.; Emmerson, B. C.; Chung, C.; et al.: Fresh osteochondral allografts. *Clin Orthop Relat Res* 437:176–185, 2005.

44. Johnson, D. P.; Wakeley, C.: Reconstruction of the lateral patellar retinaculum following lateral release: a case report. *Knee Surg Sports Traumatol Arthrosc* 10:361–363, 2002.

45. Kannus, P.; Nittymaki, S.: Which factors predict outcome in the nonoperative treatment of patellofemoral pain syndrome? A prospective follow-up study. *Med Sci Sports Exerc* 26:289–296, 1994.

46. Koeter, S.; Diks, M. J.; Anderson, P. G.; Wymenga, A. B.: A modified tibial tubercle osteotomy for patellar maltracking: results at two years. *J Bone Joint Surg Br* 89:180–185, 2007.

47. Kolowich, P. A.; Paulos, L. E.; Rosenberg, T. D.; et al.: Lateral release of the patella: indications and contraindications. *Am J Sports Med* 18:359–365, 1990.

48. Kujala, U. M.; Jaakkola, L. H.; Koskinen, S. K.; et al.: Scoring of patellofemoral disorders. *Arthroscopy* 9:159–163, 1993.

49. Lancourt, J. E.; Cristini, J. A.: Patella alta and patella infera. Their etiological role in patellar dislocation, chondromalacia, and apophysitis of the tibial tubercle. *J Bone Joint Surg Am* 57:1112–1115, 1975.

50. Larsen, E.; Lauridsen, F.: Conservative treatment of patellar dislocations. Influence of evident factors on the tendency to redislocation and the therapeutic result. *Clin Orthop Relat Res* 171:131–136, 1982.

51. Linclau, L.: Measuring patellar height. *Acta Orthop Belg* 50:70–74, 1984.

52. Maenpaa, H.; Huhtala, H.; Lehto, M. U.: Recurrence after patellar dislocation. Redislocation in 37/75 patients followed for 6-24 years. *Acta Orthop Scand* 68:424–426, 1997.

53. Maenpaa, H.; Lehto, M. U.: Patellar dislocation. The long-term results of nonoperative management in 100 patients. *Am J Sports Med* 25:213–217, 1997.

54. Mandelbaum, B.; Browne, J. E.; Fu, F.; et al.: Treatment outcomes of autologous chondrocyte implantation for full-thickness articular cartilage defects of the trochlea. *Am J Sports Med* 35:915–921, 2007.

55. Maquet, P.: Valgus osteotomy for osteoarthritis of the knee. *Clin Orthop Relat Res* 120:143–148, 1976.

56. Marks, K. E.; Bentley, G.: Patella alta and chondromalacia. *J Bone Joint Surg Br* 60:71–73, 1978.

57. McGinty, J. B.; McCarthy, J. C.: Endoscopic lateral retinacular release: a preliminary report. *Clin Orthop Relat Res* 158:120–125, 1981.

58. Meister, K.; James, S. L.: Proximal tibial derotation osteotomy for anterior knee pain in the miserably malaligned extremity. *Am J Orthop* 24:149–155, 1995.

59. Merchant, A. C.; Mercer, R. L.; Jacobsen, R. H.; Cool, C.: Roentgenographic analysis of patellofemoral congruence. *J Bone Joint Surg Am* 56:1391–1396, 1974.

60. Metcalf, R. W.: An arthroscopic method for lateral release of subluxating or dislocating patella. *Clin Orthop Relat Res* 167:9–18, 1982.

61. Mihalko, W. M.; Boachie-Adjei, Y.; Spang, J. T.; et al.: Controversies and techniques in the surgical management of patellofemoral arthritis. *Instr Course Lect* 57:365–380, 2008.

62. Mikashima, Y.; Kimura, M.; Kobayashi, Y.; et al.: Medial patellofemoral ligament reconstruction for recurrent patellar instability. *Acta Orthop Belg* 70:545–550, 2004.

63. Mikashima, Y.; Kimura, M.; Kobayashi, Y.; et al.: Clinical results of isolated reconstruction of the medial patellofemoral ligament for recurrent dislocation and subluxation of the patella. *Acta Orthop Belg* 72:65–71, 2006.

64. Minas, T.; Bryant, T.: The role of autologous chondrocyte implantation in the patellofemoral joint. *Clin Orthop Relat Res* 436:30–39, 2005.

64a. Muneta, T.; Sekiya, I.; Tsuchiya, M.; Shinomiya, K.: A technique for reconstruction of the medial patellofemoral ligament. *Clin Orthop Relat Res* 359:151–155, 1999.

65. Murphy, S. B.; Simon, S. R.; Kijewski, P. K.; et al.: Femoral anteversion. *J Bone Joint Surg Am* 69:1169–1176, 1987.

66. Neyret, P.; Robinson, A. H.; Le Coultre, B.; et al.: Patellar tendon length—the factor in patellar instability? *Knee* 9:3–6, 2002.

67. Nomura, E.: Classification of lesions of the medial patello-femoral ligament in patellar dislocation. *Int Orthop* 23:260–263, 1999.

67a. Nomura, E.; Inoue, M.: Hybrid medial patellofemoral ligament reconstruction using the semitendinous tendon for recurrent patellar dislocation: minimum 3 years' follow-up. *Arthroscopy* 22:787–793, 2006.

68. Nomura, E.; Horiuchi, Y.; Kihara, M.: Medial patellofemoral ligament restraint in lateral patellar translation and reconstruction. *Knee* 7:121–127, 2000.

68a. Nomura, E.; Inoue, M.; Kobayashi, S.: Long-term follow-up and knee osteoarthritis change after medial patellofemoral ligament reconstruction for recurrent patellar dislocation. *Am J Sports Med* 35:1851–1858, 2007.

69. Nonweiler, D. E.; DeLee, J. C.: The diagnosis and treatment of medial subluxation of the patella after lateral retinacular release. *Am J Sports Med* 22:680–686, 1994.

70. Noyes, F. R.; Stabler, C. L.: A system for grading articular cartilage lesions at arthroscopy. *Am J Sports Med* 17:505–513, 1989.

71. Noyes, F. R.; Wojtys, E. M.; Marshall, M. T.: The early diagnosis and treatment of developmental patella infera syndrome. *Clin Orthop* 265:241–252, 1991.

72. Palmu, S.; Kallio, P. E.; Donell, S. T.; et al.: Acute patellar dislocation in children and adolescents: a randomized clinical trial. *J Bone Joint Surg Am* 90:463–470, 2008.

73. Panagiotopoulos, E.; Strzelczyk, P.; Herrmann, M.; Scuderi, G.: Cadaveric study on static medial patellar stabilizers: the dynamizing role of the vastus medialis obliquus on medial patellofemoral ligament. *Knee Surg Sports Traumatol Arthrosc* 14:7–12, 2006.

74. Peterson, L.; Brittberg, M.; Kiviranta, I.; et al.: Autologous chondrocyte transplantation. Biomechanics and long-term durability. *Am J Sports Med* 30:2–12, 2002.

75. Peterson, L.; Karlsson, J.; Brittberg, M.: Patellar instability with recurrent dislocation due to patellofemoral dysplasia. Results after surgical treatment. *Bull Hosp Jt Dis Orthop Inst* 48:130–139, 1988.

76. Peterson, L.; Minas, T.; Brittberg, M.; Lindahl, A.: Treatment of osteochondritis dissecans of the knee with autologous chondrocyte transplantation. Results at two to ten years. *J Bone Joint Surg Am* 85(suppl 2):17–24, 2003.

77. Peterson, L.; Minas, T.; Brittberg, M.; Nilsson, A.; et al.: Two- to 9-year outcome after autologous chondrocyte transplantation of the knee. *Clin Orthop Relat Res* 374:212–234, 2000.

78. Sallay, P. I.; Poggi, J.; Speer, K. P.; Garrett, W. E.: Acute dislocation of the patella. A correlative pathoanatomic study. *Am J Sports Med* 24:52–60, 1996.

79. Sayli, U.; Bolukbasi, S.; Atik, O. S.; Gundogdu, S.: Determination of tibial torsion by computed tomography. *J Foot Ankle Surg* 33:144–147, 1994.

79a. Schottle, P. B.; Fucentese, S. F.; Romero, J.: Clinical and radiological outcome of medial patellofemoral ligament reconstruction with a semitendinosus autograft for patella instability. *Knee Surg Sports Traumatol Arthrosc* 13:516–521, 2005.

80. Seil, R.; Muller, B.; Georg, T.; et al.: Reliability and interobserver variability in radiological patellar height ratios. *Knee Surg Sports Traumatol Arthrosc* 8:231–236, 2000.

81. Senavongse, W.; Amis, A. A.: The effects of articular, retinacular, or muscular deficiencies on patellofemoral joint stability. *J Bone Joint Surg Br* 87:577–582, 2005.

82. Servien, E.; Verdonk, P. C.; Neyret, P.: Tibial tuberosity transfer for episodic patellar dislocation. *Sports Med Arthrosc* 15:61–67, 2007.

83. Shabshin, N.; Schweitzer, M. E.; Morrison, W. B.; Parker, L.: MRI criteria for patella alta and baja. *Skeletal Radiol* 33:445–450, 2004.

84. Shea, K. P.; Fulkerson, J. P.: Preoperative computed tomography scanning and arthroscopy in predicting outcome after lateral retinacular release. *Arthroscopy* 8:327–334, 1992.

85. Sillanpaa, P.; Mattila, V. M.; Iivonen, T.; et al.: Incidence and risk factors of acute traumatic primary patellar dislocation. *Med Sci Sports Exerc* 40:606–611, 2008.

86. Smith, T. O.; Walker, J.; Russell, N.: Outcomes of medial patellofemoral ligament reconstruction for patellar instability: a systematic review. *Knee Surg Sports Traumatol Arthrosc* 15:1301–1314, 2007.

87. Stefancin, J. J.; Parker, R. D.: First-time traumatic patellar dislocation: a systematic review. *Clin Orthop Relat Res* 455:93–101, 2007.

87a. Steiner, T. M.; Torga-Spak, R.; Teitge, R. A.: Medial patellofemoral ligament reconstruction in patients with lateral patellar instability and trochlear dysplasia. *Am J Sports Med* 34:1254–1261, 2006.

88. Tamari, K.; Tinley, P.; Briffa, K.; Breidahl, W.: Validity and reliability of existing and modified clinical methods of measuring femoral and tibiofibular torsion in healthy subjects: use of different reference axes may improve reliability. *Clin Anat* 18:46–55, 2005.

89. Teitge, R. A.: Osteotomy in the treatment of patellofemoral instability. *Tech Knee Surg* 5:2–18, 2006.

90. Teitge, R. A.; Faerber, W. W.; Des Madryl, P.; Matelic, T. M.: Stress radiographs of the patellofemoral joint. *J Bone Joint Surg Am* 78:193–203, 1996.

91. Thomee, R.; Renstrom, P.; Karlsson, J.; Grimby, G.: Patellofemoral pain syndrome in young women. I. A clinical analysis of alignment, pain parameters, common symptoms and functional activity level. *Scand J Med Sci Sports* 5:237–244, 1995.

92. Trikha, S. P.; Acton, D.; O'Reilly, M.; et al.: Acute lateral dislocation of the patella: correlation of ultrasound scanning with operative findings. *Injury* 34:568–571, 2003.

93. Trillat, A.; Dejour, H.; Conette, A.: [Diagnosis and treatment of recurrent dislocations of the patella]. *Rev Chir Orthop Reparatrice Appar Mot* 50:813–824, 1964.

94. Turner, M. S.: The association between tibial torsion and knee joint pathology. *Clin Orthop Relat Res* 302:47–51, 1994.

95. Ward, S. R.; Terk, M. R.; Powers, C. M.: Patella alta: association with patellofemoral alignment and changes in contact area during weight-bearing. *J Bone Joint Surg Am* 89:1749–1755, 2007.

96. Witvrouw, E.; Danneels, L.; Van Tiggelen, D.; et al.: Open versus closed kinetic chain exercises in patellofemoral pain: a 5-year prospective randomized study. *Am J Sports Med* 32:1122–1130, 2004.

97. Yoshioka, Y.; Cooke, T. D.: Femoral anteversion: assessment based on function axes. *J Orthop Res* 5:86–91, 1987.

98. Yoshioka, Y.; Siu, D. W.; Scudamore, R. A.; Cooke, T. D.: Tibial anatomy and functional axes. *J Orthop Res* 7:132–137, 1989.

Chapter 40

Patellofemoral Disorders: Correction of Rotational Malalignment of the Lower Extremity

Robert A. Teitge, MD

INTRODUCTION

This chapter reviews the concept of torsional malalignment of the lower limb and its importance on patellofemoral (PF) pathology. This topic was first well reviewed by Stan James, M.D., in which he introduced the term "miserable malalignment."[15] His classic description is highly recommended reading.

Critical Points INTRODUCTION

- Chapter reviews the concept of torsional malalignment of the lower limb and its importance on patellofemoral pathology.
- The treatment of patellofemoral disease remains without consensus, with little agreement on definition of terms.
- The term *malalignment* is used to refer to a limb that deviates from normal in any one plane or any combination of the three anatomic planes: coronal (frontal), sagittal, or transverse (horizontal).
- Abnormal geometry results in unusual force transmissions through the patellofemoral joint during gait; however, clinical studies rarely review limb alignment adequately.
- Over 50 independent observations have been reported in the literature to be associated with anterior knee pain, chondromalacia, patellar instability, or patellar malalignment.
- Author considers four independent but related variables that must be assessed: skeletal geometry, ligaments, articular cartilage (patella and trochlea), and musculotendinous units.

It is essential in a chapter on osteotomy for treating PF symptoms to place this operation in proper context relative to other surgical procedures. The treatment of PF disease remains without consensus. There is little agreement on definitions. Objective evidence is scant. Most studies lack precise terminology and complete physical examinations, use incomparable imaging studies, and refer to incomplete biomechanical studies. The terms *malalignment, instability, subluxation, dislocation, chondromalacia, chondropathy,* and *anterior knee pain* are inappropriately used interchangeably. Measurements lack objectivity and validation.

Confusion exists in the literature regarding the term *malalignment.* Insall and coworkers[13] in 1976 defined *patellar malalignment* as being either an increased Q-angle or a high-riding patella. No other options were considered. Then, Insall and coworkers observed that "an increased Q-angle is usually associated with increased femoral anteversion and external tibial torsion. In the presence of these abnormalities when the hip and ankle joints are normally aligned, the patella faces inward and motion of the knee occurs about an axis which is rotated medially compared with the axes of the hip and ankle joints." These authors recommended a medial tibial tubercle transfer or "patellar realignment" to treat this torsional malalignment, and it is no small wonder that the investigation reported that 61% of the patients remained symptomatic. Clearly, the underlying pathoanatomy had not been addressed. Tibial tubercle transfer has been shown to cause external rotation of the tibia on the femur rather than pull the patella medially into the trochlea.[17] In addition, this procedure has been shown to increase medial compartment loading[20] and medial facet loading. This author does not use the term "patellar malalignment" or "patellar realignment," and reserves the term *malalignment* to refer only to a limb that deviates from normal in any one plane or any combination of the three anatomic planes: coronal (frontal), sagittal, or transverse (horizontal). Limb alignment is a direct result of the shape of the bones in the limb, but malalignment may be the result of acquired cartilage or ligament loss in which the deformity exists at the joint and not the bones.

Normal alignment is presumed to be normal because it is the optimal limb geometry for the transfer of the body mass to the ground. Abnormal geometry results in unusual force transmissions through the PF joint during gait. Rarely have published PF clinical studies adequately reviewed limb alignment. The precise variation from the normal skeleton is generally not specified, ranges of motion of all joints in all planes of the lower extremity have not been adequately recorded, and ligamentous stability is not measured.

Over 50 independent observations have been reported in the literature to be associated with anterior knee pain, chondromalacia, patellar instability, or patellar malalignment (Table 40-1).

Whereas these factors may be very important, objective measurement tools are lacking. No study has ever tried to assess all these variables in a single cohort of patients, and even if this were undertaken, the lack of objective measurement techniques would make the study invalid. If these variables are indeed important, then any study would need to incorporate accurate measurements of each. The relative importance of each will need to be developed. Without this, clinicians are left with a realization that data do not exist to guide in the knowledge of pathomechanics, diagnosis, and treatment and that we depend only on unrelated clinical observations and some very basic laboratory studies.

Table 40-1 shows the variables related to PF syndrome, anterior knee pain, PF instability, chondromalacia, and PF arthritis. The contributions of these variables need to be defined, measured, and validated before any meaningful outcome studies can be completed. It is critical to simplify the confusing clinical picture created by so many variables. Toward this end, this author considers that there are only four independent but related variables to assess. Each of the conditions just discussed can be fitted into one of these four: skeletal geometry, ligaments, articular cartilage (patella and trochlea), and musculotendinous units.

BASIC ASSUMPTIONS

The geometry of the skeleton determines the direction of the load applied on the PF joint. The PF ligaments acting against the patella in the trochlea are responsible for stability. Articular cartilage reduces friction to conserve energy and to transmit force generated by a combination of body mass, momentum, gravity, and muscles. The musculotendinous units move the skeleton, stop it from moving, or hold it against gravity but are not normally responsible for preventing joint dislocation or subluxation.

TABLE 40-1 Cited Contributions to Patellofemoral Dysfunction	
Genu valgum	Genu varum
Femoral anteversion	Femoral retroversion
Excess external tibial torsion	Excessive internal tibial torsion
Outerbridge ridge	Trochlear dysplasia
Shallow trochlea	Short lateral trochlea
Increased Q-angle	Decreased Q-angle
Excessive lateral quadriceps pull	Insufficient vastus medialis obliquus
Decreased patellar surface contact area	Abnormal patellar spin
Patellar dysplasia	Patella alta
Patella baja (infera)	Meniscectomy
Laxity of ACL, PCL, MCL, or FCL	Rotatory instability
Iliotibial band contracture	Quadriceps contracture
Achilles contracture	Retinacular contracture
Retinacular laxity	Hyperpronation
Pes planus	Tibial tubercle–trochlear groove distance (TT/TG)
Patellar malalignment	Patellar instability
Patellar subluxation	Medial patellar dislocation
Lateral patellar dislocation	Chondral softening
Genu recurvatum	Patellar tilt
Patellar shift	Abnormal (mal) tracking
VMO dysplasia	J sign
A sign	Bayonet sign
Crossing sign	Trochlear bump
Patellar thickness	Knee flexion contracture
Infrapatellar contracture	VMO/VLO ratio
Rearfoot varus	Patellar glide
Quadriceps tendon width	Flexor hallucis longus tendon entrapment
Flexor hallucis dysfunction	Increased lumbosacral instability
Hip flexion contracture	Abdominal oblique: rectus femoris + psoas imbalance
Quadriceps atrophy	Pelvic abductor weakness
Increased thoracolumbar extension	Inward pointing knee
Female gender	

ACL, anterior cruciate ligament; FCL, fibular collateral ligament; MCL, medial collateral ligament; PCL, posterior cruciate ligament; VLO, vastus lateralis obliquus; VMO, vastus medialis obliquus.

Critical Points BASIC ASSUMPTIONS
<ul><li>The geometry of the skeleton determines the direction of the load applied on the patellofemoral joint.</li><li>The patellofemoral ligaments are responsible for stability.</li><li>Articular cartilage reduces friction to conserve energy and to transmit force generated by a combination of body mass, momentum, gravity, and muscles.</li><li>The musculotendinous units move the skeleton, stop it from moving, or hold it against gravity, but are not normally responsible for preventing joint dislocation or subluxation.</li><li>Assessment<ul><li>Limb alignment: physical examination, coronal standing radiographs, sagittal radiographs, and rotational CT studies.</li><li>Ligaments: physical examination, stress radiographs.</li><li>Articular cartilage: double-contrast CT arthrography with fine cuts.</li><li>Musculotendinous units: usual clinical tests of strength, orientation, flexibility.</li></ul></li><li>Patellar instability results from a loss of the patellar stabilizers and often an excess of displacement forces.</li><li>Patellar stabilizers: trochlear groove, medial and lateral patellofemoral ligaments, medial and lateral meniscopatellar ligaments.</li><li>For lateral patellar dislocation to occur, the medial patellofemoral ligament must be injured.</li><li>Arthrosis or chondromalacia exists when articular cartilage fails as the force per unit area exceeds biologic tolerance.</li></ul>

CT, computed tomography.

It has been useful to independently assess these four structures and then try to understand the cause-and-effect relationship between each. This integrated picture is then used to develop an understanding of the pathomechanics, diagnosis, and logical treatment.

This author uses physical examination, coronal standing radiographs, sagittal radiographs, and rotational computed tomography (CT) studies to assess limb alignment. Physical examination and stress radiography[43] are used to assess ligament insufficiency. Double-contrast CT arthrography with fine cuts determines the thickness of articular cartilage and the location and size of various focal defects. The usual clinical tests of strength, orientation, and flexibility (e.g., Ober test, prone rectus test, straight leg raising, Achilles contracture) are used to assess musculotendinous units.

Patellar instability results from a loss of the patellar stabilizers and often an excess of displacement forces. The patellar stabilizers are the trochlear groove and the ligaments (both the medial and the lateral patellofemoral ligaments) and the medial and lateral meniscopatellar ligaments. Brattström,[2] as early as 1964, demonstrated that in recurrent dislocation of the patella, a flattening or dysplasia of the trochlear groove is nearly always present. Dejour and colleagues[6] demonstrated that this dysplasia

is often in the proximal portion of the trochlea not seen on an axial patellofemoral radiograph. This can be measured on a true lateral knee radiograph by recognizing the floor of the groove and the anterior projections of the medial and lateral condyles. For lateral patellar dislocation to occur, the medial patellofemoral ligament (MPFL) must be injured. A number of authors including Christoforakis and associates[4] and Desio and colleagues[8] have demonstrated in the laboratory that the lateral retinaculum provides up to 19% of the resistance against lateral displacement; thus, the patella is usually more unstable after lateral retinacular release. Medial dislocation is a distinct possibility and this author reported 70 cases confirmed with stress radiography in 1990 (Annual Meeting of the American Academy of Orthopaedic Surgeons). The diagnosis of instability requires a force and displacement examination and stress radiography may provide documentation (Figs. 40–1 and 40–2), because unstressed radiographs are normal but stress application demonstrates obvious excessive displacement.

A frequent contributing cause of patellar dislocation is the existence of an abnormally high displacement force. This most often occurs when the direction of the lateral quadriceps vector is increased. This commonly occurs when the femur twists away

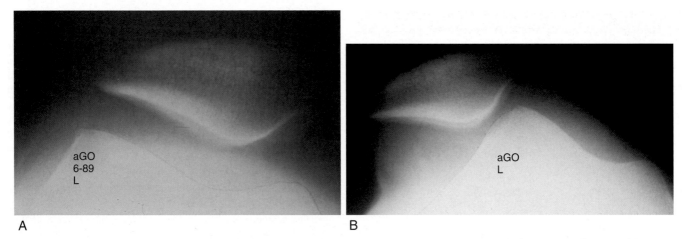

FIGURE 40–1. A, An 18-year-old patient complained of anterior knee pain and giving-way, without history of dislocation. Radiographic parameters were normal. **B,** Stress application was necessary to demonstrate dislocation.

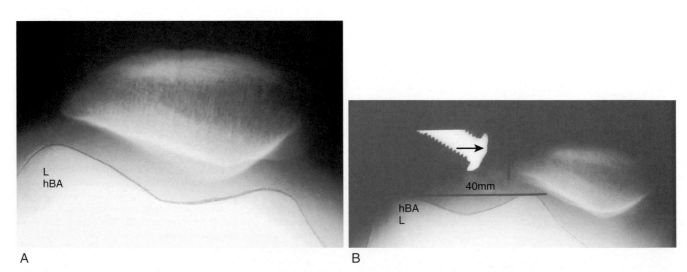

FIGURE 40–2. A, Radiograph of a 38-year-old woman with anterior knee pain after a dashboard injury. Symptoms worsened after a lateral retinacular release. Radiographic parameters were normal. **B,** Stress radiographs demonstrated medial dislocation.

from under the patella, most often in the direction of medial rotation. This is usually due to some torsional abnormality of the lower limb (Fig. 40–3). In the face of such excess displacement forces, a PF ligament reconstruction may fail.

Arthrosis or chondromalacia exists when articular cartilage fails as the force per unit area exceeds biologic tolerance. For acute fractures of articular cartilage, this may be in the range of 20 MPa. In the case of chronic overload due to a too small articular surface area or too much body weight, muscle loading or long lever arms with chronic pressure exceeding 5 MPa may lead to arthrosis. Articular fractures exist approximately 90% of the time after acute patellar dislocation.[31] Although magnetic resonance imaging (MRI) is often used to demonstrate articular cartilage lesions, Figure 40–4 gives an example of pathology clearly seen with double-contrast CT arthrography not visualized on MRI. Rotational malalignment is often a major contributing cause of pain, instability, and cartilage injury, but the evidence of how much benefit can be derived from rotational osteotomy in the presence of instability and arthrosis is unknown.

HOW DOES LONG BONE TORSION AFFECT THE PF JOINT?

The knee joint axis moves straight forward during gait, with a small (<10°) turning inward and outward.[27] The foot also tends to move in a fairly constant direction (foot progression angle).[28,37] The geometry of the lower extremity skeleton largely determines the direction of load applied at the PF joint, with the amount of load depending on the body mass, the length of the lever arms, the surface area of the PF joint, and the velocity of the moving system. If the knee joint axis is twisted out of its normal plane of flexion and extension while the quadriceps is contracting, a side directed force is created that acts on the patella, attempting to displace it. This causes an increased strain on the PF ligaments and retinaculum and an imbalanced direction of force on the PF articular surface.

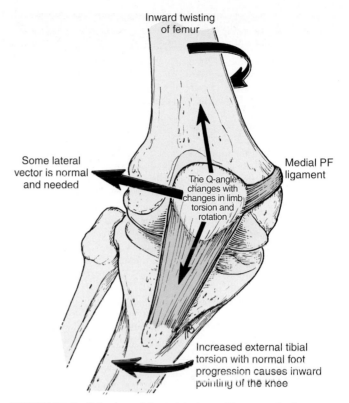

FIGURE 40–3. If the knee joint twists inward because the femur twists inward, the lateral pull on the quadriceps is increased, the lateral displacement pull on the patella is increased, the strain on the medial patellofemoral ligament (MPFL) ligament is increased, the compression on the lateral patellar facet is increased, and the compression on the medial patellar facet is decreased. The treatment must be to decrease the inward twist on the knee joint, not to move the tubercle medially. A similar increase of inward pointing of the knee joint occurs in the presence of excess external tibial torsion when the foot is pointed forward.

Labels on figure: Inward twisting of femur / Some lateral vector is normal and needed / The Q-angle changes with changes in limb torsion and rotation / Medial PF ligament / Increased external tibial torsion with normal foot progression causes inward pointing of the knee

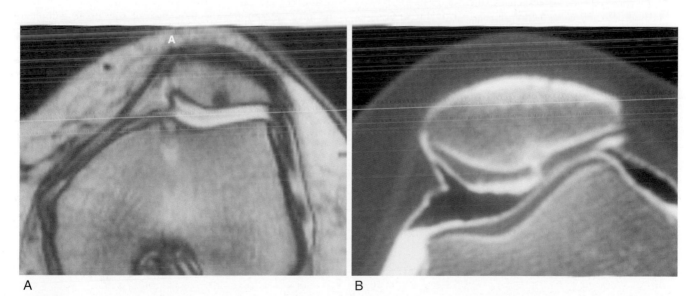

A   B

FIGURE 40–4. A, Magnetic resonance imaging (MRI) read as focal osteonecrosis. **B,** Contrast computed tomography (CT) arthrogram clearly shows a split in the articular cartilage extending down to the cystic lesion with damaged articular cartilage medial to the cartilage split. Most likely, there was an acute subluxation episode that compressed the articular cartilage until it failed with a split relieving ligament tension, with further lateral subluxation damaging the medial articular cartilage into which the contrast dye now moves.

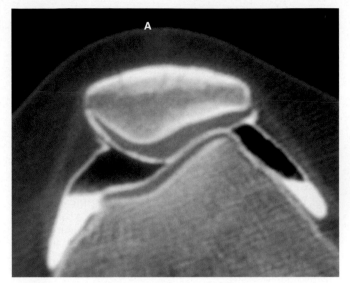

FIGURE 40–6. As the femur rotates internally beneath the patella, the lateral patellar articular cartilage is compressed. The increased crescentric density in the lateral patellar subchondral bone is indicative of chronic localized pressure.

If these side-directed vectors exceed biologic tolerance, either instability or arthrosis may result. For example, an inward pointing of the knee increases the lateral direction of pull of the quadriceps. Therefore, the pull on the MPFL (and also medial retinaculum and medial meniscopatellar ligament) is increased and the direction of pressure on the patella is altered, creating an increase on the lateral facet and a decrease on the medial facet (Fig. 40–5). The radiographic appearance of subchondral density under the patellar facets is a useful clue to the mechanical environment (Fig. 40–6).

Maximum energy conservation during gait is due to precise anatomy and joint kinematics.[34] Abnormalities in normal bony anatomy or joint motions distort the normal force vectors needed to transfer the body mass to the ground. Deviations in normal limb alignment may result in the knee joint flexion-extension axis advancing sideways while the body moves forward. These deviations include femoral anteversion or retroversion, excess internal or external tibial torsion, genu valgum or varus, hyperpronation, and Achilles contracture.

The *foot progression angle* (FPA) is generally defined as the angle between the long axis of the foot and the direction of body progression and averages 10° to 15°.[28,37] It has been shown that the FPA remains similar despite differences in the torsion of the tibia or femur.[37] It is likely that this is because proper ankle dorsiflexion cannot occur during gait if the ankle joint axis is not aligned with the direction of forward movement or because this presents the most stable position of the foot on the ground. Hip rotation must vary if the torsion of the long bones changes and the FPA stays constant. Alterations in both femoral and tibial torsion change the effective lever arm of the hip stabilizers[1] and may account for the frequency of soft tissue complaints around the hip and pelvis, as well as the increased pelvic tilt and lumbar lordosis seen in these patients. Examples of the change in the position of the hip and knee with a constant foot progression angle and changes in femoral and tibial torsion are seen in Figures 40–7 to 40–11.

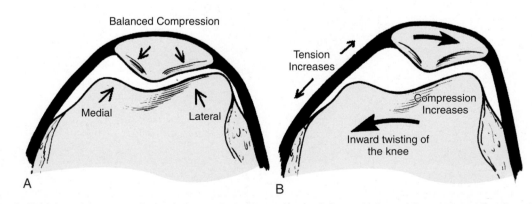

FIGURE 40–5. A, If the knee joint moves forward, the compression on the patellofemoral joint and ligaments tensioned are balanced. **B,** If the knee joint twists inward from beneath the patella, the MPFL is placed under increased tension, the compression beneath the lateral facet increases, and the compression beneath the medial facet decreases.

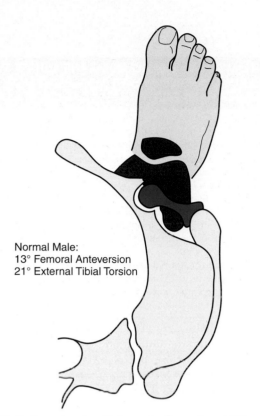

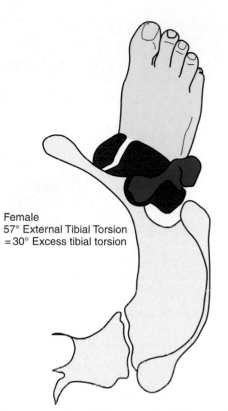

FIGURE 40–7. Normal male with femoral anteversion of 13° and external tibial torsion of 21°. Note that with a foot progression angle of 13°, the knee joint faces slightly outward.

Female
57° External Tibial Torsion
=30° Excess tibial torsion

FIGURE 40–9. Female with a 30° increase in tibial torsion. To keep the foot progression angle normal, the knee joint axis points inward nearly 30°, causing increased strain on the knee. The hip appears markedly internally rotated with the greater trochanter pointing somewhat anteriorly.

Normal Male:
13° Femoral Anteversion
21° External Tibial Torsion

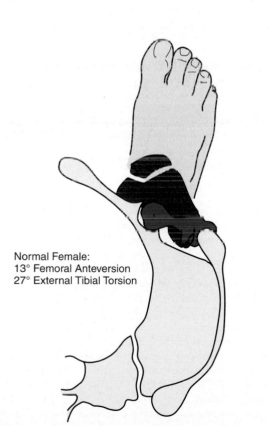

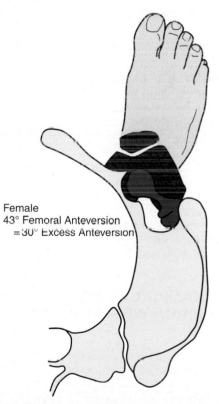

Normal Female:
13° Femoral Anteversion
27° External Tibial Torsion

Female
43° Femoral Anteversion
=30° Excess Anteversion

FIGURE 40–8. Normal female with femoral anteversion of 13° and external tibial torsion of 27°. Note that the knee joint is pointing slightly more inward and the greater trochanter is slightly more anterior than in the normal male.

FIGURE 40–10. Female with a 30° increase in femoral anteversion. The knee joint points the same direction, slightly inward, as in the normal female, but the greater trochanter points posteriorly, giving a poor mechanical advantage. At some point, the hip cannot externally rotate enough to keep the knee joint pointed forward. With fatigue of the hip abductors, the knee points more inward to compensate for hip collapse, placing greater stress on the knee.

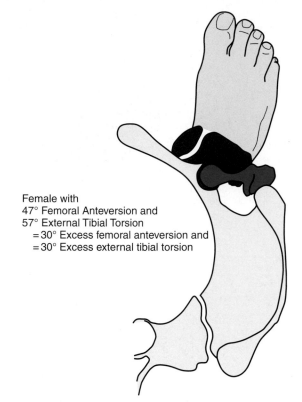

FIGURE 40–11. Female with a 30° increase in both femoral anteversion and external tibial torsion. Note that the trochanter is pointed more anterior than normal, and with the foot progression angle normal, the knee joint axis points markedly inward.

Female with
47° Femoral Anteversion and
57° External Tibial Torsion
= 30° Excess femoral anteversion and
= 30° Excess external tibial torsion

Figures 40–7 to 40–11 are drawn with an FPA of 13° (Seber average) for a normal male torsional alignment (Fig. 40–7), a normal female torsional alignment (Fig. 40–8), a female with 30° excess external tibial torsion (Fig. 40–9), a female with 30° excess femoral anteversion (Fig. 40–10), and a female with both 30° excess tibial external torsion and 30° excess femoral anteversion (Fig. 40–11). One may study the variations in knee joint progression with these common abnormal patterns. Yoshioka and associates[47–49] found identical femoral anteversion in both males and females, equal genu valgus in both males and females, but an increase in external tibial torsion and in foot external rotation in females over males. This increase in external foot rotation may account for the apparent increased genu valgus in females, the increased incidence in PF symptoms in females, and even for the increased incidence of ACL tears in females.

BIOMECHANICAL EVIDENCE RELATING LIMB TORSION WITH PF INSTABILITY AND PAIN

A change in PF contact areas and pressures was noted after alteration of femoral or tibial torsion or rotation by Lee and coworkers[22–24] Hefzy and associates,[12] and van Kampen and Huiskes.[45] Kiljowski and colleagues[18] (unpublished data) placed lower limbs (femoral head to foot) in a frame with a clamp, attaching the femoral head to a vertical post that allowed the knee flexion to be altered by sliding the femoral head up and down the post. The foot was held in a position of normal FPA and an osteotomy was performed in the shaft of the femur, allowing

rotation. PF contact pressures and MPFL strain were measured while the osteotomy changed the femoral torsion 15° and 30°, both inward and outward. At 30° knee flexion, lateral facet pressure increased an average of 30%, with a 30° increase in femoral anteversion, while medial facet pressures were decreased. Strain in the MPFL increased 57% after a 30° increase of internal femoral torsion. Fujikawa and coworkers[11] in a biomechanical study that measured PF contact pressures concluded that if an angular deformity and a torsional deformity coexist, the rotatory component causes the greater PF changes. These authors also noted that when a varus deformity was created, the greater the varus deformity, the less the PF congruence.

CLINICAL EVIDENCE RELATING LIMB TORSION TO PF INSTABILITY AND PAIN

Brattström[2] in 1964 measured trochlear depth in a group of patients with recurrent dislocation of the patella and confirmed that a shallow trochlea was always present. This author also defined the Q-angle and pointed out the change in Q-angle as a result of changes in limb rotation. He reviewed the literature on the rotational femoral osteotomy as described by Graser (1904), Fürmeier (1953), Kiesselbach (1956), and Vinditti and Forcella (1958) and concluded that the "femoral osteotomy is a big operation that demands prolonged after treatment. I have not encountered any instance of recurrent dislocation of the patella that justified my suggesting an operation of this nature to the patient." Takai and associates[41] measured femoral and tibial torsion in patients with unicompartmental arthrosis in either the medial, the lateral, or the PF compartment and found the highest correlation to be that of PF arthrosis with increased femoral anteversion (23° anteversion in the osteoarthritis group vs. 9° anteversion in the control group). Janssen[16] found a high correlation between patellar dislocation and an increase in medial femoral torsion and speculated that this medial femoral torsion was also responsible for the development of trochlear dysplasia. Lerat and colleagues[25,26] noted a significantly increased association of internal femoral torsion with both patellar instability ($P < .0001$) and patellar chondropathy ($P < .001$). Stroud and coworkers[40] followed 92 patients who at age 5 showed 30° greater medial hip rotation (measured in extension) than lateral rotation. At age 24, PF pain was noted by 30% in the increased medial rotation group compared with only 8% in the control group ($P < .001$). Winson and associates[46] found that 70% of adolescents undergoing arthroscopy for anterior knee pain had an increased internal torsion of the femur, compared with only 33% of those undergoing arthroscopy for a meniscal or cruciate injury. Turner[44] noted increased external tibial torsion in patients with PF instability (25° vs. 19°). Of perhaps great significance to those who believe that muscle strengthening is the key to treating PF symptoms, Nyland and colleagues[32] found a significant decrease in vastus medialis and gluteus medius electromyogram amplitude in athletes with clinically increased internal femoral torsion. Arnold and coworkers[1] noted that an increase in femoral anteversion of 30° to 40° and decreased abduction moment arm strength of 40 to 50% was enough to impair normal walking, and therefore, those individuals required turning the knee inward to keep the hip from collapsing. This inward pointing of the knee creates high shearing force on the PF joint.

FEMORAL AND TIBIAL TORSION MEASUREMENTS

Femoral anteversion has been measured by a variety of techniques by many authors and recently by Yoshioka and associates[47,48] (Fig. 40–12). To measure limb alignment in the horizontal (transverse) plane, a CT rotational study is obtained. This is a CT scan that overlaps cuts from the femoral head, base of the femoral neck or lesser trochanter, the knee joint (either tangent to the posterior condyles or between the medial and the lateral epicondyles), the proximal tibia at the joint and the tibial tuberosity, and the ankle joint (Fig. 40–13). These cuts allow measurement of femoral torsion, tibial torsion, knee torsion, and the tibial tubercle–trochlear groove (TT/TG) distance. CT also allows for the observation of trochlear depth or dysplasia, the position of the patella in the

trochlea (unstressed), patellar tilt, and shift and the density of the subchondral trabeculae.

To measure torsion of the femur, the recommendations of Murphy and coworkers[30] and Yoshioka and Cooke[47] are followed; these superimpose the CT cuts through the center of the femoral head and the base of the femoral neck where the circular nature of the femoral shaft becomes apparent (see Fig. 40–13A–C). A line drawn through the center of each femoral segment becomes the proximal reference. A CT cut through the distal femur where the anteroposterior (AP) dimension of the medial and lateral condyles is greatest allows a line to be drawn tangent to the posterior condylar surface. A second line can be drawn through the medial and lateral epicondyles. Yoshioka and Cooke[47] measured femoral torsion (anteversion)

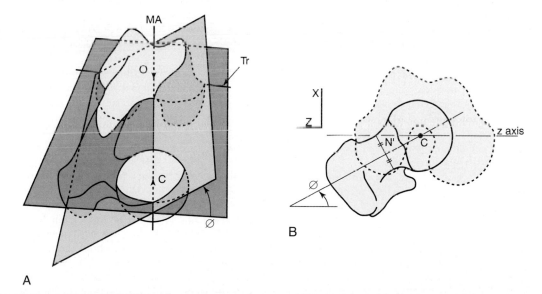

FIGURE 40–12. A, Femoral anteversion or antetorsion (angle φ here) may be measured along the center of the femoral neck from the center of the femoral head to the center of the femoral shaft at the base of the neck, and distally either along the transepicondylar axis (Tr) 7.4° or along the tangent of the posterior femoral condyles 13.1°. These differ by about 6°, with a range of 11° retroversion to 22° anteversion. **B,** This measurement by Yoshioka and associates[48] is taken directly off the bone. Murphy and coworkers[30] validated a CT measurement along these same lines. (*A, From Yoshioka, Y.; Cooke, T. D. V.: Femoral anteversion: assessment based on function axes. J Orthop Res 5:86–91, 1987, p. 88. Fig 3A; B, from Yoshioka, Y.; Siu, D.; Cooke, T. D. V.: The anatomy and functional axes of the femur. J Bone Joint Surg Am 69:873–880, 1987, p. 875, Fig. 2B.*)

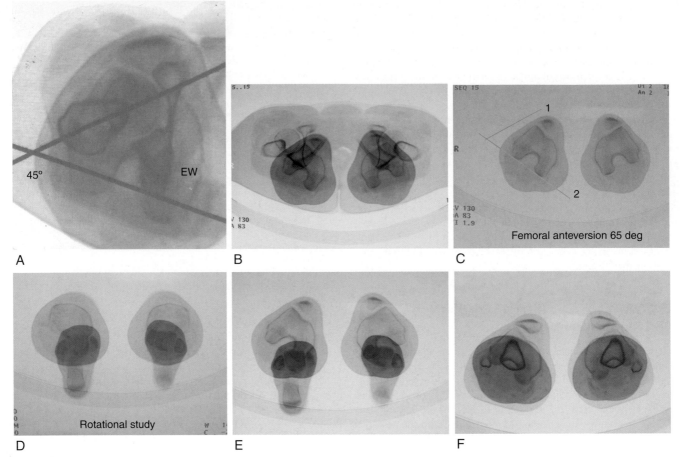

FIGURE 40–13. A, For measuring femoral torsion (anteversion), CT slices taken through the femoral head, the inferior greater trochanter, and the knee joint are superimposed. One line is drawn from the center of the femoral head through the greater trochanter, and a second is tangent to the posterior femoral condyles at the knee joint. **B,** Hip and knee overlapped, allowing references lines seen in **C** to be drawn. **C,** *Reference line 1* is taken from the center of femoral head to the center of femur at the level of the lower greater trochanter. *Reference line 2* is a tangent to the posterior surface of the femoral condyles. The epicondyles are also readily seen and can be used as a second reference. There is generally a 6° difference between these two choices of reference. **D,** Tibial torsion can be measured between the axis of the tibial plateau and the ankle joint axis. **E,** The angle between the epicondylar axis of the femur and the ankle joint axis can be used as a measure of tibial torsion. **F,** The distance between the tibial tubercle and the center of the trochlear groove (TT/TG) is also provided in the rotational study. Dejour and colleagues[6] stated that a distance > 20 mm is abnormal and correlates with objective patellar instability.

directly from the bone in a series of 32 femora and noted an average anteversion of 13.1° in both males and females when the distal measurement was the tangent across the femoral condyles, and 7.4° when measured across the epicondyles (standard deviation [SD], 8°; range, –11°–+22°). It is useful to measure both to avoid an error should dysplasia of the lateral femoral condyle with a short AP distance be present.

Yoshioka and Cooke[47] reviewed the literature measuring femoral anteversion by a variety of different techniques and noted that 12 of the 18 reviewed papers reported normal values between 8° and 16°. This author has arbitrarily chosen 13° as the goal for correction. Kuo and associates[19] observed various measurement techniques and concluded that CT was accurate, but that the plane radiographic techniques were not. It is often stated that a patient with increased femoral anteversion has a compensatory external tibial torsion. Pasciak and colleagues[33] found this not to be the case and found no relation between femoral anteversion and tibial torsion. In a review of over 300 CT rotational studies, the author of this chapter found that with increased femoral anteversion, tibial torsion may be normal, increased external, or increased internal.

The measurement of tibial torsion by CT has not been standardized. Jakob and coworkers[14] described a common sense method superimposing cuts across the proximal tibia and distal ankle joint. The author of this chapter has attempted to use the anatomic measurements of the tibia described by Yoshioka and colleagues[49] as a basis for measuring the proximal tibial reference line (Fig. 40–14). Blinded repeat measurements made by an orthopaedic radiologist produced a measurement variation of less than 1°, indicating that reproducible measurements are possible. Yoshioka and colleagues' anatomic study[49] reported a lateral torsion of 21° in males and 27° in females, a significant difference. This was the only difference in geometry noted between males and females in both the tibia and the femur. In addition, these authors noticed a gender difference of 16° between the transverse axis across the tibial plateau and the center of the foot. If this observation is confirmed, it is of major importance because it may explain the widely quoted difference between men and women in the frequency of PF disorders. It may also explain the reported increased incidence of anterior cruciate ligament (ACL) tears in women. Le Damany[21] reported 23.7° to be normal tibial torsion. Seber and associates[37]

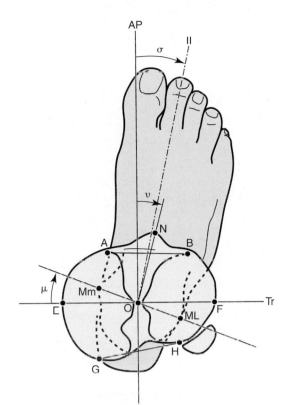

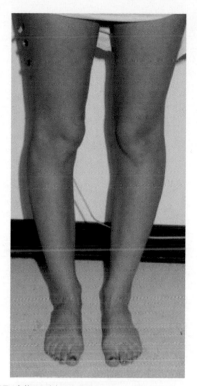

FIGURE 40–14. The tibial torsion may be measured as the angle μ, which is between the widest distance on the tibial plateau (EF) and the line connecting the malleoli (M_m M_L). Males — 21°, Females = 27°. Angle σ is the "foot rotation," the outward deviation of the foot in reference to the tibial plateau transverse axis (EF). Males = –5°, Females = +11°. *(From Yoshioka, Y.; Siu, D, W.; Scudamore R A; Cooke, T D V: Tibial anatomy and functional axes. J Orthop Res 7:132–137, 1989.)*

FIGURE 40–15. Miserable malalignment. The patient often presents with medial parapatellar pain with no localizing findings or images indicating pathology. Later, instability or arthrosis may develop.

calculated external tibial torsion to be 30° (range, 16°–50°) in a group of 50 "normal" (asymptomatic) men, but their measurement technique was unique in selecting the location for drawing the proximal tibial reference. Eckhoff and coworkers[9] noted variations between 15° and 30°. Turner[44] found 19° (SD, 4.8°) in a control group and 24.5° (SD, 6.3°) in a group with unstable patella. The CT measurements of Sayli and coworkers[35] averaged 30° to 35°. Tamari and associates[42] recently demonstrated a lack of reliability between currently used measurement methods, which is a major stumbling block in answering the question of how much of an influence altered tibial torsion plays in PF instability and when osteotomy may be useful.

In addition to the just-discussed method taken after Yoshioka and colleagues' anatomic measurements,[49] the author of this chapter also uses the femoral epicondylar axis as the proximal reference for tibial torsion, owing to the interest in the relationship of the knee joint axis to the ankle joint axis and the problem incurred when selecting a line across an oval tibial plateau. The error of twisting across the knee joint while obtaining the CT must be avoided to use this reference.

INDICATIONS

Any variation from optimal skeletal alignment may increase the vector forces acting on the PF joint causing either PF ligament failure with subsequent subluxation or cartilage failure as in

chondromalacia or arthrosis or both ligament and cartilage failure. Anterior knee pain may result from these abnormal forces or their consequences (Fig. 40–15).

An inward-pointing knee due to any cause will increase the lateral displacement force on the patella (Figs. 40–16 to 40–18). If this force is great or if the trochlear support is reduced from dysplasia or fracture, the medial ligaments may fail, resulting in lateral patellar instability. The converse is also true. Pain in the medial retinaculum is a common symptom caused by this increased stress. If the trochlear support is normal, the ligament may not fail but the articular load may increase, causing arthrosis. This increased force may be the result of abnormal femoral torsion, abnormal tibial torsion, genu valgum, hyperpronation, Achilles' contracture, or other conditions. The choice for surgery depends on the relative size of the deformity and the relative surgical risk and morbidity.

The MPFL is a rather small structure. This is because a large ligament is not needed to restrain the patella from leaving the center of the trochlea if the limb is straight, the knee joint axis points forward, the quadriceps vector is in the frontal plane, and the trochlea is normal. If the trochlea is dysplastic (shallow), the ligament may not be strong enough to withstand the normal lateral pull of the quadriceps. If there is an abnormal limb torsion (so the knee joint does not move forward in the direction the body is moving), the side-displacing force is increased and the ligament is more likely to be overcome, leading to patellar instability. An MPFL reconstruction may be useful to restore the normal patellar restraint, but in the face of continued increased displacement forces caused by a torsional limb malalignment, such a reconstruction may fail. Conversely, in the face of normal limb torsion, the side-directed force may not be sufficient to displace the patella even with insufficient ligaments. The clinical presentation may be pain, instability, arthrosis, or a combination of these problems.

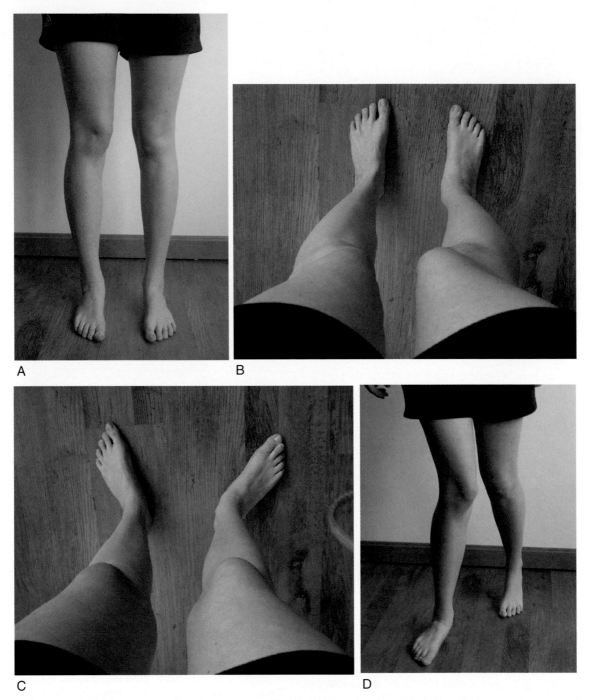

FIGURE 40–16. A 17–year-old student with rapid onset of pain and abnormal gait. It is likely that progressive overload due to torsional malalignment resulted in progressive increased foot pronation with loss of foot and ankle stability and secondary weakness of the lateral hip musculature. **A,** On standing anteroposterior (AP), the squinting patella on the right is well seen. Both femurs have 50° greater than normal anteversion. **B,** What the patient sees looking down her legs. **C,** If the knee faces forward, the foot turns out. **D,** The dynamic picture is much worse, because the anteversion puts the greater trochanter pointing posteriorly so there is no hip abduction power and the pelvis collapses. In an attempt to increase hip power and put the foot forward, the knee joint must point inward, even more when there is an increase in hyperpronation.

SURGICAL STRATEGY

The goal of operative treatment is to normalize the biomechanics through restitution of normal anatomy. The morbidity of surgery may dictate otherwise. When multiple anatomic abnormalities exist, it is not known which may be more important. If a patient has recurrent patellar lateral subluxation, articular cartilage damage, trochlear dysplasia, patella alta, an Achilles contracture, a femoral anteversion of 45°, an external tibial torsion of 55°, and a genu valgum of 10°, is it best to perform a varus, external rotational femoral osteotomy; a distalization of the tibial tuberosity; a reconstruction of the MPFL; a trochlear osteotomy; an internal rotation osteotomy of the tibia;

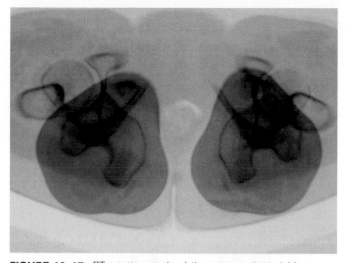

FIGURE 40–17. CT rotation study of the same patient yields anteversion of 67°. The hip cannot be rotated externally enough for the knee joint to face forward.

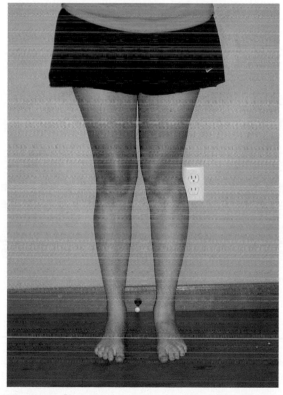

FIGURE 40–18. Six weeks postoperative, the patient shows 50° external rotational intertrochanteric osteotomy on the right hip. The right foot is less pronated than the left foot and the left knee joint is pointed slightly more inward than the right. Gait has already improved and knee pain diminished immediately after surgery.

or an Achilles lengthening? These abnormal findings are often quite subtle, but combinations are surprisingly common. The surgical approach to correct all abnormalities may be quite logical from the biomechanical view, but excessive from the surgical morbidity standpoint. A biomechanical solution with osteotomy may mean that the ligament reconstruction is not necessary, because the displacing forces are reduced. A cartilage restoration

---

Critical Points WHEN TO CONSIDER OSTEOTOMY AND SURGICAL STRATEGY

- Choice for surgery depends on the relative size of the deformity (femoral torsion, abnormal tibial torsion, genu valgum, hyperpronation) and the relative surgical risk and morbidity.
- Abnormal limb torsion: side-displacing force is increased, MPFL is more likely to be overcome, leading to patellar instability.
- MPFL reconstruction may be useful to restore the normal patellar restraint, but in the face of continued increased displacement forces caused by a torsional limb malalignment, such a reconstruction may fail.
- Surgery is indicated in most cases with torsion of the femur or tibia exceeding 30° from normal. Surgery is usually beneficial for those with torsion exceeding 20° from normal.

MPFL, medial patellofemoral ligament.

procedure is not necessary because the compressive forces are reduced and changed in direction. As yet, no biomechanical studies indicate which surgery alters biomechanics the most.

Experience suggests that for most cases with torsion of the femur or tibia exceeding 30° from normal, surgery is indicated. For those with torsion exceeding 20° from normal, surgery is thought to be beneficial. For cases with abnormality less than 20°, the accuracy of surgery or the morbidity may not justify the smaller biomechanical changes. Turner's data[44] found 19° average external torsion in a control group and 24.5° in a patellar instability group. In another study, Takai and associates[41] found 9° average femoral anteversion in a control group and 23° average in a PF arthrosis group. Therefore, it is possible that very small limb torsional differences are significant.

SURGICAL TECHNIQUE

To correct an excess of internal femoral torsion that is not associated with a genu varus or valgus, an intertrochanteric osteotomy has been used since the late 1980s. Prior to that, the author used the technique of intramedullary saw and fixation with an intramedullary nail. However, the antecurvatum of the femoral shaft is destroyed when the curved segments are rotated and the nail can split the distal fragment attempting to compensate (Fig. 40–19). In the original series of patients, cutting the femur from the intramedullary position and fixing with an

---

Critical Points SURGICAL TECHNIQUE

- Intertrochanteric osteotomy used to correct an excess of internal femoral torsion that is not associated with a genu varus or valgus.
- Standard AO/ASIF technique for hip osteotomy is used. Osteotomy is placed at the level of the proximal third of the lesser trochanter.
- AO 95° condylar blade plate is used for fixation.
- Rotational osteotomy of the tibia is performed below the level of the tibial tuberosity.
- Q-angle or TT/TG distance is not changed.
- Author uses a navigation system that indicates the changed alignment in all three planes (transverse, coronal, and sagittal).

AO/ASIF, Arbeitsgemainshaft für Osteosynthesefragen/Association for the Study of Internal Fixation; TT/TG, tibial tubercle–trochlear groove.

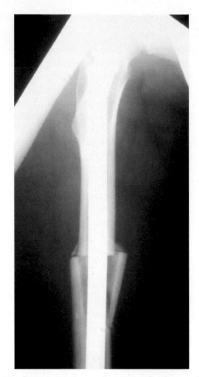

FIGURE 40–19. Postoperative radiograph of a femoral rotational osteotomy produced with an intramedullary saw. Rotation changes the anterior bow of the femur to a corkscrew shape that does not allow the nail to pass congruently, resulting in splitting of the distal fragment.

intramedullary nail, bone stability appeared to be less with more postoperative pain and blood loss. There was a higher incidence of delayed union and one death resulted from apparent fat embolism. Consequently, the intertrochanteric region using an AO 95° condylar blade plate (Figs. 40–20 and 40–21) for fixation was selected. The intertrochanteric location was chosen to minimize damage to the quadriceps, avoid scarring that may occur between the distal quadriceps and the supracondylar femur with a supracondylar location, and theoretically reduce the abrupt angular change the quadriceps would make with a supracondylar location. It should be noted these decisions are without scientific evidence. If a genu varum or genu valgum is associated with a torsional abnormality and the tibiofemoral angle is abnormal, this deformity must be corrected in the supracondylar region.

The standard AO/ASIF (Arbeitsgemainshaft für Osteosynthesefragen/Association for the Study of Internal Fixation) technique for hip osteotomy is used. This has been well described. The ability to solidly compress the two osteotomy fragments ensures stability and reduces pain. This compression remains a major advantage of the classic approach. The osteotomy is placed at the level of the proximal third of the lesser trochanter to increase the osteotomy surface contact area and to leave sufficient purchase for the 95° condylar blade plate in the proximal fragment. The blade plate is a tool that controls the correction. One needs to ensure only that the seating chisel for the blade plate enters the femoral neck at the proper height and orientation. The goal is for the blade of the blade plate to be centered in the femoral neck at such an angle that the side plate will sit on the lateral cortex of the femur without altering flexion-extension or varus-valgus. The standard AO tools aid in this goal (Fig. 40–22).

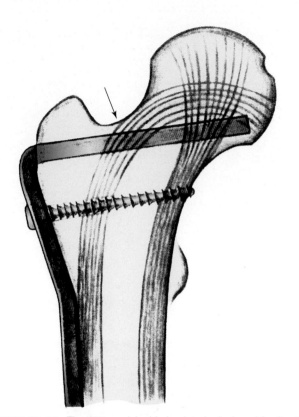

FIGURE 40–20. The 95° condylar blade plate is designed for fixation of the proximal femur. The U-shaped blade is inserted into the center of the neck and the inferior half of the head of the femur. *(From Müller, M. E.; Allgöwer, M.; Schneider, R.; Willenegger, H.:* Manual of Internal Fixation, *2nd ed. New York: Springer-Verlag, 1979; p. 91.)*

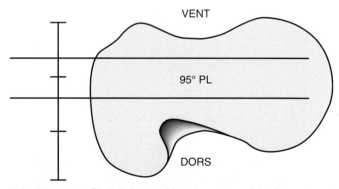

FIGURE 40–21. Blade is inserted into the center of the femoral neck and head. *(From Müller, M. E.; Allgöwer, M.; Schneider, R.; Willenegger, H.:* Manual of Internal Fixation, *2nd ed. New York: Springer-Verlag, 1979; p. 93.)*

A standard lateral approach to the hip is altered so the iliotibial track (fascia lata) is entered more anterior than usual to ensure that the trochanter or the plate over the trochanter will not put pressure on the repaired facial incision, causing a dehiscence.

After exposure of the lateral shaft of the femur by elevating the vastus lateralis anteriorly, the condylar plate guide, a mirror image of the 95° condylar plate, is placed along the lateral shaft of the femur. It is moved proximally and distally until an extension along its proximal flat surface lines up just below the center of the femoral head, as seen with x-ray image intensification (Fig. 40–23). A 2.0-mm K-wire is inserted into a 2.5-mm hole

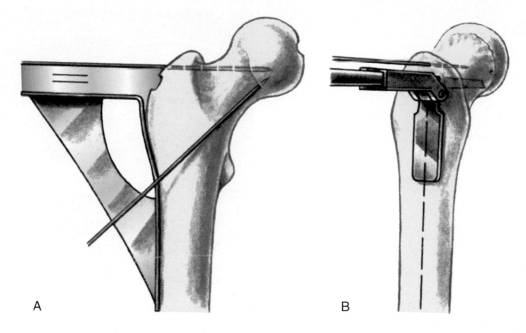

A   B

FIGURE 40–22. A, When a 95° condylar blade plate is to be used for fixation of a proximal femoral osteotomy, the site of insertion can be located with the aid of the condylar plate guide, which is a mirror image of the condylar blade plate. A K-wire inserted parallel to the top of the condylar plate guide will guide the insertion of the seating chisel. The direction of the femoral neck can be approximated with a K-wire placed along its anterior cortex. The neck must be seen for this to be precise and radiographic control with the image intensifier may be easier than opening the hip capsule. **B,** The seating guide placed in line with the axis of the femur will ensure that there is no change in flexion or extension of the hip. *(A and B, From Müller, M. E.; Allgöwer, M.; Schneider, R.; Willenegger, H.: Manual of Internal Fixation, 2nd ed. New York: Springer-Verlag, 1979; p. 93.)*

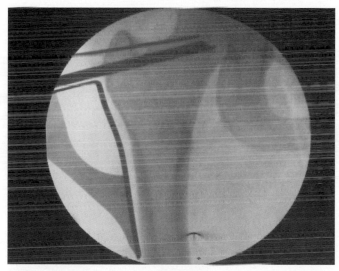

FIGURE 40–23. The condylar plate guide is placed along the lateral femoral shaft. It is moved proximal or distal until a line extending medially parallel to the top of the guide is located just below the center of the femoral head. A K-wire is inserted above and parallel to this line; this K-wire position is checked on the lateral radiograph to ensure that it is in the center of the femoral neck. Once proper positioning of the K-wire is obtained, the seating chisel for the blade of the blade plate is inserted into the femoral neck and head parallel to the K-wire and to the top of the condylar plate guide.

drilled into the femoral neck parallel to the top of the condylar plate guide and centered anteriorly and posteriorly in the neck. This hole is placed proximal enough to leave room below it to insert a seating chisel on top of the condylar plate guide.

Because of the torsional deformity, the femoral neck is often angled quite anteriorly relative to the knee joint, but its exact direction cannot be seen. Classically, one may expose the neck of the femur anteriorly or slide a K-wire along the anterior cortex of the neck, but this is usually approximate and not exactly in the center line. To find whether this 2-mm K-wire is parallel to the center line of the femoral neck, a frog-leg lateral image is obtained. This normally results in bending of the K-wire against the iliotibial band, but the portion within the femoral neck will indicate whether the direction is appropriate. It is common to need to change these K-wires when they are bent. Obtaining the frog-leg lateral radiographic projection and the ability to slide the 2.0-mm wire in and out of the 2.5-mm hole are useful.

Once the proper position of the K-wire is obtained, the seating chisel for the angled blade is inserted. A window in the lateral cortex of the greater trochanter for the seating chisel may be started with drills (Fig. 40–24). The thickness of the 95° condylar blade is 4.5 mm, allowing a 4.5-mm drill to be used. A triple drill guide is available to attach to the top of the condylar plate guide to ensure the correct drill direction.

The condylar plate guide and later the seating chisel guide are held parallel to the femoral shaft to ensure the side plate will align with the lateral femoral shaft and there will be no change in flexion or extension (Fig. 40–25). Once the proper position of a K-wire is obtained, a thin chisel is used to cut into the lateral femoral cortex at the top of the properly positioned condylar plate guide. This cut in the cortex will allow the seating chisel for the blade to be advanced without sliding proximally or distally (Fig. 40–26). The condylar plate guide is used repeatedly to check that the varus-valgus angulation is not being changed and also that the flexion-extension angle will not be changed (Fig. 40–27). The seating chisel is advanced slowly until

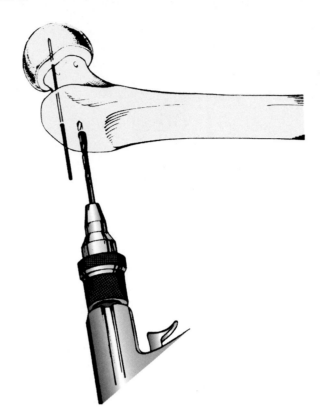

FIGURE 40–24. The window for the seating chisel may be created in the lateral cortex of the greater trochanter with a 4.5-mm drill. A triple drill guide (4.5 mm) may be attached to the top of the condylar plate guide. *(From Schauwecker, F.: Practice of Osteosynthesis, 2nd rev. ed. New York: Thieme-Stratton, 1982; p. 187.)*

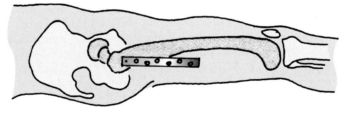

FIGURE 40–25. The seating chisel guide and condylar plate guide must be placed parallel to the shaft of the femur to avoid causing a flexion or extension change. The tendency is for the plate to be inserted horizontally (shown here), forgetting the anterior curve to the femur, thus causing an increased hip extension. *(From Schauwecker, F.: Practice of Osteosynthesis, 2nd rev. ed. New York: Thieme-Stratton, 1982; p. 163.)*

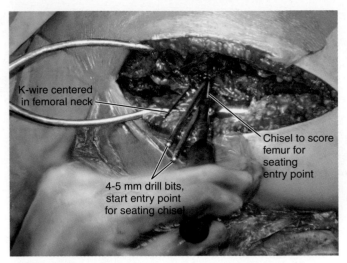

FIGURE 40–26. A triple drill guide is attached to the top of the condylar plate guide and 2- x 4.5-mm drill bits used to start the window for the seating chisel in the lateral cortex of the greater trochanter. A thin chisel is used to cut the cortex to begin the entry point for the seating chisel.

K-wire centered in femoral neck

4-5 mm drill bits, start entry point for seating chisel

Chisel to score femur for seating entry point

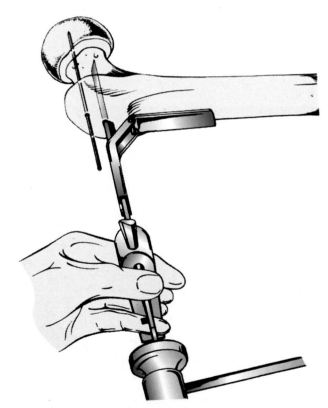

FIGURE 40–27. The seating chisel is driven into the femoral neck, parallel to the K-wire previously placed. The seating chisel guide is used to ensure that the plate will lie centered on the lateral shaft of the femur. This flexion and extension are controlled by the slotted hammer. *(From Schauwecker, F.: Practice of Osteosynthesis, 2nd rev. ed. New York: Thieme-Stratton, 1982; p. 188.)*

it approaches the center of the femoral head. It is backed out after advancing every 5 mm or so, so that it does not become incarcerated. The slotted hammer is used to prevent twisting of the seating chisel into flexion or extension as it is advanced. The depth of insertion is read off the marks etched on the seating chisel. A chisel is used to remove a small sliver of bone from the inferior edge of the entry site for the blade. This allows the shoulder of the plate to be advanced into the proximal fragment (Figs. 40–28 and 40–29).

When the seating chisel is removed, a 2.0-mm K-wire may be inserted into the chisel track and this wire will slide into the U corner (Figs. 40–30 and 40–31). This guarantees that the direction for the blade will not be lost while the osteotomy is completed.

A 2.5-mm drill hole is placed at the location for the osteotomy, usually at the upper third of the lesser trochanter, and drilled from lateral to medial and perpendicular to the femoral shaft coronal axis. A 2.5-mm K-wire, which will be used to guide the saw, is inserted into this hole.

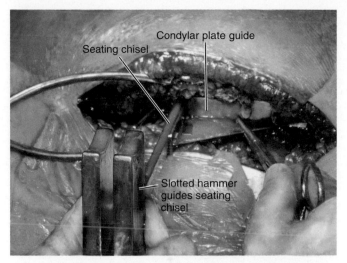

FIGURE 40–28. The condylar plate guide is placed parallel to and touching the lateral femoral cortex, and the seating chisel is kept flush and parallel with the top of the guide. The slotted hammer allows control of the twist of the seating chisel; thus, it controls flexion and extension of the osteotomy.

Two anterior-to-posterior K-wires, which are set at the desired angle of correction, are placed in the femur, one proximal and one distal to the selected site for osteotomy (Figs. 40–32 and 40–33). A 2.5-mm drill is used to create the holes for these two K-wires. These are the markers to indicate the torsional correction. For excess femoral anteversion, the need is to externally rotate the distal fragment. The proximal pin is placed first, far enough anterior and medial that it will not come into conflict with the angled blade plate that will be inserted into the proximal fragment. The distal pin is started in line with the proximal

pin in the anterior femoral cortex, but angled from medial to lateral the desired correction amount. Commercially provided triangles of various angles are available to be placed along the proximal K-wire and used as a guide to drill the 2.5-mm hole for the distal 2.5-mm K-wire reference.

Once these reference pins are in place, the osteotomy is completed with a thin saw (Fig. 40–34). The saw blade is kept perpendicular to the axis of the femur, and the image helps ensure that the orientation is proper (Fig. 40–35). Elevators are placed anterior and posterior to the bone to protect the soft tissues, and the image is used to judge the medial depth of the cut. Once the cut is completed, the soft tissues adjacent to the cut are stretched by placing a lamina spreader within the osteotomy (Fig. 40–36). This makes it easier to adjust rotation. Next, the blade plate is inserted into the proximal fragment (Fig. 40–37). The previously placed 2.0-mm K-wire in the seating chisel track makes the direction easier to follow. If the blade is properly in line with the track, it can often be pushed in by hand. After it is correctly placed in the femoral neck and head, it is necessary to impact the blade tightly into the proximal fragment (Fig. 40–38). Usually, a five-hole length side plate is sufficient. A longer-length side plate provides greater leverage but requires a longer incision and surgical approach.

The distal fragment is now externally rotated until the two torsional reference K-wires are parallel and the cortices of the osteotomy surface are well aligned circumferentially (Fig. 40–39). If the blade is not driven sufficiently far into the proximal fragment, it may allow the distal fragment to translate more laterally than the proximal fragment such that the surfaces of the osteotomy do not line up. This can be corrected by removing a small amount of bone from beneath the shoulder of the plate and impacting the plate further into the proximal fragment. Hohmann retractors or clamps may be useful to help align the axis of both fragments while maintaining the rotational correction. Once this position is reached,

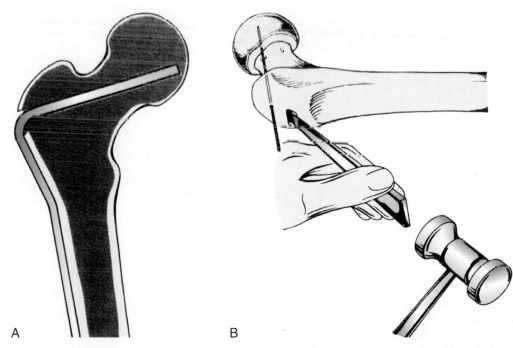

A   B

FIGURE 40–29. A, The shoulder of the condylar blade plate will prevent the plate from seating all the way into the proximal fragment. **B,** A chisel is used to remove the lower edge of the window for the blade plate so it does not block full insertion. (*A and B, From Schauwecker, F.: Practice of Osteosynthesis, 2nd rev. ed. New York: Thieme-Stratton, 1982; p. 188.*)

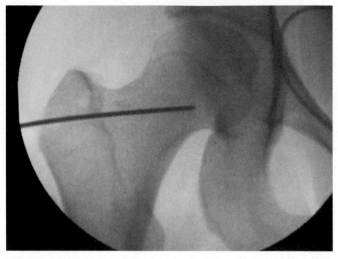

FIGURE 40–30. A 2-mm-diameter K-wire is inserted in the corner of the U-shaped chisel track so it can be located later when the osteotomy is complete and the blade is ready for insertion.

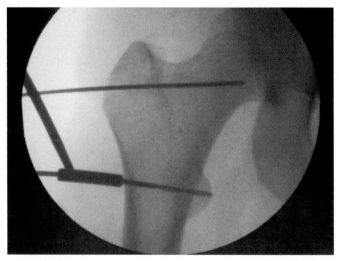

FIGURE 40–31. Once the seating chisel has been inserted, it is removed and a 2-mm K-wire is placed into the seating chisel track. A 2.5-mm wire is to be placed in the top half of the lesser trochanter and perpendicular to the femoral shaft.

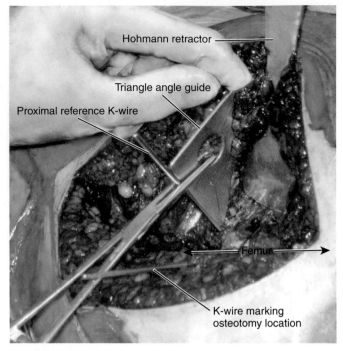

FIGURE 40–32. After the level of osteotomy is selected and marked with a K-wire (*bottom of photo*), K-wires are needed as rotational markers. The first is placed proximal to the level of osteotomy and anterior to the location for the blade plate. For a 50° correction, one side of a 50° triangle is placed along the vertical K-wire and a second K-wire will be placed distal to the osteotomy level (bottom K-wire) and parallel to the medial edge of the 50° triangle.

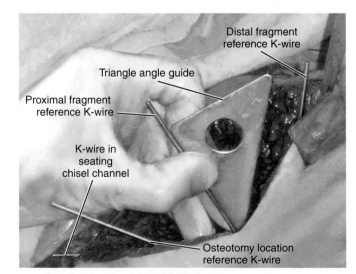

FIGURE 40–33. The K-wires (*right*) to indicate the angle of correction are seen to subtend an angle of 50°. To the *left* are the K-wires in the osteotomy site and in the seating chisel tract.

the articular tension device is attached to the femur distal to the plate (Fig. 40–40). This must be in line with the plate or the rotation will be changed as tension is applied to the plate.

A tension device placed anterior to the plate will cause external rotation of the distal fragment when tension is applied, and a tension device placed posterior to the plate will cause internal rotation of the distal fragment to be introduced. The articular tension device is color-coded, with the red indicating 120 kPa. Using the spanning wrench, an attempt is made to always exceed the 120 kPa indicator (Fig. 40–41). If the screw attaching the tension device to the femoral shaft is bent, the author is confident satisfactory compression of the osteotomy surfaces has been reached. If the blade is not tightly seated in the proximal fragment, it may pull out as tension is placed in the plate. A screw through the proximal plate into the proximal fragment is often required to prevent the blade from backing out with subsequent loss of osteotomy compression (Figs. 40–42 and

40–43). The author has not found that proximal femoral nails or locked plates provide the degree of compression that can be obtained with the angled plates and the articulated tension device.

Rotational osteotomy of the tibia should be performed below the level of the tibial tuberosity. The Q-angle or TT/TG distance is an important biomechanical arrangement that should not be changed. It makes little difference where the osteotomy

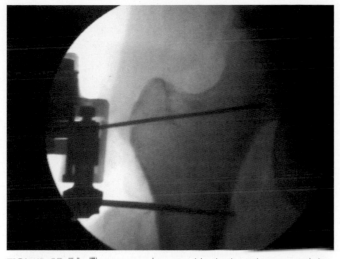

FIGURE 40–34. The saw cut is started in the lateral cortex and the saw blade is perpendicular to the shaft in both the AP and the lateral radiographic projections. The K-wires indicate that rotation must be placed prior to completing the osteotomy and should be placed now.

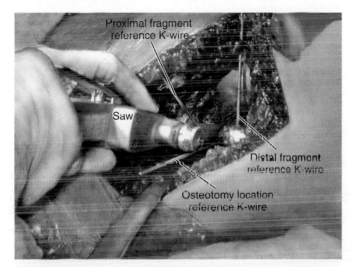

FIGURE 40–35. An oscillating saw is used to cut the femur transversely. The two rotation wires (*right*) subtend the desired angle of correction, and the lower K-wire is a guide for the saw at the osteotomy level.

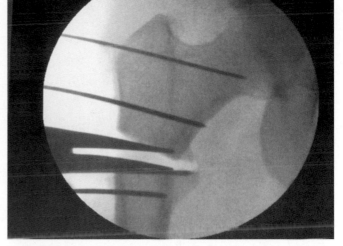

FIGURE 40–36. When the osteotomy is complete, it is useful to stretch the soft tissue with a lamina spreader. Four K-wires are shown: a 2-mm-diameter in the track of the seating chisel, 2- x 2.5-mm-diameter rotational wires above and below the osteotomy placed for rotational reference, and the fourth between to serve as a guide for the saw.

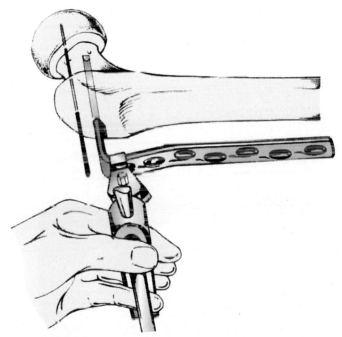

FIGURE 40–37. The blade can often be inserted by hand. The inserter handle is set so it is parallel to the blade and the insertion is parallel to the orientation K-wire. *(From Schauwecker, F.: Practice of Osteosynthesis, 2nd rev. ed. New York: Thieme-Stratton, 1982; p. 189.)*

is performed, because the goal is to realign the knee joint axis with the ankle joint axis in the transverse plane, leaving the trochlea-tubercle relationship normal (Fig. 40–44). The author prefers the proximal tibia below the tubercle for the location of the osteotomy and the angled blade plate for compression, but the geometry of the proximal tibia makes the blade insertion always a problem. With a lateral approach, the side plate will come to lie along the flat surface of the tibia so the angle the blade takes into the proximal fragment will determine rotation, but the precise direction of this is not easily referenced off the flat surface of the tibia. This lack of smooth tibial surface for reference also makes proper insertion in varus-valgus a problem when tension is applied to the plate with the articular tension device. The eccentric loading of the plate may introduce a varus or valgus deformity that must be corrected.

The locking plate allows greater ease of rotational control, but still allows a distortion of varus-valgus correction when a compression is applied to the osteotomy. Tensioning of a locked plate that is fixed in the proximal fragment may also result in the distal plate sitting well off the bone, producing an unsatisfactory prominence that can tent the anterior compartment muscle laterally or the sparse subcutaneous tissue medially. Locking plates without high compression of the osteotomy fragments definitely result in delayed union time and more postoperative discomfort than the tight compression possible with an angled blade plate.

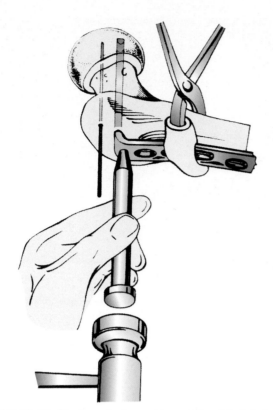

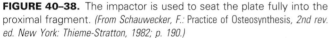

FIGURE 40–38. The impactor is used to seat the plate fully into the proximal fragment. *(From Schauwecker, F.: Practice of Osteosynthesis, 2nd rev. ed. New York: Thieme-Stratton, 1982; p. 190.)*

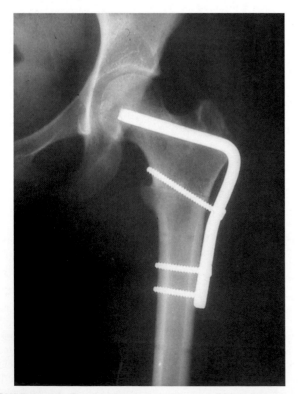

FIGURE 40–39. The desired cortical alignment. The oblique lag screw prevents the plate from backing out and contributes extra compression across the osteotomy. The holes for attachment of the articulated tension device are seen distal to the plate.

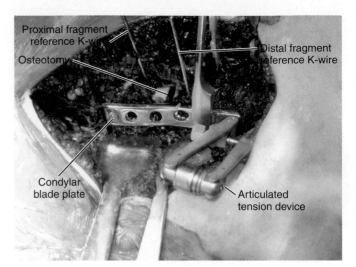

FIGURE 40–40. The distal fragment has been externally rotated so the rotational wires are parallel, the gap at the osteotomy is seen between the two K-wires. The articulated tension device has been screwed onto the femur distally. Applying tension to the plate will compress the osteotomy surfaces providing stability.

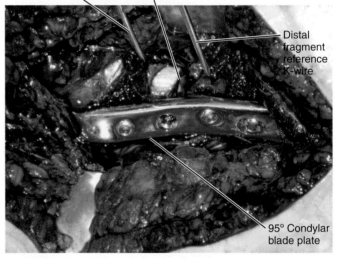

FIGURE 40–41. The osteotomy is compressed; the two rotational K-wires are parallel.

Two 2.5-mm K-wires are placed from front to back in the anterior cortex of the tibia, one proximal and one distal to the anticipated level of osteotomy. These may be parallel or subtend the desired angle of correction in the transverse plane. If they are parallel, the angle between the two after manipulation of the osteotomy fragments indicates the correction angle (Fig. 40–45). If they have been placed at an angle to each other for the desired correction, the pins are brought parallel for judging the desired correction. It is important to have these as reference points before the osteotomy is made. Currently, the author uses a navigation system (Praxim, Walpole, MA) that indicates the changed alignment in all three planes (transverse, coronal, and sagittal) (Fig. 40–46). It is impressive that small changes in all three planes are usually present and the manipulation of the

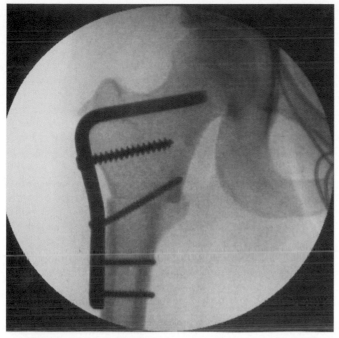

FIGURE 40–42. The blade has been inserted, and the tensioning of the plate complete and screws inserted. The top cancellous screw is used to keep the plate from backing out of the proximal fragment as it is pulled distally with the tensioning device. The distal two screws hold the plate in tension by preventing the plate from proximal migration. The second screw from the top is both an interfragmentary lag screw and adds additional rotational support. For perfect cortical contact without the medial translation of the proximal fragment, bone under the shoulder of the plate could have been removed so it would not prevent the further advancement of the blade into the proximal fragment. The surgeon felt this would have little or no effect on the limb alignment and advised against taking down the fixation at this point.

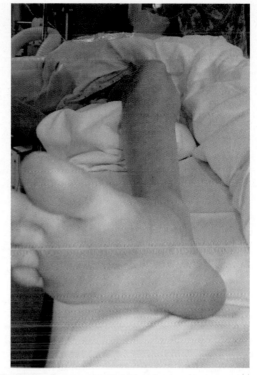

FIGURE 40–44. Excess external tibial torsion is corrected by an internal rotation osteotomy below the level of the tibial tubercle.

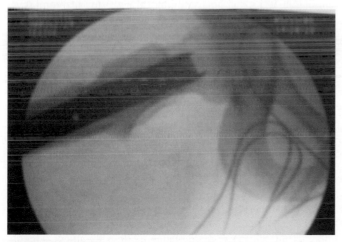

FIGURE 40–43. The blade is centered in the femoral neck as seen on the frog-leg lateral.

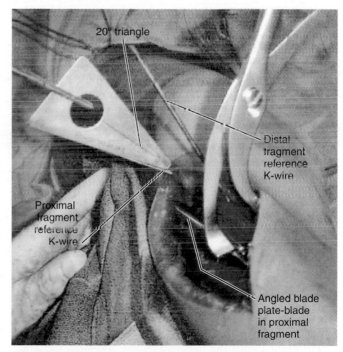

FIGURE 40–45. A blade of a blade plate has been inserted into the proximal tibial fragment in a direction to prevent changes in varus or valgus, flexion or extension. It is inserted 30° in a posteromedial direction relative to the flat surface on the lateral tibial diaphysis. Two K-wires that were placed parallel before the osteotomy now are changed to an angle of 30° with the distal wire in the distal or shaft fragment having been rotated internally 30°. A clamp is holding the side plate to the lateral tibial cortex while the tension device will be applied.

fragments to a realignment precise in all three planes is difficult to obtain and difficult to hold while fixation is applied. In the author's experience, the precision and confidence are greatly improved while the time and effort to obtain the correction is also increased. If a blade plate is used and the blade is inserted

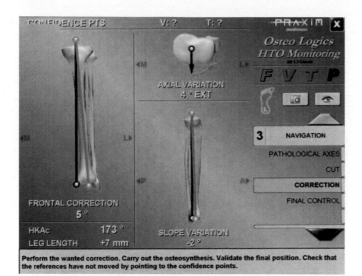

FIGURE 40–46. Computer screen from a navigation system that allows a direct and accurate reading of the change in position of fragments. This system uses infrared reflectors placed into the femur, the tibia above the osteotomy, and the tibia below the osteotomy. Three planes are represented with the correction in each plane. **Left,** the frontal correction, the sample shows that 5° of valgus has been introduced with current hip-knee-ankle line measuring 173° and with an increase in leg length of 7 mm. **Upper central figure,** The horizontal plane correction shows an example of 4° of increased external rotation. **Lower central figure,** The sagittal plane change, an example of 2° of recurvatum or extension. The *green V and T* in this program indicate which markers are being visualized by the camera and utilized by the computer. The *red P* is not being seen by the camera. V: ?, T: ? are reference points on the metaphyseal and diaphyseal reflectors that are used as a test to ensure that there has been no loss of position of these reflectors. *(From Praxim, Walpole, MA.)*

at the correct angle, the osteotomy fixation is easier to obtain but more difficult to change should an error have been made. Unfortunately, there are no imageless navigation systems the author has seen for use in the proximal femur.

COMPLICATIONS

As with all major surgery, complications are possible and include malunion with overcorrection, undercorrection or the addition of a varus or valgus deformity, flexion-extension deformity, non-union, muscle adhesions, compartment syndrome, vascular or neurologic injury, painful trochanter, and painful implants. Implant removal is generally necessary. Generalized complications are the usual expected and not listed here. This author has not performed a revision osteotomy for overcorrection or undercorrection when the blade plate was used. One revision was required in which an intramedullary nail was used for fixation. There have been no cases in which the external rotation of the femur caused the foot to turn out too far if the femur was not overcorrected (except for the one intramedullary nail case) and if an excess external tibial torsion was not already present. Such complications reported in the literature are rare owing to meticulous and slow surgical technique and use of rigid internal fixation.

The immediate goal of osteotomy is to obtain the planned correction. Failure to obtain the proper correction—that is, over- or undercorrection or secondary deformities of abnormal

varus or valgus or flexion or extension—are due to errors in planning, execution, or fixation. The technique of using CT rotational studies for measurement of femoral or tibial torsion is not yet standard. The lines selected for axis measurements may not be accurate. The population normal values need further assessment. The clinical incidence of maltorsion is unknown and symptoms that develop may occur because of activity level. It is common that patients may have abnormal torsion in both the femur and the tibia. Any relationship between these two remains unknown.

The goal of femoral or tibial osteotomy is to put the knee joint axis in line with the forward progression of the body. If an excess femoral anteversion coexists with excess external tibial torsion, then following femoral external rotation osteotomy, the foot may appear to point too far outward and an internal tibial rotational osteotomy may be necessary. This has rarely occurred in this author's experience. At times, the reverse has been noted in which, during walking after an external femoral rotational osteotomy, the foot may be less pronated and therefore appear to point less outward than before the osteotomy. In some patients, the foot is so pronated that it appears to be pointing outward when in reality the ankle joint is in proper alignment but the subtalar joint is not. This author cannot at this time predict before surgery what the gait will be after either a femoral or a tibial osteotomy or after an osteotomy of both femur and tibia. However, with accurate preoperative measurements, the patient can be informed of the existence of multiple deformities that might eventually require further correction.

Proper execution depends on the use of exacting intraoperative references. The references for rotation are K-wires placed above and below the level selected for osteotomy. When the osteotomy has been completed, it is necessary to manually manipulate the fragments into the newly desired position. The surgeons' interpretation of the angulation between the reference K-wires is a source of potential error. The rotation of the tibia and femur is equally difficult, but because of a difficulty in maintaining the reduction, malposition of the proximal femoral fragments is less common than malposition of the proximal tibial fragments. This is because the site of the femoral osteotomy is through a relatively circular bone and the exact fit of a condylar blade plate to the proximal femur. At the proximal tibia, there is no implant that matches the bony anatomy both before and after correction. This makes it difficult to use the implant to control both varus-valgus and flexion-extension changes. In addition, the triangular shape of the tibia below the tubercle imposes a reduced contact area between the two cut surfaces, which is inherently more unstable. The reference wires are useful for estimating rotation and, to some extent, for estimating flexion and extension, but are not useful to accurately estimate varus or valgus changes. C-Arm images with a marker placed over the center of the femoral head and the center of the talus with a Bovie cord or an alignment rod placed between the two are more useful, but this method of judging limb alignment is highly sensitive to uncontrolled limb rotation. The knee joint axis must be perpendicular to the x-ray beam while this measurement is being made. The more compression that can be applied to the osteotomy surfaces, the greater stability, but this requires that the pull on the plate be in line with the axis of the limb. With a plate not perfectly contoured to the newly corrected bony anatomy, it is difficult to obtain attachment of the plate to the proximal tibial fragment such that the distal portion of the plate is aligned with the limb axis.

Rotational CT studies postoperatively would be required to measure the accuracy of the postoperative correction; this has been done in a limited number of cases. These limited results suggest that the accuracy of correction is within 5° of the planned correction when a blade plate was used, but up to 10° to 12° when an intramedullary nail was used for fixation.

Fixation without compression has a higher rate of delayed union, nonunion, and loss of correction. In spite of the published suggestion of frequent complications with tibial osteotomy, these have been relatively few when solid fixation through compression has been obtained. In this author's experience, delayed union or nonunion has always been associated with inadequate fixation and compression. If this occurs without loss of correction, recompression is usually a reliable solution. This author recommends to not "take-down" a biologically active nonunion. In an unpublished review of 72 intertrochanteric osteotomies (author's series), there was one delayed union that healed uneventfully after reoperation to add compression to the osteotomy by adding tension to the implant.

RESULTS OF TORSIONAL REALIGNMENT

Meister and James[29] reviewed 7 patients who had undergone tibial rotational osteotomy for anterior knee pain at an average of 10 years previously, and rated 1 patient excellent, 5 good, and 1 fair. Bruce and Stevens[3] reviewed 14 patients with anterior knee pain caused by miserable malalignment treated with combined external femoral rotational osteotomy and internal rotational tibial osteotomy at an average of 5 years and reported that all were satisfied. Cooke and colleagues[5] reported on 7 patients with anterior knee pain associated with varus and excessive external tibial torsion treated with valgus internal rotation osteotomy in which 5 were rated as excellent. Delgado and coworkers[7] reported on 9 patients with anterior knee pain and 13 osteotomies of the femur, tibia, or both, with marked improvement seen over 2 years. Server and associates[38] reported on 25 patients undergoing internal rotational tibial osteotomy for excessive external tibial torsion and symptoms suggesting patellar subluxation, with 23 of 25 satisfied, including some athletes. Ficat and Hungerford[10] reported 1 case of recurrent patellar subluxation that responded to osteotomy of both the femur and the tibia.

Ruesch in 1995 (unpublished paper) reviewed a series of 35 femoral external rotational osteotomies performed for anterior knee pain and/or instability in 31 patients. Five patients were not located, but 26 (84%) were seen an average of 5.3 years postoperatively. Eighty-eight percent of the group presented with failed PF surgery, with 23 of the patients averaging more than 2 prior surgeries. Only 3 patients had not had prior surgery. Six of the 35 osteotomies were intramedullary fixed with intramedullary nails and 29 were intertrochanteric. Two PF rating scores were used. The average Schwartz and colleagues' score[36] was 24.6 points (of 29 points), with 15 of 35 excellent, 6 good, 5 fair, and 9 poor. The average Shea and Fulkerson score[39] was 82.5 points (of 100 points), with 20 excellent, 6 good, 1 fair, and 8 poor. The poor results mostly reflected preexisting arthrosis. However, subjectively, 77% indicated a decrease in the amount of pain, 86% less giving-way, 80% improvement in quality of life, and 42% a reduction in retropatellar crepitation. Of the 3 patients without prior surgery, the

Shea and Fulkerson score was 100 points and the Schwartz score was 28.7 points.

Latteier (the author's series; unpublished data) reviewed 72 intertrochanteric, external rotational osteotomies in 53 patients presenting with PF dysfunction. These included the patients reviewed by Ruesch described earlier. The mean follow-up was 9.7 years (range, 2–17 yr). Follow-up was obtained in 92% of the patients. Preoperative and postoperative Kujala, Lysholm, and Tegner scores were obtained. The mean Tegner activity score increased from 2.2 to 4.0 points, the mean Kyjala score increased from 53 to 86 points, and the mean Lysholm increased from 49 to 89 points. All but 1 patient showed improvement in all postoperative scores. However, in 20%, the Kujala improvement was insufficient to raise the score beyond the fair or poor range, and in 22%, the Lysholm improvement was insufficient to raise the score beyond the fair or poor range. Patients subjectively stated they improved by an average of 91%, with 55% of all respondents reporting improvement at 100%. The patient with the worst result reported improvement of 20%. Three patients would not undergo surgery again. One would not repeat the surgery because the amount of improvement was not enough, and 1 because of a femur fracture after blade plate removal 11 months after osteotomy. In the third patient, the surgery uncovered a previously unknown rare genetic coagulopathy requiring Greenfield filter, permanent anticoagulation, and advice not to have plate removal or further surgery. One patient had a delayed union treated by recompression of the osteotomy.

Each patient presents with different problems and different structural failures; thus, outcome measures fail to reveal the complete patient profile. Pain in the absence of instability or chondral disease is the most common early presentation. The only objective measurement may be that of abnormal limb torsion. Patients after surgery have reported returning to painless cross-country running after not being able to walk to classes before correction, the loss of bunions, the loss of radiating pain down the lateral side of the limb from pelvis to lateral ankle after 40 years without relief, the loss of retropatellar crepitation on stairs, the first ability to ride a bicycle and ski without pain, and the feeling of stability in landing after a jump in basketball. Such observations are not part of any PF scores and the improvements are therefore missed. Exercise that constrains the pelvis and feet such as bicycling, classic cross-country skiing, or elliptical machines is a particular problem for these patients because there is no escape for the inward-pointing knee. Strong hip abduction is a benefit for patients with femoral anteversion, because it may allow the patient to be active with a knee that points forward thus relieving pain. However, because the hip abductor is working at a mechanical disadvantage, it will often fatigue and the knee joint must point medially to gain mechanical leverage at the hip. This inward limb rotation forces an increased pronation at the foot such that medial arch strain, posterior tibial tendon strain, and bunions are more common. This chronic foot pronation may allow an increase in equinus ankle contracture, which then accentuates the increase in internal limb rotation. Excess external tibial torsion with normal femoral torsion presents a different problem. The knee points inward because this is necessary for proper ankle dorsiflexion during gait. The medial knee pain is common because the quadriceps increases the lateral vector on the patella when the foot is pointing forward. The hip abductors, however, are working at near-normal mechanical advantage so pelvic strengthening is less likely to be useful.

CONCLUSIONS

1. Miserable malalignment as described by James[15] exists and must be recognized in the patient with PF pain, instability, or arthrosis.
2. Torsional limb malalignment may present with only pain or may coexist with patellar instability and/or patellar chondrosis, and it may be a biomechanical contributor to the etiology of both instability and arthrosis, but all three conditions must be assessed independently.
3. Restoration of normal limb alignment in all three planes is thought to restore the normal direction of the force vectors that cross the knee joint.

4. The transverse (horizontal) plane is frequently overlooked and is best evaluated with a CT scan that allows the axis of the hip, knee, and ankle to be measured relative to each other.
5. Realignment of the femur and tibia by rotational osteotomy may be not only appropriate but also necessary. It is the only reasonable surgical treatment for PF symptoms due to skeletal malalignment.
6. Surgery for instability or for cartilage restoration is more likely to fail in the mechanical environment of persistent lower limb maltorsion.
7. Surgical morbidity must not be underestimated.

REFERENCES

1. Arnold, A. S.; Komattu, A. V.; Delp, S. L.: Internal rotation gait: a compensatory mechanism to restore abduction capacity decreased by bone deformity. *Dev Med Child Neurol* 39:40–44, 1997.
2. Brattström, H.: Shape of the intercondylar groove normally and in recurrent dislocation of the patella. *Acta Orthop Scand* 68 (suppl):1–148, 1964.
3. Bruce, W. D.; Stevens, P. M.: Surgical correction of miserable malalignment syndrome. *J Pediatr Orthop* 24:392–396, 2004.
4. Christoforakis, J.; Bull, A. M.; Strachan, R. K.; et al: Effects of lateral retinacular release on the lateral stability of the patella. *Knee Surg Sports Traumatol Arthrosc* 14:273–277, 2006.
5. Cooke, T. D.; Price, N.; Fisher, B.; et al: The inwardly pointing knee. An unrecognized problem of external rotational malalignment. *Clin Orthop Relat Res* 260:56–60, 1990.
6. Dejour, H.; Walch, G.; Nove-Josserand, L.; et al.: Factors of patellar instability: an anatomic radiographic study. *Knee Surg Sports Traumatol Arthrosc* 2:19–26, 1994.
7. Delgado, E. D.; Schoenecker, P. L.; Rich, M. M.; et al.: Treatment of severe torsional malalignment syndrome. *J Pediatr Orthop* 16:484–488, 1996.
8. Desio, S. M.; Burks, R. T.; Bachus, K. N.: Soft tissue restraints to lateral patellar translation in the human knee. *Am J Sports Med* 26:59–65, 1998.
9. Eckhoff, D. G.; Brown, A. W.; Kilcoyne, R. F.; et al.: Knee version associated with anterior knee pain. *Clin Orthop Relat Res* 339:152–155, 1997.
10. Ficat, R. P.; Hungerford, D. S.: Chondrosis and arthrosis, a hypothesis. *Disorders of the Patellofemoral Joint*. Baltimore: Williams & Wilkins, 1977; p. 103.
11. Fujikawa, K.; Seedhom, B. B.; Wright, V.: Biomechanics of the patello-femoral joint. Part I: a study of the contact and the congruity of the patello-femoral compartment and movement of the patella. *Eng Med* 12:3–11, 1983.
12. Hefzy, M. S.; Jackson, W. T.; Saddemi, S. R.; et al.: Effects of tibial rotations on patellar tracking and patello-femoral contact areas. *J Biomed Eng* 14:329–343, 1992.
13. Insall, J.; Falvo, K. A.; Wise, D. W.: Chondromalacia patellae. A prospective study. *J Bone Joint Surg Am* 58:1–8, 1976.
14. Jakob, R. P.; Haertel, M.; Stussi, E.: Tibial torsion calculated by computerised tomography and compared to other methods of measurement. *J Bone Joint Surg Br* 62:238–242, 1980.
15. James, S. L.: Chondromalacia of the patella in the adolescent. In Kennedy J.C. (ed.): *The Injured Adolescent Knee*. Baltimore: Williams & Wilkins, 1979; pp. 205–251.
16. Janssen, G.: Increased medial torsion of the knee joint producing chondromalacia patella. In Trickey, E.; Hertel, P. (eds.): *Surgery and Arthroscopy of the Knee, 2nd Congress of the European Society*. Berlin: Springer-Verlag; 1988; pp. 263–267.
17. Kelman, G. J.; Focht, L.; Drakauer, J. D.; et al.: A cadaveric study of patellofemoral kinematics using a biomechanical testing rig and gait laboratory motion analysis. *Orthop Trans* 13:248–249, 1989.
18. Kijowski, R.; Plagens, D.; Shaeh, S. J.; et al.: The effects of rotational deformities of the femur on contact pressure and contact area in the patellofemoral joint and on strain in the medial patellofemoral ligament. *Annual Meeting of the International Patellofemoral Study Group*. Meadowood, CA, Sept. 29, 1999.
19. Kuo, T. Y.; Skedros, J. G.; Bloebaum, R. D.: Measurement of femoral anteversion by biplane radiography and computed tomography imaging: comparison with an anatomic reference. *Invest Radiol* 38:221–229, 2003.
20. Kuroda, R.; Kambic, H.; Valdevit, A.; et al.: Articular cartilage contact pressure after tibial tuberosity transfer. A cadaveric study. *Am J Sports Med* 29:403–409, 2001.
21. Le Damany, P.: La torsion du tibia, normale pathologique, experimentale. *J Int Anat Physiol* 45:598–615, 1990.
22. Lee, T. Q.; Anzel, S. H.; Bennett, K. A.; et al.: The influence of fixed rotational deformities of the femur on the patellofemoral contact pressures in human cadaver knees. *Clin Orthop* 302:69–74, 1994.
23. Lee, T. Q.; Morris, G.; Csintalan, R. P.: The influence of tibial and femoral rotation on patellofemoral contact area and pressure. *J Orthop Sports Phys Ther* 33:686–693, 2003.
24. Lee, T. Q.; Yang, B. Y.; Sandusky, M. D.; et al.: The effects of tibial rotation on the patellofemoral joint: assessment of the changes in in situ strain in the peripatellar retinaculum and the patellofemoral contact pressures and areas. *J Rehabil Res Dev* 38:463–469, 2001.
25. Lerat, J. L.; Moyen, B.; Bochu, M.; et al.: Femoropatellar pathology and rotational and torsional abnormalities of the inferior limbs: the use of CT scan. In Muller, W.; Hackenbruch W. (eds.): *Surgery and Arthroscopy of the Knee. 2nd Congress of the European Society*. Berlin: Springer-Verlag, 1988.
26. Lerat, J. L.; Moyen, B.; Galland, O.; et al.: [Morphological types of the lower limbs in femoro-patellar disequilibrium. Analysis in 3 planes]. *Acta Orthop Belg* 55:347–355, 1989.
27. Levens, A. S.; Berkeley, C. E.; Inman, V. T.; et al.: Transverse rotation of the segments of the lower extremity in locomotion. *J Bone Joint Surg Am* 30:859–872, 1948.
28. Losel, S.; Burgess-Milliron, M. J.; Micheli, L. J.; et al.: A simplified technique for determining foot progression angle in children 4 to 16 years of age. *J Pediatr Orthop* 16:570–574, 1996.
29. Meister, K.; James, S. L.: Proximal tibial derotation osteotomy for anterior knee pain in the miserably malaligned extremity. *Am J Orthop* 24:149–155, 1995.
30. Murphy, S. B.; Simon, S. R.; Kijewski, P. K.; et al.: Femoral anteversion. *J Bone Joint Surg Am* 69:1169–1176, 1987.
31. Nomura, E.; Inoue, M.: Cartilage lesions of the patella in recurrent patellar dislocation. *Am J Sports Med* 32:498–502, 2004.
32. Nyland, J.; Kuzemchek, S.; Parks, M.; et al.: Femoral anteversion influences vastus medialis and gluteus medius EMG amplitude: composite hip abductor EMG amplitude ratios during isometric combined hip abduction-external rotation. *J Electromyogr Kinesiol* 14:255–261, 2004.
33. Pasciak, M.; Stoll, T. M.; Hefti F.: Relation of femoral to tibial torsion in children measured by ultrasound. *J Pediatr Orthop B* 5:268–272, 1996.
34. Saunders, J.; Inman, V.; Eberhart, H.: The major determinants in normal and pathological gait. *J Bone Joint Surg Am* 35:543–558, 1953.
35. Sayli, U.; Bolukbasi, S.; Atik, O. S.; et al.: Determination of tibial torsion by computed tomography. *J Foot Ankle Surg* 33:144–147, 1994.

36. Schwarz, C.; Blazina, M. E.; Sisto, D. J.; et al.: The results of operative treatment of osteochondritis dissecans of the patella. *Am J Sports Med* 16:522–529, 1988.

37. Seber, S.; Hazer, B.; Kose, N.; et al.: Rotational profile of the lower extremity and foot progression angle: computerized tomographic examination of 50 male adults. *Arch Orthop Trauma Surg* 120:255–258, 2000.

38. Server, F.; Miralles, R. C.; Garcia, E.; et al.: Medial rotational tibial osteotomy for patellar instability secondary to lateral tibial torsion. *Int Orthop* 20:153–158, 1996.

39. Shea, K. P.; Fulkerson, J. P.: Preoperative computed tomography scanning and arthroscopy in predicting outcome after lateral retinacular release. *Arthroscopy* 8:327–334, 1992.

40. Stroud, K. L.; Smith, A. D.; Kruse, R. W.: The relationship between increased femoral anteversion in childhood and patellofemoral pain in adulthood. *Orthop Trans* 13:555, 1989.

41. Takai, S.; Sakakida, K.; Yamashita, F.; et al.: Rotational alignment of the lower limb in osteoarthritis of the knee. *Int Orthop* 9:209–215, 1985.

42. Tamari, K.; Tinley, P.; Briffa, K.; et al.: Validity and reliability of existing and modified clinical methods of measuring femoral and tibiofibular torsion in healthy subjects: use of different reference axes may improve reliability. *Clin Anat* 18:46–55, 2005.

43. Teitge, R. A.; Faerber, W. W.; Des Madryl, P.; et al.: Stress radiographs of the patellofemoral joint. *J Bone Joint Surg Am* 78:193–203, 1996.

44. Turner, M. S.: The association between tibial torsion and knee joint pathology. *Clin Orthop Relat Res* 302:47–51, 1994.

45. van Kampen, A.; Huiskes, R.: The three-dimensional tracking pattern of the human patella. *J Orthop Res* 8:372–382, 1990.

46. Winson, I. G.; Miranda, J.; Smith, T. W.: Anterior knee pain in the post-adolescent decade. *Acta Orthop Scand* 61 (suppl 237):62, 1990.

47. Yoshioka, Y.; Cooke, T. D.: Femoral anteversion: assessment based on function axes. *J Orthop Res* 5:86–91, 1987.

48. Yoshioka, Y.; Siu, D.; Cooke, T. D.: The anatomy and functional axes of the femur. *J Bone Joint Surg Am* 69:873–880, 1987.

49. Yoshioka, Y.; Siu, D. W.; Scudamore, R. A.; et al.: Tibial anatomy and functional axes. *J Orthop Res* 7:132–137, 1989.

Postoperative Complications

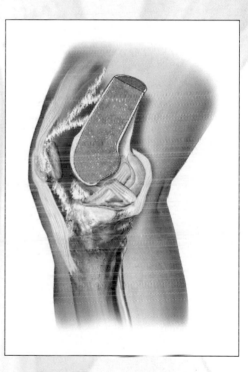

Prevention and Treatment of Knee Arthrofibrosis

Frank R. Noyes, MD ■ *Sue D. Barber-Westin*, BS

INTRODUCTION

Loss of a normal range of knee motion after an injury or ligament reconstruction is a potentially devastating complication. Although a multitude of investigations and publications have appeared since the early 1990s regarding this problem, loss of knee motion continues to be one of the most frequently reported complications after surgical procedures.[27,31,72,83,84] Although the definition and use of the term *arthrofibrosis* vary among authors, it implies a loss of knee flexion, extension, or both compared with the contralateral normal knee.

Primary arthrofibrosis is caused by an exaggerated inflammatory response to an injury or surgical procedure, followed by the production of fibroblastic cells and an increase in the deposition of extracellular matrix proteins.[147] Proliferative scar tissue or fibrous adhesions form within the joint, which can result in either localized or diffuse involvement of all of the compartments of the knee and the extra-articular soft tissues (Fig. 41–1). In the most severe cases, dense scar tissue obliterates the normal peripatellar recesses, suprapatellar pouch, intercondylar notch, and articular surfaces. Formation of dense scar tissue in the infrapatellar region may result in a patella infera and permanent limitation of normal knee flexion and extension. The consequent pain and restricted knee motion resulting from arthrofibrosis may lead to disabling events including severe quadriceps atrophy, loss of patellar mobility, patellar tendon adaptive shortening, patella infera, and articular cartilage deterioration.[105,106]

The incidence of arthrofibrosis after ligament reconstructive surgery varies according to several factors, which are discussed. Two of the most commonly noted factors are knee dislocations and major concurrent operative procedures performed with the ligament surgery such as reconstruction of other knee ligaments, complex meniscus repair, or high tibial osteotomy (Table 41–1).[7,91–103] Publications show wide disparity among authors regarding the treatment of this problem, especially the time postoperatively that intervention is warranted and what type of treatment should be implemented for losses of knee extension and flexion and loss of patella mobility.

Critical Points INTRODUCTION

- Arthrofibrosis implies a loss of knee flexion, extension, or both compared with the contralateral normal knee.
- Primary arthrofibrosis is caused by an exaggerated inflammatory response to an injury or surgical procedure, followed by the production of fibroblastic cells and an increase in the deposition of extracellular matrix proteins. Proliferative scar tissue or fibrous adhesions form within the joint, which can be either localized or diffuse.
- Incidence of arthrofibrosis after ligament reconstructive surgery varies.
- Wide disparity exists among authors regarding the treatment of this problem.
- Limitations in knee motion may occur owing to reasons other than arthrofibrosis:
  - Mechanical block from a displaced bucket-handle meniscus tear.
  - Impinged or improperly placed ACL graft.

- Cyclops lesion.
- Improper ACL graft tensioning.
- Contracture of posterior capsular structures.
- If not resolved, these problems may result in the development of secondary arthrofibrosis.
- Most individuals have some amount of hyperextension to allow the normal "screw-home" mechanism to occur: knee stabilized in extension during the stance phase, with the quadriceps muscle relaxed.
- Normal knee flexion averages 140° in men and 143° in women.
- Patients not involved in athletics tolerate small flexion deficits. Significant flexion deficits < 90° cause problems with squatting, stair-climbing, and sitting.
- Loss of just 5° of extension may produce a flexed-knee gait, fatigue the quadriceps muscle, and cause patellofemoral pain.
- Prevention of knee arthrofibrosis is paramount and preferred over the current treatment options for this complication.

ACL, anterior cruciate ligament.

It is important to note that limitations in knee flexion and extension may occur owing to reasons other than arthrofibrosis. Any acute injury causing pain and swelling may cause a short-term loss of knee motion, which usually resolves as symptoms subside. Other factors influencing the restoration of knee motion include a mechanical block from a displaced bucket-handle meniscus tear, an impinged or improperly placed anterior cruciate ligament (ACL) graft, a cyclops lesion,[65] improper graft tensioning that constrains normal knee joint motion,[20] and graft fixation at 30° or more of extension.[5] In addition, contracture of the posterior capsular structures may limit knee extension. If not resolved, these problems may result in the development of what is termed *secondary arthrofibrosis*, complicating the course of treatment.

Normal knee motion varies, but most individuals have some amount of hyperextension, which averages 5° in men and 6° in women.[30,31,74] This degree of hyperextension is required so that the normal "screw-home" mechanism can occur that allows the knee to be stabilized in extension during the stance phase, with the quadriceps muscle relaxed. Normal knee flexion averages 140° in men and 143° in women. It is generally assumed that

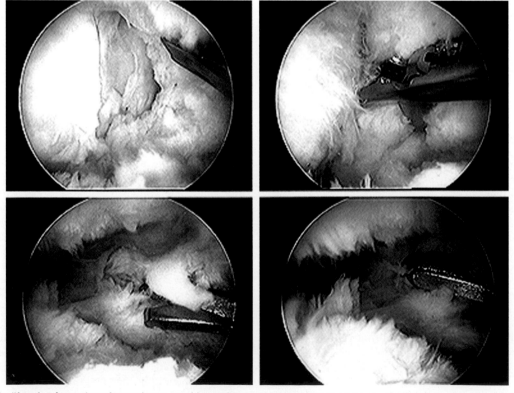

FIGURE 41–1. Proliferative formation of scar tissue requiring arthroscopic débridement and lysis of adhesions. A contracture of medial and lateral parapatellar soft tissues is shown, along with patella and trochlear cartilage deterioration.

TABLE 41–1   Incidence of Knee Motion Problems after Knee Operations: Authors' Clinical Studies

Reference*	Operation	Type of Ligament Graft, Concomitant Procedures, Patients (N)	Incidence Motion Problems Requiring Therapeutic Intervention (%)
JBJSA, 1990[93]	ACL reconstruction	Allograft, acute: 40	17
JBJSA, 1991[92]	ACL reconstruction	Allograft only, chronic: 64	8
		Allograft + EA, chronic: 40	18
JBJSA, 1992[91]	ACL reconstruction	Allograft only, chronic: 66	8
		Allograft + LAD, chronic: 49	2
CORR, 1992[102]	ACL reconstruction	Allograft only: 90	4
		Allograft + EA: 52	10
		Allograft + meniscus repair: 52	12
		Allograft + MCL repair: 13	23
AJSM, 1995[98]	ACL reconstruction	Allograft + MCL repair: 34	26
		Allograft + MCL conservative treatment: 12	17
AJSM, 1997[95]	ACL reconstruction	PT autograft, acute: 30	10
		PT autograft, chronic: 57	2
AJSM, 1997[7]	ACL reconstruction	PT autograft, men: 47	4
		PT autograft, women: 47	6
AJSM, 1997[97]	Multiple ligament reconstruction for knee dislocation	Allograft + autograft: 11 All ACL + PCL; also + MCL: 6; also + PL: 6	45
KSSTA, 2000[101]	ACL reconstruction	PT autograft only: 219	6
		PT autograft + PL procedure: 37	5
		PT autograft + meniscus repair: 194	8
		PT autograft + patellar realignment: 17	18
		PT autograft + MCL repair: 9	22
AJSM, 2000[99]	HTO, closing wedge	N: 38	0
		HTO + ACL: 3	0
JBJSA, 2004[100]	Meniscus transplantation	Transplant only: 18	0
		Transplant + OAT: 16	12
		Transplant + knee ligament procedure: 4	50
JBJSA, 2005[94]	PCL reconstruction	Isolated: 11	18
		PCL + other knee ligament: 8	25
AJSM, 2006[103]	HTO, opening wedge	HTO only: 49	0
		HTO + ACL: 4	0
		HTO + OAT: 2	0
AJSM, 2007[96]	PL anatomic reconstruction	PL only: 2	0
		PL + knee ligament procedure: 12	17

*See References for complete citations. AJSM, *Am J Sports Med*; CORR, *Clin Orthop*; JBJSA, *J Bone Joint Surg Am*; KSSTA, *Knee Surg Sports Traumatol Arthrosc*.
ACL, anterior cruciate ligament; acute, reconstruction done within 3 mo of the original knee injury; chronic, reconstruction done more than 3 mo after the original knee injury; EA, iliotibial band extra-articular procedure; HTO, high tibial osteotomy; LAD, ligament augmentation device; MCL, medial collateral ligament; OAT, osteochondral autograft transplantation; PCL, posterior cruciate ligament; PL, posterolateral; PT, patellar tendon.

at least 125° of knee flexion is required for activities of daily living.[31,74] Rowe and coworkers[120] measured knee kinematics during functional activities in a group of 20 subjects aged 49 to 80 years and reported that 90° of flexion is required for gait and slopes, 90° to 120° for stairs and sitting, and 135° for bathing. Patients not involved in athletics tolerate small flexion deficits. Significant flexion deficits of less than 90° cause problems with squatting, stair-climbing, and sitting. Athletes have a poorer tolerance for even minor losses of flexion, which affect running and jumping. Cosgarea and associates[24] reported that deficits of 10° or more of flexion were associated with decreased running speed.

All patients, regardless of their activity level, have greater problems with loss of knee extension. A loss of just 5° of extension may produce a flexed-knee gait, fatigue the quadriceps muscle, and cause patellofemoral pain.[63,66,86,89,121] Limitation of more than 20° may cause a functional limb-length discrepancy.[24] Many years ago, Perry and colleagues[114] demonstrated the effect of a loss of extension on joint contact pressures, quadriceps muscle activity, and fatigue. These investigators measured the extensor forces required to stabilize the flexed knee during simulated

weight-bearing in cadaver specimens. The quadriceps force required to stabilize the knee was 75% of the load on the head of the femur at 15° of flexion, which increased to 210% at 30° of flexion, and to 410% at 60° of flexion. The quadriceps force was equal to 20% of the average maximum quadriceps strength at 15° of flexion, but increased to 50% at 30° of flexion. Surface pressure in the tibiofemoral and patellofemoral joints also increased with greater amounts of knee flexion.

It has become evident that the prevention of knee arthrofibrosis is paramount and preferred over using the currently available treatment options for this complication. This chapter discusses the risk factors and preventive measures for loss of knee motion after knee injury and surgery. In addition, conservative medical and therapeutic treatment intervention strategies are discussed that are usually successful in resolving a transient limitation of knee motion if initiated early postoperatively. Surgical procedures for severe cases of restriction of knee motion are presented. The authors' clinical studies involving 650 ACL-reconstructed knees are included to provide support for treatment recommendations.

TERMINOLOGY AND CLASSIFICATION SYSTEMS

A variety of terms have been used to describe, define, or classify a limitation of knee flexion and extension including arthrofibrosis, flexion contracture, ankylosis, infrapatellar contracture syndrome, and motion loss. Some of the terms indicate a specific process whereas others simply imply a limitation of motion compared with the contralateral normal knee. *Ankylosis* is one such generic term that indicates stiffness of joints that occurs for any reason and may represent loss of knee flexion, extension, or both. The term *motion loss* is another general phrase used to describe deviations from the amount of flexion and extension compared with the contralateral normal knee. Conversely, *arthrofibrosis* describes a specific cause for a limitation of knee motion, which is the formation of diffuse scar tissue or fibrous adhesions within a joint.[63,111,115] *Flexion contracture* indicates a loss of extension due to any cause and is accompanied by a relative shortening of the posterior soft tissues (in either the capsule

or the muscles). Petsche and Hutchinson[115] stated that *arthrofibrosis* and *flexion contracture* are general terms, and it is necessary to indicate a specific cause for loss of motion.

Classification systems have been proposed by various authors to describe limitations in knee motion, based on either the anatomic location of scar tissue and adhesions or the amount of knee motion in the affected joint (Table 41–2).[12,33,111,132,141] Sprague and coworkers[141] first introduced a system based on the arthroscopically observed location of scar tissues and adhesions in 24 patients who had a severe limitation of knee motion. Paulos and associates[111] described three stages of knee motion restrictions due to infrapatellar contracture syndrome. Del Pizzo and colleagues[33] and Shelbourne and coworkers[132] developed classification systems based on the deviation of knee motion compared to the opposite knee. Blauth and Jaeger[12] described a system based on the total arc of motion in the affected knee.

The authors developed a classification system based on the anatomic sites at which scar tissue, adhesions, and adaptive shortening of soft tissues occur (Fig. 41–2 and Table 41–3). This system is advantageous because it highlights the areas that must be addressed surgically, as is discussed.

Critical Points TERMINOLOGY AND CLASSIFICATION SYSTEMS

- Terms used to describe limitation knee motion: *arthrofibrosis, flexion contracture, ankylosis, infrapatellar contracture syndrome, motion loss.*
- The term *arthrofibrosis* describes a specific cause for a limitation of knee motion, which is the formation of diffuse scar tissue or fibrous adhesions within a joint.
- Classification systems describe limitations in knee motion, based on either the anatomic location of scar tissue and adhesions or the amount of knee motion in the affected joint.
- Authors' classification system is based on the anatomic sites where scar tissue, adhesions, and adaptive shortening of soft tissues occur.

RISK FACTORS AFTER KNEE LIGAMENT RECONSTRUCTION

A variety of factors appear to influence the requirement for treatment intervention for knee motion limitations (Table 41–4) and the final amount of knee flexion and extension gained after ligament reconstruction. These factors are related to the severity of the injury, the timing of surgery, preoperative treatment, technical aspects of the ligament reconstruction, and the postoperative course and rehabilitation. Although it remains uncertain why some knees are more likely to form an abnormal scar response to trauma and surgery than others, knowledge of these factors may help reduce this problem.

TABLE 41–2   Classification Systems of Arthrofibrosis

Reference	Classification System
Sprague et al., 1982[141]	I: Discreet bands or a single sheet of adhesions traversing the suprapatellar pouch II: Near-complete obliteration of suprapatellar pouch and peripatellar gutters with masses of adhesions III: Multiple bands of adhesions or complete obliteration of suprapatellar pouch with extracapsular involvement

Del Pizzo et al., 1985[33]	Based on deviation from full extension and amount of flexion present:
	  Mild: <5° extension, >110° flexion
	  Moderate: 5°–10° extension, 90°–100° flexion
	  Severe: >10° extension, <90° flexion

Paulos et al., 1987[111]	Three stages of infrapatellar contracture syndrome:
	  I: Prodromal stage (2–8 wk postoperative) hardened synovium, fat pad, retinaculum marked by painful motion, restricted patellar mobility, quadriceps muscle lag
	  II: Active stage (6–20 wk postoperative) peripatellar swelling, severely restricted patellar motion, hardening anterior tissues, step-off between patellar tendon and tibial tuberosity
	  III: Residual stage (>8 mo postoperative) fat pad atrophy, patellofemoral crepitus and arthrosis, patella infera, quadriceps atrophy

Blauth & Jaeger, 1990[12]	Based on total arc of motion:
	  I (mild): >120°
	  II (moderate): 80°–120°
	  III (severe): 40°–80°
	  IV (extreme): <40°

Shelbourne et al., 1996[132]	Based on deviation from full flexion and extension of opposite, normal knee:
	  I: <10° extension, normal flexion
	  II: >10° extension, normal flexion
	  III: >10° extension, >25° loss of flexion
	  IV: >10° extension, >30° loss of flexion, patella infera

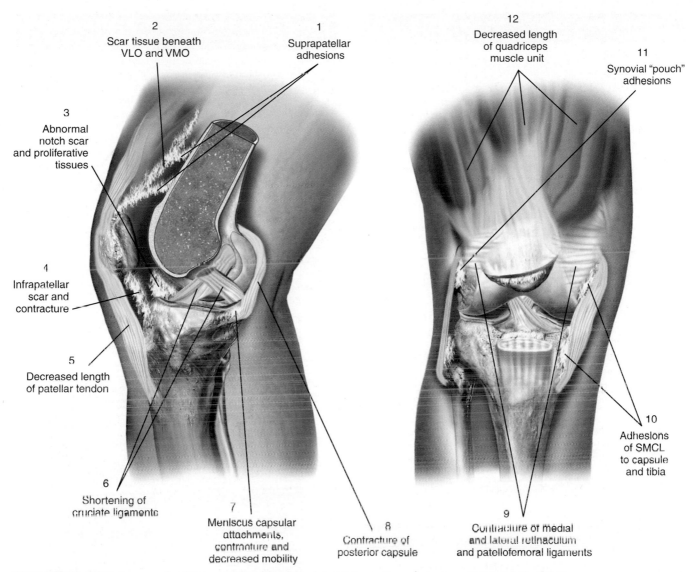

FIGURE 41-2. Multiple areas of soft tissue contracture, adhesions, and scar tissue formation with knee arthrofibrosis.

Severity of the Injury

Patients who sustain knee dislocations are at increased risk for developing motion complications (Fig. 41–3).[23,35,83,97,127,136] These injuries frequently occur from high-energy accidents that produce extreme soft tissue swelling and edema, hematomas, muscle damage, and other multiple trauma that must be resolved before consideration of knee soft tissue reconstructions. Early operative intervention when possible is advisable for multiple ligament injuries that involve the lateral and posterolateral structures where acute repair and augmentation procedures are performed (see Chapter 22, Posterolateral Ligament Injuries: Diagnosis, Operative Techniques, and Clinical Outcomes). For all other dislocations, surgery is delayed with the limb immobilized in a posterior plaster splint or bivalved cast with a posterior pad to prevent posterior tibial subluxation. Even in these severe knee injuries, it is possible to start immediate range of motion and prevent scar tissue formation that may compromise the outcome of a subsequent ligament reconstruction. Too often, these serious knee joint injuries are not treated with an early motion and function program. When surgical treatment is elected, the reconstructive and repair procedures of torn ligaments, capsular structures, and menisci are performed in a manner that allows immediate knee motion to be instituted postoperatively.[97]

Preoperative Issues

Performing ACL and other knee ligament reconstruction within a few weeks of the injury or before the resolution of swelling, pain, quadriceps muscle atrophy, abnormal gait mechanics, and motion limitations has been noted by many authors to correlate with postoperative knee motion problems.[25,54,86,129,130,134,144,152] Shelbourne and associates[134] noted an increased rate of arthrofibrosis in patients who underwent acute ACL reconstruction (within 1 week of the injury) compared with those in whom the reconstruction was delayed for at least 21 days. Similar findings were reported by Wasilewski and colleagues[152] who noted that arthrofibrosis was found in 22% of acutely reconstructed knees versus 12.5% of knees reconstructed with chronic ACL deficiency. Mohtadi and coworkers[86] found that ACL reconstructions performed less than 6 weeks postinjury had a higher rate of knee

TABLE 41–3   Authors' Anatomic Classification System of Arthrofibrosis

Loss of Flexion

Quadriceps muscle
- Shortens due to scar tissue and intramuscular changes, limiting normal muscle lengthening.

Suprapatellar pouch
- Scar tissue may form underneath quadriceps VMO, VLO, limiting muscle extensibility.
- Scar tissue from the superior pole of the patella produces patellar clunk, may extend as a band just above the femoral trochlea.
- Scar tissue and adhesions obliterate the suprapatellar pouch.

Medial and lateral capsular pouches
- Scar down and become adhesive to the medial and lateral side of the femur.

Patellar retinaculum and associated ligaments
- Scar tissue forms with thickening, shortening, limiting patellar mobility.

Patellar tendon
- Tendon shortens or may adhere to the tibia.
- Infrapatellar scar tissue inferior pole to tibia just anterior to fat pad.

Medial and lateral extra-articular ligament structures
- Scar tissue, adhesions, adaptive shortening.

Loss of Extension

Posterior capsule
- Scar tissue, adhesions, shortening of structures.

Femoral notch
- In-growth scar tissue, cyclops lesion.

Hamstrings muscle
- Shortening of musculotendinosus unit.

Cruciate ligaments
- ACL, PCL adaptive shortening.

ACL, anterior cruciate ligament; PCL, posterior cruciate ligament; VLO, vastus lateralis obliquus; VMO, vastus medialis obliquus.

TABLE 41–4   Risk Factors for the Development of Knee Arthrofibrosis

Magnitude of the injury: dislocation, multiple ligament injury
Normal or nearly normal knee motion not restored before surgery
Acute ligament reconstruction in swollen, painful knee
Technical errors in ACL graft placement, fixation, tensioning
Concurrent MCL repair or reconstruction
Infection
Immobilization
Chronic joint effusion
Quadriceps atrophy, shutdown
Poor rehabilitation, noncompliant patient
Cyclops lesion
Complex regional pain syndrome, reflex sympathetic dystrophy

ACL, anterior cruciate ligament; MCL, medial collateral ligament.

stiffness than those done more than 6 weeks postinjury (11% and 4%, respectively). Harner and associates[54] reported a 37% rate of motion complications after acute ACL reconstructions (done within 1 month of the injury) compared with a 5% rate in chronic ACL-deficient knees.

Although Bach and colleagues[6] did not observe a significant difference in knee motion complications between acute and chronic ACL-reconstructed knees, the authors stressed the need to delay surgery until patients achieved 120° of knee motion and swelling had resolved. The authors found "no advantage to

Critical Points RISK FACTORS AFTER KNEE LIGAMENT RECONSTRUCTION

- Severity of injury: knee dislocations increase risk for developing motion complications. Surgery is delayed in all cases except those with ruptures to the posterolateral structures.
- Preoperative issues: performing knee ligament reconstruction within a few weeks of the injury or before the resolution of swelling, pain, quadriceps muscle atrophy, abnormal gait mechanics, and motion limitations correlates with postoperative knee motion problems.
- Technical factors at surgery: improper ACL graft placement, overtensioning graft at surgery, performing concurrent MCL repair with ACL reconstruction.
- Postoperative course and rehabilitation: immobilization is detrimental to all of the knee joint structures and may result in a permanent limitation of knee motion, prolonged muscle atrophy, patella infera, and articular cartilage deterioration. Begin knee motion, patellar mobilization, and muscle-strengthening exercises the day after surgery. Treat joint effusion immediately.
- Postoperative infection, complex regional pain syndromes, and reflex sympathetic dystrophy may cause knee motion problems.

ACL, anterior cruciate ligament; MCL, medial collateral ligament.

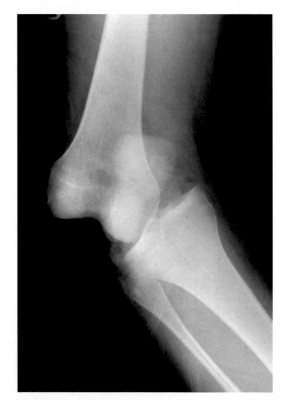

FIGURE 41–3. Acute knee dislocation results in severe disruption of soft tissues, swelling, hemorrhage, and muscle damage always resulting in motion problems and risk of arthrofibrosis.

performing urgent acute ACL reconstruction."[6] Sterett and coworkers[143] found no association between surgical timing and postoperative motion problems. However, in their series, all patients had achieved at least 0° to 120°, had good quadriceps control, and could perform a straight leg raise without an extensor lag before undergoing surgery. Eight percent of the patients in this investigation's acute subgroup required arthroscopic débridement of scar tissue. Meighan and associates[81] also found no advantage in performing early ACL reconstruction and noted an increased rate of complications in patients who underwent surgery within 2 weeks of the injury compared with those who had surgery between 8 and 12 weeks postinjury. The delayed group had a faster return of knee motion and quadriceps strength.

A few authors have not found a higher rate of postoperative motion problems after acute ACL reconstruction.[18,62,75] However, it appears that delaying surgery until knee motion is regained, swelling is resolved, and a good quadriceps contraction is demonstrated is advantageous in decreasing the risk of postoperative arthrofibrosis. The inflammatory response to the initial injury varies among patients. Whereas some have little effusion and swelling, others have an exaggerated inflammatory response characterized by pain, soft tissue edema, and redness and increased warmth to tissues surrounding the knee. These knees are placed into an initial conservative treatment program to resolve these problems first and are also carefully monitored after ACL reconstruction for a similar exaggerated inflammatory reaction postoperatively. Knees with isolated ACL ruptures that have little swelling and demonstrate normal motion early after injury may be considered for earlier reconstruction. In addition, knees with multiple ligament ruptures that include the posterolateral structures are also candidates for early surgical repair, as discussed in Chapter 22, Posterolateral Ligament Structures: Diagnosis, Operative Techniques, and Clinical Outcomes.

Technical Factors at Surgery

Improper ACL graft placement has been frequently noted as a cause of loss of knee motion.* On the tibia, grafts placed anterior to the native ACL insertion result in impingement on the roof of the intercondylar notch when the knee is extended.[59,60,78] Yaru and colleagues[154] recommended that with passive extension, there should be a 3-mm clearance between the anterior portion of the intercondylar notch and the graft to prevent impingement. Grafts placed lateral to the insertion site impinge on the lateral wall of the notch. In addition, Romano and coworkers[119] found that ACL grafts placed too far anterior in the tibial tunnel can cause knee extension deficits, and grafts placed too far medially in the tibial tunnel can cause knee flexion deficits. On the femur, an excessive anterior graft placement causes deleterious forces on the graft, leading to limitations in flexion and potential graft failure (Fig. 41–4).

Overtensioning ACL grafts may lead to abnormal knee kinematics.[84,115] In addition, the degree of knee extension during graft tensioning and fixation may affect postoperative motion.[5,20,47,82,89] Austin and associates[5] noted in a cadaver study that the amount of graft tension (44 N or 89 N) did not effect knee extension; however, tensioning the graft in knee flexion was associated with extension deficits. The authors reported that grafts tensioned and fixed at 30° of flexion had more than a 12° increase in knee flexion after ACL reconstruction compared with those tensioned and fixed at 0° of flexion. From a two-part biomechanical and clinical study, Nabors and colleagues[89] suggested that grafts tensioned in full extension result in a low incidence of knee motion loss. In their series of 57 patients who underwent patellar tendon autograft ACL reconstruction, only 1 patient had a mild (5°) loss of extension.

*See references 9, 43, 61, 63, 66, 72, 77, 85, 119, 131, 135, 154.

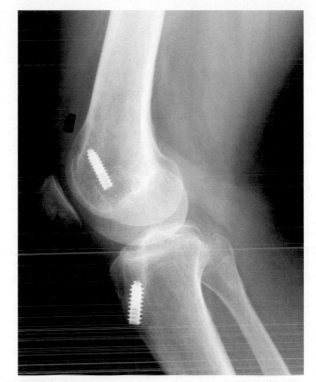

FIGURE 41–4. Lateral radiographs show excessive anterior placement of the femoral tunnel limiting knee flexion and the anterior tibial tunnel limiting knee extension. The graft failed as motion was regained postoperatively.

Concurrent medial collateral ligament (MCL) repair with ACL reconstruction has been associated with an increased risk of knee arthrofibrosis.[54,98,128] Harner and associates[54] postulated that concurrent MCL primary repair may cause a limitation of knee motion due to the disruption of the medial capsule, because the procedure does not restore the normal tissue planes, resulting in scar formation and a heightened pain response. The studies of Shelbourne and coworkers[128,133] and the authors of this chapter[98] led to the recommendation many years ago to treat the majority of combined ACL-MCL ruptures conservatively. This allows healing of the medial-side injury, followed by ACL reconstruction in appropriately indicated patients (see Chapter 24, Medial and Posteromedial Ligament Injuries: Diagnosis, Operative Techniques, and Clinical Outcomes). There are exceptions to this rule, and any surgical procedure on the medial side of the knee joint should be carefully observed postoperatively for a limitation of motion or, in acute knee injuries, the development of heterotopic soft tissue ossification requiring treatment.[126,150]

Postoperative Course and Rehabilitation

There is consensus in the literature that immobilization is detrimental to all of the knee joint structures and may result in a permanent limitation of knee motion, prolonged muscle atrophy, patella infera, and articular cartilage deterioration.[25,51,67,104–106,112,122] Early knee joint motion decreases pain and postoperative joint effusions, aids in the prevention of scar tissue formation and capsular contractions that can limit normal knee flexion and extension, decreases muscle disuse effects, maintains articular cartilage nutrition, and benefits the healing

ACL graft.[†] Modern rehabilitation programs (see Chapters 12, Scientific Basis of Rehabilitation after Anterior Cruciate Ligament Autogenous Reconstruction; 13, Rehabilitation of Primary and Revision Anterior Cruciate Ligament Reconstructions; and 14, Neuromuscular Retraining after Anterior Cruciate Ligament Reconstruction) incorporate immediate knee motion and muscle-strengthening exercises the day after surgery, both of which have been shown to be safe and not deleterious to healing grafts. Importantly, the immediate motion program must include patellar mobilization (inferior, superior, medial, and lateral directions) to avoid an infrapatellar contracture.

Patient compliance with postoperative rehabilitation is essential in recovering full knee motion. In the authors' experience, the small percentage of patients who have permanent restrictions in extension or flexion have often been unwilling to perform the required motion, strengthening, and patellar mobilization exercises postoperatively. In addition, in instances in which an early postoperative limitation of motion has been recognized, these patients are also unwilling to undergo treatment recommendations such as overpressure exercises, extension casts, and other modalities that are usually effective in resolving these problems.[101,102] Thus, in a majority of cases, the inflammatory and fibrotic response that follows surgery and initially limits knee motion is treatable if no delay occurs in instituting a gentle motion and overpressure program along with appropriate anti-inflammatory medications. There is a distinct group of patients, probably in the range of 1% to 2%, who demonstrate a pathologic exaggerated fibrous tissue proliferative response from a genetic basis, in which the treatment is prolonged and may not be successful. This unique group of patients are discussed in a later section of this chapter.

Significant lower extremity muscle atrophy represents an unresolved problem after ACL reconstruction, because the magnitude of quadriceps atrophy and strength loss may exceed 20% to 30% in the first few months postoperatively.[39,40,50,81,117] Prolonged quadriceps atrophy may affect the ability to regain normal knee motion and maintain knee extension. Chronic swelling may also cause a limitation of knee motion by inhibiting the function of the quadriceps muscle.[29,110,140,145,146] It is important that a knee joint effusion be treated to lessen its deleterious effect on quadriceps function.

Infection may result in loss of knee motion after ACL reconstruction. The rule followed in the authors' clinical practice is to always consider first that an exaggerated inflammatory response with joint swelling, synovitis, and early limitation of joint motion is caused by a joint infection until proved otherwise. Even when an infectious process appears to have been excluded, a knee joint that does not respond to the gentle modalities to regain knee motion, or that has continued pain or lack of patellar mobility, should undergo repeat aspiration, cell count, culture, and diagnostic studies. In the authors' experience, the most severe cases of arthrofibrosis that initially are presumed to be on a genetic basis are subsequently proved to have an occult unrecognized infectious etiology. In patients with an established infectious process, the principles of treatment have been discussed (see Chapter 7, Anterior Cruciate Ligament Primary and Revision Reconstruction: Diagnosis, Operative Techniques, and Clinical Outcomes), and it is important that gentle motion and overpressure programs continue to maintain the joint motion. Even in knees with swelling of soft tissues and the initial host response to an infection, it is possible

within days after instituting arthroscopic lavage, débridement, and appropriate antibiotics to initiate motion exercises and prevent a flexion contracture or patella infera. Although aggressive management of this complication usually leads to resolution of the infection, studies report permanent loss of extension and flexion in the majority of patients treated, which may be avoidable.[80,125,148,153]

Complex regional pain syndromes and reflex sympathetic dystrophy may cause knee motion problems as a result of quadriceps atrophy, chronic swelling, and an increased sensitivity to pain.[49,107] These issues are discussed in detail in Chapter 43, Diagnosis and Treatment of Complex Regional Pain Syndrome. Appropriate management using a variety of medical specialists is essential to diagnose and treat these problems.

PATHOPHYSIOLOGY

In 1972, Enneking and Horowitz[36] published one of the first studies on the pathophysiology of a joint contracture after immobilization in humans. The investigators described in a series of case reports the presence of fibrofatty connective tissue in the infrapatellar fat pad, suprapatellar pouch, and posterior recesses of the knee joint with eventual obliteration of the joint cavity. Over time, this tissue was replaced with mature fibrous connective tissue.

Tissue homeostasis is maintained by the normal level of cell growth and proliferation along with the production and turnover of the extracellular matrix.[13,15] Polypeptides known as cytokines or growth factors are responsible for the constant signaling that occurs both between local cells (paracrine) and within cells (autocrine). Cytokines exist as small proteins that signal cells in response to injury and infection. One cytokine, interleukin-1, has been found to stimulate platelets and macrophages to release a variety of growth factors, including transforming growth factor–β (TGF-β). TGF-β is thought to be one of the factors (among others[19,68,124]) mediating Dupuytren's Contracture.[3] Cytokines regulate all aspects of tissue remodeling and may act positively or negatively on tissue damage. This variability results in a wide range of potential responses to injury between patients.

Critical Points PATHOPHYSIOLOGY

- Cytokines or growth factors responsible for constant signaling occurring both between local cells and within cells.
- TGF-β is a key cytokine that initiates and ends the process of tissue repair. Its actions enhance the deposition of extracellular matrix and regulate the actions of other cytokines.
- Overexpression of TGF-β$_1$ results in progressive accumulation of matrix in tissues and an elevated number of myofibroblasts, leading to fibrosis.
- Specific ASMA-expressing myofibroblasts generate tissue contraction, are responsible for collagen overproduction during fibrotic diseases. TGF-β is capable of up-regulating ASMA and collagen in fibroblasts.
- ASMA is involved in scar formation and scar tissue contraction during the course of primary arthrofibrosis.
- Collagen type VI could play a contributory role in the deposition of extracellular matrix that leads to arthrofibrosis.
- Primary arthrofibrosis may be the result of an immune response.
- It appears that in the future, chemical agents will become available to treat fibrotic response to injury by controlling elevated levels of myofibroblast unregulators and fibrogenic growth factors

ASMA, α-smooth muscle actin; TGF-β, transforming growth factor–β.

[†]See references 4, 25, 26, 32, 37, 51, 56, 108, 113, 123, 139.

TGF-β, released by platelets, tendon fibroblasts,[137,138] and the joint capsule,[52,53] has been identified as a key cytokine that both initiates and ends the process of tissue repair. Although other growth factors are involved in tissue remodeling, TGF-β is unique in its actions that enhance the deposition of extracellular matrix and regulate the actions of other cytokines.[118,138] An overexpression of TGF-β₁ results in progressive accumulation of matrix in tissues and an elevated number of myofibroblasts, leading to fibrosis.[13,15,52,57,58,87] Border and Noble[13] believe that repeated injury or trauma may also cause autoinduction of TGF-β beyond normal levels, creating a "chronic, vicious circle of TGF-β overproduction," resulting in tissue fibrosis that may also occur in organ systems such as the kidney, liver, and lung. Investigators have documented that elevated levels of myofibroblasts and TGF-β occur rapidly, within 2 weeks after injury in experimental models, and that these changes are similar to those observed in humans with chronic elbow joint contractures.[52,57,58]

There is evidence that during the exaggerated fibrotic response that occurs in knee arthrofibrosis, a certain amount of tissue contraction or shrinkage occurs.[16,111,131] Specific α-smooth muscle actin (ASMA)–expressing myofibroblasts generate tissue contraction during wound healing and are responsible for collagen overproduction during fibrotic diseases.[28,34,38,46] TGF-β is capable of up-regulating ASMA and collagen in fibroblasts.

Unterhauser and associates[147] measured the amount of ASMA-containing fibroblastic cells in arthrofibrotic tissue to determine whether the number of these cells was increased over that found in normal tissue. Tissue biopsies were obtained from 9 patients who underwent surgery for arthrofibrosis that had developed after ACL reconstruction. The patients all had primary arthrofibrosis and underwent the débridement procedure between 4 and 12 months after the ACL reconstruction. Tissue samples were also taken from 5 patients who underwent ACL reconstruction for chronic ligament deficiency and from 8 patients who had follow-up arthroscopy after ACL reconstruction for meniscus pathology; all 13 of these control patients showed no signs of arthrofibrosis. A significantly higher expression of ASMA-positive fibroblastic cells were found in the collagen bundles and remaining fatty tissue in the study group compared with both control groups (23.4% of the total cell count vs. 2.3% and 10.8%, respectively; $P < .001$). The authors concluded that this cell type is involved in scar formation and scar tissue contraction during the course of primary arthrofibrosis. They speculated that the expression of ASMA is most likely variable according to the time from the onset of the disease to tissue biopsy and probably decreases as the disease progresses.

Unterhauser and associates[147] also reported that the fatty tissues in the arthrofibrotic knees were replaced by a dense collagenous network with parallel fiber orientation. A significantly higher total cell count and lower vessel density were measured in the arthrofibrotic knees compared with the control group who underwent ACL reconstruction. Similar findings were noted by Mariani and colleagues[76] who biopsied 17 knees with arthrofibrosis that occurred after a variety of surgical procedures. The tissue samples were obtained less than 6 months from the onset of stiffness in 9 patients, from 6 to 12 months in 5 patients, and more than 12 months in 4 patients. The histologic evaluations demonstrated collagen-producing fibroblastic tissue with differing amounts of cellularity and vascularization. This study supports the hypothesis that arthrofibrotic tissue undergoes progressive remodeling and acquires the characteristics of mature collagen, all within the first 6 months after the onset of joint stiffness. There was no association between the amount of knee motion and the time from surgery or the degree of tissue maturation. The severity of loss of motion was associated only with the location and amount of adhesive tissue in the knee joint.

Unterhauser and associates[147] concluded that the ratio of myofibroblasts to the total cells in connective tissue is a factor in the onset of arthrofibrosis. The authors suggested that future antifibrosis agents (such as decorin) be evaluated, because they inhibit the signaling pathway of TGF-β. Decorin is a human proteoglycan that inactivates the effect of TGF-β and may have a beneficial effect in arthrofibrotic tissues. Fukushima and coworkers[45] reported that injection of decorin improved both the muscle structure and the function of lacerated muscle to near-complete recovery in mice. Several other experimental models have demonstrated the effectiveness of decorin in inhibiting adhesion formation in intra-articular adhesions,[44] kidneys,[14,61] and lungs.[48] However, the effectiveness of this agent in humans with early or later-stage arthrofibrosis has not been investigated to date.[58]

In an in vivo small animal model, Bedair and associates[8] showed that an antiotension II systemic receptor blocker decreased fibrosis and enhanced muscle regeneration in acutely injured skeletal muscle and hypothesized that the blocker modulated TGF-β₁. Hagiwara and colleagues[53] reported that the joint capsule has the potential to produce TGF-β₁ and connective tissue growth factor, both of which play a role in causing fibrosis.

Zeichen and coworkers[155] compared tissue samples of 13 patients with arthrofibrosis, obtained a mean of 16 months after the inciting knee ligament surgery, with those of 8 patients undergoing primary ACL surgery. Histologic examination from the patients with arthrofibrosis showed marked synovial hyperplasia, infiltration of inflammatory cells, and vascular proliferation with an increased level of collagen types VI and III. None of the control subjects demonstrated these findings. The authors noted that this confirmed the observations of Murakami and associates[88] regarding the association between an inflammatory process and the proliferation of fibroblasts. The suggestion was made that collagen type VI could play a contributory role in the deposition of extracellular matrix that leads to arthrofibrosis.

Bosch and colleagues[17] advanced the hypothesis that primary arthrofibrosis is the result of an immune response. Tissue samples obtained from 18 patients between 4 and 48 months from the triggering event to surgical débridement demonstrated synovial hyperplasia with fibrotic enlargement of the subintima and infiltration of inflammatory cells. The authors believed their findings supported an immune response as the cause of capsulitis leading to formation of diffuse scar tissue. The clinical implication was to avoid further surgery or aggressive manipulation while patients are suffering from acute capsulitis and to wait 3 to 6 months for the inflammatory response to resolve before débridement is considered. As is discussed, too often, there is a delay in treatment that results in a permanent limitation of knee motion. Unfortunately, even though a delay in treatment may allow tissues to "quiet down," the resulting fibrotic tissue that forms becomes well organized and dense and treatment becomes more difficult. It appears that in the future, chemical agents will become available to treat fibrotic response to injury by controlling elevated levels of myofibroblast up-regulators and fibrogenic growth factors.[8,22,42,45,52,57,58,70,90]

PREVENTION

Preoperative

After an acute ACL tear and before reconstruction, the surgeon-therapist team must manage pain, effusion, quadriceps weakness, knee motion limitations, and gait abnormalities. Effusion and hemarthrosis are treated with appropriate nonsteroidal anti-inflammatory drugs (NSAIDs), cryotherapy, compression, and limb elevation. Patients work with physical therapists to learn safe and effective muscle-strengthening exercises (such as straight leg raises, bicycling, mini-squats, wall-sits, calf raises, knee extensions from 90°–30°, hamstring curls, and swimming) and must demonstrate good quadriceps control without an extensor lag before consideration for surgery. Regaining normal or nearly normal knee motion is essential and may take several weeks after an ACL rupture. The exceptions are knees with a mechanical block to motion, such as a displaced meniscus tear, in which early surgical intervention is warranted to preserve and repair the meniscus. A decision regarding future ACL reconstruction is based on the patient's activity goals and other factors (see Chapter 7, Anterior Cruciate Ligament Primary and Revision Reconstruction: Diagnosis, Operative Techniques, and Clinical Outcomes). Other exceptions are knees with concomitant posterolateral ligament ruptures who are candidates for surgical intervention within 7 to 10 days of the injury. Knees with concomitant MCL tears are treated conservatively for at least 4 to 8 weeks to allow the medial side structures to heal and regain motion and muscle strength before proceeding to ACL reconstruction (see Chapter 24, Medial and Posteromedial Ligament Injuries: Diagnosis, Operative Techniques, and Clinical Outcomes).

Critical Points PREVENTION

Preoperative

- After ACL injury, the surgeon-therapist team manages pain, effusion, quadriceps weakness, knee motion limitations, gait abnormalities, other knee ligament injuries before ACL reconstruction.

Intraoperative

- Principles of correct graft placement, tensioning, and fixation are paramount to avoid a limitation of knee motion postoperatively.
- ACL graft placed within the femoral and tibial footprint, occupying the central two thirds or more. Limited notchplasty may be required.
- Femoral tunnel: anteromedial portal or a two-incision procedure favored.
- ACL graft conditioning: approximately 44 N tension placed on the distal graft sutures, knee flexed from 0° to 120° for 30 flexion-extension cycles. Arthroscope verifies ideal graft position, no impingement against the lateral femoral condyle or notch with full hyperextension.

Postoperative

- 1st wk: control knee joint pain and swelling, regain adequate quadriceps muscle contraction, initiate immediate knee motion exercises, and maintain adequate limb elevation.
- Goal: achieve 0° to 90° of knee motion by the 7th postoperative day. Begin overpressure program immediately if goal not obtained.

ACL, anterior cruciate ligament.

Intraoperative

The principles of correct graft placement, tensioning, and fixation are paramount to avoid a limitation of knee motion postoperatively (see Chapter 7, Anterior Cruciate Ligament Primary and Revision Reconstruction: Diagnosis, Operative Techniques, and Clinical Outcomes). The ACL graft is placed within the femoral and tibial footprint, occupying the central two thirds or more of the footprint, to achieve an anatomic position that allows the graft to control the pivot shift and anterior tibial translation. To achieve an anatomic graft placement in the center of the tibial attachment may require a limited notchplasty to avoid a limitation of knee extension. For the femoral tunnel, an anteromedial portal drilling technique or a two-incision procedure is favored to obtain a central anatomic femoral footprint placement. An endoscopic transtibial drilling technique is not recommended.[55] In most chronic ACL-deficient knees, there is an overgrowth of cartilage and spur formation in the femoral notch, which necessitates a notchplasty to prevent ACL graft impingement.

The ACL graft is conditioned after femoral fixation by placing approximately 44 N tension on the distal graft sutures and flexing the knee from 0° to 120° for 30 flexion-extension cycles. The arthroscope is used to verify that the graft position is ideal and there is no impingement against the lateral femoral condyle or notch with full hyperextension. The knee is placed at 20° flexion and the tension on the graft is reduced to approximately 10 to 15 N in order to avoid overconstraining tibial anteroposterior (AP) translation. Alternatively, the graft can be tensioned to a higher load with knee extension. After graft fixation, a Lachman test is performed and anterior tibial translation of 2 to 3 mm should be elicited, indicating that the graft has not been overtightened. If the graft has a "bow-string," tight appearance with no anterior tibial translation on testing, the distal tensioning and fixation procedure is repeated with less tension placed on the graft.

In knees that undergo concomitant meniscus repair, the sutures are tied with the knee at 30° of flexion to prevent capsular shortening or increased pain with postoperative extension exercises. If an associated lateral extra-articular procedure is required, care is taken to avoiding overtensioning the iliotibial band graft and to place the graft in the correct position on the femur to allow restoration of normal knee flexion (see Chapter 7, Anterior Cruciate Ligament Primary and Revision Reconstruction: Diagnosis, Operative Techniques, and Clinical Outcomes). Posteromedial and posterolateral capsular plication procedures are performed in a manner that will not result in a limitation of knee extension, which is tested at the operative table.

Postoperative

The 1st week after ACL or other knee ligament reconstruction represents a critical time period for patients to control knee joint pain and swelling, regain adequate quadriceps muscle contraction, initiate immediate knee motion exercises, and maintain adequate limb elevation (see Chapter 13, Rehabilitation of Primary and Revision Anterior Cruciate Ligament Reconstructions). A bulky compression dressing (cotton-Ace Brand [Becton, Dickinson and Company, Franklin Lakes, NY] elastic bandage–cotton–Ace Brand elastic bandage) is used for 48 hours, followed by antiembolic compression stockings and supplemental Ace bandage. Cryotherapy is begun in the recovery

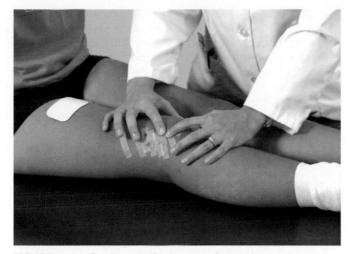

FIGURE 41–5. Patellar mobilization is performed by the therapist during physical therapy visits and at home by the patient or family member several times daily.

room after surgery. NSAIDs are used for 5 days along with pain medication to allow the immediate exercise protocol to be successfully implemented. Electrogalvanic stimulation or hi-volt electrical muscle stimulation may be used along with ice, compression, and elevation to control swelling.[109]

On the 1st postoperative day, patients perform passive and active range of motion exercises in a seated position for 10 minutes a session, approximately four to six times per day. This is accompanied by patellar glides (mobilization), which are performed in all four planes (superior, inferior, medial, and lateral) with sustained pressure applied to the appropriate patellar border for at least 10 seconds (Fig. 41–5). The goal is to achieve 0° to 90° of knee motion by the 7th postoperative day. Patients who are unable to achieve this amount of extension and flexion are immediately placed into an overpressure motion program, described in detail later in this chapter. In the authors' experience, the exercises and modalities in the overpressure program resolve the majority of knee motion limitations when initiated early postoperatively. In 650 knees that underwent ACL reconstruction, described elsewhere in this chapter, only 18 (3%) required a gentle manipulation under anesthesia and 6 (<1%) underwent surgical débridement and lysis of adhesions after the overpressure program failed to resolve knee motion limitations.

Hamstring and gastrocnemius-soleus flexibility exercises are begun immediately, as are straight leg raises in all four planes of hip movement. Partial weight-bearing is permitted as long as pain and swelling are controlled and a voluntary quadriceps contraction demonstrated. Isometric quadriceps contractions are also begun the 1st postoperative day and are performed on an hourly basis following the repetition rules of 10-second holds, 10 repetitions, 10 times per day. The remainder of the rehabilitation program is detailed in Chapter 13, Rehabilitation of Primary and Revision Anterior Cruciate Ligament Reconstructions.

DIAGNOSIS AND CLINICAL PRESENTATION

The early detection of a limitation of knee motion after ACL reconstruction is paramount for resolving the problem and preventing permanent arthrofibrosis. The establishment of specific knee flexion and extension goals according to the amount of time that has elapsed postoperatively and concurrent major operative procedures performed is required. In all knees, full passive knee extension must be obtained immediately to avoid excessive fibrous tissue proliferation in the intercondylar notch and posterior capsular contracture. In patients with physiologic bilateral knee hyperextension, the authors recommend the gradual return of 3° to 5° of hyperextension in the reconstructed knee and not more than 5° of hyperextension owing to potentially deleterious forces on the healing graft. Specific range of knee motion goals after ACL reconstruction (Table 41–5) are communicated to the patient before surgery and during postoperative assessments. Knee motion is carefully documented by the therapist in a closely supervised postoperative rehabilitation program so that detection of a knee motion problem occurs in a timely manner. Failure to meet these goals prompts entering the patient in an overpressure program using appropriate medical and therapeutic measures, to be described.

Joint aspiration with cell analysis and culture are important with any indication of joint redness, warmth, and limitation of knee motion. A serum sedimentation rate is usually not reliable after surgery, because it is elevated for a number of weeks. If surgery is required, multiple tissue specimens are sent for culture and microscopic evaluation. As already discussed, an occult infectious process is not excluded by a single negative joint aspirate, and repeat joint aspirations, culture, and blood studies are required.

The initial phase of primary arthrofibrosis occurs within the first few weeks after surgery. The condition at this time is transient, because limitations in knee flexion and extension are usually resolved with conservative measures as long as the patient complies with the recommended program. However, if knee motion deficits are untreated for a few weeks, the condition becomes more established and eventually requires operative management. Findings include shortening of the posteromedial

TABLE 41–5 Authors' Goals for Restoration of Knee Motion after Anterior Cruciate Ligament Reconstruction

Operative Procedure Details	Weeks Postoperative	Range of Knee Motion Goal*
ACL B-PT-B autograft reconstruction, isolated or with meniscus repair, patient desires to return to strenuous athletics as soon as possible	1–2 3–4 5–6	0°–110° 0°–120° 0°–135°
ACL revision reconstruction (any graft source) ACL primary reconstruction with allograft or semitendinosus autograft Complex reconstructions with concomitant operative procedures Knees with noteworthy articular cartilage lesions	1–4 5–6 7–8	0°–90° 0°–120° 0°–135°
ACL reconstruction with posterior cruciate ligament reconstruction (see Chapter 21, Posterior Cruciate Ligament: Diagnosis, Operative Techniques, and Clinical Outcomes)	1–2 3–4 5–6 7–8	0°–90° 0°–110° 0°–120° 0°–135°
ACL reconstruction with posterolateral procedure (see Chapter 22, Posterolateral Ligament Structures: Diagnosis, Operative Techniques, and Clinical Outcomes)	1–4 5–6 7–8 9–12	0°–90° 0°–110° 0°–120° 0°–135°

*In patients with physiologic bilateral knee hyperextension, the authors recommend the gradual return of 3°–5° of hyperextension in the reconstructed knee. Greater than 5° of hyperextension is not recommended owing to potentially deleterious forces placed on the healing graft.

ACL, anterior cruciate ligament; B-PT-B, bone–patellar tendon–bone.

and posterolateral capsule, blocking extension; significant ingrowth of fibroproliferative tissue into the intercondylar notch; shortening of the ACL graft, preventing normal anterior tibial translation with extension; obliteration of the suprapatellar pouch; and shortening of the quadriceps muscles, limiting flexion. A comprehensive débridement and lysis of adhesions, followed by an in-patient epidural and physical therapy program and many weeks of continued outpatient therapy, may still be successful in achieving significant gains in knee motion. The final phase of arthrofibrosis involves patellar infera and articular cartilage damage, which are exceedingly difficult to treat and the loss of knee motion is usually permanent.

Patients who present with an established arthrofibrosis condition require a comprehensive evaluation, including appropriate radiographs (Fig. 41–6), bone scans, and magnetic resonance imaging (MRI) to determine whether the condition is primary or secondary, as previously discussed. The examination may demonstrate diffuse edema, increased warmth, constant pain, limited patellar mobility (Fig. 41–7), contracture of peripatellar and infrapatellar soft tissues, tenderness in the fat pad, and limits in both extension and flexion compared with the contralateral normal knee (Fig. 41–8). Anterior knee pain, stiffness, pain with attempted knee motion, a flexed-knee gait, and severe quadriceps atrophy are common findings.

Patellar vertical height is determined using the radiographic method described by Caton and coworkers[21] and Linclau.[71] In Figure 41–9, Left, the patellar vertical-height ratio is calculated by dividing line segment A, the distance between the most ventral rim of the tibial plateau and the lowest end of the patellar articular surface, by line segment B, the maximum length of the patellar articular surface. An alternative method described

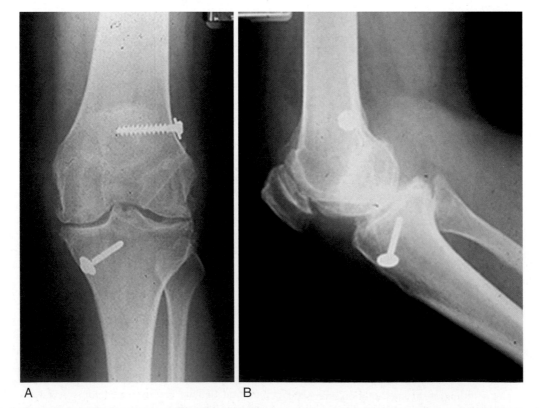

A   B

FIGURE 41–6. Anteroposterior (AP; **A**) and lateral (**B**) radiographs of a knee with a severe flexion contracture and development of advanced joint arthritis after anterior cruciate ligament (ACL) reconstruction. The patient was not a candidate for surgical soft tissue releases and subsequently underwent total knee arthroplasty.

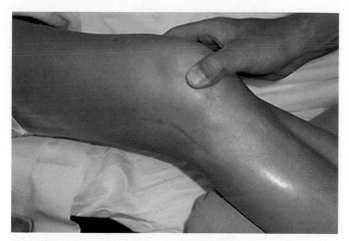

FIGURE 41–7. Limited patellar mobility is demonstrated in this patient, referred after undergoing ACL reconstruction elsewhere. The normal patellar medial glide allows at least 10–15 mm medial translation with the knee at 20° of flexion. A normal lateral glide of up to 10–15 mm is possible. A loss of either medial or lateral translation occurs with contracture of peripatellar tissues. There is usually a limitation of proximal-distal glide due to an infrapatellar contracture.

by Blackburne and Peel[11] locates the tibial reference point at an anterior central location on the tibial plateau (shown in Fig. 41–9 as line segment C). Using this method, the patellar vertical-height ratio equals C/B. The senior author conducted a study to determine normal right to left patellar vertical height ratios within the same individual in a group of 51 patients (102 knees).[106] The difference in the vertical-height ratio of the patella between these two methods ranged from 0 to 9%, with an average difference of 3%. Large variations existed in the ratios between individual patients (range, 0.75–1.46). Therefore, the diagnosis of patellar infera requires analysis of patellar height ratios compared with those of the opposite knee and subsequent radiographs compared with the same knee at different time periods (Fig. 41–10). A decrease in the vertical-height ratio of 14% to 15%, depending on the method used (Table 41–6), indicates a patella infera condition because this amount of difference is greater than 2 standard deviations of the normal difference between knees. An alternative method for the calculation of patellar height is the patellotrochlear index,[10] expressed as a percentage at knee extension (Fig. 41–9, Right).

MRI is useful in assessing the extent and location of scar tissue formation (Fig. 41–11). The infrapatellar band of scar tissue

frequently found in the patellar infera state is just anterior to the fat pad and attaches from the inferior patellar pole to the anterior aspect of the tibia. Obliteration of the fat pad, with the patellar tendon attaching directly to the anterior tibia, is a poor prognostic sign, because the patella may adhere to the proximal tibia, which markedly restricts medial-to-lateral mobility. Thick peripatellar tissues are frequently observed. The location of prior ACL or posterior cruciate ligament (PCL) grafts must be determined. Important signs of an infectious process or unexplained edema and fluid in soft tissues or bone or about fixation implants are specifically evaluated to exclude an infectious etiology.

Patients who present with arthrofibrosis secondary to a cyclops lesion or an impinged or improperly placed ACL graft require surgical débridement of the lesion or graft and scar tissue, followed by several months of physical therapy to regain normal knee motion and muscle function. The decision may then be made regarding the necessity for revision ACL reconstruction. In addition, patients with established primary arthrofibrosis require surgical management of the condition, described in detail elsewhere. These two groups of patients will not be successfully managed with conservative treatment measures. However, patients who fail to meet the knee motion goals established after ACL reconstruction (see Table 41–5) and in whom the arthrofibrosis is in the early, transient stage may usually be effectively treated with the exercises and modalities described later. The key is the early detection of the limitation of knee motion, as soon as the 7th postoperative day if 0° to 90° is not demonstrated.

CONSERVATIVE MANAGEMENT OF LIMITATION OF KNEE EXTENSION

If the patient has not achieved at least 0° by the 7th postoperative day, she or he is placed into an overpressure extension program. The goal is to produce a gradual stretching of posterior capsular tissues, but not to induce soft tissue tearing and further injury because this could lead to an inflammatory response and worsen the condition. One effective exercise involves hanging weights, in which the foot and ankle are propped on a towel or other device to elevate the hamstrings and gastrocnemius, which allows the knee to drop into full extension (Fig. 41–12A). This position is maintained for 10 to 15 minutes and repeated at least eight times per day. Initially a 10-pound weight is used, which may be progressed up to 25 pounds to the distal thigh and knee

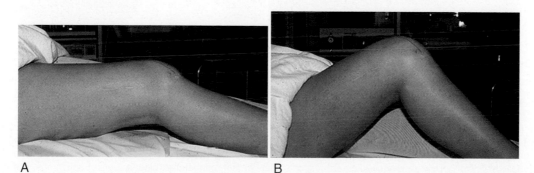

A   B

FIGURE 41–8. A severe limitation of knee extension (**A**) and flexion (**B**) demonstrated after ACL reconstruction in a patient referred for treatment 10 wk after surgery. An arthroscopic débridement, lysis of adhesions, and posteromedial and capsular releases were required. Unfortunately, the motion deficits were not resolved in the first few weeks after ACL surgery.

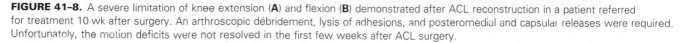

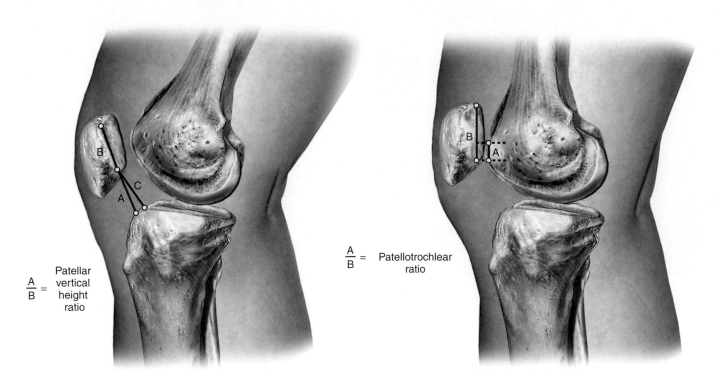

FIGURE 41–9. Methods used to determine patellar vertical-height ratio on a lateral radiograph. **Left,** The numerator (*line segment A*) is the distance between the most ventral (anterosuperior) rim of the tibial plateau and the lowest end of the patellar articular surface. The denominator (*line segment B*) is the maximum length of the patellar articular surface. An alternative numerator (*line segment C*) locates the tibial reference point on the middle of the tibial plateau. The patellar vertical-height ratio equals A/B or C/B. **Right,** The numerator (*A*) is the superiormost aspect of the trochlear cartilage that is in contact with *line segment B*. The denominator (*line segment B*) is the maximum length of the articular patellar surface. Using this method, the mean index is 32 ± 12%, >50% is a patellar infera, and <12% is a patella alta.[10]

Within the figure:

$$\frac{A}{B} = \text{Patellar vertical height ratio}$$

$$\frac{A}{B} = \text{Patellotrochlear ratio}$$

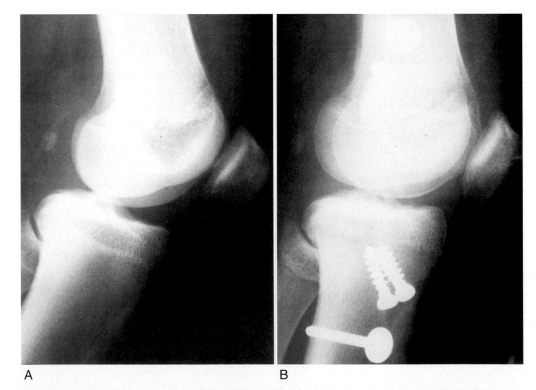

A   B

FIGURE 41–10. Lateral radiographs document a 22% decrease in patellar vertical-height ratio after a combined ACL reconstruction and medial meniscus repair in a 14-year-old female gymnast. **A,** The injured knee before the reconstruction. **B,** Four wk postoperative, the patient was referred to our center with significant quadriceps atrophy, difficulty performing knee motion exercises, and limited patellar mobility. The patient was treated with daily physical therapy and required an arthroscopic débridement, peripatellar release, lysis of adhesions, and removal of infrapatellar scar tissue. Nine months postoperative, the patient had regained full knee motion, had no pain symptoms, and had returned to recreational activities. However, the patellar infera remained unchanged. The patient is being followed for signs of patellofemoral arthritis and need for further treatment. (**A** and **B,** *From Noyes, F. R.; Wojtys, E. M.; Marshall, M. T.: The early diagnosis and treatment of developmental patella infera syndrome. Clin Orthop 265:241–252, 1991.*)

TABLE 41-6   Differences between Three Radiographic Methods of Computing Patellar Vertical-Height Ratios

Method	Knee	Patellar Ligament Length	Patellar Length	Ratio	Difference Right/Left Ratios	Difference within 2 Standard Deviations (95% of population)
Linclau[71] N = 51 pairs	Right	3.65 ± 0.46 (2.70–4.70)	3.54 ± 0.37 (2.80–4.20)	1.04 ± 0.13 (0.75–1.36)	−0.0200 ± 0.070 (−0.2100–+0.135)	15%
	Left	3.69 ± 0.46 (2.90–4.70)	3.51 ± 0.33 (2.70–4.20)	1.06 ± 0.15 (0.80–1.46)		
Blackburne & Peel[11] N = 51 pairs	Right	2.95 ± 0.45 (2.00–4.10)	3.53 ± 0.43 (2.60–4.40)	0.84 ± 0.14 (0.61–1.33)	0.0003 ± 0.060 (−0.1930–+0.190)	14%
	Left	2.95 ± 0.44 (2.10–3.90)	3.52 ± 0.39 (2.30–4.30)	0.84 ± 0.14 (0.64–1.30)		
Insall & Salvati[62a] N = 50 pairs	Right	4.90 ± 0.45 (4.10–5.90)	4.69 ± 0.43 (4.00–6.20)	1.05 ± 0.11 (0.86–1.28)	0.0140 ± 0.050 (0.1230–0.107)	11%
	Left	4.86 ± 0.44 (4.00–6.20)	4.72 ± 0.42 (4.00–6.20)	1.04 ± 0.10 (0.85–1.26)		

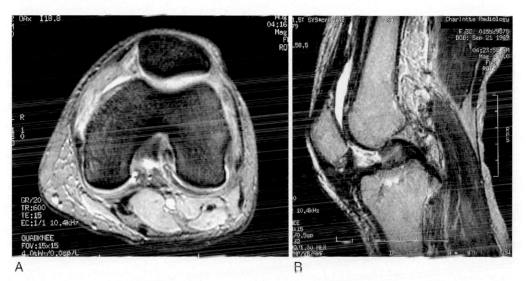

FIGURE 41-11. Magentic resonance imaging (MRI) of a knee with patella infera. **A,** Thickening of the medial and lateral peripatellar tissues. **B,** Note the infrapatellar tissues are replaced with dense fibrotic connective tissue. There is loss of the normal patellar tendon outline, because the tendon is encased with scar tissue and attached to the proximal tibia. The infrapatellar scar extends from the inferior pole to the anterior tibia. This patient required arthroscopic débridement of the suprapatellar pouch, followed by open débridement of infrapatellar scar tissue and Z-plasty lengthening of the medial and lateral parapatellar tissues. The decrease in patellar tendon length is permanent.

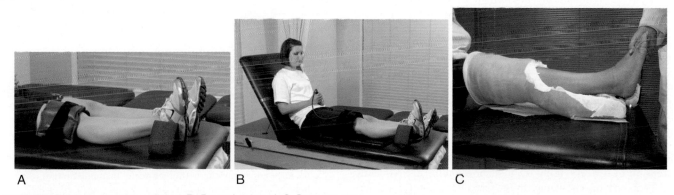

FIGURE 41-12. A, Hanging weights. **B,** Extension board. **C,** Drop-out cast.

to provide overpressure to stretch the posterior contracted tissues. Full knee extension is usually obtained by the 2nd to 3rd postoperative week. A commercial extension appliance (see Fig. 41–12B) is also an option.

If these treatment measures are not effective, a drop-out (bivalved) cast (see Fig. 41–12C) is implemented for continuous extension overpressure. The advantage of this technique is that the patient is in control of the process and can apply or delete wedge material as tolerated and may bathe. A hyperextension splint may be used in the same manner; however, the authors believe that the bivalved cast offers superior benefits. Casting is not recommended in knees that have greater than a –12° extension deficit with a hard block to terminal extension. These knees are usually 3 or more months postoperative, and dense scar tissue has formed posteriorly with posterior capsular contracture requiring surgical releases and débridement. In knees with a rigid block to extension, extension casts have the potential to produce high tibiofemoral compressive forces and articular cartilage damage. Extension casts are also not effective when there is proliferative ingrowth of fibrous tissue in the femoral notch. These cases require arthroscopic débridement.

When indicated, the cast is used within the first 4 weeks for cases resistant to the other overpressure extension modalities. The goal is to resolve all extension problems by 4 weeks postoperatively. In select knees, the extension deficit may return and, accordingly, the drop-out cast is repeated. On occasion, the drop-out cast will not be effective and it is necessary to use a cylinder cast and serial wedges to gain extension. The cast is well padded to prevent skin breakdown. An anterior wedge is used every 12 to 24 hours to gradually achieve extension. The cast is applied for 36 to 48 hours and then removed to resume knee flexion and extension motion exercises. Again, some knees do not have a rigid block to full extension requiring surgery. Once extension is regained, the cast is converted into a posterior night splint, which is used for an additional 7 to 10 days. In some knees, full extension is regained but then gradually lost over the course of several weeks. In these cases, a repeat cast application may resolve the problem.

The treatment algorithm for limitations of knee extension is shown in Figure 41–13. The goal is to resolve the loss of knee extension by 4 weeks, using the modalities outlined. Frequently, it is necessary to repeat steps in the treatment protocol, because the return in a knee extension deficit may occur. It is rare that manipulation or continuous epidural is necessary when the program is followed; however, these steps are provided for the most resistant cases. The most difficult problem is the knee joint that does not respond and, despite the overpressure program, continues to show a lack of full extension. If the lack of knee extension is 10° or less, the overpressure program will usually be successful. However, it is important to identify the knee in which there is a rigid hard block to extension and the deficit is greater than 10°. In these knees, it is better to proceed with a posterior capsulotomy through a limited medial and lateral approach, to be described.

CONSERVATIVE MANAGEMENT OF LIMITATION OF KNEE FLEXION

Because full knee flexion is present at the end of the ACL reconstruction, any limitation in the early postoperative period is due to intra-articular adhesions and contracture of peripatellar tissues and muscle spasm or pain. The early detection of a limitation of flexion (<90° by the 7th postoperative day) necessitates an overpressure flexion program. A rolling stool exercise (Fig. 41–14A) may be done in which the patient sits on a small stool close to the ground, the knee is flexed to the maximum position possible and held in that position for approximately 1 minute or as long as the patient is able to tolerate mild discomfort. Then, the patient rolls the stool forward without moving the foot position on the floor to achieve a few more degrees of flexion. The procedure is performed for 10 to 12 minutes and repeated six to eight times a day. Wall-slides are another effective exercise to achieve flexion. The patient lies on his or her back and places the foot of the reconstructed knee on a wall as shown in Figure 41–14B. The foot of the opposite leg is used to gently slide the opposite foot and flex the reconstructed knee in a gradual manner. Commercial knee flexion devices (see Fig. 41–14C and D) may also be used as available to further promote overpressure. In addition, a figure-four overpressure exercise is effective (see Fig. 41–14E). A 4-inch tubular stocking is used, double-wrapped around the foot and ankle, that allows the patient under his or her own power to flex the knee. The patient shown in Figure 41–14E had 90° of flexion, and an arthroscopic release was successful in achieving 135°. After the débridement and placement of an epidural, the surgeon sets a mark on the thigh by gentle pressure to establish the flexion goal for that day. The mark on the thigh in the photograph demonstrates the 135° flexion position, which is the overall goal. The mark on the distal portion of the patella in the photograph demonstrates the starting position, which in this case was 90°. The goal of these exercises and modalities is to gradually and passively stretch tissues in a controlled manner, while not

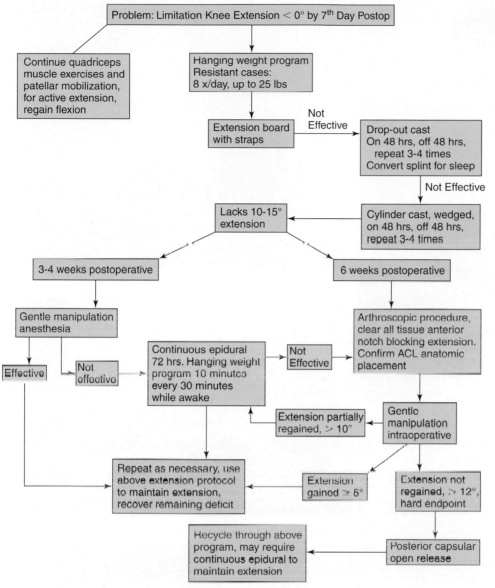

FIGURE 41–13. Treatment algorithm of limitations of knee extension.

inducing pain or tearing of tissues. Patients who have difficulty achieving 90° by the 3rd to 4th week require a gentle ranging of the knee under anesthesia (not a forceful manipulation) in which full flexion is easily obtained with only light loads applied. This stretches out early joint adhesions, markedly reduces postoperative pain, and allows the patient to regain motion.

The treatment algorithm for a limitation of knee flexion is shown in Figure 41–15. The first step is to determine whether there is associated contracture of patellar tissues, which makes the treatment more difficult. The loss of knee flexion when there is no peripatellar contracture is more easily resolved. With the treatment protocol shown, it is rare to progress to the necessity for an arthroscopic débridement and release of peripatellar tissues. When there is an associated peripatellar contracture, it is important that the condition be immediately treated because this can result in a patella infera. A conservative patellar mobilization program with oral steroids is performed for a week. If the limitation of motion and peripatellar contracture persists, a gentle

manipulation under anesthesia is performed; however, no more than "two to three fingers of pressure" is placed at the distal tibia to achieve knee flexion. If more force is necessary, it indicates that the peripatellar contracture is composed of more dense, resistant scar that requires arthroscopic débridement. An aggressive manipulation under higher forces risks damaging the patellofemoral articular cartilage, because the tight contracted tissues increase patellofemoral contact forces with knee flexion. Knee flexion is gained, but at the expense of possibly damaging the patellofemoral joint. This is also true for pushing knee flexion in the clinic when there is no patellar mobility. Again, an operative release of tight contracture peripatellar tissues is indicated instead of overzealous flexion exercises or a knee manipulation with high flexion loads.

It should be noted that there are select knees, most commonly chronic cases of arthrofibrosis, in which the peripatellar scar tissue is thick and contracted and an attempted arthroscopic release would result in too extensive a release on both the medial

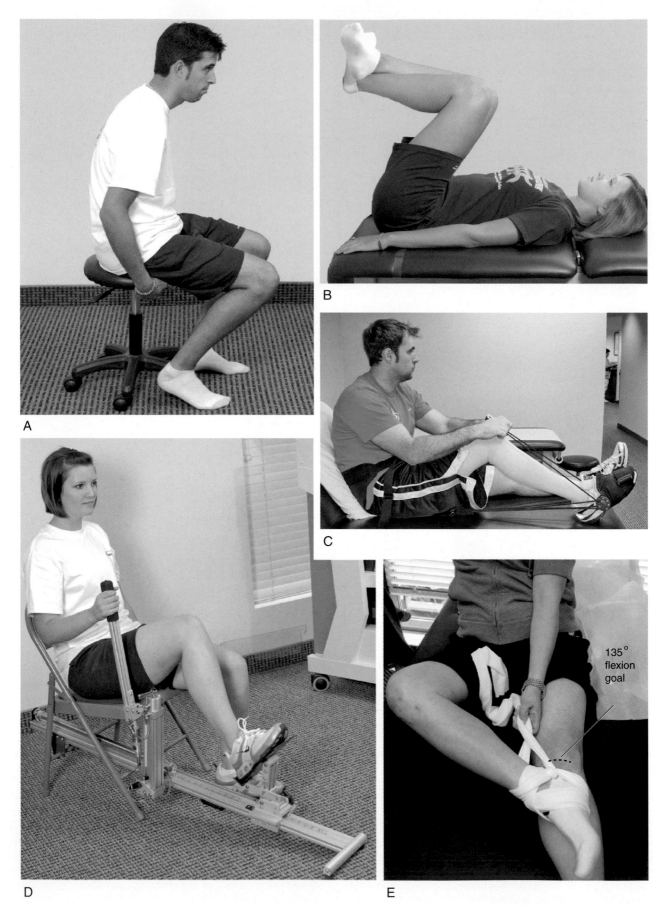

FIGURE 41–14. A, Rolling stool exercise. **B,** Wall-slides. **C,** Flexion seat. **D,** Knee flexion overpressure device. **E,** Figure-four knee flexion overpressure exercise.

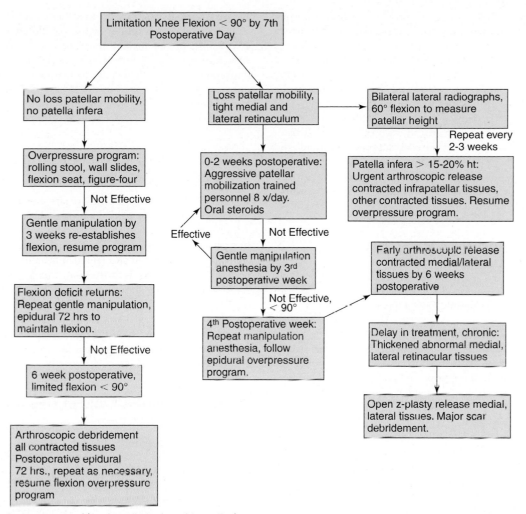

FIGURE 41-15. Treatment algorithm for a limitation of knee flexion.

and the lateral peripatellar tissues. If a major release is necessary, extending to the proximal aspect of the patella, the senior author recommends an open medial Z-plasty release in which the more normal tissue laxity is restored and the abnormal scar tissue is excised. In addition, the Z-plasty procedure prevents the occurrence of a major capsular defect with joint communication to subcutaneous tissues, which is a complication of an extensive medial or lateral arthroscopic release.

ROLE OF ORAL CORTICOSTEROIDS

There is a subset of patients who develop postoperatively an exaggerated inflammatory soft tissue response with excessive pain, joint stiffness, soft tissue edema, warmth, and redness about the knee. The inflammation is not resolved by the standard treatment methods of cryotherapy, anti-inflammatory medications, elevation, and compression. It is first recommended to use a maximum dose of an NSAID for 1 week. If this is not successful, a trial of oral steroids is indicated. It is important that before and during the treatment of these resistant cases, an occult infectious process is ruled out, with appropriate serial diagnostic tests (aspiration, sedimentation rate) performed as necessary.

A 6 day dose pack of 4-mg methylprednisolone tablets (Watson Laboratories, CA) is effective if used early in the phase. Six tablets are taken on the 1st day of treatment, five on the 2nd, four on the 3rd, three on the 4th, two on the 5th, and one on the 6th. During this treatment period, forceful and aggressive physical therapy is avoided. Gentle knee motion and lighter overpressure exercises are performed. In select cases, the 6-day dose pack may be repeated.

Critical Points ROLE OF ORAL CORTICOSTEROIDS

- Indications: knees with exaggerated inflammatory soft tissue response with excessive pain, joint stiffness, soft tissue edema, warmth, and redness about the joint.
- Inflammation not resolved by cryotherapy, anti-inflammatory medications, elevation, and compression.
- A 6-day dose pack of 4-mg methylprednisolone tablets (Watson Laboratories, CA) is effective if used early. Avoid forceful and aggressive physical therapy.
- Consider oral corticosteroids (prednisone 5 mg [UpJohn, Kalamazoo, MI]) for 4 wk if the inflammatory symptoms return or are more severe.
- In cases of severe arthrofibrosis, oral corticosteroids may be required for 2–3 months in an effort to avoid repeat surgery.

Another option is to use oral corticosteroids (prednisone 5 mg, UpJohn, Kalamazoo, MI) for 4 weeks if the inflammatory symptoms return or are more severe. The usual daily dose is 30 mg in the 1st week (two tablets taken three times a day), 15 mg in the 2nd (one tablet taken three times a day), 10 mg in the 3rd (one tablet taken two times a day), and 5 mg in the 4th. In cases of severe arthrofibrosis, oral corticosteroids may be required for 2 to 3 months in an effort to avoid repeat surgery. Complications that may arise from prolonged corticosteroid intake include pituitary adrenal suppression, fluid and electrolyte disturbance, hyperglycemia, peptic ulcers, and avascular necrosis. In the most resistant cases, it is necessary to repeat oral steroid cycling on the off days to NSAIDs, which are prescribed at their maximum dosage.

GENTLE MANIPULATION UNDER ANESTHESIA

As already described, a forceful manipulation of a knee with extensive scar tissue is harmful and ineffective in treating the limitation of knee motion. A forced manipulation may tear intra-articular and extra-articular tissues and cause excessive tibiofemoral and patellofemoral compression with the risk of fracture, damage to the articular cartilage, rupture of the patellar tendon, and even femoral fracture.[72] Therefore, any patient who has a hard-stop to knee motion (which represents a joint contracture) is treated with an arthroscopic débridement and lysis of adhesions.

A gentle manipulation under anesthesia, done with only mild pressure exerted on the distal leg, is effective if performed early after ligament surgery, within 3 to 4 weeks postoperatively. Even at 6 weeks, dense scar tissue proliferation may exist in joint soft tissues and the window of opportunity has been lost in not performing an early ranging of motion under general anesthesia. Adequate patellar mobilization must be established before flexing the knee during the procedure to prevent damage to the patellofemoral articular surface. A supervised physical therapy program is required to maintain the knee motion achieved by the manipulation, as detailed in the treatment algorithm.

OPERATIVE MANAGEMENT OF SEVERE RESTRICTION OF KNEE MOTION

Arthroscopic Soft Tissue Releases

A demonstration of an arthroscopic technique for débridement of contracted tissues in a knee with arthrofibrosis is shown in

---

Critical Points GENTLE MANIPULATION UNDER ANESTHESIA

- Forceful manipulation of a knee with extensive scar tissue is harmful and ineffective in treating the limitation of motion.
- Patients with a hard-stop to knee motion (joint contracture) treated with arthroscopic débridement, lysis of adhesions.
- A gentle manipulation under anesthesia, done with only mild pressure exerted on the distal leg, is effective if performed within 3–4 wk postoperatively.
- Supervised physical therapy program required to maintain the knee motion achieved by the manipulation.

Figure 41–16. In this patient, there was a restriction in medial-to-lateral translation (glide) of the patellofemoral joint, with a contracture of the medial and lateral retinaculum. However, approximately 50% of normal patellar mobility was still present, indicating that an arthroscopic technique could be used and an open extensive technique was not necessary. There was a limitation of motion at 0°/5°/90°. The procedure was performed after tourniquet inflation.

Open Z-Plasty, Medial-Lateral Retinacular Tissues

Figure 41–17 demonstrates the operative technique for an open Z-plasty release of the medial and lateral retinacular tissues. An arthroscopic release alone is contraindicated in this case, because the release is so extensive (extending above the proximal patella and releasing all medial and lateral soft tissues) that there would be open communication of the joint into the subcutaneous tissues. The principle shown is to preserve the function of the medial and lateral retinacular soft tissues and, as well, débride the tissues to a normal thickness. The Z-plasty open release allows an arthrotomy to thoroughly débride infrapatellar contracted tissues, protect the patellar tendon, and lengthen contracted medial and lateral patellar tissues.

Posterior Medial-Lateral Capsulotomy

The technique for a posterior medial-lateral capsulotomy involves the same exposure as that used for a medial or lateral meniscus repair (Fig. 41–18). On the medial side, the posterior capsule is sectioned at its femoral attachment proximally. On the lateral side, the capsule is sectioned in its proximal aspect just below the attachment of the lateral gastrocnemius to the posterior capsule. The dissection and posterior capsule excision are carried directly over the posterior femoral condyles and not into the posterior intercondylar region, because scar tissue may extend to the neurovascular structures. It is often impressive how dense the posterior capsular structures are, and with their release, further gains in knee extension are possible on the operating table. The remaining posterior intercondylar tissues are easily stretched with the overpressure program. The posterior capsule releases are also accompanied with an arthroscopic procedure to remove any tissue that has grown into the notch producing an anterior impingement that would also block extension.

IN-PATIENT PHYSICAL THERAPY PROGRAM

An in-patient physical therapy program, supplemented with a continuous epidural anesthetic, femoral nerve block, or appropriate analgesics may be used for 3 to 4 days in resistant patients who do not respond to other interventions or in whom limitations of knee motion return after manipulation or arthroscopic débridement. The epidural is regulated to block pain and sensory input, with the goal to retain muscle motor control to allow active knee motion and the overpressure program. The block requires close supervision by an anesthesiologist for levels and medication dosage. The catheter is replaced under fluoroscopy control if the patient expresses insufficient pain relief. If the repeat block fails, pain relief is obtained with a femoral nerve block and analgesics. A skin care and protection program is

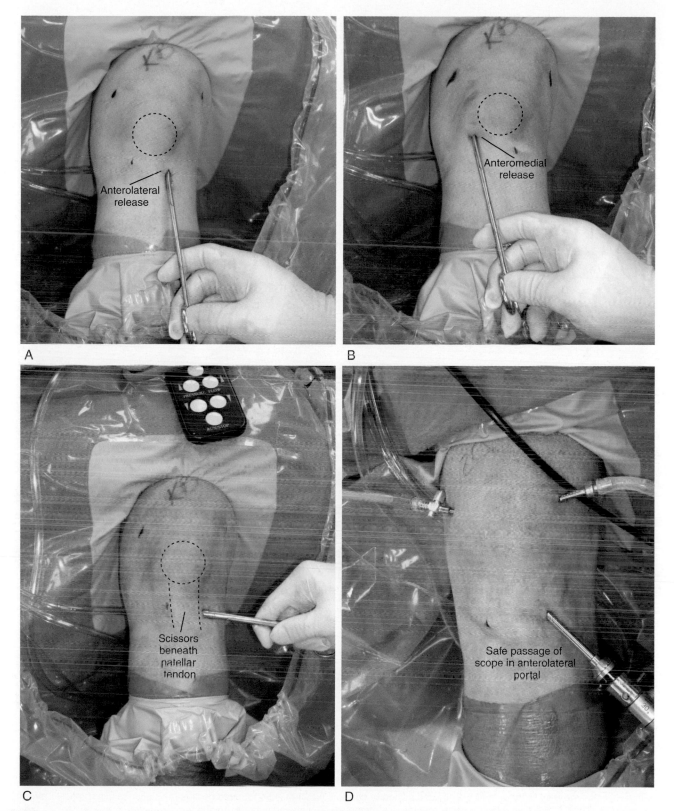

FIGURE 41–16. A, The anterolateral portal is used to transect the lateral retinaculum 15 mm. **B,** The anteromedial portal is used to transect the medial retinaculum 15 mm. **C,** The anterolateral portal is used to place a Metzenbaum scissor beneath the patellar tendon and palpate for an infrapatellar patella–tibial band of scar tissue. The scissor is bluntly pushed posterior to the patellar tendon and through the infrapatellar band to allow fluid to pass into the fatty space behind the patellar tendon. This maneuver protects the patellar tendon during removal of the infrapatellar band, to be described. If a safe plane cannot be established and verified arthroscopically, an open débridement procedure is indicated. **D,** There is now sufficient patellar mobility to pass an arthroscope beneath the patella safely without damaging the patellofemoral cartilage surfaces. If this is not possible, additional medial and lateral releases are performed. The releases at this point are conservative.

(Continued)

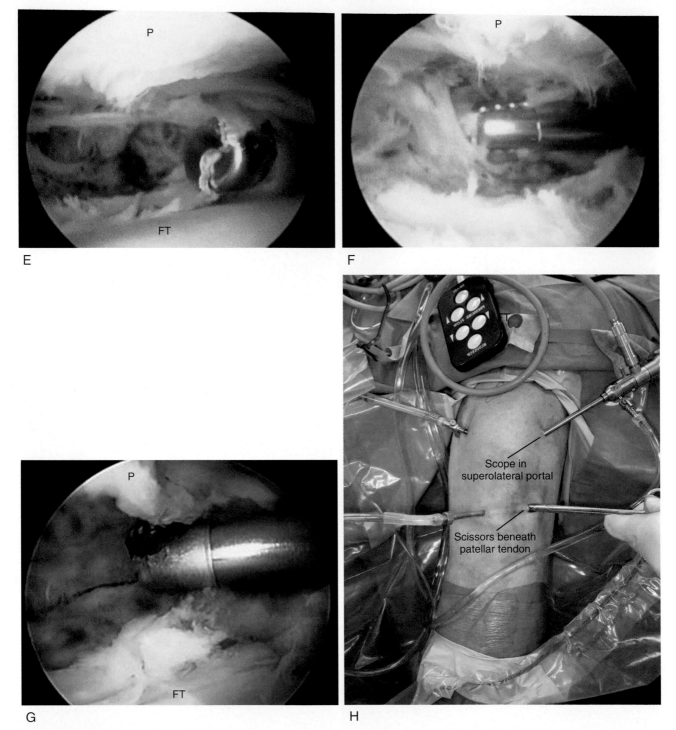

FIGURE 41–16—cont'd. E, A blunt obturator or shaver is placed into the suprapatellar pouch and translated in a superior and inferior plane to reestablish a space sufficient for the initial arthroscopic débridement. A band of scar extends from the superior patella to the trochlea, and dense suprapatellar adhesions are present. Débridement of suprapatellar scar tissues is performed using an electrocuting device. **F,** The soft tissues and synovium over the anterior femur are not removed to leave a gliding soft tissue surface. **G,** A resection of scar tissue beneath the vastus medialis obliquus (VMO) and vastus lateralis obliquus (VLO) may be required because this scar can limit muscle mobility. **H,** The scope is placed in the superolateral portal to view the infrapatellar region and débride an infrapatellar contracture.

performed by nursing personnel. The block is maintained for a minimum of 72 hours in order to allow a gradual overpressure program to stretch contracted soft tissues.

The following measures are taken in order to avoid deep venous thrombosis and pulmonary embolism. First, a careful analysis is done to detect patients at increased risk, including diabetics, obese individuals, or those with venous insufficiency, prior history of phlebitis, or venous clots or embolism. These patients are not appropriate candidates for the epidural program owing to the associated inactivity and bedrest. When the

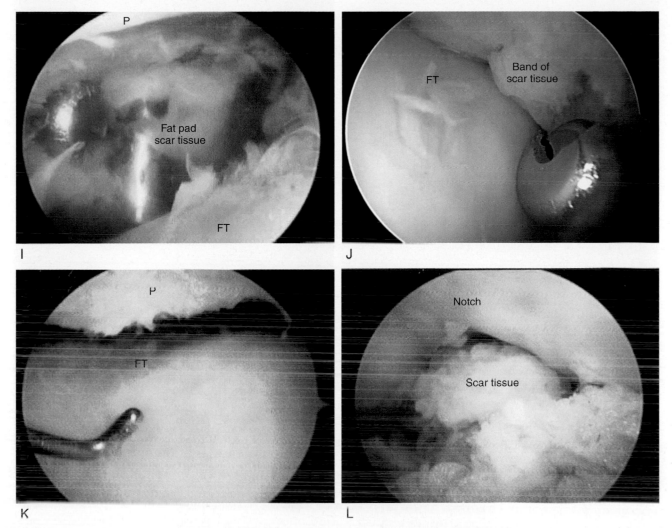

FIGURE 41-16—cont'd. **I,** An arthroscopic view through the superolateral portal shows the fat pad and instruments to remove infrapatellar scar tissue. Care is taken to not transect the anterior medial and lateral meniscus attachments. **J,** With the scope placed alternatively in the anteromedial and anterolateral portals, extensive synovium and scar are removed from the medial and lateral recesses and intercondylar notch. Scar tissue proliferation may block extension on the anterior aspect of the medial and lateral meniscus; this requires removal. **K,** The knee is placed at 30° flexion and sufficient medial and lateral parapatellar contracted tissue and retinaculum are removed to allow for a normal medial-lateral glide. This release rarely extends above the midportion of the patella. In this knee, moderate patellofemoral damage is observed. **L,** Notch ingrowth of tissue removed that may block extension. After completion of the arthroscopic procedure, and verification that no scar tissue remains, the tourniquet is deflated and meticulous electrocoagulation of bleeding points is performed. The decision to use a drain is based on the ability to control intra-articular bleeding. A gentle ranging of the knee with the patient under anesthesia is performed that is not aggressive in terms of the loads applied. The knee is placed into a bulky compression (cotton-Ace-cotton-Ace) dressing with an ice bladder incorporated into the dressing.

epidural is in place, the patient remains mobile and is encouraged to be out of the bed intermittently throughout the day. Antiembolism stockings are worn and ankle pumps are done for 5 to 10 minutes hourly. The extremity is monitored daily and a calf venous compression device is used. Aspirin (600 mg daily) is prescribed. The patient is monitored for calf tenderness or leg edema and an ultrasound examination of both lower extremities is obtained if any suggestion of a deep venous thrombosis exists.

The in-patient overpressure program is contraindicated in patients with open growth plates or disuse osteopenia owing to the increased risk of a fracture. The patient is taught before the epidural how to perform the program, and the patient uses the amount of tension applied to the foot-calf stocking for achieving knee flexion. It is important that other individuals such as the family not assist in the overpressure flexion, because this would involve a flexion manipulation by untrained personnel.

The overpressure extension (Fig. 41-19) and flexion (Fig. 41-20) exercises are described in Table 41-7. The authors recommend an active range of motion program performed by the patient instead of use of a continuous passive motion machine. As well, the patient should continue with leg lifts and isometric exercises while in the hospital. It is imperative to control soft tissue inflammation and avoid a hemarthrosis. If soft tissue swelling persists, or thigh muscle pain occurs owing to excessive stretching, an NSAID or steroidal dose pack should

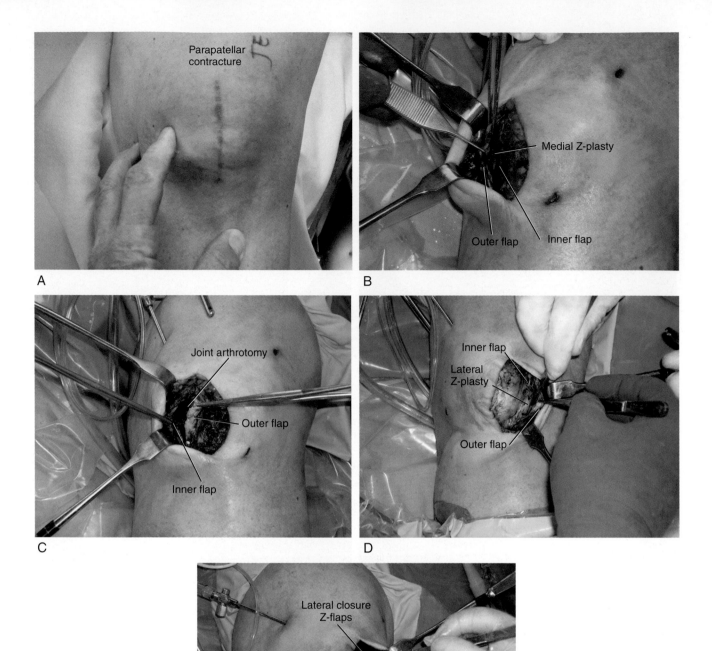

FIGURE 41–17. Z-Plasty operative technique for contracted medial and lateral peripatellar tissues. **A,** Preoperative examination under anesthesia of a patient with established arthrofibrosis discloses a complete lack of patellar mobility, absent medial and lateral glide, and an obvious patella infera with shortening of the patellar tendon. The patient's range of motion was 0°/0°/80°. **B,** Open medial Z-plasty approach. The medial retinaculum and soft tissues are split in a Z-plasty fashion to allow a loose closure and restore a normal medial patellar glide. An arthroscopic procedure was performed just prior to the open procedure to reestablish the suprapatellar pouch, remove intra-articular adhesions within the suprapatellar pouch and medial and lateral tibiofemoral gutters, and document the condition of the joint. **C,** Completion of medial Z-plasty release shows the medial soft tissue flaps that have been developed. A débridement of infrapatellar scar tissue was performed under direct visualization. **D,** A lateral Z-plasty release of contracted lateral retinacular tissues is performed in a similar fashion. **E,** The loose closure of the lateral Z-plasty release allows restoration of a normal medial glide. A medial and lateral Z-plasty release for contracted soft tissues represents a real key for the successful management of this type of contracture. There is restoration of normal patellar mobility, and most importantly, the joint soft tissues can be closed.

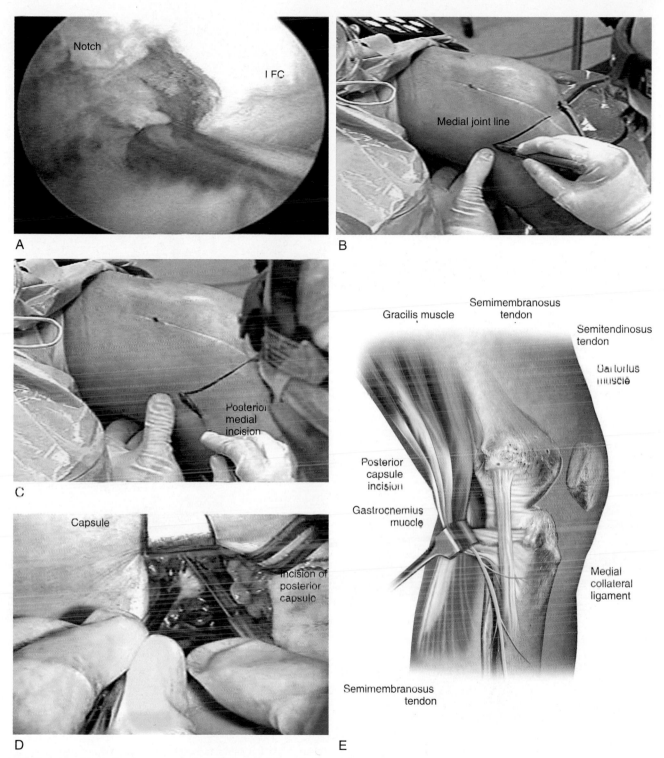

FIGURE 41–18. Operative photographs of a patient with arthrofibrosis (0°/15°/80°) requiring an arthroscopic lysis of adhesions, parapatellar releases, and posterior medial and lateral capsulotomy for the 15° flexion contracture. **A,** An arthroscopic lysis of adhesions, removal of scar tissue, and parapatellar releases is performed, as already described. All scar tissue from the notch region is removed and a notchplasty performed as required so that these tissues do not block extension. **B,** The medial joint line is marked. **C,** A posteromedial incision is made. **D,** The approach reflecting the sartorius is used as described for an inside-out medial meniscus repair (see Chapter 28, Meniscus Tears. Diagnosis, Repair Techniques, and Clinical Outcomes). **E,** A vertical posteromedial capsulotomy is made directly behind the superficial medial collateral ligament (MCL). Operative photograph: The surgeon uses a headlamp and the femoral insertion of the posteromedial capsule is identified and transected millimeter by millimeter to the edge of the medial femoral condyle, but not beyond to avoid the neurovascular structures.

(Continued)

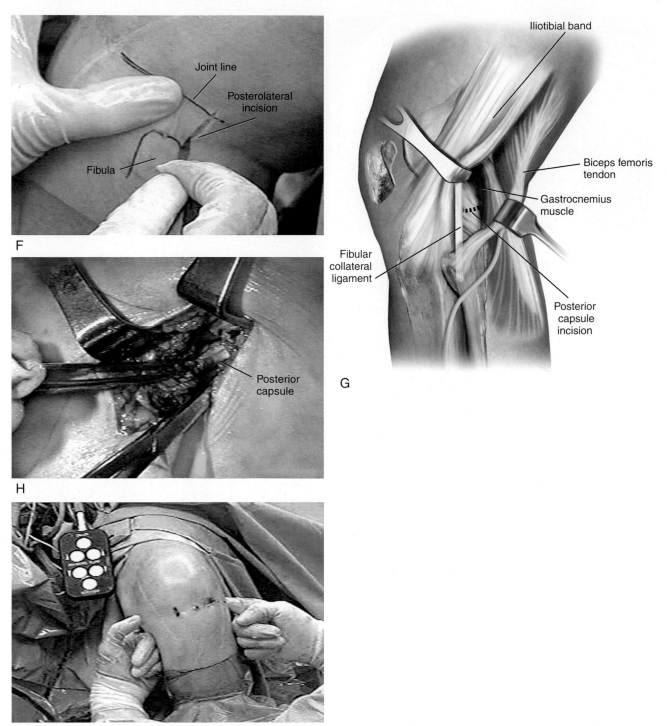

FIGURE 41–18—cont'd.   F, The posterolateral approach for a capsular release uses the same approach as that for a lateral meniscus repair (see Chapter 28, Meniscus Tears: Diagnosis, Repair Techniques, and Clinical Outcomes) with a skin incision just distal to the joint line as shown. **G,** The posterolateral capsule anterior to the gastrocnemius tendon is identified. **H,** The posterolateral capsule is carefully incised under direct visualization to the edge of the lateral femoral condyle, avoiding the neurovascular structures. **I,** A finger is placed into the posteromedial and posterolateral incisions and the central neurovascular structures can be palpated. The central posterior capsule anterior to the neurovascular structures is not released. The finger palpation confirms that the capsule directly posterior to the medial and lateral femoral condyles has been incised, removing this block to extension as the knee is extended.

be considered. After the epidural, it is routine to obtain a venous ultrasound to exclude venous clot disease.

Upon completion of the in-patient program, the exercises must be continued at home eight times a day. Close supervision by the physical therapist is required, because the gains in knee flexion and extension may be reduced rapidly if the regimen is not maintained or if pain and swelling prohibit the patient's ability to perform the exercises.

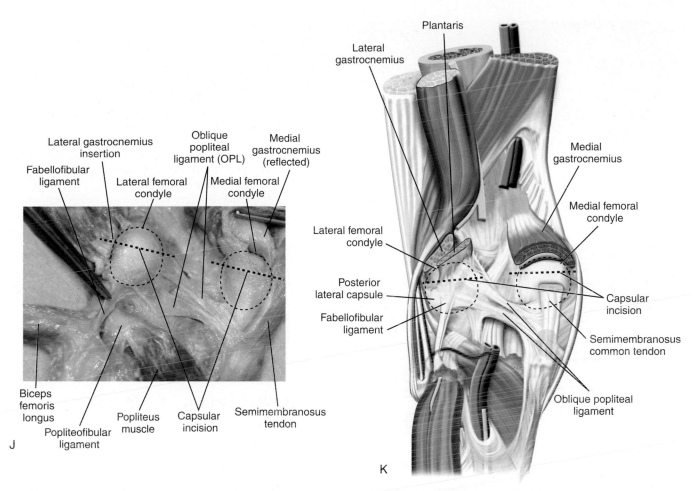

FIGURE 41–18—cont'd. **J** and **K,** The posterior capsular releases. The remaining posterior capsular tissues are gently stretched with the overpressure program to achieve extension. This is a limited cosmetic approach that does not disturb other posterior soft tissues and removes only the contracted posterior capsule as shown by the *dotted line.*

Critical Points IN-PATIENT PHYSICAL THERAPY PROGRAM

- An in-patient physical therapy program—supplemented with either a continuous epidural anesthetic, femoral nerve block, or appropriate analgesics—may be used for 3–4 days in resistant cases who do not respond to other interventions or in whom limitations of knee motion return after manipulation or arthroscopic débridement.
- Contraindicated in patients with open growth plates or disuse osteopenia owing to the increased risk of a fracture.
- Block maintained at least 72 hr to allow a gradual overpressure program to stretch contracted soft tissues.
- Take appropriate measures to avoid deep venous thrombosis.
- Patient is taught before the epidural how to perform the overpressure program.
- Recommend active range of motion program by the patient, not continuous passive motion machine.
- Leg lifts, isometric exercises performed while in the hospital.
- Exercises must be continued after discharge at home eight times a day, along with supervised therapy program.

Critical Points DEVELOPMENTAL PATELLA INFERA

- Occurs secondary to contracture of peripatellar and infrapatellar scar tissues and quadriceps weakness.
- May result in permanent shortening of the patellar tendon, patellofemoral arthritis, and severe functional limitations.
- Prevention: voluntary quadriceps contraction by 2nd postoperative day, knee motion, patellar mobilization.
- Serial lateral radiographs to measure patellar height in patients with limited patellar mobility, early arthrofibrotic response detected.
- Treatment of established patella infera: preoperative muscle strengthening, rehabilitation. Operative removal of contracted and scarred tissues.
- Final functional limitations based on residual motion deficits, joint arthritis.

DEVELOPMENTAL PATELLA INFERA

The senior author has reported on the complication of developmental patella infera (Fig. 41–21) that occurs after major knee injury or surgery, secondary to contracture of peripatellar and

infrapatellar scar tissues and quadriceps weakness.[105,106] This condition may result in permanent shortening of the patellar tendon, patellofemoral arthritis, and severe functional limitations. To prevent this problem, the steps previously described to prevent arthrofibrosis are taken before and after surgery. In addition, the patient is instructed preoperatively on the importance of achieving a voluntary quadriceps contraction as soon as possible after surgery, which is expected to occur by the 2nd postoperative day. Patellar mobility is assessed weekly by the

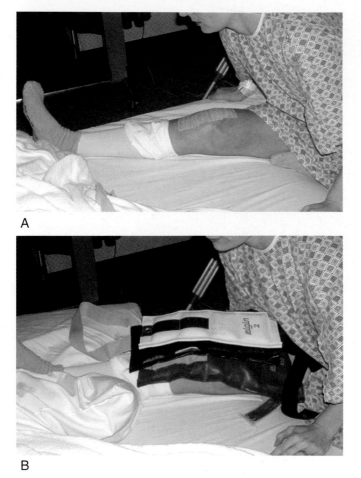

A

B

FIGURE 41–19. In-patient extension overpressure exercises include hamstring stretching (**A**) and hanging weights (**B**).

therapist to detect any early contracture. Serial lateral radiographs are taken to detect any decrease in patellar height for patients demonstrating limited patellar mobility or in whom an early arthrofibrotic response is detected (Fig. 41–22). The differences in criteria for determining the presence of patella infera according to published techniques are shown in Table 41–8.

For patients who present with an established patella infera, the treatment algorithm is shown in Figure 41–23. The first principle of treatment is the preoperative preparation of the patient to establish quadriceps muscle function, rehabilitation, and training to avoid a quadriceps shutdown after the surgical procedure. Second, to remove the contracted and scarred tissues by either arthroscopic or open surgery, as already discussed. A number of months of intensive therapy are then required. The final functional limitations are based on residual motion deficits and joint arthritis that are present. A majority of patients with established patella infera have functional limitations.[106] The patients do not desire any further surgery and are willing to live with these limitations, understanding that an eventual arthroplasty procedure may be required. A small percentage of patients with a remaining patella infera and minimal patellofemoral arthritis who have symptoms of anterior knee pain and stiffness may be candidates for restoration of a normal patellotrochlear relationship.

AUTHORS' CLINICAL STUDIES

Two studies were conducted by the authors to determine the effectiveness of the postoperative rehabilitation program and early diagnosis and treatment of knee motion limitations after ACL reconstruction in preventing arthrofibrosis. In the first study,[102] a group of 207 knees that underwent an ACL bone–patellar tendon–bone (B-PT-B) allograft reconstruction were followed for at least 1 year postoperatively to determine the final

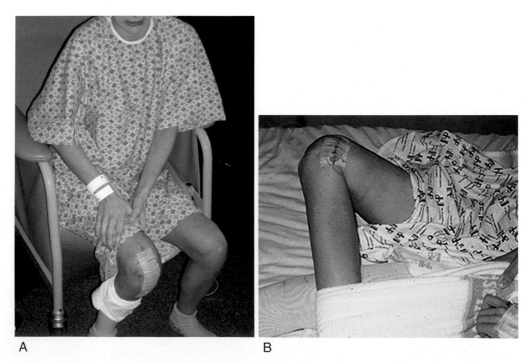

A   B

FIGURE 41–20. In-patient flexion overpressure exercises include rolling stool (**A**) and figure-four with a towel or strap in which the heel is brought up to a predetermined mark on the anterior thigh of the opposite extremity (**B**).

TABLE 41–7 In-Patient Overpressure Extension and Flexion Program

	Exercises
Extension (perform first, before flexion)	1. Determine weight to be used and pain limits before epidural is begun. 2. Use 15-20-25 lb of weight over the knee with the foot and ankle supported. Progress as tolerated. 3. Use lowest amount of weight to achieve 3° hyperextension at the 3rd day.
Flexion	1. Perform release of contracted tissues that produce a hard-stop to flexion before the overpressure program, protect patellofemoral joint. Expect soft-stop to gradually release over 72 hr, producing significant gains in flexion. 2. Mark the affected heel height on the opposite thigh before the epidural is begun to determine the extent of contracture and starting point. 3. Limit the amount of flexion gained over the first 24 hr to prevent muscle and tissue tearing. 4. Perform patellar mobilizations to avoid patella overpressure with knee flexion. 5. Figure-four position in bed, place and hold strap or towel using approximately 15–20 lb of pull on the ankle. Monitor heel-thigh mark on the opposite thigh to determine the gain in flexion. 6. Perform flexion overpressure program every 30 min for 5 min while awake. Goal is to achieve heel-height above patella. 7. Physician performs flexion overpressure test to determine whether soft or hard resistance is present and measures knee flexion angle daily. 8. Continue the overpressure program after discharge at home, eight times every 24 hr, using pain control to achieve flexion gained under the epidural.

amount of knee flexion and extension obtained and document the necessity of treatment interventions. Sixty-nine patients received the operation for an acute ACL rupture, and 138 for chronic ACL deficiency. Of the 207 knees, 90 had the ACL reconstruction alone, 52 had a concurrent iliotibial band extra-articular procedure, 52 had a concurrent meniscus repair, and 13 had a concurrent MCL repair.

The investigation found that 189 of the knees (91%) regained normal motion without requiring additional treatment intervention. The remaining 18 required extension casting, gentle manipulation under anesthesia, or (in only 3 knees) arthroscopic débridement and lysis of adhesions (Table 41–9). There was a correlation between concurrent procedures and the incidence of patients requiring addition treatment, because 4% in the ACL alone subgroup, 10% in the iliotibial band extra-articular subgroup, 12% in the meniscus repair subgroup, and 23% in the MCL subgroup required intervention. The timing of surgery had no effect on the necessity for treatment intervention.

Critical Points AUTHORS' CLINICAL STUDIES

Study #1
- $N = 207$ knees ACL B-PT-B allograft reconstruction.
- Followed at least 1 year postoperatively.
- 189 (91%) regained normal motion without additional treatment intervention:
  - 6 extension casting.
  - 9 gentle manipulation under anesthesia.
  - 3 arthroscopic débridement, lysis of adhesions.
- Correlation concurrent procedures and incidence of patients requiring treatment:
  - 4% ACL alone.
  - 10% ACL + iliotibial band extra-articular.
  - 12% ACL + meniscus repair.
  - 23% ACL + MCL.
- At follow-up, full knee motion was present in 98%, 1% had a 5° limitation of extension, 1% had a permanent contracture

Study #2
- $N = 443$ knees ACL B-PT-B autograft reconstruction.
- Followed mean, 25 mo (range, 12–86 mo) postoperatively.
- Treatment intervention required 23 knees, all successfully resolved.
- Concurrent procedures and incidence of patients requiring treatment:
  - 6% ACL alone.
  - 5% ACL + FCL reconstruction/posterolateral advancement.
  - 8% ACL + meniscus repair.
  - 18% ACL + proximal patellar realignment.
  - 22% ACL + MCL.
- 98% regained normal motion, 2% (refused additional treatment) had mild losses of extension of 5°.

ACL, anterior cruciate ligament; B-PT-B, bone–patellar tendon–bone; FCL, fibular collateral ligament; MCL, medial collateral ligament.

Extension casts were applied to 6 knees between 4 and 12 weeks postoperatively and all regained normal extension. A gentle manipulation under anesthesia was performed in 9 knees between 3 and 13 weeks postoperatively. All achieved full flexion and all but 2 achieved full extension; two knees lacked 5° of extension at follow-up. Arthroscopic débridement was done in 3 knees; the details and results are shown in Table 41–10. At follow-up, full knee motion was present in 98%, 1% had a 5° limitation of extension, and 1% had a permanent contracture.

The authors conducted a second study[101] comprising 443 knees that underwent ACL B-PT-B autograft reconstruction. The operations were performed for acute/subacute ACL ruptures in 161 patients and for chronic ruptures in 283 patients. All were followed an average of 25 months (range, 12–86 mo) postoperatively. Concurrent procedures done in 224 knees included meniscus repairs in 194 knees, proximal advancement of the posterolateral structures in 32 knees, an autograft reconstruction of the fibular collateral ligament (FCL) in 4 knees, a repair or reconstruction of the MCL in 9 knees, and a proximal patellar realignment in 17 knees.

No correlation existed between concurrent procedures and the incidence of patients requiring addition treatment in this study. The percentage of patients requiring additional treatment intervention was 6% in the ACL alone subgroup, 5% in the FCL reconstruction/posterolateral advancement subgroup, 8% in the meniscus repair subgroup, 18% in the proximal patellar realignment subgroup, and 22% in the MCL subgroup. The

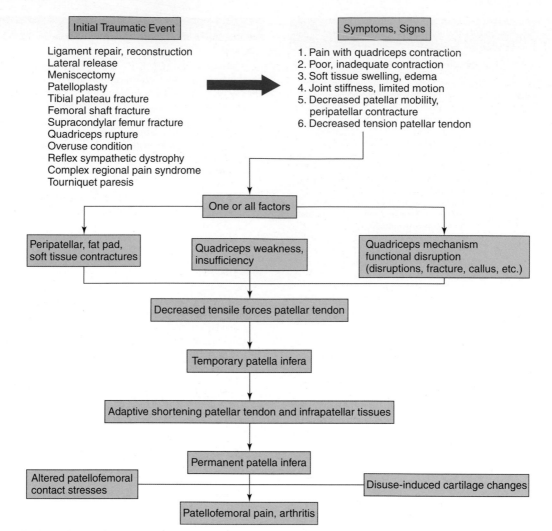

FIGURE 41–21. Pathomechanics for developmental patella infera, quadriceps insufficiency, patellar tendon shortening, and arthritis. *(From Noyes, F. R.; Wojtys, E. M.; Marshall, M. T.: The early diagnosis and treatment of developmental patella infera syndrome. Clin Orthop 265:241–252, 1991.)*

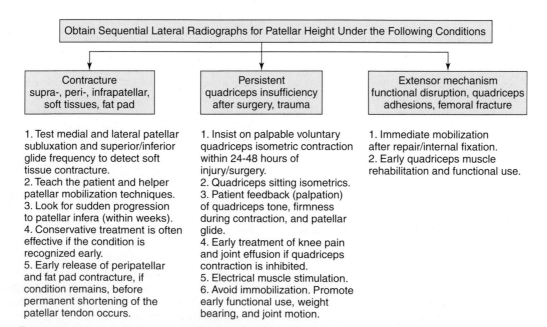

FIGURE 41–22. Treatment recommendations for avoiding developmental patella infera syndrome. *(From Noyes, F. R.; Wojtys, E. M.; Marshall, M. T.: The early diagnosis and treatment of developmental patella infera syndrome. Clin Orthop 265:241–252, 1991.)*

TABLE 41–8   Published Values for Patellar Height: Normal, Alta, Infera

Reference	Technique Source	Normal Mean ± Standard Deviation (Range)	Alta	Infera
Insall & Salvati, 1971[62a]	Authors' own	1.02 ± 0.13 (0.7–1.3)	>1.2	<0.8
Blackburne & Peel, 1977[11]	Authors' own	0.8 ± 0.13 (0.54–1.06)	>1.2	<0.5
Caton et al, 1982[21]	Authors' own	<1.2	>1.2	≤0.6
Linclau, 1984[71]	Caton et al.	1.0 ± 0.08 (0.84–1.16)	>1.2	<0.8
	Blackburne & Peel	0.8 ± 0.10 (0.61–1.01)	>1.0	<0.6
Noyes et al, 1991[106]	Caton et al.	1.04 ± 0.13 (0.75–1.36)	NA	≥15%*
	Blackburne & Peel	0.84 ± 0.14 (0.61–1.33)	NA	≥14%*
	Insall & Salvati	1.05 ± 0.11 (0.86–1.28)	NA	≥11%*

*Decrease in patellar height between the involved and the contralateral knee.
NA, not available.

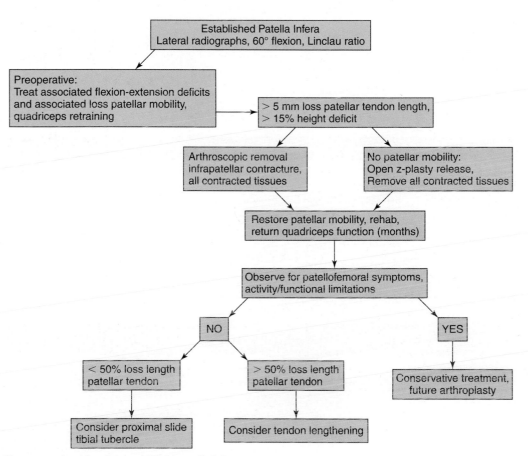

FIGURE 41–23. Treatment algorithm for established patella infera.

timing of surgery had no effect on the necessity for treatment intervention.

The investigation found that 98% of the knees regained normal motion and 2% had mild losses of extension of 5°. In 23 knees, treatment intervention was required (Table 41–11), which was successful in treating the limitation of knee flexion or extension (Table 41–12). The 2% (7 knees) who had mild losses of extension refused treatment intervention.

Extension casts were applied to 9 knees an average of 13 weeks postoperatively. All of these knees regained normal extension. A gentle manipulation under anesthesia was performed in 9 knees a mean of 6.4 weeks postoperatively, and all achieved full knee motion. Arthroscopic débridement was done in 3 knees, which also successfully restored normal knee motion. There was no statistically significant increased risk for knee

motion problems for six variables studied including gender, injury chronicity, condition of the articular cartilage at reconstruction, location of physical therapy, whether prior surgery had been performed, and whether a prior ACL reconstruction had been performed.

The data from the two investigations on 650 knees showed that 6% of the patients required and agreed to treatment intervention for a knee motion problem. At the final follow-up evaluation, 2% lacked normal knee motion (9 knees lacked 5° of extension and 2 had permanent contractures). An extension cast was applied in 2%, gentle manipulation under anesthesia was done in 3%, and arthroscopic débridement was performed in less than 1%. The percentage of all 650 knees requiring additional treatment intervention was 5% in the ACL alone subgroup, 5% in the FCL reconstruction/posterolateral

TABLE 41–9 Patients Requiring Treatment Intervention for Knee Motion Limitations after Anterior Cruciate Ligament Allograft Reconstruction

Case #	Additional Procedures at ACL Reconstruction	Extension Casting	Gentle Manipulation under Anesthesia	Arthroscopic Débridement
1	Meniscus repair, EA	Yes	Yes	
2	None	Yes	Yes	
3	Meniscus repair	Yes	Yes	
4	Meniscus repair	Yes	Yes	
5	MCL repair		Yes (x2)	Yes
6	EA	Yes		
7	Meniscus repair		Yes	
8	None	Yes		
9	Meniscus repair, EA		Yes	
10	Meniscus repair	Yes		
11	Meniscus repair	Yes		
12	None	Yes		
13	EA		Yes	
14	MCL repair		Yes	
15	Meniscus repair	Yes		
16	Meniscus repair, EA	Yes	Yes	
17	MCL repair, meniscus repair	Yes	Yes	Yes
18	None		Yes	Yes

ACL, anterior cruciate ligament; EA, iliotibial band extra-articular procedure; MCL, medial collateral ligament.

TABLE 41–10 Results of Arthroscopic Débridement for Arthrofibrosis after ACL Allograft Reconstruction

Case #	Week Release Performed after ACL Reconstruction	ROM before Release	ROM after Release	Week Manipulation Performed after Release	Complications, Final Outcome
5	9	5°–80°	5°–100°	12, 16	Knee infection: open drainage; patella infera due to noncompliance with rehabilitation program
17	32	10°–90°	5°–105°	None	Continued contracture owing to noncompliance with rehabilitation program
18	7	8°–89°	0°–100°	9	Achieved full knee motion

ACL, anterior cruciate ligament; ROM, range of motion.

TABLE 41–11 Patients Requiring Treatment Intervention for Knee Motion Limitations after Anterior Cruciate Ligament Bone–Patellar Tendon–Bone Autograft Reconstruction

Case #	Additional Procedures at ACL Reconstruction	Steroid Dose Pack	Extension Casting	Epidural, In-Patient Physical Therapy	Gentle Manipulation under Anesthesia	Arthroscopic Débridement
1	None	Yes	Yes			
2	None		Yes			
3	None		Yes			
4	Meniscus repair		Yes			
5	Meniscus repair		Yes			
6	MCL reconstruction		Yes			
7	Meniscus repair		Yes			
8	Advance PLS		Yes			
9	None	Yes	Yes			
10	Meniscus repair		Yes	Yes	Yes	
11	None	Yes	Yes		Yes	
12	Advance PLS, meniscus repair	Yes	Yes	Yes	Yes	
13	Meniscus repair, PR				Yes	
14	None	Yes			Yes	
15	PR				Yes	
16	PR	Yes			Yes	
17	Meniscus repair				Yes	
18	Meniscus repair				Yes	
19	Meniscus repair	Yes	Yes	Yes	Yes	Yes
20	MCL, meniscus repair		Yes		Yes	Yes
21	Meniscus repair	Yes				Yes
22	None			Yes		
23	None		Yes			

ACL, anterior cruciate ligament; MCL, medial collateral ligament; PLS, posterolateral structures; PR, proximal realignment.

TABLE 41–12 Results of Treatment Intervention

Case #	Treatment Intervention	Wk Postoperative Intervention Applied	ROM before Treatment*	ROM after Treatment*	Week Postoperative Full ROM Achieved
1	Extension cast	8, 15, 16	–7° (extension loss)	0/0/157	18
2	Extension cast	6, 28, 45	–5° (extension loss)	0/0/142	46
3	Extension cast	7	–3° (extension loss)	0/0/140	16
4	Extension cast	30	–3° (extension loss)	0/0/144	35
5	Extension cast	3	–7° (extension loss)	5/0/152	10
6	Extension cast	20	–3° (extension loss)	0/0/140	22
7	Extension cast	15	–5° (extension loss)	1/0/148	19
8	Extension cast	12, 36	–3° (extension loss)	5/0/146	48
9	Extension cast	20	–5° (extension loss)	0/0/137	23
10	Manipulation	7	0/–3/110	0/0/136	13
11	Manipulation	5	0/–3/95	0/0/142	12
12	Manipulation	7	0/–5/110	2/0/138	22
13	Manipulation	6	0/0/90	0/0/140	9
14	Manipulation	12	0/–3/118	5/0/140	18
15	Manipulation	4	0/0/97	0/0/136	6
16	Manipulation	5	0/0/96	0/0/147	9
17	Manipulation	5	0/–5/60	0/0/141	22
18	Manipulation	7	0/0/73	0/0/135	19
19	Scope, release	7	0/–10/121	0/0/140	17
20	Scope, release	14	0/0/90	10/0/126[†]	NA[‡]
21	Scope, release	10	0/0/126	0/0/135	16
22	In-patient rehabilitation	48	0/–20/120	3/0/138	48
23	Epidural	20	0/–3/115	0/0/137	NA[‡]

*Values are for passive hyperextension/zero point/flexion.
[†]Equal to the opposite normal knee.
[‡]Not available, patient lived out of town, but full at the 2 yr follow-up evaluation.
NA, not available; ROM, range of motion.

advancement subgroup, 10% in the meniscus repair subgroup, 10% in the extra-articular subgroup, 18% in the proximal patellar realignment subgroup, and 23% in the MCL subgroup.

OTHER AUTHORS' CLINICAL STUDIES

Several authors have reported on the outcome of the treatment of arthrofibrosis after ACL reconstruction (Table 41–13).* These studies help identify risk factors for a limitation of knee motion, discussed previously. In general, the surgical débridement procedures were done an average of 1 year after

*See references 2, 24, 25, 41, 54, 69, 79, 112, 116, 130, 132, 142.

the reconstruction, which in the opinion of authors of this chapter, is too late. In many of the series, patients were referred from other centers and the treating surgeon was unable to perform the débridement earlier. Although many authors reported that significant gains were obtained in knee motion, most found that the majority of patients had permanent residual losses of flexion and extension and more complaints of pain and limitations compared with patients who did not suffer from this complication. Table 41–13 also shows other studies of the treatment of arthrofibrosis after fractures, infection, meniscectomy, and other knee ligament reconstructions.[1,73,149,151] These studies report even poorer results in terms of restoration of normal knee motion and function.

TABLE 41–13 Clinical Studies Treatment of Arthrofibrosis

Reference	Number, Follow-up	Causes Arthrofibrosis Incidence Rate	Pretreatment ROM	Treatment	Post-Treatment ROM	Comments
Wang et al., 2006[151]	22, Mean: 44 mo (range, 24–63 mo)	Fracture 20 (17 treated with ORIF, 2 external fixators, 1 dynamic hip screw) ACL reconstruction 2	Flexion mean: 27° (range, 5°–45°) 2 patients loss extension (range, 5°–10°)	Mini-open & arthroscopic débridement, quadriceps tendon lengthening in 16, CPM	Flexion mean: 115° (range, 75°–150°) 3 patients loss extension (5°–15°)	All patients severe loss flexion pre-débridement. All but 1 satisfied with outcome.
Mayr et al., 2004[79]	223, Mean: 4.29 yr	ACL reconstruction	Extension loss: <3°: 12.1% 3°–5°: 25.5% 6°–10°: 26.1% >10°: 35.7%	Scope, débridement Mean time procedure to treatment: 17.6 mo	Extension loss: <3°: 63.7% 3°–5°: 26.8% 6°–10°: 5.1% >10°: 3.2% Mean flexion: 127°	88% x-ray signs DJD. Risk factors: acute ACL reconstruction, preoperative irritated knee (swelling, effusion, hyperthermia), limited motion pre-ACL reconstruction.

Continued

TABLE 41–13 Clinical Studies Treatment of Arthrofibrosis—Cont'd

Reference	Number, Follow-up	Causes Arthrofibrosis Incidence Rate	Pretreatment ROM	Treatment	Post-Treatment ROM	Comments
Millett et al., 1999[85]	8, Mean: 57 mo (range, 9–113 mo)	ACL reconstruction 4 Multiligament reconstruction 3 Meniscectomy post septic arthritis 1	Mean extension: 18.7° (range, 15°–20°), Mean flexion: 81° (40°–130°)	Open débridement, soft tissue release, CPM, custom drop-lock extension brace. Mean time procedure to treatment: 12.3 mos (6-19)	Mean extension: 1.25° (0°–5°) Mean flexion: 125° (range, 110°–145°)	Risk factors: acute ACL reconstruction, multiligament reconstruction. 7 had prior scope/ débridement that failed. All salvage knees.
Reider et al., 1996[116]	11, Mean: 22 mo (range, 9–67 mo)	ACL reconstruction	Mean loss extension: 19.6° (7°–35°)	Scope, débridement Mean time procedure to treatment: 12.6 mo (range, 5–38 mo)	Mean loss extension: 2° (0°–6°)	All patients immobilized in flexion for mean 6 wk after ACL reconstruction. No cases of patella infera.
Lobenhoffer et al., 1996[73]	21, Mean: 18 mo (range, 6–38 mo)	Ligament reconstruction 58% Fractures 30% Infection 12%	Mean loss ext. ension: 17° (range, 10°–30°)	Scope, open posterior capsulotomy. Time procedure to treatment: 6 mo–7 yr	Mean loss extension 2° (range, 0°–5°)	All chronic, all had at least 1 prior scope, débridement that failed.
Shelbourne et al., 1996[132]	72, Mean: 35 mo (range, 28–115 mo)	ACL reconstruction	5°/0°/143° (range, 0°/0°/ 130°–10°/5°/ 156°)	Scope, débridement, removal ACL graft if required, extention cast for types 2, 3, 4 arthrofibrosis. Mean time procedure to therapy: 12.5 mo (range, 2.4–60 mo)	Full extension: Type 1: 88% Type 2: 81% Type 3: 80% Type 4: 69% Full flexion: Types 1 & 2: 100% Type 3: 53% Type 4: 19%	Arthrofibrosis defined as any symptomatic limitation in knee motion compared with opposite knee.
Cosgarea et al., 1995[25]	22, F/U NA	ACL PT autograft reconstruction 22/188 (12%)	All loss extension ≥10°, flexion < 125°, or both	20 at least 1 operation 2 declined further treatment	NA	Risk factors: preoperative extension loss >10°, acute reconstruction <3 wk after injury, postoperative immobilization.
Aglietti et al., 1995[2]	31, Mean: 3.5 yr (range, 1.5–7 yr)	ACL autograft reconstruction	Mean loss extension: 11°; mean loss flexion: 14°	7 Arthroscopic débridement for cyclops lesions, 14 Arthroscopic débridement for global scar tissue, 10 Open débridement, 7 Posteromedial, posterolateral capsulotomy	IKDC rating motion: 8 Normal 15 Nearly normal 8 Abnormal	ACL graft malpositioned/ nonfunctional in 18. Significantly poorer results for symptoms, final overall IKDC rating global scar involvement subgroup.
Shelbourne & Johnson, 1994[130]	9, Mean: 31 mo (range, 7–73 mo)	ACL autograft reconstruction	0°/23°/112° (0°/ 15°–35°/70°– 35°)	Scope, débridement, notchplasty, manipulation, extension cast. Mean time procedure to treatment: 10.2 mo (range, 3–14 mo). All patients referred from elsewhere	2°/0°/130° (0°/ 0°–10°/120°– 150°) 1 patient failed to improve	8 patients had ACL reconstruction within 2 wk of injury, all immobilized in flexion.
Cosgarea et al., 1994[24]	43, Mean: 3.6 yr	ACL reconstruction 23 ACL repair 12 PCL reconstruction 1 MCL repair 1	14°–120°	27 One lysis adhesion 6 Two lysis adhesions 9 "Early" intervention < 6 mo post ligament surgery 34 Late intervention > 6 mo	3°–141° 84% extension deficit ≤ 5° 89% flexion deficit < 15°	Functional outcome poor compared with control group. High incidence radiographic degenerative changes (89%). Patella infera in 9%.

TABLE 41–13   Clinical Studies Treatment of Arthrofibrosis—Cont'd

Reference	Number, Follow-up	Causes Arthrofibrosis Incidence Rate	Pretreatment ROM	Treatment	Post-Treatment ROM	Comments
Klein et al., 1994[69]	46, Mean: 22 mo	ACL reconstruction 74% Meniscus operation 9%	Mean extension loss: 10.4° (range, 5°–20°) Mean flexion loss: 31.6° (range, 5°–100°)	Scope/débridement Mean time procedure to treatment: 22.8 mo (range, 4–105 mo). All but 1 patient referred from elsewhere.	Mean extension loss: 1.7° (range, 0°–15°), Mean flexion loss: 7.9° (0°–50°)	
Paulos et al., 1994[112]	76, Mean: 53 mo (range, 24–86 mo)	ACL reconstruction 63 Multiligament reconstruction 5 Other 8	Loss of ≥ 10° ext & loss ≥ 25° of flexion, Patellar entrapment	Open débridement, release, CPM, night splint for extension. Scope/débridement 3–4 mo later in 84%. Time procedure to treatment: 3 mo – 5 yr. Patients referred from elsewhere.	Mean extension: –2° (range, 0°–8°), Mean flexion: 128° (range, 125°–150°). 3 knees failed to improve.	Most common causes infrapatellar contracture syndrome: nonisometric ACL graft placement, graft impingement.
Achalandabaso & Albillos, 1993[1]	67, F/U NA	Ligament reconstruction 47 Fracture 9 PF surgery 4 Dislocated knee 4 Open meniscus surgery 3	11°–89°, All knees loss flexion. 53 knees loss extension.	62 Scope 5 Scope + open débridement Mean time procedure to treatment: 8 mo	4°–127°, D'Aubige relative improvement: 83.6% excellent 6% good 6% average 4.4% poor	Patients with extra-articular adhesions poor results.
Steadman et al., 1993[142]	44, F/U NA	ACL reconstruction 40 Other 4	17° (range, 0°–40°) to 108.9° (range, 65°–150°)	Scope/débridement 20 Multiple operations 24 Mean time procedure to treatment: 14.1 mo (range, 4–94 mo); all patients referred from elsewhere.	2.2° (range, 0°–15°) to 128.9° (range, 95°–135°) 75% had <5°–≥120°	
Harner et al., 1992[54]	27, Mean: 22.8 mo (range, 12–42 mo)	ACL reconstruction Autograft: 13 Allograft: 14 27/244 (11.1%)	13°–124°, All loss extension 2/3 loss flexion	14 Scope/débridement 6 Open débridement 1 Manipulation Mean time ACL reconstruction to treatment: 6.1 mo (range, 2.5–13)	3°–126°	Risk factors: male gender, acute ACL surgery, concomitant MCL repair.
Fisher & Shelbourne, 1993[41]	35, Mean: 28 mo (range, 6–72 mo)	ACL open reconstruction 42/959 (4%)	6°–119°, Mean loss extension: 12° (range, 3°–22°)	Scope/débridement Mean time ACL reconstruction to treatment: 9 mo (range, 3–48 mo)	0°–135° 7 patients 2°–5° residual extension loss	
Vaquero et al., 1993[149]	21, Mean: 14 mo (range, 6–35 mo)	Ligament reconstruction 6 Tibial fracture 6 Patellar fracture 3 Infrapatellar tendon operation 3 Femur fracture 1 Femur/tibia fracture 2	11.2°–54°	Scope/lysis adhesions Mean time procedure to treatment: 4 mo (range, 2–12 mo)	1.9°–113°	

ACL, anterior cruciate ligament; CPM, continuous passive motion; DJD, degenerative joint disease; F/U, follow-up; IKDC, International Knee Documentation Committee; MCL, medial collateral ligament; NA, not available; ORIF, open reduction and internal fixation; PCL, posterior cruciate ligament; PF, patellofemoral; PT, patellar tendon; ROM, range of motion.

ILLUSTRATIVE CASES

Case 1 A 42-year-old woman presented 7 months after an open reduction internal fixation of a patellar fracture and 4 weeks of immobilization with a severe patella infera, marked by a Linclau ratio of 60% of the left knee (compared with 97% on the opposite knee; Fig. 41–24A). She complained of muscle weakness, pain, and limitations with activities of daily living. She had a range of motion of 0°/10°/95° and a significant decrease in patellar mobility in both medial-lateral and superior-inferior directions. Physical examination showed an obvious patella infera, with mild patellofemoral crepitus. An isokinetic evaluation revealed a 75% deficit in quadriceps peak torque compared with the contralateral side. She underwent 2 months of rehabilitation owing to this severe quadriceps muscle weakness.

The patient was then treated with an open release of scar tissue, which completely obliterated the suprapatellar pouch. Dense scar was present in the medial and lateral gutters, the medial and lateral joint lines, and the intercondylar notch. After the procedure, the patient underwent 3 days of in-patient physical therapy on the epidural overpressure program described previously. Her knee motion improved to 0°/0°/100°.

Two months later, the patient continued to have symptoms and minimal improvement. Therefore, the decision was reached to perform a patellar lengthening procedure. Figure 41–24B–G demonstrates the tendon lengthening. A Z-plasty lengthening of the patient's patellar tendon was performed along with an augmentation using a four-strand semitendinosus-gracilis autograft.

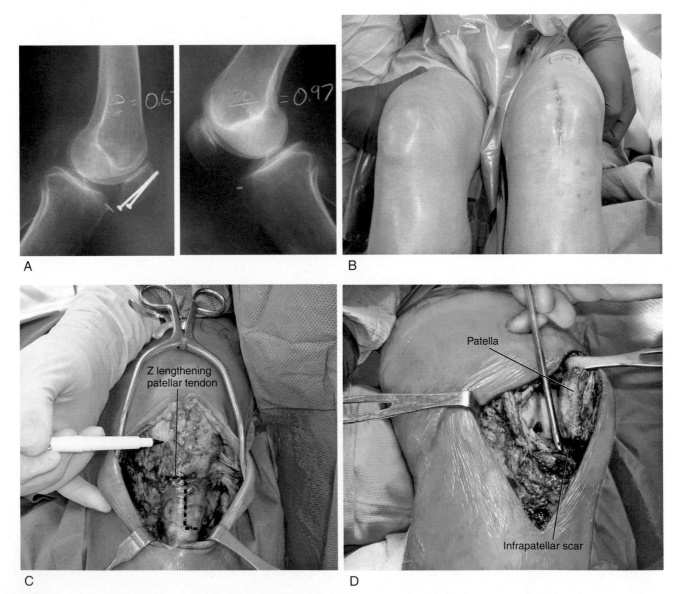

FIGURE 41–24. Case 1. **A,** Preoperative lateral radiographs demonstrate patella infera. **B,** Preoperative appearance of the left knee. The skin mobility was sufficient and did not contraindicate surgery. **C,** The line for the incision of the Z-plasty lengthening of the patient's patellar tendon. **D,** Extensive resection of infrapatellar scar tissue was required.

(Continued)

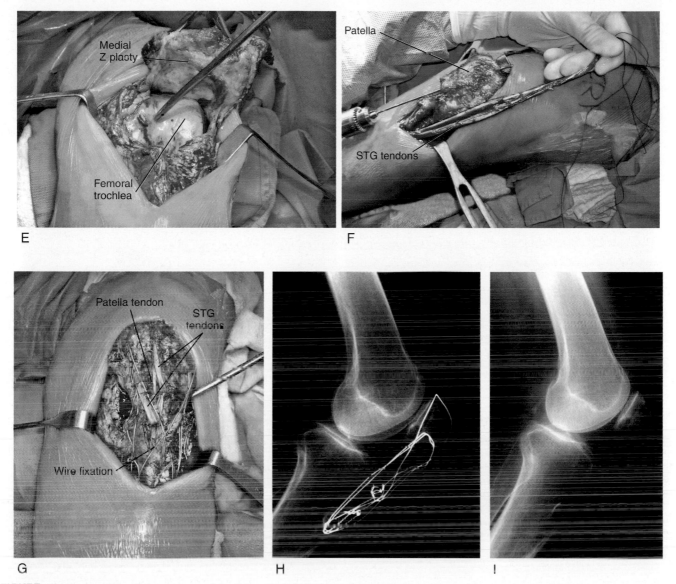

FIGURE 41–24—cont'd. **E,** Appearance of the femoral trochlea shows intact articular cartilage. An extensive medial Z-plasty release was performed. **F,** Placement of a central patellar tunnel for later passage of semitendinosus and gracilis tendons from a distal-to-proximal direction. **G,** Final appearance of patellar tendon reconstruction. The patient's patellar tendon was reapproximated after the Z-plasty lengthening. The semitendinosus and gracilis tendons were passed from the inferior to the superior pole and brought distally along the medial retinaculum to further augment the medial portion of the patellar tendon. In this case, the advantage of using the patient's own patellar tendon added significant soft tissues so that further augmentation was not required. **H,** Postoperative radiograph shows three internal fixation wires that provide stabilization and allow immediate range of motion. **I,** Radiograph shows restoration of normal patellar height after removal of internal fixation wires. The patient was asymptomatic with activities of daily living and able to perform light recreational activities. The final range of motion was normal (0°/0°/135°).

Internal fixation with wire was used to initiate immediate knee motion. The procedure was successful in restoring a normal patellar height (see Fig. 41–24H and I). The goal is to buy time until the patient eventually requires a patellofemoral arthroplasty, which is possible with normal patellar height.

Case 2 A 33-year-old woman presented with severe patellar infera (Linclau ratio, 29%) 4 months after resection of a ganglion cyst, which was growing under her patellar tendon. A portion of the patellar tendon was damaged in the procedure and the patient was treated with 5 weeks of plaster immobilization, which

resulted in severe quadriceps atrophy and severely contracted peripatellar and joint soft tissues. This represented a salvage knee condition because the patient had significant loss of function of the lower extremity. The range of motion was 0°/10°/75°. She underwent 6 weeks of intense preoperative rehabilitation for muscle strengthening and then a skin expansion procedure (Fig. 41–25A and B). Because this patient had no remaining patellar tendon to use in a Z-plasty fashion to incorporate into the reconstruction, she underwent a combined allograft-autograft patellar tendon lengthening procedure (see Fig. 41–25C–G). The patient required intensive rehabilitation for 6 months.

At the most recent follow-up evaluation, 2 years postoperative, the patient had equal Linclau ratios of 85% (see Fig. 41–25H and I) and a range of motion of 0 to 120°. She has no symptoms with activities of daily living or swimming and, while pleased with her condition, realizes that in the future a patellofemoral arthroplasty may be required.

Authors' comment: The salvage procedure of lengthening the patellar tendon was performed in this young patient to buy time before an anticipated total knee replacement. The benefit of reestablishing the normal patellar height (see Fig. 41–25H and I)

allowed a return of moderate lower limb function, with the added benefit at the time of the total joint procedure of retaining patellofemoral joint function.

Case 3 A 42-year-old woman sustained an acute ACL rupture to the right knee that was treated 4 weeks later with an anterior tibialis allograft reconstruction. Before surgery, the patient had achieved 0°/0°/100° of knee motion. Postoperatively, she experienced significant problems with quadriceps muscle atrophy and failed to gain more than 100° of knee flexion. A manipulation under anesthesia was performed 2 months postoperatively in

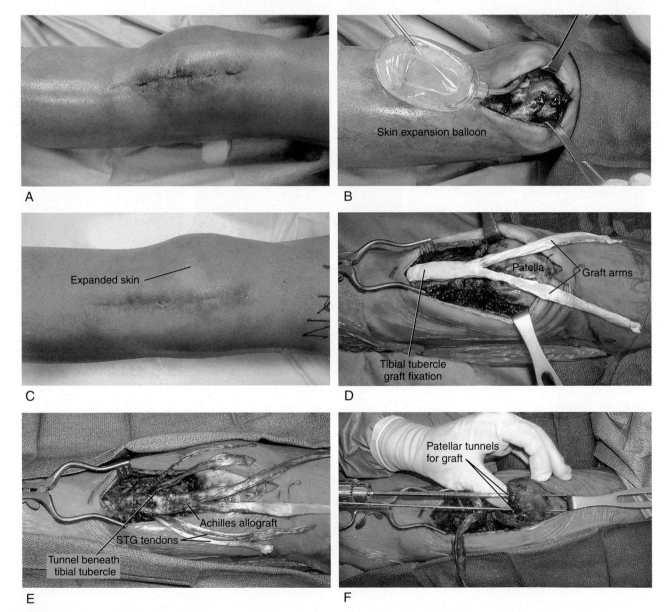

FIGURE 41–25. Case 2. **A,** Preoperative appearance of skin contracture. It is necessary to obtain more normal skin and soft tissue prior to the patellar tendon–lengthening procedure. Otherwise, there would be an increased risk of a complication of skin breakdown and infection. **B,** Placement of the skin expansion system at surgery. The expansion system may be placed either through the prior incision or through limited medial and lateral incisions using two balloons to avoid the primary incision. **C,** Appearance of expanded skin over the anterior aspect of the knee joint after 4 wk of skin expansion. The balloon was removed through a small incision before the operative procedure. Extra redundant skin and subcutaneous tissue is shown and a scar revision was performed. **D,** Operative photograph shows an Achilles tendon allograft for reconstruction of the patellar tendon. The bone portion of the graft is fixated at the tibial tubercle. The two arms of the graft are placed through separate patellar tunnels and sewn into the quadriceps tendon proximally. **E,** A semitendinosus and gracilis autograft harvest is performed. The tendons are passed beneath the tibial tubercle and the Achilles tendon–bone allograft. **F,** Placement of two patellar tunnels.

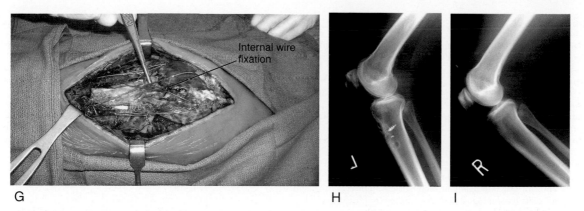

G   H   I

FIGURE 41–25—cont'd. G, Final tendon-lengthening construct. The Achilles tendon has been secured both proximally and distally. The semitendinosus-gracilis autograft tendons are placed through the proximal tibia adjacent to the tibial tubercle. Both tendon arms are passed medially and laterally and secured to the peripatellar tissues to augment the allograft tendon reconstruction. Two wire loops are placed through the tibial tubercle to the midpoint of the patella. A third wire is crossed from the tibial tubercle over the superior portion of the patella and passed beneath the quadriceps tendon patella insertion as a tension band. The height of the patella is adjusted to the normal opposite side using intraoperative fluoroscopy. **H** and **I,** Postoperative lateral radiographs of both knees show retention of the normal height of the patella in the left knee (**H**) compared with the right knee (**I**).

which 0°/0°/120° was achieved; however, the patient gradually reverted to 0°/0°/90° of motion.

The patient presented to our center 5 months postoperatively with complaints of stiffness, tightness, failure to achieve past 90° knee flexion, and a flexed knee gait. On physical examination, she had a stable knee with negative Lachman and pivot shift tests. There was significant muscle atrophy, and the patient was unable to actively perform an isometric quadriceps contraction. She ambulated with limited knee flexion. The patellofemoral joint was markedly restricted, with no medial or lateral glide and an obvious patella infera position.

Standing posteroanterior radiographs showed a decrease in the height of the patella and osteopenia (Fig. 41–26A). Lateral radiographs with the knee flexed showed an obvious patella infera, with a 60% Linclau ratio on the involved side (see Fig. 41–26B) compared with the opposite side of 87% (see Fig. 41–26C). The patient underwent Z plasty lengthening of the medial and lateral retinacular structures to restore patellar mobility, an arthroscopic suprapatellar debridement to open the synovial pouch, and removal of infrapatellar contracture. The patellar tendon shortening was permanent. The

patient underwent 3 months of intensive rehabilitation, muscle strengthening, and gait retraining and achieved 0°/0°/125° of motion, with restoration of patellar mobility.

Authors' comment. This case demonstrates the importance of maintaining normal patellar mobility postoperatively. Any limitation of patellar mobility should be treated by 3 weeks postoperatively using the programs discussed in this chapter. The lack of motion preoperatively, with inadequate rehabilitation, contributed to the postoperative problem. It is not advisable to perform a manipulation at 8 weeks postoperative in a knee in which the joint contracture is well established. Arthroscopic débridement and appropriate lysis of adhesions are instead indicated. Overpressure flexion exercises are contraindicated until release procedures are performed to restore patellar mobility, otherwise, high patellofemoral forces exist with forced flexion and possible articular cartilage damage. If treated early, loss of patellar tendon length and patella infera and associated patellofemoral cartilage damage could possibly have been avoided in this knee. The contracture of the medial and lateral parapatellar tissues was so severe that an open Z-plasty release was required.

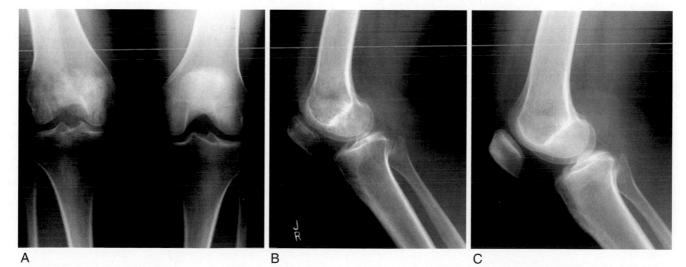

A   B   C

FIGURE 41–26. Case 3.

REFERENCES

1. Achalandabaso, J.; Albillos, J.: Stiffness of the knee—mixed arthroscopic and subcutaneous technique: results of 67 cases. *Arthroscopy* 9:685–690, 1993.
2. Aglietti, P.; Buzzi, R.; De Felice, R.; et al.: Results of surgical treatment of arthrofibrosis after ACL reconstruction. *Knee Surg Sports Traumatol Arthrosc* 3:83–88, 1995.
3. Al-Qattan, M. M.: Factors in the pathogenesis of Dupuytren's contracture. *J Hand Surg [Am]* 31:1527–1534, 2006.
4. Alm, A.; Liljedahl, S.-O.; Stromberg, B.: Clinical and experimental experience in reconstruction of the anterior cruciate ligament. *Orthop Clin North Am* 7:181–189, 1976.
5. Austin, J. C.; Phornphutkul, C.; Wojtys, E. M.: Loss of knee extension after anterior cruciate ligament reconstruction: effects of knee position and graft tensioning. *J Bone Joint Surg Am* 89:1565–1574, 2007.
6. Bach, B. R.; Jones, G. T.; Sweet, F. A.; Hager, C. A.: Arthroscopy-assisted anterior cruciate ligament reconstruction using patellar tendon substitution. Two- to four-year follow-up results. *Am J Sports Med* 22:758–767, 1994.
7. Barber-Westin, S. D.; Noyes, F. R.; Andrews, M.: A rigorous comparison between the sexes of results and complications after anterior cruciate ligament reconstruction. *Am J Sports Med* 25:514–526, 1997.
8. Bedair, H. S.; Karthikeyan, T.; Quintero, A.; et al.: Angiotensin II receptor blockade administered after injury improves muscle regeneration and decreases fibrosis in normal skeletal muscle. *Am J Sports Med* 36:1548–1554, 2008.
9. Berns, G. S.; Howell, S. M.: Roofplasty requirements in vitro for different tibial hole placements in anterior cruciate ligament reconstruction. *Am J Sports Med* 21:292–298, 1993.
10. Biedert, R. M.; Albrecht, S.: The patellotrochlear index: a new index for assessing patellar height. *Knee Surg Sports Traumatol Arthrosc* 14:707–712, 2006.
11. Blackburne, J.; Peel, T.: A new method for measuring patellar height. *J Bone Joint Surg Br* 58:241–242, 1977.
12. Blauth, W.; Jaeger, T.: [Arthrolysis of the knee joint]. *Orthopade* 19:388–399, 1990.
13. Border, W. A.; Noble, N. A.: Transforming growth factor beta in tissue fibrosis. *N Engl J Med* 331:1286–1292, 1994.
14. Border, W. A.; Noble, N. A.; Yamamoto, T.; et al.: Natural inhibitor of transforming growth factor-beta protects against scarring in experimental kidney disease. *Nature* 360:361–364, 1992.
15. Border, W. A.; Ruoslahti, E.: Transforming growth factor-beta in disease: the dark side of tissue repair. *J Clin Invest* 90:1–7, 1992.
16. Bosch, U.: [Etiology of arthrofibrosis]. *Arthroskopie* 12:215–221, 1999.
17. Bosch, U.; Zeichen, J.; Skutek, M.; et al.: Arthrofibrosis is the result of a T-cell–mediated immune response. *Knee Surg Sports Traumatol Arthrosc* 9:282–289, 2001.
18. Bottoni, C. R.; Liddell, T. R.; Trainor, T. J.; et al.: Postoperative range of motion following anterior cruciate ligament reconstruction using autograft hamstrings: a prospective, randomized clinical trial of early versus delayed reconstructions. *Am J Sports Med* 36:656–662, 2008.
19. Bowley, E.; O'Gorman, D. B.; Gan, B. S.: Beta-catenin signaling in fibroproliferative disease. *J Surg Res* 138:141–150, 2007.
20. Bylski-Austrow, D. I.; Grood, E. S.; Hefzy, M. S.; et al.: Anterior cruciate ligament replacements: a mechanical study of femoral attachment location, flexion angle at tensioning, and initial tension. *J Orthop Res* 8:522–531, 1990.
21. Caton, J.; Deschamps, G.; Chambat, P.; et al.: [Patella infera. Apropos of 128 cases]. *Rev Chir Orthop Reparatrice Appar Mot* 68:317–325, 1982.
22. Chan, Y. S.; Li, Y.; Foster, W.; et al.: Antifibrotic effects of suramin in injured skeletal muscle after laceration. *J Appl Physiol* 95:771–780, 2003.
23. Cole, B. J.; Harner, C. D.: The multiple ligament injured knee. *Clin Sports Med* 18:241–262, 1999.
24. Cosgarea, A. J.; DeHaven, K. E.; Lovelock, J. E.: The surgical treatment of arthrofibrosis of the knee. *Am J Sports Med* 22:184–191, 1994.
25. Cosgarea, A. J.; Sebastianelli, W. J.; DeHaven, K. E.: Prevention of arthrofibrosis after anterior cruciate ligament reconstruction using

the central third patellar tendon autograft. *Am J Sports Med* 23:87–92, 1995.
26. Coutts, R.; Rothe, C.; Kaita, J.: The role of continuous passive motion in the rehabilitation of the total knee patient. *Clin Orthop* 159:126–132, 1981.
27. Creighton, R.; Bach, B. R., Jr.: Arthrofibrosis: evaluation, prevention, and treatment. *Tech Knee Surg* 4:163–172, 2005.
28. Darby, I.; Skalli, O.; Gabbiani, G.: Alpha-smooth muscle actin is transiently expressed by myofibroblasts during experimental wound healing. *Lab Invest* 63:21–29, 1990.
29. deAndrade, J. R.; Grant, C.; Dixon, A. S. J.: Joint distension and reflex muscle inhibition in the knee. *J Bone Joint Surg Am* 47:313–322, 1963.
30. DeCarlo, M. S.; Sell, K.: Normative data for range of motion and single leg hop in high school athletes. *J Sports Rehabil* 6:246–255, 1997.
31. DeHaven, K. E.; Cosgarea, A. J.; Sebastianelli, W. J.: Arthrofibrosis of the knee following ligament surgery. *Instr Course Lect* 52:369–381, 2003.
32. Dehne, E.; Torp, R. P.: Treatment of joint injuries by immediate mobilization. Based upon the spinal adaptation concept. *Clin Orthop Relat Res* 77:218–232, 1971.
33. Del Pizzo, W.; Fox, J. M.; Friedman, M. J.: Operative arthroscopy for the treatment of arthrofibrosis of the knee. *Contemp Orthop* 10:67–72, 1985.
34. Eddy, R. J.; Petro, J. A.; Tomasek, J. J.: Evidence for the nonmuscle nature of the "myofibroblast" of granulation tissue and hypertropic scar. An immunofluorescence study. *Am J Pathol* 130:252–260, 1988.
35. Ekeland, A.; Vikne, J.: Treatment of acute combined knee instabilities and subsequent sport performance. *Knee Surg Sports Traumatol Arthrosc* 3:180–183, 1995.
36. Enneking, W. F.; Horowitz, M.: The intra-articular effects of immobilization on the human knee. *J Bone Joint Surg Am* 54:973–985, 1972.
37. Eriksson, E.: Rehabilitation of muscle function after sport injury—major problem in sports medicine. *Int J Sports Med* 2:1–6, 1981.
38. Estes, J. M.; Vande Berg, J. S.; Adzick, N. S.; et al.: Phenotypic and functional features of myofibroblasts in sheep fetal wounds. *Differentiation* 56:173–181, 1994.
39. Feller, J. A.; Webster, K. E.: A randomized comparison of patellar tendon and hamstring tendon anterior cruciate ligament reconstruction. *Am J Sports Med* 31:564–573, 2003.
40. Feller, J. A.; Webster, K. E.; Gavin, B.: Early post-operative morbidity following anterior cruciate ligament reconstruction: patellar tendon versus hamstring graft. *Knee Surg Sports Traumatol Arthrosc* 9:260–266, 2001.
41. Fisher, S. E.; Shelbourne, K. D.: Arthroscopic treatment of symptomatic extension block complicating anterior cruciate ligament reconstruction. *Am J Sports Med* 21:558–564, 1993.
42. Foster, W.; Li, Y.; Usas, A.; et al.: Gamma interferon as an antifibrosis agent in skeletal muscle. *J Orthop Res* 21:798–804, 2003.
43. Fu, F. H.; Bennett, C. H.; Ma, C. B.; et al.: Current trends in anterior cruciate ligament reconstruction. Part II. Operative procedures and clinical correlations. *Am J Sports Med* 28:124–130, 2000.
44. Fukui, N.; Fukuda, A.; Kojima, K.; et al.: Suppression of fibrous adhesion by proteoglycan decorin. *J Orthop Res* 19:456–462, 2001.
45. Fukushima, K.; Badlani, N.; Usas, A.; et al.: The use of an antifibrosis agent to improve muscle recovery after laceration. *Am J Sports Med* 29:394–402, 2001.
46. Gabbiani, G.; Hirschel, B. J.; Ryan, G. B.; et al.: Granulation tissue as a contractile organ. A study of structure and function. *J Exp Med* 135:719–734, 1972.
47. Gertel, T. H.; Lew, W. D.; Lewis, J. L.; et al.: Effect of anterior cruciate ligament graft tensioning direction, magnitude, and flexion angle on knee biomechanics. *Am J Sports Med* 21:572–579, 1993.
48. Giri, S. N.; Hyde, D. M.; Braun, R. K.; et al.: Antifibrotic effect of decorin in a bleomycin hamster model of lung fibrosis. *Biochem Pharmacol* 54:1205–1216, 1997.
49. Graf, B.; Uhr, F.: Complications of intra-articular anterior cruciate reconstruction. *Clin Sports Med* 7:835–848, 1988.
50. Grant, J. A.; Mohtadi, N. G.; Maitland, M. E.; Zernicke, R. F.: Comparison of home versus physical therapy–supervised

rehabilitation programs after anterior cruciate ligament reconstruction: a randomized clinical trial. *Am J Sports Med* 33:1288–1297, 2005.

51. Haggmark, T.; Eriksson, E.: Cylinder or mobile cast brace after knee ligament surgery: a clinical analysis and morphologic and enzymatic studies of changes in the quadriceps muscle. *Am J Sports Med* 7:48–56, 1979.

52. Hagiwara, Y.; Chimoto, E.; Ando, A.; et al.: Expression of type I collagen in the capsule of a contracture knee in a rat model. *Ups J Med Sci* 112:356–365, 2007.

53. Hagiwara, Y.; Chimoto, E.; Takahashi, I.; et al.: Expression of transforming growth factor–beta1 and connective tissue growth factor in the capsule in a rat immobilized knee model. *Ups J Med Sci* 113:221–234, 2008.

54. Harner, C. D.; Irrgang, J. J.; Paul, J.; et al.: Loss of motion after anterior cruciate ligament reconstruction. *Am J Sports Med* 20:499–506, 1992.

55. Heming, J. F.; Rand, J.; Steiner, M. E.: Anatomical limitations of transtibial drilling in anterior cruciate ligament reconstruction. *Am J Sports Med* 35:1708–1715, 2007.

56. Henriksson, M.; Rockborn, P.; Good, L.: Range of motion training in brace vs. plaster immobilization after anterior cruciate ligament reconstruction: a prospective randomized comparison with a 2-year follow-up. *Scand J Med Sci Sports* 12:73–80, 2002.

57. Hildebrand, K. A.; Zhang, M.; Germscheid, N. M.; et al.: Cellular, matrix, and growth factor components of the joint capsule are modified early in the process of posttraumatic contracture formation in a rabbit model. *Acta Orthop* 79:116–125, 2008.

58. Hildebrand, K. A.; Zhang, M.; Hart, D. A.: Joint capsule matrix turnover in a rabbit model of chronic joint contractures: correlation with human contractures. *J Orthop Res* 24:1036–1043, 2006.

59. Howell, S. M.; Clark, J. A.: Tibial tunnel placement in anterior cruciate ligament reconstructions and graft impingement. *Clin Orthop Relat Res* 283:187–195, 1992.

60. Howell, S. M.; Clark, J. A.; Farley, T. E.: A rationale for predicting anterior cruciate graft impingement by the intercondylar roof. A magnetic resonance imaging study. *Am J Sports Med* 19:276–282, 1991.

61. Howell, S. M.; Taylor, M. A.: Failure of reconstruction of the anterior cruciate ligament due to impingement by the intercondylar roof. *J Bone Joint Surg Am* 75:1044–1055, 1993.

62. Hunter, R. E.; Mastrangelo, J.; Freeman, J. R.; et al.: The impact of surgical timing on postoperative motion and stability following anterior cruciate ligament reconstruction. *Arthroscopy* 12:667–674, 1996.

62a. Insall, J.; Salvati, E.: Patella position in the normal knee joint. *Radiology* 101:101–104, 1971.

63. Irrgang, J. J.; Harner, C. D.: Loss of motion following knee ligament reconstruction. *Sports Med* 19:150–159, 1995.

64. Isaka, Y.; Brees, D. K.; Ikegaya, K.; et al.: Gene therapy by skeletal muscle expression of decorin prevents fibrotic disease in rat kidney. *Nat Med* 2:418–423, 1996.

65. Jackson, D. W.; Schaefer, R. K.: Cyclops syndrome: loss of extension following intra-articular anterior cruciate ligament reconstruction. *Arthroscopy* 6:171–178, 1990.

66. Johnson, K. L.; Fu, F. H.: Anterior cruciate ligament reconstruction: why do failures occur? In Jackson, D. W. (ed.): *Instructional Course Lectures*. Rosemont, IL: American Academy of Orthopaedic Surgeons, 1995; pp. 391–406.

67. Johnson, R. J.; Eriksson, E.; Haggmark, T.; Pope, M. H.: Five- to ten-year follow-up evaluation after reconstruction of the anterior cruciate ligament. *Clin Orthop Relat Res* 183:122–140, 1984.

68. Johnston, P.; Chojnowski, A. J.; Davidson, R. K.; et al.: A complete expression profile of matrix-degrading metalloproteinases in Dupuytren's disease. *J Hand Surg [Am]* 32:343–351, 2007.

69. Klein, W.; Shah, N.; Gassen, A.: Arthroscopic management of postoperative arthrofibrosis of the knee joint: indication, technique, and results. *Arthroscopy* 10:591–597, 1994.

70. Li, Y.; Negishi, S.; Sakamoto, M.; et al.: The use of relaxin improves healing in injured muscle. *Ann N Y Acad Sci* 1041:395–397, 2005.

71. Linclau, L.: Measuring patellar height. *Acta Orthop Belg* 50:70–74, 1984.

72. Lindenfeld, T. N.; Wojtys, E. M.; Husain, A.: Operative treatment of arthrofibrosis of the knee. *J Bone Joint Surg Am* 81:1772–1784, 1999.

73. Lobenhoffer, H. P.; Bosch, U.; Gerich, T. G.: Role of posterior capsulotomy for the treatment of extension deficits of the knee. *Knee Surg Sports Traumatol Arthrosc* 4:237–241, 1996.

74. Magit, D.; Wolff, A.; Sutton, K.; Medvecky, M. J.: Arthrofibrosis of the knee. *J Am Acad Orthop Surg* 15:682–694, 2007.

75. Majors, R. A.; Woodfin, B.: Achieving full range of motion after anterior cruciate ligament reconstruction. *Am J Sports Med* 24:350–355, 1996.

76. Mariani, P. P.; Santori, N.; Rovere, P.; et al.: Histological and structural study of the adhesive tissue in knee fibroarthrosis: a clinical-pathological correlation. *Arthroscopy* 13:313–318, 1997.

77. Markolf, K. L.; Hame, S.; Hunter, D. M.; et al.: Effects of femoral tunnel placement on knee laxity and forces in an anterior cruciate ligament graft. *J Orthop Res* 20:1016–1024, 2002.

78. Marzo, J. M.; Bowen, M. K.; Warren, R. F.; et al.: Intra-articular fibrous nodule as a cause of loss of extension following anterior cruciate ligament reconstruction. *Arthroscopy* 8:10–18, 1992.

79. Mayr, H. O.; Weig, T. G.; Plitz, W.: Arthrofibrosis following ACL reconstruction—reasons and outcome. *Arch Orthop Trauma Surg* 124:518–522, 2004.

80. McAllister, D. R.; Parker, R. D.; Cooper, A. E.; et al.: Outcomes of postoperative septic arthritis after anterior cruciate ligament reconstruction. *Am J Sports Med* 27:562–570, 1999.

81. Meighan, A. A.; Keating, J. F.; Will, E.: Outcome after reconstruction of the anterior cruciate ligament in athletic patients. A comparison of early versus delayed surgery. *J Bone Joint Surg Br* 85:521–524, 2003.

82. Melby, A., 3rd; Noble, J. S.; Askew, M. J.; et al.: The effects of graft tensioning on the laxity and kinematics of the anterior cruciate ligament reconstructed knee. *Arthroscopy* 7:257–266, 1991.

83. Millett, P. J.; Wickiewicz, T. L.; Warren, R. F.: Motion loss after ligament injuries to the knee. Part II: prevention and treatment. *Am J Sports Med* 29:822–828, 2001.

84. Millett, P. J.; Wickiewicz, T. L.; Warren, R. F.: Motion loss after ligament injuries to the knee. Part I: causes. *Am J Sports Med* 29:664–675, 2001.

85. Millett, P. J.; Williams, R. J.; Wickiewicz, T. L.: Open debridement and soft tissue release as a salvage procedure for the severely arthrofibrotic knee. *Am J Sports Med* 27:552–561, 1999.

86. Mohtadi, N. G.; Webster-Bogaert, S.; Fowler, P. J.: Limitation of motion following anterior cruciate ligament reconstruction. A case-control study. *Am J Sports Med* 19:620–624; discussion 624–625, 1991.

87. Murakami, S.; Muneta, T.; Ezura, Y.; et al.: Quantitative analysis of synovial fibrosis in the infrapatellar fat pad before and after anterior cruciate ligament reconstruction. *Am J Sports Med* 25:29–34, 1997.

88. Murakami, S.; Muneta, T.; Furuya, K.; et al.: Immunohistologic analysis of synovium in infrapatellar fat pad after anterior cruciate ligament injury. *Am J Sports Med* 23:763–768, 1995.

89. Nabors, E. D.; Richmond, J. C.; Vannah, W. M.; McConville, O. R.: Anterior cruciate ligament graft tensioning in full extension. *Am J Sports Med* 23:488–492, 1995.

90. Negishi, S.; Li, Y.; Usas, A.; et al.: The effect of relaxin treatment on skeletal muscle injuries. *Am J Sports Med* 33:1816–1824, 2005.

91. Noyes, F. R.; Barber, S. D.: The effect of a ligament-augmentation device on allograft reconstructions for chronic ruptures of the anterior cruciate ligament. *J Bone Joint Surg Am* 74:960–973, 1992.

92. Noyes, F. R.; Barber, S. D.: The effect of an extra-articular procedure on allograft reconstructions for chronic ruptures of the anterior cruciate ligament. *J Bone Joint Surg Am* 73:882–892, 1991.

93. Noyes, F. R.; Barber, S. D.; Mangine, R. E.: Bone-patellar ligament-bone and fascia lata allografts for reconstruction of the anterior cruciate ligament. *J Bone Joint Surg Am* 72:1125–1136, 1990.

94. Noyes, F. R.; Barber-Westin, S.: Posterior cruciate ligament replacement with a two-strand quadriceps tendon–patellar bone autograft and a tibial inlay technique. *J Bone Joint Surg Am* 87:1241–1252, 2005.

95. Noyes, F. R.; Barber-Westin, S. D.: A comparison of results in acute and chronic anterior cruciate ligament ruptures of arthroscopically assisted autogenous patellar tendon reconstruction. *Am J Sports Med* 25:460–471, 1997.

96. Noyes, F. R.; Barber-Westin, S. D.: Posterolateral knee reconstruction with an anatomical bone–patellar tendon–bone reconstruction of the fibular collateral ligament. *Am J Sports Med* 35:259–273, 2007.

97. Noyes, F. R.; Barber-Westin, S. D.: Reconstruction of the anterior and posterior cruciate ligaments after knee dislocation. Use of early protected postoperative motion to decrease arthrofibrosis. *Am J Sports Med* 25:769–778, 1997.

98. Noyes, F. R.; Barber-Westin, S. D.: The treatment of acute combined ruptures of the anterior cruciate and medial ligaments of the knee. *Am J Sports Med* 23:380–389, 1995.

99. Noyes, F. R.; Barber-Westin, S. D.; Hewett, T. E.: High tibial osteotomy and ligament reconstruction for varus angulated anterior cruciate ligament–deficient knees. *Am J Sports Med* 28:282–296, 2000.

100. Noyes, F. R.; Barber-Westin, S. D.; Rankin, M.: Meniscal transplantation in symptomatic patients less than fifty years old. *J Bone Joint Surg Am* 86:1392–1404, 2004.

101. Noyes, F. R.; Berrios-Torres, S.; Barber-Westin, S. D.; Heckmann, T. P.: Prevention of permanent arthrofibrosis after anterior cruciate ligament reconstruction alone or combined with associated procedures: a prospective study in 443 knees. *Knee Surg Sports Traumatol Arthrosc* 8:196–206, 2000.

102. Noyes, F. R.; Mangine, R. E.; Barber, S. D.: The early treatment of motion complications after reconstruction of the anterior cruciate ligament. *Clin Orthop* 277:217–228, 1992.

103. Noyes, F. R.; Mayfield, W.; Barber-Westin, S. D.; et al.: Opening wedge high tibial osteotomy: an operative technique and rehabilitation program to decrease complications and promote early union and function. *Am J Sports Med* 34:1262–1273, 2006.

104. Noyes, F. R.; Torvik, P. J.; Hyde, W. B.; DeLucas, J. L.: Biomechanics of ligament failure. II. An analysis of immobilization, exercise, and reconditioning effects in primates. *J Bone Joint Surg Am* 56:1406–1418, 1974.

105. Noyes, F. R.; Wojtys, E. M.: The early recognition, diagnosis and treatment of the patella infera syndrome. In Tullos, H. S. (ed.): *Instructional Course Lectures*. Rosemont, IL: AAOS, 1991; pp. 233–247.

106. Noyes, F. R.; Wojtys, E. M.; Marshall, M. T.: The early diagnosis and treatment of developmental patella infera syndrome. *Clin Orthop* 265:241–252, 1991.

107. O'Brien, S. J.; Ngeow, J.; Gibney, M. A.; et al.: Reflex sympathetic dystrophy of the knee. Causes, diagnosis, and treatment. *Am J Sports Med* 23:655–659, 1995.

108. O'Driscoll, S. W.; Kumar, A.; Salter, R. B.: The effect of continuous passive motion on the clearance of a hemarthrosis from a synovial joint. An experimental investigation in the rabbit. *Clin Orthop Relat Res* 176:305–311, 1983.

109. Paillard, T.: Combined application of neuromuscular electrical stimulation and voluntary muscular contractions. *Sports Med* 38:161–177, 2008.

110. Palmieri-Smith, R. M.; Kreinbrink, J.; Ashton-Miller, J. A.; Wojtys, E. M.: Quadriceps inhibition induced by an experimental knee joint effusion affects knee joint mechanics during a single-legged drop landing. *Am J Sports Med* 35:1269–1275, 2007.

111. Paulos, L. E.; Rosenberg, T. D.; Drawbert, J.; et al.: Infrapatellar contracture syndrome. An unrecognized cause of knee stiffness with patella entrapment and patella infera. *Am J Sports Med* 15:331–341, 1987.

112. Paulos, L. E.; Wnorowski, D. C.; Greenwald, A. E.: Infrapatellar contracture syndrome. Diagnosis, treatment, and long-term follow-up. *Am J Sports Med* 22:440–449, 1994.

113. Perkins, G.: Rest and movement. *J Bone Joint Surg Br* 35:521–539, 1953.

114. Perry, J.; Antonelli, D.; Ford, W.: Analysis of knee joint forces during flexed-knee stance. *J Bone Joint Surg Am* 57:961–967, 1975.

115. Petsche, T. S.; Hutchinson, M. R.: Loss of extension after reconstruction of the anterior cruciate ligament. *J Am Acad Orthop Surg* 7:119–127, 1999.

116. Reider, B.; Belniak, R. M.; Preiskorn, D.: Arthroscopic arthrolysis for flexion contracture following intra-articular reconstruction of the anterior cruciate ligament. *Arthroscopy* 12:165–173, 1996.

117. Risberg, M. A.; Holm, I.; Steen, H.; et al.: The effect of knee bracing after anterior cruciate ligament reconstruction. A prospective, randomized study with two years' follow-up. *Am J Sports Med* 27:76–83, 1999.

118. Roberts, A. B.; Sporn, M. B.: The transforming growth factors–β. In Sporn, M. B.; Roberts, A. B. (eds.): *Peptide Growth Factors and Their Receptors*. Vol. 95 of *Handbook of Experimental Pharmacology*. New York: Springer-Verlag, 1990; pp. 419–472.

119. Romano, V. M.; Graf, B. K.; Keene, J. S.; Lange, R. H.: Anterior cruciate ligament reconstruction. The effect of tibial tunnel placement on range of motion. *Am J Sports Med* 21:415–418, 1993.

120. Rowe, P. J.; Myles, C. M.; Walker, C.; Nutton, R.: Knee joint kinematics in gait and other functional activities measured using flexible electrogoniometry: how much knee motion is sufficient for normal daily life? *Gait Posture* 12:143–155, 2000.

121. Sachs, R. A.; Daniel, D. M.; Stone, M. L.; Garfein, R. F.: Patellofemoral problems after anterior cruciate ligament reconstruction. *Am J Sports Med* 17:760–765, 1989.

122. Salter, R. B.: The biologic concept of continuous passive motion of synovial joints. The first 18 years of basic research and its clinical application. *Clin Orthop Relat Res* 242:12–25, 1989.

123. Salter, R. B.; Simmonds, D. F.; Malcolm, B. W.; et al.: The biological effect of continuous passive motion on the healing of full-thickness defects in articular cartilage. An experimental investigation in the rabbit. *J Bone Joint Surg Am* 62:1232–1251, 1980.

124. Satish, L.; Laframboise, W. W.; O'Gorman, D. B.; et al.: Identification of differentially expressed genes in fibroblasts derived from patients with Dupuytren's Contracture. *BMC Med Genomics* 1:10, 2008.

125. Schulz, A. P.; Gotze, S.; Schmidt, H. G.; et al.: Septic arthritis of the knee after anterior cruciate ligament surgery: a stage-adapted treatment regimen. *Am J Sports Med* 35:1064–1069, 2007.

126. Shanker, V. S.; Gadikoppula, S.; Loeffler, M. D.: Post-traumatic osteoma of tibial insertion of medial collateral ligament of knee joint. *Br J Sports Med* 32:73–74, 1998.

127. Shapiro, M. S.; Freedman, E. L.: Allograft reconstruction of the anterior and posterior cruciate ligaments after traumatic knee dislocation. *Am J Sports Med* 23:580–587, 1995.

128. Shelbourne, K. D.; Baele, J. R.: Treatment of combined anterior cruciate ligament and medial collateral ligament injuries. *Am J Knee Surg* 1:56–58, 1988.

129. Shelbourne, K. D.; Foulk, D. A.: Timing of surgery in acute anterior cruciate ligament tears on the return of quadriceps muscle strength after reconstruction using an autogenous patellar tendon graft. *Am J Sports Med* 23:686–689, 1995.

130. Shelbourne, K. D.; Johnson, G. E.: Outpatient surgical management of arthrofibrosis after anterior cruciate ligament surgery. *Am J Sports Med* 22:192–197, 1994.

131. Shelbourne, K. D.; Patel, D. V.: Treatment of limited motion after anterior cruciate ligament reconstruction. *Knee Surg Sports Traumatol Arthrosc* 7:85–92, 1999.

132. Shelbourne, K. D.; Patel, D. V.; Martini, D. J.: Classification and management of arthrofibrosis of the knee after anterior cruciate ligament reconstruction. *Am J Sports Med* 24:857–862, 1996.

133. Shelbourne, K. D.; Porter, D. A.: Anterior cruciate ligament–medial collateral ligament injury: nonoperative management of medial collateral ligament tears with anterior cruciate ligament reconstruction. A preliminary report. *Am J Sports Med* 20:283–286, 1992.

134. Shelbourne, K. D.; Wilckens, J. H.; Mollabashy, A.; DeCarlo, M.: Arthrofibrosis in acute anterior cruciate ligament reconstruction. The effect of timing of reconstruction and rehabilitation. *Am J Sports Med* 19:332–336, 1991.

135. Simmons, R.; Howell, S. M.; Hull, M. L.: Effect of the angle of the femoral and tibial tunnels in the coronal plane and incremental excision of the posterior cruciate ligament on tension of an anterior cruciate ligament graft: an in vitro study. *J Bone Joint Surg Am* 85:1018–1029, 2003.

136. Sisto, D. J.; Warren, R. F.: Complete knee dislocation. A follow-up study of operative treatment. *Clin Orthop Relat Res* 198:94–101, 1985.

137. Skutek, M.; van Griensven, M.; Zeichen, J.; et al.: Cyclic mechanical stretching enhances secretion of interleukin 6 in human tendon fibroblasts. *Knee Surg Sports Traumatol Arthrosc* 9:322–326, 2001.

138. Skutek, M.; van Griensven, M.; Zeichen, J.; et al.: Cyclic mechanical stretching modulates secretion pattern of growth factors in human tendon fibroblasts. *Eur J Appl Physiol* 86:48–52, 2001.

139. Skyhar, M. J.; Danzig, L. A.; Hargens, A. R.; Akeson, W. H.: Nutrition of the anterior cruciate ligament. Effects of continuous passive motion. *Am J Sports Med* 3:415–418, 1985.

140. Spencer, J. D.; Hayes, K. C.; Alexander, I. J.: Knee joint effusion and quadriceps reflex inhibition in man. *Arch Phys Med Rehabil* 65:171–177, 1984.

141. Sprague, N. F.; O'Connor, R. L.; Fox, J. M.: Arthroscopic treatment of postoperative knee fibroarthrosis. *Clin Orthop Relat Res* 166:165–172, 1982.

142. Steadman, J. R.; Burns, T. P.; Peloza, J.; et al.: Surgical treatment of arthrofibrosis of the knee. *J Orthop Tech* 1:119–128, 1993.

143. Sterett, W. I.; Hutton, K. S.; Briggs, K. K.; Steadman, J. R.: Decreased range of motion following acute versus chronic anterior cruciate ligament reconstruction. *Orthopedics* 26:151–154, 2003.

144. Strum, G. M.; Friedman, M. J.; Fox, J. M.; et al.: Acute anterior cruciate ligament reconstruction. Analysis of complications. *Clin Orthop Relat Res* 253:184–189, 1990.

145. Torry, M. R.; Decker, M. J.; Millett, P. J.; et al.: The effects of knee joint effusion on quadriceps electromyography during jogging. *J Sports Sci Med* 4:1–8, 2005.

146. Torry, M. R.; Decker, M. J.; Viola, R. W.; et al.: Intra-articular knee joint effusion induces quadriceps avoidance gait patterns. *Clin Biomech (Bristol, Avon)* 15:147–159, 2000.

147. Unterhauser, F. N.; Bosch, U.; Zeichen, J.; Weiler, A.: Alpha-smooth muscle actin containing contractile fibroblastic cells in human knee arthrofibrosis tissue. Winner of the AGA-DonJoy Award 2003. *Arch Orthop Trauma Surg* 124:585–591, 2004.

148. Van Tongel, A.; Stuyck, J.; Bellemans, J.; Vandenneucker, H.: Septic arthritis after arthroscopic anterior cruciate ligament reconstruction: a retrospective analysis of incidence, management and outcome. *Am J Sports Med* 35:1059–1063, 2007.

149. Vaquero, J.; Vidal, C.; Medina, E.; Baena, J.: Arthroscopic lysis in knee arthrofibrosis. *Arthroscopy* 9:691–694, 1993.

150. Wang, J. C.; Shapiro, M. S.: Pellegrini-Stieda syndrome. *Am J Orthop* 24:493–497, 1995.

151. Wang, J. H.; Zhao, J. Z.; He, Y. H.: A new treatment strategy for severe arthrofibrosis of the knee. A review of twenty-two cases. *J Bone Joint Surg Am* 88:1245–1250, 2006.

152. Wasilewski, S. A.; Covall, D. J.; Cohen, S.: Effect of surgical timing on recovery and associated injuries after anterior cruciate ligament reconstruction. *Am J Sports Med* 21:338–342, 1993.

153. Williams, R. J., 3rd; Laurencin, C. T.; Warren, R. F.; et al.: Septic arthritis after arthroscopic anterior cruciate ligament reconstruction. Diagnosis and management. *Am J Sports Med* 25:261–267, 1997.

154. Yaru, N. C.; Daniel, D. M.; Penner, D.: The effect of tibial attachment site on graft impingement in an anterior cruciate ligament reconstruction. *Am J Sports Med* 20:217–220, 1992.

155. Zeichen, J.; van Griensven, M.; Albers, I.; et al.: Immunohistochemical localization of collagen VI in arthrofibrosis. *Arch Orthop Trauma Surg* 119:315–318, 1999.

Chapter 42

Knee Pain of Neural Origin

A. Lee Dellon, MD, PhD

INTRODUCTION

Nerves related to the knee include not only those that go in the skin about the surface of the knee joint but also mixed (motor and sensory) nerves that pass the knee on the way to their targets distal to this joint. In addition to these well-known nerves are those that innervate the knee joint. Each of these nerves is at risk of injury whenever (1) there is blunt force directed at the knee, (2) there is a stretch/traction injury to the musculoskeletal system of the knee joint, (3) there is an inversion sprain to the ankle, and (4) open or arthroscopic knee surgery has been performed. Whereas it is intuitively clear that a joint is innervated, the exact pathways of this innervation are curiously omitted from the classic and even the newer anatomy texts. For the human knee, the innervation pattern was not found to be described until 1994 during the author's search for an etiology of knee pain unrelated to musculoskeletal dysfunction.[25] The approach to knee pain described in this chapter follows closely that developed for wrist pain,[8,16,20] which preceded the author's interest in knee pain and led to a subsequent similar approach to those for shoulder pain[1,3] and ankle pain.[6,13,29]

The approach described in this chapter considers knee pain that exists after musculoskeletal treatment to be of neural origin. The physician caring for these patients must consider whether

Critical Points INTRODUCTION

Nerves are at risk of injury from
- Blunt force directed at the knee.
- Stretch/traction injury of the knee joint.
- Inversion sprain to the ankle.
- Open or arthroscopic knee surgery.

Approach: knee pain that exists after musculoskeletal treatment is of neural origin.
- Decide whether pain is coming from direct damage to the cutaneous nerves about the knee or from an injury to one of the nerves arising within the knee joint structures themselves.
- Partial joint denervation is an approach in which the joint afferents that transmit a pain message are interrupted.

the pain is coming from direct damage to the cutaneous nerves about the knee, such as a neuroma of the infrapatellar branch of the saphenous nerve, or from an injury to one of the nerves arising within the knee joint structures themselves. A further source of knee pain due to nerve injury is an injury to a nerve far away from the knee, such as the lateral femoral cutaneous nerve, or a nerve that is simply going past the knee on its way to some other distal target. The concept of partial joint denervation is presented as an approach in which those joint afferents that transmit a pain message are interrupted, thereby stopping the pain and preserving the musculoskeletal components of the joint. A Charcot type joint is not created because the deafferentation is partial instead of total.

PERIPHERAL NERVE ANATOMY RELATED TO THE KNEE

Innervation of the Human Knee Joint

The innervation of the human knee joint is remarkably constant.[25] On the medial aspect (Fig. 42-1), the femoral nerve branch that innervates the vastus medialis continues past its motor point and exits deep and distal to the vastus medialis. At this point, it lies deep to the medial retinaculum and becomes related to the medial recurrent geniculate artery and vein. This structure is termed the *medial retinacular nerve*. These structures, nerve and vessels, continue directly adjacent to the vastus medialis and superficial to the synovium to enter the ligamentous structures of the medial aspect of the knee. These fibers also continue toward the midline of the knee to innervate the undersurface of the patella (see Fig. 42-1).

On the lateral aspect of the knee (Fig. 42-2), a branch of the sciatic nerve leaves the popliteal fossa, travels laterally and anteriorly, emerges deep to the biceps tendon, and enters the space beneath the lateral retinaculum. In this location, the nerve is adjacent to the superior lateral geniculate artery and vein. This structure is termed the *lateral retinacular nerve*. These structures, the nerve and vessels, are immediately distal to the vastus lateralis and superficial to the synovium. The nerve enters the ligamentous structures of the lateral aspect of the knee (which have not yet been further defined histologically) and travels to the midline to innervate the undersurface of the patella.

Anteriorly, another source of innervation is derived from the femoral nerve innervation of the vastus intermedius. This nerve continues on the surface of the periosteum to innervate the tissues around the prepatellar bursa. Finally, posteriorly, branches from the sciatic nerve enter the posterior knee joint capsule to provide innervation (see Fig. 42-2).

Innervation of the Proximal Tibiofibular Joint

Although many patients complain of "knee pain," they may be pointing or referring to the region distal and lateral to the knee, which is the articulation between the fibular head and the tibia. This joint space is likely to be injured from fractures of the

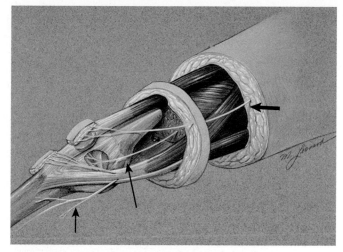

FIGURE 42-1. Medial view of the innervation of the knee. The skin overlying the patella is innervated by the medial cutaneous nerve of the thigh, a branch of the saphenous nerve (*thick arrow*). The medial joint structures are innervated by a branch of the femoral nerve, the medial retinacular nerve, which, after innervating the vastus medialis, continues distal and then anterior to this muscle to enter the ligamentous structures of the knee joint (*long thin arrow*). This nerve lies superficial to the synovium and deep to the medial retinaculum. The saphenous nerve's infrapatellar and distal branches are shown in their most common variation (*short thin arrow*). (*Reprinted with permission from Dellon.com.*)

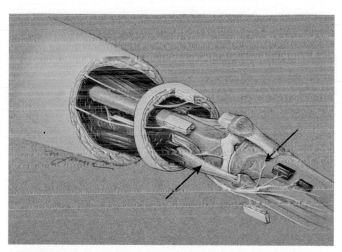

FIGURE 42-2. Lateral view of the innervation of the knee. The innervation of the skin in this area represents the terminal branches of the lateral femoral cutaneous nerve. The lateral joint structures are innervated by a branch of the sciatic nerve that comes from the popliteal fossa, goes deep to the biceps tendon to enter the joint, termed the lateral retinacular nerve (*bottom arrow*). The nerve passes just distal to the vastus lateralis and then lies superficial to the synovium and deep to the lateral retinaculum as it enters the joint. The branches of the sciatic nerve to the posterior knee joint capsule are shown next to the femur posteriorly. The branch to the prepatellar bursa is shown on the anterior surface of the femur as it exists the vastus intermedius. The innervation of the proximal tibiofibular joint is shown as branches proximal and distal to the fibular head, arising from the common peroneal nerve (*top arrow*). (*Reprinted with permission from Dellon.com.*)

Critical Points PERIPHERAL NERVE ANATOMY RELATED TO THE KNEE

- Innervation of human knee joint
- Innervation of proximal tibiofibular joint
- Common peroneal nerve
- Deep peroneal nerve
- Superficial peroneal nerve
- Proximal tibial nerve
- Lateral femoral cutaneous nerve
- Saphenous nerve

fibula or lateral tibial plateau or from high tibial osteotomy or a Maquet operative procedure. This space is innervated by the common peroneal nerve (see Fig. 42–2). As the common peroneal nerve travels from the popliteal fossa to the fibular head, it gives off a small (~1 mm in diameter) nerve that may enter this space posterior to the fibular head. The common peroneal nerve gives off a second branch to this space immediately as it curves anterior to the fibular head, at the junction with the fibular neck. This branch is also approximately 1 mm in diameter. The next branch of the common peroneal nerve goes to the tibialis anterior, which is a critical motor branch. In the operating room, the only way to identify the branch to the joint is to stimulate it electrically. No motor function will be elicited when the branch to the joint is stimulated. This is a critical step. This small branch often looks like epineurium.

Common Peroneal Nerve

The common peroneal nerve is the lateral branch of the sciatic nerve. It can most often be identified as a distinct branch even to the sciatic notch. Therefore, in the thigh, there is clearly a common peroneal nerve even though it may be referred to as the sciatic nerve. In the distal thigh, the common peroneal nerve courses laterally, approaches the fibular head, and continues anteriorly to cross the fibular neck and enter the leg. As the common peroneal nerve approaches the fibular neck, it clearly divides into the superficial and the deep peroneal nerve, increasing in size as increased epineurium is required to ensheath these two branches (Fig. 42–3). The critical anatomic sites that can cause compression have long been appreciated to occur as the common peroneal nerve crosses the fibular neck, requiring division of the fascia of the peroneus longus fascia.[35] With increasing experience, it has become evident that three other anatomic factors must be considered. A fibrous band exists beneath the peroneus longus in 20% of cadavers, but this band is present (and ranges from 5–15 mm in width) in 80% of patients requiring neurolysis.[14] The surgeon must identify the common peroneal nerve by elevating it from the fibular neck, determine whether fibrous thickening in the lateral gastrocnemius muscle fascia is present, and finally, be certain that the overall entrance into the anterior and lateral compartments is sufficiently large.

Deep Peroneal Nerve

The deep peroneal nerve arises over the fibular neck as a discrete fascicle. It can be dissected proximally by microtechnique if necessary. Immediately after crossing the fibular neck, it gives off tiny branches to the tibialis anterior and the toe extensor muscles. In so doing, the deep peroneal nerve effectively tethers the common peroneal and its distal branches from having too much excursion. This predisposes the common peroneal nerve and its branches in this region to stretch/traction injuries. The entrapment site for the deep peroneal nerve is at the ankle, the "anterior tarsal tunnel," which is a rare site for compression unless there has been a direct injury in this location. A more common site for compression is over the dorsum of the foot where the tendon of the extensor hallucis brevis represents the anatomic structure causing the compression. A portion of the tendon of the extensor hallucis brevis is excised in the region of the deep peroneal nerve[5] (see Fig. 42–3).

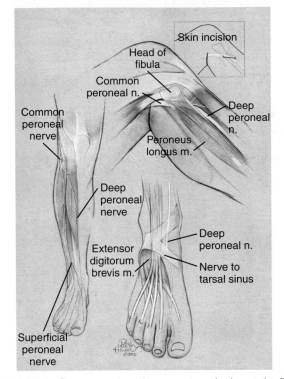

FIGURE 42–3. Common peroneal nerve enters the leg at the fibular head and divides into the deep and superficial peroneal nerves. *Inset,* The typical incision for the decompression of the common peroneal nerve. The superficial peroneal nerve entrapment site as it exits from the deep fascia is noted laterally, and the deep peroneal nerve entrapment site is illustrated beneath the extensor hallucis brevis tendon. *(Reprinted with permission from Dellon.com.)*

Superficial Peroneal Nerve

The superficial peroneal nerve arises over the fibular neck from the common peroneal nerve. It can be dissected more proximally by microdissection if required. The motor innervation to the foot everters arises within the first 1 to 2 cm distal to the neck of the fibula. The known site of entrapment for this nerve is the region where it transitions from deep to the fascia into the subcutaneous tissues in the distal third of the leg. The typical division into its dorsomedial and dorsolateral branches occurs just proximal to the ankle in approximately 75% of patients (see Fig. 42–3). In the author's experience, it is now clear that in at least 25% of cadavers and patients coming to surgery, this division can occur in the proximal third of the leg.[2,39] This creates the situation in which the superficial peroneal nerve may be found in both the anterior and, its most usually described location, the lateral compartment. Indeed, the superficial peroneal nerve may be present in just the anterior compartment or within the septum between the two compartments.[40] The anatomic variability means that any surgical approach to this nerve must open both the anterior and the lateral compartments.

Proximal Tibial Nerve

Although the tibial nerve (like the common peroneal nerve) arises at the sciatic notch as the medial component of the sciatic nerve, and is often clearly a distinct nerve in the thigh, the only well-described site for tibial nerve compression was at the medial ankle in the tarsal tunnel.[31] It is now evident that the tibial nerve can be compressed in a site more proximal than the tarsal tunnel, and this site (just distal to the knee) is best described as the proximal tibial nerve to distinguish it from the tarsal tunnel region. Tibial nerve compression in the popliteal fossa has been described related to the presence of compartment syndrome or space-occupying masses, such as a popliteal artery or a Baker cyst.[26,34] Although anatomy texts clearly depict a fibrous arch or soleal sling from which the soleus muscle arises, only recently has there been an anatomic study describing the relationship of this sling to the proximal tibial nerve.[41] This sling lies at a mean distance of 9.3 cm (range, 7–13 cm) from the middle of the popliteal fossa and causes a visible narrowing of the tibial nerve over a length of 1.5 cm in 55% of the cadavers, with a severe constriction being found in 2% of the specimens. With injury to the knee, especially one associated with postoperative bleeding into the popliteal fossa, tibial nerve compression at this proximal site must be considered as a source of symptoms of numbness in the plantar aspect of the foot, with proximal referral to the knee region.

Lateral Femoral Cutaneous Nerve

The lateral femoral cutaneous nerve has a great deal of anatomic variability related both to its location at the anterior superior iliac crest[2] and to its innervated skin territory. If the location is within the inguinal ligament instead of inferior to it, the lateral femoral cutaneous nerve is at risk for compression or stretch/traction injury during falls, while wearing tight belts, during a seatbelt injury, or during manipulation of the knee with the patient on the operating room table. From Figure 42–4, it can be appreciated that compression of the lateral femoral cutaneous nerve can produce symptoms that include numbness or pain about the lateral aspect of the knee.[37] This nerve, or the femoral nerve itself, can be injured during regional anesthesia given for knee surgery.[22]

Saphenous Nerve

The saphenous nerve is a branch of the femoral nerve that arises from the femoral nerve in the proximal thigh. Its cutaneous branches to the skin below the knee are well described and lie in a position to be injured directly from either a medial ankle arthroscopy portal or the midline incisions used for many surgical approaches to the knee. These branches can be directly injured by blunt trauma as well. Less well recognized is the nerve to the skin overlying the patellar itself. This is a branch of the femoral nerve, which may include sensory contribution from the obturator nerve joining within Hunter's canal. The medial cutaneous nerve of the thigh (see Fig. 42–1) approaches from the medial aspect of the knee compared with the vertical approach taken by the anterior femoral cutaneous nerves.[1] Even less well appreciated is that the saphenous nerve can be compressed in the distal thigh within Hunter's canal. This is called *adductor canal syndrome*, which is rare in the absence of direct trauma to this region. Entrapment of the saphenous nerve in this location can present as medial knee pain.[36]

CLINICAL EVALUATION OF KNEE PAIN OF NEURAL ORIGIN

The history of knee pain is critical to obtain. Knee pain does not arise de novo, but due to a history of some type of sports event, overuse activity, new activity, or actual direct injury to the knee. The knee injury may be blunt or open. Surgery should also be considered as a source of trauma. Many patients with knee pain due to musculoskeletal problems awake from their reconstructive knee surgery to have a different pain or paralysis. These are known complications of knee surgery that should be recognized as such and referred for appropriate treatment in a timely manner. The determination of whether the pain is made worse by certain positions of the body or leg or by certain activities is important to arrive at a correct diagnosis. Certainly, most knee pain unrelated to structural impairment will be relieved by nonoperative treatment. But when pain persists beyond a reasonable timeframe of 3 to 6 months, the diagnosis is most consistent with pain of neural origin.

The physical examination is directed to identifying one or more sources of neural origin of the pain. First, the clinician should try to distinguish whether any skin territories are dysesthetic or painful when touched lightly. If so, these areas should be outlined. The most common distribution is that of the infrapatellar

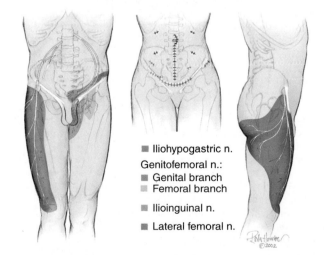

CUTANEOUS NERVES OF THE THIGH AND GROIN REGIONS

■ Iliohypogastric n.

Genitofemoral n.:
■ Genital branch
■ Femoral branch

■ Ilioinguinal n.

■ Lateral femoral n.

FIGURE 42–4. Skin territory innervated by different nerves related to the groin. The lateral femoral cutaneous nerve territory is shown in *blue* and extends distally to the knee. Compression or stretch/traction injury of this nerve can be perceived as knee pain. *(Reprinted with permission from Dellon.com.)*

Critical Points CLINICAL EVALUATION OF KNEE PAIN OF NEURAL ORIGIN

- History is critical.
- Determine whether pain is made worse by certain positions of the body or leg or by certain activities.
- If pain persists beyond a reasonable timeframe of 3 to 6 mo, diagnosis is most consistent with pain of neural origin.
- Distinguish whether any skin territories are dysesthetic; observe for trigger spot.
- Joint afferents: palpate medial and lateral retinacular nerves. To determine whether knee pain is due to an injury to one or both of the joint afferents, conduct diagnostic nerve block. Determine whether effective.
- If block is not effective, look for more rare sources of nerve pain: anterior femoral cutaneous nerve, another branch of the infrapatellar saphenous nerve, Tinel's sign over lateral femoral cutaneous nerve, or motor function of the common peroneal nerve.

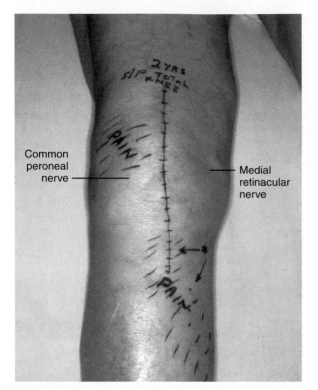

FIGURE 42-5. Demonstration of the sites to palpate a tender medial and lateral retinacular nerve in the patient with joint pain.

branch of the saphenous nerve; the second most common is the skin over the patella itself. These areas might be numb, indicating loss of sensation (Fig. 42–5). Once the pattern is identified, examine proximally along the course of the given nerve, observing for a trigger spot, which is either a true end-bulb neuroma or an in-continuity nerve lesion. The hypothesis is made that this nerve or these nerves are the source of the cutaneous pain; a diagnostic nerve block will be required to confirm this hypothesis.

The physical examination is then directed to the joint afferents. Palpation is done deeply to the spot located just distal to the vastus medialis muscle, through the medial retinaculum to elicit pain from the medial retinacular nerve. Palpation is next done deeply to the area located just distal to the vastus lateralis muscle, through the lateral retinaculum, to elicit pain from the lateral retinacular nerve (Fig. 42–5). The hypothesis is made that the knee joint pain is due to an injury to one or both of the joint afferents; a diagnostic nerve block will be required to confirm this hypothesis. The medial cutaneous nerve to the thigh and the medial retinacular nerve can be blocked at the same area. Ten minutes after the nerve blocks, the patient is instructed to walk in the hallway, climb and descend a few steps, and even to kneel on a padded chair (Fig. 42–6). A reduction of 5 points on a visual analog scale; for example, from 10 to 5, where 10 represents the worst pain, is confirmation that sufficient relief of pain has occurred to permit surgery for partial knee denervation and resection of cutaneous neuromas.

If the nerve blocks just described have not reduced the pain level to less than 5 points, or the blocks were not effective, the physical examination should proceed to include other more rare sources for the nerve pain. In the patient with a knee replacement, the remaining pain may stem from an anterior femoral cutaneous nerve found in the proximal portions of the incision or another branch of the infrapatellar saphenous nerve, which can have many branches, including more distal branches.

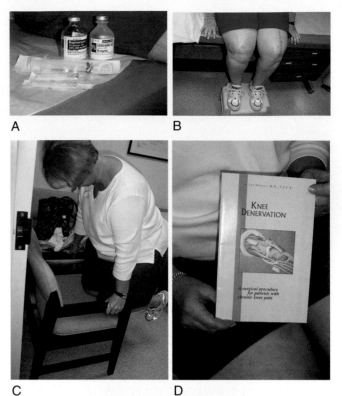

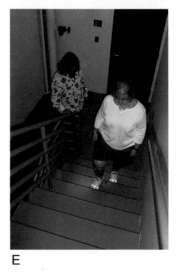

FIGURE 42-6. Demonstration of the use of local anesthesia to block the suspected joint and cutaneous afferents in the patient with knee pain. A mixture of 0.5% bupivacaine (Marcaine) and 1% lidocaine (Xylocaine), each without epinephrine (*upper left*), is used to conduct the local block at the two sites indicated in Figure 42–5 to block the joint afferents most likely to be the source of joint pain. Additional blocks would also be done of cutaneous afferents. After the block, the patient should be able to climb stairs and kneel without the previous pain (as shown). There should be a reduction of at least 5 on the 10-point Likert scale in order for this block to be considered successful enough to recommend a partial knee denervation. If there is significant residual pain after the block, additional nerves causing this pain should be identified.

Finally, the groin should be examined to search for a Tinel sign over the lateral femoral cutaneous nerve. The patient will be noted to sit with the lower extremity extended at the hip joint (Fig. 42–7). The midthigh should be examined to search for a

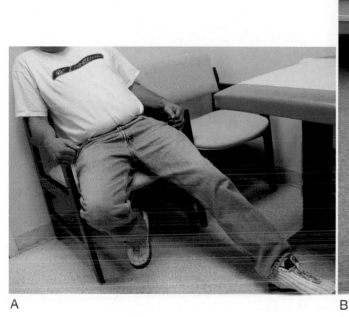
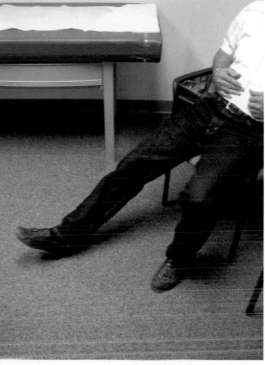

A   B

FIGURE 42–7. Clinical sign of compression of the lateral femoral cutaneous nerve (meralgia paresthetica). Two examples are shown. The patient can be observed to be sitting with the lower extremity on the painful side extended at the hip. Hip flexion increases pressure on the lateral femoral cutaneous nerve as it exits through the site of compression. Shown are a left (**A**) and a right (**B**) lateral femoral cutaneous nerve compression.

Tinel sign over Hunter's adductor canal. This is most effectively done with the patient supine, and the effected leg externally rotated at the hip, leaving the knee bent. This stretches the adductor muscle group over the saphenous nerve. Then, gentle palpation over the canal produces a distal radiating painful response (Fig. 42–8).

If the pain is below the knee joint and laterally located, examine for tenderness in the proximal tibiofibular joint space. If this is present, a nerve block can be done directly into this space without blocking the common peroneal nerve.

If pain is accompanied by complaints of the leg "giving out," the foot dragging, or a "footdrop," the motor function of the common peroneal nerve must be evaluated by manual muscle testing. The common peroneal nerve must be palpated or percussed at the fibular neck, with tenderness (even without distal radiation) considered a positive sign for nerve entrapment.

INDICATIONS FOR PARTIAL KNEE DENERVATION

Knee pain that persists for more than 6 months despite musculoskeletal nonoperative and operative treatment is considered chronic. By definition, patients with chronic pain require appropriate management. The diagnosis of knee pain of neural origin should be considered before sending a patient for pain management or, at the least, be considered and evaluated with nerve blocks by a pain-management physician. Certainly, before any consideration is given for a peripheral nerve or spinal stimulator for pain relief, the physician should contemplate treating the peripheral nerve pain generators directly by resection or decompression, as described in this chapter.

In the athlete, persistent knee pain after ligamentous repair or knee arthroscopy is an indication to determine whether the pain is due to a traction injury to the nerves that innervate the knee joint, a stress/traction injury, or compression of nerves that cross the knee. Medial knee pain can be related to a groin pull if the contracted adductor muscles create an adductor canal syndrome.

In the patient who has had knee reconstruction related to other disorders, persistent pain must be considered as related to a cutaneous neuroma or an injury to the joint afferents.

In the patient who has severe degenerative knee pain, but who is "too young" for a hemi- or total knee replacement, consideration should be given to diagnostic nerve blocks. Although partial joint denervation will not change the underlying osteoarthritic process, it may provide the patient some degree of relief until she or he ages sufficiently to enter the age bracket considered appropriate for an arthroplasty.

In the patient with persistent knee pain after total knee arthroplasty (TKA), in the absence of loosening, malalignment, or infection, pain of neural origin clearly must be evaluated, as described in this chapter.

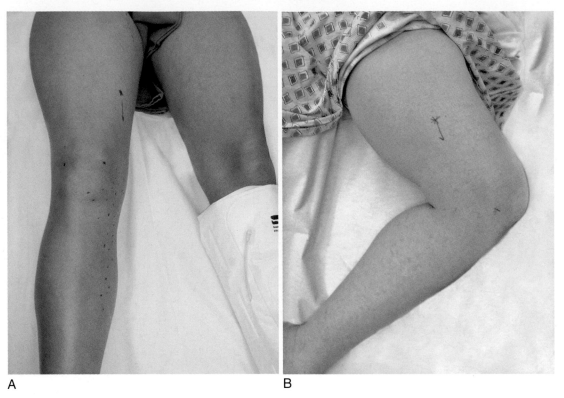

A   B

FIGURE 42–8. Location of the distally radiating Tinel's sign in the patient with compression of the saphenous nerve in Hunter's canal. **A**, Site in a right thigh. **B**, Site in a left thigh. Tinel's sign is marked and distal radiation into saphenous skin territory is noted.

Critical Points INDICATIONS FOR PARTIAL KNEE DENERVATION

- Knee pain > 6 mo.
- Persistent knee pain in athletes after ligamentous repair or knee arthroscopy.
- Persistent pain after knee reconstruction related to other disorders.
- Patient who has severe degenerative knee pain, but who is "too young" for a hemi- or total knee replacement.
- Patient with persistent knee pain after total knee arthroplasty, in the absence of loosening, malalignment, or infection.

Critical Points PREOPERATIVE PLANNING

- Identify pain as coming from either an injured joint afferent, an injured cutaneous nerve, or a nerve entrapment.
- All structural musculoskeletal problems have been treated either nonoperatively, operatively, or both.
- Treat lumbosacral disk disease if present first.
- Determine whether neuropathy exists.
- Consider general health condition of patient, vascular status of limb.
- Educate patient regarding postoperative pain, success rate, and therapy required.

PREOPERATIVE PLANNING

The first consideration is to make the correct diagnosis. The pain must be identified as coming from either an injured joint afferent as proven by a successful nerve block, an injured cutaneous nerve as proven by a successful nerve block, or a nerve entrapment as demonstrated by the history and physical examination.

The second consideration is that all structural musculoskeletal problems have been treated either nonoperatively, operatively, or both as documented in the referring letter from the orthopaedic surgeon.

The third consideration is the presence of lumbosacral disk disease. Appropriate imaging, electrodiagnostic studies, and subspecialty referral must be completed before peripheral nerve surgery is conducted.

The fourth consideration is the existence of a neuropathy, either diabetic or idiopathic. If the patient has complaints related to the feet, the presence of neuropathy should be evaluated. In addition to the history and physical examination, the author's preferred approach is to obtain nonpainful and noninvasive neurosensory testing with the Pressure-Specified Sensory Device (PSSD) (Sensory Management Services, LLC, Baltimore, MD).[4,7,38] The PSSD documents the presence of a neuropathy and a nerve entrapment, providing a basis for decompression of the common or superficial peroneal nerve or both (dorsomedial and dorsolateral foot sensibility sites). This device also documents the presence of tibial nerve dysfunction by evaluating the medial calcaneal and medial plantar nerves (heel and hallux pulp skin test sites). This is especially helpful in the patient with postarthroplasty palsy, in whom the PSSD evaluation can document whether the involved nerves demonstrate a nerve regeneration pattern and warrant further observation or, in the absence of that pattern, whether neurolysis is indicated at the 3-month timeframe.[9]

The fifth consideration is the medical condition of the patient with regard to the risks of general anesthesia.

The sixth consideration is the vascular status of the limb. The peripheral nerve surgery is done with the use of a tourniquet.

Currently, it is recommended not to use a tourniquet in the presence of a leg that has had a bypass grafting procedure.[21]

The seventh consideration is to inform the patient that after a denervation procedure, a neurectomy of a peripheral nerve, or a decompression, there may be unusual and sometimes painful postoperative sensations. These are due to either nerve regeneration in the case of a nerve decompression or collateral sprouting in the case of a resection of a cutaneous nerve. Some patients perceive that the knee area is swollen, although no visible effusion is present. Postoperatively, the patient should be prepared to participate in aquatic therapy pool sessions two to three times a week for 3 weeks and perform water-walking to desensitize the skin and help reorganize the cortical maps.[10]

The eighth consideration is to inform the patient that not all of the original knee pain may be resolved. Small nerves have many anatomic variations, and although in some patients the preoperative block suggests that all pain has been relieved, there may still be a small branch (e.g., the infrapatellar branch of the saphenous nerve) that will require a second operation to remove. A second operation may be necessary in approximately 10% of patients.

With regard to postoperative care, the patient ambulates immediately. This facilitates gliding of any nerves that have been decompressed and minimizes the risk of venous thrombosis. Once the sutures are removed, the patient begins water therapy. With regard to postoperative wound healing, in the obese individual, the lipid substances may come out of the fat cells into the subcutaneous tissue. The biologic process to absorb this often results in a firm, warm area in the fat that may appear to be cellulitis. This responds to topical warmth and anti-inflammatory medication. If it is difficult to distinguish this from a bacterial problem, a course of antibiotics may be necessary.

Finally, the patient must be told that peripheral nerve surgery will not alter the stiffness present in the knee joint. Once pain has been relieved, the patient's range of motion and strength can again be addressed by the orthopaedic surgeon and the physical therapist.

OPERATIVE TECHNIQUES

The operative techniques for partial knee denervation described later have been published previously.[17–19] For each patient, a tourniquet is used and set at a pressure of 300 mg Hg. If the leg is quite large or exceptionally muscular, this pressure can be increased to 325 mm Hg. It is critical to note that the leg is *not* completely exsanguinated. Deliberately, some venous blood is left in the region around the knee by not wrapping the Ace bandage tightly. The small amount of blood left in all the recurrent geniculate artery and veins is helpful in identifying the small joint afferents that lie next to these structures and the larger nerves such as the infrapatellar branch of the saphenous nerve. A bipolar coagulator and Loupe magnification (3.5x) are used. Intravenous antibiotic prophylaxis is given prior to inflating the tourniquet. A femoral nerve block is *not* done owing to the risk of injury to the femoral nerve, but rather bupivicaine (Marcaine) 0.5% is infiltrated into the skin edges of the incisions at the end of the surgical procedure. The dressing consists of Xeroform gauze over the incision, followed by sterile 4- x 4-inch gauze, which is held in place with Kling and covered with a stockinette. Then, an Ace wrap is applied firmly and left in place for 30 minutes to counteract the reactive hyperemia attendant to use of the tourniquet.

Critical Points OPERATIVE TECHNIQUES

- Intravenous antibiotic prophylaxis.
- Tourniquet used, leg not completely exsanguinated.
- Femoral nerve block not done owing to risk of injury to femoral nerve.
- Bupivacaine (Marcaine) 0.5% is infiltrated into skin edges of incisions at end of surgical procedure.
- Dressing: Xeroform gauze over incision, followed by sterile 4- × 4-inch gauze held in place with Kling and covered with a stockinette. Ace wrap applied firmly, left in place for 30 min.
- Operative procedures
  ○ Lateral denervation of knee joint.
  ○ Medial denervation of knee joint.
  ○ Resection of infrapatellar branch of saphenous nerve.
  ○ Resection of medial cutaneous nerve of thigh.
  ○ Neurolysis of common peroneal nerve.
  ○ Denervation of proximal tibiofibular joint.
  ○ Neurolysis of superficial peroneal nerve.
  ○ Neurolysis of proximal tibial nerve.
  ○ Neurolysis of lateral femoral cutaneous nerve.
  ○ Neurolysis of saphenous nerve in Hunter's canal.

Finally, the concept of minimizing the risk of recurrent neuroma pain must be understood. Because the sensory nerves remain alive once divided owing to their intact nucleus in the dorsal root ganglion, nerve regeneration will occur in every joint afferent or cutaneous afferent that is divided. Alteration of the microenvironment of the nerve by implanting the proximal end of a divided sensory nerve into an innervated motor environment results in the absence of formation of a true neuroma.[37] Implanting a sensory nerve into an innervated muscle after resecting the painful neuroma or after interruption of that nerve function by division of that nerve results in predictable pain relief without recurrent neuroma for upper[15,30] and lower extremity[12,28,29] peripheral nerves. The location chosen to place the divided nerve is explained for each operation described later.

Lateral Denervation of the Knee Joint

An incision is outlined lateral to the patella, beginning over the distal muscle belly of the vastus lateralis. This muscle sometimes has a slight distal split, and the surgeon must be sure to remain distal to the most distal portion of the vastus lateralis muscle. The iliotibial band (lateral retinaculum) is divided longitudinally for approximately 1.5 cm. Immediately adjacent to the muscle belly are small recurrent vessels and a 1- to 1.5-mm nerve that go from beneath the biceps tendon and the iliotibial band and across the synovium into the lateral joint and infrapatellar structures. This nerve is infiltrated with bupivacaine 0.5% down beneath the iliotibial band and the nerve and vessels are cauterized toward the patella to prevent bleeding and placed under traction and cauterized deep beneath the iliotibial band to prevent bleeding. The portion between the two cauterized sites is sent to pathology. The iliotibial band (lateral retinaculum) is repaired with two figure-eight sutures of 2-0 braided nonabsorbable material (Fig. 42–9).

Medial Denervation of the Knee Joint

An incision is outlined medial to the patella beginning over the distal muscle belly of the vastus medialis. The thin medial retinaculum is divided longitudinally for approximately 1.5 cm. Immediately

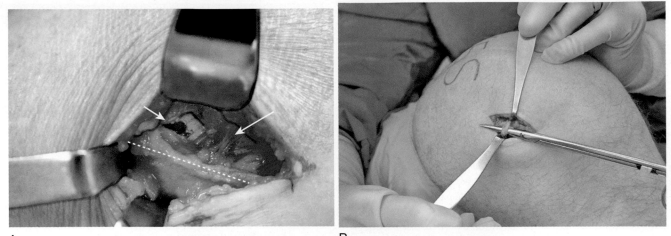

A   B

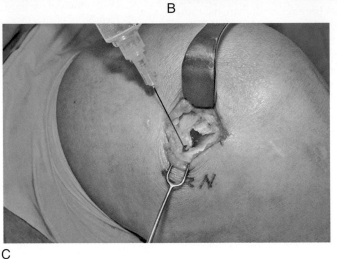

C

FIGURE 42–9. Lateral knee denervation. **A**, Incision is shown, lateral to the patella, centered over the tender site shown in Figure 42–5. The *short arrow* indicates the vastus lateralis. The iliotibial tract is incised (*dotted line*) to demonstrate the lateral retinacular nerve (*long arrow*) adjacent to the superior lateral geniculate vessels. **B**, The lateral retinacular nerve. **C**, The nerve is first infiltrated with local anesthetic, cauterized distally and proximally, and then divided proximally below the level of the iliotibial band so that the nerve drops into the popliteal fossa.

adjacent to the muscle belly are the small recurrent vessels and a 1- to 1.5-mm nerve that goes from beneath the vastus medialis and across the synovium into the medial joint and infrapatellar structures. This nerve is dissected proximally beneath the retinaculum until it exits from beneath the muscle. This nerve is infiltrated with bupivacaine 0.5% down beneath the vastus medialis and the nerve and vessels are cauterized toward the patella to prevent bleeding and placed under traction and cauterized deep beneath the vastus medialis to prevent bleeding. The portion between the two cauterized sites is sent to pathology. The medial retinaculum is repaired with two figure-eight sutures of 3-0 braided nonabsorbable material (Fig. 42–10).

Resection of the Infrapatellar Branch of the Saphenous Nerve

The saphenous nerve exits Hunter's canal in the distal thigh to become the medial cutaneous nerve of the thigh, the infrapatellar branch of the saphenous nerve, and the distal saphenous nerve. The infrapatellar branch crosses the insertion of the adductor tendons into Gerdy's tubercle beneath the deep fascia.

There may already be two branches at this level. Ultimately, several terminal branches cross from medial to lateral across the region of the tibial tuberosity to innervate the lateral knee skin. The skin proximal to this laterally is the terminal zone of innervation of the lateral femoral cutaneous nerve. Whereas the numbness is lateral, the damage to the nerve usually occurs in the axial line of the knee from an incision or medially from a scope portal. The site of the Tinel sign medially is around Gerdy's tubercle. An incision is made longitudinally across the Tinel sign. The dissection is carried deep to the fascia where one or more branches are noted by the blood in the vein that accompanies the nerve branch. A thorough search proximally and distally must be done to identify more than one branch. This is the most common location for a missed remaining painful nerve. The nerve is infiltrated with bupivacaine 0.5% proximally, the distal end cauterized to minimize bleeding, a segment resected for pathology, and the proximal end dissected. There is usually a clear tunnel where this nerve has transversed along or through the sartorius or other adductor muscle or tendon. The proximal end of the divided nerve, after cauterization to prevent bleeding, is turned blindly into these muscles and implanted there, proximal to the popliteal crease (Fig. 42–11).

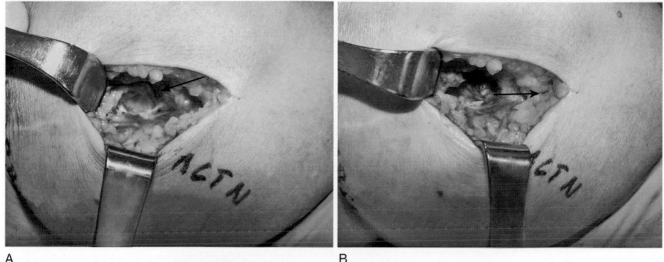

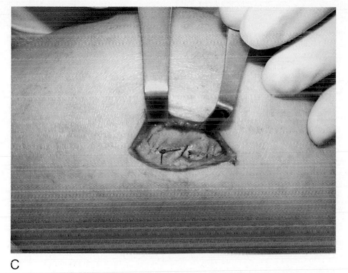

FIGURE 42–10. Medial knee denervation. **A**, Incision is shown, medial to the patella, centered over the tender site shown in Figure 42–5. The medial retinaculum is opened. The *arrow* points to the medial retinacular nerve adjacent to the recurrent medial recurrent geniculate vessels. **B**, The nerve has been resected. The *arrow* points to the direction in which, beneath the medial retinaculum, the nerve has been implanted into the vastus medialis muscle. **C**, Closure of the medial retinaculum.

Resection of the Medial Cutaneous Nerve of the Thigh

The medial cutaneous nerve goes to the skin overlying the patella. This skin is traditionally shown as being innervated by an anterior femoral cutaneous nerve coming vertically down the leg. However, the skin is innervated by a branch of the saphenous and approaches this region medially. Indeed, the same tender location for the medial retinacular nerve is the location of this nerve. The clinical clue is that the skin of the patella is dysesthetic. The nerve block medially will block both of these nerves. An incision is used to approach the medial retinacular nerve. There will be blood in the immediate subcutaneous tissue from the small vein that accompanies this nerve. The nerve is cauterized distally, and the proximal end is dissected medially across the surface of the vastus medialis. The nerve is injected with bupivacaine 0.5% proximally.

A small window is opened into the fascia of the vastus medialis. The proximal end of the nerve is implanted loosely into this muscle (Fig. 42–12).

Neurolysis of the Common Peroneal Nerve

An oblique incision is made going from the location of the popliteal fossa distally across the fibular neck overlying the palpable and tender common peroneal nerve. In the immediate subcutaneous tissue, the surgeon should be aware that the lateral cutaneous nerve of the calf can be present as a branch of the common peroneal nerve. Injury to this nerve will cause a postoperative painful incision. In addition, this nerve can become adherent to the biceps tendon, which also causes postoperative pain beneath the incision proximally.

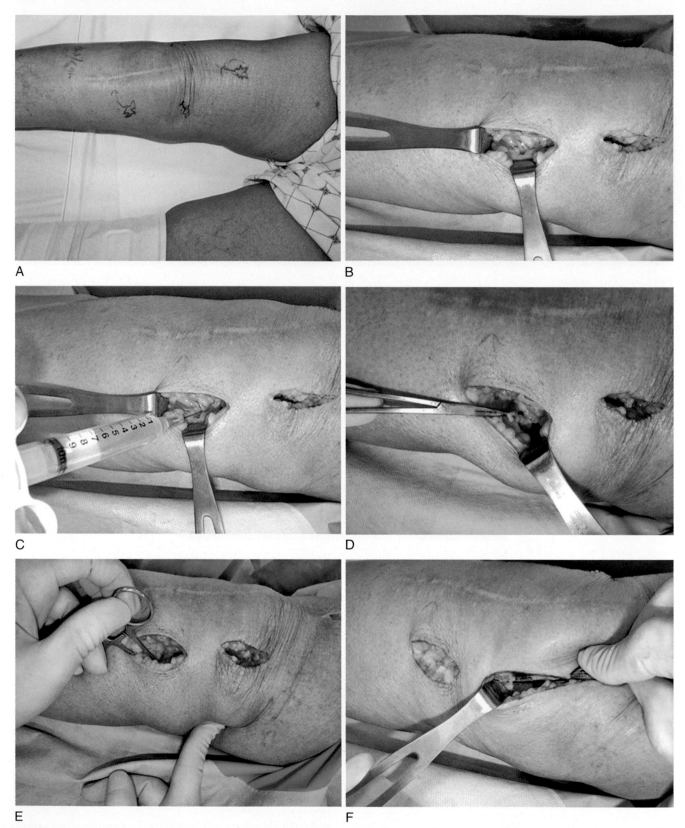

FIGURE 42–11. Resection of the infrapatellar branch of the saphenous nerve. **A,** A woman 9 years after total knee arthroplasty whose knee is shown from medial aspect demonstrating sites of pain over the anterior femoral cutaneous nerve (proximally), over the medial cutaneous nerve of the thigh (and medial retinacular nerve), and over the infrapatellar branch of the saphenous nerve. **B,** The infrapatellar branch is noted at the medial aspect of the knee, near the tibial tuberosity, at which site it is usually painful to touch. The nerve is infiltrated with local anesthetic prior (**C**) and then cauterized and divided (**D**). **E,** The proximal end of the nerve is dissected and implanted into an adductor muscle medially (location denoted by the finger at the popliteal fossa). **F,** A search must be made proximally for other infrapatellar branches. One is shown here in the incision used to resect the medial cutaneous nerve of the thigh and the medial retinacular nerves.

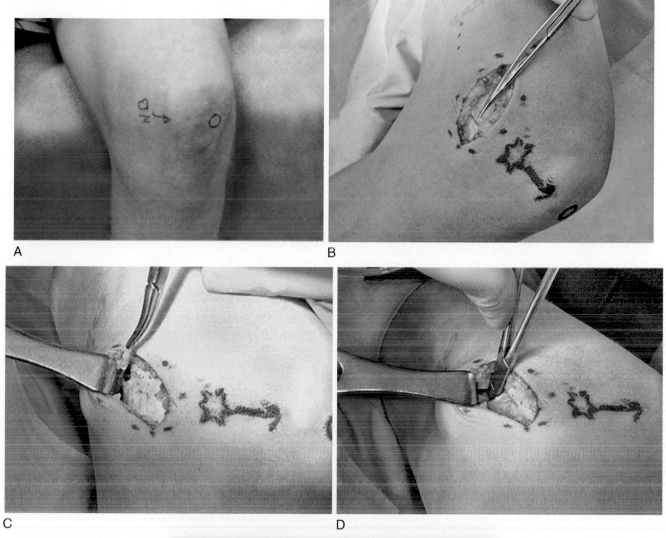

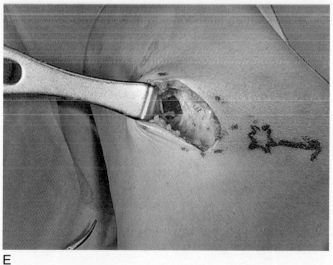

FIGURE 42–12. Resection of the medial cutaneous nerve of the thigh. A 23-year-old with a direct injury to the knee resulting in pain over the patellar region. **A,** Site of Tinel's sign and nerve block that eliminated the pain. **B,** Medial cutaneous nerve of the thigh demonstrated by the scissors' tips in the subcutaneous plane. **C,** This is superficial to the medial retinaculum. **D,** The nerve has been divided distally and dissected proximally and is held by a clamp. **E,** A window is made in the fascia over the vastus medialis into which the proximal end of the nerve will be implanted.

The deep fascia is opened. In patients who do not have a neuropathy but who sustained trauma, this fascia will be adherent to the common peroneal nerve, which will be white with an area of inflammation and swelling as the peroneus longus muscle is approached. In patients with neuropathy, and particularly those with glucose intolerance or actual diabetes, the common peroneal nerve will be yellow and resemble a neuroma. Be aware of these cases and handle the fat beneath the fascia with great care because it is usually the nerve. The dissection must release the nerve into the popliteal fossa, especially in the case of trauma or joint replacement. The usual compression site, however, is beneath the peroneus muscles. As the surgeon evaluates the common peroneal nerve approaching the fibular head and crossing the fibular neck, two or more tiny branches will be observed that go around the fibular head to innervate the proximal tibiofibular joint. Because the peroneus fascia is the main site of compression, divide the peroneus longus fascia transversely and from the fibula head distally, cauterizing the edges. If there is a septum between muscle groups, divide this septum, being careful on its deep surface. Retract the muscle; dividing the muscle is not necessary. In 20% of cadavers, but in 80% of patients, there will be another band of varying width and thickness deep to the muscle and overlying the nerve across the fibular neck.[12] This is the site of compression, and this band is resected. Then, look beneath the nerve for fibrous bands on the lateral gastrocnemius muscle; if they are present, cauterize and resect them. Check the passageway of the common peroneal nerve beneath the muscles and into the leg. If this is tight, divide the fascial origins of the muscle at the fibula by cautery. This completes the neurolysis of the common peroneal nerve (Fig. 42–13).

Denervation of the Proximal Tibiofibular Joint

In the preceding section, the small branches to the proximal tibiofibular joint were observed. The safest way to denervate this joint is to perform a complete neurolysis of the common peroneal nerve. Then, using a disposable nerve stimulator, stimulate the deep and the superficial peroneal nerves to demonstrate a "positive control." Stimulate the small branches purported to go the proximal tibiofibular joint. If no muscle twitches, these are indeed the correct nerves and they may be resected back to the common peroneal nerve and submitted to pathology. Do not inject bupivacaine into these nerves because this is likely to create a motor block and cause worry in the recovery room until it wears off (Fig. 42–14).

Neurolysis of the Superficial Peroneal Nerve

Symptoms related to compression of the superficial peroneal nerve are numbness, tingling, or pain radiating from the midlateral lower leg to the top of the foot.

The most important concept here is that the superficial peroneal nerve in at least 25% of patients will have a branch in the anterior compartment.[2,39] Therefore, in addition to opening the lateral compartment, the anterior compartment must be opened. The incision is made approximately 4 cm long, centered on the site of the positive Tinel sign. The most common location for the incision is 10 to 15 cm proximal to the lateral malleolus. In the subcutaneous tissue, look for a small bulge in the fascia or fat protruding from the fascia because this may be the transit site of the superficial peroneal nerve from deep to superficial to the fascia. There may be a small branch to the skin right at this point that must be preserved. Create a longitudinal opening in the lateral compartment. Even if a nerve is found, a longitudinal opening in the anterior compartment must be made. In addition, transversely cut the fascia to visualize all the way anteriorly. The fascial edges must be cauterized because they are well vascularized and can be a source of postoperative bleeding. The septum between the two compartments is another site in which a branch or the entire superficial peroneal nerve may be located. Do not just simply cut across this region.[40] The goal is to leave the superficial peroneal nerves surrounded only by muscle, because this guides the proximal and distal extent of the fascial releases (Fig. 42–15).

Neurolysis of the Proximal Tibial Nerve

An incision approximately 12 cm long is made medially in the calf just anterior to the medial head of the gastrocnemius muscle. The center of the incision is made at the level of the tender proximal tibial nerve, approximately 9 cm distal to the popliteal crease. The deep fascia is opened and the medial gastrocnemius

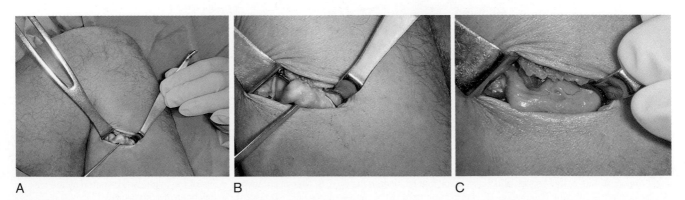

FIGURE 42–13. Decompression of the common peroneal nerve. **A**, The incision is noted on a right knee, overlying the fibular head and angling toward the popliteal fossa. **B**, The peroneus fascia has been released superficially and the muscles retracted anteriorly. The common peroneal nerve is infiltrated by fat in this patient with diabetes and is compressed by the fibrous band deep to the retracted muscle. **C**, The fibrous band has been excised. The nerve is noted to be indented at the site and to have lost its fascicular markings, consistent with severe compression.

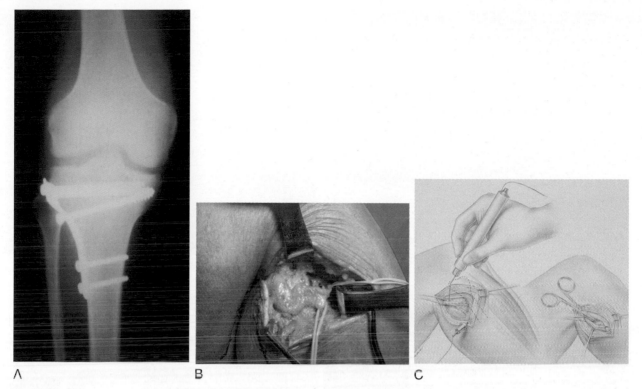

FIGURE 42–14. Denervation of the proximal tibiofibular joint. **A,** Example of surgery in the region of the proximal tibiofibular joint that can cause pain in this region, typically after a high tibial osteotomy or tibial plateau fracture. **B,** The common peroneal nerve has been decompressed, with the normal common peroneal nerve proximally, and a vessel loop placed about its major branches, the deep and superficial peroneal nerves. The *arrow* marks a branch that innervates the proximal tibiofibular joint. **C,** Electrical stimulation will give no motor response, and this small branch can be resected. There may be a more proximal branch as well.

muscle is dissected bluntly from the soleus muscle. The plantaris tendon and the popliteus muscle will be seen. The tibial nerve and the popliteal vein will be observed to pass anterior to the fascial origin or arch or sling of the soleus muscle. A large clamp placed deep to this arch demonstrates the tight area. The soleus muscle fibers may require dissection to reveal the fibrous arch. If there has been bleeding in this area, this dissection can be difficult. The soleal arch must be completely divided. Usually, a notch in the tibial nerve will be identified (Fig. 42–16).

Neurolysis of the Lateral Femoral Cutaneous Nerve

A tender spot exists just anterior to the anterior superior iliac crest. An incision approximately 4 cm long is made just cephalad to this area and deepened into the subcutaneous tissue. The inguinal ligament is identified and carefully divided, millimeter by millimeter, adjacent to the anterior superior iliac crest and the surgeon looks for the compressed lateral femoral cutaneous nerve. The nerve is narrowed, yellow, and inflamed and often does not look like a nerve. The nerve must be released into the thigh and then proximally until it enters the pelvis. Proximally, this entails dividing portions of the internal oblique fascia. Where this dissection stops, the surgeon should take care not to divide the deep circumflex iliac artery and vein. If the lateral femoral cutaneous nerve is too badly damaged by the compression, it may need to be resected with the proximal end allowed to lie within the pelvis (Fig. 42–17).

Neurolysis of the Saphenous Nerve in Hunter's Canal

A 6-cm incision is made longitudinally at the site of the Tinel sign of the saphenous nerve in the adductor canal. The dissection goes deep until the fascia connecting the vastus medialis to the adductor longus is identified. The length of this tunnel is between 6 and 8 cm. Small nerves will be in this vicinity. They need to be stimulated, because some are not saphenous branches but motor branches. Once the fascia is released, the saphenous nerve will be present as one or more branches. Deep to them will be the superficial femoral artery (Fig. 42–18).

AUTHOR'S CLINICAL STUDIES

If a patient obtains relief of knee pain after a block of any combination of joint or cutaneous afferents, there is a 90% chance that he or she should also obtain good to excellent relief of his or her knee pain postoperatively.[17, 19] Patients who achieve less than a satisfactory result either have another nerve that requires removal or have confounding problems such as a central mechanism for their chronic pain, drug addiction, or legal issues related to work or an accident.

The first group of patients selected for partial knee denervation were chosen from a group who had undergone a TKA but had persistent pain for greater than 6 months that was unrelated to loosening, malalignment, or infection.[19] In this study, the orthopaedic surgeons completed a preoperative Knee Society

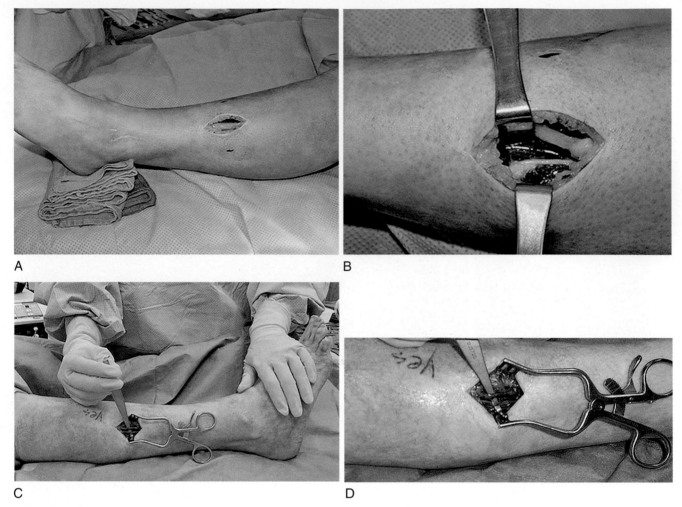

FIGURE 42–15. Neurolysis of the superficial peroneal nerve. An incision is made over the lateral aspect of the leg at the site of the Tinel sign. Whereas the superficial peroneal nerve is in the lateral compartment in 75% of patients, it can be in just the anterior compartment (**A** and **B**) or in both the anterior and the lateral compartments (**C** and **D**). For this reason, a fasciotomy of both compartments must be done for each patient. The neurolysis is continued until the nerve is distally in the subcutaneous tissue and is proximally surrounded by muscle. In some patients, a portion of the septum between the two compartments must be excised.

Function Score, range of motion, and pain assessment in 15 patients. The author independently performed the partial knee denervation, whereas the orthopaedic surgeons conducted the postoperative assessment. To be selected for surgery, each patient had to achieve a reduction of 5 points on a visual analog scale for pain after undergoing selective nerve blocks. A total of 45 nerves were resected in the 15 patients including (in each patient) both the medial and the lateral retinacular nerve and the infrapatellar branch of the saphenous nerve. All patients reported subjective improvement in the immediate postoperative period, which was maintained at a mean follow-up of 12 months (range, 6–16 mo). It was concluded that selective knee denervation is indicated in the management of intractable knee pain of neuroma origin after TKA.

The next series reported comprised 70 patients.[18] Some of these patients had persistent knee pain after TKA, but the indications were extended to include those with chronic pain after knee trauma or tibial osteotomy. In patients with TKA, aseptic loosening, sepsis, ligamentous instability, malalignment, and polyethylene wear were systematically ruled out as the source of pain by the orthopaedic surgeons. In patients with non-TKA pain,

arthrosis, synovitis, ligamentous instability, and meniscal derangement were excluded as a source of pain. All candidates for the procedure had a successful selective nerve block. Sixty of the 70 patients (86%) were satisfied with the denervation procedure as judged by direct questioning and a reduction in their preoperative pain visual analog score of 5 or more points. The average Knee Society Score improved from a preoperative mean of 51 points (range, 40–62 points) to a follow-up mean of 82 points (range, 15–100 points). Forty-nine patients (70%) had final Knee Society objective scores greater than 80 points. There was no difference in patient satisfaction whether the follow-up period was less than 2 years or more than 2 years. Selective knee denervation is indicated in the management of intractable knee pain after exhaustion of traditional approaches to any structural or infectious etiologies and after successful selective nerve block.

In 2000, a series of 344 patients were reviewed.[17] Of these, 255 had a previous TKA and 89 had knee trauma. Most patients had several nerves removed; none had only one nerve resected. All required removal of the medial and the lateral retinacular nerves, and the majority also required removal of the medial cutaneous nerve of the thigh and the infrapatellar branch of

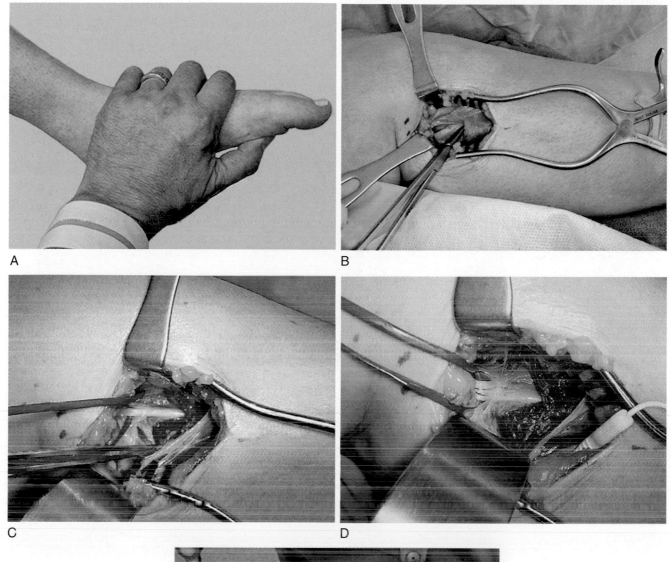

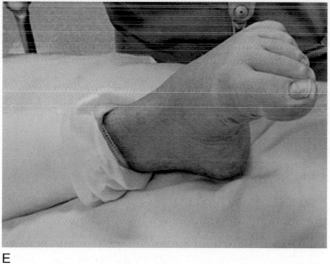

FIGURE 42–16. Neurolysis of the proximal tibial nerve. Compression of the tibial nerve proximally or distally will decrease sensibility in the plantar aspect of the foot. **A**, However, with a proximal compression versus a tarsal tunnel syndrome, the patient may lose the ability to flex the big toe. **B**, The medial incision is used to expose the space between the medial gastrocnemius muscle and the soleus. **C**, The clamp identifies the compression site of the tibial nerve by the fibrous arch of the soleus muscle. **D**, The nerve has been decompressed, and a difference in appearance of the nerve at this site is noted. **E**, In the recovery room, the patient regained the ability to flex the big toe.

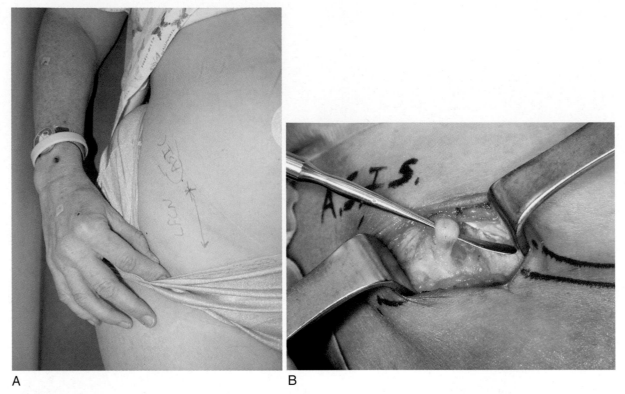

A   B

FIGURE 42–17. Neurolysis of the lateral femoral cutaneous nerve. **A**, Typical site of tenderness of the lateral femoral cutaneous nerve, just medial to the anterior superior iliac crest. **B**, A decompressed right lateral femoral cutaneous nerve is elevated by the instrument after division of the inguinal ligament from above and below. Additional neurolysis is required more proximally for the internal oblique fascia.

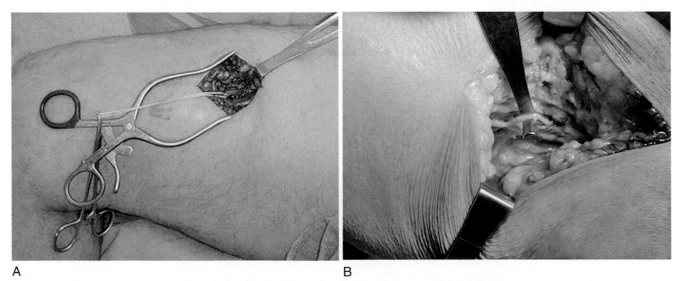

A   B

FIGURE 42–18. Neurolysis of the saphenous nerve in Hunter's canal. **A**, The location of the incision is clear. The entire fascial band from the vastus medialis to the adductor magnus has been released. The large single saphenous nerve is noted. **B**, In this view, a single small saphenous nerve branch is seen emerging from the fascia of Hunter's canal prior to its release.

the saphenous nerve. The nerves least often removed were the anterior femoral cutaneous and the distal saphenous nerve. Approximately one half of the patients, especially those who had sustained knee trauma, required a neurolysis of the common peroneal nerve. The proximal tibiofibular joint required

denervation in patients with fractures of the fibula or tibial plateau and who had undergone a Maquet procedure or a high tibial osteotomy. The results for the entire series were 70% excellent (no remaining pain), 20% good (some pain remained, but no medication was required), 5% some improvement

Study #1

- 45 nerves resected in 15 patients after total knee arthroplasty.
- All patients subjective improvement immediately postoperative, maintained 6–16 mo.

Study #2

- 70 patients after total knee arthroplasty, knee trauma, tibial osteotomy.
- 86% satisfied with results.
- Knee Society score: preoperative mean, 51 points (range, 40–62 points); follow-up mean, 82 points (range, 15–100 points).

Study #3

- 344 patients after total knee arthroplasty, knee trauma.
- All had multiple nerves resected.
- 70% excellent (no remaining pain), 20% good (some pain remained, but no medication was required), 5% some improvement (surgery helped, but pain medication still required), and 5% no improvement.

(surgery helped, but pain medication still required), and 5% no improvement. No patient was neurologically downgraded or made worse. No knee implant or hardware was exposed. No patient had to be hospitalized to treat infection. The abnormal sensibility, which is usually decreased sensibility, remains to some degree in everyone after a cutaneous nerve is removed.

A review of knee denervation patients on our office computer from January of 2000 through December of 2006 includes 405 patients. Whereas this large group of patients has not been reviewed at this time, the overall experience with the diagnosis, intraoperative management, and postoperative outcomes remains the same as that obtained in our 2000 review data.[10]

OTHER AUTHORS' CLINICAL STUDIES

In contrast to the vast literature on relief of acute knee pain with femoral, obturator, or even lateral femoral cutaneous nerve blocks (more than 120 references cited in Pubmed between 2006 and 2008), with the exception of one surgeon in Germany,[23,24] there have been no reported studies of partial knee denervation. Between May of 1995 and June of 1999, Fromberg and Hempfling[24] performed partial denervation using the "Dellon technique" described in this chapter in 45 knees. The investigations

Fromberg and Hempfling[24]

- $N = 45$.
- 70% reported "a reduction in pain" 6–18 mo postoperative.
- After 4 yr, 50% "still confirmed a positive result."

Maralcan et al.[33]

- Local anesthesia block in 32 knees of 20 patients with patellofemoral pain.
- Significant difference between the visual analog scale scores before and after local anesthetic injections.
- Confirmed that knee pain can be of neural origin from the medial and the lateral retinacular nerves.

of Fromberg and Hempfling included patients with direct knee injury as well as those who had knee joint replacement. Thirty-four patients were followed, 11 with bilateral knee pain, whose ages ranged from 25 to 86 years (mean, 34 yr). At follow-up, 6 to 18 months postoperatively, 70% of the patients reported "a reduction in pain," and after 4 years, 50% "still confirmed a positive result." Complications included 1 hematoma and 2 seromas, which resolved with conservative management.

A recent study evaluated the innervation of the patella in 30 knees of 15 formaldehyde-fixed cadavers.[33] A nerve from the vastus medialis (which is the nerve described previously[1]) entering the patella "superomedially" and a nerve "from the vastus lateralis entering the patella superolaterally" were identified. The origin of these nerves was not described. The superolateral nerve "from the vastus lateralis" was most likely the nerve described previously that originates from the sciatic nerve and crosses in front of the vastus lateralis.[25] This anatomic study in fixed cadavers confirms the author's observations reported in 1994.[25] Maralcan and co-workers[33] confirmed that these nerves were patellar pain afferents by performing a local anesthesia block in 32 knees of 20 patients with patellofemoral pain. They observed a significant difference between the visual analog scale scores before and after local anesthetic injections ($P < .01$). Their observations appear to confirm that knee pain can be of neural origin from the medial and the lateral retinacular nerves, as described previously.[17,19,25]

REFLEX SYMPATHETIC DYSTROPHY OF THE KNEE

In 1986, Katz and associates[27] defined reflex sympathetic dystrophy of the knee as diffuse pain, often accompanied with skin color changes, in patients who did not allow their knee to be touched and exhibited all the characteristics of what today is termed *complex regional pain syndrome*. These authors reported on 5 patients from a series of 662 primary total knee arthroplasties (0.8%) who demonstrated, in addition to pain, marked limitation of flexion. They stated that the traditional bone scan and osteopenia that were used as criteria for diagnosing reflex sympathetic dystrophy in the hand were difficult to aid in diagnosing this disease in patients who had TKA (Fig. 42–19). A lumbar sympathetic block was believed to be more helpful in making the diagnosis.

With the vision of hindsight, the author now maintains that this condition is related to the combination of joint and cutaneous neuromas. However, instead of attempting to treat this problem by blocking the sympathetic outflow, the author's

- Condition related to the combination of joint and cutaneous neuromas.
- Preferred treatment is to interrupt the pain stimuli from entering the dorsal columns of the spinal cord.
- $N = 40$ upper and 30 lower extremity patients with complex regional pain syndrome followed a mean of 15 mo postoperative.

Outcome

- Upper extremity patients: 55% excellent, 35% good, 10% failed.
- Lower extremity patients: 66% excellent, 30% good, 4% failed.

The clinical findings of light touch hypersensitivity (allodynia) and cold hypersensitivity (hyperalgesia) are believed to occur through a central sensitization model termed *the Raja model*.[55] In this model, pain receptors (nociceptors) up-regulate their α receptors. Because the body is constantly sending sympathetic signals, these nociceptors are being constantly stimulated, which reduces the CNS threshold for perceiving pain.[58] Once again, changes occur in the dorsal root ganglion.[22] The mechanoreceptors responsible for light touch sensation and thermoreceptors responsible for cold sensation instead produce an abnormal painful response when they stimulate the sensitized central pain neurons.

In the Raja model, treatment by sympathetic blockade is effective through the production of a temporary inhibition of norepinephrine release. By temporarily blocking the release of catecholamines, the sympathetic block relieves pain. By allowing the CNS to experience relief from pain, the central pain neurons may be desensitized (down-regulation of α receptors), resulting in a long-term improvement in the painful response to light touch.[3]

The change in regulation of α receptors also explains the change in appearance of the limb over time. Initially, an increase in α receptors causes excess stimulation that presents as a red, warm, and swollen limb (increased sympathetic function). Later, as the body adjusts and down-regulates the expression of α receptors, the same limb will take on a blue, cool, and contracted appearance.[3] This can be explained to the patient with the following analogy. The patient controls the home computer (the CNS) and his or her children control the computer speakers (the PNS). If music is playing from the computer and the children like the song, they will turn up the volume to a painful level for the patient (perceived as pain by the CNS). In response to the pain of this loud noise, the patient (CNS) turns down the volume at the computer terminal, thereby decreasing the sound to a reasonable level (and decreasing the pain signal in the body). Unfortunately, by decreasing the strength of the signal from the computer to the speakers, other signals are also being transmitted weaker than normal. So, while the pain is decreased in the body, so is the strength of the sympathetic signal sent to the extremity, changing it from abnormally warm, red, and swollen to abnormally cool, blue, and constricted.

DIAGNOSIS

Clinical Presentation

The clinical presentation of CRPS is variable and comes in different stages with diverse appearances.[54] The disease has no predilection for gender, age, or dominant extremity. The common cause is an initiating trauma to an extremity, which can be as obvious as a fracture or as minor as an ankle sprain. It can also occur in response to surgery, arthritis, and inflammatory conditions or reactions.[7] In as many as 10% of cases, no initiating trauma can be identified.[20]

The physical examination findings are subcategorized into sensory disturbances, sympathetic dysfunction, motor abnormalities, trophic changes, and psychological issues. During the initial examination and throughout the diagnostic process, the clinician should determine the answers to four questions:

1. Is the condition CRPS?
2. Is the extremity hot and swollen or cold and atrophic?
3. Is there a neural or a mechanical nociceptor focus?
4. Is the process sympathetically maintained or sympathetically independent?[36]

Critical Points DIAGNOSIS

- Hallmark finding of CRPS: intolerable, burning pain disproportionate to inciting event. Classic finding is allodynia or pain with light touch.
- Aggressive physical therapy that is painful to the patient may worsen the condition.
- Cold intolerance: cryotherapy, ice test.
- Naturally falls into three stages (acute, dystrophic, and atrophic), no specific timeline.
- One half of CRPS patients show decreased range of motion, physiologic tremor, weakness.
- Particular personality type may increase risk for CRPS. More likely that the emotional and behavioral disturbances are the result of chronic pain and loss of function.
- No laboratory test or imaging study exists to confirm diagnosis.
- Paravertebral sympathetic ganglion blockade best tool for diagnosing SMP-related CRPS and initiating treatment. Examine patient while block is in effect to determine whether a focus for the pain exists.
- Bone scan: increased uptake to limb—CRPS in acute phase or successful treatment. Normal scan may miss CRPS in dystrophic phase.
- Magnetic resonance imaging useful to rule out other causes, allow clinician to narrow the differential diagnosis.
- Classic radiographic finding for CRPS—Sudeck's atrophy, patchy periarticular osteoporosis.
- Spinal or epidural anesthesia may be used for sympathetic blockade. However, given at low concentrations, some sensory blockade occurs and can lead to false-positive results when pain is relieved and attributed to SMP rather than generalized sensory blockade.
- Conflicting study results make any use of phentolamine testing questionable. Injections are painful and poorly tolerated.
- Thermography and sweat tests are poor tests.

Sensory Disturbances

The hallmark finding of CRPS is pain disproportionate to the inciting event. The disproportionate response includes pain more intense than expected, lasting longer than expected, and expanding beyond the dermatomal region of the extremity. Pain is the body's response to impending or ongoing cell death. With CRPS, the pain may be generated in the absence of cellular insult.[36] Within hours to days after the initial noxious event, the pain becomes diffuse and expands beyond the site of the injury. As the condition progresses, the pain expands beyond dermatomal distributions in a stocking or glove pattern with a preference for distal limb involvement. Patients describe the pain as "burning and shooting" or as "deep, constant, and aching." A classic finding is allodynia, pain with light touch. This is manifested during the physical examination and described by the patients during the history as the inability to tolerate pressure from bed sheets at night, clothing, and even air currents. The pain may fluctuate in intensity in response to many influencing factors. Aggressive physical therapy that is painful to the patient may worsen the condition. As the weather changes and becomes colder, the condition may worsen. Also, owing to the sympathetic nature of the disease, as patients become excited, their pain may worsen.

Sympathetic Dysfunction

Sympathetic dysfunction is manifested through changes in skin color, swelling, temperature changes, and cold intolerance. Classically, the limb will initially appear red, warm, and dry and progress over time to a mottled, bluish, cool, and moist condition. Note that the sudomotor function is opposite of what is normally expected. A red and swollen limb will normally be moist, and a bluish and cool limb will normally be dry. Side-to-side temperature differences can average 3.5°C in 80% of CPRS patients.[77]

Patients frequently report swelling that is extra-articular and painful. It is a prominent finding early in the course of the disease that decreases over time. Initially, the skin is edematous but gradually is replaced by skin that is tight, shiny, and lacking in normal skin creases.[15]

Of particular interest is a corresponding intolerance to cold. This finding is particularly sensitive for diagnosing SMP. Cold intolerance is often first encountered in physical therapy when cryotherapy is used to control swelling and produces a significant painful response.[40] In the office, the clinician can use an ice cube test (Fig. 43–3) by applying ice to the sensitive region and asking the patient about the evoked sensations. The abnormal response the clinician seeks is a description of intolerable, burning pain. In the very early phase, the patient may describe the sensation evoked from the ice cube test as decreased cold sensation when compared with the contralateral limb. In a similar manner, cold weather can precipitate a painful flare.[40]

The natural history of sympathetic dysfunction falls into three stages. These stages do not follow a specific timeline and the patient can go forward and backward through the stages over time or in response to treatment. For this reason, the staging system has little clinical usefulness other than to understand the classic progression of the disease. The patient with CRPS may present with some or all of these symptoms, but may also present only with the symptom of disproportionate pain. The stages are acute, dystrophic, and atrophic.[71]

The acute stage usually lasts less than 6 months. During this time, the sympathetic system is hyperactive, yielding a limb with red, warm, and dry skin. The dystrophic stage begins after 3 to 9 months when the hyperactive sympathetic system finally diminishes to a period of decreased sympathetic activity. In this stage, the limb is cyanotic or mottled, cool, and moist, with thickening of the nails and coarse hair (owing to decreased blood flow to the skin). When the dystrophic stage persists long enough

to produce an overall level of atrophy in the limb, the patient enters the atrophic stage. This stage is characterized by thin, tight, shiny skin, osteoporosis from prolonged decreased weight-bearing, and joint contractures from prolonged decreased range of motion.[71]

Sympathetic hypersensitivity and denervation do not account for all the abnormalities in CRPS. For example, in CRPS type I, there is no identifiable nerve lesion, and in CRPS type II, the symptoms often spread beyond the dermatome of the damaged nerve.

Motor Abnormalities

Motor impairment is a more recently appreciated symptom of CRPS.[64] The deficits range from weakness to increased tone and hyperfunction. Even when motor abnormalities are grossly evident, electromyography tests remain normal. This finding suggests that the motor response of CRPS is centrally mediated, most likely at the spinal cord level.[77] Initially, weakness can be attributed to disuse and expected muscle atrophy. Some patients develop pseudoparalysis that may extend to limb neglect. When hyperfunction is present, it manifests as action tremors, myoclonus, hyperreflexia, muscle spasm, and voluntary guarding.[64] In longstanding illness, dystonia, apraxia, and lack of coordination may be present.[77] In 50% of CRPS cases, patients show decreased range of motion, physiologic tremor, and weakness. About 10% of chronic cases will reveal dystonia in the hand or foot of the affected extremity.[2]

Psychological Issues

The clinician may respond to patients with CRPS and their disproportionate pain by believing they are malingerers or have fictitious disorders or other psychiatric overtones. However, as with many patients with a chronic pain syndrome, comorbid psychiatric disease either develops or promotes the pain syndrome.[7,51] It is uncertain whether this is a cause or an effect of the CRPS, but in daily diaries kept by chronic pain patients, investigators found that yesterday's depressed mood contributed to today's increased pain, and yesterday's pain also contributed to today's depression, anxiety, and anger.[20]

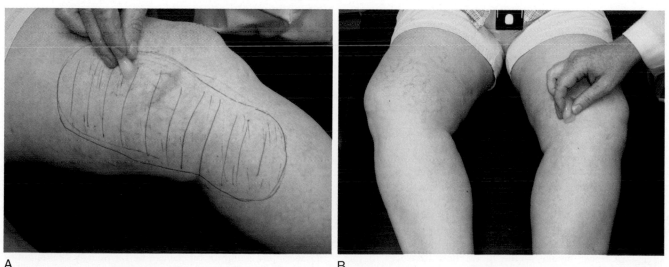

A   **B**

FIGURE 43–3. A and **B,** Ice test.

It has been suggested by some authors that a particular personality type increases the risk for developing CRPS.[18] However, this has never been proved.[10] It is more likely that the emotional and behavioral disturbances are the result of chronic pain and loss of function. These psychological disturbances have been proved to resolve when the pain resolves.[42,47]

Objective Tests

CRPS is primarily a clinical diagnosis. There is no laboratory test or imaging study that can absolutely confirm a diagnosis of CRPS. Even so, many tests are useful for lending additional credibility to clinical suspicions and ruling out other possible diagnoses.

Paravertebral Sympathetic Ganglion Blockade

Paravertebral sympathetic ganglion blockade is the best tool for diagnosing SMP-related CRPS and initiating treatment of CRPS. The patient is injected with a local anesthetic under fluoroscopic control. The local anesthetic is injected near the lumbar paravertebral sympathetic ganglion (for lower extremity disease) or the stellate ganglion (for upper extremity disease).[40,70,77] Successful block of the ganglion is monitored by documenting vasomotor and sudomotor changes in the extremity. In a technically adequate block, the skin temperature of the extremity will approach core body temperature. In addition, in a stellate ganglion block, Horner's syndrome (ptosis, miosis, and anhidrosis) will be induced. Relief of pain is due to blocking the SMP portion of CRPS. However, a placebo response as high as 33% has been documented and clinicians should be cautioned not to rely solely on this test for diagnosis.[51]

In general terms, any documented pain relief from these blocks is attributed to SMP, and any remaining pain is therefore SIP. It is worthwhile to examine the patient while the block is still providing relief to determine whether a focus for this pain syndrome exists. Prior to the block, patients may complain of diffuse pain about the knee. After a block, patients may be able to localize their pain to the medial aspect of the knee and an astute clinician may be able to localize clinical findings to a specific disorder (such as saphenous neuritis or a medial meniscal tear).

Triple-Phase Bone Scan

Diagnosis of CRPS based on bone scans is controversial because the test results vary based on the phase of the disease and by successful treatment.[25,35,81] The triple-phase bone scan has three phases: arterial, soft tissue, and bone. The radionucleotide tracer injected during a bone scan has increased uptake in CRPS in the second and third phases (soft tissue and bone; Fig. 43–4) of the test.[64] This occurs due to the increased blood flow and bone turnover in the acute phase of CRPS. During the acute phase of the disease, the reported sensitivity and specificity of this test range from 60% to 100% and 80% to 98%, respectively.[25,26,35] Unfortunately, as the disease progresses to the dystrophic phase, blood flow to the limb decreases and the affected limb will appear cold on bone scan. Finally, successful treatment of a CRPS limb with sympatholysis can result in a paradoxical increase in tracer uptake as the blood flow improves to the affected limb.[25,41] Thus, increased uptake to a limb can indicate CRPS in the acute phase or successful treatment of the disease.

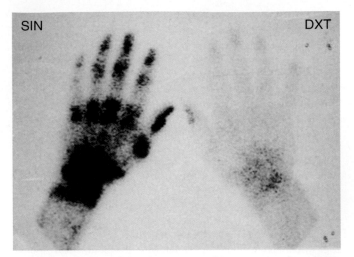

FIGURE 43–4. The left hand represents either an acute-phase CRPS or successful treatment of CRPS. The right hand represents either a normal examination or a dystrophic/atrophic-phase CRPS.

A normal scan may miss CRPS in the dystrophic phase. This tendency for change in bone scan results over time is also why this test should not be used to track the course of the disease or the success of treatment.[25]

Magnetic Resonance Imaging

Magnetic resonance imaging (MRI) is a poor test for confirming CRPS. However, it can be useful in ruling out other possible causes of pain and allow the clinician to narrow the differential diagnosis. MRI may also be useful in identifying a possible focus for the pathology that triggered the disease. Radiology literature describes the characteristic MRI findings of CRPS to be thickening of the skin, soft tissue swelling that enhances with contrast, and intra-articular effusions. Chronic changes are muscle atrophy and thinning of the skin.[65]

Hematology/Serology

There is no laboratory marker for CRPS. Increased white blood count, erythrocyte sedimentation rate, and C-reactive protein can indicate a generalized inflammatory process, but these findings are nonspecific. However, these tests along with others such as rheumatoid factor and antinuclear antibody tests can help in identifying other possible diagnoses.

Radiographs

Virtually all orthopaedic patients will have radiographs taken of the affected extremity. In the acute phase, no change in radiographic appearance will be noticed. As the disease progresses to the dystrophic and atrophic phases, films will reveal decreased cortical density of the affected extremity when compared with the contralateral limb. The classic radiographic finding for CRPS is Sudeck's atrophy, a patchy periarticular osteoporosis.[67]

Differential Spinal and Epidural Blockade

Paravertebral ganglion blocks can be technically challenging to perform. Less accurate, but easier methods to perform are spinal or epidural blocks. The blocks can be used for diagnosis because the nerve fibers respond differently to varying concentrations of local anesthetic. The lowest concentrations of local anesthetic penetrate the least myelinated sympathetic nerve fibers with the goal to relieve the SMP component. At increasing concentrations, the sensory nervous system is blocked, and even higher concentrations block the motor system. When used to test for CRPS, the initial injection is often saline to detect a placebo response. Unfortunately, even at low concentrations, some sensory blockade occurs and can lead to false-positive results when pain is relieved and attributed to SMP rather than generalized sensory blockade.[40]

Phentolamine Challenge

Phentolamine is a nonspecific α-antagonist with a short half-life of 17 minutes. When administered, any pain relieved from blocking the α receptors of the sympathetic nervous system may be attributed to SMP of CRPS. A study performed in 1991 reported favorable results in using phentolamine to diagnose CRPS; this test is still used today.[56] However, a second phentolamine study performed by another group of investigators in 1994 invalidated the results of the 1991 study.[61] In the later study, both phentolamine (an α-antagonist) and phenylephrine (an α-agonist) were used in 77 patients in a double blinded fashion. The results showed no pain relief with phentolamine testing and no worsening of pain with phenylephrine. Of the study group, 22 had pain relief with saline infusions and only 7 had relief with phentolamine. These test results make any use of phentolamine testing questionable.[61]

Regional Intravenous Sympathetic Blockade

Regional intravenous sympathetic blockade has been used for both diagnosis and treatment. These blocks are performed with either reserpine or bretylium.[64] These drugs act at the sympathetic terminals to deplete the stores of norepinephrine and inhibit its reuptake, which may last up to 2 days.[8] Upon initial release of norepinephrine, patients with SMP will note a burning pain. Pain relief has been described as lasting from 2 weeks to 6 months. Pain relief less than 5 days favors a diagnosis of SIP.

There are several reasons why these blocks are a poor choice for diagnosing CRPS. First, it is unknown to what degree these medications target sympathetic functions. Second, local anesthetic agents are often injected with reserpine or bretylium, and it is not possible to determine whether the pain relief is from the local anesthetic or a true blockade of the sympathetic nervous system. Third, these injections are painful and poorly tolerated by patients. Finally, this method requires the use of a tourniquet, which is poorly tolerated in patients with CRPS and can actually lead to exacerbation of the condition.[64,72]

Vasomotor Measurements

Sympathetic dysfunction can be measured by thermography. This test requires extensive setup and monitoring and is not useful clinically if only for cost reasons. Thermography is successful in measuring temperature changes in a limb compared with the contralateral limb and can be depicted using colorized images. Some authors have reported that use of thermography allows for early detection of CRPS.[6,30] However, this technique has several drawbacks. Thermography requires a carefully controlled environment that is free of drafts and well controlled for temperature and humidity. It requires a period of 20 minutes to 2 hours for the limb to acclimatize prior to testing. There is no agreement on the amount of temperature difference that constitutes a positive test. If the temperature is set for a difference at 0.4° C, the test is sensitive but poorly specific. If the temperature is set for 1.2° C, the test is specific but not at all sensitive.[6] Lastly, even superficial scars may cause thermographic changes.

Sudomotor Measurements

The quantitative sudomotor axon reflex test (QSART) is one method of measuring sweat output. In this test, acetylcholine is administered to the extremities and the sweat output of each extremity is measured and compared.[5,62] One criticism of this test is based on theories stating that sudomotor dysfunction is centrally mediated and this test has its mechanism of action at the postganglionic sympathetic neuron. Therefore, the results of this test may not reflect CRPS sympathetic hyperactivity.[5]

TREATMENT

Many treatments have been proposed since CRPS was first described in 1864, but unfortunately, few are supported by prospective, double-blinded, randomized, clinical trials. A lack of consensus exists regarding the preferred treatment algorithm for CRPS. As stated previously, the placebo response to treatment has been recorded in as high as 33% of patients tested. For this reason, the results of studies that are not randomized should be treated with caution.[61]

Despite the inability to state with confidence an exact treatment protocol, several principles may be noted. First, treatment should begin as soon as possible, within 3 weeks of the onset of the disease. The long term prognosis depends upon the time span from the onset of the disease to the initiation of treatment. Authors have postulated that a delay in treatment of more than 6 months is associated with a poor prognosis.[80] One study revealed that greater than 80% of patients who had treatment initiated within 1 year of the onset of CRPS had a significant improvement in their symptoms. However, delay of greater than 1 year resulted in some degree of permanent impairment in 50% of the patients.[36]

CRPS often has a painful focus that perpetuates the SMP. As such, the identification and elimination of this painful focus are critical to alleviating the SMP. Even so, SIP may remain and worsen over time. Eliminating the painful focus in the acute phase is important along with treatment of the SMP to eliminate the pain. In chronic cases with established SMP, elimination of the painful focus late in the course of the disease may be of very little help. Surgery may be poorly tolerated in the CRPS limb, and symptoms are often exacerbated postoperatively if steps are not taken to control perioperative pain.[40] However, when a painful focus is identified, surgery may be performed in a manner that minimizes the chance of exacerbating the condition. In most cases, it is worth the risk of worsening the condition to eliminate the root cause of the CRPS symptoms and potentially eliminate the condition.

Treatment often requires multiple disciplines. The cooperation of orthopaedists, pain specialists, anesthesiologists, physical therapists, neurologists, psychologists, and primary care physicians is required to provide the most effective care. The following methods are all described in conjunction with physical

encountered. A possible genetic association between CRPS and the human leukocyte antigen (HLA) system has been described by others. However, when the following patients were tested for HLA-specific antigens, none related to CRPS were detected. The following cases represent a mother and her two daughters, each of whom developed CRPS.

The primary case, a 43-year-old mother, was diagnosed with bilateral patellofemoral malalignment and severe trochlear dysplasia at the age of 13 years. The patient had repeated injuries (bilateral meniscal tears, bilateral patellar subluxations, and right patellar chondral injury) while playing tennis and softball. These injuries resulted in multiple surgical procedures (seven on the left knee, four on the right knee) to address her patellofemoral malalignment, meniscal injuries, and patellofemoral arthritis. At the age of 26 years, bilateral, staged patellectomies were performed for severe patellofemoral arthritis. She had brief relief of pain; however, 2 months after the right patellectomy, she experienced increasing pain that was generalized around the knee and along the leg. The pain was described as "severe and burning," even with the light touch of her clothing. The skin over the leg was shiny and edematous. Her family history was not significant except for a brother with diabetes mellitus and a sister with rheumatoid arthritis. There was no history of smoking. There were no lawsuit or workers' compensation claims involved. She was initially treated with multiple medications, physical therapy, and transcutaneous electrical nerve stimulation. The medications included combinations of anti-inflammatories, analgesics, anxiolytics, oral steroids, and gabapentin. Later that year, four sympathetic lumbar blocks were performed that provided only temporary relief. A surgical sympathectomy was performed. One month later, most of her symptoms had resolved, although she continued to have occasional episodes of hyperesthesia over the medial aspect of her knee.

This patient's 13-year-old daughter was diagnosed with idiopathic toe-walking at the age of 8 years. She developed tendoachilles contracture on the left side, which was treated using sequential below-knee casts in maximal dorsiflexion. After removal of the second cast, she refused to bear weight on the involved side and complained of burning pain around her ankle and foot. The skin over the foot was shiny, edematous, and cooler than the contralateral side. Prompt treatment was instituted in the form of multiple medications, physical therapy, and transcutaneous electrical nerve stimulation. Six months later, there was no improvement in her symptoms and she was admitted for continuous epidural sympathetic blockade for 5 days. The patient had complete relief of symptoms with the epidural blockade, only to have a recurrence of all her symptoms 1 month later, after a great toe injury on the same side. Again, treatment was instituted with medications, physical therapy, and hydrotherapy. The symptoms gradually diminished over a period of 3 months. She developed a normal heel-toe gait pattern during this timeframe.

The mother's 15-year-old daughter sustained an ankle sprain at the age of 11 years. She was treated with a soft ankle support brace, crutches, and partial weight-bearing. Three weeks later, she developed hyperesthesia, burning sensation, and temperature changes along her ankle and foot. There was increased swelling and shiny skin over the involved area. The pain was not resolved with anti-inflammatories, rest, and elevation and was worse with ice application. The family members promptly recognized the symptoms consistent with CRPS owing to their prior experiences and sought immediate medical attention. Treatment consisted of multiple medications, transcutaneous electrical nerve stimulation, physical therapy, and hydrotherapy. The symptoms gradually resolved over a period of 6 months.

Case 5. A 38-year-old woman sustained a fall at work and dislocated her left patella. She underwent initial conservative treatment. Within 3 months, the patient was diagnosed with CRPS owing to a burning sensation and had developed arthrofibrosis. Ice to the affected area created burning pain. She had no recurrent instability episodes. The range of motion was 5° to 110°, and severe quadriceps atrophy was noted. She was referred to pain management and placed on venlafaxine hydrochloride (Effexor) and baclofen. As well, she continued physical therapy for knee motion–strengthening exercises. Over several months, she consistently improved, but had a gradual return of her hypersensitivity 1½ years later. She was placed on Neurontin and Depakote and her symptoms abated within 1 month.

Case 6. A 26-year-old woman diagnosed with a medial meniscus tear by MRI was referred for extreme pain. The patient was taking oxycodone and acetaminophen (Percocet) and celecoxib (Celebrex). Her medial knee and tibia were exquisitely tender to palpation (Fig. 43–7). She held her leg flexed 30° and would not allow physical examination secondary to extreme pain with light touch. She had a mild effusion with no color changes, but her limb was cool to the touch. She reported being unable to tolerate the pressure of her bed sheets on her knee. She was prescribed Neurontin and referred for paraspinal ganglion blocks. Although the Neurontin helped her pain, the patient was prescribed tramadol because she could not tolerate the sedating effects. She underwent 10 blocks, which relieved her pain. She is currently in remission and being treated conservatively for patellar malalignment syndrome. She never underwent arthroscopy at our institution. This case demonstrates the importance of an immediate diagnosis, because the pain could have been mistakenly attributed to the medial meniscus tear.

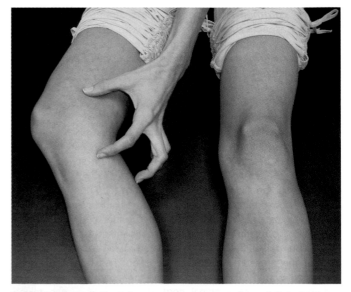

FIGURE 43–7. Patient demonstrates an area of exquisitely tender medial knee and tibia pain.

Case 7. The patient is a 46-year-old man who previously had sustained a crush injury to the left hand at work. At that time, he sustained an open, but nondisplaced, third metacarpal fracture, which was treated with immobilization.

Six weeks later, the patient complained of increasing pain and numbness in the hand and was diagnosed with carpal tunnel syndrome. A carpal tunnel release was performed. Soon thereafter, he developed a CRPS type II syndrome, with pain from the tip of the small finger up to the shoulder. He complained of a constant burning pain. The patient was begun on Neurontin and a series of stellate ganglion blocks. Neurontin was then switched to Lyrica. He received a total of 17 stellate ganglion blocks, which provided good, but only temporary, pain relief.

The patient was evaluated with computed tomography (CT) scan and MRI of the hand and wrist that showed no structural abnormalities. Electromyography showed very mild ulnar neuropathy beginning at the cubital tunnel that had not been present on the Electromyographic study obtained to diagnose his carpal tunnel syndrome. The patient was too tender to use his hand to help push himself up from a seated position. He had constant pain, which was worst in his shoulder.

Physical examination showed the extremities had mild atrophy of the interosseous muscles. There was some chronic darkening of the skin, particularly on the ulnar side of the hand. There were involuntary-type movements of the forearm and hand, particularly in the hypothenar area with spasm of the flexor digiti quinti. The patient was very tender to direct palpation over the cubital tunnel that produced radiating pain both up to the shoulder and down to the hand. He was also tender over the medial epicondyle and had pain with passive forearm pronation. His elbow had full range of motion. The patient demonstrated marked weakness with all motor functions of the left hand. Hypothenar and thenar muscles were very weak when tested manually. He had both cutaneous paresthesias and dysesthesias.

The patient was placed on alendronate sodium (Fosamax) and calcitonin (Miacalcin) and indicated that this solved most of the pain at the wrist. Physical examination at that time showed continued weakness in the ulnar distribution, particularly in the hand. He had an extremely positive Tinel sign in the proximal cubital tunnel.

The patient was seen in consultation with a diagnosis of cubital tunnel syndrome with CRPS type II. After discussion, he underwent a subcutaneous ulnar nerve transposition while under continuous stellate ganglion block. He had some immediate pain relief, but approximately 1 week postoperative, he had a flare of CRPS-type symptoms. He was given a Medrol Dosepak, which calmed his symptoms considerably. Approximately 1 month after surgery, the patient claimed to have 75% pain relief and noted that all the pain in his shoulder was gone, as was almost all the pain in the elbow. He continued, however, to have some spasm and sensitivity in the ulnar side of the hand.

With relief of the severe pain, the patient now began to have a positive Tinel sign at Guyon's canal. Whereas the proximal pain abated, the hand pain did not seem to improve. Approximately 2 months after the ulnar transposition, a release of Guyon's canal was performed, again under continuous stellate ganglion block for 2 days. Three months after the Guyon canal release, the patient claimed that approximately 90% of his original pain was gone. There was intermittent spasm of the flexor digiti quinti, where this had been continuous previously. The patient was gaining motion and strength in the hand. Two point discrimination was 6 mm in the median innervated digits and 7 to 8 mm in the ulnar innervated digits. Hand examination at this time showed some scaphotrapezial tenderness and review of old x-rays showed some mild degenerative changes in the scaphotrapezial joint.

Whereas established CRPS is often extremely difficult to treat successfully, this patient received dramatic, but not complete, relief from appropriate management of painful conditions. He had a mild flare of CRPS after his ulnar nerve transposition, but this was managed successfully with a Medrol Dosepak. This example demonstrates that painful conditions that normally would be relatively tolerable can greatly exacerbate CRPS. Appropriate management of these painful conditions when done under continuous sympathetic blockade can lead to successful outcomes, sometimes even in patients with well-established CRPS.

REFERENCES

1. Adami, S.; Fossaluzza, V.; Gatti, D.; et al.: Bisphosphonate therapy of reflex sympathetic dystrophy syndrome. *Ann Rheum Dis* 56:201–204, 1997.
2. Baron, R.: Reflex sympathetic dystrophy and causalgia. *Suppl Clin Neurophysiol* 57:24–38, 2004.
3. Baron, R.; Levine, J. D.; Fields, H. L.: Causalgia and reflex sympathetic dystrophy: does the sympathetic nervous system contribute to the generation of pain? *Muscle Nerve* 22:678–695, 1999.
4. Bengtson, K.: Physical modalities for complex regional pain syndrome. *Hand Clin* 13:443–454, 1997.
5. Birklein, F.; Riedl, B.; Claus, D.; Neundorfer, B.: Pattern of autonomic dysfunction in time course of complex regional pain syndrome. *Clin Auton Res* 8:79–85, 1998.
6. Bruehl, S.; Lubenow, T. R.; Nath, H.; Ivankovich, O.: Validation of thermography in the diagnosis of reflex sympathetic dystrophy. *Clin J Pain* 12:316–325, 1996.
7. Bushnell, T. G.; Cobo-Castro, T.: Complex regional pain syndrome: becoming more or less complex? *Man Ther* 4:221–228, 1999.
8. Campbell, J. N.; Raja, S. N.; Meyer, R. A.; Mackinnon, S. E.: Myelinated afferents signal the hyperalgesia associated with nerve injury. *Pain* 32:89–94, 1988.
9. Christensen, K.; Jensen, E. M.; Noer, I.: The reflex dystrophy syndrome response to treatment with systemic corticosteroids. *Acta Chir Scand* 148:653–655, 1982.
10. Ciccone, D. S.; Bandilla, E. B.; Wu, W.: Psychological dysfunction in patients with reflex sympathetic dystrophy. *Pain* 71:323–333, 1997.
11. Cooper, D. E.; DeLee, J. C.: Reflex sympathetic dystrophy of the knee. *J Am Acad Orthop Surg* 2:79–86, 1994.
12. Correll, G. E.; Maleki, J.; Gracely, E. J.; et al.: Subanesthetic ketamine infusion therapy: a retrospective analysis of a novel therapeutic approach to complex regional pain syndrome. *Pain Med* 5:263–275, 2004.
13. Dielissen, P. W.; Claassen, A. T.; Veldman, P. H.; Goris, R. J.: Amputation for reflex sympathetic dystrophy. *J Bone Joint Surg Br* 77:270–273, 1995.
14. Dobritt, D. W.; Gutowski, P.: Successful treatment of recurrent reflex sympathetic dystrophy with bilateral lumbar sympathectomies. *J Am Osteopath Assoc* 97:533–535, 1997.
15. Dzwierzynski, W. W.; Sanger, J. R.: Reflex sympathetic dystrophy. *Hand Clin* 10:29–44, 1994.
16. Field, M. J.; McCleary, S.; Hughes, J.; Singh, L.: Gabapentin and pregabalin, but not morphine and amitriptyline, block both static and dynamic components of mechanical allodynia induced by streptozocin in the rat. *Pain* 80:391–398, 1999.
17. Finsterbush, A.; Frankl, U.; Mann, G.; Lowe, J.: Reflex sympathetic dystrophy of the patellofemoral joint. *Orthop Rev* 20:877–885, 1991.